D0479553

HEALING
Without
MEDICATION

A Comprehensive Guide to the Complementary Techniques Anyone Can Use to Achieve Real Healing

ROBERT S. RISTER

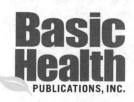

**Basic
Health**
PUBLICATIONS, INC.

The information contained in this book is based upon the research and personal and professional experiences of the author. It is not intended as a substitute for consulting with your physician or other healthcare provider. Any attempt to diagnose and treat an illness should be done under the direction of a healthcare professional.

The publisher does not advocate the use of any particular healthcare protocol but believes the information in this book should be available to the public. The publisher and author are not responsible for any adverse effects or consequences resulting from the use of the suggestions, preparations, or procedures discussed in this book. Should the reader have any questions concerning the appropriateness of any procedures or preparation mentioned, the author and the publisher strongly suggest consulting a professional healthcare advisor.

Basic Health Publications, Inc.
28812 Top of the World Drive
Laguna Beach, CA 92651
949-715-7327 • www.basichealthpub.com

Library of Congress Cataloging-in-Publication Data
Rister, Robert.
  Healing without medication : a comprehensive guide to the complementary
techniques anyone can use to achieve real healing / Robert Rister.
    p. cm.
Includes bibliographical references and index.
  ISBN 978-1-59120-017-8
1. Alternative medicine. I. Title.

R733.R576   2003
615.5—dc21
                                        2002015518

Copyright © 2003 by Robert S. Rister

All rights reserved. No part of this publication may be reproduced, stored in a retrieval system, or transmitted, in any form or by any means, electronic, mechanical, photocopying, recording, or otherwise, without the prior written consent of the copyright owner.

Editor: Linda Comac, Carol Rosenberg, and Tara Durkin
Typesetter/Book design: Gary A. Rosenberg
Cover design: Mike Stromberg

This edition published in Canada.
Licensed by Readon Publications Inc in agreement with Basic Health Publications Inc
8241 Keele Street, Units 9-10, Concord, Ontario L4K 1Z5
Tel: (905) 761-9666 Fax: (905) 761-1377 Toll Free: 1-800-401-9774
E-mail: readon@readon.com Website: www.readon.com

Printed in Canada

10   9   8   7   6   5

CONTENTS

Acknowledgments, ix

Preface, xi

How to Use This Book, xiii

Introduction, 1

Part One Health Conditions

Part Two **Healing Tools**

Part Three **Healing Partners**

ACKNOWLEDGMENTS

Writing is a lonely task, but publication is a group effort. This book would not have been possible without the dedication and generosity of individuals who cannot be adequately thanked here.

Researching this book required reading more than 10,000 scientific articles. My brother, Mark Rister, my sister-in-law, Johnna Rister, and my friend and supporter, Brian Johnson, found many of the scientific sources needed to write this book in medical and technical libraries and provided them to me in digital form. They worked days and nights to enable me to complete this book with the most current and timely information possible. I also thank my niece, Sammie, and my nephew, Chuck, for giving their parents the space they needed to help me with this book.

On a number of occasions, understanding the findings of expert medical and scientific research necessitated conversing and corresponding with the experts, doctors, and scientists themselves. I am appreciative of Hideo Anzai, Dennis Awang, Patricia Betancourth, Werner Busse, Mark Blumenthal, Jean Carper, Marcia Dean, Larry Dossey, Jim Duke, Steven Foster, Alicia Goldberg, Tara Hall, Chris Hobbs, Wayne Jonas, Penny King, Gyo Kinoshita, Thomas Kroiss, Al Radford, Laurie Radford, Ramona Ruffino, Wayne Silverman, Michael Solomon, Leslie Taylor, Kevin Vann, Andrew Vickers, Andrew Weil, Dan Wen, Helmut Wiedenfeld, Len Wisneski, Janet Zand, and the late Varro Tyler for tolerating my questions and enhancing my understanding of many of the topics covered in this book. I am especially indebted to the renowned cardiologist Demetrio Sodi-Pallares for giving me entire days of his schedule. I am also indebted to pharmacologist Artem Agafonov of the Institute of Pharmacy in St. Petersburg, Russia, for sharing his special insights into the use of natural healing where conventional medications are not available.

Books also need editors and designers, and I have been blessed with some of the best. Kramer Wetzel took on the task of reading my first drafts. My father, Raymond Rister, offered pointed and constructive criticisms throughout my writing of this book. Linda Comac contributed her exacting understanding of the usage of the English language and her zeal for factual accuracy. Carol Rosenberg and Tara Durkin scrutinized every detail of the final draft, and Gary Rosenberg created this book's distinctive look and feel.

But the tasks of writing, refining, and designing only reach readers with the help of agents, publicists, and publishers. Thanks are due to my agent Jeff Herman for his willingness to take an unproven writer and for his unfailing calm and good sense. I wish to express my appreciation to my publicist, Diane Glynn, for her many reassurances through the long process of writing this book. And I am grateful to my publisher Norman Goldfind for his readiness to invest his resources in this publication, for his unfaltering kindness, and for his unwavering friendship and support.

PREFACE

The cardinal rule of healing with medication and healing without medication is the same: "First, do no harm." This book exclusively recommends well-known remedies that are generally recognized as safe. The U.S. FDA approves the herbs, minerals, vitamins, essences, functional foods, and other nutritional products listed in this book as acceptable supplements to a healthy diet. The therapeutic techniques this book describes derive from historical use or contemporary science and can be safely used to complement necessary medical care.

Because most people take both nutritional supplements and the drugs their doctors prescribe, this book describes the application of vitamins, minerals, herbs, and supplements at very specific dosages, usually considerably below "megadose" levels. When a smaller dosage of an herb, mineral, vitamin, or nutritional supplement works just as well as a larger one, care has been taken not to encourage you to buy more supplements than you need. Every effort has been made to provide a warning when a natural treatment could interfere with a prescription drug.

Purists of natural healing and devotees of scientific method alike may disagree with some of the therapies suggested in this book. The suggested form of most of the herbs recommended in this book is a standardized extract. Critics of standardization rightly point out that herbs are more than the sum of their chemical constituents. Herbs contain hundreds or even thousands of biologically active ingredients that extend their effectiveness far beyond that of corresponding prescription drugs.

In the light of history, the critics of standardized herbs are on the right side of the issue. Herbalists schooled in their craft were careful to grow herbs in the right soil, at the right altitudes, and with the right exposure to sunlight. They harvested the herbs in their season and even at the proper time of day.

Nowadays, however, many herbs are purchased by the hundreds of tons from farmers in developing countries. Herb growers are under intense economic pressure to meet contractually specified production quotas. The old craft of herbalism is not respected. To compensate for uneven quality resulting from the industrialization of herb production, it is necessary to standardize extracts so that the final product is reliably potent. When herbs are used with prescription medications, it is especially important to know the chemical composition of the drug so that undesirable interactions between herbs and drugs can be prevented. None of this is to say that safe, effective, and reliable products made from whole herbs without standardization do not exist. They are merely hard to find, and they should be taken with caution by people who also use prescription drugs.

Devotees of scientific method will also note that this book recommends many treatments that have not been confirmed by double-blind, randomized, placebo-controlled clinical trials. Double-blind clinical experimentation is frequently described as the only valid means of scientific research. The fact is, even the most methodologically orthodox modern scientists conduct preliminary studies under more relaxed standards, and mainstream medicine itself did not promote double-blind clinical experimentation to its gold standard until about 1980.

The downside of this more scientific method is that it is bound to the outmoded concept that a single condition has a single cause and a single cure. Nutritional therapies tend to influence the individual symptoms comprising a disease. Herbs, in particular, exert multiple modes of action against multiple causes of disease. (And it is only fair to note that herbs can have multiple side effects when overdosed and can present multiple interactions with prescription drugs.)

Double-blind trials are the most scientific standard, but science is not the entirety of reliable human experience. Personal experiences count, too. This book makes every effort to avoid the suggestion that the use of a product has been confirmed by double-blind clinical testing when it has not. In the absence of proof that a traditional healing material simply does not work (which is relatively rare) or that it is unsafe (which is even rarer), nutritional supplements can be used with confidence. The practical experience of millions of people outside the medical establishment should not be ignored.

Not every condition can be healed by natural therapies alone, but all of the herbs, minerals, vitamins, essences, functional foods, nutritional supplements, healing methods, and lifestyle changes recommended in this book are sufficient in themselves to have a significant impact on the course of recovery. When healing without medication is not enough, natural therapies subdue the side effects of prescription drugs and make necessary medical treatments more bearable. Following the essential principles of healing without medication reduces the overall expense of care. And more often than not, natural healing methods are the tools of prevention and preservation necessary for vibrant health.

HOW TO USE THIS BOOK

This book describes how you can take charge of more than 200 health conditions with aromatherapy, flower remedies, functional foods, herbs, homeopathics, minerals, vitamins, nutritional supplements, simple dietary changes, and non-medical methods of healing. Health conditions are listed from A to Z. Each entry consists of 4 parts.

• The *Symptom Summary* is an inventory of the important diagnostic features of the health condition. While initial diagnosis of any serious illness should be made by a healthcare professional, the symptom summary can serve as a scorecard to help you determine whether you are getting better, getting worse, or have a new health concern.

• *Understanding the Disease Process* discusses the health alterations that set the stage for the development of disease. This book places special emphasis on the features of the pathological process that you can correct by changing your health habits.

• The *Treatment Summary* is a checklist of the tools of healing without medication. It gives you a list of changes to diet, exercise, and lifestyle you can make and the herbs, minerals, vitamins, homeopathics, and other nutritional supplements you can take organized the same way you would find them in a retail store.

• *Understanding the Healing Process* describes the limitations and possibilities of both conventional medical treatment and self-care. It offers you an in-depth understanding of how healing without medication works, and points you to sources of information you can review for yourself.

At the end of each entry you will find *Concepts for Coping*. This section offers additional information concerning choices and changes to lifestyle that will help you deal with the condition more easily and less expensively. This information will help you achieve a more comprehensive state of good health.

This book is also your guide to the medicine cabinet of natural and complementary healing. Part Two, Healing Tools, contains a series of ready reference guides to the uses and properties of aromatherapy, functional foods, herbs, homeopathics, minerals, vitamins, and other natural supplements, and to a variety of traditional and emerging healing techniques. Part Three, Healing Partners, is your guide to interactions between common prescription drugs and herbs, minerals, vitamins, and nutritional supplements. The recommendations in this book are supported by more than 2,000 scientific references listed in the notes section. Hundreds of the articles cited in this book are available in full text over the Internet and all of them can be read as abstracts on MedLine.

INTRODUCTION

There is an integrative solution for every health problem. This book is your comprehensive guide to combining the best of conventional and complementary care for more than 200 health conditions. It is also your concise reference to hundreds of healing substances and dozens of healing methods, and it is largely written from sources of information your can confirm for yourself.

Healing without Medication is not a book about alternative medicine. There is no alternative to medicine. A physician's care is essential to survival in many medical emergencies. Everyone benefits from consulting a professional before putting a label on symptoms. Modern medical practice employs a procedure for almost every set of symptoms and prescribes a drug for almost every disease.

The shortcoming of the modern healthcare system is that the care you need often is not the care you get. House calls by a conscientious personal physician have been replaced by mouse calls over a commercial and impersonal Internet. Insurance companies pay healthcare professionals and their patients little or nothing for prevention or restoration. The dizzying cost and complexity of modern medicine forces overworked doctors to become specialists in disease and leaves the general tasks of healing and prevention to patients alone.

Fortunately, everyone seeking healing has access to an enormous variety of safe and effective herbs, minerals, vitamins, and nutritional supplements, as well as a great range of nonmedical healing techniques. Many natural healing methods accomplish the same objectives as medication. As you will read in this book, forward-thinking physicians have confirmed that vigilant attention to a low-sodium diet can lead to recovery from congestive heart failure. Red yeast rice lowers cholesterol as effectively as some of the most commonly prescribed cholesterol-lowering drugs. Herbs can be more effective than antibiotics for ear infections. Acupressure can stop headaches. Magnets really do relieve pain, although not necessarily by magnetism. Dozens of conditions are effectively treated with exercise—and some conditions can be effectively treated by doing nothing at all.

Many doctors mistakenly believe that the reason people turn to holistic medicine is the high cost of healthcare, and the fact is, natural treatments carefully chosen to fit medical diagnoses are often less expensive than their prescription counterparts. The great value of natural methods, however, lies beyond controlling symptoms. Real healing is about more than keeping the numbers measured in laboratory tests within acceptable levels. It is about more than stopping pain. It is about more than avoiding decline and death.

Real healing restores the body's inherent powers of recuperation. It brings you back—or brings you for the first time—to normal activities and joy of life. The tools of mainstream medicine lay the foundation for healing, but recovery, restoration, and healing are impossible without a balanced diet, exercise, and sometimes, sensible nutritional support in the forms of herbs, vitamins, minerals, and other supplements. Scientific medicine prevents disasters. But natural healing brings your body back to its original state of resilience and vitality.

In writing this book as a layperson for lay people, I have attempted to empower you to take advantage of the best of both natural healing and modern medicine. It is my sincere hope that you will find the treatments discussed in this book to be of great efficacy. It is my deep desire that the principles explained in this book speed you on your way to good health.

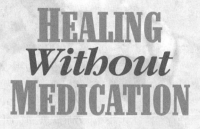

Part One
Health Conditions

Abdominal Bloating

See **Bloating**.

Abdominal Pain in Infants

See **Colic**.

Abnormal Pap Smear

SYMPTOM SUMMARY

○ Pap smear shows abnormal cell growth known as dysplasia

○ Colposcopy (doctor's cervical exam) shows gray or white patchy growth on cervical surface

○ Usually no other noticeable symptoms

UNDERSTANDING THE DISEASE PROCESS

An abnormal Pap smear detects dysfunctional cells in the cervix, the lowest part of a woman's uterus. Every year, as many as 1 million women in the United States have an abnormal Pap smear leading to a diagnosis of cervical dysplasia. The term dysplasia refers to premalignant or precancerous change to the cells of the cervix.

Cervical dysplasia can occur at any age, but it is most common in women between the ages of 25 and 35. Nearly all cases of cervical dysplasia can be treated. Left untreated, however, between 30 and 50 percent of cases progress to cervical cancer.

Most experts agree that the human papillomavirus (HPV) is the chief cause of cervical dysplasia. HPV is a group of more than 100 different strains of the same virus. Some strains of HPV cause genital warts. At least 12 different strains of HPV cause precancerous cervical lesions, the most serious among them being HVP-16 and HVP-18. Most women infected with HPV do not develop any obvious symptoms, but hormonal and nutritional factors can unleash HPV to damage cervical cells.

The papillomavirus has two modes of replication. In one mode, HPV makes a single copy of itself. In the other mode, known as runaway replication, HPV makes vast quantities of copies of itself so that it can infect new host cells. Runaway replication only takes place in the oldest and outermost layer of cells lining the cervix. Growth of the lining of the cervix, forcing older cells to the outer layers, is stimulated by the hormone progesterone. Women are most likely to transmit the virus to their sex partners when their progesterone levels are highest, during the second week of their periods.

The use of oral contraceptives is an important risk factor for cervical dysplasia. The progesterone in some versions of the Pill stimulates protein synthesis in at least one strain of papillomavirus, HPV-16.[1] High-progesterone contraceptives are presumably worse for cervical dysplasia than high-estrogen contraceptives.

Women who have more than one sexual partner in their lifetimes are the most likely to be infected with HPV.[2] Having intercourse for the first time before age 16 is also associated with increased risk of infection, especially among teens who use drugs and alcohol.[3]

Women who smoke are also more likely to develop dysplasia. Nicotine has been found in cervical tissues of female smokers. Men who smoke release nicotine and related chemicals in their genital secretions, and increase their female partner's chances of developing cervical dysplasia. Women who have HIV are especially at risk for cervical dysplasia and should have a Pap screening at least once a year.

TREATMENT SUMMARY

NUTRITIONAL SUPPLEMENTS

○ Folic acid: 4 milligrams per day for 3 months, then 2.4 milligrams per day. Use brands listing folic triglutamate (pteroyltriglutamate) as an ingredient.

○ Lutein: 5 milligrams per day.

○ Mixed carotenoids: 25 milligrams per day. The alga *Dunaliella salina* is a particularly rich source of carotenoids.

○ Vitamin B_{12}: 1 milligram per day.

○ Vitamin E: 100 IU or more per day.

○ Avoid copper supplements.

HERBS

○ Tampon soaked in 1 tablespoon goldenseal tincture, 1 tablespoon tea tree oil, and 1 tablespoon thuja oil (*not* thuja in oil) for several hours, inserted, and left for 24 hours. Use *one time* after initial diagnosis. Do not repeat.

See Part Three if you take prescription medication.

UNDERSTANDING THE HEALING PROCESS

The basic holistic approach to preventing and healing cervical dysplasia is correcting nutritional deficiencies. It is much easier to prevent cervical dysplasia than it is to treat it. The least expensive and most extensively studied natural treatment for the condition is the B vitamin folic acid. Unraveling and understanding the scientific evidence for this supplement takes a little effort.

A group of scientists suspected that folic acid could prevent cervical dysplasia in women who take oral contraceptives. They organized a clinical trial recruiting 47 women who did not yet have cervical dysplasia and who had been on the Pill for at least 6 months. These women received 10 milligrams of folic acid or a placebo daily for 3 months. At the end of the study, fewer abnormal Pap smears were found in the group of women who had been taking folic acid.[4] This study confirmed the idea that folic acid prevents cervical dysplasia in healthy women on the Pill.

A later group of scientists tested the idea that folic acid might reverse cervical dysplasia in women who already had it. One hundred fifty-four women with abnormal Pap smears were given 10 milligrams of folic acid or a placebo daily for 6 months. This study found no benefits from taking folic acid with regard to either follow-up Pap smear results or measures of the severity of HPV infection.[5]

One way to understand the results of the second study is simply that folic acid may be useful for preventing cervical dysplasia but not for treating it. Another way to understand the differences in results requires a more technical explanation. Scientists have learned that not all women inherit the same genes that control the production of the enzymes that convert folic acid to its active form, a chemical known as methylenetetrahydrofolate (MTHF). Women who have 2 copies of a defective gene involved in the manufacture of MTHF are 3 times as likely to develop cervical dysplasia as women who have no copies of the defective gene.[6] In other words, the women who need folic acid the most can use it the least. Fortunately, there exists another form of folic acid known by its chemical name, folic triglutamate (and also known by several other names listed below). This form of the vitamin does not require the same level of activity of MTHF enzymes. It is useful when the most common form of folic acid is not.

Vitamin manufactures make special supplements for women that contain folic triglutamate rather than the more common folic acid. This vitamin may be identified on the label as folic triglutamate, folic polyglutamate, pteroylglutamic acid, or pteroyltriglutamate. The best form of the vitamin for women at risk for cervical dysplasia will not be identified simply as folic acid or folate.

Certain medications increase a woman's need for folic acid. Anticonvulsants, cholesterol-lowering drugs, the diabetes drug metformin (Glucophage), over-the-counter pain relievers, and most drugs for epilepsy deplete a woman's body of this vitamin. Women who take any of these drugs should take folic acid or, if cervical dysplasia has been diagnosed, folic triglutamate supplements.

The body's absorption of folic acid is impaired during infection with HIV (the AIDS virus).[7] Women who have HIV are up to 46 times more likely to develop cervical dysplasia than women who do not have the infection.[8]

Folic acid is slightly better absorbed when it is taken on an empty stomach. If you take folic acid, you should also take vitamin B_{12}, since repletion of folic acid can lead to depletion of B_{12}. Complete vitamin B supplementation with both folic acid and B_{12} to prevent cervical dysplasia is important for women who have depression, epilepsy, or other neurological disorders.

The second category of nutrients important in preventing and treating cervical dysplasia is a *group* of vitamins related to the pigment beta-carotene found in carrots and in other orange and yellow fruits and vegetables and in dark leafy greens. One study found that women who develop cervical dysplasia have on average about two-thirds as much beta-carotene in their bloodstreams as healthy women.[9] Beta-carotene enhances the activity of the immune system in both men and women, and ensures the normal adhesion of skin cells to each other.[10] When the cells in the lining of the cervix "stick together," rapid growth to repair the lining of the cervix is not necessary and HPV multiplies slowly.

Supplementation with beta-carotene alone, however, does not heal cervical dysplasia. An Australian study of 141 women given 30 milligrams of beta-carotene or a placebo daily for 2 years found that the women given beta-carotene actually had higher rates of progression to cancer than those given a sugar pill.[11]

The failure of beta-carotene to heal cervical dysplasia is probably due to the fact that taking beta-carotene by itself keeps the body from absorbing other important, closely related vitamins. A Japanese study found that *alpha*-carotene is even more important for cervical health than beta-carotene. Women with the highest bloodstream levels of alpha-carotene are 6 times less likely to develop cervical dysplasia than women with the lowest levels of the vitamin. In this study, beta-carotene was found to be important, but the plant pigments lutein, lycopene, and zeaxanthin were more significantly associated with lower risk of developing the condition.[12]

Studies of a multiethnic group of women in Hawaii found that higher levels of yet another related vitamin, alpha-cryptoxanthin, were associated with a reduction in the risk of cervical dysplasia by nearly two-thirds.[13] The benefits of carotenoids are especially significant for African-American women. Researchers at the University of Pennsylvania reported that black women with the highest bloodstream levels of the carotene-cousin lutein were only one-third as likely to have cervical dysplasia as black women with the lowest bloodstream levels of vitamin.[14]

Considered together, these studies suggest that supplementation with mixed carotenoids is probably a very effective way to prevent cervical dysplasia. Supplementing with mixed carotenoids is at least a safe way to treat cervical dysplasia, although the data on the ability of mixed carotenoids to reverse the condition is incomplete. There has never been a reported case of side effects due to mixed carotenoids. Women who take cholesterol-lowering medications particularly need these important plant chemicals.

In addition to supplemental mixed carotenoids, certain foods provide these chemicals. Lutein is found in carrots, corn, greens, potatoes, tomatoes, and most fruits. Zeaxanthin is found in corn, honeydew melons, mangoes, orange peppers, paprika, spinach, and egg yolks (of chicken eggs). Eating these foods is another helpful way to get a healthy mix of carotenoids.

Vitamin A seems to prevent the progression of cervical dysplasia to cervical cancer. Another Japanese study found that women with the lowest bloodstream concentrations of vitamin A were 4.5 times more likely to develop cervical cancer than women with the highest bloodstream levels of the vitamin.[15] The problem with vitamin A is that there is a possibility of birth defects if it is accidentally overdosed during the first 3 months of pregnancy. Very high doses of the vitamin (more than 300,000 IU) have, on rare occasions (approximately 1 in 5 million births in the United States), caused birth defects. A daily dose of 5,000 IU per day can be used safely during pregnancy but may not prevent cervical cancer.

Vitamin E, also known as alpha-tocopherol, is possibly helpful in preventing cervical dysplasia. A survey of southwestern American Indian women found that women who were deficient in vitamin E were twice as likely to have cervical dysplasia.[16] Taking just 100 IU a day is enough to prevent deficiency in most women, although much larger amounts can be helpful in many conditions. Some experts suggest that eating vitamin E–rich foods such as egg yolks and nuts (not peanuts) provides beta- and gamma-tocopherols that may be essential for the body to absorb and use alpha-tocopherol efficiently. Be careful not to overdose vitamin E if you take blood-thinning agents such as aspirin, warfarin (Coumadin), or clopidogrel (Plavix). Taking more than 2,000 IU of vitamin E and any of these drugs on the same day can make you especially susceptible to bleeding.

All women who have had abnormal Pap smears should avoid copper supplements and multivitamin supplements containing copper. Recent study has found that copper levels are positively associated with the severity of cervical dysplasia.[17]

Goldenseal, tea tree oil, and thuja oil are traditional herbal treatments for cervical inflammation and cervical dysplasia. Naturopaths report that a vaginal pack made with a combination of all 3 herb oils causes temporary inflammation of the cervix followed by sloughing off of damaged tissue in 7–10 days. Be forewarned that any treatment strong enough to cause blistering off of abnormal cervical tissue *will* cause irritation and discomfort. Do not use vaginal packs on an ongoing basis. If they are going to help, they will help the first time. It is very important to refrain from unprotected vaginal intercourse for 2–3 weeks after using the packs to avoid reinfecting rapidly growing cervical tissue with HPV. Use condoms or other barrier contraceptives if you believe your partner may be infected with HPV.

The herbs for a vaginal pack are available in many herb stores. There is no evidence, either anecdotal or scientific, that taking any of these herbs in tinctures, tablets, or in any form other than a vaginal pack will help cervical dysplasia.

CONCEPTS FOR COPING WITH ABNORMAL PAP SMEAR

O An abnormal Pap smear does not automatically mean you have cervical dysplasia and certainly does not mean you have cervical cancer. Even though the Pap smear is a well-established technique, diagnostic errors are possible. If your doctor calls you about a second exam to confirm abnormal findings, be sure that follow-up tests are conducted at a different time during your menstrual cycle and that the doctor has ruled out the possibility of endometriosis. Avoid douches before your Pap smear, since irritant chemicals can affect interpretation of the results. Hormonal changes related to the menstrual cycle and endometriosis can also affect interpretation of results.[18]

O If you smoke, quit. Chemicals in tobacco smoke damage the DNA in cells in the cervix, and accelerate the progression of cervical dysplasia to cervical cancer.[19]

O Barrier contraceptives (foam and condoms) reduce the risk of cervical dysplasia. They reduce transmission of human papillomavirus (HPV), and prevent contact of the lining of the cervix with sperm. Release of the amino acid arginine during the decomposition of sperm is a possible contributor to carcinogenesis in the cervix.[20]

O The latest studies find that estrogen replacement therapy increases the risk of cervical dysplasia in *postmenopausal* women by about 60 percent, from approximately 1 in 500 to 1 in 200.[21]

Abscesses of the Skin

SYMPTOM SUMMARY

O Open sore or domed nodule

O Local swelling

O Draining pus

O Reddened skin around the lesion

O Warm to the touch

UNDERSTANDING THE DISEASE PROCESS

An abscess is an infection that causes pus to accumulate in the skin or in the tissues just below it. Abscesses may develop after a cut or a scrape, or they may be a complication of the infection of a hair follicle. The infectious agent responsible for an abscess is usually the bacterium *Staphylococcus aureus*, better known as staph.

Abscesses are very common, because staph bacteria are with us from birth. These microorganisms regularly colonize healthy skin without causing disease. At any given time, from 20–50 percent of people support thriving colonies of staph bacteria on their skin with no signs of infection. Staph bacteria cause inflammation only when the skin is damaged, and even then, in most people, the immune system can quickly get rid of them.[1]

Unfortunately, some people are prone to problematic staph infections. Insulin-dependent diabetics, people with chronic skin conditions such as eczema and psoriasis, intravenous drug users, and healthcare workers are especially likely to have problems with chronic staph infections.[2] Young children also have higher rates of staph infections than the rest of the population. This is due to their frequent contact with mucous secretions from other children with infected noses and throats.[3] Once a colony of staph bacteria is established, it may persist for years, and it may cause abscesses again and again.[4]

TREATMENT SUMMARY

DIET

O Avoid foods that cause allergic reactions.

O Limit consumption of simple sugars to 50 grams (2 ounces) per day. This is approximately 1 small candy bar or a 1-inch slice of cake, with no other sugars all day (and night). Restricting sugar consumption is especially important if you have diabetes. If you have diabetes, you may not be able to eat sweets at all.

O Be sure to eat a few servings of whole, natural foods, such as fruits, vegetables, legumes, and whole grains every day. Dark red and dark blue fruits (blackberries, blueberries, cherries, and raspberries) are best.

O Drink at least six 8-ounce glasses of water daily.

NUTRITIONAL SUPPLEMENTS

O Bromelain: 250–750 milligrams 3 times a day before meals.

O Coenzyme Q_{10}: 30 milligrams per day.

O Thymus extract: 500 milligrams of crude polypeptides daily.

○ Vitamin A: 5,000 IU per day.

○ Vitamin C: 1,000 milligrams 3 times per day.

○ Zinc picolinate: 30 milligrams per day.

HERBS

○ Aloe vera gel (for abscesses that have not been lanced or have not broken open): apply to skin over the abscess 2–3 times daily.

○ Astragalus: solid extract (0.5% 4-hydroxy-3-methoxy isoflavone), 100–150 milligrams 3 times a day, or dried root or tincture as recommended on the label.

○ Echinacea: 150–300 milligrams of solid extract (3.5% echinacosides) 3 times a day, or dried root, freeze-dried plant, juice, fluid extract, or tincture as recommended on the label.

○ Tea tree oil (for abscesses that have been lanced or have broken open): apply creams containing 8 to 20 percent tea tree oil or 40 percent solution to the skin with a cotton swab 2–3 times daily. Be sure to discard the cotton swab or applicator in a plastic bag so that the infection is not spread.

See Part Three if you take prescription medication.

UNDERSTANDING THE HEALING PROCESS

Abscesses are healed from the inside out. Boosting your immune system is the key to controlling infection. Because the bacterial infections that cause abscesses are active below the surface of the skin, applying either antibiotics or herbs to the surface of the skin is of limited value. Of the natural products that are applied topically, only aloe and tea tree oil have been scientifically demonstrated to heal abscesses. Poultices of barberry, coptis, and goldenseal, however, keep staph bacteria from spreading to other areas of skin.

Simply hydrating the skin by drinking water 6–8 times a day can be of great value in treating abscesses. Well-hydrated skin is supple and more resistant to reinfection. It releases accumulated white blood cells and pus more easily. Excessive amounts of sugar in your bloodstream create an acidic environment in which skin bacteria thrive. To stabilize sugar levels, your body has to produce (or you have to inject) large quantities of insulin, which is a growth factor for the skin. Stimulating growth of the layers of skin that line the infected hair follicles traps infection inside. Whole grains, fruits, and vegetables are natural sources of flavonoids. These are natural compounds that activate vitamin C in fighting infection and strengthen collagen, the principal protein from which the skin is made.[5]

Bromelain is a proteolytic or protein-dissolving enzyme refined from the stem of the pineapple plant. Its primary benefit in treating skin abscesses is dissolving the proteins that make the sloughed-off dead cells in the shaft of the hair follicle stick together.[6] Bromelain essentially "unplugs" the path to the surface of the skin through which an abscess can drain.

Bromelain also improves circulation to healthy skin. The immune system causes blood to clot around an abscess. The clotting protein fibrin forms a net around the area of inflammation to deprive it of oxygen and nutrients. This cuts off bacteria from their nutrient supply, but also traps the fluids that cause swelling. Bromelain stimulates the production of plasmin, a chemical that causes the protein chains that make up fibrin to unlink. When the fibrin chains unlink, circulation is restored.[7]

Since bromelain products are not standardized, finding the right dosage is a matter of trial and error. Start with the lower dose and work upward to the maximum until you notice changes in the "springiness" or "squishiness" of the abscess, springier and squishier being better. Allergies to bromelain are very rare but not unheard of. Reactions to this supplement are most likely to occur in people who are already allergic to pineapple, papaya, wheat flour, rye flour, or birch pollen. There has never been a report of an anaphylactic reaction, that is, a life-threatening allergic reaction, to bromelain. There have been isolated reports of heavy menstrual periods in women, nausea, vomiting, and hives when bromelain is taken in overdoses (2,000 milligrams and higher).

In laboratory experiments with mice, coenzyme Q_{10} (CoQ_{10}) increased immune response to *Staphylococcus aureus*.[8] CoQ_{10} is especially useful for persons who take statin drugs to lower cholesterol, a group including atorvastatin (Lipitor), lovastatin (Mevacor), pravastatin (Pravachol), and simvastatin (Zocor). CoQ_{10} is recommended for people who take red yeast rice (Cholestin), which is a naturally occurring statin drug. Statins interfere with the body's ability to produce both CoQ_{10} and cholesterol.

There is one report of CoQ_{10} increasing bleeding when taken with the anticlotting drug warfarin. Type 2 diabetics may find that their blood sugars are unexpectedly low when taking CoQ_{10}. If you have diabetes and you take CoQ_{10}, be sure to check your blood sugars every day.

There are no studies that directly confirm the usefulness of thymus extracts in treating staph infections, but there is considerable evidence that thymus extracts lift low immune function. Research has shown that thymus extract normalizes the ratio of helper T cells to suppressor T cells. This maintains a healthy immune response that neither destroys healthy tissue nor allows infectious microorganisms to flourish.[9]

Relatively low doses of vitamin A are sufficient to prevent immune "burnout" due to stress on the thymus.[10] Vitamin A also makes antibodies more responsive to various kinds of infections, increases the rate at which macrophages engulf and destroy bacteria, and stimulates natural killer cells.[11] The dosage of vitamin A recommended here is extremely unlikely to cause typical side effects, such as dry skin, chapped lips, headaches, and joint pain. Nonetheless, you should discontinue vitamin A immediately in the unlikely event that any of these symptoms appears. Women who are or who could become pregnant should be extremely careful not to take more than 5,000 IU of vitamin A in any single dose or in any single day, since overdoses (generally more than 300,000 IU) can cause birth defects if taken during the first 3 months of pregnancy.

Vitamin C is quickly depleted during the stress of an infection.[12] In combination with the anthocyanidin and proanthocyanidin bioflavonoids found in blue and dark-red fruits, vitamin C increases the stability of the ground substance, the "glue" between the skin and the tissues below it.[13] If you take aspirin on a daily basis, you may be deficient in vitamin C.

Dosages of vitamin C that are high enough to help fight staph infection almost always cause diarrhea at first. This side effect usually goes away in 3–4 days and can be avoided entirely if vitamin C is administered by injection (by a nutritionally oriented, qualified healthcare practitioner). Taking high doses of vitamin C without drinking 8–10 glasses of water a day can cause kidney stones. Abruptly discontinuing a high daily dosage of vitamin C can lead to symptoms of vitamin C deficiency. Before starting any high-dosage regimen of vitamin C, consult with your healthcare provider to make sure it will not aggravate any other health conditions or interfere with medications.

Zinc is an important cofactor for vitamin A. If you take tetracycline antibiotics for skin infections, chances are you are deficient in zinc. Taking tetracycline interferes with the body's absorption of zinc (and taking zinc interferes with the body's absorption of tetracycline). When zinc is deficient, the immune system's ability to produce white blood cells in response to infection is reduced, thymic hormone levels are lower, the immune response in the skin is especially reduced, and phagocytosis, the process in which bacteria are engulfed and digested, is slowed. All of these processes can be corrected by taking zinc supplements.[14] A good way to determine whether you need zinc is a taste test: chew a zinc tablet. If it doesn't taste bad, you probably need to take zinc.

Zinc picolinate is the most readily absorbed form of zinc. Do not take more than 50 milligrams of any zinc supplement daily. In rare cases, excessive intake of zinc depletes copper and causes anemia, that is, a deficiency of red blood cells, and neutropenia, a serious deficiency of white blood cells.[15]

Aloe is especially useful in treating abscesses that have been lanced (something you should never do at home). It contains a number of compounds necessary for healing wounds, including vitamin C, vitamin E, and zinc. Gels that are at least 70 percent aloe are bactericidal against both *Pseudomonas aeruginosa* and *Staphylococcus aureus*, the 2 most common causes of abscesses.[16] A small number of people are allergic to aloe, but the herb used topically has no other side effects.

Astragalus is a traditional Chinese treatment for abscesses, although Chinese tradition suggests that it is more useful for abscesses that sink in than it is for abscesses that dome out. This herb is especially useful in reversing damage to the immune system caused by chemicals or radiation.[17] In laboratory studies with test animals, astragalus increases the number and activity of monocytes and macrophages, the white blood cells responsible for controlling bacterial infection.[18]

Astragalus is an extremely useful immune stimulant, but not everyone should take it. Anyone who is on an immune suppressant—for example, people who have had organ transplants, or people who take immune suppressant drugs for multiple sclerosis, myasthenia gravis, rheumatoid arthritis, scleroderma, Sjögren's syndrome, or similar diseases—should not take astragalus. (If you develop an abscess while taking drugs for any of these conditions, you should seek medical care.) Stop taking astragalus if you notice a bruise or a bleeding cut.

There is no specific clinical evidence that echinacea

can cure the infections that cause abscesses, but there is considerable evidence that echinacea can relieve the pain of abscesses. German studies have found that *Echinacea purpurea* stimulates the immune system to produce macrophages. Echinacea increases the number of macrophages without increasing the numbers of other kinds of white blood cells that generate inflammatory hormones.[19] This targeted immune stimulation fights infection but avoids inflammation. In fact, echinacea relieves inflammation. One study found that a teaspoon of *Echinacea purpurea* juice is as effective in relieving pain and swelling as 100 milligrams of cortisone.[20]

Women who are trying to get pregnant should avoid *Echinacea purpurea*. It contains caffeoyl esters that can interfere with the action of hyaluronidase, an enzyme essential to the release of unfertilized eggs into the fallopian tube.[21]

There has been some controversy over the use of echinacea by people who have HIV. Echinacea stimulates immune function, but it also slightly increases production of T cells. These are the immune cells attacked by HIV. When there are more T cells, the virus has more cells to infect. This gives it more opportunities to mutate into a drug-resistant form. The authoritative reference work *The Complete German Commission E Monographs* counsels against the use of echinacea for treating colds in people who have HIV or autoimmune diseases, such as multiple sclerosis. Later communications between the senior editor of the Monographs and the German Food and Drug Administration revealed that the warning in the reference book was based on theoretical speculation rather than on practical experience. Still, as a precaution, people with HIV should only use echinacea for *treating* abscesses rather than preventing them.

Naturopathic physicians Michael Murray and Joseph Pizzorno write that an Australian study conducted in the 1960s found that tea tree oil accelerated the healing process and prevented scarring in staph infections. The method of application included cleaning the site, then painting the surface of the boil with tea tree oil 2 or 3 times a day.[22]

CONCEPTS FOR COPING WITH SKIN ABSCESSES

○ Apply hot, wet compresses to relieve pain. Repeated application of compresses will make it easier for your healthcare professional to lance an abscess. You can make a hot compress by soaking a clean towel in 2 cups of hot water to which you have added a teaspoon of powdered barberry, coptis, or goldenseal. These herbs contain berberine, which stops the multiplication of infectious bacteria outside the area of the abscess and prevents spread of the infection. (Do not take these herbs internally in these dosages to treat skin infections.) Apply the hot towel (as hot as you can stand) to the abscess. When the compress has cooled to body temperature, reheat the towel and reapply. Be sure to dry your skin after you have finished using the compress.

○ Elevate an abscess to a height higher than your heart to avoid swelling.

○ Avoid external friction, such as that caused by tight-fitting clothes.

○ Never squeeze bumps or cut open abscesses yourself, especially if they are located on the face. When an abscess is ready to be lanced by a doctor or nurse, it will feel "squishy" and may begin draining on its own.

○ Change your washcloth every time you wash, and change sheets and towels daily.

○ Wash your hands frequently, especially after changing a dressing or applying ointment.

○ If you take antibiotics, also take 1 or 2 capsules of *Acidophilus* or *Lactobacillus* every day. These probiotics help restore the friendly bacteria in your intestine that are destroyed by antibiotic treatment.

○ Flulike symptoms when you have an abscess are a possible symptom of sepsis. See a physician immediately if you feel like you are coming down with the flu when you have an abscess, particularly if the abscess gets redder or hotter.

Achilles Tendonitis

SYMPTOM SUMMARY

○ Pain and inflammation felt at the back of the leg from the calf to the heel

○ Difficulty lifting the heel above the toes

UNDERSTANDING THE DISEASE PROCESS

Achilles tendonitis is a painful and often debilitating

inflammation of the Achilles tendon, a cord running down the back of the lower leg and connecting the calf muscles to the heel bone. The Achilles tendon derives its name from the Greek mythological character Achilles, a mighty warrior whose mother Thetis bathed him in the magical waters of the river Styx at birth to make him invulnerable to harm. According to the legend, as Thetis dipped her son into the mystic river she held him by the heel. The unprotected heel became Achilles' only vulnerability. Many years later, Achilles was mortally wounded when an arrow struck him in the heel.

The Achilles tendon connects the strong leg muscles to the foot and makes it possible to rise up on the toes, facilitating the act of walking. This cord is vital to the ability to walk upright. Inflammation of the Achilles tendon can make walking almost impossible. Dancers, runners, and baseball, football, and tennis players are particularly at risk for Achilles tendonitis because their activities involve sudden stops and starts. Women who wear heels at work and switch to sneakers for exercise and people with "flat feet" are also susceptible to the condition.

The injury causing Achilles tendonitis occurs at any point along the Achilles tendon from the heel to the calf muscle. It can develop slowly over a period of months or years, or it can strike "weekend warriors" (those who are physically active only on weekends) who fail to warm up before exercise only once. Overdoing exercise at the beginning of a new fitness program is a frequent precipitating event for tendonitis because the muscles are not flexible enough to withstand the new forces being placed upon them.

The Achilles tendon is prone to inflammation because of its relatively poor blood supply. When blood circulation to the tendon is not increased gradually through warm-up exercises, the heel releases inflammatory hormones known as bradykinins to dilate the blood vessels and increase the flow of oxygen to the back of the leg.[1] The lack of circulation to the tendon makes other inflammatory hormones released in response to injury very slow to clear. An injured Achilles tendon can accumulate 100 times the concentration of inflammatory interleukin-6 found in surrounding tissues, and retain this level of the inflammatory chemical for at least 96 hours.[2]

Continuous stress on the Achilles tendon can cause more problems than just pain and inflammation. In severe cases, overstress may cause the rupture of the tendon. Rupture results in severe pain and traumatic damage. Walking may become impossible and the tendon may take a long time to heal, even requiring reparative surgery.

TREATMENT SUMMARY

NUTRITIONAL SUPPLEMENTS

To accelerate the healing process, take:

❍ Vitamin E: 800 IU per day.

For relief of pain, take the following or any one of the herbs mentioned below:

❍ SAM-e: 400 milligrams 3 times a day.

HERBS

❍ Boswellic acid extracts: 400 milligrams per day.

❍ Capsaicin cream, applied to the tendon daily. If you are sensitive to capsaicin, substitute diluted essential oils of peppermint, eucalyptus, rosemary, or wintergreen.

❍ Devil's claw (as an alternative to aspirin or NSAIDs): 405–520 milligrams up to 8 times a day.

❍ Willow bark (as an alternative to aspirin or NSAIDs): 1 teaspoon in a cup of hot water or tea, as desired.

❍ Yucca (leaf): 2–4 grams (1–2 teaspoons) per day.

If you use aspirin or NSAIDs on a regular basis, take:

❍ DGL (deglycyrrhizinated licorice): Chew and swallow 1–2 380 milligram tablets of DGL 20 minutes before meals 3 times a day.

See Part Three if you take prescription medication.

UNDERSTANDING THE HEALING PROCESS

Some of the latest research in sports medicine has shown that vitamin E spun into fibers and applied directly to the Achilles tendon greatly accelerates the healing process. Vitamin E absorbs free radicals of oxygen that activate inflammatory hormones, and accelerates the process of recovery in the injured tendon.[3] Strictly speaking, scientists have not studied whether over-the-counter capsules of vitamin E can accelerate the healing process, but trainers report that the vitamin is helpful and the likelihood of side effects in active individuals is minimal. In the unlikely event that you are prescribed clopidogrel (Plavix) or warfarin (Coumadin) after developing Achilles tendonitis or if you take aspirin on a daily basis, reduce your dosage of vitamin E to 200 IU per day.

A number of nutritional supplements and herbs help relieve the pain of Achilles tendonitis. Since not every supplement (or every medication) relieves pain in every case of Achilles tendonitis, you may have to experiment to find which supplement is most effective for you.

SAM-e, best known as a treatment for depression, also relieves pain. Various studies have found SAM-e as good or better for pain relief as Advil, Motrin, Naprosyn, and Nuprin. A study involving 20,641 people with osteoarthritis of the finger, hip, knee, and spine found that SAM-e alone was as effective as their ordinary pain relievers.[4] Another study involving 734 subjects found that it was more effective than Naprosyn (naproxen sodium).

The advantage of SAM-e is that it very seldom causes side effects. In the longest-running study involving the supplement, various minor side effects occurred in 20 out of 97 patients from time to time during the first 18 months of the intervention. In the final 6 months of the study, however, no patients experienced any side effects from SAM-e. Patients received relief of morning stiffness, pain at rest, and pain on movement, and depression as well.[5]

Although the use of herbal treatments for Achilles tendonitis is not especially well documented, several herbs are likely to be helpful if used on an occasional basis. Animal studies shows that boswellic acid extracts (produced from the Ayurvedic herb guggul) stop inflammation, increase glycosaminoglycan synthesis needed to repair injured tissue, and improve blood flow, the latter especially important in the treatment of Achilles tendonitis.[6] When used at a dosage of 400 milligrams per day, there are no reported side effects from this product. The Ayurvedic formula Yogaraj Guggulu has the same effect.

Some people should avoid boswellin, boswellic acid extracts, and guggul (guggulu). Both boswellic acid extracts and Yogaraj Guggulu alter the body's production of thyroid hormone. They should be avoided by people who have Graves' disease or other forms of hyperthyroidism. Boswellic acid supplements should be avoided by persons taking beta-blockers, especially propanolol (Inderal, Inderide), or calcium channel blockers, especially diltiazem (Cardizem), for high blood pressure, since boswellic acid can make these drugs less available to the body.[7]

Capsaicin, devil's claw, and willow bark offer pain relief. Capsaicin is the chemical that gives hot peppers their heat. As anyone who has cooked with chiles knows, capsaicin can cause burning, redness, and inflammation, especially to the eyes and mouth. The first time it is applied in a cream to the skin over a painful injury, capsaicin causes these symptoms, but the nerve fibers serving the back of the leg become insensitive to it—and to pain.[8]

Capsaicin works best when there is good circulation to the skin to which it is applied.[9] Do not apply capsaicin to your legs if you have diabetes and never apply capsaicin to ulcerated skin. It is also important to keep capsaicin out of your nose and eyes. Allergic reactions to capsaicin are rare but are not unknown, and there have been cases of hypothermia in people who used capsaicin in an especially cold room. It is theoretically possible that capsaicin absorbed into the bloodstream could reduce the bioavailability of aspirin; if you use capsaicin, use pain relievers other than aspirin.

Devil's claw relieves knee pain, but only if it is taken in an enteric-coated form that protects its analgesic compounds from being digested in the stomach. Do not use devil's claw with NSAIDs such as aspirin and Tylenol and avoid it entirely if you have duodenal or gastric ulcers.

Willow bark is a natural substitute for aspirin. It contains a pain reliever less potent than the salicylates found in aspirin but that does not generally cause bleeding or stomach irritation. Do not use willow bark during pregnancy, if you have tinnitus (ringing in the ears), or if you are allergic to aspirin. Do not give willow bark or aspirin to children who have colds or flu.

Natural health experts Dr. Michael Murray and Dr. Joseph Pizzorno suggest that yucca reduces inflammation in various forms of joint pain through a unique pathway, stopping the production of bacterial toxins in the intestines. They base their suggestion on the scientific observation that bacterial endotoxins stop proteoglycan synthesis, and that yucca contains natural soaps that break up the fat components of the bacterial endotoxins.[10] Although research has not yet confirmed their theory, many sufferers of osteoarthritis report that yucca seems to help if it is used over a period of several months.

CONCEPTS FOR COPING WITH ACHILLES TENDONITIS

O The best defense against Achilles tendonitis is to be sure to do jumping jacks, light jogging, and leg stretches, or get a massage before engaging in vigorous physical activity and to wear low-heeled, well-fitted shoes. Never continue exercise if you feel a sharp pain in your heel.

○ The standard treatment for minor tendon pain is known by the acronym RICE:

• **Rest** the tendon by staying off your feet as much as possible.

• Apply **ice** packs to the affected area for 20 minutes at a time at least 3 times a day for several days to reduce inflammation.

• **Compress** the ankle and foot with a firm (but not tight) elastic bandage.

• **Elevate** the leg to reduce swelling.

○ Ice packs are universally recommended in treating injury and swelling, but not everyone feels better after applying a cold pack to the Achilles tendon. Use other methods if applying ice increases rather than decreases pain.

○ Avoid wearing high heels. In women who wear high-heeled shoes on a daily basis, the Achilles tendon and muscles gradually adapt to a shortened position because the heel does not stretch all the way to the ground. When this occurs, switching to sneakers or flat shoes forces the Achilles tendon to stretch. If high heels must be worn every day, stretching exercises should be performed *every* day to keep the Achilles tendon at its full length.

○ When Achilles tendon pain occurs even with proper stretching and warm-ups, it is helpful to consult a podiatrist to check for hyperpronation and adequate arch support. Inserting an orthotic into the shoe may be enough to maintain a good arch and foot alignment and eliminate pain.

Acne

SYMPTOM SUMMARY

○ Small, flesh-colored, white, or dark bumps that give skin a rough texture, including:

• Blackheads—enlarged pores of the skin blocked by a dark plug with an irregular surface

• Whiteheads—normal-sized pores of the skin blocked by accumulated secretions but not inflamed

• Papules—pores of normal size each with a ruptured wall blocked by accumulated secretions and inflammation

• Pustules—ruptured pores with collections of pus (dead bacteria and white blood cells) draining at the surface

• Nodules—inflamed, tender accumulations of pus within the skin

• Cysts—nodules greater than 5 millimeters (0.2 inches) in diameter that fail to discharge pus

• Large, deep pustules—nodules that break down surrounding tissues

UNDERSTANDING THE DISEASE PROCESS

Acne is a condition of chronic inflammation of the pores of the skin. More than 85 percent of young people aged 12 to 14 get acne.[1] The skin condition can also appear or reappear in adults in their 20s and 30s, or even into their 40s and 50s.

Across all age groups, acne is the most common of all skin problems. Among teenagers, acne that is bad enough to cause scarring is more common among boys than among girls. The persistence of acne into adulthood, however, is more common among women than among men.[2]

Acne vulgaris is the technical term for the most common form of acne. This type of acne causes whiteheads, blackheads, papules, and pustules. Acne conglobata is the technical term for the more serious form of the disease. This type of acne causes cysts and makes scars. Both types of acne usually appear on the face, as does acne rosacea, reddening of the skin of the nose that is aggravated by changes in temperature (see ROSACEA). Acne vulgaris and acne conglobata can occur on the back, chest, and shoulders. More often than not, acne vulgaris clears up even if it is not treated. Nonetheless, any kind of acne can severely affect self-image, especially in teenagers.

Acne begins with the accumulation of sebum, an oil secreted by the skin. Sebum is essential to healthy skin. Its primary function is lubrication of the hair shaft, allowing hair to move with the skin. This vital oil also helps prevent excessive evaporation and absorption of water.

Sebum keeps the skin soft and supple. It minimizes wrinkling. It enables the skin to act as a raincoat, protecting the body from water absorption through the skin. Sebum also prevents the evaporation of essential fluids from the skin. Because fat is a poor conductor of heat, sebum lessens the amount of heat lost from the body's surface in cold weather.

Sebum itself does not cause acne. Neither do the two strains of bacteria associated with acne, *Propionibacterium acnes* (also known as *Corynebacterium acnes*) and *Staphylococcus albus*. In healthy skin, these bacteria feed on excess sebum, keeping it from blocking pores. In the process of digesting sebum, they release a chemical related to hydrogen peroxide as they digest its fatty acids. This potent oxidant does no damage to the skin as long as it is free to flow to the surface, where ordinary washing with soap and water carry it away. Acne only occurs when the opening of the follicle is blocked and the peroxide is trapped, so that it inflames the skin.

Several hormonal processes cause pores to narrow and trap inflammatory peroxides. One of them is stress, contributing to acne in both males and females of all ages. Stress causes microscopic packets in the ends of the nerve cells controlling the muscles and skin to break open and release two stress hormones, adrenaline and substance P. These chemicals help nerve signals jump from cell to cell. Once in the bloodstream, substance P eventually reaches the skin where it signals the cells that make sebum not just to grow in numbers but also to increase productivity. Under conditions of stress, greatly increased numbers of sebum glands pour out greatly increased amounts of oily sebum.[3] This is the reason people who have acne have more severe outbreaks when they are under stress.

Another hormonal process that influences acne at all ages is insulin resistance. Insulin moves sugar from the bloodstream into cells. When skin cells are unable to respond to insulin, sugar accumulates in the fluids between them. Some of this sugar flows into the follicle and feeds bacteria. The insulin resistance that causes acne is peculiar in that it is localized to the skin. It is a kind of "skin diabetes" that does not result in other complications. People who have acne do not generally have systemic problems with blood sugars or full-blown diabetes, and people who have diabetes are not at special risk for acne.[4]

The primary hormonal imbalance that causes acne, however, is an excess of the male-associated sex hormone testosterone. This hormone is produced by the bodies of both men and women, but in vastly greater quantities in men. Most people have some understanding of how testosterone causes the hairiness, muscularity, and aggression of male secondary characteristics, but the role of testosterone in women requires some explanation. Women's bodies contain testosterone throughout their lives, but only in vanishingly small quantities until puberty. About the time of a woman's first period, the adrenal glands begin to make massive quantities of dehydroepiandrosterone (DHEA) from cholesterol. Most of the young woman's DHEA is processed by the adrenal glands into the stress hormones so well known in adolescence. Some of the DHEA goes to the ovaries and uterus to form the female hormones estrogen and progesterone. Trace amounts of DHEA accumulate as a byproduct, dehydroepiandrosterone sulfate. When a woman's adrenal glands and ovaries turn this byproduct into testosterone, she begins to experience sexual desire. About the time a young woman becomes interested in sex, she also becomes at risk for acne.[5]

Like sebum and acne bacteria, testosterone itself does not aggravate acne. Testosterone becomes a problem only when it is chemically processed by the enzyme 5-alpha-reductase into a more potent form of the hormone, dihydrotesterone. This form of testosterone stimulates the production of the tough protein keratin that lines the interior of the pore.[6,7] As keratin builds up in the cells lining the shaft of the pore, it narrows the pore's opening. The narrowed pore traps peroxide-producing bacteria, dead skin cells, and pus inside.

Testosterone levels are especially high in both boys and girls aged 10–14. They are also elevated in women who have ovarian cysts, in men who take the body-building aid androstenedione, and in women who use oral contraceptives. All of these groups are especially susceptible to acne.

Acne also results from exposure to industrial pollutants, including machine oils, chlorinated hydrocarbons, and coal tar derivatives. Acne is a frequent side effect of treatment with steroids for asthma or rheumatoid arthritis, lithium carbonate for bipolar disorder, and isonicotinic acid (isoniazid) for tuberculosis. Overdoses of vitamin B supplements (specifically vitamin B_6 and B_{12}) can cause acne.[8] Even more frequently, acne results from the overuse of pore-clogging cosmetics or pomades, or is a complication of skin irritation caused by overwashing and nervous, repetitive rubbing of the skin.

Prescription medications for acne often make the condition worse before it gets better. Most drugs for acne require several weeks to several months to take effect. Any medication for acne must be used regularly to work.

TREATMENT SUMMARY

DIET

○ Avoid caffeine, cola drinks, and refined sugars.

○ In general, avoid overeating starchy or sugary foods.

○ Avoid shellfish and iodized salt.

○ Drink at least 6–8 glasses of water every day.

NUTRITIONAL SUPPLEMENTS

○ Brewer's yeast: 1 tablespoon of powdered yeast or 3,000 milligrams of brewer's yeast capsules 2 times per day. (Persons who are susceptible to gout should take chromium supplements instead of brewer's yeast.) Yeast beta-D-glucan, 20 milligrams 3 times a day, can be substituted for brewer's yeast.

○ Selenium: 200 micrograms per day.

○ Vitamin A: 100,000 IU per day for up to 3 months. Women who are or who may become pregnant should strictly limit their intake of vitamin A to 5,000 IU per day or less.

○ Vitamin C: 1,000 milligrams per day.

○ Vitamin E: 400 IU per day.

○ Zinc picolinate: 50 milligrams per day.

Women who experience outbreaks of acne before their menstrual period may benefit from:

○ Vitamin B_6 (pyridoxine): 50 milligrams per day, or 1 complete B vitamin supplement tablet 3 times per day.

Anyone who has acne who engages in vigorous physical exercise on a regular basis, especially teenagers, should be sure to take vitamins C and E, plus:

○ Alpha-lipoic acid, 100 milligrams daily.

HERBS

○ Avoid avena, chrysin, muira puama, pine pollen, Siberian ginseng, stinging nettle, and Tribestan. All of these herbs either increase testosterone production or elevate testosterone levels in the bloodstream.

○ Tea tree oil (5 to 15 percent strength), use topically.

○ Calendula soap.

OTHER HELPFUL NATURAL PRODUCTS

○ Alpha hydroxy acid (lotions containing 5 to 10 percent glycolic acid).

○ Azelaic acid (creams in 20 percent strength), used topically.

○ Pantothenic acid creams (available from compounding pharmacies).

See Part Three if you take prescription medication.

UNDERSTANDING THE HEALING PROCESS

For most people who have acne, the cardinal rule of skin care should be "Wash less." Washing the surface of the skin does *not* remove embedded oils or cellular debris, but it can make the skin dry and wrinkle-prone. Rubbing too hard can injure the skin so that infection sets in. Washing with soap and water in the morning and in the evening is enough.

In taking care of acne, it is particularly important not to try to dry out oily skin. Drying the skin with alcohol or alcohol-based astringents or gels does not eliminate the pus that clogs pores. It only tightens the skin and makes the natural elimination of sebum and dead skin cells more difficult. Dry skin ages more quickly.

Caffeine, colas, and sugary soft drinks induce an adrenaline surge. This triggers the release of substance P. In turn, substance P signals the glands to make more sebum. It is especially important to avoid caffeinated, sugary soft drinks and coffee during times of stress.

It is also important not to overeat even unrefined carbohydrates. Healthy carbohydrates, such as those found in fruit, vegetables, legumes, and whole grains, do not trigger a sugar surge, but they do become sugar once they are digested. High sugar levels can be reduced only by the production of (or injection of) insulin. The same insulin that reduces blood sugars stimulates the growth of the skin, pushing a layer of skin cells to the surface. This blocks the exit of the pores.

Avoiding carbohydrates has other benefits in taking care of acne. Reducing consumption of high-carbohydrate foods reduces the amount of sugar available to bacteria. It slows the conversion by alpha-reductase of testosterone into its more potent form, dihydrotesterone. For this reason cutting out carbohydrates has special benefit for men and boys with acne, and for women who suffer acne as a side effect of testosterone treatments. Doctors conducting clinical research have found that a high-protein diet (in this study, 44 percent protein, 35 percent carbohydrate, and 21 percent fat) slows the conversion of testosterone into dihydrotesterone. The effects of the diet were measurable in fewer than 2 weeks. A high-carbohydrate diet (10 percent protein, 70 percent carbohydrate, and 20 percent fat) had the opposite effect, accelerating the conversion of testosterone into its acne-inducing form, also in fewer than 2 weeks.[9]

Most naturopathic physicians also advise avoiding iodine found in shellfish and iodized salt, since it is essential to the production of thyroid hormones that enable the release of sugar into the bloodstream. Of all the diet recommendations for acne care, the easiest is just to drink more water. Keeping the skin adequately hydrated keeps it supple, helping sebum to flow to the surface.

Some readers may wonder why certain dietary suggestions are not made here. There is no evidence that high-fat foods, in and of themselves, cause acne. Cholesterol is a building block for testosterone, but the body's supply of cholesterol is mostly made by the liver. Eliminating fatty foods generally has very little effect on either the amount of cholesterol in circulation or the progress of acne. Among high-fat foods, chocolate and nuts are frequently singled out as causes of acne. They are not. The tyrosine in chocolate, gelatin, and nuts can aggravate herpes, but does not affect acne.

Another recommendation that is not made here is to take fiber. Fiber absorbs waste estrogen in the intestines, which prevents the hormone from being absorbed through the intestinal wall back into the bloodstream, where it can be converted into testosterone. While taking fiber does not hurt, there is no evidence that it produces specific improvements in acne. Nonetheless, if you choose to use fiber, always take fiber supplements separately from other supplements and medications. Fiber keeps medicine from being fully absorbed.

High-chromium yeast enhances the ability of insulin to carry sugar out of the bloodstream and into cells.[10] A preliminary clinical study reported rapid improvement in acne patients who took brewer's yeast for acne.[11] Yeast beta-D-glucan stimulates the activity of macrophages, the white blood cells that are responsible for eliminating bacterial infections.[12]

Yeast is also thought to enhance the elasticity of the skin, and is used in many cosmetics. There are no reports of side effects from using yeast. Yeast may even increase the effectiveness of antibiotic treatments for acne.

Selenium is an important cofactor for vitamin E. Adult male acne patients have low levels of the antioxidant glutathione peroxidase, which normalizes with vitamin E and selenium treatment. Glutathione peroxidase puts a brake on inflammatory reactions throughout the body, especially in the skin. Selenium depresses the parts of the immune system that cause allergic reactions, but encourages the parts of the immune system that respond to bacterial infection. There is also evidence that selenium compounds control the breakdown of thyroid hormones into forms that do not aggravate acne.[13]

Selenium from yeast is the best form of selenium for treating acne. Taking selenium at the same time as vitamin C reduces the absorption of selenium, and you should never take more that 1,000 milligrams of selenium a day. The first sign that you have overdosed selenium is usually a garlicky breath odor. Excessive use of selenium can also cause hair loss, fatigue, irritability, and hyperreflexia or "jumpiness." Horizontal streaking, blackening, and fragility of the nails when you take selenium is a sure sign you are taking too much or you are taking a product that has been improperly standardized.

Both men and women with acne benefit from taking selenium with vitamin E.[14] Taking these two nutrients together is especially important for acne that has reached the pustule stage.[15] Vitamin E is also an important cofactor for vitamin A. In laboratory studies with animals, the amount of vitamin A in the bloodstream stays low regardless of intake until vitamin E levels are normal. Vitamin E supplementation is useful even if you do not take vitamin A, since it complements the vitamin A available from the diet.

Vitamin A is the naturally occurring analog of the prescription drug tretinoin (Accutane). Like its chemical cousin, vitamin A reduces the production of sebum and slows the rate at which skin cells produce keratin. Together, these actions keep pores open and reduce the probability of infection.

The drawback to using vitamin A as a supplement is that a dose that is big enough to stop acne is big enough to cause side effects. Problems from using even up to 300,000 IU of vitamin A per day are rare, but they are significant. The first signs of vitamin A overdose are dry skin and chapped lips, especially in dry weather. Later signs of toxicity are headache, mood swings, and pain in muscles and joints. In massive doses, vitamin A can cause liver damage. In the first 3 months of pregnancy, it can cause birth defects. Women who are or may become pregnant should not use more than 5,000 IU of vitamin A per day, which is not enough to improve acne. Discontinue high-dosage vitamin A at the first sign of toxicity, and never use it for more than 3 months at a time.

Vitamin C does not have a scientifically demonstrated direct effect on acne, but it makes other vitamins more available. Studies at the Northern Ireland Centre for Diet and Health have found that taking vitamin C increases the amount of available vitamin E in the bloodstream by about 10 percent. Taking vitamin E increases the amount of available vitamin C in the bloodstream by about 60 percent.[16]

Vitamin C also may protect against the side effects of prescription acne drugs. Tetracycline antibiotics for acne, especially minocycline (Cyclimycin, Minocin, or Trimomin), cause a condition known as "blue smile," a discoloration of the tongue and teeth. Scientists at the Baylor College of Dentistry in Dallas have found that giving vitamin C to lab rats at a dosage approximating 1,000 milligrams per day in humans prevents staining of teeth during minocycline therapy.[17]

Several clinical studies report that zinc is only slightly less effective than antibiotics in controlling acne. The key to using zinc effectively is buying the right kind of zinc. Researchers using an effervescent (fizzy) form of zinc sulfate found it to be about as effective as the antibiotic tetracycline. Researchers using a plain form of zinc sulfate found that it appeared to have a somewhat beneficial effect on pustules but not on blackheads, whiteheads, nodules, or cysts.[18] The most recent clinical study found that acne patients given a moderate dose of zinc gluconate (30 milligrams) per day were about half as likely to be completely cured after 90 days as those given the minocycline. Among patients who did not achieve total remission, however, zinc treatment eliminated over 90 percent as many lesions as treatment with the antibiotic after 30 days and over 80 percent as many lesions as the antibiotic after 90 days.[19]

The bottom line of these studies is, if you have acne, take zinc and be prepared to wait a couple of months for results. The best-absorbed form of zinc is zinc picolinate. Do not take more than 50 milligrams of any zinc supplement daily. In rare cases, excessive intake of zinc depletes copper to cause anemia, that is, a deficiency of red blood cells, and neutropenia, a serious deficiency of white blood cells.[20] If you take tetracycline antibiotics for skin infections, chances are you are deficient in zinc. Taking tetracycline interferes with the body's absorption of zinc (and taking zinc interferes with the body's absorption of tetracycline).

One other supplement is helpful if you exercise and you have acne. Aerobic exercise helps acne by increasing circulation to the skin, but anaerobic exercise (huffing and puffing to the point of exhaustion) *without antioxidant supplementation* may aggravate acne. Strenuous exercise depletes glutathione. This naturally occurring antioxidant slows inflammatory reactions and is essential to the normal function of estrogen and testosterone. Laboratory studies with animals have found that supplementation with alpha-lipoic acid keeps glutathione from breaking down, especially in the liver and in the bloodstream.[21]

Also in laboratory experiments with animals, vitamin B_6 (pyridoxine) deficiencies cause increased sensitivity to testosterone.[22] Women who have flare-ups of acne along with PMS often improve after taking vitamin B_6.[23] Women who develop acne during testosterone treatment usually benefit from taking B_6.

A study conducted at the Royal Prince Alfred Hospital in New South Wales, Australia, found that a 5 percent tea tree oil solution was as beneficial as a 5 percent benzoyl peroxide cream in reducing the number of pimples. Benzoyl peroxide got faster results, but tea tree oil had fewer side effects.[24] Tea tree oil is antibacterial against 27 of 32 strains of *Propionibacterium acnes*, the infectious agent most commonly associated with the disease.[25] Tea tree oil may be used at a strength of up to 15 percent for especially severe cases of acne. There are very few reports of problems with tea tree oil, although it can cause allergies and should be kept away from small children.

Calendula and marigold are the same herb. The botanical term calendula is used to name bath products and the common term marigold is used to refer to the plant as a healing herb. Calendula soaps are a very useful complement to tea tree oil. They kill *Staphylococcus aureus*,[26] a bacterium not affected by tea tree oil. The essential oil in the herb is a potent anti-inflammatory agent, offering about the same degree of pain relief as the over-the-counter nonsteroidal anti-inflammatory agent indomethacin (Indocin),[27] but without side effects on the digestive tract. Marigold oil applied to the skin with a cotton swab has the same analgesic effect. About 1 in 500 people is allergic to calendula. Test the soap or oil on a small area of skin before using it on a large patch of skin.

There are several other natural products you can use to treat acne. Alpha hydroxy acids are commonly found in and isolated from fruits of all sorts. Exactly how they help control acne is not fully understood, but they function in at least two ways. They act as a humectant, increasing the water content of the skin and moisturizing the outer layer of the epidermis. This makes the skin softer and more flexible. Secondarily, alpha-hydroxy acids reduce skin cell adhesion and accelerate skin cell proliferation within the basal cell layers.

Alpha hydroxy acids encourage the growth of blood vessels to oxygenate the skin. They activate an internal clock inside skin cells at the surface reminding them of the time to die and be sloughed off, providing room for the growth of new, healthy skin. The growth of skin underneath the follicle forces it open and allows the release of dead skin cells and irritants.[28]

Azelaic acid is a naturally occurring hydrocarbon, found in wheat, rye, and barley. It is one of the acids used in "facial peels" performed in a doctor's office. This organic product prevents the process of hyperkeratosis, or overgrowth of skin cells, forcing follicles shut. By reducing the rate at which skin cells grow in the linings of pores, it keeps pores open.[29] It is antibacterial, controlling both *Propionibacterium acnes*, the microorganism that flourishes in clogged pores, and *Staphylococcus aureus*, the bacterium that also causes abscesses, boils, and impetigo.[30] Physicians at the University of California at San Francisco have found that a cream containing 20 percent azelaic acid is as effective in treating acne as benzoyl peroxide gel (5 percent concentration), tretinoin cream (0.05 percent concentration), erythromycin cream (2 percent concentration), and oral tetracycline given at a dosage of 500–1,000 milligrams per day, provided it is used to treat pimples and mild to moderate inflammatory acne. However, azelaic acid is less effective than Accutane for the treatment of acne conglobata, the form of the condition that produces large, deep pustules.[31]

Azelaic acid cream should be applied twice daily for at least 2–3 months. It can be used for up to 1 year. Improvement should be detectable within 1–2 months.[32] To ensure adequate penetration, the cream should be rubbed thoroughly (but not too vigorously) into clean skin for 2–3 minutes. An advantage of azelaic acid over antibiotics is that azelaic acid does not cause bacteria to become antibiotic-resistant. Azelaic acid seldom produces adverse effects, the most common being short-term itching and burning sensations. About 10 percent of people who use azelaic acid will experience burning and itching during the first 2–4 weeks it is used.

Alpha Hydroxy Acid Ingredients

Recognizing which products contain alpha hydroxy acids requires reading the label. Alpha hydroxy acid ingredients may be listed as any of the following:

- alpha hydroxy and botanical complex
- alpha hydroxycaprylic acid
- alpha hydroxyethanoic acid + ammonium alpha hydroxyethanoate
- alpha hydroxyoctanoic acid
- citric acid
- glycolic acid
- glycolic acid + ammonium glycolate
- glycomer in crosslinked fatty acids alpha nutrium (three AHAs).

- hydroxycaprylic acid
- lactic acid
- L-alpha hydroxy acid
- malic acid
- mixed fruit acid
- sugar cane extract
- tri-alpha hydroxy fruit acids
- triple fruit acid

Of these, the most frequently used in cosmetics are glycolic acid and lactic acid.

Pantothenic acid (vitamin B$_5$) creams, which are available from compounding pharmacists, are of potential value in treating acne. The body uses pantothenic acid to make coenzyme A, which releases energy from carbohydrates, fats, and proteins. A clinical study in China of 45 males and 55 females between 12 and 30 years of age found that applying a cream made with pantothenic acid began to eliminate pimples in 1–2 weeks. The cream contained 10 grams of pantothenic acid diluted to a 20 percent concentration. It was applied 4–6 times per day. The physicians supervising the study noted no side effects.[33]

Obtain a pantothenic acid cream from a compounding pharmacy when other treatments fail. The commercially available MSM Cream (sold by General Vitamin) is also helpful but does not have the same concentration of pantothenic acid used in the Chinese study.

CONCEPTS FOR COPING WITH ACNE

○ Avoid touching your hands to your face. Squeezing and picking at pimples will make them worse.

○ Wear your hair so it stays out of your face. Keeping your hair out of your face keeps oils from reaching facial skin.

○ Avoid heavy makeup, moisturizing creams, and oily hair preparations.

○ Always use a clean towel to dry your face, to avoid reinfecting your skin with acne-causing bacteria.

○ If you experience periodic outbreaks of acne not related to stress (in both sexes) or your menstrual cycle (in women), the problem may be cumulative stress to your skin from the way you wash your face. Do not scrub too hard—rough treatment of your skin opens pores to bacteria.

○ If you have been prescribed tetracycline or minocycline antibiotics, be sure to take them at least 1 hour before or 2 hours after meals to avoid stomach upset. Never take antibiotics with milk. It is best to take these medications with water at bedtime.

○ Do not try to get a tan to "dry out" acne. Exposure to sun does not help acne and can cause wrinkles.

○ Several Oriental formulas treat special cases of acne. In women who have not yet reached menopause, Dong Quai and Peony Formula increases the production of estrogen when it is needed but not when it could cause premenstrual syndrome. During the first 14 days of the menstrual cycle, the formula stimulates ovulation and stops outbreaks of acne by causing the ovaries to produce more estrogen and less testosterone. Dong Quai and Peony Formula is available in the United States and Canada under the following trade names:

- Dang Gui & Peony (Qualiherb)
- Kampo4Women MenopauEase (Honso)
- Tangkuei & Peony Formula (Lotus Classics)
- Tang-Kuei and Peony Formula (Golden Flower Chinese Herbs, Sun Ten)
- Toki-shakuyaku-san (Honso, Tsumura)

○ White Tiger Formula with Ginseng treats acne in people who also have outbreaks of eczema. This Chinese herbal formula is available in the United States and Canada as:

- Bai Hu Jai Ren Shen Tang (Lotus Classics, Qualiherb, Sun Ten)
- Byakko-ka-ninjin-to (Honso, Tsumura)
- Ginseng & Gypsum (Qualiherb)
- Ginseng & Gypsum Combination (Lotus Classics, Sun Ten)

○ Homeopathic medicine offers a number of treatments for acne. While homeopathic preparations are generally more effective than a placebo, the full benefit of homeopathy is found through interaction with a homeopathic physician who can match the symptoms of the whole person to a specific remedy. Because homeopathy treats people rather than diseases, homeopathic remedies match not only specific symptoms, but "central delusions," the essential ways people misperceive their life issues, that lead to illness.

If you choose to try homeopathy without the assistance of a homeopathic physician, start with a single dose of the lowest strength (6C, 6X, or 12C) of the remedy matching the symptoms to be treated, and then wait for a response. If there is an improvement in symptoms, let the remedy continue to work until there is no more improvement, then take another dose. If there is no improvement, try a different potency (30X or 30C). Sometimes homeopathic medicines work for a few minutes, and sometimes they work for an entire day before another dose is needed.

- Antimonium tartaricum treats acne in people who tend to get frequent infections and who are generally irritable. The specific manifestations of acne may be bluish marks that remain on the skin after pimples have cleared up, or large pustules that are tender to the touch.

• Calcarea carbonica treats acne in people who have a tendency to sweat (especially in the hands and feet), are overweight, tend to become anxious when on a tight schedule, and who have cravings for sweets. For this person, acne outbreaks are frequent and coincide with other infections.

• Hepar sulphuris calcareum is usually recommended for people who are sensitive to cold and who respond to cold with irritability. Skin eruptions may be sensitive to the touch and easily infected, but slow to come to a head.

• Pulsatilla, sometimes labeled as silverweed, is helpful when acne is aggravated by eating too many sugary foods. The person often has a fair complexion and is inclined toward soft emotions. Homeopathic physicians often recommend it to women whose acne breaks out near menstrual periods.

• Silicea (silica), a homeopathic remedy made from the most common material in the earth's crust, relieves deep-seated acne with swollen lymph nodes and fatigue. People who benefit from this remedy are generally chilly but may wake up in the middle of the night drenched with sweat. They may have to endure deep depression stemming from deprivation in life.

• Sulfur treats inflamed and itchy outbreaks of dirty-looking skin. Homeopaths tend to recommend it to patients who suffer a general lack of order and neatness in their lives.

Acne Rosacea
See **Rosacea.**

Acoustic Trauma

SYMPTOM SUMMARY

○ Hearing loss
  • Lose hearing of high pitches first
  • Usually partial but may be progressive
○ Ringing in the ears (tinnitus)

UNDERSTANDING THE DISEASE PROCESS

Nearly everyone has had the experience of acoustic trauma, the loss of hearing after exposure to loud noise. The term acoustic trauma refers to the damage to hearing caused by a single experience or a few experiences of very loud sounds.

Damaging sounds such as explosions, gunshots, rock concerts, listening to music through headphones turned too loud, and the din of noisy machinery can temporarily or permanently damage hearing. Acoustic trauma is especially destructive of the ability to hear high pitches.

Loud noises hurt hearing by injuring microscopic hairs called stereocilia. These hairs lie on the organ of Corti, the membrane that vibrates so that sound is perceived. Every sound causes a surge of fluid through the cochlea, the spiral channel in the inner ear. The swooshing fluids flow past the stereocilia, which transmit the sensation of sound to nerves reaching the brain. Low pitches can be heard even if the surge of fluid passes through just a small part of the cochlea. The highest pitches can only be heard if the surge of fluid passes all the way to the end of the cochlea. The stereocilia must be firmly attached to the organ of Corti and rigid enough to be moved by the fluid for sound to be perceived.

A very loud noise causes a very strong rush of fluid strong enough to damage the stereocilia. These tiny hairs can be literally torn out by their roots. Even if they are not, the stereocilia can experience metabolic exhaustion trying to repair themselves. In the latter case, the hairs swell with fluids, become limp, and stop moving with the flow of fluid through the cochlea. This causes a threshold shift, that is, sounds have to be louder and lower to be heard at all. If the hairs have a chance to recover, the threshold shift is temporary. Nevertheless, if there is constant exposure to noise, the stereocilia never get a chance to recover, and the threshold shift and related hearing loss are permanent.

How loud is too loud? Sounds louder than 90 decibels (dB, a measurement of the loudness or strength of vibration of a sound) may cause such intense vibration that the inner ear is damaged, especially if the sound is prolonged. Ninety decibels is about the loudness of a large truck about 5 yards (5 meters) away. A jackhammer emits sounds of about 120 decibels from 3 feet (1 meter) away, and a jet engine emits sound of about 130 decibels from 100 feet (30 meters) away. Motorcycles, snowmobiles, and similar engines range around 85–90 decibels, and a rock concert may approach 100 decibels. A general rule is if you need to shout to be heard, the sound is in the range that can damage hearing.

TREATMENT SUMMARY

NUTRITIONAL SUPPLEMENTS

○ Vitamin A: 300,000 IU *weekly* for 6 weeks. Women who are or who could become pregnant should strictly limit their intake of vitamin A to 5,000 IU per day or less.

○ Vitamin B$_{12}$: 250 milligrams daily for 6 weeks.

○ Vitamin E: 100 IU daily for 6 weeks.

HERBS

○ Ginkgo: 80 milligrams of an extract containing 24% ginkgo flavonglycosides, taken 3 times a day for 6 weeks.

UNDERSTANDING THE HEALING PROCESS

The rule to remember when dealing with acoustic trauma is the sooner, the better. The very best way to deal with acoustic trauma is to wear hearing protection so that it never occurs. If you can't avoid exposure to loud noise, then you must take immediate steps to treat it. Ideally, treatment should begin within 12 hours of trauma.

Vitamin A in very high doses for very short periods sometimes can greatly improve hearing loss. A Swiss study in 1952 found that survivors of explosions sometimes regained hearing after treatment with 300,000 IU of vitamin A per *week* for 6 weeks. The effect of the vitamin was greatest for people whose acoustic trauma was the most recent. Vitamin A helped recover the ability to hear high pitches more than it helped recover the ability to hear low intensity sounds, such as whispers.[1]

The drawback to using vitamin A as a supplement is that a dose that is big enough to help heal acoustic trauma is big enough to cause side effects. Problems from using even up to 300,000 IU of vitamin A per *day* (nearly 7 times as much as was used in the Swiss study) are rare, but they are significant. The first signs of vitamin A overdose are dry skin and chapped lips, especially in dry weather. Later signs of toxicity are headache, mood swings, and pain in muscles and joints. In massive doses, vitamin A can cause liver damage. In the first 3 months of pregnancy, it can cause birth defects. Women who are or who could become pregnant should

strictly limit their intake of vitamin A to 5,000 IU per day or less. Discontinue vitamin A at the first sign of toxicity, and do not use it for longer than the recommended 6 weeks.

A study by the Israeli Army found that about half of the 86 soldiers in the study who suffered hearing loss related to acoustic trauma also suffered vitamin B$_{12}$ deficiency. (The study also found that about a quarter of soldiers who do *not* have hearing loss suffer vitamin B$_{12}$ deficiency.) The researchers concluded there is a relationship between vitamin B$_{12}$ deficiency and dysfunction of the auditory pathway. Some of the soldiers given vitamin B$_{12}$ supplements regained some of their hearing.[2]

The people who are most likely to be deficient in vitamin B$_{12}$ are vegetarians who take either antibiotics or any kind of medication for gastroesophageal reflux disease (GERD) on a regular basis. Vitamin B$_{12}$ is nontoxic even when it is taken in a dosage 1,000 times greater than the RDA.

Vitamin E is an important cofactor for vitamin A. In laboratory studies with animals, the amount of vitamin A in the bloodstream stays low regardless of intake until vitamin E levels are normalized. Vitamin E supplementation is useful even if you don't take vitamin A, since it complements the vitamin A available from the diet. The very low dosage of vitamin E recommended here is just enough to activate the vitamin A needed for treating acoustic trauma. It will not hurt you to take more, but you should be careful to watch for bruising and bleeding if you take any amount of vitamin E with the blood thinners warfarin (Coumadin), clopidogrel (Plavix), or aspirin. If bruising or bleeding occurs, stop taking vitamin E immediately.

There is some ambivalence in the medical literature concerning the efficacy of ginkgo in treating acoustic trauma. An often-cited experiment with guinea pigs found that ginkgo reduces noise-related hearing loss only when it is given intravenously, but this study only tracked ginkgo's effects on the animals for 3$\frac{1}{2}$ hours.[3] Another study found positive benefits of ginkgo in treating laboratory rats.[4] A clinical study with human volunteers in Switzerland found considerable benefit in the emergency treatment of acoustic trauma with *injections* of ginkgo, but this treatment program also used repeated treatments in a hyperbaric (high pressure) oxygen chamber and prednisone shots.[5] Low doses of ginkgo do not help problems related to acoustic trauma.[6] You probably need to take 240 milligrams of ginkgo a day to get any benefit at all.

Like vitamin E, ginkgo also can increase the risk of bleeding or bruising if you take the blood thinners warfarin (Coumadin), clopidogrel (Plavix), or aspirin. If bruising or bleeding occur, stop taking ginkgo immediately. Don't take more than 240 milligrams a day, because high dosages of ginkgo can cause nausea, diarrhea, stomach cramps, or headaches in some individuals.

CONCEPTS FOR COPING WITH ACOUSTIC TRAUMA

❍ Wear ear protection. Earmuffs, the kind that go over your ears and are worn by luggage handlers around jet planes, cost around $10 a pair. Foam earplugs are 25–50¢ a pair. Both earmuffs and earplugs are available where sporting goods are sold. Used before exposure to loud sounds, earmuffs and earplugs can prevent a potential hearing loss.

❍ Sometimes acoustic trauma requires medical care, and in a few instances acoustic trauma requires emergency care. See your doctor when:

• A child does not respond to any sound, such as a whistle or a clap. This is a medical emergency. Go to an emergency room.

• A child does not respond to sound after an earache, headache, upper respiratory infection, or recent air travel. This is also a medical emergency. Go to an emergency room.

• Hearing loss is accompanied by a discharge from the ear, earache, dizziness, or sense that things are spinning around you. You do not need emergency care, but arrange to see your doctor as soon as possible.

• You can't hear a (regular, not digital) watch ticking when it is held next to your ear. Arrange to see your doctor as soon as possible.

• You hear a ringing in both ears all the time that began after a recent exposure to a loud noise. Arrange to see your doctor as soon as possible.

Acquired Immune Deficiency Syndrome

See **HIV and AIDS**.

Acrodermatitis Enteropathica

See **Zinc Deficiency**.

Actinic Keratosis

SYMPTOM SUMMARY

❍ Begins as flat, scaly, dry skin, then becomes slightly elevated

❍ Easier to feel than to see at first

❍ May be pink, red, gray, or the same color as adjacent skin

❍ May develop gritty or sandpaperlike texture over a period of several years

❍ Usually located on the face, back of the hands, forearms, or other areas exposed to the sun

❍ Small hornlike growths appear in older people with this condition

UNDERSTANDING THE DISEASE PROCESS

Actinic refers to the sun and keratosis is a growth of skin. An actinic keratosis (plural, actinic keratoses) is a sunlight-induced injury to the skin that can lead to skin cancer. The cancers to which actinic keratosis leads will strike 1 out of 8 people who get the condition at some point in their lives. Those most at risk for developing sun-related skin cancers are people with HIV, transplant recipients who are on antirejection drugs, psoriasis patients who have been treated with psoralens and UVA light, and people who have Epstein-Barr virus (EBV) or chronic fatigue syndrome. Actinic keratoses are more common on fair skin than on dark skin. Every year, there are 900,000 new cases of sun-related skin cancer just in North America.[1]

The cells that are affected by actinic keratosis are pluripotent, that is, they are cells that can form skin, hair, or sweat glands. Ultraviolet light causes the C and T bases (of the A, G, C, and T of DNA) of basal cells to be transposed.[2] This DNA damage deactivates gene p53, which ordinarily makes sure dividing cells "rest for repairs" if there are other defects in their genetic material.[3]

Many skin cells with damaged DNA simply rise to the surface of the skin during their life cycle and are sloughed off. When the skin cells that form hair shafts and sweat glands are damaged by the sun, however, they begin to multiply in an unregulated manner and form actinic keratoses. If these blemishes are allowed to develop unchecked, that can turn into aggressive squamous cell carcinomas, cancers with the potential to spread throughout the body.

TREATMENT SUMMARY

NUTRITIONAL SUPPLEMENTS

○ N-acetyl cysteine (NAC): 100 milligrams per day.

○ Selenium: 200 micrograms per day.

○ Vitamin C: 1,000 mg per day.

○ Vitamin E: 400 IU per day.

If you exercise vigorously out of doors, be sure also to take:

○ Alpha-lipoic acid: 100 milligrams daily.

UNDERSTANDING THE HEALING PROCESS

The key nutrients for preventing the progression of actinic keratosis to squamous cell carcinoma are antioxidants. Laboratory experiments with skin cells have found that providing the cells with selenium, vitamin C, and vitamin E *before* exposure to ultraviolet light greatly reduces the amount of DNA damage.[4] Even after exposure to sunlight, selenium and vitamin E help the skin make glutathione, which in turn stops the process through which sunlight causes apoptosis, the initiation of skin cell death.[5] N-acetyl cysteine (NAC), vitamin C, and vitamin E work together to protect p53, the gene that ensures that cells repair defects in their DNA before multiplying.[6]

Additional supplements may be needed for people who exercise in the sun. Strenuous exercise depletes glutathione. This naturally occurring antioxidant slows inflammatory reactions and is essential to the normal function of estrogen and testosterone. Laboratory studies with animals have found that supplementation with alpha-lipoic acid keeps glutathione from breaking down, especially in the liver and in the bloodstream.[7]

While the antioxidant supplements that fight basal cell carcinoma are largely free of side effects, there are some precautions to be observed in their use. NAC may cause headaches if taken with sildenafil (Viagra), and in rare cases can cause cysteine-crystal kidney stones. Smokers should not take NAC. Diabetics who have high blood sugars may find that taking NAC causes false readings in urine tests for ketones. Selenium is better absorbed if it is not taken at the same time as vitamin C. Vitamin C taken in the form of vitamin C with bioflavonoids can interfere with the liver's ability to process statin drugs for controlling cholesterol, calcium channel blockers such as nifedipine (Procardia) for hypertension, or cyclosporine for preventing transplant rejection. Vitamin E should be used with caution by those who take blood thinners such as aspirin, clopidogrel (Plavix), ticlopidine HCl (Ticlid), or warfarin (Coumadin).

CONCEPTS FOR COPING WITH ACTINIC KERATOSIS

○ Do not try to remove actinic keratoses by "rubbing them off." Some of the damaged cells will remain in the skin only to multiply again, and breaking the skin increases the risk of infection.

○ Don't go overboard and try to avoid the sun completely. Sun avoidance depletes the body's supply of vitamin D and, ironically, can increase the risk of certain kinds of skin cancer.

○ Don't try to tan. Sun exposure and sunbathing produce gradual skin damage even if sunburn is avoided. Ten to forty years can pass between the time of sun exposure and the development of skin cancer.

○ People who have had any form of skin cancer should have a skin exam every 6 months to 1 year.

○ Put on sunscreen with an SPF of 15 or higher every day before leaving the house. White clothing that has become wet (for example, a wet T-shirt) is not a substitute for sunscreen. Wet white clothing offers no protection against the sun.

Acute Bacterial Prostatitis

See **Prostatitis**.

ADD/ADHD
(Attention Deficit Disorder/Attention Deficit Hyperactivity Disorder) in Children

SYMPTOM SUMMARY

Attention deficit:

❍ Difficulty maintaining attention to work or play

❍ Does not complete tasks

❍ Does not listen when spoken to

❍ Easily distracted

❍ Failure to pay attention to details, makes careless mistakes at school or work

❍ Has difficulty organizing tasks or time

❍ Unable to follow instructions unless they are given one at a time

Hyperactivity:

❍ Has trouble engaging in quiet activities, such as reading

❍ Runs or climbs in inappropriate situations

❍ Talks excessively

❍ Thumping, fidgeting, squirming, moving constantly

❍ Wanders through classroom or workplace

Impulsivity:

❍ Blurts out answers before questions have been completed

❍ Difficulty waiting turns

❍ Interrupts others

Associated symptoms:

❍ Behavior not shaped by consequences

❍ Disregard for personal safety

❍ Failure to meet developmental milestones or, in adults, rites of passage

❍ Inability to delay gratification

❍ Learning disabilities

❍ Social isolation, although may relate well one-on-one

UNDERSTANDING THE DISEASE PROCESS

Attention deficit disorder (ADD) and attention deficit hyperactivity disorder (ADHD) are loosely defined and poorly understood groupings of psychiatric symptoms that begin in childhood and continue into adulthood. Although these conditions can be diagnosed with a brain-scanning method known as positron emission tomography (PET), usually a label of ADD or ADHD is applied after repeated problems with disagreeable behaviors. These include inability to focus, mood swings, temper tantrums or sudden anger, problems completing assignments or making choices, lack of organization, and impulsivity.

ADD and ADHD damage children, families, and classrooms. They interfere with personal relationships, disrupt families, and make it difficult for classmates of the ADD or ADHD child to learn. Overwhelmingly, ADD and ADHD are treated with potent psychoactive drugs, but not without potential danger to the child. In the words of a distinguished natural health expert, "Parents and children express desperation for interventions that will work, but without the adverse effects inflicted by the pharmaceutical management model."[1] An integrated explanation of ADD and ADHD with a comprehensive management model is beyond the scope of this book, but presented here is a collection of holistic methods to relieve the symptoms of ADHD with a minimum of unproductive effort.

TREATMENT SUMMARY

DIET

❍ Be sure to provide a protein food with every meal. Never allow a child with ADHD to eat a meal or snack consisting solely of sweets or highly refined carbohydrates.

NUTRITIONAL SUPPLEMENTS

❍ Essential fatty acids: 1 tablespoon of flavored flaxseed oil per day, or 3 maxEPA softgels.

❍ Vitamin B_6: 20 milligrams per day.

See Part Three if the child takes prescription medication.

UNDERSTANDING THE HEALING PROCESS

The nearly universal treatment for ADD and ADHD is the drug methylphenidate (Ritalin). This drug acts on the central nervous system in much the same way as cocaine. The second-line choices of medication include methamphetamines (Desoxyn or the Desoxyn Gradumet), or pemoline (Cylert), the latter causing liver damage in about 3 percent of children treated with it and sometimes even causing death. The potential dangers of these drugs combined with the absence of hard and fast scientific methods of diagnosing ADD and ADHD make many parents search for alternative treatments.

Unfortunately, one of the problems in evaluating research on the nutritional treatment of ADHD is that some commentators on both sides of the issue tend to distort the facts. A proponent of strict dietary measures derided a study that found that sugar does not affect ADHD with the comment "the authors thanked Pepsi Cola and Royal Crown for funding their study," but inspection of the original article reveals they did not. Critics may offer distorted interpretations of measurement standards used in articles they do not like. In reviewing food allergy studies, a medication-oriented physician complained that holistically oriented researchers tested amounts of chemicals *smaller* than those found in everyday foodstuffs. He offered the opinion that since the amounts of chemicals tested were small, the findings of the food allergy scientists were irrelevant, based on the untenable theory that a small amount of a chemical might cause an allergy but a large amount would not. In light of the distressing biases in many review articles on both sides of the drug treatment of ADD and ADHD, only simple treatments are listed here.

Sugar is often thought to be a cause of aggressive and destructive behavior, and parents of hyperactive children usually attempt to ban it from the daily diet. It is important to consider that *occasional* acting out connected with consumption of sugar is often simply a feature of an exciting event, such as a birthday party or Halloween. The times children may eat large amounts of candies and high-sugar foods are the times when even normal children are hyperactive. Children with ADHD and their harried parents may come to associate sugar-containing foods with events like parties, especially if they are not allowed to have sugared foods under normal circumstances. As a result of their parents' expectations, children may behave in an excited, hyperactive manner, especially if they are inclined to do so anyway.

An *ongoing* pattern of acting out combined with an increased *appetite* for sugar, however, is more likely to be part of the body's attempt to cure ADHD. At least some scientific studies indicate that most children with ADHD have an abnormal response to table sugar, causing levels of glucose to build up in their bloodstreams far in excess of what would be expected.[2] However, the very latest research finds that the resulting cascade of biochemical reactions in the brain primarily relates to social orientation.[3] Children with ADD or ADHD become more interested in social activity as sugar "pushes" the amino acid tryptophan into the brain, where it becomes serotonin. This mood-lifting hormone stimulates social interaction and lifts depression. Craving sugar all the time may, if there are no psychological issues related to defying parental rules about sugar, indicate chronic mild depression. It is important not to treat ADD or ADHD when the real problem is depression (see DEPRESSION).

If your ADHD child craves sugar, first make sure he or she consumes protein at every meal. Protein provides the amino acid the brain needs to make serotonin, and reduces the physical appetite for sugar. If there is no improvement, then consider eliminating sugar.

Numerous studies link food allergies to ADHD. Chocolate, eggs, milk, peanuts, and over 3,000 food additives are believed to cause allergies that worsen ADD and ADHD. Up to 88 percent of children with ADHD test positive for allergies to food dyes, and there is general agreement that more than half of children with ADD or ADHD get better when they are put on allergen-free diets.[4]

Unfortunately, eliminating allergies never cures hyperactive children. Even the one study that obtained an 82-percent success rate with an extremely restricted diet found that its measures of success were subjective rather than objective.[5] That is, parents felt good about all the effort but basic observable behaviors did not change even after allergens were eliminated from the children's diets.

A sensible way to deal with possible food allergies is to eliminate potentially offending foods one at a time. For example, don't give your child chocolate (and make sure he or she does not get chocolate at school or from friends) for a test period of 1 week. If your child appears better off, then quietly stop offering chocolate at home. Repeat the process for wheat, meat, fish, eggs, dairy products, refined sugar, citrus fruits, preservatives, coffee, and tea, eliminating just one food at a time and waiting to see if there are any changes. If you can make the changes in the foods you offer your child into a game, or associate them with a story, so much the better.

The next step in dietary modification is eliminating food additives. The least-complicated way to eliminate food additives is to cook from scratch—a difficult undertaking for families in which both parents work. Another approach is to avoid foods sold in cellophane packages. If time constraints in your household make it impossible to avoid all prepared foods, try avoiding the commercial antioxidants BHT and BHA, typically found in foods prepared with fat and stored without refrigeration, such as bread and baked goods. Then eliminate products made with emulsifier, such as pudding cups, canned soups, and ice cream, and foods containing salicylates, raisins, prunes, curry powder, paprika, thyme, dill, oregano, and turmeric. Try each elimination for a week and if there is improvement in symptoms, continue it.

Nutritional supplementation is much easier than dietary elimination. The most important nutritional supplement for the ADD or ADHD child are the omega-3 (also known as n-3) fatty acids. Children who are deficient in these essential fatty acids are often thirsty, but do not make additional trips to the bathroom (that is, their volume of urination is increased).[6] Children with ADD or ADHD who need fatty acid supplements also tend to have dry skin.[7] The clinical studies of essential fatty acids in the treatment of ADHD consistently show higher ratings of effectiveness by parents than by teachers[8] and somewhat less effective than an amphetamine similar to Adderall.[9]

The benefits of essential fatty acid supplementation only occur, however, when zinc levels are neither deficient nor excessive.[10] A good measure of whether your child needs zinc is to give him or her an uncoated zinc tablet. If they complain that it tastes bad, they probably are not deficient in zinc. If they do not complain about the bitter taste, give them 30 milligrams of zinc picolinate a day until they do complain. At this point, the zinc deficiency has been corrected. Appropriate zinc supplementation will make both essential fatty acids and amphetamines such as Ritalin and Adderall work better.

The second most useful supplement is vitamin B_6 (pyridoxine), preferably in its activated form, pyridoxal-5'-phosphate (PLP). A very small-scale, preliminary study found that vitamin B_6 was as effective as Ritalin in controlling "hyper" behaviors, and that the benefits of vitamin B_6 supplementation continued for nearly a month after its daily use was discontinued. Vitamin B_6 had an additional advantage in that it increased bloodstream levels of the hormone serotonin, associated with improved social orientation in ADHD.[11]

The caveat in interpreting these results is that, with the widespread use of Ritalin, follow-up studies were never funded. Children who have not reached the age of 3 should not be given vitamin B_6, since it can, in rare cases, cause seizures. Children over the age of 3 who have seizures should never be given more than 25 milligrams of the vitamin per day. Higher doses can interfere with seizure medications. Finally, a very common side effect of vitamin B_6 is the formation of "neon yellow" urine. There have been cases in which older children overdosed the vitamin to achieve this effect.

Several other supplements have special applications in the treatment of childhood ADHD. Iron, which is also used in treating restless legs syndrome (see RESTLESS LEGS SYNDROME), may be helpful for children who "can't sit still." Magnesium may be helpful for children who have tics and twitches—but be careful not to overdose, as overdoses of magnesium can cause diarrhea. Phosphatidylserine is frequently recommended for treating poor attention span, but changes may take 3–4 months.

CONCEPTS FOR COPING WITH ADD AND ADHD

○ While it is commonly believed that most children learn more when they study in silence, children and teens with ADD or ADHD may actually learn better with loud music playing. Doctors at Schneider Children's Hospital in New Hyde Park, New York, found that ADD-ADHD children did better on an arithmetic learning task if they were exposed to music, but only if they started the study session with music. The researchers believe that "optimal stimulation" may enhance learning in ADD-ADHD children. Children who did not have ADD or ADHD learned equally well with or without music playing in the background.[12] It is important to make sure that headphones are not turned so loud as to cause damage to hearing.

○ Flower essences are beginning to receive serious scientific attention as potential treatments for ADD and ADHD.[13] The use of Bach flower remedies is well established in the holistic treatment of anxiety (see ANXIETY).

○ Allergies often go hand in hand with ADHD, particularly if acting out is worse at school than at home, or vice versa. Many schools are reservoirs of dust, mold, and

Treating ADHD in Adults

In adults, "undirected" behaviors play much the same role in the brain as alcohol or cocaine. The unproductive behaviors associated with adult ADHD allow the brain to produce "reward" chemicals that have the same physiological effect as the chemicals produced by purposeful behavior in healthy individuals. Changes in diet and nutritional supplementation play a much clearer role in treating adult ADHD and related disorders, such as addiction.

TREATMENT SUMMARY

DIET

O Eliminate table sugar, sweets, pastries, and soft drinks sweetened with cane sugar or corn syrup.

O Eat fruit in moderation. Do not eat dried fruit, citrus, or grapes.

O Avoid bread, potatoes, and rice.

O Unless you have been diagnosed as having cirrhosis, eat a protein food (preferably lean meat or soy) 3 times a day.

NUTRITIONAL SUPPLEMENTS

O 5-HTP: 400 milligrams daily.

O L-glutamine: 500–600 milligrams daily. (This is the minimum dose that is commercially available in the United States. A smaller dose would be sufficient.)

O DL-phenylalanine (a mixture of D- and L-phenylalanine): 1,500 milligrams daily.

O Pyridoxal-5'-phosphate (activated vitamin B_6): 200 milligram extended-release tablet.

See Part Three if you take prescription medication.

One of the most important things you can do if you are an adult with ADHD is to avoid sugar. In physically inactive adults, sugar soothes the depression that follows embarrassing behaviors, only to cause agitation that leads to more embarrassing behaviors. You can break this cycle by avoiding sugar. Eliminate table sugar, sweets, and pastries. Be especially careful to eliminate soft drinks sweetened with high-fructose syrup. Especially among adults who have ADHD and who drink alcohol, this form of sugar, more than any other, contributes to reactive hypoglycemia and the soar and crash cycle of sugar consumption.

The most important nutritional supplements any adult with ADHD can take are those that help restore control over personal behavior. The supplement 5-HTP is a source of a form of the amino acid tryptophan that can easily enter the brain. The brain converts tryptophan into serotonin, which reduces carbohydrate craving and improves the quality of sleep. L-glutamine helps the brain produce a chemical known as gamma-aminobutyric acid (GABA), which induces sleep. D-phenylalanine, a component of DL-phenylalanine, decreases alcohol craving by increasing the production of the reward chemical enkephalin in the brain. L-phenylalanine increases production of another reward chemical, dopamine, as well as a stimulant hormone, noradrenaline. This reduces depression. Pyridoxal-5'-phosphate, the activated form of vitamin B_6, helps the gastrointestinal tract absorb amino acids. It is not unusual for adults with ADHD to have a vitamin B_6 deficiency.

Compared to the long-term effects of ADHD, any potential side effects of these five supplements are quite mild, but people who take prescription drugs must use caution. Avoid 5-HTP if you take antidepressants or St. John's wort. The combination can cause an unhealthy elation or euphoria known as serotonin syndrome (see DEPRESSION). L-glutamine does not react in any detrimental ways with prescription drugs, although people with bipolar disorder should only use it under supervision. In very rare cases, L-glutamine has aggravated manic symptoms. People taking one of the older-style antidepressants such as imipramine (Tofranil) should not take phenylalanine. The combination can also cause elation or euphoria with impaired judgment. If you have high blood pressure, check your blood pressure every day when taking phenylalanine. Discontinue the supplement if your blood pressure is unusually elevated (by more than 10 mm/Hg for either the higher or lower number). Pyridoxal-5'-phosphate can interact with prescription drugs for arrhythmia, asthma, epilepsy, Parkinson's disease, and tuberculosis, increasing their toxicity.

environmental toxins. A "yes" answer to any two of these five questions suggests that allergies may be making your child's ADHD worse:

- Does your child seem to feel, behave, and remember differently at school?

- Does your child's appearance change between the time he or she is dropped off and picked up at school?

- Is your child's handwriting or art work different at home?

- Does asthma or another breathing problem appear at school but not at home?

- Does your child regularly experience a racing pulse at school but not at home?

Addison's Disease
(Adrenocortical Insufficiency)

SYMPTOM SUMMARY

- ○ Cravings for salty foods
- ○ Cravings for sugar (in children who have the disease)
- ○ Dark sores in the mouth
- ○ Depression
- ○ Excessive sweating
- ○ Extreme weakness
- ○ Hallucinations
- ○ Headaches
- ○ Impaired short-term memory, episodes of amnesia
- ○ Involuntary movements of the eyelids
- ○ Loss of interest in sex
- ○ Menstrual irregularity
- ○ Nausea, vomiting, loss of appetite, chronic diarrhea
- ○ Patchy, dark coloration of the skin in some areas, paleness in others
- ○ Tanning without sun exposure
- ○ Tremors
- ○ Unintentional weight loss

UNDERSTANDING THE DISEASE PROCESS

Addison's disease is a relatively rare hormonal disorder that will affect about 300,000 people in North America at some time in their lives. It occurs in all age groups and afflicts men and women equally. The condition causes weight loss, muscle weakness, fatigue, and low blood pressure. It sometimes causes darkening of the skin in both sun-exposed and unexposed parts of the body.

Addison's disease occurs when the cortexes of the adrenal glands, located just above the kidneys, do not produce enough of the hormone cortisol. For this reason, the disease is sometimes called chronic adrenocortical insufficiency, or hypocortisolism. Cortisol's job is to help the body respond to stress. Cortisol also helps regulate the immune system's inflammatory response, balance the effects of insulin in breaking down sugar for energy, and maintain blood pressure.

Because cortisol is so vital to health, the amount of cortisol produced by the adrenals is precisely balanced. Like many other glands, the adrenals are regulated by the hypothalamus inside the brain and the pituitary gland, a bean-sized organ at the base of the brain. First, the hypothalamus sends releasing hormones to the pituitary gland. The pituitary gland responds by secreting other hormones that regulate growth, thyroid and adrenal function, and sex hormones such as estrogen and testosterone. One of the pituitary gland's most important tasks is to secrete adrenocorticotropin (ACTH), a hormone that stimulates the adrenal glands. When the adrenals receive the pituitary's signal in the form of ACTH, they respond by producing cortisol. Completing the cycle, a surge of cortisol then signals the pituitary to lower secretion of ACTH.

In some cases of Addison's disease, the adrenal glands also fail to produce enough aldosterone. This hormone is one of a class of hormones called mineralocorticoids. These hormones maintain blood pressure as well as salt and water balance by helping the kidney retain sodium and excrete potassium. When aldosterone production falls too low, the kidneys are not able to regulate salt and water balance. Both blood volume and blood pressure fall.

Most cases of Addison's disease result from the gradual destruction of the adrenal cortex, the outer layer of the adrenal glands, by the body itself. The immune system makes antibodies that slowly destroy the cortex.

This kind of immune destruction can be triggered by tuberculosis or fungal infections. Addison's disease can also occur when cancer attacks the adrenal glands. A temporary form of Addison's disease sometimes results when people with asthma stop using their inhalers or when benign tumors are surgically removed from the pituitary gland.

An Addisonian crisis, heralded by sudden penetrating pain in the lower back, abdomen, or legs and severe vomiting and diarrhea, followed by dehydration, low blood pressure, and loss of consciousness, is a medical emergency. During an Addisonian crisis, low blood pressure, low blood sugar, and high levels of potassium can be life threatening if not immediately treated. Fortunately, medical treatment for this complication of the disease is very straightforward (IVs of saline and glucose plus injections of cortisone are administered) and usually results in rapid improvement.

TREATMENT SUMMARY

NUTRITIONAL SUPPLEMENTS

O DHEA: 50 milligrams per day.

See Part Three if you take prescription medication.

UNDERSTANDING THE HEALING PROCESS

There are no alternatives to hormone replacement therapy for Addison's disease. Untreated Addison's disease is nearly always fatal. With hormone replacement therapy, however, a person with Addison's disease can expect to live a normal life span.[1] Standard hormone replacement for Addison's disease, however, fails to support the body's production of normal levels of the hormone testosterone, which is essential for sex drive in both men and women and for other aspects of quality of life.

The New England Journal of Medicine reports a double-blind study of 24 women with Addison's disease who were given either 50 milligrams of DHEA or a placebo every day for 4 months. Every woman in the study was DHEA-deficient at the beginning of treatment. The researchers found that taking DHEA reduced anxiety and depression and heightened overall sense of well-being in the treated women. DHEA also restored normal sex drive.[2]

Experts in treating adrenocortical insufficiency speculate that DHEA can also restore sex drive in men with Addison's disease, but this idea has not been subjected to clinical testing. An editorial in *The New England Journal of Medicine* suggests that men with Addison's disease can probably benefit from taking DHEA on an ongoing basis.[3]

Women who take DHEA should get regular breast exams, and men who take DHEA should get regular prostate exams. About half of people who take DHEA for Addison's disease will notice slightly oilier skin and hair and increased growth of hair—detrimental only to those wearing hair weaves or extensions or who are averse to getting haircuts.

CONCEPTS FOR COPING WITH ADDISON'S DISEASE

O Know how to recognize an Addisonian crisis. Symptoms include:

- Sudden penetrating pain in the lower back, abdomen, or legs;

- Severe vomiting and diarrhea;

- Low blood pressure;

- Loss of consciousness;

- Pale skin;

- Excessive sweating.

These symptoms require immediate medical treatment. They are treated with an emergency injection of cortisol and IVs of saline and glucose.

O If you have Addison's disease, you should carry identification alerting emergency medical personnel to the need to inject 100 milligrams of cortisol if you are found injured or unconscious. Carry a syringe and cortisol with you at all times.

O To avoid a "crash and burn" crisis:

- Alternate active periods with rest;

- Avoid strenuous physical activity in hot, humid weather;

- Don't be afraid to eat salty foods, especially when you sweat a lot;

- Don't skip meals;

- Make sure you drink plenty of fluids.

Age Spots

SYMPTOM SUMMARY

○ Regions of dark pigmentation on the skin resembling freckles

- Dark brown or black spots
- Do not change color after exposure to sun (as freckles do)
- Usually appear after age 40

UNDERSTANDING THE DISEASE PROCESS

Age spots, also known as liver spots, lentigos, or lentigines, are rounded regions of dark brown or black pigment on sun-exposed skin. Age spots differ from freckles in that they do not get darker after surrounding skin tans or burns. Like freckles, however, they are more common in people with fair skin. Age spots may occur anywhere on the body but they are most likely to appear on regions of skin that are exposed to the sun on a daily basis. For most people, these regions are the face, hands, arms, and lower legs.

The processes that cause age spots can be understood at a molecular level. Essentially, for many of us, the skin slowly becomes "tired" as we age. UV radiation from the sun, air pollution, the growth of colonies of bacteria on the skin, prescription medications, inflammatory disorders, and nutritional stress team together to generate massive quantities of free radicals. These oxidizing chemicals are essential to both respiration and immunity, but they can accumulate on the surfaces of skin cells, locking sodium inside. The cell membrane loses its electrical charge so that nutrients are kept out. The sodium trapped within the cell has a caustic effect on lipids, proteins, and DNA. It creates age spots, wrinkles, and other manifestations of aging skin.[1]

Of all the natural processes that damage the skin, the most destructive is excessive exposure to sunlight. Sun damage occurs even when there is not enough exposure to sun to cause sunburn. Dermatologists report that it is not unusual to see patients with numerous age spots despite regularly applying a sufficient quantity of sunscreen before exposing themselves to the afternoon sun's ultraviolet rays.

The problem is that sunscreens offer good protection against some kinds of ultraviolet rays but not against others. The sunlight that reaches the earth's surface consists of both UVA (long-wavelength) and UVB (short-wavelength) ultraviolet light. Sunscreens generally block UVB, but sunscreens with SPFs lower than 30 allow UVA rays to reach the skin.

At least 95 percent of all the solar radiation reaching the earth consists of UVA. This part of the UV spectrum is present from sunrise to sunset. In contrast, UVB only reaches significant levels between 10:00 A.M. and 3:00 P.M. UVB rays are more abundant in summer sun, but the amount of UVA radiation in sunlight does not vary according to the season. There is just as much UVA in winter sun as in summer sun. Exposure to UVA for even 1 hour a day 5 days a week for 5 weeks at any time of year can cause substantial damage to the skin. Eighty-five percent of UVA radiation penetrates to the lowest level of the skin where new skin cells are formed, compared to only 15 percent of UVB.

UVA exposure activates a system of enzymes known as the metalloproteinases. These enzymes break down connective proteins in the skin. As the metalloproteinases do their work, the stratum corneum underlying the skin thickens while the skin's outer layers dry out and become more fragile. Tiny cracks develop. Portions of the outermost layers of skin detach and flake off easily. To slow down this process, the skin produces large amounts of the brown pigment melanin that absorbs UV rays.

Skin that is forced to produce massive amounts of protective pigments develops freckles and age spots. Spots on the skin that are strictly related to aging are rare—the number of pigment-producing cells in the skin actually drops by 10–20 percent every 10 years across the entire surface of the body. Sun-related age spots, or lentigos, are the result of the overproduction of protective pigments in the bottommost layer of the epidermis in skin that is exposed to UVA over a period of years.

TREATMENT SUMMARY

DIET

○ Avoid sugar.

○ Drink 6–8 eight-ounce glasses of water daily.

○ Eat 2–3 servings of yellow or orange vegetables daily.

○ Eat three 3-ounce servings of cold-water fish (such as

herring, mackerel, sardines, tuna, or wild salmon) weekly, or take DHA and EPA supplements or 1 tablespoon of flaxseed oil daily.

NUTRITIONAL SUPPLEMENTS

○ Alpha-lipoic acid: 100 mg daily.

○ Mixed carotenoids: 25 milligrams per day, starting 8–10 weeks before exposure to summer sun.

○ Vitamin C: 2,000 milligrams per day.

○ Vitamin E: 800 IU per day.

See Part Three if you take prescription medication.

UNDERSTANDING THE HEALING PROCESS

The easiest way to treat age spots is to apply alpha-lipoic acid, DMAE, and vitamin C esters directly to the skin. These relatively expensive treatments sometimes produce visible results within a few weeks. When you use topical creams, age spots will not completely disappear in less than a month, but they should lighten appreciably.

The least expensive way to treat age spots is to take the same supplements in oral form. Be forewarned that using supplements in tablet form may not give you any results at all for several months. Age spots may take as long as a year to disappear and you will need to protect your skin from the sun to keep them from reappearing. If expense is a concern, however, oral supplementation *will* work, only more slowly.

Whatever treatments you choose, you can increase the speed at which your skin is rejuvenated by appropriate diet, smoking cessation, and use of sunscreens. Of course, you can also remove age spots with prescription hydroquinone or retin-A, or with facial peels—at greater expense and with greater pain and inflammation. These drugs may also require several weeks to begin to lighten age spots and 6–12 months to remove them.

Sugar is the enemy of circulation in the skin. Excessive levels of sugar in the bloodstream "sugar-coat" cells in a process known as glycation. In the skin, sugar forms cross-links in the collagen making the skin less supple and impeding circulation. Drinking adequate amounts of water lowers the concentration of sugar in the bloodstream and reduces glycation.

Orange and yellow vegetables make the skin less sensitive to the sun. The scientific study of hereditary diseases causing severe sun sensitivity shows that beta-carotene slightly raises the minimum level of UV exposure causing tissue damage, so people who take beta-carotene are more likely to tan than to burn.[3] Orange vegetables such as carrots and sweet potatoes are an excellent source of beta-carotene. While synthetic beta-carotene is better absorbed, natural sources of this vitamin have a greater positive effect on the immune system.[4] The carotenes in palm oil are 4–10 better absorbed that synthetic *trans*-beta-carotene.

Eating very large quantities of carrots, in the range of 450–1,000 grams (1–2 pounds) per day can cause a condition known as carotenodermia, in which the skin turns yellow and then orange. To reverse the condition, stop eating carrots. Eating large quantities of carrots daily for several years can cause depletion of white blood cells (neutropenia)[6] and menstrual disorders.[7]

Omega-3 fatty acids from cold-water fish moderate the skin's susceptibility to inflammation. Fatty acid deficiency increases the rate at which skin cells multiply,[8] makes them more permeable to water, induces the formation of abnormal keratinocytes,[9] and accelerates the production of natural steroid hormones in the skin.[10]

Alpha-lipoic acid counteracts skin damage done by excessive sugar in the diet. In a study of diabetics with a condition called peripheral diabetic neuropathy (damage to the sensory nerves of the skin caused by poor circulation), German researchers found that a relatively large dose (600 milligrams) of alpha-lipoic acid given by injection increased blood circulation in the skin by approximately 70 percent.[11] Although this clinical trial and similar studies do not conclusively establish that alpha-lipoic acid is useful in treating age spots, many dermatologists use the supplement to treat age spots as well as bags under the eyes, enlarged pores, and sallow or dull skin.

Mixed carotenoids, a group of vegetable pigments found in orange and yellow vegetables and the algae *Dunaliella salina*, have been tested in several clinical trials as a preventative for sunburn. In one study, 20 young women took 30 milligrams daily of beta-carotene or placebo for 10 weeks before a 13-day stretch of controlled sun exposure at a resort on the shores of the Red Sea. Participants taking beta-carotene before and during the sun exposure experienced less skin redness than those taking placebo, even when both groups used sunscreen. Two other studies conducted without a control group reported similar results. One study involving 20 participants and another study involving 22 participants found that supplementation with mixed carotenoids for 12–24 weeks increased tolerance for summer sun. The evidence is that it is necessary to take mixed carotenoids for several months to gain any benefit. A study lasting 23 days and another study lasting 4 weeks did not find any advantage of taking mixed carotenoids over taking a placebo in reducing sensitivity to sun. Protecting the skin from sun damage, of course, prevents both age spots and wrinkles.

Experiments with animals have confirmed that applying vitamin C and vitamin E directly to the skin protects against UV damage. One study found that topical vitamin C protected more against UVA rays, topical vitamin E protected more against UVB rays, and that applying vitamins C and E together worked better than applying either by itself. The sun-protective value of the vitamins was even greater when they were applied with sunscreen. Dr. Steve Bratman reports a study in which 20 women aged 55–60 with sun-damaged skin on the neck were given either 5 percent vitamin C or a placebo. The results at 3 and 6 months, according Dr. Bratman, showed that use of vitamin C improves cosmetic appearance, especially wrinkles, and the general health of the skin as evaluated under a microscope.[12] It is important to note that these studies focused on the use of topical vitamin C rather than on vitamin C supplements. And once again, the studies focused on physiological processes that are the same across several manifestations of aging skin, rather than specifically on age spots.

CONCEPTS FOR COPING WITH AGE SPOTS

For dry skin:

○ Don't use buffing pads or granular cleaning products.

○ Don't wash skin with hard soap.

○ Choose moisturizers formulated with dimethicone, glycerin, or hyaluronic acid.

○ Just splash your face with warm water in the morning, and use a "superfatted" cleansing bar (a "beauty bar" with lanolin or olive oil) or a mild, soap-free liquid cleanser to wash your skin at night.

○ Lock in skin moisture with moisturizers while your face and body are still damp.

○ Protect sun-exposed skin with a sunblock with a SPF of at least 30.

○ Soften fine lines and wrinkles with oil-based foundations and cream or cream-powder blushers.

For oily skin:

○ Don't scrub your skin. Removing oils deprives your skin of its protective layer.

○ Don't use astringents more than twice a week.

○ Don't use moisturizers if you don't need them.

○ Don't wash your skin more than twice a day, unless you exercise.

○ Cleanse your face twice a day with a mild liquid cleanser.

○ Protect sun-exposed skin with a sunblock with an SPF of at least 30.

○ Use Clinac O.C. rather than an astringent to soak up excessive oil.

○ Use oil-free or oil-blotting foundation and powder.

Age-Related Cataracts
See **Cataracts.**

Age-Related Cognitive Decline
See **Alzheimer's Disease, Memory Loss.**

Age-Related Macular Degeneration
See **Macular Degeneration.**

Age-Related Memory Impairment
See **Memory Loss.**

AIDS
See **HIV and AIDS.**

Alcohol Withdrawal

SYMPTOM SUMMARY

- Generalized anxiety
- Anger
- Headache
- Insomnia accompanied by bad dreams
- Jitters or shakes
- Nausea
- Panic attacks
- Vomiting

In some cases:

- Delirium tremens
- Hallucinations
- Seizures

UNDERSTANDING THE DISEASE PROCESS

Alcoholics and alcohol abusers who choose to stop drinking almost invariably go through a physiological crisis. While there are many ways to understand alcohol withdrawal, the model developed by Kenneth Blum, one of the world's leading authorities on addiction, is one of the more helpful. Blum has found evidence that genetic abnormalities in alcoholics cause what he calls a "reward deficiency syndrome." The normal brain reacts to pleasant everyday events with a "reward cascade" of brain chemicals that create a sense of satisfaction and well-being. In an alcoholic's brain, the flow of chemicals in the reward cascade is minimal unless the alcoholic drinks.

When the other effects of chronic alcohol use become so overwhelming that the alcoholic chooses—or is forced—to stop drinking, he or she experiences sensory deprivation. The reward cascade is disrupted, resulting in anger, anxiety, and other bad feelings, which may be accompanied by headache, insomnia, jitters, nausea, and vomiting.

TREATMENT SUMMARY

NUTRITIONAL SUPPLEMENTS

- 5-HTP: 400 milligrams daily.
- L-glutamine: 500–600 milligrams daily. (This is the minimum dose that is commercially available in the United States. A smaller dose would be sufficient.)
- DL-phenylalanine (a mixture of D- and L-phenylalanine): 1,500 milligrams daily
- Pyridoxal-5'-phosphate (activated vitamin B_6): 200-milligram extended-release tablet.

See Part Three if you take prescription medication.

UNDERSTANDING THE HEALING PROCESS

If you have decided to quit drinking, you will need more support than just nutritional supplementation, particularly during the first week. The symptoms of alcohol withdrawal begin in as little as a few minutes to at most 48 hours, and peak on the third and fourth day. Only the most mildly addicted alcohol abusers should attempt to stop drinking outside of a residential treatment facility. You can obtain a referral to a doctor who will see you on an outpatient basis through your local chapter of Alcoholics Anonymous, which also offers other help.

If you are only mildly addicted to alcohol, however, nutritional supplementation can help you a great deal when you stop drinking. Kenneth Blum and his associates have formulated a nutritional supplement program created to maintain the flow of reward chemicals in the brain. In a hospital setting, it can boost the rate of success in alcohol treatment programs to nearly 75 percent.[1] For most recovering alcoholics, this program of nutritional supplementation makes it possible to stop using alcohol without having to take tranquillizers.[2]

The supplement 5-HTP is a source of a form of the amino acid tryptophan that can easily enter the brain. The brain converts tryptophan into serotonin, which reduces carbohydrate craving and improves the quality of sleep. L-glutamine helps the brain produce a chemical known as gamma-aminobutyric acid (GABA), which induces sleep. D-phenylalanine, a component of DL-phenylalanine, decreases alcohol craving by increasing the production of the reward chemical enkephalin in the brain. L-phenylalanine increases production of another reward chemical, dopamine, as well as a stimulant hormone, noradrenaline. This reduces depression. Pyridoxal-5'-phosphate, the activated form of vitamin B_6, helps the gastrointestinal tract absorb amino acids. Alcoholics usually have a vitamin B_6 deficiency.

SAAVE is Dr. Blum's prescription nutritional supplement containing all of these nutritional supplements except 5-HTP. (In its original form, SAAVE used L-tryptophan instead of 5-HTP.) You can take SAAVE or a similar prescription formula, which may be covered by insurance, or you can take the supplements individually.

Compared to the "side effects" of alcohol cessation, any potential side effects of these five supplements are quite mild, but people who take prescription drugs must use caution. Avoid 5-HTP if you take antidepressants or St. John's wort. The combination can cause an unhealthy elation or euphoria known as serotonin syndrome (see DEPRESSION). L-glutamine does not react in any detrimental ways with prescription drugs, although people with bipolar disorder should only use it under supervision. In very rare cases, L-glutamine has aggravated manic symptoms. People taking one of the older-style antidepressants such as imipramine (Tofranil) should not take phenylalanine. The combination can also cause elation or euphoria with impaired judgment. If you have high blood pressure, check your blood pressure every day when taking phenylalanine. Discontinue the supplement if your blood pressure is unusually elevated (by more than 10 mm/Hg for either the higher or lower number). Pyridoxal-5'-phosphate can interact with prescription drugs for arrhythmia, asthma, epilepsy, Parkinson's disease, and tuberculosis, increasing their toxicity. For more information on potential drug-supplement interactions, see Part Three.

CONCEPTS FOR COPING WITH ALCOHOL WITHDRAWAL

○ Most alcoholics have low levels of vitamins C and E and selenium that do not increase during recovery without supplementation. These antioxidants have relatively little effect on your ability to withdraw from alcohol but are very important for your general health. During your first 3 months of sobriety, take:

- Selenium: 800 micrograms per day;
- Vitamin C: At least 500 milligrams per day, preferably 500 milligrams with each meal; and
- Vitamin E: At least 200 IU per day.

○ Silymarin (milk thistle), preferably taken in the form of a phytosome (120 milligrams 2–3 times a day), can greatly reduce your risk of complications from liver disease[3] and increase your immune resistance.[4] Take silymarin on an ongoing basis.

○ If you experience the "munchies" on a regular basis

while in recovery from alcoholism, your brain is manipulating your appetite so that tryptophan will pass more easily across the blood-brain barrier. (See DEPRESSION for a complete discussion of this phenomenon.) Instead of binging on sugars and junk food, eat lean meat, fish, or soy at every meal and take 100–200 milligrams of 5-HTP daily. Increased protein and 5-HTP supplementation will also supply your brain with the tryptophan it needs to make mood-lifting serotonin.[5]

○ Avoid the settings in which you once drank alcohol heavily—bars, clubs, and restaurants. Heavy social drinkers are especially susceptible to visual cues to drink.[6]

○ Staying away from caffeine will help you stay sober. Most alcoholics have some degree of liver damage. A study at the Bromley Hospital in Kent, England, found that alcoholics take twice as long to "come down" from a caffeine buzz as nonalcoholics.[7] For many people, caffeine aggravates anxiety and depression that can restore an urge to drink.

○ As strange as it may sound, many alcoholics can get drunk just from looking at a drink. Psychologists at the University of Pittsburgh found that the sight of an alcoholic beverage reduced alcoholic men's reaction times more than the sight of a glass of water.[8]

Alcoholism and Alcohol Abuse

SYMPTOM SUMMARY

○ Frequent infections

○ Neglect of food intake

○ Night blindness

○ Numbness and tingling

○ Slow healing of cuts and scrapes

In men:

○ Liver damage causing decreased testosterone levels and testicular atrophy, enlargement of the breasts, and erectile dysfunction

In women after menopause:

○ Liver damage causing increased estrogen levels and increased risk of estrogen-related cancers

UNDERSTANDING THE DISEASE PROCESS

Alcoholics and other heavy drinkers experience a variety of nutritional problems. Some of these nutritional deficiencies are caused by an impaired ability to absorb nutrients. Others are caused by the fact that alcoholics tend not to eat. Alcohol stimulates appetite, but some of the same genetic alterations that predispose people to alcoholism also induce anorexia.

Some problem drinkers have an abnormality in the brain's production of the enzyme tyrosine hydroxylase. This chemical allows the brain to convert the amino acid tyrosine into the mood-lifting hormone norepinephrine. Chronic use of alcohol depletes the enzyme, and sets off not one or two but three vicious cycles.[1]

The first problem is that depletion of the enzyme by excess alcohol causes depression, and depression leads the alcoholic to drink. Since physical activity helps the remaining tyrosine hydroxylase work more effectively, alcoholics with this defect tend to be driven to remain active and alert. Their bodies burn more calories.

The second problem is that depression leads to sugar cravings. Higher sugar levels clear alcohol out of the bloodstream, and the result is a craving for both alcohol and sugar. Finally, many alcoholics consume alcohol and sugar almost to the total exclusion of other nutritious foods—and even when these alcoholics do eat healthy food, their bodies have trouble absorbing nutrients.

TREATMENT SUMMARY

DIET

O Eliminate table sugar, sweets, pastries, and soft drinks sweetened with cane sugar or corn syrup.

O Eat fruit in moderation. Do not eat dried fruit, citrus, or grapes.

O Avoid bread, potatoes, and rice.

O Unless you have been diagnosed as having cirrhosis, eat a protein food (preferably lean meat or soy) 3 times a day.

NUTRITIONAL SUPPLEMENTS

To help you control your drinking:

O 5-HTP: 400 milligrams daily.

O L-glutamine: 500–600 milligrams daily. (This is the minimum dose that is commercially available in the United States. A smaller dose would be sufficient.)

O DL-phenylalanine (a mixture of D- and L-phenylalanine): 1,500 milligrams daily.

O Pyridoxal-5'-phosphate (activated vitamin B_6): 200 milligram extended-release tablet.

To remedy nutritional deficits:

O L-carnitine: 500 milligrams twice a day.

O Magnesium: 250 milligrams with breakfast and in the afternoon.

O Selenium: 200 micrograms per day.

O Vitamin A: Only 5,000 IU per day.

O Vitamin B: Any complete supplement (providing the RDA of all B vitamins), 3 times a day.

O Vitamin C: 1,000 milligrams twice a day with meals.

O Vitamin E: 400 IU per day.

O Zinc picolinate: 30 milligrams per day.

See Part Three if you take prescription medication.

UNDERSTANDING THE HEALING PROCESS

One of the most important things you can do to manage your health if you drink heavily is to avoid sugar. Alcohol aggravates the crash that follows a sugar high, making you want to drink to boost your blood sugar levels temporarily only to have them crash again. You can break this cycle by avoiding sugar. Eliminate table sugar, sweets, and pastries. Be especially careful to eliminate soft drinks sweetened with high-fructose syrup. In alcoholics, this form of sugar, more than any other, contributes to reactive hypoglycemia and the soar and crash cycle of sugar consumption.

The most important nutritional supplements any problem drinker can take are those that help restore control over drinking. The supplement 5-HTP is a source of a form of the amino acid tryptophan that can easily enter the brain. The brain converts tryptophan into serotonin, which reduces carbohydrate craving and improves the quality of sleep. L-glutamine helps the brain produce a chemical known as gamma-aminobutyric acid (GABA), which induces sleep. D-phenylalanine, a component of DL-phenylalanine, decreases alcohol craving by increasing the production of the reward chemical enkephalin in the brain. L-phenylalanine increases production of another reward chemical, dopamine, as well as a stimulant hormone, noradrenaline. This reduces depression. Pyridoxal-5'-phosphate, the activated form of vitamin B_6, helps the gastrointestinal tract absorb amino acids. Alcoholics usually have a vitamin B$_6$ deficiency.

Compared to the long-term effects of heavy drinking, any potential side effects of these five supplements are quite mild, but people who take prescription drugs must use caution. Avoid 5-HTP if you take antidepressants or St. John's wort. The combination can cause an unhealthy elation or euphoria known as serotonin syndrome (see DEPRESSION). L-glutamine does not react in any detrimental ways with prescription drugs, although people with bipolar disorder should only use it under supervision. In very rare cases, L-glutamine has aggravated manic symptoms. People taking one of the older-style antidepressants such as imipramine (Tofranil) should not take phenylalanine. The combination can also cause elation or euphoria with impaired judgment. If you have high blood pressure, check your blood pressure every day when taking phenylalanine. Discontinue the supplement if your blood pressure is unusually elevated (by more than 10 mm/Hg for either the higher or lower number). Pyridoxal-5'-phosphate can interact with prescription drugs for arrhythmia, asthma, epilepsy, Parkinson's disease, and tuberculosis, increasing their toxicity. For more information on potential drug-supplement interactions, see Part Three.

The next group of supplements offers you a degree of protection against the worst long-term effects of heavy drinking. Excessive alcohol consumption impairs the liver's ability to synthesize the amino acid L-carnitine. This amino acid is critical for the ability of the heart and the skeletal muscles to make energy from fatty acids during times of oxygen deprivation or other kinds of stress.[2] It also helps protect the brain from tissue degeneration similar to that in Alzheimer's disease. L-carnitine helps protect against alcohol-induced fatty liver disease. It helps your liver process dietary fat, increases the production of HDL ("good") cholesterol, and lowers triglycerides.[3]

L-carnitine is nontoxic. People with HIV and AIDS who take didanosine (ddI), stavudine (d4t), or zalcitabine (ddC) cocktails and anyone treated with the antibiotics pivampicillin, pivcephalexin, or pivmecillinam (primarily used in Europe and Latin America) is likely to be deficient in L-carnitine and especially needs this supplement.

Some researchers believe that magnesium deficiencies cause the alcohol withdrawal symptom known as delirium tremens (DT), a terrifying combination of uncontrollable shaking and hallucinations.[4] Magnesium deficiency is likely to be the major reason heavy drinkers are a high risk for heart disease.[5]

Don't overdose magnesium. In addition to its role as a dietary supplement, magnesium is part of the active ingredient in milk of magnesia, the laxative. You should also avoid taking magnesium while you are on any antibiotic. Magnesium reduces the body's absorption of most antibiotics. Eating green beans, rhubarb, spinach, or sweet potatoes within 2 hours of taking magnesium keeps your body from absorbing the supplement, so unless you eat green beans, rhubarb, spinach, or sweet potatoes for breakfast or on your coffee break, take magnesium with breakfast and in the afternoon.

Selenium, vitamin C, and vitamin E are antioxidants that prevent destruction of liver cells. Taking these antioxidants before you drink moderates the toxic effects of alcohol on the liver and helps prevent fatty liver.[6] Selenium is better absorbed if it is not taken at the same time as vitamin C.

Vitamin A and zinc deficiencies produce the major complications of alcohol abuse: poor night vision, slow healing of wounds to the skin, depressed production of testosterone and estrogen, and poor immune function. Alcohol interferes with the intestines' ability to absorb vitamin A and zinc, and the liver's constant need to manufacture the detoxifying enzymes alcohol dehydrogenase and acetaldehyde dehydrogenase depletes the vitamin A and zinc that make it through the intestines. Tissue damage makes it impossible for the liver to store these nutrients or to process them in large quantities. Only consistent, low-dose supplementation can correct this problem as long as you drink.

People who drink heavily should take no more than 5,000 IU of vitamin A per day. This dosage will not cause birth defects and is safe for women who may become pregnant (although alcohol is not safe for the baby). The first signs of vitamin A overdose are dry skin and chapped lips, especially in dry weather. Later signs of toxicity are headache, mood swings, and pain in muscles and joints. In massive doses, vitamin A itself can cause liver damage. Discontinue vitamin A at the first sign of toxicity.

Do not take more than 50 milligrams of any zinc supplement daily. In rare cases, excessive intake of zinc depletes copper to cause anemia, that is, a deficiency of red blood cells, and neutropenia, a serious deficiency of white blood cells.[7]

The liver's constant need to make detoxifying enzymes also stresses its ability to activate various types of vitamin B. High levels of alcohol in the bloodstream cause the kidneys to excrete folic acid,[8] and a deficiency of thiamine results in a greater urge to drink.[9] Vitamin B_{12} can help correct numbness and tingling. Vitamin B deficiencies are most severe in heavy drinkers who also use diuretics, especially furosemide (Lasix), or medications for asthma, bipolar disorder, or seizures. Women who drink heavily and use oral contraceptives also tend to have vitamin B deficiency.

Don't take a vitamin B tablet with coffee, tea, or herb tinctures. Tannins in coffee, tea, and tinctures can deactivate thiamine. Ask you doctor before taking vitamin B and any prescription drug for arrhythmia, asthma, epilepsy, Parkinson's disease, or tuberculosis. Vitamin B_6 (pyridoxine) can increase their toxicity.

CONCEPTS FOR COPING WITH ALCOHOLISM AND ALCOHOL ABUSE

○ Any kind of steroid drug, whether an anabolic steroid or cortisone shot, increases cravings for alcohol.

○ The "munchies" are your body's way of fighting depression. Eating carbohydrates increases the amount of sugar in your bloodstream. This "pushes" an amino acid use to make antidepressant serotonin into your brain. If you have frequent attacks of carbohydrate cravings, consider taking steps to deal with depression (see DEPRESSION).

Allergies

SYMPTOM SUMMARY

○ Cough

○ Headache

○ Itching of the nose, eyes, mouth, throat, or skin

○ Runny nose

○ Impaired sense of smell

○ Sneezing

○ Sore throat

○ Tearing

○ Wheezing

UNDERSTANDING THE DISEASE PROCESS

The sneezing, wheezing, coughing, and tearing caused by seasonal allergies are among the most common of all health problems. Animal dander, dust mite droppings, pollen, grass, mold spores, and the infamous ragweed trigger annual episodes of hay fever, sinusitis, and itchy eyes for nearly 50 million people in North America alone.[1] Many people with allergies of the eye, ear, nose, and throat are also allergic to certain foods. They may experience symptoms from eating allergens in such foods as dairy products, eggs, nuts, shellfish, or wheat.

Even when the air is filled with pollen and dust, the overwhelming majority of airborne particles cause no harm. The nose is an efficient filtration system, trapping potentially offending allergens in mucus. The tiny hairs known as cilia in the linings of the nasal passages, however, beat rhythmically to transport mucus away from the nose and into the throat. Some of the captured allergenic particles arrive in the lower throat where their tough outer coats are partially digested. Allergenic particles are partially dissolved even before they reach the base of the throat.

Once its tough outer coat is dissolved, a liberated allergen makes contact with a specialized white blood cell known as a mast cell. The allergy particle attaches to a recognition site known as an immunoglobulin, specifically immunoglobulin E (IgE). This immune receptor site identifies it as a foreign substance and a potential toxin or infection. Mast cells break open to release histamine to cause tissue to swell up around the allergen. Some of the fluid swelling the tissues around the allergen leaks out and "runs" into the mucus.

At this point IgE sends out a chemical message to attract white blood cells known as basophils, eosinophils, neutrophils, and monocytes to infiltrate the linings of the nose and throat and isolate the allergen. The basophils release other chemicals to dissolve the healthy tissue surrounding the allergen so it can be swept away with mucus. IgE is a memory system known as a "perpetual mediator," so every repeated exposure to the allergen produces a swifter and greater response.

While allergies are often treated as an inconvenience rather than an illness, they can have profound influences on productivity and quality of life. A nationwide study conducted in the early 1990s confirmed what was already well known, that allergy sufferers lose sleep and have difficulty concentrating and are tormented by having constantly to blow their noses.[2] Another study published in 1997 found a significant impairment in verbal learning, decision-making speed, and psychomotor speed in people who suffer from allergies, resulting in either chronic absence from work or substantial decreases in work productivity.[3]

TREATMENT SUMMARY

NUTRITIONAL SUPPLEMENTS

O Bromelain: 500 milligrams 3 times a day.

O N-acetyl cysteine (NAC): 500–1,000 milligrams daily.

O Quercetin: 250–600 milligrams 3 times a day, taken at the same time as bromelain.

O Vitamin C: 2,000 milligrams daily.

HERBS

O Stinging nettle (*Urtica dioica*): 300 milligrams 3 times a day, taken with food.

O Various Chinese and Japanese herbal formulas.

See Part Three if you take prescription medication.

UNDERSTANDING THE HEALING PROCESS

If you buy an over-the-counter allergy medication, chances are you will be taking a first-generation antihistamine such as diphenhydramine (Benadryl), brompheniramine (Dimetane, Dimetapp Allergy, Nasahist B, ND-Stat, Oraminic II), clemastine (Antihist-1, Tavist, Tavist Allergy), or chlorpheniramine (Aller-Chlor, Chlor-Trimeton Allergy, Teldrin), which are found in products marketed under over 100 brand names. These drugs work by attaching to the cholesterol-derived coat of nerve cells. They deaden nerve fibers in the nose, throat, and sinuses that tell the mast cells to break open and release histamine. They also deaden fibers in the brain, causing discernible drowsiness in about 1 out of every 4 people who use them.[4] First-generation antihistamines can cause dizziness, irregular heartbeats, lassitude, euphoria, blurred vision, double vision, muscle tremors, and general klutziness, and even when they do not cause these symptoms, they increase your risk of accidents while driving or, as the warning label says, operating heavy machinery.

Medical science attempted to address these problems by creating a second generation of antihistamines that are not attracted to cholesterol and do not cross the blood-brain barrier into the brain. Most of the antihistamines in this class are chemically similar to the active chemicals in anti-inflammatory herbs, such as comfrey. The problem is that these antihistamines (and, for that matter, comfrey) have to be used with extreme caution by people who take certain prescription drugs. While certirizine (Zyrtec), fexofenadine (Allegra), loratadine (Claritin), and the now banned astemizole (Hismanal) and terfenadine (Seldane) do not cause drowsiness, they can cause serious and potentially deadly cardiac arrhythmias when mixed with certain prescription drugs. These side effects can occur when the antihistamines are taken with the antibiotics erythromycin (sold as Benzamycin, Staticin, and under 2 dozen other trade names) and troleandomycin (TAO), or when they are taken with certain treatments for yeast infections such as itraconazole (Sporanox) or ketoconazole (Nizoral), or when they are taken by someone with liver disease.

Nasal sprays present their own problems. These topical decongestants reduce the flow of blood to the mucous membranes of the nose. This deprives mast cells, nerve cells, and other tissues of their normal supply of oxygen and nutrients, making them too weak to create an allergic reaction. Continuous use of nasal decongestants can cause atrophy of nasal tissues. Discontinuing nasal decongestants can result in a rebound reaction in which the linings of the nose and sinuses swell in response to their newly restored blood flow. There are also less commonly prescribed anticholinergic drugs that paralyze the nerves that control memory, but also interfere with memory, coordination, visual perception, and reaction time.

In general, medications control the symptoms of allergies but lower quality of life. Fortunately, there are natural therapies that can be used by themselves to control mild symptoms, without side effects. They can be used with over-the-counter and prescription medications to make it possible to control symptoms with a lower dose.

Bromelain is a protein-dissolving enzyme refined from the stem of the pineapple plant. In everyday language, bromelain turns sticky mucus into runny mucus. It dissolves the proteins that make the sloughed-off dead cells in mucus stick together.[5]

Bromelain also helps restore circulation to clogged sinuses and nasal passages. The tissue damage inflicted by the immune system in response to an allergen activates the clotting system in the blood supplying the affected membrane. Fibrin forms around the area of inflammation to deprive it of oxygen and nutrients, trapping the fluids that cause swelling. Bromelain stimulates the production of plasmin, a chemical that causes the protein chains that make up fibrin to unlink. This restores circulation. Bromelain also counteracts the bradykinin system that makes the healthy capillaries near the site of inflammation "leak" fluid. Stopping the release of bradykinins keeps them from causing swelling and pain [6]

Since bromelain restores circulation and nasal decongestants cut off circulation, you do not want to use both products at the same time. The first time you use bromelain, you may have to find the right dosage through trial and error. Start with the lower dose and work upward to the maximum if you do not notice changes in the thickness of mucous discharge. Allergies to bromelain are very rare but are not unheard of. Allergic reactions to this supplement are most likely in people who are already allergic to pineapple, papaya, wheat flour, rye flour, or birch pollen. There has never been a report of an anaphylactic reaction to bromelain. There have been isolated reports of heavy menstrual periods, nausea, vomiting, and hives when bromelain is taken in very large overdoses (2,000 milligrams and higher).

N-acetyl cysteine (NAC) is an amino acid derivative and a potent antioxidant. Like bromelain, NAC does not stop the production of mucus, but it helps reduce the viscosity of mucus so it may be more easily coughed or sneezed out of the respiratory tract.[7] NAC has been documented as an effective mucolytic (mucus-dissolving) agent in people who have asthma, chronic bronchitis, cystic fibrosis, pneumonia, and sinusitis. It has not been scientifically documented for the specific indication of hay fever, but there are anecdotal reports that it is helpful and it makes scientific sense to believe them.

No one in good general health should take NAC on an ongoing basis. At least one long-term study suggests that the antioxidant effect of NAC can actually interfere with some of the actions of the immune system against bacteria. You should only use NAC during your allergy season, or, if you have allergies all year round, for no more than 3 months at a time. Smokers who have had bronchitis for 2 years or less should not take NAC unless they are quitting. There is some evidence that NAC may activate eosinophils, the white blood cells that may

cause smoker's cough to develop into emphysema.[8] NAC may cause headaches if taken with sildenafil (Viagra). There have been a few reports of people overdosing NAC and developing cysteine-crystal kidney stones. Diabetics with very poor blood sugar control may find that taking NAC causes false readings in urine tests for ketones. However, if you do not use Viagra, do not have uncontrolled diabetes, and do not have a history of cysteine-crystal kidney stones, NAC and bromelain together can be your most effective decongestant.

Quercetin is a flavonoid compound found in a wide variety of vegetables and herbs. It stops inflammation caused by the neutrophils. It also blocks the action of hyaluronidase, an enzyme that breaks down collagen in the linings of the walls of capillaries so that they can leak fluid and cause swelling around a point of allergic irritation. Keeping collagen intact also keeps mast cells from releasing their packets of histamine—without having any effect on the nervous system.

Japanese scientists studied mast cells taken from the nasal passages of volunteers who had yearly bouts of hay fever. Quercetin significantly reduced allergen-stimulated release of histamine, twice as effectively as the placebo. Quercetin's effect was almost twice that of sodium cromoglycate (Nalcrom) at the same concentration.[9]

For best results, take bromelain and quercetin together 5–10 minutes before meals. Bromelain increases the absorption of quercetin.[10] Use quercetin with caution if you take certain prescription drugs listed in the entry for Quercetin in Part Two.

Vitamin C prevents the secretion of histamine by mast cells and accelerates its degradation.[11] Laboratory experiments have found exponential increases in the release of histamine when vitamin C is deficient.[12] If you tend to get colds after you have allergies, taking 2,000 milligrams of vitamin C at the first sign of symptoms will make your cold less severe and help you get over it more quickly. Clear or white mucus is a sign of an allergy, while yellow or green mucus is a sign of a cold. Be sure to take vitamin C if your mucus turns yellow.

The very best form of vitamin C for treating allergies is an inhaler. One clinical trial gave hay fever sufferers a nose spray containing either vitamin C or a placebo. After 2 weeks, 74 percent of the volunteers given vitamin C solution were found to have decreased nasal secretions, blockage, and edema. Improvement was seen in only 24 percent of volunteers given a placebo. One of the revelations of the test was that vitamin C was most effective in an alkaline environment. Diets high in carbohydrates and refined sugars produce acidity, so if you are going to take vitamin C, your best results will come if you also restrict sugars and refined carbohydrates.[13]

Therapeutic dosages of vitamin C for treating seasonal allergies have not been scientifically established, but experts agree that 2,000 milligrams a day is adequate. Very few people experience any side effects with this dosage, and those who do are only likely to have diarrhea or abdominal swelling for a few days after beginning the vitamin. Take vitamin C with caution if you also take certain prescription drugs. Vitamin C taken in the form of vitamin C with bioflavonoids can interfere with the liver's ability to process statin drugs for controlling cholesterol, calcium channel blockers such as nifedipine (Procardia) for hypertension, or cyclosporine for preventing transplant rejection.

Stinging nettle acts as an antihistamine, strangely, by providing histamine. Freeze-dried stinging nettle leaf contains histamine and serotonin, two chemicals released in small amounts during an allergic reaction. Providing the body with large amounts of these chemicals, however, sets up a local anti-inflammatory reaction.[14] (Doctors inject histamine to treat cluster headaches associated with hay fever, allergic arthritis, penicillin reactions, and "cold" hives.[15]) Clinical tests have confirmed that stinging nettle has an antihistamine effect in treating hay fever—without inducing drowsiness.[16] Never take stinging nettle on an empty stomach. The serotonin it contains can cause mild stomach cramps.

There are many herbs that can relieve allergic irritation, including chamomile, ginger, horseradish, and rooibos. Use these herbs as desired for additional relief. Several Asian herbal formulas provide specific relief in treating allergies.

❍ The Chinese herbal formula Ge Gen Tang, also known as Kudzu Decoction or *kakkon-to*, offers specific relief for allergies that cause tension in the shoulders or the back of the neck. Brand names available in North America and the companies that manufacture them include:

- Ge Gen Tang (Chinese Classics, Golden Flower Chinese Herbs, Honso, Kan Traditionals, Lotus Classics, ProBotanixx, Qualiherb, Sun Ten)

- Kakkon-to (Tsumura)
- Kakkonto Formula 026 (Kampo Institute)
- Kampo4Cold/Flu Pueraria Formula (Honso)
- Kudzu Releasing Formula (Kan Traditionals)
- Pueraria Combination (Lotus Classics, Qualiherb, Sun Ten)
- Pueraria Formula (Golden Flower Chinese Herbs)
- Pueraria Plus Formula (Chinese Classics)
- Shu Jin 1 (ProBotanixx)
- Huang Qi Jian Zhong Tang, also known as Astragalus
- Decoction to Construct the Middle or *ogi-kenchu-to*, offers relief of especially severe allergic symptoms in people who also have eczema or chronic digestive problems such irritable bowel syndrome or peptic ulcer disease. Brand names of this formula available in North American include:

- Astragalus Formula (Golden Flower)
- Huang Qi Jian Zhong Tang (Lotus Classics, Qualiherb, Sun Ten)
- Ogi-kenchu-to (Honso, Tsumura)

❍ Finally, sufferers of "cedar fever," a seasonal allergy affecting millions of people in Texas, may be surprised to learn that winter cedar allergies are also a major problem in Japan. The formula *mao-bushin-saishin-to* offers specific relief for cedar fever. North American brand names include:

- Ma Huang & Asarum Combination (Sun Ten)
- Ma Huang & Asarum (Qualiherb)
- Ma Huang Fu Zi Xi Xin Tang (Qualiherb, Sun Tang)

CONCEPTS FOR COPING WITH ALLERGIES

❍ Allergy-causing pollens are carried by the wind. To reduce your exposure to pollen, close windows and run the air conditioner in the home and car. Stay indoors when pollen counts are high, especially on sunny, breezy days.

❍ The timing of your sneezing season gives you some idea of what you are allergic to, even without allergy testing. In most of North America, spring allergies are most commonly due to tree pollen. Allergy-invoking trees that are common to many areas include birches, elms, junipers, maples, and oaks. Summer allergies are usually due to grasses—Bermuda, Johnsongrass, timothy, and bluegrass are the most frequent offenders. Ragweed is the most common source of fall allergies.

❍ Don't hang laundry out to dry during your allergy season. Pollen and molds can stick to cloth surfaces.

❍ Outdoor air is most heavily saturated with pollen and mold between 5 and 10 A.M., so early morning is a good time to limit outdoor activities.

❍ A HEPA (High Energy Particulate Air) filter or an electrostatic precipitator may help clean pollen and mold from the indoor air.

❍ Wear a dust mask when mowing the lawn, raking leaves, or gardening.

❍ Dust mites live in bedding, curtains, carpets, upholstered furniture, and stuffed animals. Wash all bedding in hot (130°F or 55°C) water every week. Vacuum at least twice a week to remove dust mites from the carpet and furniture. Cover pillows, box spring, and mattress with allergy-proof encasings. Your vacuum cleaner should be fitted with a HEPA filter.

❍ Mold thrives in warm, damp, dark places, especially bathrooms, basements, and garbage cans. Keep all rooms clean and dry to prevent the growth of mold. Reduce indoor humidity by running your air conditioner or dehumidifier during the high-humidity seasons. If you use a humidifier in the winter, make sure the humidity remains around 40 percent. Keep garbage cans covered.

❍ There is no such thing as a nonallergenic cat or dog. Dander is a collection of microscopic skin cells shed by animals. It can stick to carpet, upholstery, and drapes long after a pet has left the room. Vacuum drapes and upholstery when you vacuum carpets, and keep pets out of your own sleeping quarters.

❍ Allergy shots have been used to treat inhalant allergies since 1912, when Dr. Noon injected boiled grass pollen into hay fever sufferers. The method has been refined so that it is now used to treat allergies to virtually every airborne allergen with a medically acceptable rate of success. Allergy vaccines work by "confusing" your immune system so that it eventually turns off the IgE system that causes allergic reactions. Overall, allergy shots have provided effective relief for millions of patients. They do not cause cancer, kidney disease, autoimmune disease, or any other illness in the millions of patients who receive them. They are not, however,

inexpensive. They can only be taken under professional supervision. While you may get some benefit after taking shots for only a few months, you typically would need to take shots for 3–5 years to have an 80 percent chance of protection.

❍ Chinese-trained acupuncturists often have good results in treating allergies, some studies reporting cure rates of up to 70 percent 3 years after treatment.[17] Six to eight treatments are usually required—and some of the acupuncture points used in the treatment of the most difficult cases may be in the nose itself.

❍ Homeopathic medicine offers a number of treatments for allergies. While homeopathic preparations are generally more effective than a placebo, the full benefit of homeopathy is found through interaction with a homeopathic physician who can match the symptoms of the whole person to a specific remedy. Because homeopathy treats people rather than diseases, homeopathic remedies match not only specific symptoms, but "central delusions," the essential ways people misperceive their life issues, that lead to illness.

If you choose to try homeopathy without the assistance of a homeopathic physician, start with a single dose of the lowest strength (6C, 6X, or 12C) of the remedy matching the symptoms to be treated, and then wait for a response. If there is an improvement in symptoms, let the remedy continue to work until there is no more improvement, then take another dose. If there is no improvement, try a different potency (30X or 30C). Sometimes homeopathic medicines work for a few minutes, sometimes they work for an entire day before another dose is needed.

• Arsenicum album treats people who suffer violent reactions to many different foods and pollens and who tend toward anxiety, compulsivity, and overattention to details and order.

• Calcarea carbonica treats allergies that occur with digestive problems, such as gas and heartburn, and possibly back pain, dizziness, fatigue, nightmares, and swollen lymph glands and tonsils. People who benefit from this remedy often have a fear of heights or claustrophobia.

• Calcarea phosphorica relieves allergies occurring with stomach pains, headaches, and "munchies." The individual who benefits most from this remedy may have wanderlust, a strong desire to travel, especially when life's problems seem to close in. It is also used for children who are picky eaters and who tend to complain a lot.

• Carbo vegetabilis relieves allergies in people who have bloating, flatulence, and a frequent need to burp. This remedy is appropriately prescribed when symptoms worsen when eating, talking, or lying down.

• Gelsemium treats aches and pains, droopy eyelids, trembling, weakness, and back pain—symptoms of allergy that are more like the flu. The person who needs this remedy tends to have symptoms that worsen when under pressure to perform, either to meet a deadline or in a stressful situation, such as public speaking.

• Hepar sulphuris calcareum treats allergies in "touchy" people, especially people whose allergies are worst after exposure to chills and drafts. The personality type associated with this remedy tends to release tension in angry bursts punctuating long periods of gloominess.

• Ignatia relieves allergies in people who tend to have muscle cramps and mood swings. People who need this remedy often have paradoxical symptoms: joint pain improved by lifting or stressing the joint, sore throat improved by swallowing, heartburn improved by eating peppers and onions, and so on.

• Lycopodium treats allergies in people whose symptoms are worse on the right side of the body (the right eye, the right nostril, and so on). People who get ravenously hungry and feel bloated after eating benefit from this remedy.

• Natrum carbonicum is recommended for allergies in people with sensitive stomachs, especially if there is lactose intolerance.

• Natrum muriaticum treats allergies in people who experience a variety of symptoms: back pain, neck pain, headaches, canker sores, fever, and fatigue. People who benefit from this remedy tend to crave salt and to have strong thirst. This remedy is more appropriate for summer allergies than for winter allergies.

• Nux moschata treats allergies occurring with a feeling of giddiness. Dry mouth, dry eyes, and tingling or numbness in the fingers or toes are other indications this remedy may be helpful.

• Nux vomica treats allergies in people whose symptoms are made worse by their tobacco habit. It is appropriate for people who are sensitive to multiple substances and who have runny nose and headaches compounded by heartburn and constipation.

• Petroleum treats allergies in people who are sensitive to fumes. A person who will respond well to this remedy is likely to have inflamed or cracked skin, especially around the fingertips.

• Phosphorus treats allergies in people for whom a simple experience lights an emotional fire. People who need this remedy tend to be impressionable and to have strong anxieties and fears. They may react to pollens or allergenic foods by "spacing out" or by having headaches, nausea, or diarrhea.

• Sulphuricum acidum treats intense reactions to fumes.

Alopecia Areata

SYMPTOM SUMMARY

○ Sudden hair loss in one or more small, round, smooth patches on the scalp or beard

○ (Rarely) Total hair loss on the scalp or entire body

UNDERSTANDING THE DISEASE PROCESS

Alopecia areata is an autoimmune disease that causes loss of hair. The latest scientific understanding of the condition is that people with alopecia areata have an excess of macrophage migration inhibitory factor. This is a hormone that causes a special class of circulating white blood cells to become "stuck" around hair follicles.[1] These CD4+ cells secrete inflammatory hormones normally reserved for combating bacterial infections, and eventually stop growth of the follicle. Affected follicles become very small and grow no visible hair above the surface of the skin for months or years.

Alopecia areata most commonly affects the scalp, but any hair-bearing site can be affected by itself or together with the scalp. Most frequently, the condition starts in childhood. According to the National Alopecia Areata Foundation, approximately 1 in 50 people in the United States, or 4.5 million people in the United States alone, experiences this form of hair loss at some point in their lives.

Some people with alopecia areata develop only a few bare patches that regrow hair within a few months to a year. Others have extensive patchy loss of hair, and some lose all the visible hair on the scalp (alopecia totalis) or even the entire body (alopecia universalis). In all cases of autoimmune hair loss, however, the hair regrows if it receives the appropriate signal from the immune system. Without a change in immune balance, however, hair does not regrow.

TREATMENT SUMMARY

AROMATHERAPY

○ 2–3 drops each of cedarwood, lavender, rosemary, and thyme mixed in a tablespoon of grape seed or jojoba oil and applied to bald areas of the scalp nightly.

HERBS

○ Khellin: 100 milligrams daily.

See Part Three if you take prescription medication.

UNDERSTANDING THE HEALING PROCESS

The easiest and most promising natural treatment for alopecia areata is a combination of essential oils. A clinical trial at the Aberdeen Royal Infirmary in Scotland enrolled 84 individuals who massaged either essential oils or a non-treatment oil into their scalps every night for 7 months. At the end of the study, 44 percent of the treatment group experienced new hair growth compared to only 15 percent in the control group. The treatment oil contained essential oils of cedarwood, lavender, rosemary, and thyme.[2]

Khellin is a gentler alternative to treatment with prescription anthralin creams or ointments. Anthralin was originally a coal tar derivative. It is irritating to the skin to which it is applied, hands, and eyes. It also leaves a brown stain. Khellin is activated by exposure to ultraviolet light, so it is essential to expose the scalp to sun or a sun lamp for at least 30 minutes a day while taking the herb.[3]

Khellin can cause nausea and stomach upset, but this side effect usually subsides after the first week of treatment. About two-thirds of people who take the herb experience no unpleasant side effects of any kind.

CONCEPTS FOR COPING WITH ALOPECIA AREATA

○ Acupuncture treatments sometimes produce dramatic improvements in alopecia universalis. In successful acupuncture treatment, hair usually returns the same way it fell out, in clumps. It may be necessary to take acupuncture treatments for 6 months to a year to get results. An argument could be made that hair might return on its own during that period, but acupuncture has been used to treat cases in which hair loss has been total for as long as 7 years.

○ Steroids such as cortisone are often effective but carry the risk of serious side effects, such as lowered immune resistance and weight gain. If you choose to take cortisone injections, a licorice extract called glycyrrhizin will slow the rate at which your body breaks down the cortisone, extending its healing effects but also increasing the risk of side effects.[4] Take 250–500 milligrams of glycyrrhizin 3 times per day. Do not use deglycyrrhizinated licorice (DGL), since it does not enhance the effects of steroids. Discontinue the supplement if you observe slow healing of a cut or scrape or unexplained weight gain, or if you develop an infection. Do not take glycyrrhizin if you have high blood pressure.

○ Many doctors treat alopecia areata with minoxidil. An alternative to minoxidil is diphencyprone (DPC), a chemical also used in developing film. Workers at Kodak found that it caused hair to sprout in unwanted places if they failed to wash after using it. While DCP is not a prescription drug, it is in no way a natural treatment, and applying it requires the use of protective garments and special ventilation under professional supervision. The advantage of DCP is that hair does not fall out immediately when treatment is discontinued, as is the case with minoxidil. In alopecia universalis (total hair loss), DCP produces cosmetically acceptable results only about 17 percent of the time, but when hair loss is less than 50 percent, DCP is 100 percent effective. Hair typically begins to reappear after 3 months of treatment, but it is sometimes necessary to take the drug for as long as 2 years before hair regrowth occurs. When hair loss is less than 50 percent, hair restoration typically takes about 10 months. Side effects are common, including blistering (45 percent of users), freckling (12 percent), vitiligo (2 percent), and swollen lymph glands (2 percent). Hair that grows back during DCP treatment usually lasts 2–3 years before resumption of treatment is necessary.[5] DCP must be applied weekly to be effective. It is available from dermatologists.

○ Several treatments attempt to change the immune balance of the scalp by inducing skin allergies, including topical applications of nickel sulfate[6] or primula leaf oil.[7]

In this method, irritation to the skin is essential to stimulating hair growth. Small-scale studies suggest this method may help most people with alopecia, but dosages have not been established.

○ Zinc supplementation does not help most cases of alopecia areata. However, when alopecia follows extreme low-calorie diets or gastroplasty, a surgical shrinking of the stomach to treat obesity, zinc may be very helpful. In one study, *all* gastroplasty patients who had experienced hair loss regained their hair after taking 200 milligrams of zinc sulfate 3 times a day for 6 months.[8] This dosage of zinc is potentially high enough to interfere with the immune system's resistance to infection, so it is essential to treat infections promptly.

Altitude Sickness

SYMPTOM SUMMARY

○ Headache
  • Interrupts sleep
  • Also occurs on awakening in the morning
  • Aggravated by lying down
  • Aggravated by standing up
  • Aggravated by lifting
  • Aggravated by coughing or sneezing
  • Accompanied by nausea and vomiting

○ Constant dry cough

○ Shortness of breath, even at rest, but worse during exercise

○ Confusion

○ Coughing up blood

○ Fatigue

○ Insomnia

○ Loss of appetite

○ Nausea

○ Rapid pulse

○ Vomiting

May also cause:

○ Drooping eyelid on one side

○ Loss of consciousness

○ Pupil dilated in only one eye

○ Swelling around the eye socket

○ Swelling in the ankles or legs

○ Swollen face

○ Visual distortion

UNDERSTANDING THE DISEASE PROCESS

Altitude sickness is a condition of oxygen deprivation that can affect travelers, hikers, skiers, and mountain climbers who have ascended too rapidly to an elevation of 7,000 feet (2,000 meters) or higher. Altitude sickness affects the heart, lungs, and central nervous system. Its symptoms can range from the minor discomfort of fatigue, headache, and nausea to life-threatening accumulations of fluid in the lungs and brain.

Changes in altitude can affect the body in ways other than just oxygen deprivation. Gases inside enclosed spaces expand at lower pressures. Gas in the bowel expands 20 percent at 8,000 feet (2,700 meters), making abdominal bloating much more intense at higher elevations than at sea level. Changes in gas pressure in the uterus can hasten labor in pregnant women.

TREATMENT SUMMARY

DIET

○ Drink lots of water.

○ Avoid alcohol.

○ Unless you are diabetic or dieting, eat as many carbohydrates as you want. Increasing your consumption of fat may also help.

NUTRITIONAL SUPPLEMENTS

Start 2–3 weeks before travel:

○ Alpha-lipoic acid: 600 milligrams daily.

○ Vitamin C: 1,000 milligrams daily.

○ Vitamin E: 400 IU daily.

HERBS

Also start 2–3 weeks before travel:

○ Ginkgo: 70–80 milligrams, twice a day.

UNDERSTANDING THE HEALING PROCESS

Generally speaking, the faster you go up, the worse the

symptoms of altitude sickness. Getting really comfortable with mountain air can take weeks. Ideally, you should plan to limit your activities for the first 2 days at 7,000 feet (2,000 meters), and an additional 1–2 days for every 1,000 feet (300 meters) you ascend beyond 7,000 feet (2,000 meters). People who are physically fit can usually function well without transition time at lower mountains, below 10,000 feet (3,000 meters), but others will experience at least fatigue and headache. For most of us, an enjoyable quick weekend trip to a high-mountain ski resort or other destination requires medication or additional preparation.

Physicians usually offer one of two medications to sufferers of altitude sickness. Acetazolamide (Acetazolam or Diamox) eliminates fluid and increases the oxygen content of the blood. Eliminating fluid, of course, requires more frequent urination—not a plus on the ski slopes. Acetazolamide can also cause drowsiness, numbness in the fingers and toes that can delay recognition of frostbite, and a flat taste when drinking carbonated beverages. Dexamethasone (Deronil, Dexasone, Dexone) is an anti-inflammatory steroid that prevents swelling, but it can also cause dizziness, headache, nausea, and vomiting, the very symptoms it is taken to prevent.

Diet and supplements are not as fast in relieving the symptoms of altitude sickness, but they do not cause side effects. Your body loses more fluids at higher altitude. Replacing fluids by drinking lots of water does not have a direct effect on mountain sickness, but it does prevent headaches caused by dehydration. Alcohol also dehydrates, and slows your rate of breathing. Avoid it.

Provided you aren't diabetic, a high-mountain vacation is your time to indulge in potatoes, pasta, and sugary desserts. Burning carbohydrate calories increases your rate of respiration, which makes you take more breaths, increasing your oxygen supply. Doctors at the Walter Reed Army Medical Center took 15 healthy volunteers aged 18–33 to a height of 15,000 feet (4,600 meters), asked them to fast for 5 hours, and then gave them a 500-calorie sugared drink. The researchers found that consuming carbohydrates increased the oxygen saturation of hemoglobin (the volunteers' PulsOx levels) from 79–84 percent.[1] Other tests suggest that a high-fat diet may be equally beneficial,[2] although the benefits of either diet wear off over 4–5 days as the body becomes naturally adjusted to altitude.[3]

If you can plan ahead, it helps to take antioxidants, preferably for 2–3 weeks before your travel. A study of mountaineers climbing Mt. Everest found that taking alpha-lipoic acid and vitamins C and E made climbing Mt. Everest as easy as ascending to Canada's Lake Louise, increasing both oxygen saturation and calorie intake, and reducing the frequency of headache, nausea, and fatigue.[4] To reduce problems with exposure to the cold, take ginkgo. A French expedition to the Himalayas found that mountaineers who took ginkgo had warmer skin, fingers, and toes that mountaineers who did not. More important, no one in the French study who took ginkgo suffered acute headache, compared to 40 percent of those who did not. Only 3 mountaineers taking ginkgo experienced acute breathing problems, compared to 18 who did not.[5]

If you are diabetic, exercise special caution when taking alpha-lipoic acid at high altitude. The combination of low oxygen, high activity, and alpha-lipoic acid can make you prone to hypoglycemia, especially if you take insulin.

CONCEPTS FOR COPING WITH ALTITUDE SICKNESS

○ Children adapt better to high altitudes than adults, but paradoxically are also more susceptible to high altitude pulmonary edema (HAPE). Blood-stained phlegm, blue lips, and white tongue with red spots of varying sizes, along with shortness of breath and a fast pulse indicate a medical emergency in a child recently transported to high altitude. HAPE can be fatal within a few hours unless treated by descent or oxygen. HAPE is most likely to occur on the second night at a new mountain.

○ Most high-mountain airports are at a higher elevation than the cities they serve. Do not remain at the airport any longer than necessary when starting a mountain vacation.

○ Take aromatherapy instead of sleeping pills. Like alcohol, sleeping pills can slow your rate of breathing. Instead, add a few drops of essential oil of lavender to any warm beverage or, if you are staying indoors, a teaspoon of essential oil of lavender to your bath. Lavender oil is relaxing and relieves muscle pain.

○ Avoid trace-mineral supplements if you are planning an extended stay at a high altitude. Accumulation of excessive cobalt can contribute to chronic mountain sickness.[6]

○ Altitude sickness can interfere with sleep, but once

you have adjusted to your elevation, you will probably sleep better. Laboratory experiments with animals indicate that the brain makes more melatonin at high altitude, the concentration of melatonin peaking after 7 days and falling back to normal levels thereafter.[7]

○ Seek medical attention if you experience blurred vision at altitudes greater than 13,000 feet (4,200 meters). At this elevation, the retina can rupture and bleed, especially after strenuous physical exertion, such as cross-country skiing.[8]

Alzheimer's Disease

SYMPTOM SUMMARY

Early stages:

○ Getting lost on familiar routes

○ Losing interest in activities once enjoyed

○ Misplacing familiar objects

○ Personality changes

○ Repeating statements frequently

○ Trouble finding names for familiar objects

More advanced stages:

○ Decreased knowledge of recent events

○ Delusions, depression, and agitation

○ Forgetting events in personal history

○ Hallucinations, arguments, striking out, and violent behavior

○ Problems choosing proper clothing

UNDERSTANDING THE DISEASE PROCESS

Alzheimer's disease (AD) is the leading cause of dementia in most Western countries. Although it can strike at any age, AD is most common in the elderly, affecting approximately 1 in 20 people over the age of 70 in the United States. People with Alzheimer's develop a steadily progressive loss of memory and gradually lose their ability to take care of themselves. The affects of the disease on the patient and family are devastating both emotionally and financially. The average cost of caring for a single AD patient in the United States in 2000 was $47,000 per year.[1]

While changes in memory style are a normal part of aging, the cognitive decline in Alzheimer's disease is severe. Many people who have the disease are unaware of their difficulties, but others retain insight, resulting in anxiety and frustration. In the early and middle stages of the disease, the person with AD may be unable to work, easily get lost and confused, and requires daily supervision, but social graces and superficial ability to use language may be preserved. In the final stages of AD, patients almost always become rigid, incontinent, and bedridden. Help is needed with the simplest tasks, such as eating, dressing, and toilet function.

The scientifically proven risk factor for AD in the general public is old age. (AD is a frequent long-term complication of Down syndrome.) There is considerable evidence, however, that inflammatory diseases play a role. The neurofibrillary tangles in brain tissue characteristic of AD contain dying nerve cells and macrophages, the white blood cells activated by bacterial infection or inflammation. A study published in *The New England Journal of Medicine* noted that people who use aspirin and NSAIDs on a daily basis for 2 years or more are 5 times less likely to develop AD than people who use these kinds of pain relievers occasionally or not at all.[2]

Another likely risk factor for the development of AD is exposure to aluminum. In the bloodstream, aluminum ions are configured with their carriers so that they are electrostatically attracted to helical filament tau (PHFt), the protein that "tangles" the neurofibrillary tangles that destroy brain tissue.[3] Although everyone accumulates aluminum in their bodies as they age, autopsies have found that people with AD accumulate unusually large quantities of aluminum in the brain.[4] While it is probably too late to do much good by restricting exposure to aluminum once symptoms have developed, at least one study has found that removing aluminum from the body with chelation therapy with desferrioxamine (not EDTA) slowed the development of symptoms in 48 AD patients.[5]

As this book is being written in 2002, twenty-one scientific studies support the observation that women who take estrogen replacement therapy are less likely to develop AD. The problem with these studies is that women who take estrogen replacement therapy tend to be generally healthier than women who do not.[6] Estrogen replacement therapy after Alzheimer's disease has already begun to develop has not yet been shown to ameliorate the disease, and studies by the Women's

Health Initiative to determine if supplemental estrogen will help AD patients will not be completed until 2010.

TREATMENT SUMMARY

DIET

O Avoid dietary sources of glutamate, including red meats, cheeses, and pureed tomatoes.

O Eliminate aspartame, hydrolyzed vegetable protein, and MSG from your diet.

NUTRITIONAL SUPPLEMENTS

For people with AD who have had symptoms for under 6 months:

O Vitamin B_{12} (methylcobalamin): 1,000 micrograms twice a day.

For people with AD who are approaching the need of nursing-home care:

O Vitamin E: 2,000 IU per day (consult a doctor before beginning therapy).

At any stage of AD:

O Acetyl-L-carnitine: 1,000 milligrams 3 times a day.

O Phosphatidylserine: 300–600 milligrams per day.

HERBS

O Ginkgo: 70–80 milligrams, 3 times a day.

For women who have Alzheimer's disease:

O *Toki-shakuyaku-san* (Japanese herbal formula): As directed on label.

See Part Three if you take prescription medication.

UNDERSTANDING THE HEALING PROCESS

While the data do not yet support the assertion that "An aspirin a day keeps Alzheimer's away," if you have a family history of AD and do not yet have the disease, see your healthcare advisor about taking a baby aspirin every day. Do not take aspirin if you are allergic to it or if you have peptic ulcers, kidney disease, or gout, or if you take any prescription blood thinner. If you have a family history of AD, it may also be helpful to avoid aluminum: antacids, aluminum-based antiperspirants, aluminum cooking ware, aluminum foil, baking powder, ordinary table salt, and nondairy creamers. Unprocessed fruits and vegetables, fruits, nuts, and seeds are excellent sources of magnesium, which competes with and prevents aluminum from entering your body.

If you are in the early stages of Alzheimer's disease or are a caretaker for someone with the disease, various supplements may be helpful at different stages of the disease. Vitamin B_{12} deficiency is very common among the elderly. Inadequate levels of B_{12} can cause numbness, burning feet, depression, and impaired memory function that can mimic AD. The best course of action for someone in the early stages of AD who has any of the symptoms of vitamin B_{12} deficiency is to have a blood or urine test to confirm the deficiency (a urinary methylmalonic acid or homocysteine screening test is easiest), and then to take 1,000 micrograms of the methylcobalamin form of the vitamin twice a day.

Supplementation with vitamin B_{12} and folic acid sometimes completely reverses symptoms of AD patients who have been diagnosed with the disease within 6 months.[7] Vitamin B_{12} supplementation rarely helps AD patients who have had the disease for more than a year.[8] Some recent research suggests that these vitamins are most important when brain tissue is under attack by excitotoxins, chemicals including aspartame, hydrolyzed vegetable protein, and MSG. Scientists believe that in the absence of adequate levels of vitamin B_{12} and folic acid, small amounts of excitotoxins that ordinarily would not be harmful can cause brain damage.[9]

For this reason, it may be helpful for *anyone* at risk for Alzheimer's disease to eliminate aspartame, hydrolyzed vegetable protein, and MSG from the diet. This includes not using diet drinks sweetened with Nutra-Sweet and also eliminating foods that contain glutamate, such as instant soup mixes, red meats, cheese, and pureed tomatoes. The glutamate in whole tomatoes is bound in a way that it takes longer to digest and never reaches nerve tissue unless tomatoes are eaten in massive quantities.

At the other end of the spectrum of Alzheimer's disease, advanced patients may benefit from massive vitamin E therapy—begun under a doctor's supervision. A single clinical study reported in *The New England Journal of Medicine* found that a very high dosage, 2,000 IU per day, delays the need to put an AD patient into a nursing home by an average of 85 days.[10] It would seem logical that smaller dosages of vitamin E earlier in the disease would delay symptoms, but this has not been proven, and there are even indications that it is not a good idea. AD patients who are still ambulatory are more likely to take a fall if they take vitamin E, possibly because they have just enough additional mobility to find themselves in hazardous situations.[11]

Do not give an AD patient more than 800 IU of vitamin E a day without consulting a healthcare practitioner to make sure there are no potential bleeding conditions that could cause complications. Be forewarned that some people taking a dosage of 2,000 IU per day experience diarrhea and will need additional toilet assistance.

Other supplements are helpful at all stages of the disease. Acetyl-L-carnitine (ACL) is a modification of the amino acid derivative L-carnitine, chemically modified so that it is more easily absorbed by the brain. ACL seems to slow the life cycle of brain cells so that fewer die. AD patients under the age of 65 who take ACL sometimes improve. AD patients over the age of 65 who take ACL generally get worse more slowly.[12]

Any dosage of ACL high enough to slow the progression of Alzheimer's disease can cause mild stomach upset, abdominal cramps, and diarrhea. It sometimes causes intense dreams, and some AD patients taking it will become agitated. ACL can make seizures more frequent in epileptics, and can induce a manic state in people who have bipolar disorder.

Phosphatidylserine (PS) is a major component of the membranes lining nerve cells, particularly at their junctures with other nerve cells. Experiments with animals indicate that PS somehow encourages the regrowth of nerve networks within the brain. At its peak performance state, usually around the age of 30, the human brain may have up to 10,000 connections per each of its approximately 100 billion nerve cells, yielding as many as 1,000 trillion cell-to-cell connections, that is, a quadrillion nerve pathways. In Alzheimer's disease up to 90 percent of these connections are lost.[13] By the end of life, an Alzheimer's patient may have virtually nothing remaining of the CA_1 region of the hippocampus, the region of the brain in which memories are formed.[14]

PS seems to stimulate nerve growth factor in the cerebral cortex and the hippocampus, the two regions of the brain most affected by AD.[15] Loosely controlled clinical testing in the United States has found that it helps sufferers of age-associated memory loss recover their abilities of verbal association and recall.[16] It helps restore hormone rhythms that help AD patients deal with emotional stress.[17] In advanced Alzheimer's dis-

ease, PS will often improve sociability, attention to personal welfare, and cooperation with caregivers.[18]

A dosage of 300 milligrams per day helps memory, and a dosage of 600 milligrams per day lowers anxiety. PS is completely nontoxic and does not interfere with medications. Since European brands of PS are extracted from cow brain, there has been concern about mad cow disease, but functionally equivalent formulations made from soy are also available.

Any dosage of ginkgo greater than 160 milligrams per day seems to offer real, but modest, benefits to AD patients. Ginkgo has a variety of anti-inflammatory effects in the brain. A study published in the *Journal of the American Medical Association* found that taking ginkgo offered benefits roughly equivalent to delaying the course of the disease by 6 months.[19] The most recent research has found that ginkgo leads to improvement in very mild cases of Alzheimer's disease, but at best leads to stabilization in more advanced cases.[20]

Never take a whole-leaf preparation of ginkgo. The whole leaf of the herb can contain toxins that can be especially detrimental to AD patients. Always take ginkgo extract. Do not take ginkgo with high dosages of vitamin E, since the combination can increase the risk of bleeding.

While the research into the use of estrogen replacement therapy in treating AD is still ongoing, some researchers have investigated treatment with estrogen-preserving herbal formulas such as the Japanese herbal formula *toki-shakuyaku-san*. One of these researchers is Nobuyoshi Hagino, M.D., of Japan's Dokkyo School of Medicine and the University of Texas Health Science Center at San Antonio. He is among the clinical researchers who discovered that estrogen therapy can ease symptoms in women who have Alzheimer's disease. In a 1995 study, women with mild Alzheimer's who were given conjugated equine estrogens regained some ability to function in daily life and communicate with family and friends.

In a follow-up study, Dr. Hagino's research team found that Kampo medicine was even more effective than estrogen. Patients given Japanese herbal formulas showed significant improvement in conversation, reading, writing, removing/putting on clothes, and long-term memory. Best of all, unlike estrogen, the Kampo medicines caused no side effects. Kampo uses a combination of minimally processed herbs. Unlike a prescription medication that consists of one or occasionally two active chemical compounds, Japanese herbal formulas utilize combinations of whole herbs that contain dozens, and often hundreds, of active ingredients. This synergy makes the primary ingredients more effective and prevents the toxic reactions that lead to side effects. As a result, bodily imbalances are corrected without additional, medication-induced problems.[21]

Toki-shakuyaku-san is available under these brand names in the United States and Canada:

- Dang Gui & Peony (Qualiherb)
- Kampo4Women MenopauEase (Honso)
- Tangkuei & Peony Formula (Lotus Classics)
- Tang-Kuei and Peony Formula (Golden Flower Chinese Herbs, Sun Ten)
- Toki-shakuyaku-san (Honso, Tsumura)

There are no reports of side effects from the use of *toki-shakuyaku-san* in treating Alzheimer's disease in women. Men should not use the formula.

This is not an exhaustive list of herbs and supplements with the potential to help in AD, but these are the principal supplements that are widely available, relatively inexpensive, and free of potential side effects. Vitamin C is frequently recommended but has not been clinically studied for treatment of AD. High dosages of thiamine may be helpful for AD patients who have been heavy drinkers or who take the diuretic furosemide (Lasix), but the dosages of the vitamin required to make a difference in AD (7,000–9,000 milligrams daily) can be dangerous to anyone who later has to be put on an i.v. Very high doses of phosphatidylcholine (lecithin) also help some AD patients, but they are also likely to cause diarrhea and the needed 15,000–25,000 milligrams per day can be quite expensive. There are some theoretical reasons to believe DHEA could be as helpful as estrogen in women with AD, but this possibility has not been scientifically tested.

CONCEPTS FOR COPING WITH ALZHEIMER'S DISEASE

○ Memory loss in the elderly is not always due to Alzheimer's disease. Sometimes memory "problems" have more to do with the overwhelming amount of information in daily life. Other times memory loss is real, but more benign. Psychologists and psychiatrists employ sophisticated cognitive testing methods to detect and accurately measure the severity of cognitive decline. Never assume Alzheimer's disease without a professional evaluation.

○ The old adage, "Use it or lose it," applies to the brain. The more dense the brain circuitry is earlier in life, the more that can be lost later in life before function becomes seriously compromised. The *Journal of the American Medical Association* reported a study of nuns that found those who wrote in journals in the most complex language early in life were the least likely to develop AD later in life.[22] In the very early stages of AD, working crossword puzzles, maintaining social ties, and attempting intellectual tasks can slow intellectual decline.

○ Avoiding head trauma also helps lower the risk of developing AD. One study has found that injury to the head increases the risk of AD predicted by genetics 10-fold.[23]

○ Communicating with AD patients requires adjustments in the manner and complexity of speech. Here are some suggestions on how to talk with someone with Alzheimer's disease:

- Ask one question at a time.
- Allow time for responses.
- Avoid using negative statements, for example, "You know who this is, don't you?"
- Use proper names rather than pronouns.
- Don't talk about the person as if he or she wasn't there.
- Speak slowly and clearly.
- Use nonverbal communication such as pointing and touching.
- Use short, simple, and familiar words in a relaxed tone of voice.
- Use positive, friendly facial expressions.

○ Because bathing is an intimate experience, Alzheimer's patients may perceive it as unpleasant or threatening and in turn show various forms of resistance such as screaming and hitting. The first step in making bathing easier is to find out whether the AD patient prefers tub baths or showers, and which time of day is best. Then it is helpful to create a safe and pleasant atmosphere respecting the AD patient's needs for modesty. Allowing him or her to hold a towel in front of the body, in or out of the shower, can restore their sense of dignity. Don't worry about the frequency of bathing—it is not necessary to bathe every day.

○ "Accidents" sometimes occur because the Alzheimer's patient cannot find the bathroom. Provide a visual cue, such as a colored rug in front of the bathroom door or a colored lid on the toilet seat, to make the bathroom stand out. Identify when toileting is likely to occur and encourage the person to go to the toilet at those times. Also, make sure clothing is easy to remove.

○ Simplify choices in clothing. Lay out one or two outfits. Don't show the AD patient a closet full of clothes. Shirts and blouses that open in the front are usually easier to manage than pullovers. Velcro is preferable to buttons, snaps, and zippers that may be too difficult to handle. Make sure shoes do not have slippery soles.

○ Like everyone else, AD patients need to brush after every meal. The instruction "Brush your teeth" may be too difficult. Instead, try "Hold your toothbrush, put paste on your brush," and so on, so that the AD patient can accomplish each step. Refusing to open the mouth may be a sign of discomfort and indicate the need for more frequent oral care. Try using oral hygiene aids available from your dentist to prop the mouth open.

Amblyopia in Childhood

SYMPTOM SUMMARY

○ Eyes that turn in or out

○ Eyes that do not appear to work together

○ Inability to judge distances

UNDERSTANDING THE DISEASE PROCESS

Amblyopia, or "lazy eye," is reduced vision in an eye that has not been used enough during early childhood. The condition is most frequently noticed when the child starts school, although it can occur at any time from infancy through early adulthood. The average age at diagnosis among children given regular eye exams is 5.3 years.

Amblyopia most often results from a misalignment of the child's eyes, such as crossed eyes, due to a defect of the muscles. This condition is commonly known as strabismus. Amblyopia can also result from ansiometropia, a difference in image quality between the two eyes, one eye focusing better than the other due to differences in the lens itself. Slightly more than one-third of

children with amblyopia have strabismus only, a similar number have ansiometropia only, and about 25 percent have both defects.[1]

Ansiometropia is more difficult to treat than strabismus. In all three cases, one eye becomes stronger, suppressing the image of the other eye. If the condition persists, the weaker eye may become useless.

TREATMENT SUMMARY

NUTRITIONAL SUPPLEMENTS

○ CDP-choline: 500 milligrams daily for 10 days *every 6 months.*

See Part Three if you take prescription medication.

UNDERSTANDING THE HEALING PROCESS

The most common treatment for amblyopia is an eye patch. The better-seeing eye is covered, forcing the "lazy" one to work, thereby strengthening its vision. Alternatively, the better-seeing eye may be treated with atropine eyedrops to blur its vision, but this approach does not usually achieve success as quickly as patching the eye.[2] To avoid permanent loss of sight in the "lazy" eye, treatment usually must begin by age 10.

Two scientific studies confirm the usefulness of CDP-choline as an aid to conventional treatment of amblyopia. Also known by its scientific name cytidine-5'-diphosphocholine, this chemical is a major component of cell membranes throughout the body, helping them to maintain both form and function. An Italian study found that children aged 5–9 who were given 500 milligrams of CDP-choline every day for 10 days at the beginning of therapy began to have improved vision in 10 days, while children who only wore an eye patch began to have improved vision after 1 month. CDP-choline is not a substitute for the use eye patches, but even children whose eyes are *not* patched will experience *temporary* improvement in vision if they receive the supplement.[3]

CDP-choline is chemically similar to soy lecithin. Children who are allergic to soy may be allergic to some CDP-choline products. Taking too much of this supplement will cause gas and diarrhea.

CONCEPTS FOR COPING WITH AMBLYOPIA IN CHILDHOOD

○ It may be helpful to introduce the patch as a game in

which the child plays a fantasy character wearing an eye patch. It is usually better to start the child wearing the patch in a setting in which the child is the focus of adult attention.

○ Rewarding the child for keeping the patch on (for example, with games or videos) is usually more effective than punishing the child for taking the patch off.

○ Tincture of benzoin applied around the edge of the patch will make it difficult for the child to remove it. You can loosen the glue and remove the patch with warm water.

○ Treat skin irritation early. Some children will experience skin irritation where the patch is attached to the face. This may be due to a minor allergy to the adhesive; switching tape or patch brands may help eliminate the problem.

○ It is not necessary for the child to wear the patch all the time. Most elementary students do not do as well in school when they wear their patches all day.

Amenorrhea

SYMPTOM SUMMARY

○ Failure of menstruation to begin by age 16 (primary amenorrhea), or

○ Cessation of menstruation in a woman who has had regular periods for 3 months or more (secondary amenorrhea)

UNDERSTANDING THE DISEASE PROCESS

Amenorrhea is the absence of menstrual periods. More specifically, amenorrhea is the absence of menstruation in a woman who is not pregnant or breastfeeding and who has not reached menopause. Failure to have a period usually results from a deficiency of the female reproductive hormones that stimulate menstruation.

The most common cause of the hormone deficiency leading to missed menstrual periods is inadequate nutrition. Anorexia almost always causes amenorrhea. Many women who are not anorexic but who miss their periods have lower dietary intakes of fat, especially saturated fat, as well as protein and total calories, compared with women who menstruate regularly.[1] Women with amenorrhea also tend to obtain a greater proportion of their calories from high-fiber carbohydrates.[2] In preliminary studies of normal-weight women with no obvious eating disorders, those who reported missed periods had diets described as "close to normal" but significantly low in fat. These women also tended to have low percentages of body fat.[3]

Amenorrhea also can result from excessive exercise. Women athletes and performers tend to diet to avoid weight gain. Combined with the increased nutritional demands of intensive exercise, dieting can lead to nutrient deficiencies and lowered body-fat percentages that lead to amenorrhea and bone loss.[4] Ballet and track and field sports are most frequently associated with missed menstrual periods,[5] with as many as two-thirds of women long-distance runners and ballet dancers experiencing the condition.[6] In one study of women bodybuilders, 81 percent experienced amenorrhea.[7] Amenorrhea also has been linked to smoking and stress, but smoking cessation and relaxation do not necessarily cure it.

The primary reason for treating amenorrhea is that it can cause bone loss that cannot be remedied by taking calcium and vitamin D.[8] Amenorrhea also can result from potentially life-threatening disorders of the hypothalamus, ovaries, or pituitary gland. For this reason, a physician should always be consulted the first time menstrual periods are missed 2 months or more.

TREATMENT SUMMARY

DIET

○ Avoid low-fat or no-fat diets. If you are vegan or vegetarian, be sure to include some source of concentrated fat in every meal.

○ Do not eat more than 1 serving of dark green, yellow, or orange vegetables daily.

NUTRITIONAL SUPPLEMENTS

○ Acetyl-L-carnitine: 2,000 milligrams per day.

○ Micronized progesterone: 200–300 milligrams per day, used under a doctor's supervision.

○ Vitamin B_6: 200–600 milligrams per day.

○ Avoid beta-carotene and mixed carotenoids.

HERBS

○ *Vitex agnus-castus* (chaste tree fruit): 40 drops of

tincture, or either 40 or 100 milligrams in capsule form, daily.

UNDERSTANDING THE HEALING PROCESS

Women who develop amenorrhea after adopting a low-fat diet sometimes can reverse the condition simply by increasing fat intake for 3 to 4 months.[9] Some women athletes with amenorrhea resume menstruation when they train less often and add additional calories, protein, and fat to their diets. Women with excessive carotene levels in their blood appear to be at higher risk of amenorrhea than women with normal levels,[10] and simply consuming less beta-carotene may help restore normal periods.[11] Beta-carotene is especially abundant in carrots, collards, spinach, sweet potatoes, and yellow squash.

Progesterone is the hormone that causes the lining of the uterus to thicken during the first half of the menstrual cycle. Medically supervised progesterone therapy is extremely useful in treating amenorrhea. In addition to progesterone, there are several other helpful supplements.

A preliminary clinical study found that 2,000 milligrams of acetyl-L-carnitine (ACL) given daily to amenorrheic women who had low bloodstream levels of estrogen and progesterone restored normal periods in 3–6 months in about half the women who took it. This dosage of ACL is high enough to cause mild stomach upset, abdominal cramps, and diarrhea. It can make seizures more frequent in epileptics, and can induce a manic state in people who have bipolar disorder.

Supplementation with vitamin B_6 can help treat amenorrhea in women who have high levels of the hormone prolactin. This is the hormone that enables milk production, so B_6 is most likely to help women who fail to resume normal menstruation after they stop nursing. It may also help amenorrheic women whose stores of the vitamin have been depleted as a side effect of using oral contraceptives or prescription drugs for asthma or epilepsy.

More likely to be of help, however, is the traditional herbal remedy *Vitex agnus castus,* also known as chasteberry or chaste tree fruit. The herb corrects "luteal phase defect," a condition in which the endometrium of the uterus fails to regrow after it is sloughed off.[12] It also corrects abnormally high levels of prolactin. A small-scale clinical trial found that 10 out of 15 women began having normal periods after taking vitex for 6 months.[13]

In rare cases, vitex can cause itching. Pregnant women should never take vitex, since it can cause miscarriage. Men should never take vitex, since it can cause testicular atrophy.

No supplement other than progesterone is likely to help every woman who has amenorrhea, but when supplements don't work, sometimes acupuncture does. An eighteenth-century classic of Chinese medical literature entitled *Secret Gynecological Prescriptions* explains the origins of amenorrhea this way: "Worry injures good breath, pensiveness cancels good diet, and since lungs and spleen are injured the vital energy chi stagnates, the woman becomes irritable and resentful and develops palpitations and oppression and eventually amenorrhea." In the original theory of Chinese medicine, acupuncture was thought to release the energies of deprivation, irritation, and resentment and restore normal energy flows to the uterus.

Whatever one may make of the theory, at least two modern clinical studies indicate the technique works. In a preliminary trial conducted in Germany, acupuncture was found to be helpful for women who have widely separated menstrual cycles.[14] In another study done in Austria, amenorrheic women showed a trend toward normalizing hormone levels following acupuncture.[15]

CONCEPTS FOR COPING WITH AMENORRHEA

O Sexually active heterosexual women who miss their periods may be pregnant. When appropriate, a pregnancy test should always be performed before extensive medical examination to determine the cause of amenorrhea.

O Women who have amenorrhea should limit their consumption of coffee to 1–2 cups per day. Caffeine can contribute to osteoporosis.

O A hallmark of overexercise is the willingness to exercise even when exhausted, injured, or ill. Exercise under these circumstances is anxiety driven and should be reassessed.

American Trypanosomiasis

See **Chagas Disease**.

Amyotrophic Lateral Sclerosis (ALS)

SYMPTOM SUMMARY

○ Muscular weakness, followed by a decrease in muscle strength and coordination

○ Gradual onset

○ Progressively worsens

○ Usually involves one limb (such as the hand or foot)

○ Later affects shoulder and upper arm or hips and upper thigh

○ Tripping, falling, inability to pick up or hold objects

○ Muscle cramps

○ Muscle stiffness

○ Muscle twitching (referred to in the literature of the disease as fasciculations)

○ Paralysis

○ Hoarseness, changes in quality of voice

○ Speech impairment, slowed speech

○ Difficulty swallowing

○ Difficulty breathing

○ Swelling in ankles, feet, and legs

○ Muscle atrophy

○ Muscle spasms

○ Urgent urination, more frequent urination

○ Urinary incontinence during periods of intense excitement

UNDERSTANDING THE DISEASE PROCESS

ALS is a devastating neuromuscular condition also known as Lou Gehrig's disease or amyotrophic lateral sclerosis in the United States and motor neuron disease or MND in most other English-speaking countries. The medical term for ALS comes from a combination of Greek words: *a*—without; *myo*—muscle; *trophic*—nourishment; *lateral*—side (of the spinal cord); *Sclerosis*—hardening or scarring.

ALS is a condition in which the nerves controlling muscles shrink and disappear. Lack of nervous stimulation leads to a loss of muscle tissue. Muscle strength and coordination decrease. The symptoms of ALS begin with the voluntary muscles, that is, muscles under conscious control, such as those in the arms and legs. More and more muscle groups become involved, and eventually there may be damage to the involuntary muscles, such as those that control breathing.

The precise causes of ALS are unknown. There is substantial evidence, however, that in ALS an excess of a neurotransmitter called glutamate clogs the synapses between nerve cells, preventing the transmission of nerve messages. The excess of glutamate eventually causes the death of the nerves. There is also evidence that people with ALS have a hereditary defect in their natural antioxidant defense systems. Nerve cells are unable to counteract free radicals that damage cell membranes, proteins, and DNA by oxidizing them, the same chemical process that turns iron into rust. Other physiological processes may contribute to ALS, but these two are susceptible to nutritional intervention.

TREATMENT SUMMARY

DIET

○ Avoid dietary sources of glutamate, including red meats, cheeses, and pureed tomatoes.

○ Eliminate aspartame, hydrolyzed vegetable protein, and MSG from your diet.

NUTRITIONAL SUPPLEMENTS

○ Vitamin C: 1,000 milligrams daily.

○ Vitamin E: 800 IU daily.

○ Avoid supplementation with branched-chain amino acids (L-isoleucine, L-leucine, and L-valine) and L-threonine.

UNDERSTANDING THE HEALING PROCESS

There are no good treatments for ALS. However, dietary restrictions and some natural products are likely to slow the progress of the disease.

People with ALS tend to have higher than normal levels of glutamate in their bloodstreams.[1] Glutamate opens a channel on the surface of the nerve cell that allows calcium to flow in. The nerve cell becomes very excited, firing impulses repeatedly, until a cascade of chemical reactions produces free radicals that eventually destroy the lining of the nerve.[2]

Aspartate, found in aspartame, has an effect similar to glutamate on nerve tissue, at least during embryonic development.[3] Monosodium glutamate, or MSG, should be completely eliminated from the diet. Hydrolyzed vegetable protein, a brown powder used to enhance the flavor of prepared soups and sauces is another source of concentrated glutamate that must be eliminated from the diet. Red meats, cheeses, and pureed tomatoes are likewise concentrated sources of glutamate and should be avoided. The glutamate in whole tomatoes is bound in a way that it takes longer to digest and never reaches nerve tissue unless tomatoes are eaten in massive quantities.

Vitamin C is an important cofactor for preserving vitamin E, which is an important antioxidant. Since several of the disease processes at work in ALS involve the oxidation of nerve tissue, investigators have been hopeful that supplemental vitamin E might cure or slow down the progress of the disease. The results of the most recent study of patients treated with both vitamin E and the drug riluzole found that vitamin E did not reverse any symptoms of ALS, but at least made it less likely for a patient to progress from a milder to a more severe form of the disease.[4] Studies in 2002 and 2003 by the same investigative team will seek to more clearly define the benefits of vitamin E supplementation.

Take vitamin C with caution if you also take certain prescription drugs. Vitamin C taken in the form of vitamin C with bioflavonoids can interfere with the liver's ability to process statin drugs for controlling cholesterol, calcium channel blockers such as nifedipine (Procardia) for hypertension, or cyclosporine for preventing transplant rejection. Consult your physician before taking vitamin E if you take any medication for thinning the blood, such as aspirin, clopidogrel (Plavix), or warfarin (Coumadin).

There was initial hope that branched-chain amino acids (L-isoleucine, L-leucine, and L-valine) could be very helpful in ALS, but later research indicates they should be avoided. In a pilot study, researchers at the Mount Sinai School of Medicine in New York found that treatment of ALS patients with a cocktail of the branched-chain amino acids L-isoleucine, L-leucine, and L-valine offered significant benefit in terms of maintenance of muscle strength in the hands and feet and continued ability to walk. A follow-up study at the University of Ver-

mont College of Medicine found that ALS patients may lose pulmonary function during treatment with the triple combination of amino acids or L-threonine. The researchers conducting the follow-up study believed the negative effects of amino acids found in their study could have been a fluke. However, since the rate of loss of breathing capacity was 2.5 times faster in ALS patients receiving amino acid treatment, L-isoleucine, L-leucine, L-threonine, and L-valine supplements cannot be recommended for ALS at this time.

There are no indications that coenzyme Q_{10}, creatine, genistein, guanidine, or vitamin B_{12} can cause harm in people with ALS, and animal studies indicate they could be helpful. Unfortunately, the studies supporting their use are very preliminary, and they cannot be recommended for regular use on the basic of existing evidence.

CONCEPTS FOR COPING WITH ALS

In the early stages of ALS, avoid heavy exercise, which tears down already-weakened muscles. Light exercise may help maintain strength in muscles that are not yet affected by the disease.

Controlling blood sugars is especially important for ALS sufferers who also have diabetes. High blood sugars interfere with the transport of oxygen to the brain.

Anal Fissures

SYMPTOM SUMMARY

- Bright red blood on the surface of stool, not mixed in with stool
- Bright red blood on toilet tissues
- Fresh blood in the toilet bowl after having a bowel movement
- Pain during bowel movement

UNDERSTANDING THE DISEASE PROCESS

Anal fissures are small splits in the lining of the anus. These tears in the wall of the anus may cause painful bowel movements, blood on the toilet tissue, streaks of blood on the outside of the stool, or accumulations of blood in the toilet bowl. In some cases, pieces of dried blood may be expelled during bowel movement.

Liquid blood from anal fissures is bright red rather than dark red. Darker blood may be a symptom of other, more serious health problems.

Anal fissures are very common in infants. Up to 80 percent of infants will have had an anal fissure before their first birthday. The incidence of the condition rapidly decreases with age until middle adulthood, when anal fissures again become a relatively common complaint. In small children, fissures result from excessive wiping, irritation from stool in the diaper, and scratching in response to an allergy or pinworms (see PARASITES, INTESTINAL). In adults, anal fissures in the back of the canal are almost always caused by straining due to constipation (see CONSTIPATION). Fissures in the front of the canal may result from inflammatory bowel disease, previous anal surgery, sexually transmitted diseases, or cancer.[1] Fissures that are a complication of Crohn's disease frequently develop into fistulas, misplaced canals between the rectum and vagina or skin near the anus.

TREATMENT SUMMARY

DIET

O Anal fissures in infants may be a symptom of an allergy to cow's milk. Use other protein sources to the extent possible.

O Try drinking small quantities (1/4 cup) of raw cabbage juice throughout the day.

O Gradually increase the amount of fiber in your diet so that you eat 5–9 servings of fruit and vegetables every day. Raw fruits and vegetables are preferable. Almonds, dried beans and peas, raw root vegetables (carrots, jicama, radishes, and turnip roots), dried pumpkin and sunflower seeds, whole-grain breads, oranges, apricots, prunes, and unpeeled apples are especially good sources of soluble fiber.

O Avoid sugar.

O Drink 8 or more glasses of water every day.

O Avoid large, heavy meals. Eating smaller portions more often reduces the size of bowel movements.

O Avoid milk, wheat products, and beef.

NUTRITIONAL SUPPLEMENTS

O Fiber: 1–2 tablespoons of insoluble (psyllium) or soluble (orange pulp) fiber taken with a glass of water daily. Do not take fiber at the same time you take nutritional supplements or medications.

O Vitamin C: at least 1,000 milligrams daily. Do not take more than 3,000 milligrams a day unless you are carefully following other treatment suggestions.

HERBS

O Dioscorea (wild yam): 400 milligrams in capsule form daily.

O Slippery elm bark: 1 teaspoon in 1 cup of water as often as desired.

O Witch hazel creams (such as Venetone): apply to the anus 1–2 times daily.

O Extracts of horse chestnut and red oak and essential oils of cypress and/or frankincense are also soothing.

See Part Three if you take prescription medication.

UNDERSTANDING THE HEALING PROCESS

Anal fissures begin with trauma to the anal canal during defecation. They persist because of a cycle of pain due to hard stools and reflex spasms by which the body attempts to stop pain by stopping defecation. Hemorrhoid treatments such as calendula, citrus bioflavonoids, *Collinsonia* root (stone root), diosmin, hesperidin, mesoglycans, oxerutins, and Preparation H (made from shark oil) are not especially helpful in treating anal fissures. Healing begins when the cycle of pain and retention is broken by a high-fiber diet to soften stools with warm sitz baths to relieve pain.[9]

As its name suggests, a sitz bath is a warm bath in which the patient sits, immersing the buttocks in warm water for up to 20 minutes at a time. Several herbs can be added to the bathwater for added relief of anal fissures. Burnet, horsetail, and oak bark are anti-inflammatory. A dropper of valerian tincture is widely reported to relieve spasms. Essential oils of calendula, chamomile, or yarrow may be added to the bath to relieve inflammation.

A study published in *The New England Journal of Medicine* found that 40 out of 44, or over 90 percent of children aged 11 months to 6 years who had allergies to cow's milk also had anal fissures. Anal fissures and constipation resolved when cow's milk was replaced with soy milk for a period of 15 days. Replacing cow's milk with soy milk also lowered the frequencies of bronchitis, hay fever, and skin allergies.[10]

There is no specific scientific confirmation that raw

Answers to Questions You May Be Hesitant to Ask Your Doctor

Anal fissures are not a medical emergency, and medical exams to rule out more serious conditions should be conducted in a doctor's office rather than an emergency room when the amount of bleeding is small. The procedure used to examine the anal canal may be classified as surgery if it is performed in an emergency room, even though no incisions are involved. This greatly increases its cost.

Anal fissures are frequently confused with hemorrhoids. Since anal fissures do not involve blood vessels, treatments for hemorrhoids that involve strengthening blood vessels will not help. A simple medical exam can give you the correct diagnosis.

This procedure involves anoscopy, a visual inspection of the anal canal. First the doctor inserts a lubricated, gloved finger into the rectum to determine if anything will block the insertion of the scope. Then the doctor inserts a lubricated plastic anoscope a few inches into the rectum. The anoscope enlarges the rectum so that the doctor can view the entire canal using a light. As the doctor withdraws the scope, the lining of the canal can be carefully examined.

It is helpful to clear the rectum of stool before visiting the doctor's office. In adults, a laxative or enema is helpful. Parents of small children need to know that their children may have to be restrained during the examination, and parents of older children need to ensure that the door to the exam room is not inadvertently opened. It is comforting to explain to children that the exam may feel like passing a bowel movement. It usually does not hurt.

Steroid suppositories are frequently prescribed for treating anal fissures. Consisting of a small amount of cortisone in a soluble base, these suppositories are inexpensive, relatively easy to apply, and accelerate the healing process. The amount of steroid absorbed into the bloodstream is so small that is not likely to have any side effects. Together with dietary changes and simple herbal treatment, steroid suppositories will resolve some cases of anal fissures in a few weeks.

Chronic anal fissures are, unfortunately, more difficult to treat. Many people consent to surgery for anal fissures with the misunderstanding that the doctor will "stitch up" the fissure. This is not usually the case. Surgery for fissures cuts the muscle around the anal sphincter, allowing it to relax and heal. This procedure is known as posterior *sphincterotomy*.

In a study at Mount Sinai Medical Center in New York City, about 5 percent of posterior sphincterotomy patients experienced complications. These included retained urine, bleeding, formation of fistulas, flatulence, incontinence, and itching and burning.[2] The latest research shows that both posterior sphincterotomy and its nonsurgical alternative, "the anal stretch" (placing a metal bar up through the anus to stretch the rectum) are less effective than a simpler procedure, lateral internal sphincterotomy.[3]

An even better approach may be simply removing and stitching up the fissure, a procedure called *fissurectomy*. German surgeons have found than only 3 percent of patients have any postoperative complications after fissurectomy and none of 534 patients treated in this way had permanent complications.[4] Since surgery for anal fissures is never an emergency, be sure your surgeon explains the procedure and its alternatives to you before you have an operation.

Another way of immobilizing the sphincter muscle is injection with botulinum toxin (Botox). When this method was first introduced, it caused fecal incontinence in approximately 2 percent of cases, and the condition can be permanent.[5] More recent studies have found that proper placement of the injection into the anus can greatly reduce the occurrence of complications.[6] Another way of treating anal fissures is with various topical nitrate compounds or nitroglycerin. These act in the same way as nitroglycerin pills for heart pain or Viagra for erectile dysfunction, enlarging blood vessels and increasing circulation. Various studies find that nitrates cause headache in 20 to 100 percent of cases,[7] but the headache can be relieved by sucking on a menthol cough drop or drinking strong peppermint tea.[8]

cabbage juice can heal anal fissures, although it is helpful in healing lesions of the mucosal lining in other parts of the digestive tract. It is possible that cabbage juice provides a bioavailable form of glutamine that the body uses to make a hexosamine moiety or "glue" that provides the "stickiness" of mucosal proteins.[11] These proteins protect the lining of the anus and help it heal.

Vitamin C accelerates the healing process and is probably important in preventing the formation of fistulas.[12] Since large doses of vitamin C can cause loose bowels, it is important to use only 1,000 milligrams a day during the first few weeks of the healing process. Very few people experience any side effects with this dosage, and those who do are only likely to have diarrhea or abdominal swelling for a few days after beginning the vitamin.

Studies with laboratory animals indicate that dioscorea (wild yam) stimulates the secretion of cholesterol into the bile. The cholesterol-laden bile enters the intestine and lubricates the stool.[13] Other animal studies have shown that dioscorea reduces intestinal inflammation, especially inflammation associated with the use of NSAID pain relievers such as ibuprofen and indomethacin.[14] These studies confirm the experience of natural healers who have used wild yam for thousands of years to treat various kinds of inflammation, especially in women.

Since dioscorea acts by altering the production of estrogen, it should be used with caution by women who take estrogen replacement therapy. Tinctures are easier to use but do not give the same degree of pain relief as capsules or teas.

Slippery elm bark contains an abundance of complex carbohydrates. Taken by mouth, this herb triggers a reflex causing the stomach to produce large quantities of mucus to coat and protect the entire digestive tract[15]. Since slippery elm bark is a food as well as an herb, it is completely nontoxic.

CONCEPTS FOR COPING WITH ANAL FISSURES

○ Rest assured that bright red bleeding is almost never a sign of cancer. Extensive medical examination when blood on toilet tissue is the major symptom seldom reveals occult colon polyps.[16]

○ Be sure to treat constipation (see CONSTIPATION) or pinworms (see PARASITES, INTESTINAL).

○ Avoid excessive cleansing, which may cause anal itch. Scrubbing is not necessary. After a bowel movement, wash with a washcloth and warm water or any kind of wipes that do not contain alcohol.

○ Use only white toilet tissue. Colored dyes in toilet tissue can exacerbate anal itch.

○ Homeopathic physicians sometimes recommend Schuessler cell salts for anal fissures. The treatment is typically Bioplasma, a mixture of all twelve cell salts, or calcarea fluorica, also recommended for hemorrhoids. Homeopaths sometimes employ magnesia phosphoric (for anal spasms), natrum phosphoricum (for inflammation), or silicea (silica) (to strengthen the lining of the rectum). Scientific testing of these remedies is only in a planning stage, but thousands of users report that they help. Schuessler cell salts do not pose any potential side effects.

For infants:

○ Change diapers frequently.

○ Wipe baby's bottom with a moist cloth or cotton ball.

○ Treat contributing conditions such as pinworms.

For adults:

○ Sit down less.

○ After bowel movement, wipe gently with soft tissues.

○ Apply petroleum jelly to the first half inch to inch of the mucosal lining of the anus after voiding and cleaning.

○ Especially if you smoke, avoid aspirin and other NSAIDs, such as ibuprofen and Tylenol.

Anal Itch

SYMPTOM SUMMARY

○ Itching around the anus, worsens at night

UNDERSTANDING THE DISEASE PROCESS

Anal itch, known in medical literature as *pruitis ani*, is among the most common gastrointestinal complaints. Rectal mucus containing allergens or other irritants contacts the skin around the anus and causes very mild inflammation. This irritation is experienced as itching.

Anal itch is almost never caused by failure to keep the area clean enough. It is more likely to be caused by excessive cleaning that removes protective oils from the skin.

Most of the time, anal itch is perpetuated by efforts to relieve it. Scratching aggravates the problem by causing very fine abrasions through which these irritants can enter the skin. Washing the skin with soap, especially with soaps containing deodorants or perfumes, also makes the itch worse.[1]

Itching around the anus is usually not a serious medical problem, but it can be an early symptom of two uncommon conditions, Bowen's disease and Paget's disease. In Bowen's disease, a condition related to basal cell carcinoma, anal itch would be accompanied by occasional bleeding of the skin itself and the development of small skin growths. Bowen's disease usually does not become an invasive cancer. In the more serious bone condition Paget's disease, anal itch would likely be accompanied by pain in the lower back or face and/or hearing changes. Anal itch may also accompany yeast infections.

TREATMENT SUMMARY

DIET

❍ Eliminate food allergies.

HERBS

❍ Dioscorea (wild yam): 400 milligrams in capsule form daily.

❍ Slippery elm bark: 1 teaspoon in 1 cup of water as often as desired.

❍ Witch hazel (hamamelis) ointment: apply sparingly 2–3 times a day.

See Part Three if you take prescription medication.

UNDERSTANDING THE HEALING PROCESS

The most important thing to remember about the process of healing anal itch is not to scratch. Apply a moistened, alcohol-free tissue or a warm, moist washcloth to the affected area if immediate relief is required. Over the longer term, identifying food allergies and eliminating the offending food from the diet heals most cases of anal itch. Frequently offending foods include citrus, coffee, milk, and peanuts.

Studies with laboratory animals indicate that dioscorea (wild yam) stimulates the secretion of cholesterol into the bile.[2] The cholesterol-laden bile enters the intestine and traps some of the allergens from digested food.

Since dioscorea increases the production of estrogen, it should be used with caution by women who take estrogen replacement therapy. Tinctures are easier to use but do not give the same degree of relief of inflammation as capsules or teas.

Slippery elm bark contains an abundance of complex carbohydrates. Taken by mouth, this herb triggers a reflex causing the stomach to produce large quantities of mucus to coat and protect the entire digestive tract.[3] This dilutes the mucus reaching the skin around the anus and reduces irritation. Since slippery elm bark is a food as well as an herb, it is completely nontoxic.

Witch hazel is an astringent used to treat weeping or sweaty skin that aggravates anal itch. In North America, it is used in several over-the-counter preparations for hemorrhoids, including Tucks medicated wipes.

CONCEPTS FOR COPING WITH ANAL ITCH

❍ After a bowel movement, wipe gently with soft tissues.

❍ Avoid excessive cleansing. Do not use soap of any kind on the anal area. Scrubbing is not necessary. Cold water is more likely to be soothing than warm water.

❍ If you are very sore, using a hairdryer on a low setting is the most comfortable way of drying the perianal area.

❍ After a bowel movement, wash with a washcloth and warm water or any kind of wipes that do not contain alcohol. Blot the area clean; don't rub the area clean.

❍ Use medicated lotions sparingly. Apply them with a fingertip rather than with a cotton swab.

❍ Keep the skin around the anus clean with corn starch powder. Women should not use talcum powder, since it can cause ovarian inflammation.

❍ Relieve irritation with a sitz bath, immersing the buttocks in warm water for up to 20 minutes at a time. Do not add antiseptics, bath salts, bath oils, bubble bath, essential oils, or herbs. Be especially careful to avoid chamomile baths. Despite the fact that chamomile is sometimes recommended as a treatment for anal itch, allergies to chamomile are not an uncommon cause of anal itch.[4]

❍ If you have irresistible urges to scratch, try distraction.

Suck ice chips. Sit on a tennis ball. Rock back and forth. Lie on your side, try to relax, and then change sides.

○ Use only white toilet tissue. Colored dyes in toilet tissue can exacerbate the condition.

○ Make sure all traces of detergent are rinsed out when you launder underwear.

○ A high-fiber diet makes stools softer, easier to pass, and less likely to leak out and cause perianal irritation.

○ Homeopathic physicians treat anal itch that is worse at night or that seems to be caused by food allergies with antimonium (6C strength). Severe itching and a crawling sensation around the anus are usually treated with ignatia (6C), and itchiness due to pinworms or that is worse after a bowel movement is treated with teucrium (6C). There have been no scientific tests to confirm the usefulness of homeopathic treatment of anal itch, but the method has been used for nearly 300 years. There are no likely side effects from using homeopathic preparations.

Anaphylaxis, Preventing Recurrences of

SYMPTOM SUMMARY

○ Difficulty breathing

○ Swelling in the throat

○ Anxiety

○ Blueness of the skin, nails, or lips

○ Cough

○ Diarrhea, nausea, and/or vomiting

○ Flared nostrils

○ Hives

○ Nasal congestion

○ Reddened skin

○ Sensation of heartbeat

○ Slurred speech

○ Tightness at the sides of the chest as breathing becomes difficult

○ Wheezing

UNDERSTANDING THE DISEASE PROCESS

Anaphylaxis is a severe and sudden allergic reaction that can cause death within minutes. Any occurrence of anaphylaxis is a medical emergency for which you should not attempt self-care, other than the use of an EpiPen and calling for an ambulance. There are steps you can take, however, to reduce the risk and severity of future attacks.

TREATMENT SUMMARY

NUTRITIONAL SUPPLEMENTS

Nutritional supplements are used to lower the risk of anaphylaxis, not to treat anaphylaxis.

○ Glycyrrhizin: 250–500 milligrams daily for up to 6 weeks at a time.

○ Green tea catechins: 250–500 milligrams daily.

○ Vitamin C: 2,000 milligrams per day.

See Part Three if you take prescription medication.

UNDERSTANDING THE HEALING PROCESS

Once you have had an anaphylactic reaction, your doctor will typically give you a prescription for an EpiPen so you or an informed bystander can give you a shot of adrenaline at the first signs of anaphylaxis. If your allergies are uncontrolled, your doctor may also recommend that you take antihistamines and low doses of steroid drugs prophylactically to prevent another attack. There are no natural treatments that offer you the same level of protection against anaphylaxis as these standard medical measures until your allergies are controlled (see ALLERGIES). There are several natural treatments that offer you some protection against severe allergic reactions and help your medications work better.

Glycyrrhizin is a licorice extract. It increases the half-life of cortisol and other steroids, making it more likely that you will have adequate levels of the steroid in your system to fend off an anaphylactic reaction the next time you encounter the allergen.[1] In the People's Republic of China, glycyrrhizin is given instead of adrenaline to treat anaphylaxis.

The drawback of using glycyrrhizin for this purpose is that it *will* increase any side effects you experience from cortisone. When you take both glycyrrhizin and any corticosteroid drug, you are more likely to experience weight gain, puffiness, and elevated blood pressure.

(Glycyrrhizin does not affect your body's responses to the other commonly prescribed preventative agent, diphenhidramine, better known as Benadryl.) Do not take glycyrrhizin for more than 6 weeks at a time. Preferably, use it during your peak allergy season. Do not take glycyrrhizin if you have high blood pressure.

A safer but less researched complement in allergy care is green tea. Catechins from green tea (and, to a lesser extent, from the black tea more commonly drunk in English-speaking countries) have been shown in laboratory tests with animals to significantly reduce the risk of allergic anaphylaxis.[2] The protective effect of the catechins is enhanced by caffeine. This stimulant stops the breakdown of norepinephrine, a hormone in the same class as the epinephrine in EpiPens.

Green tea catechin tablets do not contain caffeine. They are safe to use if you have high blood pressure. They work better if you also consume caffeine, but you should not take caffeine if you have high blood pressure.

Many, but not all, of the destructive physiological reactions in anaphylaxis are mediated by histamine. Vitamin C is a natural antihistamine. Vitamin C prevents the secretion of histamine by mast cells and accelerates its degradation.[3] Laboratory experiments have found exponential increases in the release of histamine when vitamin C is deficient.[4] Research with animals indicates that taking relatively large doses of vitamin C offers protection against anaphylaxis without interfering with the production of infection-fighting antibodies.[5]

CONCEPTS FOR COPING WITH THE RISK OF ANAPHYLAXIS

❍ Your first line of protection against an anaphylactic allergic reaction to food is to avoid eating the food. But if you accidentally eat a food that causes severe allergies, you are less likely to have an anaphylactic reaction if the food is more completely digested in the stomach. Avoid antacids, but don't avoid bitter foods. The sensation of bitter taste triggers a reflex reaction increasing the production of acid in the stomach and enhances digestion, especially when the meal includes fatty foods.

❍ Nuts and seeds are common but overlooked potential triggers for anaphylactic reactions. Both sesame seeds[6] and hazelnuts[7] cause severe problems among children in locations where they are common foods.

❍ Especially in children and adolescents, exercise can induce anaphylaxis. Exercise also can increase a young person's sensitivity to certain foods.[8] For this reason, it is important to be especially vigilant to avoid allergy-provoking foods on days when the child is engaged in vigorous physical activity.

❍ Insect stings are another frequent cause of anaphylactic reactions. To avoid getting stung, stay away from areas with bees, use fragrance-free toiletries, do not wear dark or floral clothing, wear closed-toe shoes, and avoid eating outdoors in picnic areas or near garbage cans where containers for sugary drinks are thrown away.

❍ Desensitization shots (venom therapy) are strongly recommended for anyone who has ever had a whole-body reaction to a bee or wasp sting. Not everyone is protected against full-body reactions once they have reached the maintenance dose; some people will require larger than normal doses of venom therapy before they are fully protected against stings.[9] Don't be careless around bees and wasps just because you have had the shots.

Anemia, Iron-Deficiency

SYMPTOM SUMMARY

❍ Fatigue, followed by

- Headaches
- Irritability
- Lightheadedness
- Pale skin
- Restless legs syndrome
- Ringing in the ears
- Shortness of breath after exercise

In rare cases:

❍ Pica (desire to eat ice, clay, cardboard, dirt, or starch)

UNDERSTANDING THE DISEASE PROCESS

Anemia is a shortage of red blood cells, an unusually low concentration of oxygen-carrying hemoglobin in the blood, or a low value of a laboratory index called the hematocrit, which measures the volume of red blood cells in a sample of blood after they have been placed in a centrifuge. These three values are measured with a "complete blood count," more commonly referred to as a CBC. There are several deficiency diseases that cause anemia, but iron-deficiency anemia is easily identified by the fact that it causes red blood cells to appear pale and small when examined under a microscopic.

The Crohn's and Colitis Foundation of America estimates that between 30 and 70 percent of people who have inflammatory bowel disease will develop iron-deficiency anemia. The condition is also a common complication of bleeding ulcers, heavy periods, hemorrhoids, peptic ulcer disease, too-frequent donations of blood, and daily use of aspirin. It can also result from inadequate nutrition. Iron-deficiency anemia in men in North America, Australia, New Zealand, and Europe is almost always caused by blood loss.

Iron-deficiency anemia develops in three stages. The first is negative iron balance. In this stage, the body's demands for iron exceed its ability to absorb it from food. Negative iron balance can result from blood loss, pregnancy (in which the demands for red blood cell production by the fetus outpace the mother's ability to provide iron), growth spurts during adolescence, or inadequate iron in the diet. During the depletion of iron, there may be a general feeling of fatigue, but a blood test will not show iron deficiency.

The second step in the development of iron-deficiency anemia is iron-deficient erythropoiesis, or the production of red blood cells without sufficient iron. Red blood cells produced during iron-deficient erythropoiesis tend to be small and pale. They fail to carry adequate amounts of hemoglobin. This sets off changes in the bone marrow to cause the third stage of iron-deficiency anemia, hypoproliferation. When hemoglobin levels fall too low, the marrow begins to produce cigar- or pencil-shaped poikilocytes instead of round, full erythrocytes.

Very advanced iron-deficiency anemia causes easily recognized cracks and fissures at the corners of the mouth and spooning of the fingernails. Most of the time, however, this condition can only be diagnosed with a blood test. Measurement of ferritin levels is essential to determine that iron deficiency, rather than some other problem, is the cause of the anemia.

TREATMENT SUMMARY

DIET

○ If you are not a vegetarian, eat 3–4 servings of lean meat, poultry, or fish daily. If you are vegetarian, eat dried fruit, leafy green vegetables, and molasses as often as possible.

○ Cook in iron pots and pans. Use vinegar and juices in cooking as much as possible.

NUTRITIONAL SUPPLEMENTS

In addition to medically prescribed iron supplements:

○ Vitamin A: 5,000 IU per day for women of reproductive age; 10,000 IU per day for all others.

○ Vitamin C: 500 milligrams, every time you take an iron supplement.

See Part Three if you take prescription medication.

Form of Iron	Amount of Iron Supplement Needed to Provide 30 milligrams of Elemental Iron (Usual Dose for Women)	Amount of Iron Supplement Needed to Provide 60 milligrams of Elemental Iron (Usual Dose for Men)
Ferrous fumarate (Femiron, Feostat, Fumerin, Hemocyte, Ircon)	183 milligrams (Two 100-milligram chewable tablets or one 200-milligram coated tablet)	366 milligrams (Four 100-milligram chewable tablets or two 200-milligram coated tablets)
Ferrous gluconate (Fergon, Ferralet, Simron)	518 milligrams (Two tablets, coated or regular)	1,036 milligrams (Four tablets, coated or regular)
Ferrous sulfate (Feosol, Fer-In-Sol, Mol-Iron, Slow Fe)	186 milligrams (One extended-release tablet every day or one enteric-coated tablet every other day)	372 milligrams (Two extended-release tablets every day or one enteric-coated tablet every day)
Polysaccharide-iron complex (Niferex, Nu-Iron)	300 milligrams (Two capsules every day, or alternate taking one enteric-coated tablet one day and two enteric-coated tablets the next day)	600 milligrams (Four capsules or three enteric-coated capsules every day)

FORMS AND DOSAGES OF SUPPLEMENTAL IRON

UNDERSTANDING THE HEALING PROCESS

Iron-deficiency anemia is a condition you cannot diagnose for yourself. If you have iron-deficiency anemia, your physician will usually prescribe an iron supplement. If your doctor does not have a specific recommendation, you can find an appropriate form and dosage in the table below.

About 1 in 5 people who takes iron supplements will experience constipation, diarrhea, nausea, and/or vomiting. Iron injections are available if the gastrointestinal side effects of iron capsules and tablets are too uncomfortable for you.

At least 11 clinical studies have found that taking vitamin A enhances your body's ability to absorb iron supplements.[1] Vitamin C does not increase iron absorption, but taking vitamin C and iron together results in an increase in levels of ferritin, the iron-binding protein, in the blood. The dosages recommended here are not likely to cause side effects or to interfere with medications.[2]

CONCEPTS FOR COPING WITH IRON-DEFICIENCY ANEMIA

O Iron-deficiency anemia is most likely to strike children around their first birthdays.[3] Babies who are iron-deficient tend to lag behind in development throughout childhood and may be linked to later development of attention deficit disorder, so early recognition of the problem is essential. Symptoms of iron deficiency in infants include lethargy, irritability, swollen tongue, brittle nails, and sores at the corners of the mouth. Breastfeeding provides enough iron for a baby, but cow's milk does not. Iron-fortified formula or iron-rich foods are necessary if a baby is not breastfed.

O The most easily absorbed form of iron in food is heme-iron, particularly abundant in liver but also found in red meat, poultry, and fish. Your body can absorb the iron in liver nearly as well as it can absorb the iron in a supplement tablet. In contrast, your body can only absorb about 5 percent as much iron from the best plant sources of the mineral, dark leafy greens, dried fruits, and molasses. High-fiber plant foods contain phytate, which reduces iron absorption even more. Any food to which *iodized* salt is added loses available iron.[4]

O Cook in iron pots and pans. Some iron leaches out of the cooking ware into the food. More iron leaches out if food is cooked in an acid liquid containing lemon juice, wine, or vinegar. If you cook with iron utensils, be sure not to serve the food on unglazed dinnerware. The acid media that extract iron from cooking ware also extract lead from improperly fired pottery.

O Coffee interferes with the absorption of iron,[5] but your overall absorption of iron is not affected by drinking up to 4 cups a day if you also take vitamin C.[6] Black tea, on the other hand, reduces iron absorption whether or not you take vitamin C.[7]

O Fiber reduces absorption of iron. Never take iron supplements with a meal including high-fiber foods.

Anemia, Pernicious and Megaloblastic

SYMPTOM SUMMARY

O Abdominal pain

O Burning of the tongue

O Fatigue

O Loss of appetite

O Menstrual irregularities

O Numbness and tingling in the hands and feet

O Occasional constipation and diarrhea

O Weight loss

UNDERSTANDING THE DISEASE PROCESS

Pernicious anemia is a particularly destructive form of vitamin B_{12} deficiency that causes blood cells to be broken down faster than they can be replaced. This form of anemia is called "pernicious" because it develops slowly over a period of at least 3–6 years and the damage it causes is well advanced before symptoms occur.

True pernicious anemia is most common in people who have some other disease that causes the immune system to attack healthy tissues: Addison's disease, Graves' disease, hypoparathyroidism, myxedema, or vitiligo. In pernicious anemia, the immune system generates cytotoxic T cells that attack the parietal glands in the lining of the stomach. This prevents the parietal glands from producing intrinsic factor to liberate vitamin

B_{12} from food. In the absence of adequate vitamin B_{12}, the bone marrow cannot convert homocysteine to methionine. In turn it cannot use folic acid to make the building blocks of red blood cell DNA. Up to 90 percent of the materials that otherwise would be used to make red blood cells are destroyed before they can enter the bloodstream. The few red blood cells that are formed are extremely large megaloblasts, taking up materials that should go into the manufacturing of platelets and white blood cells. Low counts of platelets and white blood cells can also result. In addition to the symptoms listed above, pernicious anemia often causes mood swings and depression before other symptoms are obvious.[1]

Several other conditions deplete vitamin B_{12} and cause similar symptoms. For example, anemia is a frequent complication of chemotherapy. While the treatment of anemia due to these causes is the same as that for pernicious anemia, the condition is usually referred to as megaloblastic anemia, after the extremely large megaloblasts (red blood cells) the bone marrow produces. The good news about both pernicious and megaloblastic anemia is that once vitamin deficiency is remedied, there is usually lifetime remission.[2]

TREATMENT SUMMARY

NUTRITIONAL SUPPLEMENTS

In addition to medically prescribed vitamin B_{12}:

O Glycyrrhizin: 250–500 milligrams daily for up to 6 weeks at a time.

Use with caution:

O Folic acid: dosage varies; see text below.

See Part Three if you take prescription medication.

UNDERSTANDING THE HEALING PROCESS

If you have pernicious anemia, your treatment should begin with an injection of vitamin B_{12} by a healthcare professional. Once your symptoms begin to improve, you only need to take 1,000–2,000 micrograms (1 or 2 milligrams) of vitamin B_{12} a day to prevent recurrences of deficiency. Even if your body can no longer produce intrinsic factor, the 1–2 percent of the B_{12} supplement actually absorbed is enough to prevent future problems. Lifetime injections are not necessary.[3]

If you are taking injections of steroids to improve digestive function, a licorice derivative called glycyrrhizin

can help make them more effective. It increases the half-life of cortisol and other steroids, making them work longer to undo the damage done to the parietal glands of your stomach that caused pernicious anemia.[4] The downside of using glycyrrhizin for this purpose is that it *will* increase any side effects you experience from cortisone. When you take both glycyrrhizin and any corticosteroid drug, you are more likely to experience weight gain, puffiness, and elevated blood pressure. Do not take glycyrrhizin for more than 6 weeks at a time. Preferably, use it during your peak allergy season. Do not take glycyrrhizin if you have high blood pressure. Deglycyrrhizinated licorice (DGL) is another licorice derivative that does not aggravate side effects of steroid treatment, but it will not help pernicious anemia.

Once your symptoms have improved, it is possible to develop a new vitamin B_{12} deficiency that will not be as evident if you take more than 800 micrograms of folic acid daily. Folic acid supplementation can mask many of the symptoms of B_{12} deficiency long enough that permanent nerve damage can result. Never take 800 micrograms of folic acid on a daily basis except under the supervision of a qualified healthcare practitioner.

CONCEPTS FOR COPING WITH PERNICIOUS AND MEGALOBLASTIC ANEMIA

O People who adopt a vegan diet sometimes develop megaloblastic anemia after a period of 3–6 years, as their body's stores of vitamin B_{12} are slowly depleted. Megaloblastic anemia is very rare among vegans who eat strictly "organic" produce, because it contains microscopic animal life that is an adequate source of vitamin B_{12}. Non-animal sources of the vitamin popular with vegans include tempeh and seaweed. These foods contain highly variable amounts of B_{12}. Spirulina and nori contain both vitamin B_{12} and an anti-folate that can interfere with the use of B_{12} once it is absorbed. They are not an adequate source of vitamin B_{12} for children on a vegan diet.[5] Rather than relying on tempeh, seaweed, and spirulina, it is better to take 10–20 micrograms of B_{12} daily to prevent the possibility of megaloblastic anemia.

O Artichokes, asparagus, bananas, garlic, leeks, and onions contain inulins (not to be confused with insulins), complex sugars that feed symbiotic bacteria in the intestine that make vitamin B_{12}. Eating these foods can slightly increase your supply of the vitamin.

○ Some older people develop megaloblastic anemia because their stomachs no longer produce enough acid to digest food. In the absence of gastritis, chronic heartburn, or peptic ulcer disease, they can benefit from taking 600–650 milligrams of betaine HCl (a pill containing stomach acids) just before meals.

○ The common diabetes medication metformin (Glucophage) can cause vitamin B_{12} deficiency. To prevent vitamin deficiency, take 150–250 milligrams of calcium citrate when you take your diabetes medication.

○ Everyday use of medications for gastritis and heartburn can interfere with the absorption of vitamin B_{12} from food. They do not interfere with the absorption of vitamin B_{12} from supplement tablets.

Aneurysm

SYMPTOM SUMMARY

○ Swelling with pulsation at the site of the aneurysm matching the heartbeat (does not always occur). *Call for an ambulance if you observe this symptom.*

○ If the aneurysm ruptures:
- Rapid pulse
- Dizziness
- Extreme pain

UNDERSTANDING THE DISEASE PROCESS

An aneurysm is a ballooning or "blow-out" of an artery due to weakening of the blood vessel wall. Aneurysms may be caused by a birth defect or genetic disorder, but they are more commonly a complication of atherosclerosis. The most common aneurysm is abdominal aortic aneurysm (AAA), which occurs in the large artery that carries blood from the heart to the abdomen and legs. The risk of AAA is much higher in men, and increases with age. Any aneurysm is a potentially life-threatening condition that requires medical care.

TREATMENT SUMMARY

NUTRITIONAL SUPPLEMENTS

As a preventive measure:

○ Copper: no more than 1 milligram daily.

○ Any antioxidant formula containing beta-carotene and vitamins C and E among other antioxidants, as directed on the label.

See Part Three if you take prescription medication.

UNDERSTANDING THE HEALING PROCESS

Once an aneurysm has occurred, it must be surgically corrected. Two nutritional measures, however, may lower the risk of aneurysm and may enhance survivability if an aneurysm does occur.

Studies with animals have confirmed that copper is important for maintaining the flexibility of the heart muscle. At least in animals, adequate levels of copper in heart tissue help the muscle "spring back" from the severe pressure changes caused by an aneurysm.[1] No study has proven that copper supplementation has a similar effect in humans, but avoiding copper deficiency is a conservative measure. It is important to avoid overdosing, since copper as well as zinc, magnesium, and calcium accumulate in the cholesterol plaques that cause aneurysm.[2]

The Finnish Alpha-Tocopherol, Beta-Carotene Cancer Prevention (ATBC) Study involving 29,133 men found that daily supplementation with modest amounts of beta-carotene and vitamin E probably lowers the risk of aneurysm in men, but the data do not allow for statistical certainty.[3] Some analysts believe that the best results are likely to be obtained from supplementing with a balanced blend of antioxidants, that is, alpha-carotene as well as beta-carotene, gamma-tocopherol as well as alpha-tocopherol, and alpha-lipoic acid as well as vitamin C. High doses are not as important as a balanced blend.

Taking antioxidants may be more relevant to *recovery* from aneurysm. A recent Dutch study found that giving aneurysm patients vitamins C and E (and mannitol, which is used only in surgery) before operating to repair the aneurysm reduced inflammation and boosted white blood cell counts.[4]

CONCEPTS FOR COPING WITH ANEURYSM

○ See also ATHEROSCLEROSIS.

Angina

SYMPTOM SUMMARY

○ Chest pain or pressure:

- Under or slightly to the left of the breastbone

- May radiate to shoulder, arm, jaw, neck, back, or other areas

- Tightness, crushing, squeezing, choking, or aching

- Sometimes mistaken for gas or indigestion

- Usually not sharply localized

- Precipitated by physical activity, heavy meals, or emotional stress

- Relieved by rest or nitroglycerin

- Short duration, 1–15 minutes

UNDERSTANDING THE DISEASE PROCESS

Angina is a muscle cramp in the heart. About 10 percent of cases of angina involve Prinzmetal's variant angina, a condition in which the same physiological changes that trigger the cerebral artery spasms that cause migraine headaches trigger coronary artery spasms that cause angina. The overwhelming majority of cases of angina, however, result from coronary artery disease (CAD).

In CAD, cholesterol plaques narrow arteries so that they cannot transport as much oxygenated blood. During exercise, emotional excitement, or after a heavy meal, the heart pumps faster and harder. Narrowed arteries cannot bring the heart the oxygen it needs, and there is an angina attack. Sweating, shortness of breath, and intense chest pain, usually radiating into the left arm or neck, are the hallmarks of an angina attack.

The most common form of angina is called "stable" angina. In stable angina, repeated attacks occur after similar events, such as overexertion, overeating, or stress. In this form of angina, attacks gradually get worse over time. The more serious "unstable" angina may appear suddenly or occur frequently or without apparent cause. Unstable angina is far more likely to lead to heart attack. A third kind of angina known as Prinzmetal's variant angina is essentially a migraine of the coronary artery. Nerve impulses cause the muscles lining the coronary arteries to tighten and shut off circulation to the heart. People who have Prinzmetal's variant angina typically have "clean" arteries but circulatory problems in microscopic blood vessels supplying the heart.

An angina attack is not a heart attack. Angina is a signal that some of the heart muscle is not getting enough oxygen temporarily. This pain does not mean that heart muscle is suffering permanent damage. In heart attack, blood flow to part of the heart is permanently cut off. The pain is more severe and, unlike angina, does not go away with rest. Also unlike angina, heart attack may be accompanied by indigestion, nausea, sweating, and general weakness. If you have angina, you should pay attention to the pattern of your attacks—what they feel like, what triggers them, and how long they last—so that you will know to seek emergency medical care should experience a different pattern of pain that could be caused by a heart attack.

TREATMENT SUMMARY

DIET

○ Different people need different diets. People with angina need to follow the diet that corrects their underlying condition: a low-fat, low-cholesterol diet for people with angina who have proven occlusion of the coronary arteries (see ATHEROSCLEROSIS); a hypoallergienic diet for Prinzmetal's angina (see MIGRAINE); or sugar-restricted diet for those with hypoglycemia (see HYPOGLYCEMIA). Angina sufferers who have had a heart attack should try a low-sodium diet (see CONGESTIVE HEART FAILURE).

NUTRITIONAL SUPPLEMENTS

○ Coenzyme Q_{10}: 150–300 milligrams daily.

○ L-carnitine: 500 milligrams 3 times a day.

Diabetics with angina can especially benefit from:

○ Pantethine: 300 milligrams 3 times a day.

People with Prinzmetal's variant angina can especially benefit from:

○ Magnesium aspartate or magnesium citrate: 200–400 milligrams 3 times a day.

HERBS

Anyone who has angina can benefit from taking:

○ Hawthorn in any one of the following forms, 3 times a day:

- Solid extract (standardized to contain 1.8 percent vitexin-4'-rhamnoside): 100–250 milligrams.
- Leaf and flowers as a tea: 1–2 teaspoons (3–5 grams).
- Fluid extract: 1–2 milliliters ($\frac{1}{2}$ to 1 teaspoon).

Angina sufferers whose EKG's show S-T depression (who do not have Prinzmetal's variant angina) also benefit from:

○ Arjuna (*Terminalia arjuna*): Extract, as directed by dispensing herbalist.

○ Pushkarmoola (*Inula racemosa*): Extract, as directed by dispensing herbalist.

See Part Three if you take prescription medication.

UNDERSTANDING THE HEALING PROCESS

Angina is a serious condition that requires conventional medical treatment. Eventually, however, it can be controlled with the help of natural products. The goals of the natural treatment of angina are assisting the flow of blood and providing energy to the heart.

Coenzyme Q_{10} (CoQ_{10}) is synthesized by every cell in the body to capture electrons released as the mitochondria, the energy-making centers of the cell, release energy by combining sugar with oxygen. A solid, wax-like substance, CoQ_{10} is made by the same chemical process that makes cholesterol, and, like cholesterol, CoQ_{10} is especially abundant in the healthy heart. Since the heart muscle makes and uses energy 24 hours a day, it needs a large quantity of CoQ_{10}. Heart tissue biopsies of people with various heart diseases show a 50–75 percent deficiency of CoQ_{10} compared to normal.[1]

As people age, the heart makes less CoQ_{10}. Certain cholesterol-lowering drugs also reduce the heart's supply of this vital enzyme. Replacing CoQ_{10} is important in treating angina.

In one study, 12 patients with angina were given 150 milligrams of CoQ_{10} daily for 4 weeks. Taking CoQ_{10} reduced the average frequency of angina attacks by 53 percent. CoQ_{10} treatment also allowed the angina patients to last longer on a treadmill before experiencing chest pain or abnormal EKGs.[2] A review of more than 100 research studies conducted between 1974 and 2000 finds consistent benefit from CoQ_{10} for angina sufferers.[3]

L-carnitine also increases the heart's energy supply. L-carnitine carries fatty acids into the mitochondria, where they can be used for fuel. Most of the body's supply of L-carnitine is made in the kidneys and the liver. Stresses on these organs (such as diabetes or chronic alcohol abuse) diminish the supply of L-carnitine for the heart. When the heart has an inadequate oxygen supply, it quickly uses up its supply of L-carnitine and is then less able to produce energy.

Administering massive doses of L-carnitine—2,000 milligrams of L-carnitine for every 100 pounds (45 kilograms) of body weight—after a heart attack has been shown to reduce heart damage.[4] A Japanese study found that taking 900 milligrams of L-carnitine daily allowed angina patients to last 2.4 minutes longer in their stress tests. An Italian study in which men with angina were given 1,000 milligrams of L-carnitine daily found they not only could last longer under stress, but they could also work harder, as measured by a bicycle ergometer.[5] Approximately 1 in 30 people will experience nausea, heartburn, or gas when taking L-carnitine, but it is generally very free of side effects. People with seizure disorders, however, should consult with their physicians before taking this supplement.

Pantethine is a vitamin B derivative that helps transport useful fatty acids into cells. It lowers total cholesterol, LDL, and triglycerides, and raises HDL without interfering with the production of L-carnitine. In one study involving diabetics, taking 600 milligrams of pantethine daily lowered triglyceride levels by 37 percent.[6] Generally, pantethine lowers total cholesterol by 15–25 percent and triglycerides by 25–40 percent. Taking much more than 600 milligrams per day can increase your susceptibility to sunburn, especially if you take the blood pressure medication lisinopril (Prinivil or Zestril).

Magnesium deficiency plays a major role in spasms of the coronary arteries, the source of chest pain in Prinzmetal's variant angina.[7] Magnesium also reduces peripheral vascular resistance, shunting blood from the hands and feet to the heart. Noted naturopathic physicians Michael Murray and Joseph Pizzorno recommend magnesium as treatment during a heart attack. They state that magnesium can:

○ "Improve energy production within the heart;

○ Dilate the coronary arteries resulting in improved delivery of oxygen to the heart;

○ Reduce peripheral vascular resistance resulting in reduced demand on the heart;

○ Inhibit platelets from aggregating and forming blood clots;

○ Reduce the size of the blockage; and

○ Improve heart rate and arrythmias."[8]

Magnesium is the primary element in milk of magnesia, and magnesium supplements can cause diarrhea. Usually the effect is short term and takes place during the first 2 or 3 days the supplement is taken.

Herbs used to treat angina open circulation. Hawthorn is both extraordinarily safe and extraordinarily effective in treating angina. This herb contains a variety of flavonoids. Some increase blood flow through the coronary arteries. Some increase left ventricular pressure, making each heartbeat stronger. Some accelerate the heart rate—and some decelerate it.[9] But the most important property of hawthorn is its ability to protect the heart from the effects of oxygen deprivation.

Heart cells, like many other tissues, are able to adapt to oxygen deprivation. They shift their energy production from pathways requiring the use of oxygen to pathways requiring the use of fatty acids. However, when their oxygen supply is restored, as it is when an angina attack ends, they are sometimes damaged and sometimes destroyed.

At the end of an angina attack, the neutrophils of the immune system release a compound known as human neutrophil elastase (HNE), allowing the arteries to stretch back to a more normal size. The process of relaxing the artery, however, releases massive quantities of free radicals that disrupt the cholesterol coats of heart cells and interfere with the action of L-carnitine. At least one of the flavonoid compounds in hawthorn counteracts HNE.[10]

Hawthorn has several other beneficial effects. Animal studies have found that hawthorn stimulates the liver to use LDL cholesterol to make bile salts, cholesterol salts that are flushed out of the liver and into the stool.[11] Other studies with laboratory animals have found that the hawthorn compound monoacetyl-vitexin rhamnoside relaxes the linings of the arteries, permitting greater blood flow, through a complicated chemical process.[12] And at least one animal study suggests that hawthorn can prevent irreversible tissue damage during heart attack.[13]

There are very few precautions for the use of hawthorn. It is almost completely nontoxic. Like many other natural treatments for angina, however, it can cause diarrhea during the first few days you take it.

Arjuna has been used in Ayurvedic medicine for over 2,500 years as a "cardiac tonic." Ayurvedic physicians offer it as arjunatvagadi (arjuna in water), pardhadyaristam (grapes and arjuna fermented and boiled), arjunaghrtam (arjuna paste), and arjunatvak (arjuna powder). Animal experiments have shown that arjuna slows and strengthens the heartbeat and protects the heart from tissue destruction during oxygen deprivation. In a study of the use of the herb in treating angina, patients given the herb were found to have greater endurance in treadmill tests, without the complication of lowered blood pressure. Over a period of 3 months, 66 percent of stable angina patients and 20 percent of unstable angina patients showed improved EKGs.[14]

Arjuna is usually dispensed by a practitioner of Ayurvedic medicine. There have been no reports of side effects from arjuna products given by herbalists or physicians trained in Ayurveda. Dosage varies with the individual preparation.

Pushkarmoola is another Ayurvedic herb that grows in the foothills of the northwestern Himalayas. Traditional South Asian medicine uses pushkarmoola in the treatment of angina with shortness of breath. A small-scale study in India found that pushkarmoola was more effective than nitroglycerin in effecting favorable EKG changes (elevation of the S-T segment) and in relieving chest pain.[15] And a study involving 200 patients found that combining pushkarmoola with the traditional Indian herb guggul (Commiphora mukkul) in treatment for 6 months relieved shortness of breath in 60 percent of angina patients who had shortness of breath as a symptom at the beginning of the study. One in four patients experienced a complete remission of pain and showed a normal EKG by the end of 6 months' treatment.[16]

Like arjuna, pushkarmoola is also available from practitioners of Ayurveda. There are no reports of side effects from pushkarmoola products given by herbalists or physicians trained in Ayurveda.

CONCEPTS FOR COPING WITH ANGINA

○ If your doctor has prescribed a nitroglycerin patch, you will benefit from taking 2,000–3,000 milligrams of L-arginine daily (preferably in 2 or 3 doses of 700–1,000 milligrams each). Clinical testing has found that the supplement prevents the development of nitrate tolerance, and ensures that the medication keeps working.[17]

○ Men who use nitroglycerin for angina must never take sildenafil (Viagra). The combination of blood vessel relaxants can be deadly.

○ While hawthorn and Ayurvedic herbs are the most useful herbs for treating angina, several others are generally useful for dealing with the causes of angina. However, they also interact with medications commonly prescribed for the condition.

• Bromelain is thought to break up cholesterol plaques in arteries. There is at least some laboratory evidence that bromelain can be absorbed into the linings of red blood cells and protect them from the action of immune cells associated with plaque formation,[18] although this is not a major force in the formation of plaques. There are relatively few potential risks in using bromelain, although it should be avoided by people taking warfarin (Coumadin) or clopidogrel (Plavix).

• Coleus contains compounds that alter cellular chemistry so that arterial muscles relax and platelets do not stick together. It should be avoided, however, by people on medication for high blood pressure, since the combination of coleus and medication can cause orthostatic hypotension (passing out when rising from a seated or supine position) or sensitivity to cold. A typical dose of coleus is 50 milligrams of capsules that contain 18 percent forskolin, 2 or 3 times a day.

• Garlic is scientifically documented to lower total cholesterol and triglycerides, increase HDL ("good") cholesterol, and prevent the formation of blood clots. In combination with prescription blood thinners—such as Coumadin (warfarin), heparin, Plavix (clopidogrel), Ticlid (ticlopidine), Trental (pentoxifylline)—or aspirin, garlic increases risk of bleeding. Always tell your doctor you are taking garlic if you are prescribed any blood-thinning medication. The standard daily dosage of garlic is any number of capsules that deliver 10 milligrams of allicin.

• Ginger lowers cholesterol and reduces the tendency of blood to clot. Like garlic, ginger should be used with caution by people who take Coumadin (warfarin), heparin, Plavix (clopidogrel), Ticlid (ticlopidine), Trental (pentoxifylline), or aspirin. A quarter-inch slice of ginger root or 250 milligrams of ginger extract in capsules is an appropriate daily dose.

• Khella (*Ammi visnaga*), another herb used in Ayurvedic medicine, relaxes and dilates coronary arteries. It improves exercise tolerance and stabilizes heart rhythm. Taken with the common prescription drug lisinopril (Prinivil or Zestril), however, khella greatly increases sensitivity to sunburn. Take capsules of 250–300 milligrams of the herb standardized to contain 12 percent khellin daily.

Angioedema
See **Hives**.

Animal Bites

SYMPTOM SUMMARY

○ Skin break with no bleeding

○ Puncture wound

○ Crushing injury

UNDERSTANDING THE DISEASE PROCESS

An animal bite is a wound to flesh caught between the teeth of the upper jaw and the teeth of the lower jaw of an animal. Pets are the source of most animal bites. According to a study sponsored by the Columbia University College of Physicians and Surgeons, dogs attack more than a million Americans annually, and over half of those incidents involve children.

TREATMENT SUMMARY

Nutritional supplements and herbs do not substitute for immediate wound care, described below.

NUTRITIONAL SUPPLEMENTS

○ Vitamin C: 1,000 milligrams daily.

HERBS

○ Aloe: apply to wounds daily until healed.

○ Forskolin (a standardized extract of coleus): 5–10 milligrams 3 times daily.

○ Gotu kola (*Centella asiatica*): 60–120 milligrams of asiaticides daily. Should not be used by women who are trying to become pregnant.

○ Sangre de grado: apply to the skin immediately after

injury to form a protective crust (sometimes called a "second skin") and prevent infection.

UNDERSTANDING THE HEALING PROCESS

When a familiar household pet that is in good health causes a superficial bite, it is usually enough to wash out the wound carefully with soap and water and apply an antiseptic such as hydrogen peroxide. When a strange animal causes a bite or the attack results in a puncture wound or a large gash, proper cleansing of the wound is critical. Depending on the location, severity, and type of the wound, stitches may be necessary. In either case, consult a physician promptly if there is subsequent drainage, swelling, or pain. Report any vicious animals who are allowed to roam freely to the animal warden or health department.

Vitamin C accelerates healing. The latest research on the use of vitamin C in the treatment of wounds has found that it keeps the basal layers of skin from contracting when the upper layers are injured. This allows regrowth of skin with a minimum of scarring.[1] A series of laboratory experiments found that supplementation with relatively high dosages of vitamin C increases the strength of skin growing over the wound and accelerates closure.[2]

Aloe is anti-inflammatory, moisturizing, and emollient. It contains a number of antioxidant compounds promoting skin growth, including vitamins C and E and zinc. Unlike hydrocortisone creams used to relieve inflammation, aloe encourages skin healing while relieving pain. Wounds treated with aloe vera gel heal as much as 3 days faster than wounds treated with unmedicated dressings or with chemical antiseptic gels.[3]

Forskolin stops a chemical signaling system by which inflammatory hormones shut down fibroblasts, the cells that generate the extracellular connective tissue matrix.[4] Keeping fibroblasts at the site of the wound encourages the production of collagen and connective tissues across the region of damaged skin.

Gotu kola helps to prevent scarring. Keloids and hypertrophic scars, such as those caused by surgery, result from an extended period of inflammation that may go on for months or years without resolution. During this inflammatory phase, large numbers of swollen bundles of collagen are intermingled with cellular debris. This stage continues until sufficient numbers of fibroblasts are recruited in the wound to create well-defined collagen fibers. A clinical study found that 22 out of 27 patients' scars resolved with several months use of gotu kola.[5] The unprocessed resin of sangre de grado stimulates the production of collagen in wounds. This accelerates the formation of a protective crust over the wound.[6]

CONCEPTS FOR COPING WITH ANIMAL BITES

○ If the person bitten has not had a tetanus shot in the past 5 years, consult a healthcare provider.

○ People who have diabetes or other conditions causing circulatory problems should consult a physician after any bite, even if it seems minor.

○ Unknown animals may carry rabies, especially bats, coyotes, foxes, ground hogs, raccoons, and skunks. Any wild animal or unfamiliar domestic animal that bites a human should be examined promptly by a knowledgeable veterinarian. If the animal cannot be found, immunization for rabies may be necessary.

○ Pet reptiles commonly bite. Some research suggests that the scent of fat (in the pet's food or after the owner has cooked with fat) increases the risk of a bite, especially by lizards.[7]

○ Clinical studies show that antibiotic treatment does not prevent infection, but the potential damage to hands and fingers is so great that preventive antibiotic treatment is usually a good idea.[8] If you take antibiotics, take 1 or 2 capsules of *acidophilus* or *Lactobacillus* daily. This helps maintain the production of vitamin K in the intestine.

Ankylosing Spondylitis
See **Bechterew's Disease**.

Anorexia

SYMPTOM SUMMARY
○ Weight loss of 25 percent or greater
○ Cavities
○ Constipation

- Depression
- Dry hair
- Frequent colds and infections
- Hair loss
- Loss of fatty tissue
- Low blood pressure
- Missed menstrual periods
- Sensitivity to cold
- Yellowed skin

UNDERSTANDING THE DISEASE PROCESS

Anorexia nervosa is an eating disorder involving compulsive dieting and exercise to lose weight. It leads to dangerous weight loss and osteoporosis at a very early age. It can delay sexual maturity in teenage girls and cause lower estrogen levels and menstrual irregularities in women. The overwhelming majority of anorexics are women aged 12–30. About 10 percent of teenagers with anorexia are males, however, as are about 25 percent of adult anorexics.[1]

Anorexia is often thought of as a psychological disorder somehow connected with the value Western culture places on slimness. Psychological studies confirm that women with anorexia have lower self-esteem and poorer mental health than women who do not have eating disorders.[2] Young men with anorexia are less likely to disclose their psychological state.[3] These studies point out the need for intensive mental health support, but do not answer the question of whether low self-esteem causes anorexia or anorexia causes low self-esteem.

At least part of the cause of anorexia may be physical. In the early 1990s, scientists found that the brains of people with anorexia have a defect in the enzyme tyrosine hydroxylase.[4] This chemical allows the brain to convert the amino acid tyrosine into the stimulant hormone norepinephrine. A deficiency of tyrosine hydroxylase usually only results in mild depression, so that people with anorexia are able to go about many aspects of their lives normally. Physical exercise makes the enzyme work more efficiently,[5] so it is possible that compulsive exercise by anorexics is not merely an attempt to burn calories, but a healing stimulus arising within the brain itself. Unfortunately, the improvement in the action of the enzyme accomplished through vigorous exercise almost never stimulates appetite enough to compensate for calories burned.

TREATMENT SUMMARY

DIET

- Avoid both alcohol and stimulants, including caffeine and nicotine.

NUTRITIONAL SUPPLEMENTS

For anorexics who take Luvox, Paxil, Prozac, Zoloft, or other selective serotonin reuptake inhibitors (SSRIs):

- Tyrosine: dosage chosen in consultation with a nutritionally oriented physician.

- Folic acid and vitamin B_{12}: 800 milligrams of each daily.

For anorexics who do not take Luvox, Paxil, Prozac, Zoloft, or other selective serotonin reuptake inhibitors (SSRIs):

- Tyrosine: dosage chosen in consultation with a nutritionally oriented physician.

- 5-HTP: 100–200 milligrams 3 times a day.

- Zinc picolinate: 30 milligrams daily.

HERBS

- St. John's wort: 300 milligrams of an extract containing 0.3 percent hypericin 3 times a day.

UNDERSTANDING THE HEALING PROCESS

Anorexia is a potentially life-threatening condition. Effective treatment usually combines a weight-gain program with treatment for depression. Because experience with nutritional supplements as a treatment for anorexia is very limited, no one should rely on self-care alone for this condition.

The first priority in treating anorexia is to supply macronutrients, carbohydrates, proteins, and fats. Of the three, protein is the easiest and fat is the most difficult to restore.[6] Fat is important to physical beauty, since the smooth contours of the skin are made possibly by underlying layers of fat. Intentionally including fat in the diet helps recovery. A daily multivitamin with minerals is also helpful, since most people with anorexia suffer deficiencies of calcium, copper, folate, magnesium, vitamin B_{12}, and zinc.[7] Just replacing the minimum requirements for these nutrients, however, has no influence on the underlying illness. Other supplements are necessary to overcome the disease.

Since anorexia is a depressive illness, alcohol is unhelpful. Alcohol is the world's first choice among depressants. As is well known, alcohol can cause uncontrolled mood swings and emotional outbursts in which poor choices are made. It depresses appetite and makes the liver less able to process nutrients that it actually receives.

Caffeine is the world's first choice among stimulants. Caffeine can contribute to heartburn, however, and can also interfere with nutrient absorption. Moreover, excessive use of caffeine can aggravate depression. One study found that among healthy college students, moderate and high coffee users scored higher on a depression scale (and had lower GPAs) than students who drank relatively little coffee.[8] Two studies have found that people experiencing major depression tend to consume high amounts of caffeine, the equivalent of 6 or more cups of coffee a day.[9,10] Another two studies positively correlate caffeine intake with the degree of mental illness in psychiatric patients.[11,12]

Nicotine, like alcohol, caffeine, and sugar, is commonly considered a stimulant. In the short term, nicotine *is* a stimulant, triggering the release of norepinephrine and epinephrine (adrenaline), and heightening the sensitivity of sensory receptors throughout the body. In the long run, however, nicotine causes desensitization of the brain to norepinephrine in much the same manner as chronic stress. Since underproduction of norepinephrine is a cause of anorexia, smoking must be eliminated.

Both animal and human studies suggest that tyrosine supplements can improve appetite, mental status, and exercise tolerance in anorexia nervosa.[13,14] However, the dosage of tyrosine required is very high, approximately 100 milligrams for every kilogram (2 pounds) of body weight. A person weighing 100 pounds would need 5,000 milligrams of tyrosine daily to get this effect. Since high dosages of tyrosine can cause insomnia and nervousness, it is necessary to seek supervision from a physician or other licensed healthcare practitioner before taking the supplement.

Drugs in the same class as Luvox, Paxil, Prozac, and Zoloft seem to work better when the body has adequate supplies of folic acid. A 10-week double-blind placebo-controlled trial of folic acid in 127 individuals with severe major depression being treated with Prozac found that women who took Prozac with the vitamin supplement got better faster than those who took Prozac alone. It is

possible that the 500-microgram dose of the vitamin used in the study was not enough to produce a beneficial effect in men.[15] Vitamin B_{12} works in tandem with SAM-e (s-adenosyl-l-methionine). Vitamin B_{12} supplementation is necessary when supplementing with folic acid, which is frequently deficient in persons who have depression.

5-HTP and St. John's wort probably should not be combined with conventional antidepressants. Prescription antidepressants linger in the bloodstream for a long time, and there have been several reports of "serotonin syndrome" (anxiety, elevated blood pressure, and mania) occurring when St. John's wort and medications such as Prozac are taken together.[16] Otherwise, they may be helpful. Both supplements enhance the brain's production of serotonin, a mood-lifting hormone that acts in harmony with norepinephrine.

5-HTP is a source of the amino acid tryptophan in a form that readily enters the brain. The brain turns tryptophan into the mood regulator serotonin. A clinical study involving 60 people with mild to moderate depression compared 5-HTP against Luvox (fluvoxamine), an antidepressant in the same family as Prozac. The study found that 5-HTP was slightly more effective than the prescription drug. More important, while Luvox caused the full range of side effects usually associated with SSRIs, 5-HTP only caused mild stomach upset in a few of the people who took it.[17]

5-HTP is a relatively safe supplement, but some people should avoid it. The most common side effects of 5-HTP are heartburn, nausea, and various kinds of stomach upset including bloating, flatulence, and stomach rumbles. This complication is due to the fact that the digestive tract makes its own serotonin, which may be overabundant until it adjusts to the supplemental supply. About 2 in 5 people who use the supplement experience these effects during the first 2 weeks of using it. To avoid this complication, begin by taking a 50 milligram dose once or twice a day, gradually building up to a 100-milligram dose after 3 or 4 weeks.

There are no reports of adverse effects on the central nervous system from taking even high doses of 5-HTP. Theoretically, however, large doses of 5-HTP taken with the migraine medications naratriptan, sumatriptan, or zolmitriptan or any prescription medications for depression could cause "serotonin syndrome." This condition has never been observed from supplementation with 5-HTP, but as a precaution, avoid using 5-HTP if you take any prescription drugs for depression or migraine. Persons who have angina, uncontrolled high blood pressure, Prinzmetal's angina, or who have had a heart attack should also avoid 5-HTP.

There are reports that combining 5-HTP with the Parkinson's disease drug carbidopa can cause symptoms similar to those of the skin disease scleroderma (see SCLERODERMA).[18,19]

St. John's wort is an extraordinarily well-researched herb. Nearly 180 studies document the efficacy of St. John's wort in treating anxiety, anorexia, depression, and sleep disturbances. In the European Union, St. John's wort is an antidepressant prescribed by doctors and paid for by health insurance.

Various clinical studies have compared St. John's wort against the tricyclic antidepressants Elavil (amitriptyline) and Tofranil (imipramine) and to the SSRIs Paxil (fluoxetine) and Zoloft (sertraline). Clinical studies repeatedly find that St. John's wort is as effective as mainstream antidepressant drugs, with fewer side effects and a lower cost. Following is just a sampling of the scientific studies that find that St. John's wort is nearly as effective as any prescription antidepressant you may receive as part of anorexia treatment.

A psychiatric clinic in Darmstadt, Germany conducted a double-blind comparison trial of St. John's wort and Elavil. The 135 depressed patients were given either the herb or the prescription medication for 6 weeks. At the end of the trial, patients who had been taking St. John's wort had an average score on the Hamilton Depression Rating Scale of 8.8, compared to an average score of 10.7 for the patients treated with Elavil (that is, the patients taking St. John's wort were less depressed). The St. John's wort also had fewer and milder side effects.[20]

A randomized, double-blind clinical comparison trial of St. John's wort and Tofranil conducted by the Remotiv-Imipramine Study Group in Germany involved 324 outpatients with mild to moderate depression at 40 outpatient clinics. After 6 weeks of treatment with either St. John's wort or Tofranil, the average score on the Hamilton Depression Rating Scale was 12.00 for patients taking St. John's wort and 12.75 for patients taking Tofranil. Adverse events such as agitation, anxiety, dizziness, retching, tiredness, and erectile dysfunction occurred in 63 percent of patients taking Tofranil but in only 39 percent of participants taking St. John's wort. The most important difference between St. John's wort

and Tofranil, however, was the patient's experience of anxiety while in treatment. The mean score on the anxiety-somatization subscale of the Hamilton measurement system was 3.79 in the St. John's wort group and 4.26 in the Tofranil group. Patients who took St. John's wort were significantly less likely to experience anxiety than patients who took Tofranil.[21]

Another German study compared St. John's wort with Prozac. Researchers enrolled 240 mildly to moderate depressed individuals in a randomized, double-blind, parallel group comparison in which 114 patients received Prozac and 126 patients received St. John's wort. After 6 weeks of treatment, the mean Hamilton Depression Rating Scale decreased to 11.54 in the group taking St. John's wort and 12.20 in the group taking Prozac. Eight percent of patients taking St. John's wort experienced adverse reactions, compared to 23 percent of patients on Prozac. The researchers concluded that St. John's wort and Prozac were equally effective in treating mild to moderate depression but that St. John's wort was a safer choice.[22]

A double-blind clinical study at St. John's Episcopal Hospital in Far Rockaway, New York, tested the comparative benefit of St. John's wort and Zoloft. Thirty outpatients were given a low dose of either St. John's wort or Zoloft for a week, and then a standard dose of either St. John's wort or Zoloft for 6 weeks. A clinical response defined as a 50 percent reduction in scores on the Hamilton Depression Rating Scale was noted in 47 percent of patients receiving St. John's wort and 40 percent of patients receiving Zoloft. The difference between the two drugs was too small to say with statistical confidence which was more effective.[23]

Exactly how St. John's wort works is not known. The most recent research suggests that the chemical hyperforin in the herb modifies the expression of genes in parts of the brain that are physically changed by stress, specifically the hippocampus, locus coeruleus, and striatum.[24] These parts of the brain respond to adrenaline released in states of stress, excitement, and joy. Restoring them to normal function may counteract other processes that cause depression.

Although the clinical evidence for St. John's wort is impressive, critics of herbal medicine correctly point out that it will not reliably treat severe depression. A well-publicized study published in the *Journal of the American Medical Association* in 2001 reported that only 24 percent of severely depressed patients given a relatively high dose of St. John's wort (1,200 milligrams of hypericin per day) went into remission during an 8-week trial, compared to 19 percent of patients who were given a placebo.[25] However, the news reports did not clarify that a response rate of less than 50 percent is typical for aggressive drug treatment of major depression, nor did the news reports compare side effects of standard medical treatments for major depression with side effects of St. John's wort. Nonetheless, anytime there is a risk of suicide, reliance on St. John's wort is inappropriate.

Do not take St. John's wort unless you have been off prescription antidepressants for at least 4 weeks. Prescription antidepressants linger in the bloodstream for a long time, and there have been several reports of "serotonin syndrome" (anxiety, elevated blood pressure, and mania) occurring when St. John's wort and medications such as Prozac are taken together.[26] Natural medicine specialist Dr. Steve Bratman notes that the antimigraine drug sumatriptan (Imitrex) and the painkilling drug tramadol also raise serotonin levels and might interact similarly with the herb. St. John's wort may make the skin more sensitive to sun, especially if you also take oral contraceptives, sulfa drugs, tetracycline, the blood pressure medication lisinopril (Prinivil or Zestril), or the arthritis drug piroxicam (Feldene).

Most important of all, St. John's wort may reduce the effectiveness of chemotherapy drugs,[27] clozapine or olanzapine for schizophrenia, cyclosporine for organ transplants,[28] digoxin for heart disease,[29] oral contraceptives, protease inhibitors for HIV,[30] theophylline for asthma,[31] and warfarin[32] used as a blood thinner. If you are taking St. John's wort and one of these medications at the same time and then stop taking the herb, blood levels of the drug may rise. Increasing bloodstream concentrations of the drug may be dangerous in some circumstances.

The Eating Disorders Clinic at St. Paul's Hospital in Vancouver, British Columbia, found that giving females 100 milligrams of zinc gluconate a day doubled the rate at which they gained weight.[33] Another uncontrolled study found similar results. The way zinc helps anorexia is not understood, but may have some relationship to its effects on the immune system.

CONCEPTS FOR COPING WITH ANOREXIA

○ Human growth hormone sometimes dramatically accelerates recovery from anorexia, although clinical tri-

als have not enrolled enough patients to produce statistically significant results. Its benefits in stabilizing the heart, however, are even more significant than those in stimulating weight gain.

○ Marijuana is sometimes suggested as a treatment for anorexia, but the only clinical study of its use found that symptoms were actually worse with marijuana treatment.[35]

○ Parents may consider psychological coping strategies from the anorexic child's perspective. Some requests that could be made by an anorexic child include:

• "Do not see me as an eating disorder. Anorexia is not my identity."

• "Eat with me daily, and provide a variety of foods."

• "Encourage me to go out with my friends." (This assumes they are going to safe places.)

• "Do not try to be a second therapist to me."

• "Don't make me talk about what's going on in therapy. Let counseling be private."

• "Let me listen to my body. Don't try to reward me with food."

Anthrax, Cutaneous

SYMPTOM SUMMARY

○ Blister or ulcer with a black scab, extensive swelling surrounding the site of infection

○ Fatigue or malaise

○ Swollen lymph nodes

UNDERSTANDING THE DISEASE PROCESS

Cutaneous anthrax is a skin infection caused by the bacterium *Bacillus anthracis*. Anthrax is a relatively well-known infection among cattle and sheep in the southwestern United States, and skin infections with anthrax have been reported throughout history among farmers, veterinarians, and tannery and wool workers. Anthrax is also a modern agent of bioterrorism.

Anthrax infects the skin through a cut or scrape. An itchy lesion similar to a bug bite develops about 2 weeks after exposure. It may be followed by a black ulcer that is usually painless, although painful lymph nodes may develop at this stage of the disease. A scab forms over the site of infection. The scab dries and falls off in 2 or 3 weeks.

About 1 in 5 people with the skin form of anthrax will develop a more serious infection without medical treatment. In these people, the bacterium can spread to the lungs to cause the same symptoms as inhalational anthrax. Death in anthrax infection comes about as a result of toxic shock when macrophages, the white blood cells that ordinarily would attempt to surround and digest the bacterium, are made to burst on contact with the anthrax toxin. The toxin only affects macrophages, and the action of the toxin is only on the immune system. In experimental animals with artificially depleted immune systems, anthrax toxin does not cause death.[1]

TREATMENT SUMMARY

DIET

O Absolutely avoid apple peelings (the rest of the apple is okay), black tea, cinnamon, grapefruit, green tea, lemon zest, onions, orange juice with pulp, and red wine.

NUTRITIONAL SUPPLEMENTS

O DHEA: 50 milligrams per day.

O Melatonin: 3 milligrams 1 hour before bedtime. Do not take during the day or you will not be able to get to sleep.

O Absolutely avoid hesperidin, quercetin, rutin, and St. John's wort.

*These nutritional recommendations do not substitute for medical care. Continue antibiotic treatment as long as your doctor orders it. **See Part Three if you take prescription medication.***

UNDERSTANDING THE HEALING PROCESS

Prior to 2002, the only scientific research of nutritional treatments for anthrax was a single study conducted by scientists at the Agency for Defense Development in South Korea. Their laboratory experiments with animals found that DHEA, melatonin, or a combination of both supplements conditioned macrophages to release less of an inflammatory hormone called TNF-alpha. Lowering levels of TNF-alpha reduced the risk of toxic shock and increased chances of survival when anthrax had entered the bloodstream.[2] Extending the logic of the

study to humans, it seems likely that DHEA and melatonin would be helpful in reducing the risk of complications in cutaneous anthrax, although there have never been (and it is unlikely there ever will be) any clinical trials. Effective dosages have not been scientifically established. Theoretically, these supplements would also protect against developing toxic shock in the lungs in the case of an airborne attack with the anthrax bacillus.

Avoiding grapefruit, green tea, onions, and red wine, as well as hesperidin, quercetin, rutin, and St. John's wort has no direct effect on the course of anthrax infection. However, avoiding these otherwise healthy foods and useful supplements enables the body to respond more completely to ciprofloxacin (Cipro), as well as nearly 20 alternative antibiotics in the same class. The quercetin in grapefruit, green tea, onions, and red wine, the rutin in apple peelings and black tea, and the hesperdin in lemon zest and orange juice with pulp compete with Cipro for receptor sites on the cells that receive it. Cinnamon stimulates the body's production of TNF-alpha, which is the agent of toxic shock.

CONCEPTS FOR COPING WITH ANTHRAX

O Garlic, the ancient preventive treatment for airborne infections, could be helpful in an anthrax attack. Garlic contains chemical compounds that reduce the activity of TNF.[3]

Anxiety
(Generalized Anxiety Disorder)

SYMPTOM SUMMARY

O Excessive worry occurring more days than not for at least 6 months accompanied by 3 or more of the following 6 symptoms (only 1 symptom is required for a diagnosis of anxiety in children):

- Difficulty concentrating or mind going blank
- Easily fatigued
- Irritability
- Muscle tension
- Restless or feeling keyed-up or on edge
- Sleep disturbance

UNDERSTANDING THE DISEASE PROCESS

Generalized anxiety disorder (GAD) is a chronic condition characterized by excessive worry. Described over a century ago by Sigmund Freud,[1] chronic, free-floating anxiety is still poorly understood, since a certain level of anxiety and apprehension is a normal feature of modern life. Epidemiologists estimate that between 4 and 6 percent of the population experiences generalized anxiety disorder at some point in life. Anxiety disorders strike without regard to age, sex, race, or social class, but, in the United States, are more common in the Northeast.[2] One study found that slightly more than half (56 percent) of people who develop GAD recover within a year.[3] Unfortunately, nearly as many sufferers of GAD reported the presence of symptoms for more than 5 years, and 10 percent experienced symptoms of GAD for more than 20 years. Most of these people dated the onset of "being a nervous person" at age 10 or younger, anxiety continuing through inevitable stresses throughout life.[4]

The mental health profession defines *treatable* anxiety in adults as a presentation of any 3 of the 6 symptoms listed above in which the anxiety or worry is not about gaining weight (as in anorexia), having a serious illness (as in hypochondriasis), having multiple physical complaints (as in somatization disorder), being away from home or close relatives (as in separation-anxiety disorder), being embarrassed in public (as in social phobia), or having a panic attack (as in panic disorder). Generalized anxiety causes distress, is difficult to control, and has an impact on life beyond the objects of worry.

The biology of GAD is not very well understood. In part, the condition relates to imbalances in the production and use of the neurotransmitter serotonin. Unlike depression, in which the serotonin supply of the brain is insufficient, anxiety results from excessive amounts of serotonin in the sensory-processing sectors of the brain, the locus coeruleus[5] and the nucleus paragigantocellularis.[6] Drugs that reduce anxiety act in part by stopping excessive responses to serotonin.

Another physiological pathway for anxiety in the brain concerns the gamma-aminobutyric acid (GABA) receptors. GABA has an effect on the brain similar to that of drugs like alprazolam (Xanax), chlordiazepoxide (Librium), clonazepam (Klonopin), and diazepam (Valium). People who suffer chronic anxiety do not respond to GABA normally, so that calming chemicals do not have their normal effect on the brain.

TREATMENT SUMMARY

DIET

○ Increase your consumption of fiber-rich sources of complex carbohydrates, including fruits and vegetables, legumes, whole grains, and raw nuts. Try to avoid presweetened breakfast cereals, colas, ice cream, pastries, puffed rice, and white bread. Eliminate caffeine, nicotine, and other stimulants.

NUTRITIONAL SUPPLEMENTS

○ A high-potency multivitamin and multimineral supplement including calcium, magnesium, and zinc, daily.

HERBS

○ Kava: 70 milligrams of kavalactones 3 times a day.

○ Avoid yohimbe.

If sensitivity to loud noises is a problem, add:

○ Gotu kola (*Centella asiatica*): 30 milligrams of extract standardized for 70 percent triterpenic acid content, 3 times a day.

See Part Three if you take prescription medication.

UNDERSTANDING THE HEALING PROCESS

Anything you take for anxiety, whether a prescription drug or a nutritional supplement, is likely to work by activating tranquilizer receptor sites in the brain. Kava, for instance, interacts with the brain in the same way as drugs such as Librium, Valium, and Xanax, although recent research suggests it probably has much broader healing effects. Clinical studies indicate that herbs and medications are approximately as effective in controlling anxiety. The advantage of diet and nutritional supplements over prescription tranquilizers is the absence of side effects.

The excessive consumption of refined carbohydrates produces a "sugar surge." When the sugar concentration of the bloodstream increases, the amino acid tryptophan more readily enters the brain. The brain converts tryptophan into serotonin, which overstimulates the portions of the brain involved in chronic anxiety.

Eating highly refined carbohydrates also increases the risk of panic attacks. A "sugar surge" is rapidly followed by hypoglycemia. The body's response to low blood sugars is to release cortisol, a stress hormone that signals the liver to break down stored glycogen. This stress hormone also induces panic attacks. Complex carbohydrates in fruits and vegetables, legumes, whole grains, and nuts are absorbed into the bloodstream without a "surge" that causes the release of stress hormones.

Symptoms of chronic anxiety are heightened after consumption of caffeine.[7] Consumption of caffeine in the range of 700–800 milligrams of caffeine per day (the equivalent of 6–8 cups of coffee) can induce "caffeinism," a clinical syndrome similar to panic disorder, which causes depression, headache, irritability, nervousness, and palpitatations.[8] Even 125–250 milligrams of caffeine, the equivalent of 1–2 cups of coffee, may be too much for people who suffer chronic anxiety.[9]

Nervous people the world over smoke cigarettes. On a physiological level, nicotine would seem almost to be beneficial in the treatment of anxiety. It stimulates the production of adrenal hormones, which in turn activate the enzyme tryptophan oxygenase, which deprives the brain of the amino acids it needs to make serotonin.[10] Cortisol also makes the serotonin receptors in the brain less sensitive to the serotonin that is available. When the brain is not exposed to excessive serotonin, anxiety centers are not activated.

In the short term, nicotine in fact probably does relieve anxiety. At least one study found that smoking relieved anxiety in women, although it caused aggression in men.[11] In their more honest moments, many mental health workers would assert that it is only commonsensical that smoking is a socially tolerated behavior (at least in some communities) that relieves anxiety. Some renegade researchers have even dared to suggest that smoking acts on dopamine, norepinephrine, and serotonin in the brain in a therapeutic way in anxiety disorders.[12]

Moreover, at least one clinical experiment gave 5-HTP, a chemical precursor of serotonin, to study participants who suffered acute anxiety. This was roughly the chemical equivalent of stopping smoking. This treatment induced a cluster of stimulation symptoms, including jitteriness, insomnia, diarrhea, and a sensation of jumping out of one's skin during the first few days of treatment. However, participants in the study who managed to withstand the unpleasant symptoms caused by the first few days of treatment enjoyed a marked reduc-

tion in panic attacks and anxiety thereafter.[13] It is highly probably that people with generalized anxiety disorder who are able to give up smoking enjoy lessened anxiety and numerous other health benefits. The problem is getting through the first few days of not smoking cigarettes.

Fortunately, it is easier to take supplements than to give up sugar, caffeine, and smoking. Simply taking a balanced vitamin and mineral supplement can greatly reduce anxiety. A double-blind study involving 80 healthy male volunteers given a multivitamin and multimineral supplement including calcium, magnesium, and zinc for 28 days found that treatment reduced anxiety and perception of stress.[14] There is no downside to taking multivitamin and mineral supplements. Taking up to 2 or 3 times the RDA of commonly recognized nutrients does not interfere with any prescription drugs.

Kava plays the same role in treating anxiety in Polynesian culture that alcohol plays in European and North American culture. In Polynesian society, numerous health benefits are attributed to this herb. Recent research even suggests that people who use kava are less likely to develop cancer.[15]

Kavalactones bind to the same receptor sites in the brain as benzodiazepine tranquilizers such as Librium and Valium. They also modify the brains' responses to GABA, dopamine, histamine, and endorphins,[16] as well as to the stress hormone norepinephrine.[17] They release tension in the skeletal muscles, and, in laboratory experiment with animals, prevent epileptic seizures.[18]

One clinical test found that, over a period of six months, kava offers about the same degree of relief as using the benzodiazepam tranquilizers alprazolam (Xanax) and oxazepam (Ox-Pam).[19] A small clinical study at a gynecological hospital in Germany found that one month's treatment with kava was effective in relieving anxiety associated with menopause.[20] A later clinical study at the University of Jena in Germany involved 101 outpatients suffering from agoraphobia, other specific phobias, adjustment disorders, and/or generalized anxiety disorder. The participants in the study were given kava or a placebo for 25 weeks. The researchers concluded that kava was as effective as either tricyclic antidepressants—such as amitriptyline (Elavil, Limbitriol), imipramine (Tofranil), or doxepin (Adapin, Sinequan), or benzodiazepine tranquilizers (such as Librium, Valium, or Xanax) with "none" of the side effects associated with the commonly prescribed drugs.[21] More recent

Kava Ban?

In November 2001 the German government moved to ban kava on the grounds that it was used by twenty-four people who later developed liver damage; however, in nineteen of these cases, kava was used in addition to prescription drugs. In explaining why the ban of kava may not be appropriate, the American Botanical Council stated:

The Commission E monograph (published in June, 1990) notes no known side effects of kava use, but does note: "Extended continuous intake can cause a temporary yellow discoloration of skin, hair, and nails. In this case, further application of this drug must be discontinued. In rare cases, allergic skin reactions can occur. Also, accommodative disturbances, such as enlargement of the pupils and disturbances of the oculomotor equilibrium, have been described." These last effects are usually associated with dosage levels higher than those recommended for therapeutic use.[24]

A later, closer examination of a total of thirty-six cases reported to the German Ministry of Health found that only one could be tied to possible side effects from the use of kava.[25] In the highly unlikely event you experience symptoms such as yellow discoloration of the skin and nails, or unusual twitches around the eyes or difficulty focusing the eyes, discontinue kava immediately. Otherwise, use kava for up to three months at a time to reduce the frequency of panic attacks, alternating use of the herb with three month breaks.

research has found that kava is especially useful in controlling the racing pulse that is associated with anxiety.[22] Researchers at Duke University believe that controlling racing pulse may reduce the risk of heart attack associated with generalized anxiety disorder.[23]

Do not take kava in addition to prescription tranquilizers, especially Xanax. Taking kava with antipsychotic medications can cause abnormal movements, called a dystonic reaction. Kava reduces the effectiveness of L-dopa in the treatment of Parkinson's disease.

A different herb, gotu kola, is useful in dealing with the "startle reflex" caused by loud noises and other sudden environmental changes. Dr. Michael Davis of Yale University explains that the one part of the brain, the stria terminalis circuit, underlies "free-floating" symptoms of generalized anxiety while another part of the brain, the central nucleus pathway, generates responses to specific fearful stimuli.[26] For this reason, chemicals such as those found in kava ameliorate general anxiety whereas chemicals such as those found in gotu kola modify specific anxieties. A study at the Royal Ottawa Hospital and Department of Psychiatry in Canada found that a single dose of gotu kola increases the amplitude of the sound necessary to cause a startle response, that is, sounds have to be louder to be distracting. The study found that the herb had no effect on mood, heart rate, or blood pressure, only reducing anxiety.[27]

Yohimbe acts on the same nerve fibers as caffeine, and is used in experimental settings to induce panic attacks. Men who are subject to panic disorder should not use this herb.

Another natural treatment for anxiety is acupuncture. A small-scale study at the University of the Rühr in Bochum, Germany found that a series of 10 acupuncture treatments produced clinically significant responses in 86 percent of the anxiety patients treated. The researchers cautioned that improvements were not evident after just 5 treatments. A full course of acupuncture is necessary for results.[28]

CONCEPTS FOR COPING WITH ANXIETY

O There are a large number of herbal products that help relieve anxiety.

• Avena (oats) is relaxing and anti-inflammatory, and also stimulates sexual desire by helping the body conserve testosterone by slowing the production of a competing hormone. Make avena tea from green or yellow seeds, not straw, or take up to 3 teaspoons of tincture 4 times a day. Follow the manufacturer's directions for capsules.

• Chamomile tea relaxes muscles and relieves indigestion. Be sure to make the tea with hot, not boiling, water.

• Lavender relieves pain and relaxes. It is used as an essential oil that may be applied to the skin, added to a warm bath, or mixed with almond, olive, or sesame oil and used in massage. Do not take essential oil of lavender internally.

• Linden, or *Tilia,* eases muscle tension and lowers blood pressure. Make linden tea from 1–2 teaspoons of dried *flowers* steeped in 1 cup of water for 10 minutes.

• Motherwort (*Leonurus cardiaca*) is a traditional remedy for anxiety associated with rapid heart rate. Since the herb has definite effect on the heart rate, you should not take it if you also take beta-blockers such as atenolol (Tenormin) or propanolol (Inderal).

• Vervain, or *Verbena,* is traditionally used to treat people with anxiety who also have liver disease. It is taken as capsule, tea, or tincture.

❍ There are also a large number of nutritional supplements to treat combinations of other symptoms and anxiety.

• Inositol is useful in treating anxiety in people who also have problems with obsessive-compulsive disorder (OCD), binge eating, or panic attacks. Some recent research suggests that inositol sensitizes receptor sites in the brain to a biochemical message that a task is complete, relieving OCD.[29] A preliminary study at the University of the Negev in Israel found that inositol is more effective than antidepressants in controlling binge eating and bulimia.[30] And another study at the same institution found that inositol was 40 percent more effective than fluvoxamine (Luvox) in reducing the number of panic attacks suffered by people who experienced both generalized anxiety and panic attacks. Unlike Luvox, inositol did not cause nausea or fatigue.[31] If you suffer any of these conditions in addition to generalized anxiety disorder, try taking eight 500-milligram capsules a day. Improvement in symptoms usually takes 2–4 weeks. It is possible to take up to thirty-six 500-milligram capsules daily for additional effect.

• Magnesium may be very useful in treating anxiety coupled with Tourette's syndrome.[32] Studies in Turkey have found that intravenous magnesium significantly reduces postsurgical pain.[33] If you experience both anxiety and either Tourette's syndrome or pain after surgery, try taking up to 350 milligrams of supplemental magnesium daily (100 milligrams for children under the age of 12). Discontinue if you experience diarrhea.

Tips for Dealing with Short-term Stress to Relieve Anxiety

• Rehearse. Focus your energy by going through the steps of what you need to do with the task or situation facing you.

• Choose to stop nonproductive comments running through your head by replacing them with productive ones.

• If you have some rituals for success, use them.

• Take a break by physically distancing yourself from the anxiety-provoking situation if you can.

Relaxation Techniques:

• Stand up and stretch, or if you can't stand up, stretch as many muscle groups as possible while staying seated.

• Try tensing and releasing various muscle groups. Starting with your toes, tense up for perhaps 5–10 seconds and then let go. Relax and then go up the body to another muscle group.

• Breathe deeply. Close your eyes; then, fill your chest cavity slowly by taking 4 or 5 short, deep breaths. Hold each breath until it begins to feel uncomfortable, and then let it out slowly.

• Repeat a calming word to yourself (but not the imperative "Relax!"). This word can be any word that you associate with calm circumstances, such as "smooth," "peace," and so on.

• Scientists at the University of the Negev have also found that supplemental vitamin B_6 (pyridoxine) relieves various symptoms of schizophrenia, including anxiety.[34] Up to 100 milligrams per day may be helpful, but since vitamin B_6 interacts with many prescription drugs, be sure to check Part Three for drug interactions and consult with your prescribing physician before taking the supplement.

❍ The Bach flower remedies are a well-established part of natural medicine's repertoire for treating anxiety. Researchers conducting a double-blind, placebo-controlled, randomized clinical study in Germany concluded that these widely used treatments are (1) a placebo but (2) nonetheless effective, inasmuch as patients receiving either a "placebo" flower remedy or a Bach flower remedy all enjoyed lowered anxiety.[35] One way to interpret the results is that all flower remedies help lessen anxiety, or that the remedies' effectiveness is not limited to their traditional categories.

○ Smoking cessation increases the anxiety-provoking effects of caffeine (although only slightly).[36] If you are trying to quit smoking, reduce your consumption of coffee.

Aphthous Ulcers
See **Canker Sores**.

Apophysitis, Tibial
See **Osgood-Schlatter's Disease**.

Arrhythmia
See **Irregular Heartbeat**.

Arsenic Exposure

SYMPTOM SUMMARY

○ Areas of dark pigmentation in the skin

○ Muscle weakness

○ Symmetrical calluses on the palms of both hands or the soles of both feet

○ Tingling or numbness in the hands and feet

○ White bands across the fingernails

○ Yellowing of the skin

UNDERSTANDING THE DISEASE PROCESS

Arsenic is a naturally occurring toxin that is ubiquitous in the modern environment. Exposure to arsenic is global and life-long. In the United States, arsenic is a widespread contaminant of drinking water, especially on Long Island and in the cotton-growing counties of the rural South and Southwest. People who work in factories that make glass or semiconductors or in power plants are at special risk. In some Third World countries entire populations are at high risk for arsenic poisoning; 50 million people suffer this condition in Bangladesh alone.

Arsenic contamination has been known to occur in imported "herbal" remedies (maya yogarraj guggulu from India and "herbal balls" for cataracts imported from China), a depilatory imported from Iran, wine produced from grapes in vineyards sprayed with arsenic, and, disconcertingly, in some baby cereals made in the United States.[1] For many years, most cotton fields in the United States were sprayed with arsenic to defoliate the plants and make cotton easier to pick. Long-term exposure to arsenic is a major contributing factor to atherosclerosis, heart attack, stroke,[2] and bladder cancer,[3] as well as cancers of the liver, kidneys, and skin. Exposure to arsenic greatly increases the damage done by radiation. Uranium miners, for instance, are 10 times more likely to develop lung cancer if they have been exposed to arsenic.[4] Even a relatively short-term exposure to arsenic, such as the time needed to discover arsenic in a drinking water supply, can increase the risk of lung cancer by over 1,000 percent.[5]

Arsenic damages tissues through the massive release of free radicals of oxygen. Cells exposed to arsenic produce about 3 times as many damaging free radicals as other cells. These reactions occur within minutes of arsenic exposure and can lead to gene mutations and death of the cell.[6] Arsenic causes cells throughout the body to lose the ability to release energy from glucose, by blocking the enzyme succinic dehydrogenase.

The symptoms of arsenic poisoning are distinctive and readily recognizable to any physician aware of the possibility of the condition. Symptoms of arsenic poisoning include white bands across the nails, yellowing of the skin, and calluses that appear in mirror images on both hands or both feet. In some cases, arsenic poisoning will cause hair that has gone gray to regain its natural color.[7]

TREATMENT SUMMARY

NUTRITIONAL SUPPLEMENTS

○ Vitamin C: at least 1,000 milligrams per day.

○ Vitamin E: 400 IU per day.

○ High-potency multivitamin and multimineral supplement.

HERBS

○ Silymarin (milk thistle) phytosomes: 70–210 milligrams 3 times daily.

See Part Three if you take prescription medication.

UNDERSTANDING THE HEALING PROCESS

Fortunately, cell damage from arsenic exposure is not inevitable. The scientific team that identified the free-radical action of arsenic on healthy tissues also found that antioxidants such as vitamin C and vitamin E cut the production of free radicals in half. This gives other mechanisms in the cells a chance to offset the genetic damage cause by arsenic.[8] There has not yet been clinical research to establish effective doses of antioxidant vitamins for cancer protection. The doses recommended here are estimates. It is also possible that future research will show that other antioxidants will be more effective.

A high-potency multiple vitamin and mineral supplement will provide the liver with the B-complex vitamins, calcium, chromium, copper, iron, and zinc it needs to detoxify small quantities of arsenic. Sulfur-containing foods such as eggs, garlic, and onions provide the sulfur needed for sulfation, the process by which the liver is able to bind arsenic before it reaches the general bloodstream. If you cannot eat these foods, take supplemental cysteine, methionine, and taurine. Silymarin, the active ingredient in milk thistle, protects the liver itself against chemical damage. Some people experience diarrhea when they first start taking silymarin, but this side effect usually stops after 2–3 days.

CONCEPTS FOR COPING WITH ARSENIC EXPOSURE

○ Hair analysis offers a good measure of arsenic exposure.

○ Chelation therapy is effective against arsenic exposure, but the chelating agent most physicians knowledgeable of the condition will use is not EDTA but British anti-Lewisite.

○ If you have a deck or playground built with arsenic-treated wood:

• Replace arsenic-treated decks, swing sets, and picnic tables with products built with arsenic-free wood.

That is the safest—if least economical—solution. At a minimum, homeowners should seal the existing wood at least once a year.

• Don't store children's toys under decks. Arsenic leaches off wood when it rains and could coat the toys. Children and pets should be kept away from the dirt beneath and immediately surrounding the deck.

• Cover any picnic table made with arsenic-treated wood with a tablecloth before using it.

• Demand wood treated with arsenic-free preservatives when buying new wood at your local home improvement center.

Arterial Disease
See **Aneurysm; Atherosclerosis; High Cholesterol; Peripheral Vascular Disease; Reynaud's Phenomenon.**

Arthritis
See **Gout; Osteoarthritis; Rheumatoid Arthritis.**

Ascites
See **Cirrhosis of the Liver.**

Asthma

SYMPTOM SUMMARY

○ Wheezing

• Begins suddenly

• Aggravated by heartburn

• May be worse at night or in the early morning

• Worse after exercise

• Worse during exposure to cold air

• Resolves spontaneously

○ Cough with or without phlegm

○ Shortness of breath that is worse after exercise

○ Intercostal retractions (movement of diaphragm muscles pulls skin between ribs when breathing)

Less common symptoms:

○ Breathing out takes much longer than breathing in

○ Coughing up blood

○ Nasal flares

○ Tightness in the chest

○ Temporary cessation of breathing

Symptoms that need emergency care:

○ Extreme difficulty breathing

○ Bluish color to lips or face

○ Severe anxiety

○ Rapid pulse

○ Sweating

○ Severe drowsiness or confusion

UNDERSTANDING THE DISEASE PROCESS

The National Centers for Disease Control report that in the United States alone there are 17 million people with asthma, 4–5 million of them children. Every year in the United States alone, asthma results in 20 million visits to the doctor, 1 million trips to the emergency room, and 500,000 hospitalizations. Doctors write 35 million prescriptions for inhalers annually. Worst of all, the number of deaths from asthma attacks has multiplied six-fold over the past 20 years.

The number of children who have asthma has also risen steadily during the last 20 years. Scientists are puzzled that similar increases in asthma have not occurred in the developing world, even in especially polluted places, such as Mexico City. A paper published in *The New England Journal of Medicine* even found that in Philadelphia, asthma rates increased as air pollution rates decreased.[1] Scientists are also puzzled that asthma rates go up as smoking rates go down,[2] and they have found that early childhood infections do not generally doom children to a life with asthma.[3] Neither are houses especially dirtier or cats especially more prevalent since 1980.[4]

What has changed in the last two decades in which asthma rates have skyrocketed is children's exercise patterns. Spontaneous deep breathing is the body's first line of defense against an asthma attack. As children become more involved with computers and television, they are less involved in vigorous physical activity, and do not develop lungs that can resist asthma attacks. In other words, asthma may actually be no more common today than it was in the recent past. People simply have fewer defenses against it.

At any age, the best protection against getting asthma is logging off the Internet, turning off the television, and getting vigorous exercise. If you already have asthma, however, this may not be easy. Your body has a chronically unbalanced immune response to the environment. Every healthy immune system responds to dander, dust mites, pollen, and airborne chemicals. The immune system sends out a group of white blood cells known as CD4+. One group of CD4+ cells, known as Th1, ordinarily responds to an "invader" by causing the rupture of histamine sacs to cause swelling and inflammation to isolate it. Another group of CD4+ cells, known as Th2, comes along later to magnify the offending substance.

People with asthma have too many Th2 cells. Their immune systems cause swelling and inflammation not just of a few cells around an inhaled airborne particle but of the entire bronchial passage. The second group of CD4+ cells even recruits white blood cells that would ordinarily be engaged in fighting tumors and viruses to produce still more inflammation. They secrete inflammatory leukotrienes that attract more white blood cells, making the reaction worse and worse until their supplies of attractants are suddenly exhausted, ending the attack.

TREATMENT SUMMARY

DIET

○ Drink 6–8 glasses of water every day.

○ Avoid salty foods.

○ Eat cold-water fish 3–4 times a week, or, if you are vegetarian or otherwise do not eat fish, take 1 tablespoon of flaxseed oil every day.

NUTRITIONAL SUPPLEMENTS

○ Magnesium: 200 milligrams 3 times a day.

○ Vitamin B$_6$: 100 milligrams per day.

○ Vitamin C: 500–1,000 milligrams 3 times a day.

○ Vitamin E: 200–400 IU per day.

HERBS

○ Boswellin or boswellin with curcuminoids: 150–250 milligrams 3 times per day.

○ *Tylophora:* 400 milligrams of dried leaf or two 40-milligram capsules daily.

See Part Three if you take prescription medication.

UNDERSTANDING THE HEALING PROCESS

Drinking 6–8 glasses of water every day is especially important if your worst attacks of asthma occur after heavy exercise. Dehydrated cells in the linings of the bronchial passageways are especially susceptible to inflammation and rupture by white blood cells. While proper hydration will not prevent asthma attacks not related to exercise, it may greatly reduce their severity. Just as it is important to drink water, it is helpful to avoid salt.

Several studies from Australia suggest that asthmatics who eat fresh cold-water fish several times a week gain relief from wheezing and experience increased lung capacity. One study found that children who ate fish more than once per week had lower rates of airway hyperresponsiveness than did children who ate fish less often.[7] Another study found that consumption of fresh fish, and particularly oily fish, was protective against wheezing.[8] It should be noted that at least one study reports contrary findings: In Japan, where fish is a staple food, eating fish is associated with increased asthma in children, although the difference may be that Japanese children who eat fish more frequently tend to eat salted fish.[9]

At least 10 studies have shown that other sources of essential fatty acids reduce the production of inflammation-inducing leukotrienes, but most failed to show that taking flaxseed oil or similar products reduced the frequency of asthma attacks. The reason may be that they did not study the effects long enough. A study conducted at Harvard Medical School found that children on inhalers increased lung capacity by an average of 10 percent over the course of 9 months, whereas children on inhalers who were given essential fatty acids increased lung capacity an average of 23 percent.[10]

Essential fatty acids increase the effectiveness of the medications zafirlukast (Accolate) and montelukast (Singulair), which operate by reducing the immune system's response to other, "bad" fatty acids. Don't expect results from eating fish or taking fish oil or other kinds of n-3 fatty acids immediately. Any essential fatty acid supplement can cause bloating, burping, diarrhea, or flatulence, although these effects are likely to be mild. People with a history of partial seizures (blanking out or unexplained loss of emotional control should not use borage seed oil, since it can lower the amount of stress precipitating an attack. Hempseed oil is also helpful, but not always legal. It will not give you a marijuana high, but it can cause a false positive reading for marijuana use in some home-testing kits.

Magnesium relaxes muscles. Intravenous magnesium sulfate is part of standard treatment for severe asthma in the emergency room, and often begins to relieve symptoms as soon as it is administered.[11] It is preferable, of course, to take magnesium before emergencies arise. A large British study of dietary magnesium intake and asthma symptoms in 2,633 people found that asthmatics who had a greater dietary intake of magnesium had significantly greater lung capacity and significantly less airway hyperreactivity.[12] Taking magnesium just for a few weeks will not reduce your need for an inhaler,[13] because the body pools magnesium very slowly.[14]

Vitamin B₆ is important for children with asthma and for adults who take theophylline (Theo-Dur). In a study of 76 children with asthma, taking 100 milligrams of vitamin B₆ twice a day resulted in fewer attacks, less wheezing, cough, and chest tightness, and decreased use of inhalers.[15] In adults, vitamin B₆ does not necessarily improve lung capacity,[16] but taking the vitamin results in less wheezing.[17] Asthma patients of all ages who use theophylline have lower levels of the active form of vitamin B₆, pyridoxal-5'-phosphate (PLP), and benefit from taking vitamin B₆ in this form.

Women who use oral contraceptives and people who take prescription medications for bipolar disorder, unipolar depression, tuberculosis, or seizures are at special risk for vitamin B₆ deficiency. If you take Theo-Dur for asthma *and* have any history of seizure disorder or unexplained loss of consciousness, you should not take vitamin B₆.

The antioxidant vitamins C and E are especially important in preventing asthma attacks. The immune system uses free radicals of oxygen to break open the histamine sacs in mast cells that cause airway irritation. Vitamins C and E absorb free radicals of oxygen and thwart this process. Conversely, asthma attacks deplete the body's supplies of these vitamins.

Generally speaking, the more nearly normal your bloodstream levels of vitamin C, the greater your lung capacity and the less frequently you will have shortness of breath.[18] Not every clinical study has found that taking vitamin C helps, but the studies that did not show that it helps only tested taking vitamin C for a very short period, usually 2 weeks. Take vitamin C on an ongoing basis for maximum benefit. Vitamin E helps your body preserve vitamin C, and also has a number of beneficial effects on the bloodstream.

Boswellin is a standardized form of the Ayurvedic herb boswellia, also known as mukul or Indian frankincense. It acts in the body in a way that complements zafirlukast (Accolate) and montelukast (Singulair). Bronchial constriction is caused by leukotrienes, which are made from n-6 fatty acids. Accolate and Singulair make cells insensitive to leukotrienes. Boswellin deactivates an enzyme so that leukotrienes are never made in the first place.[19] And if enough of the enzyme 5-lipoxygenase is active so that leukotrienes are made, boswellin keeps them from being attracted after the release of histamine.[20]

Physicians conducting a double-blind, placebo-controlled clinical study gave 40 asthmatics 300 milligrams of boswellin 3 times a day for 6 weeks. Seventy percent experienced improvement in lung capacity and fewer incidents of wheezing, compared to 27 percent in the control group.[21] Boswellin is not known to interact with any prescription drugs, but it should be used with caution by people who have peptic ulcer disease.

Tylophora asthmatica is another Ayurvedic medicine for asthma, bronchitis, and rheumatoid arthritis. Taken in large doses, it induces vomiting. Taken in small doses, it seems to increase the body's production of anti-inflammatory steroids.[22] The unique advantage of *Tylophora* is that its benefits continue even after its use is discontinued. Indian researchers had 110 asthmatics chew and swallow one *Tylophora* leaf per day for 6 days. At one week, 62 percent of individuals taking *Tylophora* had moderate to complete symptom relief. Relief from asthma continued for 4 weeks after the trial.[23]

The drawback to using *Tylophora* is that for it to be effective, you have to experience a little discomfort. A significant percentage of participants in the Indian study complained of nausea, although there was a positive correlation between nausea and degree of improvement.

CONCEPTS FOR COPING WITH ASTHMA

○ Identify your personal asthma triggers. When you recognize an offending substance (tobacco smoke, paint fumes, or wafting waves of visible pollen, for instance), measure your breathing capacity with a flow meter. The lower your flow, the more of a problem the substance will be for you. If your flow reads in the red zone, go to an emergency room immediately.

○ Don't hang laundry out to dry during your allergy season. Pollen and molds can stick to cloth surfaces.

○ Pollen and mold peak outdoors between 5 and 10 A.M., so early morning is a good time to limit outdoor activities. You can clear pollen and mold from indoor air with a HEPA (High Energy Particulate Air) filter or an electrostatic precipitator.

○ Wear a dust mask when mowing the lawn, raking leaves, or gardening.

○ Dust mites live in bedding, curtains, carpets, upholstered furniture, and stuffed animals. Wash all bedding in hot (130°F or 55°C) water every week. Vacuum at least twice a week to remove dust mites from the carpet and furniture. Cover pillows, box spring, and mattress with allergy-proof encasings. Your vacuum cleaner should be fitted with a HEPA filter.

○ Mold thrives in warm, damp, dark places, especially bathrooms, basements, and garbage cans. Keep all rooms clean and dry to prevent the growth of mold. Reduce indoor humidity by running your air conditioner or dehumidifier during the high-humidity seasons. If you use a humidifier in the winter, make sure the humidity remains around 40 percent. Keep garbage cans covered.

○ There is no such thing as a nonallergenic cat or dog. Dander is a collection of microscopic skin cells shed by animals. It can stick to carpet, upholstery, and drapes long after a pet has left the room. Vacuum drapes and upholstery when you vacuum carpets, and keep pets out of your own sleeping quarters.

○ Don't smoke, and don't allow others to smoke in your home. Speak with family and friends who smoke before they visit. Offer them gum, mints, or food to help them get by without smoking, or ask them to smoke outside. Explain that you can't tolerate smoking if you visit someone who smokes. If necessary, be ready to leave. Don't allow babysitters to smoke around your child, particularly where your child sleeps.

❍ Many holistically oriented parents of children with asthma claim they "can't do without" ephedra in managing their children's condition. While restrictive legislation in many states and bad press across the country has more to do with misapplication of ephedra and confusion of the herb ephedra with its chemical constituent ephedrine, pure ephedra is no longer available in most places. Alternatives to banned ephedra products include many Chinese and Japanese Kampo patent medicines that combine ephedra with other herbs to eliminate potential side effects, or which use other nonstimulant herbs. These products include:

• Minor Construct the Middle Decoction (known in Traditional Chinese Medicine as Xiao Jian Zhong Tang and in Japanese herbal medicine as *sho-kenchu-to*): An ephedra-free formula useful for children and especially helpful for asthmatic adults who have high blood pressure. Brand names in the United States and Canada include:

  • Minor Cinnamon and Peony Combination (KPC Herbs, Lotus Classics, Qualiherb, Sun Ten)

  • Xiao Jian Zhong Tang (KPC Herbs, Lotus Classics, Qualiherb, Sun Ten)

• Minor Blue-Green Decoction (known in Traditional Chinese Medicine as Xiao Qing Long Tang and in Japanese herbal medicine as sho-seiryu-to): Especially useful for children who have both asthma and runny nose. This formula contains about 10 percent ephedra. Brand names in the United States and Canada include:

  • Minor Blue Dragon Formula (Chinese Classics)

  • Minor Blue Dragon (Health Concerns, Qualiherb)

  • Minor Blue Dragon Combination (Lotus Classics)

  • *Sho-seiryu-to* (Honso, Tsumura)

• Mysterious Decoction (known in Traditional Chinese Medicine as Shen Mi Tang and in Japanese herbal medicine as *shinpi-to*). Used to treat asthma with moderate amounts of phlegm. Contains about 25percent ephedra. Brand names in the United States and Canada include:

  • Ma Huang & Magnolia Combination (KPC Herbs, Lotus Classics, Qualiherb, Sun Ten)

  • Shen Mi Tang (KPC Herbs, Lotus Classics, Qualiherb, Sun Ten)

❍ Five scientific studies have found that yoga improves exercise tolerance, reduces need for inhalers, and increases lung capacity. It isn't necessary to master the postures of yoga to help asthma, since it is breathing practice that helps.[24]

❍ Acupuncture can also help asthma, but it is more likely to be useful for people who are physically active than for people who are sedentary. Chinese studies indicate that acupuncture is least likely to help diabetics who have asthma.[25]

❍ Aromatherapy with essential oil of rosemary can be helpful in relieving *mild* asthma. Do not attempt to use aromatherapy to treat a severe asthma attack.

❍ Many naturopathic physicians recommend adrenal glandulars for people who are coming off steroid inhalers. Glandulars do not substitute for inhalers. They are only believed to keep the adrenal glands from becoming "lazy" as a result of steroid therapy. Products usually combine dessicated adrenal gland with zinc, licorice, and both American and Chinese (*Panax*) ginseng to extend the effect both of the adrenal gland preparation and the steroid inhaler.

❍ Eating onions is a traditional remedy for asthma. Onions are an excellent source of quercetin, which interferes with the production of histamine, the chemical that causes airways to close. Onions offer a dosage of quercetin large enough to help asthma but small enough not to interfere with the action of antibiotics.

❍ Forty-eight scientific studies of the benefits of massage in treating asthma present contradictory results, but it appears the greatest benefits of massage are in treating children with asthma aged 4 to 8. According to a study published in *The Journal of Pediatrics,* nightly massages for children of this age lessen anxiety and probably reduce the frequency of nighttime asthma attacks. Teenagers also benefit from massage, but only through increased lung capacity after receiving massage for 30 days.[26]

❍ Biofeedback training is another drug-free option for assisting asthma management. In this technique, sensors are applied to the jaw to measure how much electricity each muscle is making. A video screen shows the viewer how much each muscle is relaxed, and eventually the user learns to relax the jaw muscles and open breathing passages without referring to the screen. Biofeedback can be done at home. Studies have found that biofeedback reinforcing slow, deep, diaphragmatic breathing decreases the need to use inhalers, reduces emergency room visits, and increases lung capacity.[27]

○ Another biofeedback method only requires a mirror. Stand in front of the mirror with your chest exposed. Breathe in to a count of 4 and breathe out to a count of 6. Breathing in is a contraction mode and is shorter; breathing out is a relaxation mode and is longer. Look at the mirror and see the jaw, shoulders, and chest muscles relax with each exhaled breath. By making the exhalation longer than the inhalation, you are in a state of relaxation for a longer period of time. Practicing this relaxation exercise 10 minutes a day every day is enough to allow an asthmatic to reduce the severity of the next attack.

○ Allowing your child to cut physical education classes on account of potential asthma attacks can be the beginning of a vicious cycle. Children with asthma become out of breath with less exertion than other children. If the child reduces his or her level of activity to avoid this uncomfortable sensation, the next round of breathlessness comes at even lower levels of activity. The cycle continues until the child becomes sedentary and possibly too embarrassed to begin exercising again.

○ Exposure to secondhand tobacco smoke is clearly not beneficial to children with asthma, but there is some evidence that it is not a major factor in the development of the disease. Good diet, low in saturated fats, may compensate for exposure to environmental tobacco smoke.[28]

○ The most commonly used homeopathic remedy for asthma is natrum sulphuricum (Nat Sulph). It does not interact with prescription drugs and does not cause side effects. Homeopaths sometimes treat childhood asthma with ipecac—but only in minute doses. (Do not use syrup of ipecac for asthma.) Ipecac is believed to help rattling cough accompanied by gagging and vomiting. Pulsatilla is traditionally recommended for "shy" children with asthma. Never substitute homeopathic preparations for inhalers or other prescription medications except under the supervision of a holistically oriented physician.

○ Homeopathic medicine offers a number of treatments for asthma. While homeopathic preparations are generally more effective than a placebo, the full benefit of homeopathy is found through interaction with a homeopathic physician who can match the symptoms of the whole person to a specific remedy. Because homeopathy treats people rather than diseases, homeopathic remedies match not only specific symptoms, but "central delusions," the essential ways people misperceive their life issues, that lead to illness.

If you choose to try homeopathy without the assistance of a homeopathic physician, start with a single dose of the lowest strength (6C, 6X, or 12C) of the remedy matching the symptoms to be treated, and then wait for a response. If there is an improvement in symptoms, let the remedy continue to work until there is no more improvement, then take another dose. If there is no improvement, try a different potency (30X or 30C). Sometimes homeopathic medicines work for a few minutes, and sometimes they work for an entire day before another dose is needed.

• Arsenicum album treats people who suffer violent reactions to many different foods and pollens and who tend toward anxiety, compulsivity, and over-attention to details and order. There may be a wheezing cough that produces a clear, runny fluid.

• Carbo vegetabilis relieves allergies in people who have bloating, flatulence, and a frequent need to burp. This remedy is appropriately prescribed when symptoms are worse when eating, talking, or lying down. There may be a hollow sensation in the chest. Coughing fits may lead to choking.

• Chamomilla treats asthma triggered by windborne pollen. It is especially appropriate for treating asthma in hyperactive children.

• Ipecacuanha treats coughing fits that lead to vomiting.

• Natrum sulphuricum relieves asthma that is triggered by contact with mold. People who benefit from this remedy tend to overindulge in alcohol, sweets, or spicy food.

• Pulsatilla is typically recommended for asthmatics who cough up large quantities of yellow phlegm. The person who benefits from this remedy is likely to be subject to mood swings.

• Spongia tosta, also recommended for croup, treats asthma with a barking cough that produces little or no phlegm. Symptoms successfully relieved by this treatment usually start during the first few hours of sleep.

Atherosclerosis

SYMPTOM SUMMARY

❍ Often there are no noticeable outward symptoms until a complication occurs. Symptoms associated with some, but not all, cases include:

- High blood pressure
- Weak pulse
- Chest pains
- Leg cramps
- Weakness
- Dizziness
- Diagonal crease in the ear lobe

❍ Can be detected with a stethoscope as a bruit, a "whoosh" heard when the stethoscope is held over the area of a blockage

UNDERSTANDING THE DISEASE PROCESS

Atherosclerosis, also known as hardening of the arteries, is one of the most common diseases in the Western world. The "hardening" of the arteries occurs when calcium deposits accumulate in fatty streaks in their lining. Atherosclerosis can block the flow of blood in the coronary arteries and contribute to heart attack. Atherosclerosis can also block the flow of blood to the legs and cause intermittent claudication.

A common misconception of atherosclerosis is that it is analogous to clogs in a pipe, that too much cholesterol flowing through the "pipes" eventually coats them and stops the flow of blood. The realities of atherosclerosis are far more subtle. Atherosclerosis is usually, but not always, associated with higher cholesterol levels. At least one study has found that the bodies of women past the age of menopause who have atherosclerosis make less cholesterol than the bodies of women who do not have atherosclerosis, only the elimination of cholesterol is defective.[1]

Some forms of cholesterol contribute to the formation of atherosclerosis while others are protective. Cholesterol is a fat and the blood is primarily water, so cholesterol has to be attached to a specialized protein called a lipoprotein to be soluble. Particles of low-density lipoprotein (LDL) cholesterol are larger and more like-

ly to get caught in the lining of the artery. Particles of high-density lipoprotein (HDL) are smaller and less likely to get caught in the lining of the artery.

LDL cholesterol is frequently referred to as "bad" cholesterol and HDL as "good" cholesterol; however, both forms are essential to the normal function of the body. LDL cholesterol, in particular, is a primary source of energy for the macrophages, immune cells that engulf and digest infectious bacteria. And not just any LDL causes atherosclerosis. Only the smallest and oldest of the LDL particles, those most easily seeded with free radicals, are oxidized and initiate hardening of the arteries.[2]

Even these distinctions do not adequately explain the role of cholesterol in the formation of atherosclerotic plaques. Simply getting stuck in the lining of an artery does not change cholesterol into an artery-clogging plaque. Cholesterol particles of varying sizes are normally passed through the linings of the arteries to feed underlying tissues. For cholesterol to form a plaque, it has to be damaged, either by oxygen or by free radicals, before it is eaten with food or after it is produced by the liver. To monocytes, immune system cells patrolling the bloodstream, the damaged cholesterol appears to be an infected cell. The damaged cholesterol triggers the release of chemical factors that cause the monocyte to adhere to the lining of the artery and transform itself into a macrophage, a cell that is capable of absorbing dozens of times its normal size in cholesterol and infected tissue. The macrophage, rather than the cholesterol itself, clogs the artery. The more HDL is present near the oxidized LDL, however, the less likely the macrophage is to attach itself and create a plaque.[3] HDL opens up the arteries in exactly the same way as a nitroglycerine tablet, by encouraging the release of nitric oxide, but without any side effects.[4]

Infection and inflammation are other triggers for atherosclerosis. When any kind of healthy cell is injured, LDL is oxidized. The chemically altered LDL cholesterol attracts monocytes, the monocytes morph into macrophages to remove and recycle the injured tissues, and the macrophages form a plaque. Atherosclerosis can occur after a blood vessel is injured by high blood pressure, exposure to oxidant chemicals, infection with the bacterium *Chlamydia pneumoniae* or the herpesvirus, toxic concentrations of the bloodstream chemical homocysteine, or contact with glycosylated or "sticky" red blood cells coated with sugar byproducts in uncontrolled diabetes. LDL cholesterol that literally has become rancid (as that found in spoiled cooking fats) is also a major source of injury to the arterial wall. Oxidized LDL cholesterol circulating through the bloodstream also attracts macrophages. These misinformed white blood cells attack healthy arterial tissue to get rid of the bad cholesterol.

Saturated fat has long been known as a contributing factor to atherosclerosis. The pioneering study of the subject published in 1979, however, compared a diet consisting of more than 50 percent saturated fat (more than 1,000 calories per day just from saturated fat) to a diet containing 25 percent saturated fat. Making this dietary change was enough to lower total cholesterol by 15 percent.[5] Nearly 25 years of subsequent study have consistently found that lowering the amount of saturated fat consumed in the diet consistently lowered cholesterol, by allowing the liver to "catch up" to the amount of cholesterol it has to process. The activity of macrophages is the same whether the fat in the diet is saturated (such as the fat found in fatty meats and butter) or unsaturated (such as the fat found in canola oil). Inflammation in the lining of the artery, however, is greater when the diet includes saturated fat.[6]

Atherosclerotic plaques frequently become calcified, and these calcium deposits are associated with a high risk of adverse clinical events. Ordinarily, the flow of calcium in and out of a lining of an artery is delicately balanced so that there is no accumulation. Scientists speculate that in atherosclerosis some macrophages are transformed by a hormone (macrophage colony stimulating factor) to become osteoclasts, that is, cells that make bone.[7]

TREATMENT SUMMARY

DIET

○ Use olive oil in cooking as frequently as possible.

NUTRITIONAL SUPPLEMENTS

○ Vitamin E: 800 IU per day.

HERBS

○ Red yeast rice: Cholestin, as directed on label.

See Part Three if you take prescription medication.

UNDERSTANDING THE HEALING PROCESS

Medical science's understanding of atherosclerosis is surprisingly limited. Over half of people who have atherosclerosis do not have any of the risk factors for the disease: high cholesterol, high blood pressure, history of smoking, diabetes, obesity, or a sedentary lifestyle.[8] The understanding of the relationship between atherosclerosis and obesity is especially limited. While people who are overweight are at the greatest risk for developing hardening of the arteries, people who are underweight or of normal weight are at the greatest risk for dying of complications of the disease.[9]

On the other hand, alternative therapies that seem to be useful in treating atherosclerosis are numerous. An astonishing range of naturally occurring substances slow the oxidation of LDL cholesterol and the progress of atherosclerosis: cranberry extract,[10] the polyphenols in crème de cacao,[11] germanium (a component of computer chips),[12] hibiscus (the herb responsible for the tart taste of Red Zinger tea),[13] lycopene from tomatoes,[14] melatonin,[15] perilla leaf[16] (used in making some kinds of sushi), and even an oyster extract,[17] among many others. Because there are so many possible supplements for treating atherosclerosis, only the most available and least expensive alternatives to commonly prescribed statin drugs are listed here. (For general information about lowering cholesterol levels, see HIGH CHOLESTEROL.)

The statin drugs such as atorvastatin (Lipitor), lovastatin (Mevacor), pravastatin (Pravachol), or simvastatin (Zocor) lower cholesterol levels, but lowering cholesterol is not how they protect blood vessels. Their protective effect against atherosclerosis lies in their ability to stop inflammation. Statin drugs are expensive. Additionally, they can cause serious side effects: constipation, diarrhea, flatulence, nausea, muscle destruction, accelerated worsening of cataracts, and hepatitis. The longer they are taken, the less effective they are.[18]

Olive oil, vitamin E, and red yeast rice are inexpensive and widely available alternatives to statin drugs. The Mediterranean diet is rich in olive oil. Many studies have found that the Mediterranean diet is associated with significant reductions in the risk of death from complications of atherosclerosis. The Lyon Diet Heart Study compared a diet rich in olive oil with a standard low-fat diet for patients with heart disease. Atherosclerosis patients on the Mediterranean diet showed a 76 percent reduction in angina, pulmonary embolism, heart attack, and stroke after 27 months of the study. This finding was considered so significant that the study was stopped so that all participants could add olive oil to their diets.[19] No clinical study has ever found any other diet to protect more against death from heart attack.[20]

Clinical studies suggest that only a few people who take vitamin E on a regular basis can expect their arteries to clear as a result. However, taking vitamin E may keep atherosclerosis from getting worse.[21] The very latest scientific speculation suggests that vitamin E may be extremely important in *preventing* atherosclerosis, since vitamin E is oxidized before LDL is oxidized, in effect protecting it from the physiological processes that cause the formation of atherosclerotic plaques. Vitamin E is more important in the earlier stages of atherosclerosis than in the later stages of the disease.[22]

Some studies suggest that 100–200 IU of vitamin E per day may be as effective in treating atherosclerosis as 400–800 IU, which is the most widely sold dosage of the vitamin. However, since dosages for preventing atherosclerosis have not been determined, 800 IU is better for people who are currently in good health.

The use of red yeast rice in China was first documented in the Tang Dynasty in A.D. 800. It has been used to make rice wine and as a food preservative for maintaining the color and taste of fish and meat. The medicinal properties of red yeast rice were described in detail in the ancient Chinese pharmacopoeia, *Ben Cao Gang Mu-Dan Shi Bu Yi,* published during the Ming Dynasty (A.D.1368–1644).

Red yeast rice (Cholestin) contains a naturally occurring form of lovastatin (Mevacor), a commonly prescribed cholesterol-lowering medication. The first clinical study of red yeast was conducted in China. Physicians gave 324 people with high cholesterol (average total cholesterol, 230 mg/dL; average LDL, 130 mg/dl; average HDL, under 40 mg/dl) either red yeast or a placebo for 8 weeks. Total cholesterol dropped by 23 percent, LDL cholesterol by 31 percent, and triglycerides by 34 percent. Serum HDL levels increased by 20 percent.[23]

A second study gave 65 adults with high cholesterol either 2.4 grams of red yeast rice daily or a placebo. Participants in this study were asked to follow a 30-percent fat, 10-percent saturated fat diet with no more than 300 milligrams of cholesterol daily. After 8 weeks, the participants in the study who had been given red yeast rice had an average 18-percent reduction in total choles-

terol, 23-percent reduction in LDL cholesterol, and 16-percent reduction in triglycerides. In this study, there were no changes in HDL levels.[24]

Unlike lovastatin, red yeast rice has never been known to cause serious side effects. Red yeast products have only caused headaches and stomach upset. Some precautions, however, are prudent. Like lovastatin, red yeast should be avoided by women who are or who may become pregnant, by nursing mothers, and by anyone with kidney or liver disease. It should not be taken with antibiotics, cyclosporine (a medication for preventing rejection of transplants), niacin, or protease inhibitors.

If you have been prescribed any of the statin drugs atorvastatin (Lipitor), lovastatin (Mevacor), pravastatin (Pravachol), or simvastatin (Zocor), ask your doctor about using red yeast rice. This natural supplement costs significantly less than the prescription drug.

CONCEPTS FOR COPING WITH ATHEROSCLEROSIS

O Any cholesterol-reduction program is easier if you lose weight. Losing weight causes fat cells to produce more of a hormone known as adiponectin. As fat cells get smaller, this hormone makes it easier for fatty acids to leave the bloodstream for storage as body fat. While this makes losing weight harder, it makes lowering cholesterol easier.[25]

O Coenzyme Q_{10} helps the heart operate more effectively when its oxygen supply is limited. This supplement is especially useful for persons who take statin drugs, such as atorvastatin (Lipitor), lovastatin (Mevacor), pravastatin (Pravachol), or simvastatin (Zocor). It is recommended for people who take red yeast (Cholestin), which is also a statin. Statins interfere with the body's ability to produce both coenzyme Q_{10} and cholesterol.

O Natural health practitioners have recommended folic acid to lower homocysteine levels for many years. Some of the latest research supports the use of folic acid, but not because it lowers homocysteine levels, rather, because it reduces inflammation of the arterial wall.[26]

O European, especially German, physicians frequently recommend garlic as a means of reducing the risk of atherosclerosis.[27] No fewer than 37 placebo-controlled clinical studies consistently find that using garlic for 1–3 months lowers total cholesterol levels by as much as 25 mg/dl (depending on the preparation of garlic used, 12–25 mg/dl in 3 months). However, no study has found that garlic helps lower cholesterol for as long as 6 months and no study has found that garlic prevents or cures atherosclerosis.[28] What may be much more important, however, is preliminary evidence that garlic stops the oxidation of LDL cholesterol.[29]

○ Hibiscus, an herb found in Red Zinger tea, stops the oxidation of LDL cholesterol. Two of the plant chemicals found in hibiscus are stronger antioxidants than vitamin E.[30]

○ Smokers benefit from taking vitamin C. A study at the University of California at Berkeley found that taking 500 milligrams of vitamin C a day greatly lowered the concentration of bloodstream levels of F(2)-isoprostane levels, an index of oxidant stress. A mixture of antioxidants including alpha-lipoic acid, vitamin E, and vitamin C also lowered levels of this dangerous prooxidant, but not as effectively as vitamin C alone.[31] Since vitamin E is important in fighting other factors influencing atherosclerosis,[32] smokers should take both vitamins C and E.

○ Very preliminary research indicates that transcendental meditation lowers blood pressure and reduces or reverses atherosclerosis. Since transcendental meditators also tend to give up red meat and quit smoking, it is not clear how much improvement in health is due to meditation itself.[33]

○ Untreated gum disease increases the risk of atherosclerosis by 50 to 100 percent.[34]

○ If you live in a city with particularly polluted air, a HEPA air filter may be helpful in preventing the progression of atherosclerosis. Laboratory studies with rabbits have found that exposure to air pollution (such as sand, grit, dust, and soot) activates the immune system and increases the number of macrophages available to make cholesterol plaques.[35]

○ Type 2 diabetics sometimes have the option of controlling their blood sugars with or without insulin. While there are many drawbacks to the use of insulin, insulin therapy tends to open arteries. In as little as 3 months, as much as 25 percent more blood can flow through arteries of type 2 diabetics who have begun insulin treatment.[36]

Athlete's Foot

SYMPTOM SUMMARY

○ Mild to severe scaling between the toes

○ Itch

○ Red rash

○ Blisters covering the toes and sides of the feet

UNDERSTANDING THE DISEASE PROCESS

Athlete's foot is a chronic fungal infection of the skin of the feet, particularly between the toes. In the medical literature it is referred to as tinea pedis. The three species of fungi that most frequently cause athlete's foot are *Epidermophyton floccosum, Trichophyton mentagrophytes,* and *Trichophyton rubrum.* These organisms only survive in warm, moist conditions. They live in the stratum corneum, the outermost layer of the skin.

The fungi that cause athlete's foot are not readily infectious. They need precise conditions of warmth and moisture to survive, so they are not easily spread from person to person. The body's defense against athlete's foot fungus is to shed skin faster than the fungus can multiply, eventually ridding itself of the infection. When the feet cannot shed skin faster than the infection spreads, treatment is necessary. This is especially true when the fungus causes the skin to crack, leading to painful bacterial infections, especially in people who have poor circulation to their feet.

TREATMENT SUMMARY

HERBS

To treat athlete's foot infection:

○ Tea tree oil, in creams containing 8–20 percent tea tree oil or 40 percent solution, massaged into the feet 2–3 times daily. Use tea tree foot powders or sprays after drying the feet.

To prevent secondary bacterial infections:

○ Black walnut hull, one 500 milligram capsule daily.

○ Peppermint foot lotion, alternating with tea tree oil lotions for especially reddened skin on the feet.

See Part Three if you take prescription medication.

UNDERSTANDING THE HEALING PROCESS

Antifungal ointments containing clotrimazole (Gyne-Lotrimin), econazole (Eco-Derm), ketoconazole (Nizoral), or miconazole (Daktarin) can generally cure athlete's foot. They cannot, however, strengthen the skin against secondary infections, nor are they always successful in eradicating the fungus. One combination product, Lotrisone (clotrimazole plus betamethasone) was found to cause unusual hair growth and developmental retardation in children after it had been on the market for several years.[1]

Doctors typically reserve oral antifungal drugs for especially severe cases. The drawback to any antifungal drug taken orally is that it kills both pathogenic and friendly yeasts and bacteria of all kinds throughout the body, including friendly bacteria in the lower digestive tract. About 20 percent of the time, oral antifungal agents do not kill all of the fungus. The remaining infection is then antibiotic-resistant. The people who are most likely to benefit from systemic antifungal drugs are those who have severe athlete's foot infections occurring with skin allergies.[2]

Tea tree oil relieves athlete's foot infections, bacterial inflammation, and foot odor. It allows the skin to "catch up" with the fungus and eliminate it by shedding. Tea tree oil is not as effective as the antifungal agent tolnaftate in eliminating the fungus. In a clinical trial involving 104 patients with athlete's foot, only 30 percent of subjects applying tea tree oil were culture-negative, compared to 85 percent in the tolnaftate group. However, more patients achieved relief of scaling, inflammation, itching, and burning from tea tree oil than from tolnaftate.[3]

Black walnut hull was traditionally used in baths and compresses to relieve skin inflammation of all kinds. It contains tannins that "tan" the skin, cross-linking keratin proteins to form a protective barrier against bacterial infection. There is no direct scientific evidence to support the use of black walnut hull capsules in the treatment of skin infection in humans. However, toxicological studies of black walnut involving horses find that giving the herb orally makes the veins and arterioles in "excited feet" less likely to constrict in response to adrenaline, maintaining healthy circulation in times of stress. In horses, black walnut hull opens circulation in capillaries not previously filled with blood.[4] Oak bark, more commonly used as a bath additive, would have a similar effect.

Peppermint oil is a broad-spectrum antifungal,[5] although its use specifically in treating athlete's foot has not been clinically tested. Its use in relieving pain, however, is well accepted. Peppermint oil stimulates the nerves that perceive cold while simultaneously depressing nerves that perceive pain. The effect is cooling and soothing. After the initial cooling effect, there is a period of warmth. Its net effect in treating athlete's foot is to relieve inflammation and to assist other treatments in controlling fungal infection.

CONCEPTS FOR COPING WITH ATHLETE'S FOOT

○ To prevent reinfection with athlete's foot:

- Dry feet thoroughly after bathing or showering. *Trichophyton mentagrophytes* can penetrate the skin in 2–4 days at temperatures ranging from 50–90°F (15–27°C) if the humidity of the air around the skin is 100 percent. If the humidity of the air around the skin is lowered to just 80 percent, the fungus does not penetrate the skin at all.[6]

- Remove bath mats and shower grids. If the bathroom is kept at 80°F (27°C) or higher, they harbor fungi.

- Disinfect the floor of the tub and shower daily. All of the major household cleaners have been tested and found effective for controlling athlete's foot.

○ People who take the diuretic furosemide (Lasix) for congestive heart failure frequently have symptoms resembling athlete's foot even without fungal infection. Flaking and crusting will be absent although there can be intense burning and redness. This is due to a vitamin B_{12} deficiency. Taking 1,000 milligrams of vitamin B_{12} a day sometimes stops the burning and redness in as little as 2 days. It is necessary to continue supplementation at lower dosage, 100–250 milligrams a day, as long as you take furosemide (Lasix).

Atopic Dermatitis
See **Eczema.**

Atrial Fibrillation
See **Irregular Heartbeat.**

Attention Deficit Disorder

See **ADD and ADHD**.

Attention Deficit Hyperactivity Disorder

See **ADD and ADHD**.

Autism

SYMPTOM SUMMARY

○ Difficulties in or absence of speech

○ Hyperactivity, mental retardation, obsessive-compulsive disorder, seizures

○ Inability to form normal social relationships

○ Ritualistic and compulsive behaviors, such as humming or rocking

UNDERSTANDING THE DISEASE PROCESS

Autism is a developmental disorder that is usually first observed in the first 3 years of life. Children with autism are unable to develop normal social relationships. They typically withdraw into a world of their own. Children and adults with autism frequently engage in ritualistic and compulsive behavior, such as rocking or humming. They may be unwilling or unable to speak. People with autism frequently suffer from other disorders of the central nervous system, such as attention deficit, hyperactivity, mental retardation, obsessive-compulsive disorder, or seizures.

The causes of autism are not exactly known. Not everyone with the genetic makeup associated with autism develops the disease. The trigger for autism may be a viral infection, an enzyme deficiency such as phenylketonuria (PKU), or a chromosome disorder, such as fragile X syndrome.

TREATMENT SUMMARY

DIET

○ Reduce dairy products in the diet.

○ If there is a sensitivity to gluten (which can be deter-

mined by a saliva test), avoid *all* foods made with wheat or any other grain containing gluten. Sources of hidden gluten include caramel, gum, hydrolyzed plant protein (HPP), hydrolyzed vegetable protein (HVP), malt, maltodextrin, modified food starch, mono- and diglycerides, natural flavoring, soy sauce, texturized vegetable protein (TVP), and vinegar. Spelt, a wheatlike grain, has no gluten and is a good alternative to wheat in a variety of foods.

NUTRITIONAL SUPPLEMENTS

The dosages of magnesium and vitamin B_6 that are helpful in autism are high enough potentially to cause other health problems. Under a physician's supervision, give your child:

○ Magnesium: 10–15 milligrams of magnesium daily for every kilogram of body weight. For example, a child weighing 65 pounds (30 kilograms) would receive 300–450 milligrams of magnesium daily.

○ Vitamin B_6: 30 milligrams of vitamin B_6 daily for every kilogram of body weight. For example, a child weighing 65 pounds (30 kilograms) would receive 900 milligrams of vitamin B_6 daily.

Other supplements not requiring medical supervision:

○ Folic acid: 500 micrograms per day for a child aged 2–6; 1,000–1,500 micrograms per day for an older child or adult.

○ Vitamin B_{12}: 500 micrograms per day for a child aged 2 to 6, 1,000–1,500 micrograms per day for an older child or adult.

○ Vitamin C: 1,000 milligrams per day for a child aged 2–6; 2,000–3,000 milligrams for an older child or adult.

Autistic children who have sleep problems may benefit from:

○ Melatonin: 0.1 milligram 1 hour before bedtime, daily.

See Part Three if you take prescription medication.

UNDERSTANDING THE HEALING PROCESS

Most medical treatments for autism target symptoms rather than the disease itself. Prescriptions include anticonvulsants such as Dilantin (phenytoin) for seizures and the antidepressant Tofranil (imipramine) for attention deficit hyperactivity disorder (ADHD). An exception to this rule is the use of selective serotonin reuptake inhibitors (SSRIs) such as Prozac (fluoxetine) for compulsive behaviors.[1]

Serotonin is both a brain chemical that regulates mood and a neurotransmitter that controls the digestive system. In persons with autism, there seems to be some kind of defect in both the brain's and digestive system's ability to synthesize serotonin from the amino acid tryptophan. Monoamine oxidase (MAO) and other enzymes break down the serotonin the brain manages to make, at an unusually high rate. Additionally, there is an abnormality in the enzyme tryptophan oxygenase so that tryptophan is converted into forms the brain cannot use. At the same time, the presence of these chemicals in the bloodstream keeps tryptophan from entering the brain.[2] SSRIs attempt to correct these imbalances, as do several of the vitamin treatments discussed below.

Autistic persons are likely to be allergic to milk and gluten. In one study, 19 autistic children were treated with either milk-free and gluten-free diets or gluten-free and milk-reduced diets. After 1 year, there was an observable increase in social contact and a decrease in self-mutilation and "dream-state" periods.[3]

Your doctor can order a test for gluten sensitivity that measures gluten antibodies in saliva. For information, ask your physician to contact Great Smokies Diagnostic Laboratory in Asheville, North Carolina, 1-800-252-9303.

A series of studies have found that magnesium and vitamin B_6 used together are of considerable benefit in treating autism, considerably more than either supplement used by itself.[4] Supplementation with magnesium and vitamin B_6 reduces the excretion of homovanillic acid, which is a rough measure of the presence of the stress hormones epinephrine and norepinephrine in the brain. Presumably the combination of supplements reduces stress. Approximately 35 percent of children will respond to this combination within 2 weeks.[5]

The dosages of magnesium used in these studies are high. Like milk of magnesia, magnesium taken in high dosages is likely to cause loose stools. In extreme cases, magnesium overdose can cause diarrhea resulting in dehydration. The symptoms of dehydration may be harder to detect in an autistic child. There has even been a case of death caused by excessive use of magnesium supplements in a developmentally and physically disabled child.[6] For this reason, physician supervision is required if you plan to give your child high-dosage magnesium supplements.

Folic acid, vitamin B_{12}, and vitamin C together increase the body's production of tetrahydrobiopterin (BH_4). In turn, BH_4 increases the activity of tryptophan hydroxylase, an enzyme used by the brain to synthesize serotonin. Since serotonin deficiencies are observed in most autistics, the combination of these vitamins may relieve symptoms.

Consult your physician before giving your child folic acid if he or she also takes prescription medication for seizures. Folic acid can lower bloodstream levels of seizure medications and seizure medications can lower bloodstream levels of folic acid. This is especially true of phenytoin (Dilantin).

Some treatments for acid reflux deplete the body's supply of vitamin B_{12}. Autistics who are given either over-the-counter or prescription medicine for acid reflux, GERD, or heartburn are likely to benefit from supplemental vitamin B_{12}.

A recent study at the San Gerardo Hospital in Milan found that none of the autistic children studied had a normal day-night sleep rhythm.[7] A study published in Japan found that restoring normal sleep patterns with melatonin greatly reduced "excitability," although it had no effect on compulsive behaviors or "obstinacy."[8] In older children, giving the melatonin as late as possible (for instance, at 11 P.M. rather than at 9 P.M.) may prolong morning sleep and reduce sleep disruptions.[9]

Autistic children who are prone to seizures should never be given melatonin. In some cases, melatonin aggravates depression. If your child becomes especially withdrawn after being given melatonin, lower the dosage or discontinue the supplement.

Iron deficiency is relatively common in children with autism.[10] Since inadequate iron can interfere with growth and development in many ways, be sure to ask your physician to check your child's bloodstream iron levels.

CONCEPTS FOR COPING WITH AUTISM

Parent-administered and experimental treatments attempt to treat the underlying disease, although sometimes on shaky science. The most popular experimental treatment for autism in recent years is secretin. Like serotonin, secretin is a neurotransmitter, a polypeptide that relays messages from the central nervous system to the liver, pancreas, and stomach. Secretin travels from the brain to the digestive tract to:

O Stimulate the pancreas to release digestive fluids that are rich in bicarbonate, neutralizing the acidity of the intestine.

O Stimulate the stomach to produce pepsin, an enzyme that aids digestion of protein.

O Stimulate the liver to produce bile, which emulsifies fats and helps in the digestion of cholesterol.

Since many autistics have chronic problems with digestion, it is a logical question to ask whether secretin deficiencies have some relationship to the condition. An experimental study with lab rats in the early 1980s found that secretin increased the delay time before animals jumped to avoid an aversive stimulus.[11] A follow-up study in 1995 found that injections of secretin decreased responses to novel items, limited movement in an unrestrained environment, and eased respiration.[12] Then the first reports of secretin treatments of autistic children appeared in 1998. Pediatricians at the University of Maryland School of Medicine reported results of intravenous secretin therapy in 3 autistic children, stating:

"Within 5 weeks of the secretin infusion, a significant amelioration of the children's gastrointestinal symptoms was observed, as was a dramatic improvement in their behavior, manifested as improved eye contact, alertness, and expansion of expressive language. These clinical observations suggest an association between gastrointestinal and brain function in patients with autistic behavior."[13]

These preliminary findings inspired a series of tests of intravenous secretin. Objective evidence of the value of secretin remains elusive, and the reason may be that there are profound differences in perspective between researchers studying autistic children and parents of autistic children. In the most recent study of the supplement, for example, researchers at Harvard Medical School and the University of California at San Francisco gave 20 children aged 3–6 with autism and gastrointestinal symptoms (chronic diarrhea, acid reflux, or constipation) a single injection of intravenous secretin and then gave the children 4 psychological evaluations over a period of 5 weeks. The researchers then attempted to measure the benefits of treatment in structured play ses-

sions with developmentally appropriate toys. In the highly structured test environment, the researchers were unable to find any decreases in atypical behaviors, increases in prosocial behaviors, or significant changes in language skills. In the highly unstructured environment of daily life with an autistic child, however, 14 of 20 sets of parents noted moderate to high improvement in their child's language and behavior, and 17 of 20 sets of parents felt that their child would obtain at least some additional benefits from another infusion of secretin.[14]

Even though there are many indications that secretin will eventually be useful in the treatment of autistic children, the optimal forms and dosages and possible side effects are not completely studied. At the time this book is being written, it is premature to recommend secretin as a supplemental treatment for autism, especially since the clinical studies used intravenously administered secretin rather than orally administered secretin. Moreover, all preparations of secretin are not of equal therapeutic value. Biological labs that provide this enzyme offer secretin extracted from tissues of humans, pigs, and rats. Since most of the secretin on the market is prepared for medical research rather than for medical treatment, caution in choice of supply is advised for parents who choose to try the treatment despite its risks.

Back Pain

SYMPTOM SUMMARY

O Pain in the lower back and buttocks, sometimes extending to the knees

O May or may not be immediately preceded by injury

UNDERSTANDING THE DISEASE PROCESS

Lower back pain is among the most common health problems. It is the leading cause of job-related disability, the second most common cause of missed work days, and the leading cause of disability in people aged 18 to 45. Back pain is most likely to occur between the ages of 30 and 50, during the most productive period of most people's lives. Fortunately, most cases of lower back pain are self-limited. That is, they go away no matter how they are treated. For some people, lower back pain becomes chronic, meaning it does not go away and causes problems indefinitely.

Lower back pain usually develops over a period of years from accumulated abuses of the spine, many of which are not painful when they are incurred. Even when there is a single, identifiable acute injury that causes the lower back to hurt, the overall condition of the back, not just the condition of the spine, determines the speed of recovery and whether back pain becomes permanent.

The lower back is also known as the lumbar spine, the last five vertebrae of the backbone. The vertebrae are the bones of the spine, separated by disks, which are flat, round ligaments that hold the vertebrae together. As the vertebrae are stacked on each other, they form a column in the front and a tube in the back. The tube contains the spinal cord and other nerves. The column is held together by facet joints that allow it to bend as the body bends. Like other joints, the facet joints can be attacked by arthritis.

Many of the problems that cause chronic lower back pain are the result of degeneration of the disks. The disks act as a shock absorber. As they are exposed to various kinds of wear and tear, healthy tissues are replaced by weaker scar tissues so that eventually the disks may fail. The most dramatic form of disk failure is a herniated disk, in which a tear in the ligaments connecting the vertebrae allows the contents of the disk to pour into the canal containing the spinal nerves. To make room for itself, the nerve secretes inflammatory chemicals that expand the canal, and also cause intense pain.

More often, however, a disk is merely degenerated so that it cannot absorb shocks between vertebrae. The bones of the spinal column become misaligned. Muscles around the spine go into spasm, tightening up to keep the spinal column from moving and injuring the all-important spinal nerves.

Pain caused by injury to the disks or vertebrae is usually limited to the lower back. It may spread to the buttocks, but seldom extends below the knees. Pressure on the nerves in the lower back generally causes sciatica, in which the sciatic nerves first become numb and later cause pain throughout the regions of the body they serve, extending to the lower foot. Compression of the entire spinal canal can cause numbness in both legs all the way to the feet. This loss of sensation is worse with activity, such as walking, and improves after rest.

The cauda equina syndrome, in which a ruptured disk expands to fill the entire spinal canal so that there is loss of control over urination or bowel movement, is a medical emergency. Always seek emergency medical care if you become incontinent while having lower back pain or numbness in the legs.

What the Studies Show

A study at a Canadian university found that 1 in 9 people in the province of Saskatchewan is disabled by lower back pain in any 6-month period,[1] and there is no reason to assume that the rates of back pain are any lower elsewhere in the developed world. Men are considerably more likely to have surgery for back pain than women, although symptoms severe enough to merit surgery are found with equal frequency in both sexes. Smoking cigarettes and driving a North American- or German-made car increase the risk of back pain, but smoking cigars or pipes, height, weight, wearing high heels, and participation in sports do not.[2] The best indicator of whether back pain will persist or go away seems to be how widely pain radiates through the body. One study found that people who have pain radiating to the legs and arms are more than 6 times more likely to develop persistent back problems than people who do not.[3]

TREATMENT SUMMARY

NUTRITIONAL SUPPLEMENTS

○ Calcium citrate: 1,000 milligrams a day.

○ Taurine: 500 milligrams 3 times a day.

○ Vitamin D: variable dosage, see below.

○ Vitamin K: 5 milligrams every other week, especially if taking antibiotics.

○ If you take aspirin or NSAIDs on a regular basis, you should also take a vitamin B supplement every day.

HERBS

○ Capsaicin cream, applied to the back daily. If you are sensitive to capsaicin, substitute diluted essential oils of peppermint, eucalyptus, rosemary, or wintergreen.

○ Devil's claw (as an alternative to aspirin or NSAIDs): 405–520 milligrams up to 8 times a day.

○ Willow bark (as an alternative to aspirin or NSAIDs): 1 teaspoon in a cup of hot water or tea, as desired.

See Part Three if you take prescription medication.

UNDERSTANDING THE HEALING PROCESS

Healing lower back pain requires strengthening the spine through adequate nutrition and careful exercise, and relieving pain. Dealing with emotional stresses is also important. Emotional stress causes the release of hormones that, in turn, cause microscopic packets in the ends of nerve cells controlling the muscles and skin to break open and release adrenaline and substance P, a chemical that helps pain signals jump from cell to cell.

Nutritional supplements do not have a direct or immediate effect on back pain. They prevent further injury to bone. Over the course of months and years, this reduces back pain, but you will not see immediate results (as you will from the use of the recommended herbs).

The two most important nutrients in strengthening the disks are calcium and vitamin D. Appropriate dose varies according to the contributing causes of the condition. When back pain occurs in conjunction with sunlight deprivation, such as working overtime or being confined to a sickbed, it is usually necessary to take 800–4,000 IU of the vitamin daily for 6 weeks, tapering off to a dosage of 200–600 IU a day thereafter to prevent deficiency. Healing of micro fractures in the disks, leading to reductions in pain, usually begins in 3–4 weeks. If your body is provided with vitamin D, it can use calcium efficiently. Usually 1,000 milligrams of any calcium supplement is sufficient. Calcium citrate is best.

Take calcium and vitamin D together, since vitamin D enhances the body's absorption of calcium. Don't take calcium supplements with meals including foods rich in oxalic acid (beans, rhubarb, spinach, or sweet potatoes) or phytic acid (matzo, nuts, and soy), since these foods interfere with the absorption of calcium. Do not take calcium *carbonate* if you take thyroid hormone (synchronic or desiccated thyroid). Other forms of calcium do not interfere with the body's absorption of thyroid hormone. Finally, avoid taking calcium supplements at the same time you take antibiotics, since calcium can form insoluble complexes with the antibiotics that are eliminated with stool.

Taurine increases absorption in the segment of the intestines known as the ileum, where 80 percent of bile acids reenter the bloodstream.[4] When fats are not lost in the stool, calcium and vitamin D are better absorbed. There are no side effects from using taurine. Taurine is most likely to be helpful if you have a tendency to have diarrhea; it is the least essential of the supplements recommended for back pain.

Vitamin K is necessary for the bones to make osteocalcin, a protein that controls the uptake of calcium. Deficiencies of osteocalcin result in increased risk of fractures, especially in the hips.[5] Vitamin K is synthesized by bacteria in the intestine, so vitamin K levels go down during antibiotic treatment. However, taking vitamin K supplements as infrequently as every other week is usually sufficient.[6]

The B vitamins thiamine, pyridoxine, and cobalamin (B_1, B_6, and B_{12}) make it possible to use lower doses of aspirin and other nonsteroidal anti-inflammatory drugs (NSAIDs) for the same degree of pain relief.[7] Lowering doses of aspirin or NSAIDs reduces stomach upset. Vitamin B supplements may be especially useful for sufferers of back pain who take the diuretic furosemide (Lasix) or who are heavy drinkers of coffee or tea. The drawback to using B vitamins is that they reduce the need for pain relievers, but they do not eliminate it. B vitamins enhance nerve function so that if the vitamins are taken for 3 days and the aspirin or NSAIDs are eliminated entirely, overall pain is worse.[8] Do not discontinue aspirin or NSAIDs without also discontinuing vitamin B.

Capsaicin, devil's claw, and willow bark offer pain relief. Capsaicin is the chemical that gives hot peppers their heat. As anyone who has cooked with chiles knows, capsaicin can cause burning, redness, and inflammation, especially to the eyes and mouth. The first time it is applied in a cream to the skin over a painful back, capsaicin causes these symptoms, but the nerve fibers serving the back become insensitive to it—and to back pain.[9]

Keep capsaicin away from your nose and eyes. Allergic reactions to capsaicin are rare but are not unknown, and there have been cases of hypothermia in people who used capsaicin in an especially cold room. It is theoretically possible that capsaicin absorbed into the bloodstream could reduce the bioavailability of aspirin; if you use capsaicin, use pain relievers other than aspirin.

Devil's claw relieves joint pain, but only if it is taken in an enteric-coated form that protects its analgesic compounds from being digested in the stomach. Do not use devil's claw with NSAIDs such as aspirin and Tylenol and avoid it entirely if you have duodenal or gastric ulcers.

Willow bark is a natural substitute for aspirin. It contains silicon, a less potent pain reliever than the salicylates found in aspirin that does not generally cause bleeding or stomach irritation. Do not use willow bark during pregnancy, if you have tinnitus (ringing in the ears), or if you are allergic to aspirin. Do not give willow bark or aspirin to children who have colds or flu.

CONCEPTS FOR COPING WITH BACK PAIN

❍ Listen to your back. Be aware when it is starting to give out, and don't try to be a hero or a martyr to pain. The most serious back injuries occur when you ignore pain.

❍ Good posture helps prevent back pain. Sit up straight, avoid crossing your legs, move without bobbing backward and forward. Rolling the pelvis when lifting or stretching helps prevent back strain.

❍ Some of the latest research finds that chiropractic care is most useful for back pain that can be localized to a single disk or set of disks.[10] Back pain sufferers who seek out chiropractic care are more likely to be given an effective exercise program and less likely to rely on bed rest than those who get back treatment from medical doctors.[11]

❍ Not one but ten medical studies have found that bed rest does not cure back pain.[12] Bed rest during the early stages of acute back pain can even make the condition worse,[13] although this doesn't mean that someone with a ruptured disk should go jogging, or even try to sit up in bed. While anyone with back pain needs to exercise, the benefits of exercise are usually more dramatic for women than for men and for people in sedentary occupations than for people in active occupations.[14]

❍ Sleep, however, remains as necessary for back pain sufferers as everyone else. If you usually sleep on your back, try sleeping on your stomach. Placing pressure on the stomach allows the spine to assume its normal S-shape and relieves stress on disks in your lower back.

❍ Children's backpacks can be a painful burden. The American Chiropractic Association makes a number of suggestions for helping children avoid back pain from backpacks.

• A child's backpack should never exceed 10 percent of the child's weight. If it is heavier, the child will tend to lean forward and use the muscles of the lower back rather than the shoulders. Ask teachers if heavy books can be left at school.

• Backpacks should be carried with both shoulder straps. Slinging the backpack to one side can cause spasms in the neck and lower back.

• Backpacks should have padded straps. Without pads, straps can dig in to the shoulders and cause redness and pain. Shoulder straps should be adjustable so that they can be secure but not too snug. Loose shoulder straps can cause the backpack to shift around so that the spine is stressed.

• A backpack should never extend more than 4 inches (10 centimeters) below the child's waist. A backpack that is slung too low places additional weight on the child's shoulders so that he or she leans forward and stresses the lower back.

• Backpacks with carrying compartments make it possible to place bulky or pointed objects where they will not come into contact with the child's back.

❍ The American Chiropractic Association also has suggestions for hikers who carry backpacks:

• Choose a backpack that matches your dorsal length—the distance from your shoulders to the bottom of your ribcage—rather than your total height.

• Place shoulder straps at the center of each collarbone. Shoulder straps are for stability, not to carry more weight.

• Be sure your hip belt is fitted over your hips, where your pants normally ride.

• When packing your backpack, place your heaviest items in the bottom and your lightest items at the top. This makes the pack more stable and reduces back pain.

❍ Parents with small children can reduce stress on the back by using light-weight baby carriers. It helps to alternate carrying the child with the right and then left arm, or to carry baby with a sling or a backpack on alternating days. If you need to carry your child a long way, use a stroller. It takes a minute or so to place your child in the stroller, but using the stroller can prevent considerable back strain.

❍ New mother's backs have to carry the weight of enlarged breasts with weakened abdominal muscles. Even though the idea of exercise after delivery may not be appealing, it is a good idea to begin back exercises as soon as torn tissues have healed.

○ Do as many exercises as you can—slowly. Useful exercises include:

• Abs squeeze. Squeeze your abdominal muscles every time you pick up your baby.

• Chest stretch. Stretch your chest muscles by interlocking your fingers behind your back for 20–30 seconds.

• Pelvic tilt. Lie on your back *with knees bent* and tilt your pelvis forward until you feel a slight tension. As your abdominal muscles grow stronger, curl your upper body forward with each repetition.

• Rowing exercise. Use a seated rowing machine with a stretch band.

○ Always lift with your abdominal muscles rather than with the muscles in your back.

○ Mattresses matter. People with ankylosing spondylitis, an arthritic inflammation of the spine, especially need a flat mattress and a low pillow for comfort. Other back pain sufferers benefit from mattresses that are firm but not hard. If you don't have a firm mattress, don't spend money on a new mattress without trying it out. Many people get relief from back pain by placing plywood beneath their mattresses.

○ Recent studies have found that massage is the best form of physical therapy for your back, better than both acupuncture and exercise.[15]

○ When it comes to exercise, don't let pain be your guide. Frequent exercise of all the major muscle groups is essential to preventing recurrent pain attacks. While back pain does not necessitate physical therapy or the supervision of a personal trainer on an ongoing basis, it is usually a good idea to obtain a few hours of professional instruction before beginning a regular exercise routine.

○ One to two weeks before beginning acupuncture for back pain, start taking 500 milligrams of DL-phenylalanine 2–3 times a day. DL-phenylalanine increases the analgesic effect of acupuncture in both laboratory tests with animals and in clinical trials.[16]

Bacterial Vaginosis
See **Vaginosis.**

Bad Breath
See **Halitosis.**

Balanitis and Balanoposthitis

SYMPTOM SUMMARY

○ Inflammation of the tip of the penis, followed by:

• Foul-smelling discharge

• Small red ulcers under or on the foreskin

• Non-erectile swelling of the entire penis

• Painful foreskin and penis

UNDERSTANDING THE DISEASE PROCESS

Balanitis is an inflammation of the glans or tip of the penis. In the related condition balanoposthitis, the glans becomes inflamed and irritated, usually as a result of infection with the bacterium *Mycobacterium smegmatis*. The foreskin exudes a mixture of dead skin cells, glandular secretion, and dead bacteria known as smegma. If the condition goes unchecked, painful, small red ulcers may form under the foreskin. In severe cases, the entire penis may become infected.

Balanoposthitis is far more common in uncircumcised than circumcised men. The appearance of the disease in circumcised men usually indicates a serious underlying health problem such as immune deficiency or diabetes. Standard medical treatments for the disease include circumcision and laser surgery.[1]

TREATMENT SUMMARY

HERBS

○ Any cream containing glycyrrhizin (for example, Simicort), applied under the foreskin after the area is cleaned and dried.

See Part Three if you take prescription medication.

UNDERSTANDING THE HEALING PROCESS

Glycyrrhizin is a chemical extracted from licorice that kills the *Mycobacterium smegmatis* and other microorganisms that can cause infections under the foreskin, including *Staphylococcus aureus* and the common yeast *Candida albicans.*[2] In addition to controlling bacterial and fungal infections, glycyrrhizin reduces inflammation, making it useful in treating balanitis caused by allergy or chemical irritation. Glycyrrhizin creams do not cause side effects, and they can be combined with prescription creams containing hydrocortisone for enhanced pain relief.

CONCEPTS FOR COPING WITH BALANITIS AND BALANOPOSTHITIS

❍ The bacteria and fungi that cause infections under the foreskin cannot grow in the presence of oxygen. Pulling back the foreskin every day for thorough washing and drying greatly reduces the severity of the infection. If you cannot wash under the foreskin, see a physician promptly. It may be necessary to slit the foreskin to allow drainage of fluids.

❍ When you take antibiotics for this condition, it is helpful to supplement 1–2 capsules of acidophilus or *Lactobacillus* daily. These naturally occurring bacteria produce vitamins in the digestive tract and compete with infectious bacteria for nutrients.

Baldness
See **Hair Loss, Male-Pattern**.

Barber's Itch

SYMPTOM SUMMARY

❍ Severe, deep pustules in the hair follicles of the beard, usually only on one side of the face

UNDERSTANDING THE DISEASE PROCESS

Barber's itch is the common term for tinea barbae, a fungal infection of the bearded areas of the face. In years past, the condition was called "barber's itch" because it was commonly acquired from infected hair-cutting instruments used in barber shops. Since the disease is limited to the follicles of the beard, it only affects postpubertal males.

The most common infectious agents in barber's itch are *Trichophyton mentagrophytes* and *Trichophyton verrucosum*. Most men who get barber's itch live in rural areas and acquire it from contact with dander from horses or cows. The condition is frequently mistaken for allergic contact dermatitis or eczema.[1] It is sometimes inappropriately treated by surgical drainage, which can cause scarring.

TREATMENT SUMMARY

HERBS

To treat primary infection:

❍ Tea tree oil, in creams containing 8–20 percent tea tree oil or 40 percent solution, massaged into the skin 2–3 times daily. Use tea tree foot powders or sprays after drying the face (or shaving).

To prevent secondary bacterial infections:

❍ Black walnut hull, one 500-milligram capsule daily.

❍ Peppermint oil, alternating with tea tree oil.

See Part Three if you take prescription medication.

UNDERSTANDING THE HEALING PROCESS

Antifungal ointments containing clotrimazole (Gyne-Lotrimin), econazole (Eco-Derm), ketoconazole (Nizoral), or miconazole (Daktarin) can generally cure barber's itch. They cannot, however, strengthen the skin against secondary infections, nor are they always successful in eradicating the fungus. Doctors typically prescribe oral antifungal drugs for especially severe cases. The drawback to any antifungal drug taken orally is that it kills both pathogenic and friendly yeasts and bacteria of all kinds throughout the body, including friendly bacteria in the lower digestive tract. About 20 percent of the time, oral antifungal agents do not kill all of the fungus. The remaining infection is then antibiotic-resistant.

Tea tree oil stops infections by *Trichophyton mentagrophytes* without causing antibiotic resistance. It allows the skin to "catch up" with the fungus and eliminate it by shedding.[2] Tea tree oil is not as effective as the antifungal agent tolnaftate in eliminating the fungus. In a clinical trial involving 104 patients with *Trichophyton* causing a related condition, athlete's foot, only 30 percent of subjects applying tea tree oil were culture negative, compared to 85 percent in the tolnaftate group. (Tonaftate is the active ingredient in Tough Actin' Tinactin.) However, more patients in the test achieved relief of scaling, inflammation, itching, and burning from tea tree oil than from tolnaftate.[3]

Black walnut hull was traditionally used in baths and compresses to relieve skin inflammation of all kinds. It contains tannins, which "tan" the skin, cross-linking keratin proteins to form a protective barrier against bacterial infection. There is no direct scientific evidence to support the use of black walnut hull capsules in the treatment of skin infection in humans. However, toxicological studies of black walnut hull involving horses find that giving the herb orally makes the veins and arterioles in "excited feet" less likely to constrict in response to adrenaline, maintaining healthy circulation in times of stress. In horses, black walnut opens circulation in capillaries not previously filled with blood.[4] Oak bark, more commonly used as a bath additive, would have a similar effect.

Peppermint oil is a broad-spectrum antifungal,[5] although its use specifically in treating barber's itch has not been clinically tested. Its use in relieving pain, however, is well accepted. Peppermint oil stimulates the nerves that perceive cold while simultaneously depressing nerves that perceive pain. The effect is cooling and soothing. After the initial cooling effect, there is a period of warmth. Its net effect in treating athlete's foot is to relieve inflammation and to assist other treatments in controlling fungal infection.

CONCEPTS FOR COPING WITH BARBER'S ITCH

O Experience in treating other kinds of fungal skin infections indicates that the men who are most likely to benefit from systemic antifungal drugs are those who have severe follicular infections occurring with skin allergies. For everyone else, the most effective program combines treatment with prevention of reinfection.

O Dry the face thoroughly after bathing or showering.

O If shaving is impossible, keep the beard trimmed and blow dry after showering.

O It is especially important to avoid matting the beard. *Trichophyton mentagrophytes* can penetrate the skin in 2–4 days at temperatures ranging from 50–90°F (15–27°C) if moisture is trapped on the skin.

Barotitis Media

SYMPTOM SUMMARY

O Intense pain in the middle ear after changes in atmospheric pressure

O Pain in the teeth as pressure decreases on the way up in an airplane

O Vertigo

UNDERSTANDING THE DISEASE PROCESS

Barotitis media, also called aerotitis media, is an inflammation of the ear caused by changes in atmospheric pressure. This condition most commonly occurs during air travel. Most jets maintain cabin pressure equivalent to the atmosphere at 5,000–8,000 feet (1,700–2,700 meters). The lowered air pressure causes free air in the ear canal to expand by about 25 percent. During a sudden increase in air pressure, as on descent back to the ground, air must move from the nose and throat into the middle ear to maintain equal pressure on both sides of the eardrum.

Barotitis media is a bigger problem for young fliers. Very young children cannot perform the Vasalva maneuver, that is, yawning and swallowing air to push air into the nose and throat and against the inner ear.[1] If the Eustachian tube is clogged by a cold or allergies, the pressure in the middle ear is lower than the pressure in the airplane cabin. Negative pressure in the middle ear causes fluid and sometimes blood to build up in the ear canal.

TREATMENT SUMMARY

DIET

O Drink water before and during the flight.

HERBS

Start 3 days before a flight.

For children:

O Echinacea: 300-milligram capsule or 1 teaspoon of alcohol-free extract 3 times a day.

For adults:

O Echinacea: 600-milligram capsule or 2 teaspoons of extract 3 times a day.

O Ginkgo: 210–240 milligrams daily.

UNDERSTANDING THE HEALING PROCESS

The simplest way to handle barotitis media is not to fly when you have a cold or allergies. If this is not possible, your first line of defense is to drink water before and during the flight. Drinking water partially compensates for the low humidity found in most aircraft cabins. Low humidity induces swelling in the nasal passages and the Eustachian canal. Washing your face while on the plane will also help.

Chewing gum, drinking water, or eating hard candy helps equalize air pressure around the inner ear. Children should be encouraged to drink water or chew gum immediately before landing, and babies should be given their bottles to drink.

Two herbs will be helpful provided you begin taking them at least 3 days before departure. Echinacea both stimulates the immune system and reduces inflammation in the inner ear. One study found that a teaspoon of *Echinacea purpurea* juice is as effective in relieving pain and swelling as 100 milligrams of cortisone.[2]

While 3 days of echinacea is extremely unlikely to cause any problems, some people shouldn't use echinacea on an ongoing basis. Women who are trying to get pregnant should avoid *Echinacea purpurea.* It contains caffeoyl esters that can interfere with the action of hyaluronidase, an enzyme essential to the release of unfertilized eggs into the fallopian tube.[3]

There is laboratory evidence that *Echinacea angustifolia* contains chemicals that deactivate CYP3A4. This is a liver enzyme that breaks down a wide range of medications, including anabolic steroids, the chemotherapy drug methotrexate used in treating cancer and lupus, astemizole (Hismanal) for allergies, nifedipine (Adalat) and captopril (Capoten) for high blood pressure, and sildenafil (Viagra) for impotence, as well as many others. *Echinacea angustifolia* might help maintain levels of these drugs in the bloodstream and make them more effective, or it might also cause them to accumulate to levels at which they cause side effects. Switch to a brand of echinacea that does not contain *Echinacea angustifolia* if you experience unexpected side effects while taking any of these drugs.[4]

Echinacea stimulates immune function, but it also slightly increases production of T cells.[5] These are the immune cells attacked by HIV. When there are more T cells, the virus has more opportunities to mutate into a drug-resistant form. The authoritative reference work

The Complete German Commission E Monographs counsels against the use of echinacea for treating colds by people who have HIV or autoimmune diseases such as multiple sclerosis. Later communications between the senior editor of the Monographs and the German Food and Drug Administration revealed that the warning in the reference book was based on theoretical speculation rather than practical experience.[6] Still, as a precaution, people with HIV should only use echinacea for a short-term basis to prevent barotitis media.

Ginkgo improves circulation in the ear. Many fliers attest to its practical value in preventing stopped-up ears after a quick descent. Ginkgo can increase the risk of bleeding or bruising if you take the blood thinners warfarin (Coumadin), clopidogrel (Plavix), or aspirin. If bruising or bleeding occur, stop taking ginkgo immediately. Don't take more than 240 milligrams a day because high dosages of ginkgo can cause nausea, diarrhea, stomach cramps, or headaches in some individuals.

CONCEPTS FOR COPING WITH BAROTITIS MEDIA

○ Children who do not have an ear infection often develop one after flying. However, existing ear infections are not made worse by flying.[8]

Basal Cell Carcinoma

SYMPTOM SUMMARY

○ A pink growth with a slightly elevated center, from which tiny blood vessels may be radiating, or

○ A shiny bump or nodule that is translucent pink, red, or white, or

○ An open sore that bleeds, oozes, or crusts and remains open for 3 or more weeks, or

○ Reddened skin or irritation on the arms, chest, face, or legs that persists for 3 or more weeks, with or without itching, or

○ A waxy, white, or yellow scarlike area, sometimes with a crust (this is a sign of an especially aggressive variety of this form of cancer).

○ In all forms of basal cell carcinoma, very mild trauma, such as washing or drying with a towel, may cause bleeding.

○ Basal cell carcinomas are less common on black or dark brown skin, but will usually contain concentrated black or brown pigment.

UNDERSTANDING THE DISEASE PROCESS

Basal cell carcinoma is the most common of all cancers. This sunlight-induced cancer of the skin will strike 4 out of 10 men and 3 out of 10 women in the United States at some point in their lives. According to the National Centers for Disease Control, every year there are 900,000 new cases of basal cell carcinoma just in North America.

Basal cells are skin cells that are pluripotent, that is, cells that can form skin, hair, or sweat glands. Ultraviolet light causes the C and T bases (of the A, G, C, and T of DNA) of basal cells to be transposed.[1] This DNA damage deactivates gene p53, which ordinarily makes sure that dividing cells "rest for repairs" if there are other defects in their genetic material.[2] Many skin cells with damaged DNA simply rise to the surface of the skin during their life cycle and are sloughed off. When the skin cells that form hair shafts and sweat glands are damaged by sun, however, they are trapped and form basal cell tumors.

Basal cell cancers occur almost exclusively on sun-exposed skin. In people with healthy immune systems, this kind of cancer is slow growing and rarely metastasizes, but can cause cosmetic disfigurement. Loss of vision is possible if the cancer is allowed to grow unchecked near the eye. Basal cell cancers growing near nerves can cause nerve damage and spread into the body. Since bleeding is common in advanced basal cell skin cancer, infection is a constant possibility.

TREATMENT SUMMARY

NUTRITIONAL SUPPLEMENTS

○ N-acetyl cysteine (NAC): 400 milligrams per day *during the summer.*

○ Selenium: 200 micrograms per day.

○ Vitamin C: 1,000 mg per day.

○ Vitamin E: 400 IU per day.

If you exercise vigorously out of doors, be sure also to take:

○ Alpha-lipoic acid: 100 milligrams daily

UNDERSTANDING THE HEALING PROCESS

Basal cell carcinomas are cancers. When they are identified, they require medically supervised removal. Early treatment is the most effective. A great deal of scientific evidence, however, indicates that the appearance of new basal cell carcinomas can be prevented.

The key nutrients for preventing basal cell carcinoma are antioxidants. Laboratory experiments with skin cells have found that providing the cells with selenium, vitamin C, and vitamin E *before* exposure to ultraviolet light greatly reduces the amount of DNA damage.[3] Even after exposure to sunlight, selenium and vitamin E help the skin make glutathione, which in turn stops the process through which sunlight causes apoptosis, the initiation of skin cell death.[4] N-acetyl cysteine (NAC), vitamin C, and vitamin E work together to protect p53, the gene that ensures that cells repair defects in their DNA before multiplying.[5]

Additional supplements may be needed for people who exercise in the sun. Strenuous exercise depletes glutathione. This naturally occurring antioxidant slows inflammatory reactions and is essential to the normal function of estrogen and testosterone. Laboratory studies with animals have found that supplementation with alpha-lipoic acid keeps glutathione from breaking down, especially in the liver and in the bloodstream.[6]

While the antioxidant supplements that fight basal cell carcinoma are largely free of side effects, there are some precautions to be observed in their use. No one in good general health should take NAC on an ongoing basis. At least one long-term study suggests that the antioxidant effect of NAC can actually interfere with some of the actions of the immune system against bacteria. You should only use NAC during your allergy season, or, if you have allergies all year round, for no more than 3 months at a time. Smokers who have had bronchitis for 2 years or less should not take NAC unless they are quitting. There is some evidence that NAC may activate eosinophils, the white blood cells that may cause the progression of smoker's cough to emphysema.[7]

Selenium is better absorbed if it is not taken at the same time as vitamin C. Vitamin C taken in the form of vitamin C with bioflavonoids can interfere with the liver's ability to process statin drugs for controlling cholesterol, calcium channel blockers for hypertension such as nifedipine (Procardia), or cyclosporine for preventing transplant rejection. Vitamin E should be used with caution by those who take blood thinners such as warfarin (Coumadin) or clopidogrel (Plavix).

CONCEPTS FOR COPING WITH BASAL CELL CARCINOMA

○ Sun exposure and sunbathing produce gradual skin damage even if sunburn is avoided. Ten to forty years can pass between the time of sun exposure and the development of skin cancer.

○ Put on sun screen with an SPF of 15 or higher everyday before leaving the house.

○ Don't go overboard and try to avoid the sun completely. Sun avoidance depletes the body's supply of vitamin D and, ironically, can increase the risk of skin cancer.

○ People who have had a basal cell carcinoma should have a skin exam every 6 months to 1 year.

○ Do not try to remove basal cell carcinomas by "rubbing them off." Some portion of the cancer will remain in the skin, and breaking the skin increases the risk of infection.

Bashful Bladder Syndrome

SYMPTOM SUMMARY

○ Inability to initiate urination in a public restroom

UNDERSTANDING THE DISEASE PROCESS

Bashful bladder syndrome, also known as avoidant paruresis, is a relatively common condition in which a man steps up to a public urinal and nothing happens. Urination may be impossible even though the bladder is uncomfortably full. Bashful bladder syndrome varies in severity. In mild cases, men need to use a stall rather than a urinal. In more severe cases, a man may only be able to urinate when the restroom is completely empty. In the most severe cases, urination is completely impossible away from home. Travel becomes impossible, and sufferers have bought homes near their places of employment so they can go home whenever they need to urinate. For reasons that have not been explained, more than 90 percent of men who have bashful bladders are first-born children.[1]

In about 15 percent of men over 40, bashful bladder is a complication of prostate enlargement.[2] For almost all men under 40 and the majority of men over 40, however, bashful bladder is a treatable anxiety disorder. A combination of practice and stress reduction can make bashful bladder bearable.

TREATMENT SUMMARY

○ Desensitization practice, described below

UNDERSTANDING THE HEALING PROCESS

Although antianxiety treatments help, the best way to overcome bashful bladder syndrome is practice. First, drink 2 or 3 glasses of water. Then, in the privacy of your home, practice starting and stopping your urine stream. This exercise strengthens the sphincter muscles that control urination and increases your conscious control of urination. (If you are unable to start and stop your stream of urine at will after several private practice sessions, you may have an anatomical problem that could be medically corrected. See a urologist.)

After you have practiced stopping and starting urination at home, enlist the help of a friend or therapist. Locate a public building, such as a medical center, with numerous restrooms. Drink several glasses of water, and then go to the building. With your associate watching the door of a restroom designed for multiple users, practice stopping and starting your urine stream and then fully relieving your bladder. After several practice sessions, tell your helper to wait a few minutes and then come in to the restroom. If you experience severe anxiety when your helper enters, ask him to leave and then finish urinating. At your next session, your helper should come in at a time of his own choosing. After three or four successful sessions with the help of a confederate during which you have been able to allow him to stand at the stall next to you while you relieve yourself, you should try urinating in a public restroom at a public event, such as a football game or a concert.

CONCEPTS FOR COPING WITH BASHFUL BLADDER SYNDROME

O Some therapists use biofeedback to teach pelvic floor retraining, conscious control over the muscles controlling the bladder. Before you begin a biofeedback program, however, you should have a medical examination to make sure there is no anatomical obstruction blocking your bladder.

O Natural health expert Artem Agafonov reports that in Eastern Europe bashful bladder syndrome is treated by exercising (not urinating) in public while wearing a minimum of clothing. Men who are able to appear in public with minimal attention to modesty tend to "forget" to have a bashful bladder.

O Physicians frequently prescribe antidepressants such as Paxil or Zoloft to treat bashful bladder. While they may facilitate urination, they can interfere with orgasm. The less frequently prescribed blood pressure medication atenolol also relaxes the bladder but interferes with sexual intercourse.

O If you have not yet overcome the condition, travel with bashful bladder syndrome is not impossible. The International Paruresis Association maintains a partial list of gas stations and restaurants that offer private restrooms with locked doors. Nationwide, Exxon stations usually offer private, locked bathrooms.

O Young men with bashful bladder syndrome are frequently misdiagnosed as having prostate infections. Consider taking steps to treat bashful bladder if difficulty in urination persists even when there are no signs of infection.

Bechterew's Disease

SYMPTOM SUMMARY

O Lower back pain that comes and goes, usually most severe in the morning or after a period of inactivity

O Fatigue

O Fever

O Hip deformity causing limited range of motion

O Loss of appetite and weight loss

O Occasional inflammation of the iris of the eye

O Pain and limited expansion of the chest due to peripheral arthritis involving shoulders, hips, and knees

O Stiffness and limited motion of the lower spine

O Tenderness over sites of inflammation

O Upper lobe pulmonary fibrosis (mimicking tuberculosis)

UNDERSTANDING THE DISEASE PROCESS

Bechterew's disease is also known as Marie Strumpell disease or ankylosing spondylitis, *ankylosing* referring to stiffening, *spondyl* referring to the spine, and -*itis* referring to inflammation. The condition is best understood as a form of rheumatoid arthritis of the spine. It most frequently strikes young men.

Bechterew's disease causes inflammation, pain, and stiffness in the sacroiliac, intervertebral, and costovertebral joints. As the joints and ligaments become increasingly stiff, movement becomes increasingly difficult. If the disease is allowed to run its course untreated, the spine may become completely rigid.

TREATMENT SUMMARY

All treatments for rheumatoid arthritis are helpful for Bechterew's disease. See RHEUMATOID ARTHRITIS.

CONCEPTS FOR COPING WITH BECHTEREW'S DISEASE

O Morning stiffness is less intense if you sleep on a single pillow or no pillow at all.

O Swimming is an excellent exercise for Bechterew's disease. Any exercise program for Bechterew's disease should include deep breathing and stretches for the back.

O The medical literature reports a case in which adopting a vegan diet (no meat, eggs, milk, or animal products of any kind) produced remission of Bechterew's disease, with improvement in symptoms noticed on the third day. The patient resumed consumption of meat 6 weeks later, and complaints worsened. Returning to the vegan diet resulted in significant relief of pain and morning stiffness.[1]

Bedsores

SYMPTOM SUMMARY

Stage I:

○ Persistently reddened skin that does not blanch (turn white) when pressed with a finger

○ Tenderness

○ Itch

○ Skin warm to touch

Stage II:

○ Blister or open sore that does not extend through the full thickness of the skin

○ Red or purple discoloration

○ Oozing

○ Mild swelling

Stage III:

○ Ulcer has invaded the layer of fat just below skin surface

○ Sore may be black or white

○ Foul odor may be present

Stage IV:

○ Invasion of a muscle, tendon, joint, or bone

○ Sore may be black or white

○ Surrounding area reddened and warm to the touch

Signs of infection include:

○ Fever (may not be present)

○ Foul odor

○ Pus

○ Swelling and redness

UNDERSTANDING THE DISEASE PROCESS

Bedsores, also called pressure sores or decubitus ulcers, are injuries to the skin or tissues beneath the skin caused by continuous pressure. Most bedsores form on the buttocks, tailbone, shoulder blades, the heel of the foot, or behind the ankle or knee, all places where the weight of the body presses the skin firmly to the bed beneath it. This pressure creates a "no-reflow" phenomenon that temporarily cuts off the skin's blood supply. Injury to skin cells at first only causes an area of redness and irritation. If circulation is not restored over a period of days, however, skin cells die. Bacteria that do not require an air supply can flourish, however, and invade skin, muscle, and bone. Bedsores can become serious or even life-threatening if they are left untreated.

Bedsores are a common health problem in hospitals and nursing homes. According to one report, in the United States approximately 9 percent of all hospitalized patients have bedsores, as do 9 percent of patients in home care and 23 percent of all nursing-home residents. The risk of developing bedsores is greatest in persons who have cardiovascular disease or diabetes, stroke patients, men, and persons who consume limited protein.[1]

TREATMENT SUMMARY

DIET

○ Be sure to consume at least 3 servings of a high-protein food daily.

○ Consume at least 1,200 calories for every 100 pounds of body weight every day.

NUTRITIONAL SUPPLEMENTS

○ Calcium: 1,000 milligrams per day, not taken with food (to avoid interfering with iron absorption).

○ Vitamin C: 1,000 milligrams daily.

○ Vitamin E: 400 IU daily.

○ Zinc picolinate: 30 milligrams.

HERBS

○ Aloe: apply to bedsores daily until healed.

See Part Three if you take prescription medication.

UNDERSTANDING THE HEALING PROCESS

Bedsores heal more quickly at earlier stages. A bedsore at stage I may heal in 2–3 days. Deeper stage IV bedsores may require 6 weeks to 3 months. The speed of healing also depends on the patient's age, overall health, nutrition, and mobility. Strictly speaking, no scientific study has shown that good nutrition can prevent bedsores, although good nutrition certainly accelerates healing.

Medical surveys link the slow healing of bedsores

with deficiencies of calcium, vitamin C, vitamin E, protein, and zinc.[2] Vitamin C is especially important, since vitamin C deficiencies are a special problem of persons confined to nursing homes. It is also important to consume enough calories. As a general rule, 1,200 calories a day for every 100 pounds of body weight (28 calories per kilogram) are needed to give the body the energy it needs to overcome decubitus injuries.[3]

Vitamin C also has a special role in the healing of bedsores. The latest research on the use of vitamin C in the treatment of wounds has found that it keeps the basal layers of skin from contracting when the upper layers are injured. This allows regrowth of skin with a minimum of scarring.[4] A series of experiments with animals found that supplementation with relatively high dosages of vitamin C increases the strength of skin growing over the wound and accelerates closure.[5]

Be forewarned that vitamin C interferes with some prescription drugs. Vitamin C taken in the form of vitamin C with bioflavonoids can interfere with the liver's ability to process statin drugs for controlling cholesterol, calcium channel blockers such as nifedipine (Procardia) for hypertension, or cyclosporine for preventing transplant rejection. Neither calcium nor vitamin E is likely to cause problems in the dosages recommended here, but zinc should not be taken with antibiotic drugs. It can interfere with their absorption or possibly cause rheumatoid inflammation of joints.

Aloe is an anti-inflammatory, moisturizer, and emollient. It contains a number of antioxidant compounds promoting skin growth, including vitamins C and E and zinc. Unlike hydrocortisone creams used to relieve inflammation, aloe encourages skin healing while relieving pain. Wounds treated with aloe vera gel heal as much as 3 days faster than wounds treated with unmedicated dressings or with chemical antiseptic gels.[6]

CONCEPTS FOR COPING WITH BEDSORES

Many bedsores can be prevented by using simple measures to relieve pressure and to decrease the skin's vulnerability to injury. Preventive strategies include:

○ Inspect the skin at least once a day. Early detection can keep stage I bedsores from progressing.

○ Relieve pressure on the skin. Change position every two hours when in bed and every hour when seated in a chair. Relieve pressure on the buttocks, tailbone, heels, and back of the knees with a foam egg-crate mattress, water mattress, or sheepskin. If you cannot afford these, try an air mattress. Use pillows to raise the arms, legs, buttocks, and hips.

○ Reduce friction. Never drag tender skin across the bed sheets. Encourage the use of a trapeze to lift the body off the sheets or lift the patient off the bed yourself. Keep the bed free of crumbs and dirt that can rub and irritate the skin. Wash gently, avoiding rubbing or scrubbing the skin. Use sheepskin boots and elbow pads to reduce friction on heels and elbows.

○ Avoid using irritating antiseptics, hydrogen peroxide, povidone iodine solution, or other harsh chemicals to clean or disinfect the skin. Betadine can be diluted with sugar (1 part Betadine to 4 parts sugar) and applied to dry wounds.

○ Avoid massaging the skin over bony areas.

○ Avoid doughnut-shaped cushions. They can cut off circulation.

○ Use pillows or wedges to keep the ankles and knees from touching each other.

○ Do not raise the head of the bed more than 30 degrees, unless your doctor instructs you otherwise. Raising the bed more than 30 degrees may cause the patient to slip off the bed, rupturing small blood vessels.

○ Keep the skin clean and dry. Clean the skin with saline rather than with soaps. As necessary, use absorbent pads to draw moisture away from vulnerable areas.

○ Never place pillows under the knees. This cuts off circulation.

○ Try to exercise. Even bedridden patients often can stretch and do isometric exercises. Exercise increases circulation.

○ The principles of preventing decubitus ulcers in persons who are bound to a wheelchair are essentially the same as those for preventing bedsores.

Bedwetting

SYMPTOM SUMMARY

○ Nighttime urination without waking up in a child who has been toilet trained

UNDERSTANDING THE DISEASE PROCESS

Bedwetting, or nocturnal enuresis, is the loss of urine during sleep. A major problem for children, bedwetting is almost never done on purpose. Scientists estimate that approximately 50 percent of children who wet the bed have a hormonal deficiency. During the day, the kidneys are supposed to produce urine, but at night, the brain should produce an antidiuretic hormone (ADH) to shut down the kidneys. The brains of many children who wet the bed don't produce enough ADH at night, which causes their bladders to fill. When it happens to adults, they usually wake up and go to the bathroom, but bedwetters sleep through the night and wet the bed.[1]

ADH causes the cells lining the filtration apparatus of the kidneys to expand so that less fluid can pass through.[2] Insufficient ADH production, however, is only one of the causes of nocturnal enuresis. The bladder can be scarred by infection so that it does not hold enough urine. It can be irritated so that it is difficult for the child to hold urine in. Or a child can be an especially sound sleeper, not feeling the urge to urinate.

Nocturnal enuresis tends to run in families[3] and is more common in second- and third-born children,[4] but a few episodes of nighttime bedwetting are almost universal when children have recently become toilet trained. One out of every five 5-year-olds wets the bed. Only 1 child in 20, however, still has this problem at age 10, and only 1 in 100 experiences nocturnal enuresis by age 15. When bedwetting persists through adolescence and into adulthood, it is usually the result of a sleep disorder rather than a lack of ADH.[5] Daytime wetting may be related to a urinary infection, and is a reason to see a doctor.

TREATMENT SUMMARY

DIET

○ Avoid dietary sources of glutamate, including red meats, cheeses, and pureed tomatoes.

○ Eliminate aspartame, hydrolyzed vegetable protein, and MSG from the diet.

○ Limit fluids, especially caffeinated cola drinks, at bedtime (but not during the day).

○ If your child is on desmopressin, be sure to offer a low-salt diet: no chips, no pickles, no lunch meat.

NUTRITIONAL SUPPLEMENTS

○ Any children's vitamin containing vitamin B.

HERBS

○ Shut the Sluice Pill: as directed on the label.

See Part Three if you take prescription medication.

UNDERSTANDING THE HEALING PROCESS

The good news about bedwetting is that it usually is not associated with other behavioral or emotional problems,[6] and it usually disappears by the time the child is 8 years old. One of the most helpful things you can do to stop bedwetting is also one of the simplest. Make sure your child has many opportunities to urinate during the day and immediately before bedtime. Scientific study has found that simply encouraging a child to go to the bathroom more often—and doing nothing else—significantly reduces the number of episodes of nighttime bedwetting.[7]

Another relatively simple intervention is eliminating food sources of glutamate. These roughly correspond to a pepperoni pizza: red meat, cheese, and pureed tomatoes. (The glutamate in whole tomatoes is bound in a way that it takes longer to digest and never reaches nerve tissue unless tomatoes are eaten in massive quantities.) Hydrolyzed vegetable protein, a brown powder used to enhance the flavor of prepared soups and sauces, is another source of concentrated glutamate that must be eliminated from the diet. Glutamate is essential to the startle response in the brain. Some of the latest research shows that when a noise or movement in the middle of the night causes an especially strong urge to urinate, glutamate is involved.[8] Reducing dietary consumption of glutamate will diminish the startle response and may lessen bedwetting. Aspartate, provided by aspartame (NutraSweet), performs a function in the brain similiar to that of glutamate. Diet soft drinks sweetened with aspartame should also be avoided.

However, limiting fluids in general, especially during the day, is not a good idea. Fluid deprivation can cause dehydration. Limiting fluids at night is only modestly beneficial in controlling bedwetting, although some children do much better if they are not given caffeinated soft drinks before bed.

Most other methods of controlling bedwetting require nighttime effort on the part of parents. Alarm systems to wake the child when urination starts do not stop bedwetting by themselves. When the alarm sounds, the child still must get up and go to the bathroom. Parental intervention is usually required the first time the alarm goes off.

Responding to the alarm can be encouraged by appropriate small rewards for going to the bathroom when the alarm goes off and taking away those rewards for not going to the bathroom when the alarm goes off. Alarm systems without rewards are about 70 percent effective, but alarm systems with rewards are up to 98 percent effective.[9] The complication with the reward system, of course, is that the parent must be up when the alarm goes off. It is also important to note that the reward is *not* for a dry bed, it is for getting up to go to the bathroom when the alarm goes off.

Kegel exercises to control the bladder, often very helpful for adults, are of little use in children, and they should not be attempted at all if the child wets during the day or frequently has to rush to the bathroom. Older children, however, frequently benefit from them.[10]

Prescription drugs for bedwetting also have their limitations. The antidepressant imipramine (Tofranil), available as a generic, is a relatively inexpensive treatment for bedwetting, but since it is a psychoactive drug, it can cause major alterations in the child's mood and activity levels. Imipramine helps about 1 out of 4 children who are given it.[11]

Desmopressin nasal spray (DDAVP, Stimate) contains a man-made form of ADH, causing most people to make less urine during sleep. Drinking more fluid just before bedtime cancels out its effect, and eating salty foods makes the kidneys process more fluid to get rid of the salt.[12] Desmopressin only helps slightly more than 1 in 5 children under the age of six, although 4 out of 5 children 6 and older will have dry nights when they use the drug.[13]

Anticholinergic drugs such as hyosciamine sulfate (Donnatal, Spasmolin, and other trade names) and oxybutynin (Ditropan and Ditropan XL), based on chemicals originally found in the herb henbane, relax the bladder and help it hold more urine. This stops urgent trips to the bathroom both day and night. They can be extremely helpful for children whose bedwetting is due to bladder instability, but for many children with bedwetting they are of no value. They can cause nervousness and dry mouth.

European physicians frequently prescribe vitamin B for people of all ages who experience nocturnal enuresis. A relatively old German study found that vitamin B_6, in particular, reduces bedwetting.[14] There are no potential side effects from taking up to 1,000 percent of RDAs of the B vitamins.

The primary Chinese herbal treatment for bedwetting, the aptly named Shut the Sluice Pill, likewise is not enough to cure bedwetting—but together with other measures, it can increase chances of successful treatment. This herbal combination is made with dioscorea (wild yam). It contains phytochemicals that reduce inflammation on the lining of the bladder and make it less likely for an urge to urinate to occur during sleep or during the day. This decreases the number of uninhibited bladder contractions and gives the child greater control over urination, complementing the action of alarm systems or desmopressin. Shut the Sluice Pill is made by Jade Pharmaceuticals, and is sold under the trade names Sang Piao Xiao and Firm Vessel. It is also available from practitioners of Traditional Chinese Medicine.

CONCEPTS FOR COPING WITH BEDWETTING

○ Children who start wetting the bed after age 5 usually have had a bladder infection, usually undetected. See a physician if your 6-year-old or older child suddenly starts wetting the bed. Urine with a strong smell is a sign of bladder infection, which also should be treated by a doctor.

○ Wetting the bed can be a sign of high blood sugars. If you child is constantly hungry and thirsty and frequently wets the bed, or if your child seems to be making an unusually large amount of urine, make an appointment with a doctor without delay, to rule out the possibility of diabetes.

○ Protect your child from secondhand smoke. The production of antidiuretic hormone is less in the presence of secondhand smoke.[15]

○ Protect the bed by using a waterproof mattress or a fitted mattress cover under the bottom sheet. Mattress covers must be securely tightened at the corners to prevent the remote possibility of suffocation. For children over 6, place clean pajamas and sheets next to the bed so the child can change if he or she wakes up.

○ Diapers humiliate older children and do not train them to notice the urge to urinate at night.

○ To reduce the time required to make the bed at night after accidents, make up the bed in layers: plastic, sheet, plastic, sheet, and so on. This way the parent (and, later, the child) can simply remove the top layer of plastic and the sheet, place them in the tub, and go back to sleep. Noted natural health expert Phyllis Balch points out that that works better than using pull-up diapers, which can make a child who wants to be a "big kid" feel like a baby. Using pull-ups also implies, Balch writes, that the diaper will catch the urine and wetting the bed is not a problem that needs to be solved.[16]

○ Children should not use desmopressin nose sprays when they have viral infections, especially chicken pox or shingles. Blood clots can result.[17]

○ An interesting side effect of desmopressin is enhanced memory ability. The effect begins 15 minutes after taking the medication and lasts for several hours.

○ Some recent research has found that *teenagers and adults* with nocturnal enuresis can be treated with nicotine gum. Nicotine stimulates the production of vasopressin, without changing the total volume of urine produced by the kidneys and without disturbing the balance of electrolytes in the bloodstream.[18]

Bee and Wasp Stings

SYMPTOM SUMMARY

○ Bite, sting, or wound

○ Localized pain, redness, swelling, and stinging

○ Stinger visible in the skin

Symptoms indicating a need for emergency medical attention:

○ Difficulty breathing

○ Wheezing

○ Swelling in the throat

UNDERSTANDING THE DISEASE PROCESS

Bee and wasp stings are a common hazard of outdoor activities in warm weather. The stinger of a bee has shafts that become embedded in the recipient's flesh. In these shafts, there is a venom sac that releases a toxin into surrounding tissues. The bee itself dies after the stinger is torn from its body.

Bee and wasp venom contains a variety of enzymes, including mast cell degranulation peptide. This protein causes mast cells in the skin to release histamine, which in turn causes an allergic reaction that causes the skin to swell and isolate the foreign body left by the insect. The severity of the reaction depends on the number of mast cells in the skin available to release histamine. Once the mast cell degranulates, that is, when it has broken open, the histamine it releases may cause redness, itching, swelling, and pain.

Most bee and wasp stings do not require medical care. However, about 5 percent of adults in Europe and the United States suffer whole-body reactions to bee and wasp stings, and about 1 person in 100 has a risk of severe, potentially fatal anaphylactic reactions. Researchers have recently discovered that people at risk for anaphylactic reactions have high bloodstream levels of the enzyme tryptase, an activator of mast cells. Blood tests are being developed to detect tryptase so that people at risk for severe reactions can carry EpiPens for emergency treatment. Until the tests are widely available, anyone who has ever had a severe reaction to a bee or wasp sting needs to carry emergency equipment.

TREATMENT SUMMARY

NUTRITIONAL SUPPLEMENTS

○ Papain: applied to the area of the sting as soon as possible.

○ Simicort cream: applied after first aid to area of inflammation.

If you have a tendency for severe allergic reactions, also take:

○ Glycyrrhizin: 250–500 milligrams daily for up to 6 weeks at a time.

○ Green tea catechins: 250–500 milligrams daily.

○ Vitamin C: 2,000 milligrams per day.

See Part Three if you take prescription medication.

UNDERSTANDING THE HEALING PROCESS

Reactions to bee and wasp stings occur in minutes and usually last several hours. Two herbal products help speed up the healing process. Papain, a digestive enzyme extracted from papaya, is applied directly to the sting to relieve swelling. Licorice creams such as Simicort perform many of the same functions as steroid creams but without their side effects. One of the components of licorice, glycyrrhetinic acid, potentiates the effects of the natural anti-inflammatory hormone cortisol by inhibiting the enzyme 11-beta-hydroxysteroid dehydrogenase, which converts cortisol to an inactive form.[1] Licorice-based creams soothe and relieve pain.

There are also several herbal treatments that offer some protection against severe allergic reactions and help emergency medications work better. Glycyrrhizin is a licorice extract taken internally rather than as a cream. It increases the half-life of cortisol and other steroids, making it more likely that you will have adequate levels of the steroid in your system to fend off an anaphylactic reaction the next time you are stung.[2] In the People's Republic of China, glycyrrhizin is given instead of adrenaline to treat anaphylaxis.

The drawback of using glycyrrhizin for this purpose is that it *will* increase any side effects you experience from cortisone prescribed by your doctor to prevent allergic reactions. When you take both glycyrrhizin and any corticosteroid drug, you are more likely to experience weight gain, puffiness, and elevated blood pressure. (Glycyrrhizin has no effects on your body's responses to the other commonly prescribed preventative agent, diphenhydramine, better known as Benadryl.) Do not take glycyrrhizin for more than 6 weeks at a time. Preferably, use it during your peak allergy season. Do not take glycyrrhizin if you have high blood pressure.

A safer but less researched complement in allergy care is green tea. Catechins from green tea (and, to a lesser extent, from the black tea more commonly drunk in English-speaking countries) have been shown in laboratory tests with animals to significantly reduce the risk of allergic anaphylaxis.[3] The protective effect of the catechins is enhanced by caffeine. This stimulant stops the breakdown of norepinephrine, a hormone in the same class as the epinephrine in EpiPens.

Green tea catechin tablets do not contain caffeine. They are safe to use if you have high blood pressure. They work better if you also consume caffeine, but you should not take caffeine if you have high blood pressure.

Many, but not all, of the destructive physiological reactions in anaphylaxis are mediated by histamine.

Vitamin C is a natural antihistamine. Vitamin C prevents the secretion of histamine by mast cells and accelerates its degradation.[4] Laboratory experiments have found exponential increases in the release of histamine when vitamin C is deficient.[5] Research with animals indicates that taking relatively large doses of vitamin C offers protection against anaphylaxis without interfering with the production of antibodies against infection.[6]

CONCEPTS FOR COPING WITH BEE AND WASP STINGS

○ To avoid getting stung, stay away from areas with bees, use fragrance-free toiletries, do not wear dark or floral clothing, wear closed-toe shoes, and avoid eating outdoors in picnic areas or near garbage cans where containers for sugary drinks are thrown away.

○ Desensitization shots (venom therapy) are strongly recommended for anyone who has ever had a whole-body reaction to a bee or wasp sting. Not everyone is protected against whole-body reactions once they have reached the maintenance dose; some people will require larger than normal doses of venom therapy before they are fully protected against stings.[7] Don't be careless around bees and wasps just because you have had the shots.

First aid for bee and wasp stings for people who are hypersensitive:

○ Administer adrenaline and call for emergency medical assistance.

○ If the victim has coughing, wheezing, or shortness of breath, keep the airway open. Do not allow the victim to lie down.

First aid for bee and wasp stings for people who are not allergic:

○ Remove the stinger as quickly as possible. Scraping and pinching off are equally effective. Pinching off the stinger does not result in a bigger welt.[8] Do not use tweezers, however, since tightly pinching the stinger will release more venom into the skin.

○ If the victim has coughing, wheezing, or shortness of breath, keep the airway open. Do not allow the victim to lie down.

○ Wash the site with lukewarm water and soap. Cover it with an ice pack or a fizzy paste of baking soda and vinegar. Papain (an herbal ingredient in meat tenderizer) also relieves swelling, but should not be applied with baking soda and vinegar.

❍ To avoid swelling, remove rings, watches, and jewelry that may restrict circulation. Do not raise the site of the bites above the level of the victim's heart.

❍ Do not apply a tourniquet.

❍ Do not give aspirin or other pain relievers to the victim unless prescribed by a doctor.

Behcet's Disease
See **Multisystem Vasculitis**.

Belching and Burping

SYMPTOM SUMMARY

❍ Air coming up from the stomach with a characteristic sound. Belches are louder than burps.

UNDERSTANDING THE DISEASE PROCESS

Belching, or *eructation,* is the passing of gas upward from the stomach, usually with a characteristic sound. A burp is a small belch. Belching, although not life-threatening, can cause social embarrassment.

In ancient times, the unavoidability of belching was recognized both by scholarship and by imperial decree. The great physician Hippocrates wrote, "Belching is necessary to well-being." The Roman Emperor Claudius decreed that "All Roman citizens shall be allowed to pass gas whenever necessary." Unfortunately, no such authorities ease the social pain of uncontrollable belching and burping in public settings today.

Physiologists studying the phenomenon of belching frequently refer to it as "gas without gas," since dozens of studies have failed to yield a consistent explanation of the condition. Although it would seem logical that belching is the release of swallowed air, x-rays of patients with chronic belching problems frequently reveal flat bellies and no gas. Swelling of the peritoneal cavity in conditions such as ascites and extreme obesity would seem to be a likely cause of belching, but it is not.

And patients with mechanical bowel obstruction and gas problems that are visible on x-rays usually complain of cramps, not gas.

What physiologists know about the condition is that the average audible belch releases between 20 and 80 milliliters ($1/10$–$1/3$ cup) of air and that people who have a problem with belching belch from 40 to 200 times a day. Making a belch requires a simultaneous contraction of the abdominal muscles and relaxation of the sphincter at the top of the stomach. Suppressing a belch, or the sound of a belch, requires leaning forward. This is more difficult while wearing a seatbelt or shoulder harness. Obese people find suppressing belches more difficult than thin people, but are less likely to have them.[1]

TREATMENT SUMMARY

DIET

❍ Use Angostura bitters, caraway, chamomile, cilantro (coriander leaf), cinnamon, cloves, dill, fennel, ginger, juniper berries, orange or lemon zest, parsley leaf, parsley seed (in teas), peppermint, radish, rosemary, sage, spearmint, star anise, and turmeric as desired in cooking or teas.

HERBS

❍ Peppermint: tea made with 1 teaspoon of peppermint or 1 tea bag in $2/3$ cup of hot water allowed to steep in a closed container for 10 minutes.

See Part Three if you take prescription medication.

UNDERSTANDING THE HEALING PROCESS

If you see a doctor about belching, he is likely to order a breath test for the presence of hydrogen. Because bacteria are largely responsible for the production of gas, an increase in exhaled hydrogen in the breath test will suggest a food intolerance, usually to milk sugar. When foods are not digested, bacteria ferment them and produce excess gas. Food intolerance suggests that belching is not due to swallowed air or eating too fast, rather it is due to an inability to digest a food.

Breath testing is simple, noninvasive, and relatively inexpensive. It can be done at home or in the doctor's office. But if finances are a barrier to taking this test, another approach to the problem of belching is eliminating and then testing various foods. In a food challenge test, it is necessary to completely eliminate the test food from the diet for 4 days. Then make a meal of that food and nothing else and note the results. Since milk is the most frequent cause of belching, it is the first food that should be tested.

Belching is occasionally a symptom of a serious health condition. It may be caused by chronic cholecystitis (gallbladder inflammation), GERD (gastroesophageal reflux disease), hiatal hernia, or peptic ulcer. In rare cases, belching set off by drinking cold beverages can induce irregular heartbeat.[2] Seek medical help if belching accompanies loss of breath, racing pulse, chest pain, repeated vomiting, or abdominal pain.

Various carminative (gas-relieving) herbs have been used for centuries to relieve belching, bloating, and flatulence. These herbs include Angostura bitters, caraway, chamomile, cilantro (coriander leaf), cinnamon, cloves, dill, fennel, ginger, juniper berries, orange or lemon zest, parsley leaf, parsley seed (in teas), peppermint, radish, rosemary, sage, spearmint, star anise, and turmeric. Any of these herbs used in cooking or teas is likely to reduce gas formation and therefore reduce belching.

Of all the carminative herbs, the best scientific evidence for the relief of belching exists for peppermint. Scientists at the Cedars-Sinai Medical Center Burns and Allen Research Institute in Los Angeles have made extensive tests on the usefulness of peppermint oil in treating esophageal spasms, the uncoordinated muscle movements that make belches possible. Using a pressure gauge called a manometer, the research team measured pressure at the bottom and at the top of the esophagus before and after participants took peppermint oil. The scientists found that peppermint oil eliminated simultaneous contractions—muscle movements that allow the escape of air through the mouth—in all patients. Peppermint oil made contractions of the esophageal muscles more uniform and relieved chest pain in 2 of 8 patients in the test.[3]

Peppermint is the best-documented natural remedy for belching, but not everyone should take peppermint. Peppermint stimulates the release of bile, so it should be avoided by people who have gallstones, gallbladder inflammation, or severe liver damage. Anyone who has an allergy to menthol should avoid peppermint. If you cannot take peppermint, try increasing your use of other carminative herbs.

CONCEPTS FOR COPING WITH BELCHING AND BURPING

○ Eat slowly to avoid swallowing air.

○ Don't drink carbonated beverages or any beverages through a straw. This will reduce the amount of air getting into your stomach.

○ Avoid chewing gums sweetened with sorbitol or xylitol. These sweeteners contain complex carbohydrates that are not absorbed through the lining of the intestine. Instead, they remain in the gut where they are fermented by intestinal bacteria. The action of chewing gum also causes the swallowing of air, increasing the volume of gas.

○ Contrary to common belief, drinking beer does not cause belching. Hops, in fact, relieve stress-related digestive problems, although they are more effectively taken as an herb than in beer.

○ The Southwestern herb marrubio (horehound) is a bitter that relieves belching caused by eating fatty foods. Marrubio is traditionally taken as a tea, made by steeping 1 teaspoon of the chopped herb in 1 cup of hot water in a closed vessel for 10 minutes. The tea is strained before it is drunk.

○ Peppermint liqueurs also relieve belches and burping. Prepare a homemade peppermint liqueur by leaving 8 ounces of peppermint leaves in a bottle of vodka for 10 days, shaking the bottle every 2–3 days. Strain the mixture before storage. Take $1/2$–1 teaspoon of the liqueur between meals.

○ Lactaid is an over-the-counter product that may reduce belching caused by eating or drinking dairy foods and other products containing milk sugars, including convenience foods and medications. It treats an enzyme deficiency for milk sugar rather than an allergy to milk. To determine if Lactaid may be helpful to you, eat a normal breakfast and include a large, 12-ounce glass of milk of any kind. Over the next 6 hours, keep track of any discomforts you may have. (If you experience any kind of severe reaction, consult a physician.) The next day, prepare an identical breakfast with another 12-ounce glass of milk. Swallow a Lactaid tablet with your first sip of milk. If your symptoms are not as bad on the second day, Lactaid may be beneficial for you.

Bell's Palsy

SYMPTOM SUMMARY

❍ Pain behind or in front of one ear, followed 1–2 days later by face feeling stiff or pulled to one side

❍ Change in facial appearance

- Easy to frown, hard to smile
- Drooping face
- Difficulty closing one eye
- Drooling
- Impairment of taste
- Hypersensitivity to sound in the affected ear
- Difficulty eating and drinking
- Inappropriate secretion of tears ("crocodile tears") when laughing or talking

UNDERSTANDING THE DISEASE PROCESS

Bell's palsy is a condition causing drooping of one side of the face. It results from inflammation or damage to the nerve controlling facial expression, cranial nerve VII. This nerve makes it possible for the eyelids to close and the corners of the mouth to go up in a smile on one side of the face. It also controls the production of tears and saliva and the senses of taste and smell on the side of the face it serves. The unaffected side of the forehead may wrinkle but the affected side of the forehead will not.

People often remember exposure to a cold draft just before developing Bell's palsy.[1] A stormy day after a clear day also often initiates the disease.[2] Environmental stress may be the only common denominator for the disease, because there are many other risk factors.

Diabetes is a risk factor for Bell's palsy, as is a family history of the disease. The condition may follow infection with the virus that causes shingles or infection with syphilis, tuberculosis, or HIV. Bell's palsy can occur with autoimmune diseases such as rheumatoid arthritis, sarcoidosis, and Sjögren's syndrome, or result from poor circulation. Chronic ear infections contribute to Bell's palsy, since cranial nerve VII leaves the skull near the middle ear. In New England and in the Middle Atlantic states, about 1 in 3 cases of Bell's palsy can be attributed to infection with *Borrelia burgdorferi,* the bacterium that causes Lyme disease. The most common medical designation for Bell's palsy, however, is "idiopathic," that is, the doctor can find no underlying condition responsible for symptoms.

Anywhere from 1 in 1,000 to 1 in 250 people develops Bell's palsy in any given year.[3] It most commonly strikes people over 70 years old, but it can occur at any stage of life. Bell's palsy usually goes away on its own in 6–12 months. Chronic, slow worsening of symptoms may be due to a tumor affecting the cranial nerve and calls for medical examination.

TREATMENT SUMMARY

NUTRITIONAL SUPPLEMENTS

❍ Vitamin B_{12}: Given by injection by a nutritionally oriented health practitioner

If you have had shingles, also take:

❍ Essential fatty acids (black currant seed oil, borage seed oil, evening primrose oil, etc.): 5,000 milligrams daily

❍ Pyruvate: 3,000 milligrams daily

❍ Vitamin E: 400 IU daily

See Part Three if you take prescription medication.

UNDERSTANDING THE HEALING PROCESS

No treatment for Bell's palsy, whether conventional or alternative, is more effective than vitamin B_{12}. A clinical trial in Malaysia found that standard medical treatment with steroids brought about complete recovery in average of 10 weeks, although recovery times ranged from a few days to nearly half a year. Adding vitamin B_{12} to steroid treatments accelerated the healing process to 1 to 3 weeks, while using vitamin B_{12} by itself also brought about complete healing in an average of 2 weeks. The vitamin-only treatment group had the smallest number of patients requiring more than 3 weeks for recovery.[4]

The only drawback to using vitamin B_{12} to treat Bell's palsy is that it must be given by injection. Vitamin B_{12} is nontoxic even when it is taken in a dosage 1,000 times greater than the RDA.

If you have had shingles, three other supplements may also help accelerate your recovery. Laboratory experiments have shown that vitamin E, sodium pyruvate (a sports supplement), and membrane-stabilizing free fatty acids work together to stop lesions in herpes simplex, the herpesvirus responsible for genital herpes.[5] It is likely, although not scientifically proven, that will act the same way in treating complications of other forms of herpesvirus, such as the shingles virus, most commonly associated with Bell's palsy.

Be careful not to overdose vitamin E if you take blood thinning agents such as aspirin, warfarin (Coumadin), or clopidogrel (Plavix). Taking more than 2,000 IU of vitamin E and any of these drugs on the same day can make you especially susceptible to bleeding. Overdosing pyruvate can cause abdominal bloating, gas, and diarrhea. Any essential fatty acid can cause burping, flatulence, and runny stools if taken in overdose.

CONCEPTS FOR COPING WITH BELL'S PALSY

O Use artificial tears in your affected eye several times a day to prevent drying and infection.

O Head injury can cause recurrences of Bell's palsy. Be sure to wear a helmet when cycling or playing contact sports.

O Bell's palsy is an extremely common condition in the Chinese city of Kumming. Acupuncturists there have become adept at treating disease symptoms. In their technique, needles are inserted and withdrawn from a succession of points served by cranial nerve VII on the *unaffected* side of the face. Patients usually begin to improve after 2 weeks of acupuncture treatment.[6]

Benign Prostatic Hyperplasia (BPH)

SYMPTOM SUMMARY

O Urinary hesitancy (slowed or delayed start of urine stream)

O Blood in urine

O Difficulty urinating

O Incontinence

O Increased frequency of urination

O Nocturia, getting up to urinate 2–3 times or more per night

O Painful urination

O Urinary urgency (strong and sudden urge to urinate)

O Weak urine stream

O Especially severe cases may completely stop urination and require urgent medical care, but fewer than half of men who have prostate enlargement show any signs of the disease.

UNDERSTANDING THE DISEASE PROCESS

Almost every man eventually develops the condition of noncancerous enlargement of the prostate known as benign prostatic hyperplasia (BPH). The incidence of BPH ranges from fewer than 5 percent of men at age 30 to over 90 percent of men over the age of 85.[1] The prostate surrounds the urethra, the channel that carries urine from the bladder. When the prostate becomes enlarged or inflamed, it can "choke" the urethra, resulting in difficulty starting the flow of urine, decreased force of the urinary stream, increased nighttime urination, and intermittent stopping and starting of urination.

The prostate is located in the male pelvis, behind the pelvic bone, in front of the rectum, and surrounded by several blood vessels carrying blood away from the genitals back toward the heart as well as the nerves that make erections possible. Usually a little larger than a walnut, the prostate varies in size and measures from 1 to 2 inches (2.5–5.0 cm) long by 2 to 3 inches (5.0–7.5 cm) wide.

The function of the prostate is to create and release the seminal fluid carrying the sperm in ejaculation. The prostate is covered by a thin sheet of tough muscle known as the fibromuscular stroma. Although this is the largest part of the prostate, it contains no glandular elements. This tough tissue forces the prostate to grow in a direction that allows semen to drain down into the penis and not up into the bladder. Just inside the stroma there are three zones of tissue around the urinary canal. The outermost or peripheral zone contains glands that make seminal fluid. These glands drain fluid through a system of ducts that look something like the branches of a tree into the central zone, which contains a single cylindrical opening to the urinary canal. Just beyond the central zone lies the preprostatic tissue, which opens and closes the passageway for semen during sex. At the innermost part of the prostate lies the transitional tissue, a protective barrier between the prostate and the urinary canal and the only tissue affected by BPH. The zones of the prostate form concentric circles around the urinary canal. This is the reason why the transitional tissue becomes enlarged.

A man's body produces both testosterone, the male sex hormone, and estrogen, the female sex hormone, although it produces vastly more testosterone than estrogen. A byproduct of testosterone stimulates the growth of the tissue of the inner prostate surrounding the urinary canal, while estrogen stimulates the growth of the fibromuscular stroma. Androstenedione and the stress hormones produced by the adrenal glands also cause the inner circle of the prostate to grow, although they are not as strong as testosterone in this regard. As a man ages, the body's production of testosterone decreases while production of estrogen remains the same. More and more of the body's enzymes for removing and recycling sex hormones are required for removing estrogen, so that testosterone byproducts slowly build up in the prostate itself. Combined with the action of stress hormones (and androstenedione), the buildup of testosterone in the innermost lining of the prostate causes it to grow. Since estrogen also makes the stroma grow, the prostate cannot swell outward. It has to expand inward and blocks the urinary canal.[2]

For many years, scientists believed that excesses of testosterone, androstenedione, and the stress hormones were the only cause of BPH, but recent research suggests that the immune system also plays a role. Swollen prostate tissue is invaded by a class of white blood cells known as memory T cells. It is possible that the actual injury to prostate tissue is carried out by these cells. Every time the bloodstream experiences a surge of prostate-specific hormones, white blood cells that "remember" the last round of prostate enlargement multiply and converge on the prostate, infiltrating the inner lining and causing swelling and inflammation.[3]

TREATMENT SUMMARY

DIET

○ If you eat red meat, restrict consumption to 1 serving a day and gradually replace meat with cold-water fish, up to 3 times a week. If you do not eat red meat, include nuts and seeds and fish oil or DHA from microalgae in your daily diet.

HERBS

If erectile function is not affected:

○ Saw palmetto: 160 milligrams twice a day. (Combi-nations of saw palmetto and stinging nettle offer additional relief.)

If erectile function is a problem:

○ Flower pollen extract (for example, Cernilton): 60–100 milligrams 3 times a day.

○ Pygeum: 100 milligrams a day.

See Part Three if you take prescription medication.

UNDERSTANDING THE HEALING PROCESS

A peculiarity of prostate problems is that there are fundamentally different diets for prevention and for treatment. Typically, men are advised to avoid fatty red meats, eggs, and sugar. This is because these foods contain or encourage the release of omega-6 fatty acids, which in turn are used in the production of prostaglandins, inflammation-regulating hormones. As their name suggests, prostaglandins were first found in the prostate, although they influence inflammatory processes throughout the body. The hormones made from omega-6 fatty acids are essential to prevent bleeding after cuts and scrapes and to power the immune system's creation of inflamed tissue to surround the microorganisms causing infection. They also increase swelling in the lining of the prostate. When they cause inflammation, they are "remembered" by T cells that perpetuate the enlargement of the prostate gland.

Other prostaglandins manufactured from omega-3 fatty acids found in cold-water fish and seed oils act as a brake on the process of inflammation and decrease swelling in the inner lining of the prostate. It would seem logical that one way to control BPH would be to avoid meat and to eat fish or follow a vegetarian diet including seeds, such as pumpkin seeds. This simply is not true.

Recent scientific studies certainly confirm that reducing consumption of omega-6 fatty acids *prevents* BPH. A study of 3,523 men by the American Urological Association found that consumption of omega-6 fatty acids, those predominating in red-meat and high-sugar diets, is moderately associated with an increased risk of BPH. The study also found, however, that increased consumption of omega-3 fatty acids *also* increased the risk of developing BPH. Other measures of fat in the diet did not show a difference in rates of BPH, but total calorie consumption did. Men who consumed the fewest calories overall were the least likely to develop BPH.[4] The authors of the study speculated that the reason calories and fatty acids made a difference is that increasing calories and fatty acid consumption also increases the production of free radicals, chemical attractants for the white blood cells that remember inflammation. The study implies, but cannot prove, that taking vitamins C and E in addition to eating modestly on an ongoing basis is the insurance against BPH.

Treating BPH with nutrition requires a different approach. The only clinical study of the administration of fatty acids to men with BPH was conducted just before the beginning of World War II. Doctors gave a mixture of *both* omega-6 and omega-3 fatty acids to men with enlarged prostate for 3 weeks. At the end of the study, all 19 men in the study had improved flow of urine and 12 of the 19 men were in remission from all symptoms of the disease.[5] This does not mean that a daily breakfast of steak and eggs plus an occasional tuna fish sandwich is the best diet for men to avoid BPH. The equivalent of 2 or 3 eggs a week (and no red meat at all) is probably enough to avoid an omega-6 fatty acid deficiency. Men who follow strict vegan diets or who eat fish or take fish oils on a daily basis and who are concerned about BPH should have a blood test that includes a fasting lipid profile measuring the ratio of arachidonic acid (AA) to eicosapentaenoic acid (EPA). If the AA/EPA ratio is lower than 1.5—a very rare condition in the United States—reducing the consumption of fish oils or considering the consumption of meat or sugar is indicated. Men with an AA/EPA ratio below 1.5, however, are extremely unlikely to have BPH. Men with an AA/EPA ratio above 1.5, on the other hand, are extremely likely to develop BPH.

If you eat meat, add 2 or 3 servings of cold-water fish a week or 2–3 grams of pharmaceutical-grade fish oil or DHA from microalgae to your diet. Reduce your consumption of red meat to no more than 1 serving a day and your consumption of eggs to no more than 1 a day. Simultaneously reducing omega-6 fatty acid consumption from meat and eggs and increasing omega-3 fatty acid consumption from fish or other sources reduces inflammation in the prostate. Until you have your AA/EPA tested, err on the side of eating too little red meat.

Soy products are also frequently recommended for BPH. Scientific testing shows that consumption of soy reduces the weight of the prostate without lowering sex drive—in rats.[6] Since rats do not get BPH (humans and dogs are the only animals that get BPH), it is premature to suppose that soy helps this condition. Even strong supporters of the use of soy products in the diet maintain that rates of BPH in countries where soy products are an important part of the diet have not been confirmed by hard evidence,[7] and it is possible that lower incidence of BPH in these countries is related to eating fewer calories rather than to eating more soy.

In most of the world, the treatment doctors most commonly prescribe for BPH are herbal. In Germany and Austria, 90 percent of all prescriptions for BPH are for herbs. In Italy, plant medicines account for a little more than 50 percent of all medications prescribed for BPH, while only 1 man in 20 receives the drug most commonly prescribed for BPH in the United States, Proscar (finasteride).[8]

By far the best known—although not necessarily the most effective—herbal remedy for BPH is saw palmetto. There is abundant clinical evidence that taking saw palmetto relieves the symptoms of prostate enlargement. Saw palmetto is fully as effective as Proscar. Clinical studies in Germany have found that a combination of saw palmetto and stinging nettle improved urine flow just as much as Proscar and had fewer adverse effects on sexual performance.[9] Like Proscar, saw palmetto changes the metabolism of testosterone and stops the unchecked multiplication of cells in the fibrous sheath around the prostate.[10] Clinical studies published in 2002 confirm that it is more effective than another medication often prescribed for the condition, tamsulosin (Flomax); saw palmetto is more likely to shrink the prostate, and men treated with saw palmetto are less likely to experience problems with ejaculation.[11] There are even reports that balding men who take saw palmetto begin to regrow their hair (see HAIR LOSS, MALE-PATTERN). Roughly 90 percent of men with mild to moderate BPH experience some improvement in symptoms during the first 4–6 weeks of taking saw palmetto.

The problem with saw palmetto is that it frequently interferes with erectile function. If you have erectile dysfunction (ED), you should not take saw palmetto, and you should make sure any supplement you take for BPH does not contain saw palmetto. Stinging nettle acts on the prostate through the same mechanism as saw palmetto, and should also should be avoided in the case of ED.

The herbal alternatives for BPH when ED is a problem are flower pollen and pygeum. In Germany, where saw palmetto is very commonly prescribed for BPH, pollen is described by a medical association as providing "half the pain and twice the sexual pleasure" for men with the condition. Pollen especially reduces dribbling and decreases urgency or urination in about 75 percent of men who take it.[12] There are no side effects from pollen, although some men may be allergic to it. Tested in 18 clinical studies involving 1,562 men, pygeum is somewhat less effective than saw palmetto in increasing urine flow and stopping nighttime urination, but still helpful to a majority of men taking it.[13] Side effects of pygeum are rare, although it can cause diarrhea, constipation, dizziness, gastric pain, and visual disturbances.

CONCEPTS FOR COPING WITH BENIGN PROSTATIC HYPERPLASIA

❍ Don't drink beer. A 17-year study of 6,581 men in Hawaii found that an alcohol intake of at least 25 ounces per month directly correlated to the diagnosis of BPH.[14] Beer (although not other forms of alcohol) stimulates the production of the hormone prolactin. This hormone in turn stimulates the prostate to absorb more than the usual amount of testosterone, stimulating the growth of tissue in the prostate's inner zone. Beer also contains phytoestrogens that stimulate growth of the fibrous outer layer surrounding the prostate, increasing pressure on the inner zone.

❍ There are many homeopathic remedies for BPH. Except for sabal serrulata, it is usually best to start with a single dose of the lowest strength (6C, 6X, or 12C) of the remedy matching the symptoms to be treated, and then wait for a response. If there is an improvement in symptoms, let the remedy continue to work until there is no more improvement, then take another dose. If there is no improvement, try a different potency (30X or 30C). Sometimes homeopathic remedies work for a few minutes; sometimes they work for an entire day before another dose is needed.

- Apis mellifica is recommended for men who experience burning or stinging pain that is most intense at the end of urination. Homeopathic physicians sometimes recommend it when heat makes symptoms worse and cold relieves them.

- Causticum stops "leaking" caused by coughing or sneezing. It also treats anorgasmia, loss of sexual pleasure during the climax of sexual intercourse.

- Clematis relieves dribbling and slow flowing urine.

- Lycopodium is recommended by homeopaths when pressure is felt in the prostate before and after urination, especially when impotence is also a problem. Other indications for this remedy include bloating and gas.

- Pulsatilla is indicated when there is a yellow discharge from the penis, or when there is pain that extends from the penis back to the pelvis.

- Sabal serrulata is a homeopathic remedy made from saw palmetto (but the homeopathic preparation acts differently from the herb). It treats nighttime urination, especially in older men. Unlike most homeopathic remedies, lower potencies of sabal serrulata may be more effective than higher potencies.

- Staphysagria treats burning in the urinary tract that continues even when urine is not being passed.

- Thuja is indicated when there is a forked or divided stream of urine. It also relieves cutting or stabbing pain associated with urination.

Benign Senescent Forgetfulness (BSF)
See **Memory Loss**.

Biliary Cirrhosis
See **Cirrhosis of the Liver**.

Bipolar Disorder
(Manic Depression)

SYMPTOM SUMMARY

❍ Bipolar disorder causes alternating periods of depression, mania, and possibly psychosis.

Depression:

A depressive episode is diagnosed if 5 or more of the following symptoms last most of the day, nearly every day, for a period of 2 weeks or longer.

❍ Change in appetite and/or unintended weight loss or gain

- Chronic fatigue
- Chronic pain or other persistent bodily symptoms that are not caused by physical illness or injury
- Difficulty concentrating and making decisions, as well as memory loss
- Feelings of guilt, helplessness, hopelessness, or worthlessness
- Lasting anxious, empty, or sad mood
- Loss of interest in activities once enjoyed, including sex
- Restlessness or irritability
- Sleeping too much, or inability to sleep
- Thoughts of death or suicide, or suicide attempts

Mania:

Hypomania is a short-term condition, a milder form of mania. A manic episode is diagnosed if elevated mood occurs with 3 or more of the following symptoms, most of the day, nearly every day, for 1 week or longer. If the mood is irritable, 4 additional symptoms must be present.

- A period of behavior that is different from usual, lasting up to 1 week
- Abuse of drugs, particularly cocaine, alcohol, and sleeping medications
- Denial that anything is wrong
- Excessively "high," overly good mood
- Extreme irritability
- Inability to concentrate
- Increased energy, activity, and restlessness
- Increased sexual drive
- Little need for sleep
- Poor judgment
- Provocative, intrusive, or aggressive behavior
- Racing thoughts and rapid speech, jumping from one idea to another
- Spending sprees
- Unrealistic beliefs in one's abilities and powers

Psychosis:

- Delusions (false, strongly held beliefs not influenced by logical reasoning or explained by a person's usual cultural concepts)
- Hallucinations (hearing, seeing, or otherwise sensing the presence of things not actually there)

Psychotic symptoms in bipolar disorder tend to reflect the mood state at the time. Delusions of grandiosity, such as believing one is the president or has special powers or wealth, may occur during mania. Delusions of guilt or worthlessness, such as believing that one is ruined and penniless or has committed some terrible crime, may appear during depression.

UNDERSTANDING THE DISEASE PROCESS

Bipolar disorder results in mood swings from depression to elation without reference to life events. In some cases, either depression or mania predominates, and there are few shifts of mood. In other cases, mood swings are cyclic. In the United States, approximately 1 in every 60 people has bipolar disorder.[1] It usually becomes evident between the ages of 25 and 35 and is a lifetime condition.

Children and adolescents as well as adults can develop bipolar disorder. It is more likely to affect the children of parents who have the illness. Unlike many adults with bipolar disorder, whose episodes tend to be more clearly defined, children and young adolescents with the illness often experience very fast mood swings between depression and mania many times within a day. Children with mania are more likely to be irritable and prone to destructive tantrums than to be overly happy. Mixed symptoms also are common in youths with bipolar disorder. Older adolescents who develop the illness may have more classic, adult-type episodes and symptoms.

The causes of bipolar disorder are not known, but are believed to be of biological rather than psychological origin. Treatment of the condition is largely a matter of "what works," rather than a rigorously scientific intervention into a known biochemical process. It is especially important to avoid setting off a swing from depression to mania or vice versa by inappropriate pharmaceutical or natural treatment.

TREATMENT SUMMARY

DIET

○ Eliminate all refined and processed foods, especially breakfast cereals, peanut butter, and white bread.

NUTRITIONAL SUPPLEMENTS

○ Fish oil: 10 grams per day (preferably 6–7 grams EPA plus 3–4 grams DHA).

○ *Avoid* L-phenylalanine, SAM-e, and tryptophan.

○ *Avoid* L-glutamine during hypomania.

HERBS

○ Kampo formulas may be of considerable value if chosen to conform to the full pattern of symptoms.

○ *Avoid* St. John's wort.

See Part Three if you take prescription medication.

UNDERSTANDING THE HEALING PROCESS

Bipolar persons experiencing a manic episode usually require hospitalization. Confinement prevents them from aggressive and impulsive behaviors that may be of long-term detriment to their careers, finances, or personal relationships. Manic patients are typically hospitalized for 2 weeks and kept sedated until carbamazepine or lithium levels build up in their bloodstreams to levels sufficient to control symptoms.

Several studies have found increased levels of vanadium in hair samples from manic patients. These values fall toward normal levels with recovery.[2] Exactly how the vanadium ion influences the manic stage of manic-depression is not known, but scientists believe it may upset the balance of sodium and potassium in brain cells, altering their electrical charge and especially altering the activity of brain cells that inhibit behavior. Lithium counteracts the effects of vanadium.[3]

Fresh fruits and vegetables, fats, and oils are especially low in vanadium. Meat and dairy products, seafood, and whole grains contain moderate amounts of vanadium, while breakfast cereals, peanut butter, and white bread are especially high in vanadium.[4] Persons who take lithium may especially benefit from eliminating refined carbohydrates such as these from their diet.

Fish oil, a natural source of omega-3 fatty acids, is the newest and most promising natural treatment for bipolar disorder. In 1999, Andrew Stoll, an assistant professor of psychiatry at Harvard Medical School, and his colleagues announced the results of a 4 month double-blind clinical trial involving 30 men and women aged 18–65 with bipolar disorder. Half of the patients were given fish oil, and the other half were given an olive oil placebo. Eight patients in the study received no medication other than fish oil or a placebo.

The researchers attempted to measure changes in mood in the different groups. Patients ended their participation in the study and treatment was considered to have failed if the mood symptoms emerged or continued more than 30 days. Patients were also evaluated on Young Mania Rating Scale, Hamilton Depression Rating Scale, Clinical Global Impression Scale and Global Assessment Scale ratings, taken before and after treatment.

Overall, 9 of the 14 patients who received fish oil had relief of mood swings, while only 3 out of 16 patients who received the placebo experienced improvement. Of the 8 patients who received no other medications at all, the 4 patients who received fish oil remained in remission for a significantly longer time than the 4 patients who received the placebo.

The researchers do interpret their results as reason to recommend quitting other medications and taking fish oil. Patients who were only given fish oil had not responded to prescription medications offered to them before the study.[5]

Exactly how fish oil and other sources of omega-3 fatty acids relieve bipolar disorder is not known, but the researchers speculate that the incorporation of the polyunsaturated omega-3 fatty acids into the fatty layers of the cell membrane protecting brain cells alters the cell's physical and chemical properties.[6] Brain cells become less likely to forward the tremendous numbers of electrical signals that characterize a manic episode, in the same manner as lithium and Depakote (valproic acid), but without their side effects.[7]

Fish oil is generally regarded as safe when taken in usual doses, although some people experience fishy belches. Large doses such as those recommended for bipolar disorder can cause loose stools. Fish oil counteracts clotting factors in the blood, and should be used only under a doctor's supervision by people who take Coumadin, heparin, or other blood thinners.

There are at least three reports of manic episodes triggered by the use of SAM-e.[8] This suggests that L-phenylalanine and tryptophan could cause similar problems, although there are no reports of adverse effects from using these supplements. There is also a reported case of a high dose (2 grams) of L-glutamine triggering manic episodes.[9]

Herbal treatments may also help. Bipolar disorder was recognized in Traditional Chinese Medicine (TCM) over 1,700 years ago. Many of the herbal prescriptions devised by the master physician Zhang Zhong-jing in the second century AD treat various symptoms of the condition. In the teachings of TCM, bipolar disorder (*kuang dian*) results from an accumulation of emotional energies as "phlegm," causing not only physical phlegm in the chest and sinuses but also an "energy phlegm" that blocks the normal flows of emotional energy.

Over time, energy phlegm becomes a "fire toxin." Modern Kampo physician Giovanni Maciocia theorizes that anger, frustration, and resentment become energetically "fiery" over time. These energies begin to poison the immune system with physical, mental, and even spiritual results. Persons suffering from fire toxins of the triple burners lose their sense of direction in life and become depressed. Since the energies of the liver can no longer house what Chinese Kampo medicine calls the Ethereal Soul, sleep becomes disturbed and nightmares proliferate. In extreme cases, there may be symptoms Western medicine associates with the manic phase of bipolar disorder.[10]

Although Chinese medicine's theory of bipolar disorder is even less precise than that of modern medicine, Kampo herbal formulas frequently yield impressive results, especially in treating hypomania. The appropriate formula should only be chosen with the help of an experienced practitioner of TCM or Kampo. The most commonly used formula is Coptis Formula to Relieve Toxicity, available as a patent medicine from practitioners of TCM under the following trade names:

- CoptiDetox (Kan Traditionals)
- Coptis & Scute Combination (Lotus Classics, Sun Ten)
- Coptis & Scute Formula (Chinese Classics)
- Coptis & Scutellaria (Qualiherb)
- Huang Lian Jie Du Tang (Chinese Classics, Kan Traditionals, Lotus Classics, Qualiherb, Sun Ten)
- Oregedokuto Formula 016 (Kampo Institute)
- Oren-gedoku-to (Honso, Tsumura)

Like some prescription antidepressants, St. John's wort may cause a switch into mania in some individuals with bipolar disorder, especially if no mood stabilizer is being taken.[11]

The Danger of Suicide

Some people with bipolar disorder become suicidal. *Anyone who is thinking about committing suicide needs immediate attention, preferably from a mental health professional or a physician. Anyone who talks about suicide should be taken seriously.* Risk for suicide appears to be higher earlier in the course of the illness. Recognizing bipolar disorder early and learning how best to manage it may decrease the risk of death by suicide. Signs and symptoms that may accompany suicidal feelings include:

- Abusing alcohol or drugs
- Feeling helpless, that nothing one does makes any difference
- Feeling hopeless, that nothing will ever change or get better
- Feeling like a burden to family and friends
- Putting affairs in order (for example, organizing finances or giving away possessions to prepare for death)
- Talking about feeling suicidal or wanting to die

If you are feeling suicidal or know someone who is:

- Call a doctor, emergency room, or 911 right away to get immediate help.
- Make sure you, or the suicidal person, are not left alone.
- Make sure to put away medication, weapons, or other items that could be used for self-harm.

CONCEPTS FOR COPING WITH BIPOLAR DISORDER

○ People with bipolar disorder often have abnormal thyroid function. Because too much or too little thyroid hormone alone can lead to mood and energy changes, it is important that thyroid levels are carefully monitored by a physician. Low thyroid hormone levels are common in women with bipolar disorder who experience rapid cycling, shifts from depression to mania occurring over a period of days or hours.[12]

❍ Like other serious illnesses, bipolar disorder is also hard on spouses, family members, friends, and employers. Here are some considerations to keep in mind if you know someone with bipolar disorder.

• Often people with bipolar disorder do not realize how impaired they are, or they blame their problems on some cause other than mental illness.

• A person with bipolar disorder may need strong encouragement from family and friends to seek treatment. Family physicians can play an important role in providing a referral to a mental health professional. Sometimes a family member or friend may need to take the person with bipolar disorder for a proper mental health evaluation and treatment. There may be times when the person must be hospitalized against his or her wishes.

• Ongoing encouragement and support are needed after a person obtains treatment, because it takes time to find the best treatment plan for each individual.

• It is not unusual for people with bipolar disorder to consent to take drugs in the future while they are in good control. Follow-through during a manic relapse, however, requires intense supervision.

• Family members of someone with bipolar disorder often have to cope with the person's serious behavioral problems, such as wild spending sprees during highs or extreme withdrawal from others during lows, and the lasting consequences of these behaviors.

• Many people with bipolar disorder benefit from joining support groups such as those sponsored by the National Depressive and Manic Depressive Association (NDMDA), the National Alliance for the Mentally Ill (NAMI), and the National Mental Health Association (NMHA). Families and friends can also benefit from support groups offered by these organizations.

Bladder Cancer

SYMPTOM SUMMARY

❍ Blood in the urine, turning it red or rusty-colored

❍ Feeling a need to urinate but nothing comes out

❍ Painful or urgent urination

UNDERSTANDING THE DISEASE PROCESS

Bladder cancer is the most common cancer of the urinary tract. It most often strikes older male smokers, but it is more deadly in women. The early stages of bladder cancer in women are often misdiagnosed as a bladder infection so that treatment is deferred until it is too late. The women at greatest risk for bladder cancer live in rural communities. Nitrates from farm fertilizers contaminate drinking water and greatly increase a woman's risk of the disease, more than diet, failure to take enough vitamins C and E, or smoking.[1]

TREATMENT SUMMARY

In addition to medically prescribed treatments:

HERBS

❍ Milk thistle: 80–120 milligrams of silymarin phytosomes, 3 times a day

Consult your doctor before taking silymarin if you are receiving chemotherapy for bladder cancer.

UNDERSTANDING THE HEALING PROCESS

There is little reliable data supporting the use of natural methods for healing bladder cancer. Recent Japanese research has found that, at least in laboratory animals, silymarin stops the multiplication of bladder cancer cells and blocks the formation of tumors.[2] Since silymarin does not interfere with standard medications used in the treatment of bladder cancer and may protect the liver from damage during chemotherapy, it is given a qualified recommendation.

CONCEPTS FOR COPING WITH BLADDER CANCER

❍ The best prevention strategy for bladder cancer is reduction in the consumption of cigarettes. Cigarette use increases the risk of bladder cancer by 2–5 times. When cigarette smokers quit, their risk declines in 2–4 years.[3]

❍ Women who live on farms or in farm communities should drink bottled water.

❍ Eating broccoli, cabbage, cauliflower, and kale on a regular basis may lower your risk of developing or redeveloping bladder cancer. A study of 47,909 men found that eating broccoli and cabbage on a regular basis (5 or more servings per week) was associated with as much as a 68 percent reduction in the rate of bladder cancer.[4]

○ Eating meat is not associated with elevated risk of bladder cancer.[5] Eating grilled meat, however, does increase the risk of bladder cancer.[6] Grilled meats contain carcinogenic heterocyclic amines (HCAs), from creatine, a protein that is destroyed by microwave cooking. If you must eat grilled meat, heat the meat in a microwave for at least 60 seconds before putting it on the grill. Marinades made with cherry juice also prevent the formation of HCAs.

Bladder Infections
See **Cystitis**.

Blepharitis

SYMPTOM SUMMARY

○ Eyelids that are:
- Burning
- Crusted, tending to stick together in the morning
- Itching
- Reddened
- Swollen

○ Lump under the eyelid

○ Loss of eyelashes

UNDERSTANDING THE DISEASE PROCESS

Blepharitis is a condition of excess oil production on the inner surfaces of the eyelids, creating an environment favorable for the growth of bacteria. These bacteria produce hydrogen peroxide as they digest the oils, and the peroxide in turn causes burning and irritation. Small amounts of oil or dry mucus can float on the surface of the eyelid, causing a feeling of having dirt or sand in the eyes. The combination of oils and bacterial debris can block hair follicles so that eyelashes are not replaced as they fall out.

TREATMENT SUMMARY

CLEANING

○ Liquid tears or similar product: 3–4 times a day as directed.

DIET

○ Avoid excessive protein intake (more than 6 servings of protein foods daily). Eat 3 ounces of cold-water fish 3 times weekly, or take 1 tablespoon of borage seed oil, black currant oil, or flaxseed oil daily.

NUTRITIONAL SUPPLEMENTS

○ Biotin (for children): 3 milligrams twice a day.

○ Folic acid: 4–5 milligrams per day.

○ Vitamin B complex: 100 milligrams daily.

○ Zinc picolinate: 25 milligrams per day while taking folic acid.

OTHER HELPFUL NATURAL TREATMENTS

○ Honey: crude honey diluted with a small amount of warm water, dabbed on the eyelid and left for 3 hours at a time, daily.

○ Pyridoxine ointment: applied to the eyelid daily (can be prepared by any pharmacy, 50 milligrams of pyridoxine per gram of ointment in a water-soluble base).

UNDERSTANDING THE HEALING PROCESS

The most essential step in healing blepharitis is cleaning the eyelids every day, in the morning and at bedtime. Any crusts or scales on the lids should be softened with a clean, warm, moist washcloth and then removed by scrubbing the lids with a clean paper towel. The first time you remove crusts in this manner you will probably experience discomfort, but it is essential that you clean your eyelids every day to bring the condition under control.

Never use an antibiotic ointment on your eyelids without cleaning them first. If you do not clean the eyelids before applying ointment, you are medicating mucus rather than the lids themselves. Since the crusts created by blepharitis can block tear ducts, use liquid tears several times a day to help keep the eye clean.

If your blepharitis is persistent, consider dietary changes. There is a long-held belief in naturopathic medicine that excessive protein consumption, especially of fatty meats and eggs, aggravates conditions such as blepharitis. It is possible that incomplete digestion of proteins or poor intestinal absorption of protein breakdown products results in elevated levels of certain amino acids in the bowels. Bacteria in the bowels metabolize these amino acids into cadaverine, putrescine, and spermidine. These compounds enter the bloodstream and remove a biochemical "brake" on skin cell growth.[1] Multiplying unchecked, affected cells create tiny rashes and produce excessive amounts of sebum. Bacteria feed on sebum.

While this theory is unproved in the case of blepharitis, limiting the consumption of fatty meats and eggs is of general benefit to health. Supplementing the diet with cold-water fish 3 times a week or taking a tablespoon of flaxseed or hempseed oil daily counteracts another effect of excessive protein consumption, the inflammatory arachidonic acid cascade.[2]

Blepharitis in infants and children is greatly influenced by supplementation with biotin. A large part of the body's supply of this vitamin is produced by bacteria in the colon, which have not had a chance to be established in very young children. Supplemental biotin given to infants or taken by nursing mothers is effective against sticky eyelids.[3] In adults, however, biotin by itself is of no value in treating the condition.

Adults are more responsive to vitamin B supplements. Supplementation with vitamin B_{12} (cyanocobalamin) is helpful in controlling the production of the oily sebum on which the bacteria that cause blepharitis feed.[4]

Folic acid supplementation is helpful in treating blepharitis and will also help clear up oily skin caused by seborrheic dermatitis.[5] Since folic acid may interfere with the absorption of zinc, take 25 milligrams of zinc picolinate daily while taking folic acid.

Spreading a thin layer of honey on the inner eyelid once a day often relieves blepharitis in 2–3 weeks. In the United States, this technique is most often associated with ophthalmologist Mark Elder, but clinicians in the United Arab Emirates actually performed a systematic test of honey treatment for a closely related condition, seborrheic dermatitis. The clinical trial involved 30 patients with chronic lesions on the scalp, face, and chest. Twenty patients were males and 10 were females. All the participants in the study suffered itching and hair loss as well as scaling and dry white plaques with crusts and fissures.

Half of the patients were asked to apply diluted crude honey (90 percent honey diluted in warm water) on the lesions with gentle rubbing for 2–3 minutes every other day. The honey was left for 3 hours before gently rinsing with warm water. Patients were followed for 4 weeks. They were examined daily for itching, scaling, hair loss, and lesions. All of the patients who used honey showed a significant response. Itching was relieved and scaling disappeared within 1 week. Skin lesions healed and disappeared completely within 2 weeks. In addition, patients who used honey reported reversal of hair loss.

After the end of the 4-week test period, all of the patients were instructed to use honey for 6 months. Fifteen complied. None of the patients who continued to use honey relapsed, while 12 out of 15 patients who did not continue using honey experienced a return of the lesions 2–4 months after stopping treatment.[6]

Treatment with pyridoxine (vitamin B_6) creams, available from compounding pharmacies, is helpful in treating blepharitis and seborrhea that causes greasy scales on the face. In one study, all patients with these symptoms who took a pyridoxine cream cleared completely within 10 days. The creams were not helpful, however, for seborrheic dermatitis complicated by infection, and did not clear lesions on the neck, chest, or groin.[7]

CONCEPTS FOR COPING WITH BLEPHARITIS

O Personal hygiene for blepharitis has to be ongoing. The condition tends to come back when treatment is discontinued.

O A cleansing formula such as OcuClenz is best for initial treatment of blepharitis. You can also use Johnson & Johnson Baby Shampoo, *1 drop* diluted in 3–4 drops of water on a paper towel, to scrub your eyelashes at bedtime.

O Keep not just your eyelids but your hands and face clean. Women should not use cosmetics during the first 6–8 weeks of treating blepharitis. Makeup can be used after the condition is under control, but it must be thoroughly removed every night at bedtime with a baby oil or Vaseline on a Q-tip. Removal is repeated until the last Q-tip shows no makeup. Men and women alike need to shampoo thoroughly and daily, especially if there is dandruff.

O Many medications cause blepharitis (and oily skin in general) as a side effect. These include dopamine for Parkinson's disease; hydralazine for congestive heart failure and high blood pressure; isoniazid (INH) for tuberculosis; penicillamine for kidney stones, rheumatoid arthritis, and Wilson's disease; and oral contraceptives.

Blindness, Night

See **Night Vision, Impaired**

Bloating

SYMPTOM SUMMARY

○ Feeling of fullness and tightness in the abdomen, usually accompanied by excessive release of gas (more than 20 times a day)

UNDERSTANDING THE DISEASE PROCESS

Abdominal bloating is caused by gas you cannot pass. Everyone gets gas. The production of digestive gas, or flatus, is a normal byproduct of eating. Approximately 17 milliliters of air, a little more than a tablespoon, goes down with every bite of food and every swallow of liquid. This gas builds up to a volume between $1/2$–2 liters, anywhere from a pint to a half-gallon, every day. If gas cannot be released 6–20 times a day, the result is abdominal bloating, an uncomfortable feeling of tightness and tension due to gas pressing against the walls of the abdomen.

In healthy people, social discomfort is an important factor in bloating. Fear of releasing foul-smelling flatus inhibits normal release of gas. Approximately 99.999 percent of the volume of flatus is odor-free. However, very small traces of the sulfur-containing gases hydrogen sulfide, dimethyl sulfide, and methanethiol are sufficient to cause intense odor. These sulfur-containing gases are derived from sulfur-containing foods such as beans, broccoli, cabbage, cauliflower, or Brussels sprouts.

Another important factor in bloating is inflammation of the intestinal wall. Inflammation may cause sudden release of large amounts of flatus, or it may keep flatus from being released at all. Of course, without the production of excess gas, twin problems of bloating and flatulence never occur. Gas may be released from carbonated beverages or formed in the large intestine as the result of bacterial action on undigested food, particularly dairy products. Approximately 1 in 3 people in the United States lacks an enzyme needed to digest milk sugars. Fruits and vegetables can also cause problems. Even healthy people cannot digest large quantities of fructose sugars from fruit or the complex polysaccharides found in high-fiber vegetables.

Abdominal bloating is usually not a serious medical problem. Abdominal bloating accompanying severe steady pain in the upper abdomen, however, may be a sign of bowel obstruction, or, in women, of ovarian cancer. Bloating with yellowing of the skin or eyes in either sex at any age may be a sign of hepatitis. Either combination of symptoms requires urgent medical attention. Bloating with alternating constipation and diarrhea is usually a sign of irritable bowel syndrome (IBS), which also benefits from professional care.

TREATMENT SUMMARY

DIET

○ Use cinnamon, dandelion greens, the Mexican herb epizote (in frijoles or bean dishes), fennel seeds, and flaxseed powders (not whole flaxseeds) in your favorite recipes to reduce gas formation.

○ Avoid common gas-producing foods such as apples, apricots, bagels, baked beans, barley, beets, black-eyed peas, bog beans, bran, breakfast cereals, broccoli, Brussels sprouts, cabbage, cauliflower, chickpeas, chili, corn, cucumbers, dairy products (in people who are lactose intolerant), eggs, eggplant, fava beans, leeks, lentils, lettuce, lima beans, nuts, oat flour, onions, pasta, peanut butter, peanuts, peas, peppers, pinto beans, pistachios, popcorn, prunes, raisins, sesame seeds, soybeans, soy milk, tofu, whole-wheat flour, and whole-grain breads. The no-calorie sweeteners sorbitol and xylitol may also cause gas.

HERBS

Take any one of the following herbs.

○ Angelica (European angelica or *Angelica archangelica*):
  • Essential oil, 10 drops in $1/4$ cup of water after meals, *or*
  • Fluid extract, $1/2$–1 teaspoon after meals.

○ Aniseed:
  • Tea made with 1 teaspoon of crushed seed or 1 tea bag in 1 cup of hot water steeped 10–15 minutes, up to 3 times a day after meals.

○ Caraway:
  • Oil, 1–2 drops in $1/4$ cup of water or on a sugar cube taken after meals.

○ Chamomile:

• Tea made with 1 teaspoon of crushed herb or 1 tea bag in 1 cup of hot water steeped 10–15 minutes, up to 4 times a day, after or between meals.

○ Fennel:

• Tea made with 1 teaspoon of crushed seed or 1 tea bag in 1 cup hot water steeped 10–15 minutes, up to 3 times a day after or between meals.

• Fennel-seed candies after meals.

○ Ginger:

• Capsules (400–500 milligrams), one before meals, *or*

• Chewable tablets (67.5 milligrams), one after each meal, *or*

• Ginger juice with other fruit juices, as desired.

○ Lavender:

• Prepare an infusion from 1 teaspoon of chopped herb drawn in ⅔ cup of hot water for 10 minutes, strained before drinking, *or*

• Place 1–4 drops of lavender oil on a sugar cube and eat the cube.

○ Peppermint:

• Tea made with 1 teaspoon of peppermint or 1 tea bag in ⅔ cup of hot water allowed to steep in a closed container for 10 minutes.

See Part Three if you take prescription medication.

UNDERSTANDING THE HEALING PROCESS

Over-the-counter remedies for abdominal bloating are usually less than satisfactory. Many people use simethicone, sold in the United States as Di-Gel, Extra Strength Gas-X, and Mylanta II. Simethicone relieves abdominal bloating by combining small gas bubbles to form large ones that in theory are easier to expel. In practice, simethicone mostly converts a lot of small flatus into a few large ones. Motility products such as cisapride (Propulsid) and metoclopramide (Reglan) do little to relieve the intestinal inflammation that blocks the passage of gas, but instead stimulate the muscles lining the intestines to push gas downward. The net effect can be to change painless abdominal bloating into painful abdominal bloating. Worse, cisapride and metoclopramide can cause dizziness, diarrhea, and vomiting.

There are two basic, effective ways to control abdominal bloating. One is to avoid offending foods. The other is to calm the digestive tract to minimize the production of gas and to help the intestine release it slowly. Herbal remedies are the best for treating bloating once gas has been produced.

Angelica is an appropriate remedy for people who do not care for herbal teas. It stimulates the production of gastric juices and assists the digestion of meats and fatty foods. It also prevents spasmodic flatulence.

Aniseed is a traditional remedy for bloating and flatulence and also for bronchitis, colds, coughs, fevers, and sore throat. It is an ingredient in paregoric, an opium mixture once given to colicky babies. It is particularly useful in controlling spasmodic flatulence. Aniseed acts by increasing secretions in the digestive tract that encourage passing gas in smaller, unnoticed quantities, slowly relieving abdominal bloating without embarrassment.[1] Foods prepared with aniseed, such as aniseed cookies and ouzo, have the same effect as the herb, but would have to be consumed in large quantities to control abdominal bloating.

Many recipes from the Caucasus, the Near East, the Himalayas, Mongolia, and Morocco include caraway oil to prevent flatulence from gassy foods. The combination of caraway oil plus peppermint is so well regarded in Europe that it is a doctor-prescribed remedy for abdominal bloating paid for by health insurance. Caraway oil relieves bloating, cramps, and nervous stomach. In folk medicine, caraway oil is used to induce menstruation, so it should be avoided by women who have heavy periods.

Chamomile has been used for centuries to treat abdominal bloating. When chamomile is placed in hot water, it releases chamazulene. This chemical stops the release of free radicals involved in food allergy reactions.[2] The essential oil blocks the release of histamine, protecting the digestive tract from irritation.[3]

Essential oils are lost by boiling or evaporation, so it is important to brew chamomile teas with hot but not boiling water and in a teapot or other closed container. Allergic reactions to chamomile are rare but possible. Most European regulatory boards advise that chamomile should not be used during pregnancy.

Fennel promotes the passage of food through the intestines while stopping muscle spasms that prevent the escape of gas. Never take pure fennel oil by mouth. It can cause acid stomach and intestinal irritation. In women, daily consumption of fennel seed may increase estrogen levels. Women who have estrogen-sensitive disorders (such as fibroids or fibrocystic breast disease) should not take fennel on a regular basis.

Ginger counteracts biochemical changes that occur after eating high-fat meals. Specifically, it deactivates Platelet Activating Factor (PAF), a hormonal agent of gastrointestinal inflammation.[4] It increases the rate at which food passes through the intestines, reducing the amount of bacterial fermentation in the gut.[5] This reduces the buildup of gas.

Ginger inhibits the body's synthesis of the stress hormone thromboxane, one of the chemical triggers for the formation of a thrombus, or blood clot.[6] For this reason, it should not be taken by people who suffer anemia or sickle-cell anemia or who have low levels of blood clotting factors due to liver disease. It also should be avoided by people who take blood thinners.

Lavender encourages the secretion of bile from the gallbladder, making it easier to digest fats. People who have gallstones should avoid the herb, since it increases flow through the bile duct.

Lavender is also mildly sedating. In laboratory studies with animals, the essential oils of lavender counter the anxiety-inducing effects of caffeine.[7] This property makes the herb especially useful for people whose bloating is worse under conditions of emotional duress or after drinking coffee.

Peppermint is probably the world's most widely used remedy for bloating and gas. It is especially helpful for bloating associated with a "nervous stomach." The essential oil slows the rate at which the intestines contract to expel both stool and gas, making emissions smaller, less noisy, and less frequent.[8]

Peppermint also stimulates the release of bile, so it should be avoided by people who have gallstones, gallbladder inflammation, or severe liver damage. Anyone who has an allergy to menthol should also avoid peppermint.

Peppermint Liqueurs

In addition to peppermint teas, it is possible to prepare a homemade peppermint liqueur by leaving 8 ounces of peppermint leaves in bottle of vodka for 10 days, shaking the bottle every 2–3 days. Strain the mixture before storage. Take ½–1 teaspoon of the liqueur between meals.

CONCEPTS FOR COPING WITH ABDOMINAL BLOATING

○ Reduce the formation of gas by eating slowly to avoid swallowing air.

○ Don't drink carbonated beverages or any beverages through a straw. This will reduce the amount of air getting into your stomach.

○ Keep a flatulographic record (in other words, a "flatus chart") to identify offending foods. Write down a list of the foods you eat and note whether you experience abdominal bloating and flatulence. A diary of what you eat with notes of excessive bloating will help you identify the foods you need to avoid.

○ If you find abdominal bloating to be a problem while taking a psyllium-based laxative such as Metamucil, switch to a soluble-fiber laxative such as Citrucel.

○ Angostura bitters are made from gentian, an herb that is so bitter that it induces a gastric reflex to release digestive juices. People who can stand the taste find that taking the bitters greatly reduces bloating and gas after eating meat and fatty foods. People who have gallstones should avoid Angostura and other kinds of bitters, because all bitters stimulate the flow of bile.

○ Avoid chewing gums sweetened with sorbitol or xylitol. These sweeteners contain complex carbohydrates that are not absorbed through lining of the intestine. Instead, they remain in the gut where they are fermented by intestinal bacteria. The action of chewing gum also causes the swallowing of air, increasing the volume of gas.

○ Contrary to common belief, drinking beer does not cause bloating. Hops in fact relieve stress-related digestive problems, although they are more effective as an herb than in beer.

○ Pepto-Bismol helps control odor, although it does not necessarily stop the buildup of gas. Bismuth subsalicylate, the "pink" in Pepto-Bismol, reduces odor by taking hydrogen sulfide out of the flatus. Hydrogen sulfide is the chemical responsible for rotten egg smell. Do not take Pepto-Bismol if you are sensitive to aspirin or NSAIDs such as ibuprofen (Motrin), indomethacin (Indocin), and ketoprofen (Orudis). Do not take Pepto-Bismol every day, since the bismuth in the product could build up to toxic levels.

○ Activated charcoal is sometimes recommended for people who cannot take Pepto-Bismol. Like Pepto-Bismol, activated charcoal traps obnoxious odors, but does not reduce the volume of gas.[9] Charcoal may make social situations less unpleasant but is unfortunately not helpful for relieving abdominal tension. If you would like a free sample of charcoal for odor control, write to Requa, Inc., Dept. P, P. O. Box 4008 Greenwich, CT 06830. Do not take charcoal within 2 hours of taking any medication or nutritional supplement.

O Bean-O is an over-the-counter product that may reduce bloating caused by eating fiber-rich foods such as beans, bran, and broccoli. It contains an enzyme, alpha-galactosidase, which helps break down the complex sugars found in gassy foods into simple sugars that the body can comfortably digest. These additional sugars add 2–6 percent to total calories of carbohydrate foods. Bean-O has no effect on proteins or gluten. Despite these drawbacks, many people find Bean-O to be the answer for persistent gas problems. There is also a version for pets called CurTail. For additional information and/or a free sample, call toll-free 1–800–257–8650 between 8:30 A.M. and 5:30 P.M. EST.

O Lactaid is an over-the-counter product that may reduce abdominal bloating caused by eating or drinking dairy foods and other products containing milk sugars, including convenience foods and medications. It treats an enzyme deficiency for milk sugar rather than an allergy to milk. To determine if Lactaid may be helpful to you, eat a normal breakfast and include a large, 12-ounce glass of milk of any kind. Over the next 6 hours, keep track of any discomforts you may have (if you experience any kind of severe reaction, consult a physician). The next day, prepare an identical breakfast with another 12-ounce glass of milk. Swallow a Lactaid tablet with your first sip of milk. If your symptoms are not as bad on the second day, Lactaid may be helpful.

O The Flatulence Filter, a portable seat cushion containing activated charcoal, traps disagreeable orders. Tests at the Minneapolis Veterans Affairs Medical Center found that it traps over 90 percent of the sulfur gases that cause the foul smell of flatulence, including hydrogen sulfide, methanethiol, and dimethyl sulfide.[10] The cushion is available for purchase by calling UltraTech Products at 1-800-316-8668 (outside the United States, 1-410-631-4776) or by writing UltraTech Products, Inc., 11191 Westheimer #123, Houston, Texas 77042, USA.

O The Southwestern herb marrubio (horehound) is a bitter flavoring that also relieves gas caused by eating fatty foods. Marrubio is traditionally taken as a tea, made by steeping 1 teaspoon of the chopped herb in 1 cup of hot water in a closed vessel for 10 minutes. The tea is strained before it is drunk.

O Homeopathic physicians frequently recommend lycopodium for abdominal bloating that is relieved by burping or passing gas. People who respond well to lycopodium usually have a fondness for sweets. How lycopodium works has not been scientifically established, but the club moss used to make the homeopathic preparation is also a source of anticholinergic chemicals that have a calming effect on the muscles lining the intestines. The higher-potency (30C) homeopathic is used for acute symptoms and the lower-potency (6C) homeopathic is used for prevention.

O If you experience severe abdominal bloating after traveling abroad, you may have a persistent infection known as giardiasis. See GIARDIASIS for further information.

Blood Pressure, High
See **Hypertension**.

Blood Sugar, High
See **Diabetes**.

Blood Sugar, Low
See **Hypoglycemia**.

Boils and Carbuncles

SYMPTOM SUMMARY

Boils, also known as furuncles:

O Located within hair follicles

O Usually begin as itch before lesions develop

O Form small, firm, tender red nodules in the skin after initial itch

O Usually smaller than a pea, may occasionally be as large as a golf ball

○ Swollen

○ Red or pink

○ May grow rapidly

○ May develop white or yellow centers (pustules)

○ May weep, ooze, and crust several days after onset

○ Tender, mildly to moderately painful

○ Pain increases as pus and dead tissue fills the area

○ Pain decreases as the area drains

○ May be accompanied by fatigue or fever

A carbuncle consists of several boils that grow together.

UNDERSTANDING THE DISEASE PROCESS

Boils and carbuncles most typically result from infection with *Staphylococcus aureus* (staph) and closely related bacteria. These microorganisms can colonize healthy skin without causing disease. At any given time, anywhere from 20–50 percent of the population supports thriving colonies of staph bacteria with no symptoms of disease. Staph causes infection only when the outer layer or stratum corneum of the skin is damaged.

Boils are very common, because staph bacteria are with us from birth. These microorganisms can colonize healthy skin without causing disease. At any given time, from 20–50 percent of people support thriving colonies of staph bacteria on their skins with no signs of infection. Staph bacteria cause infection only when the skin is damaged, and even then most people's immune systems can quickly get rid of them.[1]

Unfortunately, some people are prone to problematic staph infections. Insulin-dependent diabetics, people with chronic skin conditions such as eczema and psoriasis, IV drug users, and healthcare workers are especially likely to have problems with chronic staph infections.[2] Young children also have high rates of staph infections. This is due to their frequent contact with mucous secretions from other children with infected noses and throats.[3] Once a colony of staph bacteria is established, it may persist for years.[4]

Boils begin when damage to the hair follicle allows the bacteria to enter deeper into the tissues of the hair follicle and the subcutaneous tissue. Boils may occur in the hair follicles anywhere on the body, but they are most common on the armpits, buttocks, face, neck, and thighs. They may begin as tender red subcutaneous nodules but eventually become fluctuant, that is, they feel like a water-filled balloon. Boils may drain spontaneously, producing pus and a solid core. More often, they are opened in an eager attempt to relieve pain.

Boils that grow together are known as carbuncles. This continuous area of inflammation may have several drainage points, but also may grow so deep that it does not drain on its own. Carbuncles can develop anywhere, but they are most common on the back of the neck. Women are less susceptible to carbuncles than men. Carbuncles that persist longer than 2 weeks, recur, are located on the middle of the face or on the spine, or that are accompanied by fever require treatment by a healthcare provider because of the risk of complications from the spread of infection.

TREATMENT SUMMARY

DIET

○ Avoid foods that give you allergic reactions.

○ Limit consumption of simple sugars to 50 grams (2 ounces) per day. This is approximately one small candy bar or a 1-inch slice of cake, with no other sugars all day (and night). Restricting sugar consumption is especially important if you have diabetes, in which case you may not be able to eat sweets at all.

○ Be sure to eat a few servings of whole, natural foods, such as fruits, vegetables, legumes, and whole grains every day. Dark red and dark blue fruits (blackberries, blueberries, cherries, and raspberries) are best.

○ Drink at least six 8-ounce glasses of water daily.

NUTRITIONAL SUPPLEMENTS

○ Bromelain: 250–750 milligrams 3 times a day before meals.

○ Coenzyme Q_{10}: 30 milligrams per day.

○ Thymus extract: 500 milligrams of crude polypeptides daily.

○ Vitamin A: 5,000 IU per day.

○ Vitamin C: 1,000 milligrams 3 times per day.

○ Zinc picolinate: 30 milligrams per day.

HERBS

○ Aloe vera gel (for boils and carbuncles that have not been lanced or have not broken open): Apply to skin over the area of infection 2–3 times daily.

○ Astragalus: solid extract (0.5% 4-hydroxy-3-methoxy isoflavone), 100–150 milligrams 3 times a day, or dried root or tincture as recommended on the label.

○ Echinacea: 150–300 milligrams of solid extract (3.5% echinacosides) 3 times a day, or dried root, freeze-dried plant, juice, fluid extract, or tincture as recommended on the label.

○ Tea tree oil (for boils and carbuncles that have been lanced or have broken open): apply creams containing 8–20 percent tea tree oil or 40 percent solution to the skin with a cotton swab 2–3 times daily. Be sure to discard the cotton swab or applicator in a plastic bag so that the infection is not spread.

See Part Three if you take prescription medication.

UNDERSTANDING THE HEALING PROCESS

Boils and carbuncles are healed from the inside out. Boosting your immune system is the key to controlling infection. Because the bacterial infections that cause boils and carbuncles are active below the surface of the skin, applying either antibiotics or herbs to the surface of the skin is of limited value. Of the natural products that are applied topically, only aloe and tea tree oil have been scientifically demonstrated to heal infections of the kinds that typically cause boils and carbuncles. Poultices of barberry, coptis, and goldenseal, however, keep staph bacteria from spreading to other areas of skin.

Simply hydrating the skin by drinking water 6–8 times a day can be of great value in treating boils and carbuncles. Well-hydrated skin is supple and more resistant to reinfection. It releases accumulated white blood cells and pus more easily. Excessive amounts of sugar in your bloodstream create an acidic environment in which skin bacteria thrive. To stabilize sugar levels, your body has to produce (or you have to inject) large quantities of insulin, which is a growth factor for the skin. Stimulating growth of the layers of skin that line infected hair follicles traps infection inside. Whole grains, fruits, and vegetables are natural sources of flavonoids. These are natural compounds that activate vitamin C in fighting infection and strengthen collagen, the principal protein from which the skin is made.[5]

Bromelain is a protein-dissolving enzyme refined from the stem of the pineapple plant. Its primary benefit in treating boils and carbuncles is dissolving the proteins that make the sloughed-off dead cells in the shaft of the hair follicle stick together.[6] Bromelain essentially "unplugs" the path to the surface of the skin through which a boil can drain.

Bromelain also improves circulation to healthy skin. The immune system causes blood to clot around an area of infection. The clotting protein fibrin forms a net around the area of inflammation to deprive it of oxygen and nutrients. This cuts off bacteria from their nutrient supply, but also traps the fluids that cause swelling. Bromelain stimulates the production of plasmin, a chemical that causes the protein chains that make up fibrin to unlink. When the fibrin chains unlink, circulation is restored.[7]

Since bromelain products are not standardized, finding the right dosage is a matter of trial and error. Start with the lower dose and work upward to the maximum until you notice drainage from the boil. Allergies to bromelain are very rare but not unheard of. Reactions to this supplement are most likely in people who are already allergic to pineapple, papaya, wheat flour, rye flour, or birch pollen. There has never been a report of an anaphylactic reaction, that is, a life-threatening allergic reaction, to bromelain. There have been isolated reports of heavy menstrual periods in women, nausea, vomiting, and hives when bromelain is taken in overdoses (2,000 milligrams and higher).

In laboratory experiments with mice, coenzyme Q_{10} increased immune response to *Staphylococcus aureus*.[8] Coenzyme Q_{10} is especially useful for persons who take statin drugs, such as atorvastatin (Lipitor), lovastatin (Mevacor), pravastatin (Pravachol), or simvastatin (Zocor). It is recommended for people who take red yeast (Cholestin), which is also a statin. Statins interfere with the body's ability to produce both coenzyme Q_{10} and cholesterol.

There is one report of coenzyme Q_{10} increasing bleeding when taken with the anticlotting drug warfarin. Type 2 diabetics may find that their blood sugars are unexpectedly low when taking coenzyme Q_{10}. If you have diabetes and you take coenzyme Q_{10}, check your blood sugar levels every day.

There are no studies that directly confirm the usefulness of thymus extracts in treating staph infections, but there is considerable evidence that thymus extracts lift low immune function. Research has shown that thymus extract normalizes the ratio of helper T cells to suppressor T cells. This maintains a healthy immune response that neither destroys healthy tissue nor allows infectious microorganisms to flourish.[9]

Relatively low doses of vitamin A are sufficient to prevent immune "burnout" due to stress on the thymus.[10] Vitamin A also makes antibodies more responsive to various kinds of infections, increases the rate at which macrophages engulf and destroy bacteria, and stimulates natural killer cells.[11] The dosage of vitamin A recommended here is extremely unlikely to cause side effects, such as dry skin, chapped lips, headaches, and joint pain. Discontinue vitamin A immediately if any of these symptoms appear. Women who are or who could become pregnant should strictly limit their intake of vitamin A to 5,000 IU a day or less.

Vitamin C is quickly depleted during the stress of an infection.[12] In combination with the anthocyanin and proanthocyanin bioflavonoids found in blue and dark-red fruits, it helps increase the stability of the ground substance, the "glue" between the skin and the tissues below it.[13]

Dosages of vitamin C that are high enough to help fight staph infection almost always cause diarrhea at first. This side effect usually goes away in 3–4 days and can be avoided entirely if vitamin C is administered by injection (by a nutritionally oriented qualified healthcare practitioner). High dosages of vitamin C can also cause kidney stones. Abruptly discontinuing a high daily dosage of vitamin C can lead to symptoms of vitamin C deficiency. Before starting any high-dosage regimen of vitamin C, consult with your healthcare provider to make sure it will not aggravate any other health conditions or interfere with medications.

Zinc is an important cofactor for vitamin A. When zinc is deficient, the immune system's ability to produce white blood cells in response to infection is reduced, thymic hormone levels are lower, the immune response in the skin is especially reduced, and phagocytosis, the process in which bacteria are engulfed and digested, is slowed. All of these processes can be corrected by taking zinc supplements.[14] A good way to determine whether you need zinc is a through taste test. Try chewing a zinc tablet. If it doesn't taste bad, you probably need to take zinc.

Zinc picolinate is the most readily absorbed form of zinc. Do not take more than 50 milligrams of any zinc supplement daily. In rare cases, excessive intake of zinc depletes copper to cause anemia, that is, a deficiency of red blood cells, and neutropenia, a serious deficiency of white blood cells.[15] Don't take zinc if you are on antibiotics. Zinc can interfere with their absorption or possibly cause rheumatoid inflammation of joints.

Aloe is especially useful for treating boils that have been lanced (something you should never do at home). It contains a number of compounds necessary for healing wounds, including vitamin C, vitamin E, and zinc. Gels that are at least 70 percent aloe are bactericidal against both *Pseudomonas aeruginosa* and *Staphylococcus aureus,* the two most common causes of boils.[16] A small number of people are allergic to aloe, but the herb used topically has no other side effects.

Astragalus is a traditional Chinese treatment for boils, although Chinese tradition suggests that it is more useful for boils that sink in than it is for boils that dome out. This herb is especially useful in reversing damage to the immune system caused by chemicals or radiation.[17] In laboratory studies with test animals, astragalus increases the number and activity of monocytes and macrophages, the white blood cells responsible for controlling bacterial infection.[18]

There is no specific clinical evidence that echinacea can cure the infections that cause boils and carbuncles, but there is considerable evidence that echinacea can relieve the pain of boils and carbuncles. German studies have found that *Echinacea purpurea* stimulates the immune system to produce macrophages. These are the white blood cells specifically responsible for removing infectious bacteria. Echinacea increases the number of macrophages without increasing the numbers of other kinds of white blood cells that generate inflammatory hormones.[19] This targeted immune stimulation fights infection but avoids inflammation. In fact, echinacea relieves inflammation. One study found that a teaspoon of *Echinacea purpurea* juice is as effective in relieving pain and swelling as 100 milligrams of cortisone.[20]

Women who are trying to get pregnant should avoid *Echinacea purpurea.* It contains caffeoyl esters that can interfere with the action of hyaluronidase, an enzyme essential to the release of unfertilized eggs into the fallopian tube.[21]

Naturopathic physicians Michael Murray and Joseph

Pizzorno write that an Australian study conducted in the 1960s found that tea tree oil accelerated the healing process and prevented scarring in staph infections. The method of application included cleaning the site, then painting the surface of the boil with tea tree oil 2 or 3 times a day.[22]

CONCEPTS FOR COPING WITH BOILS AND CARBUNCLES

❍ Apply hot, wet compresses to relieve pain. Repeated application of compresses will make it easier for your healthcare professional to lance a boil. You can make a hot compress by soaking a clean towel in 2 cups of hot water to which you have added a teaspoon of powdered barberry, coptis, or goldenseal. These herbs contain berberine, which stops the multiplication of infectious bacteria outside the area of the boil and prevents the spread of the infection. (Do not take these herbs internally in these dosages to treat skin infections.) Apply the hot towel (as hot as you can stand it) to the boil. When the compress has cooled to body temperature, reheat the towel and reapply. Be sure to dry your skin after you have finished using the compress.

❍ Avoid external friction, such as that caused by tight-fitting clothes.

❍ Never squeeze or lance boils yourself, especially if they are located on the face. When a boil is ready to be lanced by a doctor or nurse, it will feel "squishy" and may begin draining on its own.

❍ Change your washcloth every time you wash, and change sheets and towels daily.

❍ Wash your hands frequently, especially before and after changing a dressing or applying ointment.

❍ If you take antibiotics, also take 1 or 2 capsules of *acidophilus* or *Lactobacillus* every day. These probiotics help restore the friendly bacteria in your intestine that are destroyed by antibiotic treatment.

❍ Flulike symptoms when you have a skin infection are a possible indication of sepsis. See a physician immediately if you feel like you are coming down with the flu when you have a boil or carbuncle, particularly if the area of infection gets redder or hotter.

❍ Homeopathic physicians frequently treat boils with Schuessler cell salts, particularly calcarea sulphurica (Calc Sulf) and silicea (silica).

Bone Loss

See **Osteomalacia; Osteoporosis; Paget's Disease**.

BPH

See **Benign Prostatic Hyperplasia (BPH)**.

Breast Cancer

SYMPTOM SUMMARY

In women:

❍ Lump or mass in the breast found by breast exam:
  - Firm or hard; irregular borders; usually painless

❍ Change in size or shape of one breast

❍ Change in color or feel of the skin of the breast, areola (pigmented skin around the nipple), or nipple of one breast
  - "Orange peel" texture
  - Highlighted veins on the surface of the breast
  - Puckered or scaly
  - Redness

❍ Enlargement, itching, or retraction (pulling in) of nipple

❍ (Advanced disease) Bone pain, swelling in one arm, weight loss, ulceration of the skin of the breast

In men:

❍ Any breast lump, pain, or tenderness

UNDERSTANDING THE DISEASE PROCESS

According to the National Cancer Institute, 1 in 8 American women will develop breast cancer at some time in her life. Women in other countries have lower risks of developing breast cancer: 1 in 9 women in Canada, 1 in 12 women in the United Kingdom, 1 in 14 women in Australia, and fewer than 1 in 30 in Japan.

Lifetime risk, however, does not tell the whole story.

At her fiftieth birthday, an Aleutian, Hawaiian, or white woman in the United States who does not have breast cancer has about a 1 in 300 chance of developing the disease before her fifty-first birthday. A healthy 50-year-old African-American or Hispanic woman in the United States has about a 1 in 400 chance of developing breast cancer over the next year. A 50-year-old Asian-American woman in good health has less than a 1 in 500 chance of developing breast cancer over the next 12 months. (And a man has less than a 1 in 125,000 chance of developing breast cancer in any given year.) [1] If you are a healthy woman or man who is concerned about breast cancer, you might interpret these statistics as evidence that cancer is not likely to strike soon. But a better interpretation would be that you have time to make changes in your lifestyle that increase the chances you will never have breast cancer.

The cellular changes that lead to breast cancer in women take place over a period of years or decades. Cells that become cancerous tend to get stuck in the "S (synthesis) phase" of their life cycle,[2] in which they double their DNA to have enough DNA for both an existing breast cell and a new breast cell. More DNA presents more opportunities for mutations that can lead to cancer. Like healthy cells in the breast, cancerous cells grow and multiply during the 3 or 4 days preceding menstruation in response to the hormones estrogen, progesterone, and testosterone.[3] The more these hormones are produced by the body, or supplied to the body by contraceptive pills or hormone replacement therapy, the more cancerous cells grow.

Even when cancerous changes have occurred in the breast, the body has several lines of defense that keep tumors from forming. The p53 gene, for instance, ordinarily makes sure dividing cells "rest for repairs" if there are other defects in their genetic material. Women who have a defect in this gene are many times more likely to develop breast cancer than women who do not.[4] Defects in the gene can be hereditary, but are more likely to be caused by smoking.[5] The p53 gene is especially important for preventing the progression of breast cancer in women who have been exposed to polychlorinated hydrocarbons,[6] such as DDT, DDE, and PCBs.

TREATMENT SUMMARY

DIET

○ Limit consumption of bacon, butter, liver, margarine, red meat, and sugar.

○ Maximize consumption of cruciferous vegetables (broccoli, cabbage, and Brussels sprouts), yellow and orange vegetables, tomatoes, and turmeric.

NUTRITIONAL SUPPLEMENTS

For women who drink alcohol on a regular basis:

○ Any vitamin B supplement that includes folic acid, daily.

See Part Three if you take prescription medication.

UNDERSTANDING THE PREVENTIVE PROCESS

The important thing to understand about lowering your risk of breast cancer is that extreme measures are unnecessary. The relationship between breast cancer and lifestyle factors you can control is far more complex than commonly believed. Some lifestyle choices that increase the risk of other kinds of cancers lower the risk of breast cancer. Australian women have nearly 50 percent lower risk of developing breast cancer than American women, and the most likely explanation is that Australian women get more sun.[7] The skin uses sunlight to make vitamin D, which suppresses hormonal signals that make breast cancer cells grow.[8] Even smoking less than 10 cigarettes a day cannot be clearly linked to an increased risk of breast cancer.[9]

The latest research suggests that dietary fat is a risk factor for the *first* occurrence of breast cancer only among women who have had fibrocystic breast disease.[10] A 10-year study of over 60,000 women recently concluded that there is no difference between the "Western" dietary pattern (including red and processed meats, refined grains, fat, and sweets) or the "healthy" dietary pattern (fruit and vegetables, fish and poultry, low-fat dairy, and whole grains) in predicting breast cancer risk.[11] Even extreme low-fat diets intended to lower the risk of recurrent breast cancer get very poor results. A recent study at the University of California at San Diego found that the average weight loss after a year on a rigorous high-fiber, low-fat diet was 0.04 kilograms (a little more than an ounce, and less than the weight loss in a control group of women who did not diet), and the risk of breast cancer was nil.[12]

The relationship between weight and risk of breast cancer is also complex. An analysis of studies including over 337,000 women found that before menopause, overweight women are *less* likely to develop breast cancer. A woman with a body mass index (BMI) of 31 (for example, a woman 5'4" tall weighing 181 pounds) is 50 percent less likely than a woman with a BMI of 21 (5'4", 122 pounds) to develop breast cancer. After menopause, overweight women are *more* likely to develop breast cancer. A postmenopausal woman with a BMI of 28 (5'4", 163 pounds) has about a 25 percent increased risk of developing breast cancer.[13]

Higher antioxidant levels, however, are associated with a lower risk of breast cancer. In a study of 304 women in Australia, the highest levels of the antioxidants alpha-carotene, beta-carotene, lycopene, vitamin A, and vitamin E were associated with approximately a 50 percent reduction in the risk of breast cancer (when other variables were accounted for).[14] The study did not find that vitamin C reduced the risk of breast cancer, but vitamin C is an important cofactor for vitamin E, helping the body conserve it.

Another antioxidant, curcumin, the yellow pigment in curry powder, stops the development of breast cancer cells in at least three ways. Laboratory studies find that curcumin makes breast cancer cells less responsive to the most abundant form of estrogen and stops estrogen from activating genes that control cell growth. Curcumin also has an effect on breast cancer cells that are not activated by estrogen. The plant chemical deactivates a hormone cancer cells need to break out of the tissue matrix that contains them and stimulates a hormone that makes them stay put.[15]

Curcumin is also a well-known activator of the p53 gene. It helps p53 deactivate defective cells at G2, a second gap or resting phase in the process of cell division just before the cell divides. Scientists at New York's Memorial Sloan-Kettering Cancer Center have found that at least in the test tube, green tea is a perfect complement for curcumin, since it activates p53 at G1, the first gap in the process of cell division.[16]

Indole-3-carbinol, a chemical found in broccoli, Brussels sprouts, cabbage, and cauliflower, makes estrogen less active in breast tissue. The latest thinking is that this chemical could become a substitute for Tamoxifen, which also reduces the activity of estrogen in breast tissue but increases the risk of developing cancers that are not stimulated by estrogen.[17]

Alpha-carotene, beta-carotene, curcumin, green tea polyphenols, indole-3-carbinol, lycopene, vitamin A, and vitamin E are all available as dietary supplements. (Women who are or who could become pregnant should strictly limit their intake of vitamin A to 5,000 IU

per day or less, since a massive overdose of the vitamin in the first 3 months of pregnancy could cause birth defects.) No one knows whether taking these nutrients as supplements would also lower the risk of breast cancer, and it is possible that the risk of certain other cancers could be increased by taking antioxidants on a long-term basis—for more than 5 years—especially by women who smoke. At this time, the best preventive measure for breast cancer in women is a diet with daily servings of colorful vegetables and avoiding extreme consumption of fat.

There is an important exception to this rule for women who drink. Several studies in the United States and China have found that folic acid lowers the risk of breast cancer in women who drink more than 1–2 drinks per day, and one study has found taking a multivitamin containing folic acid lowered risk of breast cancer by 26 percent in these women. Taking folic acid supplements seems to be better for lowering breast cancer risk than consuming large amounts of folic acid in food.[18]

CONCEPTS FOR COPING WITH BREAST CANCER

❍ There is very preliminary evidence that the Adjuvant Nutritional Intervention in Cancer (ANICA) protocol, developed at a private clinic in Denmark, may reduce the risk of cancer's spread, prevent weight loss, lessen the need for painkillers, and reduce the risk of death in women who already have breast cancer.[19] Unfortunately, rigorous clinical study of the ANICA protocol has not yet been done. The supplements (given in European dosages) in ANICA include:

- Beta-carotene: 32.5 IU per day.
- Coenzyme Q_{10}: 90 milligrams per day.
- Essential fatty acids: 5 grams per day.
- Selenium: 387 micrograms per day.
- Vitamin C: 2,850 milligrams per day.
- Vitamin E: 2,500 IU per day.

This supplement program is not likely to harm any woman with breast cancer, although the dosage of vitamin E is high enough to intensify the effects of certain prescription drugs. Do not take any antioxidants, including these, while you are taking radiation or chemotherapy without the express consent of your physician.

❍ If you smoke, try to smoke fewer than 10 cigarettes per day. Some epidemiological evidence suggests that there is very little effect from smoking just a few cigarettes per day. However, smoking 10–20 cigarettes a day increases the risk of breast cancer by up to 5 times. Smoking more than 30 cigarettes a day increases the risk of breast cancer by up to 10 times. Passive smoking (exposure to cigarette smoke without smoking) is a greater risk factor than smoking just a few (fewer than 10) cigarettes a day, increasing the probability of developing breast cancer by up to 4 times.[20]

○ Grilling or frying beef, chicken, fish, lamb, and pork produces a class of cancer causing compounds known as heterocyclic amines. Baking, poaching, stewing, or microwaving does not. The highest concentrations of the cancer-causing compounds are found in pan drippings. Women who are injured most by exposure to heterocyclic amines are those who are overweight, had their first period at an early age, or started menopause at a late age.[21]

○ Eating eggs may have some relationship to breast cancer risk. An analysis of the medical records of over 351,000 women found that eating fewer than 2 eggs a week was associated with a slight decrease in the risk of breast cancer, while eating more than 1 egg a day was associated with a slight increase.[22]

○ With relation to breast cancer, soy foods may either help or hurt. Women who began eating soy as girls probably have lower breast cancer rates as a result. Scientists publishing research in the *The American Journal of Clinical Nutrition* state that genistein, a chemical component of soy products, alters the physiology of the breast so that its cells go through a normal life cycle with normal amounts of DNA, provided soy is consumed before adulthood.[23] Consuming soy products after adulthood has not been reliably shown to change estrogen levels or reduce the risk of breast cancer.[24] And at least one study suggests that using soy can increase the risk of breast cancer.[25] Some current medical research suggests that seaweed, not soy, may be the reason Japanese women have lower rates of breast cancer.[26]

○ Once breast cancer occurs, choice of food does make a difference. Including any amount of bacon, butter, lard, and margarine approximately doubles the risk of recurrence of breast cancer, and the risk of recurrence doubles for each daily serving of bacon, liver, or red meat.[27]

○ Several chemicals in garlic kill breast cancer cells in the laboratory, but eating garlic has not yet been conclusively found to lower the risk of breast cancer.[28]

○ Sugar is not conclusively associated with the development of cancer, but fasting insulin is associated with the spread of cancer.[29] What this means is that once breast cancer has occurred, anything that increases fasting insulin levels, such as excessive sugar consumption, increases the risk that cancer will spread, and anything that lowers fasting insulin levels, such as regular exercise including weight training, lowers the risk that cancer will spread.

○ Working the night shift may increase a woman's risk of breast cancer. The bodies of women who are exposed to light at night make more melatonin, which in turn stimulates the production of estrogen. Risk of breast cancer in women who sleep during the day may be as much as $2\frac{1}{2}$ times greater than for women who sleep at night.[30]

○ Stress hormones are associated with the proliferation of cancer cells. A woman's body makes the greatest quantities of stress hormones at 1:00 P.M. and at 1:00 A.M.[31] Therefore, the highest priority should be relaxation at these times.

○ The Pill is a risk factor for breast cancer, but a relatively small one. Oral contraceptives contain estrogen and increase the risk of breast cancer, although studies including over 150,000 women have found that the Pill only increases the overall risk of breast cancer by about 7 percent.[32] That is, taking the Pill raises a woman's lifetime risk of developing breast cancer from 1 in 8 to 1 in $8\frac{1}{2}$.

○ Breast cancer strikes about 1,500 men in the United States annually.[33] It must be distinguished by medical examination from gynecomastia, a far more common and benign condition of breast inflammation and enlargement caused by hormonal fluctuations. The causes of male breast cancer are not very well understood, but one study finds that it is 400 times more common in men who are constantly exposed to electromagnetic fields.[34]

Breast Care Problems
See **Galactorrhea; Lactation, Insufficient; Mastitis.**

Brittle Nails

SYMPTOM SUMMARY

❍ Peeling of the fingernail in horizontal layers, starting at the nail's free end

❍ Lengthwise splits in the nail

UNDERSTANDING THE DISEASE PROCESS

As many as 4 million people a year buy home healthcare products for brittle nails, a condition known in the medical literature as onychoschizia. About 1 in 5 people has brittle nails, one survey finding the problem in 27 percent of women and 13 percent of men.[1] Brittle nails typically peel from the nail's free end, breaking off in horizontal layers. Less often, the nail splits vertically. Brittle nails are more common in women than in men.

Brittleness is usually caused by trauma to the nail: repeated exposure to detergents and water, failure to wear gloves when using solvents or excessive use of nail polish remover, or simply excessive washing and drying. Brittle nails can also be caused by an underlying medical problem, such as malnutrition, hypothyroidism, chronic lung infections, psoriasis, Raynaud's phenomenon, or Sjögren's syndrome. They may be a side effect of medication with carbamazepine or phenytoin for bipolar disorder or seizures.

Brittle nails may be a temporary complication of antibiotic therapy. They are a common problem among dialysis patients, and they can also be caused by overdosing selenium supplements. Since brittle nails can be a symptom of a serious health condition, self-treatment is only appropriate when brittle nails are the only symptom.

TREATMENT SUMMARY

NUTRITIONAL SUPPLEMENTS

❍ Biotin: 300–600 micrograms daily.

❍ Avoid high doses of pantothenic acid (vitamin B_5).

See Part Three if you take prescription medication.

UNDERSTANDING THE HEALING PROCESS

A small-scale but carefully controlled clinical study confirms the usefulness of biotin supplements in treating brittle nails. Researchers used an electron microscope to examine nail clippings taken from 8 women who were given 2.5 milligrams of biotin daily for 6–9 months. They also examined nail clippings from 10 women who were not given biotin. Microscopic examination of the nails confirmed that nails were thicker and stronger in the women who took biotin.[2] A later, larger but uncontrolled study got similar results.[3]

It may be necessary to take biotin for up to 6 months to get results. There are no adverse interactions between biotin and prescription drugs reported in the medical literature. Be sure to take biotin if you take antibiotics, since antibiotics kill the intestinal bacteria that make this vitamin.

High doses of pantothenic acid (vitamin B_5) compete with biotin for transport sites in the lining of the large intestine. Avoid high-dose vitamin B_5 therapy when taking biotin.

Gelatin is frequently recommended as a treatment for brittle nails, as are ceratin, collagen, cysteine, methionine, millet, vitamin A, brewer's yeast, zinc, and the herb horsetail. So far, there is no systematic evidence that any of these remedies help most cases of brittle nails, although they will not harm brittle nails. Zinc supplements are useful in a rare condition called acquired acrodermatitis enteropathica, in which brittle nails are only one symptom, along with perioral and perianal dermatitis, diarrhea, mouth sores, and hair loss. Usually brittle nails are a later symptom of the condition. In acrodermatitis enteropathica, zinc sulphate supplements work best.

CONCEPTS FOR COPING WITH BRITTLE NAILS

❍ Brittle nails are more of a problem in low humidity and high heat, such as in desert climates or in overheated houses in winter. In low humidity or high heat conditions, apply lotions containing alpha hydroxy acids or lanolin to the nails anytime you get your hands wet.

❍ Buff the nails in the direction the nail grows, not in a back and forth motion.

❍ Do not use metal instruments to push back the cuticle.

❍ If the fingernails are weak but the toenails are strong, the problem is external pressure, not a nutritional deficiency.

❍ Nail polishes with nylon fibers strengthen brittle nails.

❍ Shape and file the nails with a very fine file. Round

tips in a gentle curve. Filing snags and irregularities every day helps prevent further damage.

○ Try to wear gloves when performing chores that involve getting the hands wet. Heavy-duty vinyl gloves worn with a thin cotton liner are best.

○ There are some reports that the supplement methyl-sulfonylmethane (MSM) can help build both harder nails and shinier hair. A typical dosage would be 3,000 milligrams per day.

Bronchial Asthma
See **Asthma**.

Bronchitis, Chronic

SYMPTOM SUMMARY

○ Cough that produces sputum, may be blood-streaked

○ Coughing up blood

○ Ankle, foot, or leg swelling affecting both ankles, legs, or feet

○ Fatigue

○ Frequent colds, increased risk of pneumonia

○ Headaches

○ Reddish face, palms, or mucous membranes inside the mouth and nose

○ Shortness of breath aggravated by altitude, exertion, or mild activity

○ Vision abnormalities

○ Wheezing

UNDERSTANDING THE DISEASE PROCESS

Chronic bronchitis is a condition of long-term overproduction of mucus that can be coughed up. Chronic bronchitis is defined by the presence of a mucus-producing cough most days of the month, 3 months of the year for 2 successive years without other underlying disease to explain the cough. It may precede or accompany emphysema. According to the National Center for Health Statistics, in 1998, 9 million people were diagnosed with chronic bronchitis in the United States alone.

By far, the most common cause of chronic bronchitis is cigarette smoking. The condition also occurs in people whose bronchial tubes may have been irritated initially by bacterial or viral infections. Air pollution and industrial dusts and fumes are contributing factors in many cases. Once the bronchial tubes have been irritated over a long period of time, excessive mucus is produced constantly. The linings of the bronchial tubes become thickened, an irritating cough develops, and airflow may be hampered. The bronchial tubes then provide an incubator for infections.

Someone with chronic bronchitis may continue to cough and produce large amounts of mucus for several weeks after a cold seemed to have been cured. Over the years, colds become more damaging. The cycle of coughing and expectoration lasts longer after each cold. Without realizing it, one begins to take this coughing and mucus production as a matter of course. Eventually coughing is a year-round condition—before colds, during colds, after colds, although the cough is usually worse in cold, damp weather. A person with chronic bronchitis may expectorate an ounce or more of yellow mucus every day.

TREATMENT SUMMARY

DIET

○ Don't go on a low-fat, high-carbohydrate diet, but do avoid egg yolks, beef, and fried foods.

NUTRITIONAL SUPPLEMENTS

○ Bromelain: 125–250 milligrams 3 times a day.

○ Essential fatty acids:

• EPA and DHA (not to be confused with DHEA): 1,000 milligrams per day, *or*

• Eat 2–3 servings of cold-water fish weekly, *or*

• Take 1 tablespoon of any vegetarian source of essential fatty acids (borage seed oil, black currant oil, evening primrose oil, flaxseed oil, and so on) daily.

○ N-acetyl cysteine (NAC): 400 milligrams a day *if you do not smoke.*

HERBS

Choose a single form of the herb best suited to relieving the symptoms that bother you the most:

To relieve cough (antitussives):

○ Lobelia:

- Ointments: apply to the chest 2–3 times a day, *or*
- Vinegar extract (acetract): no more than $\frac{1}{2}$ teaspoon 3 times a day. Take less if you experience nausea. Do not give to children.

○ Marshmallow:

- Tea: a rounded teaspoon of the herb in a cup of water as often as desired, *or*
- Tincture: 1–3 teaspoons up to 4 times a day.

To treat sore throat (demulcents):

○ Elecampane:

- Tea: no more than $\frac{1}{4}$ teaspoon in a cup of water allowed to brew for 15 minutes, up to 3 times a day. *Strain before drinking.*

○ Ivy leaf (Hedera):

- Extract: a dropperful by itself or in a small amount of water, 2–3 times a day.

○ Marshmallow:

- Tea: a rounded teaspoon of the herb in a cup of water as often as desired, *or*
- Tincture: 1–3 teaspoons up to 4 times a day.

○ Plantain:

- Cough syrup: $\frac{1}{2}$ teaspoon 3 times a day, *or*
- Tea: $\frac{1}{4}$–$\frac{1}{2}$ teaspoon of the herb brewed in hot water for 15 minutes.

○ Scutellaria (Chinese skullcap):

- Fluid extract: $\frac{1}{2}$–2 teaspoons 1–3 times per day.

○ Slippery elm:

- Tea: 1 teaspoon in 1 cup of water as often as desired.

To break up phlegm (expectorants):

○ Anise:

- Aromatherapy: 10–20 drops of essential oil in a basin of hot water, vapors inhaled for several minutes once or twice a day. *Never drink essential oils of anise.*
- Tea: bagged anise tea brewed in 1 cup of hot but not boiling water.

○ Horehound (also known as marrubio):

- Cough lozenges containing horehound: as often as desired.

- Tea (from the chopped herb available in hierberías): 1 teaspoon brewed in a cup of hot but not boiling water for 10 minutes, strained before drinking, 2–3 times a day.

○ Horseradish:

- Apply as a plaster once or twice a day.

○ Mullein:

- Tincture: $\frac{1}{4}$–$\frac{3}{4}$ teaspoon up to 4 times a day.

○ Mustard:

- Apply as poultice or plaster once or twice a day.

To stop coughing fits (spasmolytics):

○ Lobelia

- Ointments: apply to the chest 2–3 times a day.
- Vinegar extract (acetract): no more than $\frac{1}{2}$ teaspoon 3 times a day. Take less if you experience nausea. Do not give to children.

○ Thyme:

- Tea: $\frac{1}{4}$–$\frac{1}{2}$ teaspoon of the kitchen herb in 1 cup of hot water, 2–3 times daily
- Tincture: $\frac{1}{3}$–1 teaspoon, 2–3 times daily.

AROMATHERAPY

○ Add 5–10 drops of eucalyptus oil to the water in a vaporizer operated in your bedroom as you sleep.

See Part Three if you take prescription medication.

UNDERSTANDING THE HEALING PROCESS

Smoking cessation has a dramatic effect on chronic bronchitis. Medical examination of the 29,133 participants of the Alpha-Tocopherol Beta-Carotene Cancer Prevention Study found that just quitting smoking reduced the number of days the lungs formed phlegm by 84 percent and the number of coughs by 78 percent.[1] Clearly, the most important step in treating chronic bronchitis is to quit smoking. In the meantime, there are several natural interventions that help.

Low-fat, high-carbohydrate diets are not advisable for people who have chronic bronchitis. High carbohydrate consumption increases the body's consumption of carbon dioxide. Several studies indicate that people with chronic bronchitis have difficulty eliminating carbon dioxide,[2,3] and a high-carbohydrate diet places additional stress on the lungs.

On the other hand, certain kinds of fats should be

avoided. The biochemical process that makes the lungs sensitive to allergens is made possible by the chemical thromboxane.[4] The body's production of thromboxane is greater when the diet includes egg yolks, beef tallow (often used in cooking fast-food French fries), and fried foods, and less when the diet includes fish oils. A study of 8,006 male smokers in Hawaii found that those who ate 2 or more servings of fish per week were found to lose lung capacity at less than half the rate of those who did not. The protective effect of fish oils was greatest for the smokers who smoked the most.[5] Another study published in the prestigious *New England Journal of Medicine* suggests that smokers are protected from the development of bronchitis, emphysema, and pneumonia when their diets include n-3 polyunsaturated fatty acids from any source.[6] EPA, DHA, and flaxseed oil are good sources of n-3 polyunsaturated fatty acids.

Don't expect results from eating fish or taking fish oil or other kinds of n-3 fatty acids immediately. Any essential fatty acid supplement can cause bloating, burping, diarrhea, or flatulence, although these effects are likely to be mild. People with a history of partial seizures (blanking out or unexplained loss of emotional control) should not use borage seed oil, since it can lower the amount of stress precipitating an attack. Hempseed oil is also helpful, but not always legal. It will not give you a marijuana high, but it can cause a false positive reading for marijuana use in some home-testing kits.

Bromelain is a chemical found in pineapple that can break up mucus. Bromelain treatment makes the mucus more fluid. In one study of the use of bromelain in the treatment of chronic bronchitis, patients given the supplement coughed less frequently and had greater lung capacity.[7]

Allergies to bromelain are very rare but not unheard of. Allergic reactions to this supplement are most likely to occur in people who are already allergic to pineapple, papaya, wheat flour, rye flour, or birch pollen. There has never been a report of an anaphylactic reaction to bromelain. There have been isolated reports of heavy periods, nausea, vomiting, and hives when bromelain is taken in overdoses (2,000 milligrams and higher).

N-acetyl cysteine (NAC) is an amino acid derivative that can break the chemical bonds that make mucus sticky. A study involving 10 chronic lung disease patients and 10 healthy controls found that NAC increases the activity of infection-fighting white blood cells.[8] A total of 8 double-blind, placebo-controlled scientific studies concur that regular use of NAC can significantly reduce the frequency of severe attacks of bronchitis.[9]

Not everyone with chronic bronchitis should take NAC. Smokers who have had bronchitis for 2 years or less should not take NAC unless they are quitting. There is some evidence that NAC may activate eosinophils, the white blood cells that may cause the progression of smoker's cough to chronic obstructive pulmonary disease.[10] NAC may cause headaches if taken with sildenafil (Viagra), and, in rare cases, can cause cysteine-crystal kidney stones. Diabetics who also have cystic fibrosis may find that taking NAC causes false readings in urine tests for ketones.

People who have chronic bronchitis are frequently deficient in antioxidant vitamins such as vitamin A, vitamin C, vitamin E, coenzyme Q_{10}, and beta-carotene. It would seem logical that taking supplemental antioxidants would help chronic bronchitis, but this is not necessarily the case. There is considerable evidence that consuming *low* doses of these antioxidants *in the form of fruits and vegetables* helps in various kinds of chronic obstructive pulmonary disease, including bronchitis, even among elderly long-term smokers,[11] whereas taking specific supplements (notably beta-carotene and vitamin C) does not.[12]

Many people are unaware that free radicals are not solely harmful, but they are involved in many defense reactions of the cells. High levels of antioxidants may disturb these reactions with unpredictable and unexpected consequences. Therefore, if you take antioxidants, take the smallest possible dose. Better yet, get your antioxidants from the most available and most balanced natural sources, fruits and vegetables.

There are a number of herbs that help relieve bronchitis. The best way to use them is to treat the symptoms that are the most bothersome to you. Anise and the related herb star anise contain an antimicrobial chemical, anethole.[13] The essential oil is especially deadly to molds and yeast infections.[14] Since anise stimulates production of secretions, it should be used to treat dry coughs rather than productive coughs.

Elecampane mostly consists of the sugar inulin (not to be confused with insulin), the same carbohydrate found in Jerusalem artichokes. The inulin in elecampane coats and soothes the throat. The herb also contains small amounts of volatile oils that act as counterirritants, desensitizing the throat to pain.

It is important not to use too much elecampane. The

volatile oils in the herb can irritate the mouth and the bowel. There has been a single report in the medical literature of a potentially life-threatening allergic reaction to foods containing the same carbohydrates as elecampane. This experience has been cited as a reason not to use elecampane, but this allergy was to inulin, possibly to Jerusalem artichokes, rather than to any herb. There is no evidence whatsoever that the man who experienced a severe allergic reaction after eating foods containing inulin took any herb, including elecampane.[15] Nonetheless, if you are allergic to Jerusalem artichokes, do not take elecampane. There is also a report in the medical literature of a severe allergic reaction to Inutest, a highly refined form of inulin used to measure kidney function. Although this report also has been cited as a reason not to use elecampane, Inutest is not made from elecampane, and the allergic reaction to Inutest occurred after it was *injected* into a sensitive patient.[16]

Horehound, also known as marrubio, is a traditional remedy for bronchitis in the southwestern United States and Mexico. It is also widely used in the Arab world. Unlike over-the-counter remedies for bronchitis, it lowers blood pressure.[17] It relieves the pain of sore throat.[18] Complications from using horehound are rare, but since it is a bitter and bitters stimulate production of stomach acids, people with gastroesophageal reflux disease (GERD), chronic heartburn, or peptic ulcers should use the herb in moderation.

Horseradish and mustard contain volatile oils that have antibacterial properties. They also open bronchial passages. While both herbs can be taken internally, they are more typically used in plasters and poultices.

Ivy leaf, also known as Hedera, is a common remedy for bronchitis in the Azores. Researchers have identified at least 6 chemicals in ivy leaf that stop bronchial spasms.[19] These compounds are not water soluble so the herb must be taken as an extract, although it can be mixed with water to make the extract easier to swallow. Ivy leaf is used to stop "coughing fits" caused by phlegmy coughs rather than dry coughs. Some samples of the herb can contain very small amounts of a nausea-inducing chemical known as emetine, so the herb should not be used by pregnant women or small children.

Lobelia contains the phlegm-dissolving plant chemical lobeline. This chemical acts on the same centers in the brain as nicotine, giving somewhat of the same sense of satisfaction as smoking.[20] Unlike nicotine, this plant chemical makes breathing deeper and stronger. It also stimulates the flow of blood to the heart by activating nerves in the carotid sinus.[21] In overdose, however, it can also activate the vagus nerve, which has roughly the same effect as a punch in the stomach. Too much lobeline, and too much lobelia, can cause nausea and vomiting.

Lobelia makes the brain less sensitive to amphetamines,[22] so it should not be taken by anyone who takes amphetamine or dextroamphetamine (Adderall), methamphetamine (Desoxyn), methylphenidate (Ritalin), or pemoline (Cylert). There is a widely held misconception that lobelia is toxic, but a systematic search of the medical literature failed to find any reports of lobelia poisoning.[23] Ear infections make it more likely that lobelia will cause stomach upset.

According to the herbal reference work *The Complete German Commission E Monographs,* marshmallow contains healing sugars that line and soothe the throat and stop dry cough.[24] Marshmallow teas are more effective at stopping coughs than marshmallow cough drops or tinctures.[25] Marshmallow does not interact with medications, but it is nearly pure sugar and should be used with caution by people who have diabetes.

Mullein contains chemicals that kill bacteria and stop pain.[26] Taken at the same time as a flu treatment such as amatadine (Symmetrel), it greatly increases the probability that the flu treatment will work.[27] The combination of mullein and zanamivir (Relenza) has not yet been tested. Mullein does not generally cause any side effects, although some people may be allergic to it.

Plantain is both soothing and astringent. It contains both mucilages, slimy complex carbohydrates that coat the throat, and tannins, the same chemicals that are found in tea and that tighten the lining of the throat. One of its chemical components is aucubin, a chemical that locks itself to the proteins in the lining of the throat[28] and possibly forms a protective barrier against protection. Another of its components is pectin, a sugar closely related to the pectin used in making jams and jellies, that in its purified form is as potent a stimulator of the immune system as gamma globulin.[29] Plantain is more useful in helping phlegm come up rather than in relieving dry cough. There are no interactions of plantain with prescription drugs, although it should not be taken at the same time as prescription drugs because it can interfere with their absorption.

Scutellaria is one of Traditional Chinese Medicine's most important herbs for treating respiratory infections.

It contains a variety of anti-inflammatory chemicals that are antioxidant in some situations, protecting red blood cells, and prooxidant in others, activating the immune process.[30] It contains several chemicals that are effective in treating bronchitis secondary to infection with respiratory syncitial virus (RSV).[31] That is, unlike most other herbs and medications, scutellaria is antiviral rather than only antibacterial.

Slippery elm makes the lining of the throat "slippery" and reduces inflammation from eating and drinking. The complex carbohydrates in slippery elm are completely digestible and the product is wholly nontoxic. Teas can be made with $1/2$–2 teaspoons of the bark depending on personal preferences. Slippery elm is also found in many herbal cough lozenges.

Thyme releases an essential oil known as thymol, which travels through the bloodstream to be exhaled through the lungs. Of all the herbs studied in the treatment of bronchitis, thyme has the longest half-life, lasting in the body for up to 20 hours.[32] There are reports that the essential oil of thyme, combined with essential oils of cinnamon, cloves, lavender, and mint, may reduce repeated infections in people who have bronchitis. The most common use of thyme, however, is treating coughing spasms in children.

Never take the essential oil of thyme by mouth. The essential oil should only be used in aromatherapy. The chopped herb can be used in teas. There are also commercially available fluid extracts and tinctures of thyme that are safe for use with either children or adults. In Europe, thyme is frequently combined with an extract made from a carnivorous plant, the sundew, to make cough drops such as Ricola.

Eucalyptus oil is a standard ingredient in cough drops and in oils added to humidifiers and vaporizers. While it does not increase breathing capacity, a study of 246 people with chronic bronchitis found that eucalyptus oils stop the worsening of cough that commonly occurs in the winter (in wet climates where heaters are used) or summer (in desert climates).[33]

Homeopathic physicians often recommend ipecacuanha or ipecac (the homeopathic preparation, *not* the antidote for poisons sometimes found in the medicine cabinet) for children's bronchitis or for bronchitis that is worse at night, in a warm room, or when eating. Homeopathic preparations of pulsatilla are used to treat bronchitis with green or yellow phlegm that interferes with going to sleep at night.

CONCEPTS FOR COPING WITH BRONCHITIS

○ Hydrotherapy (alternating hot and cold packs) loosens phlegm.

○ Ask your doctor about getting vaccinated against flu and pneumonia.

○ If you rely on antibiotics for treating bronchitis attacks and you smoke, quit smoking. Some antibiotics for bronchitis, such as erythromycin, are only proven effective for nonsmokers.[34]

○ Avoid exposure to colds and influenza at home or in public, and avoid respiratory irritants such as secondhand smoke, dust, and other air pollutants.

○ Avoid tight belts, bras, and girdles.

○ If you must use a vacuum cleaner, be sure it has a disposable dust bag. Use extreme caution not to break the bag when discarding it.

○ When cooking, always use your exhaust fan, or make sure there is good ventilation.

○ If you drive and gas up your car yourself, try to get upwind from the pump so that you do not inhale the gas.

○ If walking is difficult for you, a urinal by the bedside can be extremely helpful. There are urinal containers made especially for women.

○ If being constantly short of breath makes daily activities difficult, try these energy-saving shortcuts:

  • Don't engage in physical activities until an hour or more after eating. Digestion draws blood, with its oxygen, away from muscles leaving them less able to cope with extra demands. This is the very same reason that children are taught not to go swimming right after meals.

  • If you feel breathless, use pursed-lip breathing.

  • Making a bed is one of the most demanding of household tasks. If you must do it yourself, try making half the bed while you are still in it. Pull the top sheet and blanket up on one side and smooth them out. Exit from the unmade side, which is then easy to finish.

  • If you find taking a shower or bath demanding, try taking a bath or shower while sitting on a bath stool. A terrycloth robe will eliminate the effort of drying: just blot.

  • If you must go up and down stairs and cannot

afford a mechanical chair lift (they are very expensive), have a table or chair at the top of the stairs on which you can lean or sit.

Bruises

SYMPTOM SUMMARY

○ Blue or red markings on the skin that do not change color when pressure is applied

UNDERSTANDING THE DISEASE PROCESS

Bruises form when a blood vessel is damaged. When the wall of a capillary, vein, or artery is broken, blood flows out into the blood vessel's surroundings. If the escaped blood is captured under the skin, there is a bruise.

Everyone bruises from time to time, but some people bruise easily. Easy bruising can be due to problems with blood clot formation. Strong anticoagulant drugs like warfarin (Coumadin) and heparin (Calciparine or Liquaemin in the United States or Calcilean, Calciparine, Hepalean, or Heparin Leo in Canada) can cause excessive bruising when dosages are too high. This is a sign to call a doctor. Over-the-counter remedies such as aspirin, garlic, ginkgo, and vitamin E can also cause bruising when taken in excess.

Another factor in bruising is thin skin, caused by aging or steroid medications. Finally, easy bruising can be due to fragile blood vessel walls. Blood vessel fragility can be treated with herbs and nutritional supplementation. Conventional medical treatment does nothing to speed healing of a bruise.

TREATMENT SUMMARY

NUTRITIONAL SUPPLEMENTS

For preventing bruises:

○ Citrus bioflavonoids containing diosmin and hesperidin: 500 milligrams twice a day.

○ Vitamin C: at least 1,000 milligrams a day.

For accelerating the healing of bruises:

○ Bromelain: taken according to label directions, on an empty stomach.

○ Chymotrypsin and trypsin: taken according to label directions, on an empty stomach.

○ Escin (horse chestnut extract) creams: applied topically to the bruises.

See Part Three if you take prescription medication.

UNDERSTANDING THE HEALING PROCESS

An obvious but often forgotten rule for treating bruises is to give the skin time to recover without being injured again. Nutritional therapies can both help prevent future bruises and help existing bruises heal more quickly.

A French study found that the citrus bioflavonoids diosmin and hesperidin increased capillary strength and decreased the occurrence of at least 6 kinds of bruising: petechiae (pinpoint dots of blood), purpurae (larger areas of bleeding beneath the skin, up to a centimeter in diameter), hematomas (masses of clotted blood), and ecchymoses (areas of bruising larger than a centimeter in diameter), metrorrhagia (excessive menstrual bleeding) and conjunctival hemorrhage (bleeding from bloodshot eyes). There were no measurable results after only 2 weeks, but there were significant differences between the volunteers taking citrus bioflavonoids and the volunteers taking a placebo after 4 weeks. The French research team reported that there were no side effects from the treatment.[1]

If you are taking tamoxifen (Nolvadex) for breast cancer, you should avoid both citrus bioflavonoids and citrus juices. Although citrus bioflavonoids have been used to treat hemorrhoids during pregnancy, most authorities recommend that pregnant women and nursing mothers take no more than 20 milligrams of diosmin and hesperidin daily.

Scientists are unsure of the interaction between citrus bioflavonoids and vitamin C. Citrus bioflavonoids and vitamin C were once thought to be synergistic, but some recent studies suggest that diosmin and hesperidin may actually interfere with the body's ability to absorb vitamin C. To be sure vitamin C requirements are met, take at least a small dose of vitamin C (500 milligrams) when taking citrus bioflavonoids. To help prevent bruising, take a larger dose of vitamin C (at least 1,000 milligrams) a day.

Two studies in the late 1950s found that taking vitamin C reduced the frequency of bruises among collegiate athletes. In a study of 27 wrestlers, 71 percent who did not take vitamin C were injured, compared with only 38 percent of those who did. A follow-up study of football players found that taking vitamin C prevented severe bruises.[2] Vitamin C is also useful in preventing bruises in the elderly. A 2-month trial involving 94 elderly people with vitamin C deficiency found that taking vitamin C supplements decreased their tendency to bruise.[3]

While citrus bioflavonoids and vitamin C are the only supplements that have been scientifically tested for preventing bruises, many other nutritional supplements have similar activity. OPCs (oligomeric proanthocyanidins) such as those found in grape seed extract protect collagen by stopping an enzyme that breaks it down.[4] Anthocyanosides, such as those found in high concentrations in bilberry, also strengthen fragile capillaries by protecting collagen. Additionally, anthocyanosides reduce capillary flow.[5] These supplements are likely to help prevent bruises.

A study reported in the journal *Practitioner* in the late 1960s found that boxers with bruises on their faces and upper bodies healed more quickly when given bromelain. Seventy-four boxers were given bromelain until their bruises disappeared. Seventy-two boxers were given a placebo. Fifty in the bromelain group had no signs of bruising after 4 days, compared to only 10 taking the placebo.[6] A German report of a doctor's experience in using bromelain to treat bruises in 59 patients confirmed that the supplement relieves pain and swelling and restores mobility.[7] Scientists believe bromelain acts by breaking down proteins that are trapped in the bruise after trauma.

Since the concentration of bromelain varies from product to product, it is necessary to follow dosing instructions on the label. If bromelain is taken with food, it will digest the food and not reach bruises. People who take any kind of blood thinner, prescription (Coumadin, heparin, or warfarin) or otherwise (garlic or ginkgo), should not take bromelain.

Like bromelain, the enzymes chymotrypsin and trypsin break down proteins that trap fluids in bruises. A working paper from a German pharmaceutical research group confirms their efficacy in treating karate fighters. Also like bromelain, chymotrypsin and trypsin vary considerably in strength from product to product. They must be taken in the doses suggested on the label, between meals.

The special value of escin creams is its ability to relieve tenderness, especially if the cream is applied immediately after the bruise is formed.[8] Extensive studies of the value of escin creams in the treatment of vari-

cose veins have found them to be very safe, although standards for their use in treating children and pregnant women have not been established.

The herb shepherd's purse (*Capsella bursae pastoris*) is a traditional topical treatment for bruises. It should not be used during pregnancy since it may induce premature labor.

CONCEPTS FOR COPING WITH BRUISES

○ Aside from common bruises due to trauma, bleeding under the skin is a possible sign of a serious medical condition and should be evaluated by a healthcare practitioner.

○ Especially for aging skin, avoid pulling on the skin and other trauma, such as bumping.

○ For a hematoma, on the first day apply cold compresses and pressure to help reduce bleeding and swelling. After the first day, apply hot compresses to help the skin absorb blood.

○ Until the beginning of the twentieth century, leeches were used to drain blood from bruises. A modern ointment called Hirudex contains the anticoagulant in leech saliva and also relieves bruising—without the necessity of applying a leech to the skin.[9]

Bruxism

SYMPTOM SUMMARY

○ Abnormal alignment of the teeth
○ Clenched jaws
○ Earache
○ Jaw pain
○ Loud grinding of the teeth during sleep
○ Muscle contractions in the jaw

UNDERSTANDING THE DISEASE PROCESS

Bruxism is grinding, gnashing, or clenching of the teeth. The condition occurs in about 10–20 percent of the population. The typical age of onset is 17–20 years, and the problem usually resolves itself by age 40.[1] Bruxism can result in broken, chipped, or loose teeth, as well as receding gums.

While clenching the teeth is a common reaction to

stress, bruxism is not necessarily related to anxiety or stress levels. While the disease is more common among people who drink heavily, snore loudly, smoke, or live under conditions of emotional stress,[2] these conditions probably share one of the important neurological causes of the condition, a disturbance in the production of the neurotransmitter dopamine.[3] A more important underlying cause of bruxism may be a deficiency in the production of the neurotransmitter GABA (gamma-aminobutyric acid) in the brain.[4] This may be particularly true when bruxism occurs as a side effect of prescription antidepressants. GABA, an important inhibitor of nerve activity, may block the extraneous nerve impulses that cause grinding teeth.

TREATMENT SUMMARY

SUPPLEMENTS

O Vitamin B_6 (pyridoxine): 50 milligrams 3 times per day.

HERBS

Take either, but not both, of the following:

O Kava, 210 milligrams of kavalactones taken 30 minutes before bedtime.

O Valerian:

- 2–3 grams of the dried herb, *or*
- 270–450 milligrams of an alcohol-free extract, *or*
- 600 milligrams of an ethanol extract.
- Take valerian 30 minutes to 1 hour before bedtime. Combinations of valerian and hops or valerian and lemon balm (melissa) are also effective.

See Part Three if you take prescription medication.

UNDERSTANDING THE HEALING PROCESS

Since GABA is known to play a central role in anxiety and there is some evidence that it plays an important role in bruxism, it would seem logical to take this amino acid as a supplement; however, there is no scientific evidence that GABA taken orally is absorbed into the bloodstream so that it can reach the brain and do any good. Fortunately, vitamin B_6 and the herbs kava and valerian are known to have a favorable effect on GABA utilization in the brain.

Although there is no direct evidence that vitamin B_6 stops bruxism, it is known to be a necessary cofactor in the metabolism of a variety of neurotransmitters whose production is dependent on a process known as amino acid decarboxylation. Once absorbed into the body, vitamin B_6 is converted to pyridoxal-5'-phosphate, a coenzyme in the reaction converting glutamic acid to GABA. As mentioned above, GABA is an important inhibitor of nerve activity.[5]

The use of oral contraceptives increases vitamin B_6 requirements. It is depleted during treatment with carbamazepine for bipolar disorder; cycloserine or ethionamide for tuberculosis; hydralazine for high blood pressure; penicillamine for arthritis, Wilson's disease, and certain skin conditions; phenelzine for cocaine addiction, eating disorders, headaches, and panic attacks; and valproic acid for seizure disorders. If you take any of these prescription drugs and experience bruxism, you should take supplemental vitamin B_6. On the other hand, if you take levodopa for Parkinson's disease, theophylline for asthma, or valproic acid for seizures, you should not take vitamin B_6 supplements, since the vitamin interferes with the body's use of these medications.

Some of the more recent research on kava suggests it acts on the same GABA receptor sites in the brain as the benzodiazepine tranquilizers (a group of drugs including Librium and Valium), which are frequently recommended for bruxism.[6,7] A clinical test found that, over a period of 6 months, kava offers about the same degree of relief as using the benzodiazepine tranquilizers alprazolam (Xanax) and oxazepam (Ox-Pam).[8]

Do not take kava in addition to prescription tranquilizers, especially Xanax. Taking kava with antipsychotic medications can cause abnormal movements, called a dystonic reaction. Kava reduces the effectiveness of L-dopa in the treatment of Parkinson's disease. (See the inset "Kava Ban?" on page 77.)

Valerian reduces the amount of time it takes to fall asleep.[11] Since most bruxism occurs during the first half hour of sleep, valerian reduces the time spent grinding the teeth. Several studies also suggest that valerian affects GABA, binding to GABA receptors in the brain, and providing the benefits of benzodiazepine medications such as Librium and Valium.[12] Unlike these prescription tranquilizers, however, valerian does not cause morning sleepiness.[13]

Valerian has an additive effect when used with barbiturates or benzodiazepine tranquilizers. Do not use both the herb and these prescription medications.

CONCEPTS FOR COPING WITH BRUXISM

❍ Rubber tooth guards are sometimes prescribed to prevent disfigurement of the teeth. Professional fit is necessary to avoid causing the development of an overbite.

Buerger's Disease

See **Raynaud's Phenomenon**.

Bulimia

SYMPTOM SUMMARY

❍ Compulsive consumption of large quantities of high-calorie food, followed by some combination of:

- Forced vomiting
- Use of laxatives
- Compulsive exercise

UNDERSTANDING THE DISEASE PROCESS

Bulimia is also known as bingeing and purging. In this condition, there is an intensely emotional cycle of compulsive overeating followed by drastic attempts to avoid weight gain. The sufferer of bulimia usually forces himself or herself to vomit, although some bulimics take drugs to induce vomiting or laxatives. Diuretics and extreme exercise are other ways bulimics attempt to avoid gaining weight. Binge eating is similar to bulimia except there is no purging cycle.

TREATMENT SUMMARY

NUTRITIONAL SUPPLEMENTS

❍ Inositol: 4,000 milligrams (eight 500-milligram capsules) daily.

See Part Three if you take prescription medication.

UNDERSTANDING THE HEALING PROCESS

There are few supportive therapy options in the treatment of bulimia. Inositol is useful in treating anxiety in people who also have bulimia, binge eating problems, obsessive-compulsive disorder (OCD), or panic attacks. Some recent research suggests that inositol sensitizes

receptor sites in the brain to a biochemical message that a task is complete, stopping the need to keep eating.[1] A preliminary study at the University of the Negev in Israel found that inositol is more effective than antidepressants in controlling binge eating and bulimia.[2]

CONCEPTS FOR COPING WITH BULIMIA

❍ Women with bulimia tend to have low levels of melatonin, although there is no proof that taking melatonin will relieve the disease.[3]

❍ Imagery therapy, in which the patient envisions normal eating habits, sometimes blunts the need to overeat after just one session. It is most effective when bulimia follows a personal tragedy or traumatic event.[4]

Bunions

SYMPTOM SUMMARY

❍ Development of a firm bump on the outside edge of the foot, at the base of the big toe

❍ Inflammation, pain, redness, or swelling at or near the metatarsophalangeal joint at the base of the big toe

❍ Corns or other irritations caused by the overlap of the first and second toes

❍ Restricted or painful motion of the big toe

UNDERSTANDING THE DISEASE PROCESS

A bunion is an enlargement of the joint at the base of the big toe. This swelling forces the toe to bend toward the others, slowly forming a bump of bone on the foot. Since much of the body's weight rests on the joint at the base of the big toe, bunions can become acutely painful if untreated.

TREATMENT SUMMARY

HERBS

For inflammation:

❍ Glycyrrhizin (Simicort cream): applied to site of inflammation once or twice daily.

UNDERSTANDING THE HEALING PROCESS

Glycyrrhizin, an extract of licorice, is a natural anti-inflammatory. Applied to an inflamed bunion, it can reduce pain, redness, and swelling after a few hours.

CONCEPTS FOR COPING WITH BUNIONS

❑ Italian researchers have found that magnets relieve pain of bunions, especially after surgery.[1] Thick magnets imbedded in ceramics or neodymium are more effective than thin magnets imbedded in plastic or rubber. Magnets that are strong enough to relieve pain sometimes cause mild tingling sensations. The best magnets are labeled as having a field of at least 300 gauss (300 G) or 0.8–1.0 Tesla (0.8–1.0 T).

❑ For general relief of bunions:

• Apply a commercial, nonmedicated bunion pad to the bunion. Medicated pads may be allergenic.

• Avoid shoes with heels more than 2 inches (5 cm) tall.

• If your bunion becomes inflamed and painful, apply ice packs several times a day to reduce swelling the first day, then use Simicort to keep inflammation to a minimum.

• Wear shoes with a wide and deep toe box that conform to the shape of your foot. Always fit the larger foot and have your feet sized every time you buy shoes.

Burns

SYMPTOM SUMMARY

❑ First-degree burn

• Skin is reddened but unbroken

• Pain dissipates within a few minutes or hours

❑ Second-degree burn

• Skin blisters and underlying tissues swell, but lower layers of skin are intact

• Pain lingers

❑ Third-degree burn

• Skin is white or charred

• All layers are burned

• Pain is minimal at first due to destruction of nerve tissue, but is usually intense during recovery

UNDERSTANDING THE DISEASE PROCESS

Burns are an ongoing fact of life. Every year nearly 125,000 people in the United States alone suffer burns severe enough to require medical attention. Tens of millions more experience minor burns they care for themselves.

Burns are graded by degree. First-degree burns cause redness but do not break the skin, so there is minimal danger of infection. Second-degree burns cause not only redness but also swelling, lingering pain, and blistering. Third-degree burns involve the all the layers of the skin. Third-degree burns initially cause little pain in the skin itself because of the destruction of nerve tissue. The skin appears either white or charred. Pain in surrounding tissues can be intense.

TREATMENT SUMMARY

SUPPLEMENTS

❑ Vitamin C: 1,000 milligrams daily.

HERBS

❑ Aloe: apply to wounds daily until healed.

❑ Forskolin (a standardized extract of coleus): 5–10 milligrams 3 times daily.

❑ Gotu kola (*Centella asiatica*): 60–120 milligrams of asiaticides daily. Should not be used by women who are trying to become pregnant.

❑ Lavender oil: inhaled lavender oil used as aromatherapy, or several drops of lavender oil diluted in a tablespoon of water applied as a compress to the skin 2–3 days after a first-degree burn.

❑ Sangre de grado: apply to the skin immediately after injury to form a "second skin" and to prevent infection.

See Part Three if you take prescription medication.

UNDERSTANDING THE HEALING PROCESS

If you receive a first- or second-degree burn no larger than the palm of your hand, cool the skin by immersing it in cool water or by applying a cool compress for at least 10 minutes. Never apply ice directly to burned skin. Remove hot tar, melted plastic, or melted wax from the skin with water, not ice. If you receive a first- or small second-degree chemical burn, rinse affected skin under running water for at least 20 minutes. Do not apply butter or ointments. Seek medical care if there are signs of infection, such as odor, pus, or extreme redness.

Second-degree burns larger than the palm of your hand—or of any size on the hands, feet, face, or genitals—and third-degree burns require immediate medical attention. Call for emergency assistance or have someone immediately take you to the doctor. While waiting for help, cut away clothing from the burned area, and remove wristwatches, bracelets, and constrictive clothing that could impede circulation to affected skin. To prevent swelling, elevate burned extremities. *Loosely cover the skin with clean cloth. Do not apply water or anything else to serious burns. Do not treat second- or third-degree burns with the remedies recommended in this book unless your doctor directs you to do so.*

The latest research on the use of vitamin C in the treatment of skin injuries has found that it keeps the basal layers of skin from contracting when the upper layers are injured. This allows regrowth of skin with a minimum of scarring.[1] A series of experiments with animals found that supplementation with relatively high dosages of vitamin C increases the strength of skin growing over the wound and accelerates closure.[2]

Take vitamin C with caution if you also take certain prescription drugs. Vitamin C taken in the form of vitamin C with bioflavonoids can interfere with the liver's ability to process statin drugs for controlling cholesterol, calcium channel blockers such as nifedipine (Procardia) for hypertension, or cyclosporine for preventing transplant rejection.

Aloe is anti-inflammatory, moisturizing, and emollient. It contains a number of antioxidant compounds promoting skin growth, including vitamins C and E and zinc. Unlike hydrocortisone creams used to relieve inflammation, aloe encourages skin healing while relieving pain. Burns[3] and cuts[4] treated with aloe vera gel heal as much as 3 days faster than burns and cuts treated with unmedicated dressings or with chemical antiseptic gels. Allergies to aloe are extremely rare. There are no known drugs that cause adverse reactions when used with aloe.

Forskolin stops a chemical-signaling system by which inflammatory hormones shut down fibroblasts, the cells that generate the extracellular connective tissue matrix.[4] Keeping fibroblasts at the site of the wound encourages the production of collagen and connective tissues across the region of damaged skin.

Gotu kola helps to prevent scarring. Keloids and hypertrophic scars, such as those caused by surgery, result from an extended period of inflammation that may go on for months or years without resolution. During this inflammatory phase, large numbers of swollen bundles of collagen are intermingled with cellular debris. This stage continues until sufficient numbers of fibroblasts are recruited in the wound to create well-defined collagen fibers. A clinical study found that 22 out of 27 patients' scars resolved after using gotu kola for several months.[5]

The nineteenth-century French chemist René-Maurice Gattefossé accidentally discovered the healing effects of lavendar oil when he plunged the hand he burned in a laboratory accident into a container of lavender oil. The oil caused the pain to subside quickly, and his hand to heal rapidly and without scarring. It was not until 1999, however, that scientists were able to explain the therapeutic action of lavender oil on the skin in terms of its effects on energy storage in skin cells. Lavender oil modulates the production of cyclic adenosine monophosphate (cAMP) in such a way that the inflammation process stops and the maturation process of skin cells is initiated. The same mechanism explains its sedative and muscle-relaxant effects when used in aromatherapy.[7]

The unprocessed resin of sangre de grado stimulates the production of collagen in skin injury. This accelerates the formation of a protective crust over burned skin.[8]

CONCEPTS FOR COPING WITH BURNS

O When dealing with a burn, the first priority is to prevent further injury. Remove the victim from the fire or other source of the burn. Douse flames and flush chemicals off the skin with water. If clothing is on fire, lay the victim down and put out flames with water or by covering with a blanket or coat. Alternatively, have the victim turn over *slowly.*

O Do not try to remove burned clothing or objects that adhere to a burn. Leave these to medical personnel.

O Electrical burns are frequently deeper and more severe than they first appear.

O Use cool, wet compresses, not ice, to relieve pain of minor burns. Avoid prolonged cooling of large areas of the body.

O Do not use butter, margarine, grease, or petroleum jelly to cover a burn.

○ Avoid breaking blisters, which increases the risk of infection. See a doctor if blisters becomes infected.

Bursitis

SYMPTOM SUMMARY

○ Joint pain and tenderness

○ Swelling over affected joint

○ Warmth over affected joint

UNDERSTANDING THE DISEASE PROCESS

Bursitis is a condition of inflammation of one or more bursae. Everyone has hundreds of bursae scattered throughout the body. The bursae decrease friction between two surfaces that move in different directions, where ligaments, muscles, and tendons glide over bones. Dr. Jonathan Cluett compares them to a ziplock bag with a small amount of oil and no air inside. As long as nothing gets inside the bag, it provides a slippery surface with almost no friction. When the bag is puffed up with air, it blocks motion rather than aiding it.

In bursitis, the bursae fill with fluid released in response to inflammation. Bursitis most commonly occurs at the back of the heel (retrocalcaneal bursitis), below the kneecap (infrapatellar bursitis), or in the hip (olecranon bursitis) or elbow (trochanteric bursitis).

Bursitis can result from infection, gout, trauma, or rheumatoid arthritis, but its most common cause is chronic overuse of the joint. "Miner's elbow" (from swinging a pick) and "housemaid's knee" (from scrubbing floors) are classical forms of the condition. In the modern world, the occupational group most likely to suffer bursitis are housekeepers and janitors, who repetitively push and pull vacuums over floors, as well as landscapers, carpet layers, and roofers. For people in sedentary occupations, attacks of bursitis usually follow unusual exercise or strain and last for a few days to a few weeks.

At a microscopic level, stress and strain on a bursa causes a breakdown of the collagen fibers holding the bursa together. The immune system senses the presence of injured tissues and sends neutrophils to release hormones that cause swelling to hold the fibers of the bursa in place. When the total damage is too great, however, fluid accumulates in the bursa and there is intense pain.[1]

TREATMENT SUMMARY

NUTRITIONAL SUPPLEMENTS

○ Vitamin B_{12}: injection from a nutritionally oriented healthcare practitioner, followed by supplementation with 1,000–2,000 micrograms (1–2 milligrams) of B_{12} plus 800 micrograms of folic acid every day under the supervision of a healthcare practitioner.

HERBS

For pain relief, select from:

○ Bromelain: 250–500 milligrams 3 times a day.

○ Devil's claw: 405–520 milligrams up to 8 times a day.

○ Feverfew: 70–100 milligrams of dried extract daily.

○ Ginger (fresh): 2 tablespoons included in vegetable dishes, fruit salad, or used to make a tea.

○ Willow bark: 1 teaspoon in a cup of hot water or tea, as desired.

If you take steroid injections:

○ Glycyrrhizin: 250–500 milligrams daily for up to 6 weeks at a time.

See Part Three if you take prescription medication.

UNDERSTANDING THE HEALING PROCESS

The first step in healing bursitis is resting the affected joint. In severe cases, it may be necessary to immobilize the joint with a splint. When rest is not enough, it may be helpful to remove fluid from the bursa by aspiration, that is, removing fluid with a needle and syringe after the area has been treated with a local anesthetic. It is important to resume using the joint as soon as pain resolves, since muscles can atrophy from prolonged disuse or immobility.

In the 1950s, researchers reported that injections of vitamin B_{12} can relieve pain in bursitis of the shoulder and stop calcification around the joint.[2] The way vitamin B_{12} works to stop inflammation was not understood until over 30 years later. Studies of other kinds of inflammation have revealed that vitamin B_{12} binds to proteins that otherwise act as a kind of loading dock for a specialized subset of white blood cells known as neutrophils, which release chemical agents of pain and swelling.[3]

There are no well-established protocols for treating bursitis with vitamin B_{12}. The people most likely to benefit from taking vitamin B_{12} are those who use the diuretic furosemide (Lasix), or people with neuropathy (experiencing burning, numbness, or tingling of the skin that cannot be linked to any obvious cause). The best approach is to get an injection of the vitamin from a nutritionally oriented healthcare practitioner, and then to prevent future deficiencies by taking 1,000–2,000 milligrams of the vitamin every day.

Once your symptoms have improved, it is possible to develop a new vitamin B_{12} deficiency that will not be as evident if you take more than 800 micrograms of folic acid daily. Folic acid supplementation can mask many of the symptoms of B_{12} deficiency long enough that permanent nerve damage can result. Never take 800 micrograms of folic acid on a daily basis except under the supervision of qualified healthcare practitioner.

Bromelain can start relieving pain and swelling almost as soon as you start taking it, provided you take it in an enteric-coated form (unavailable in the United States).[4] For those of us who have to take uncoated bromelain tablets, it is best to experiment with the smallest dose and increase by 250 milligrams a day until the highest recommended dose is reached. It may be necessary to take the highest recommended dose of uncoated bromelain for a week before obtaining relief.

Allergies to bromelain are very rare but not unheard of. Allergic reactions to this supplement are most likely in people who are already allergic to pineapple, papaya, wheat flour, rye flour, or birch pollen. There has never been a report of an anaphylactic reaction to bromelain. There have been isolated reports of heavy periods, nausea, vomiting, and hives when bromelain is taken in very large overdoses (2,000 milligrams and higher).

Devil's claw relieves joint pain, but only if it is taken in an enteric-coated form that protects its analgesic compounds from being digested in the stomach. Do not use devil's claw with NSAIDs such as aspirin and Tylenol and avoid the herb entirely if you have duodenal or gastric ulcers.

Clinical trials with women who have arthritis found that taking 70–86 milligrams of feverfew every day for 6 weeks increased grip strength. Feverfew likewise can cause stomach irritation. Do not use it with NSAIDs and avoid the herb if you have ulcers.

Two tablespoons of fresh ginger every day is likely to relieve pain and swelling even when pain relievers are discontinued, but the effect takes 1–3 months.

Willow bark is a natural substitute for aspirin. It contains salicin, a less potent pain reliever than the salicy-lates found in aspirin but one that does not generally cause bleeding or stomach irritation. Do not use willow bark during pregnancy, if you have tinnitus (ringing in the ears), or if you are allergic to aspirin. Do not give willow bark or aspirin to children who have colds or flu.

If you are taking injections of steroids to relieve pain, a licorice derivative called glycyrrhizin can help make them more effective. It increases the half-life of cortisol and other steroids, making them work longer to undo the damage done to your joints.[5] The downside of using glycyrrhizin for this purpose is that it *will* increase any side effects you experience from cortisone. When you take both glycyrrhizin and any corticosteroid drug, you are more likely to experience weight gain, puffiness, and elevated blood pressure. Do not take glycyrrhizin for more than 6 weeks at a time. Preferably, use it during your peak allergy season. Do not take glycyrrhizin if you have high blood pressure. DGL is another licorice derivative that does not aggravate side effects of steroid treatment, but it will not help bursitis.

CONCEPTS FOR COPING WITH BURSITIS

❍ To prevent recurrences of bursitis, you should take the pain relief supplements listed in the section above. Other helpful measures include:

• Protect the joint. Rest the joint during an attack of bursitis. When you resume activity, keep pressure off the affected joint by wearing an elastic bandage, splint, or brace.

• Use cushions. If a bandage, splint, or brace interferes with your work, use protective cushions. Pads for the knees are available at hardware stores.

• Take breaks. Alternate repetitive tasks with breaks to relieve pressure.

❍ Raisins soaked in gin are a commonly recommended remedy for bursitis and many other conditions of joint inflammation. Research indicates, however, that relief is due to the gin, not the raisins. Drinking beverage alcohol stops the flow of neutrophils to sites of inflammation and keeps them from releasing hormones that cause pain and swelling.[6]

❍ The Instituto Superior de Ciencias Médicas "Dr. Carlos Juan Finlay" in Camagüey, Cuba, has done extensive research in the use of acupressure and acupuncture in treating a particularly troublesome form of bursitis, frozen shoulder.[7] Their research involving 60 patients found that using either treatment over a period of 10 weeks increased range of motion for all participants in the study and reduced pain in 59 out of 60 participants in the study. Acupuncture alone began to show results in an average of 7 weeks. Acupressure plus acupuncture got results in an average of 4 weeks.

The Cuban study did not consider acupressure used by itself, but it is likely that acupressure will begin to help relieve pain and restore motion in a couple of months. One of the points to massage to relieve frozen shoulder can be found by extending the arm horizontally away from the body. The depression made beneath the shoulder is one of the areas to massage to relieve shoulder pain. (It is not necessary to extend the arm horizontally during massage.) Other points are at the front of the shoulder where it joins the arm and at the outside of the crease in the arm on the opposite side of the elbow.

Cachexia
See **Wasting**.

Cancer
See **Actinic Keratosis; Basal Cell Carcinoma; Bladder Cancer; Breast Cancer; Colorectal Cancer; Lung Cancer; Pancreatic Cancer; Prostate Cancer**.

Canker Sores

SYMPTOM SUMMARY

○ Burning or tingling sensation on the mucous membranes of the mouth, followed by red spots that become open ulcers
- Usually small (not wider than $1/2$ inch, or 1 centimeter)
- Often appearing in groups
- Painful
- Center appears white or yellow
- May have red halo
- May be covered with gray membrane just before healing

UNDERSTANDING THE DISEASE PROCESS

Canker sores are areas of inflammation on the lining of the mouth that have a characteristic white or yellow center with a fibrous texture and usually a red halo. They range in size from a pinhead to a pea. Canker sores start out as small, circular, reddish swelling that usually rupture within a day. Later, they are covered by a thin gray film. Because canker sores are located in the mouth, there is considerable opportunity for saliva, food, and drinks to irritate them.

The medical literature refers to canker sores as aphthous stomatitis. Physiological factors for the disease include stress, food sensitivity, and nutrient deficiencies. Stress encourages the formation of inflammatory hormones and is associated with recurrent outbreaks of canker sores, although stress is not enough to cause canker sores by itself.[1] In the 1970s, British researchers found that a majority of people who suffer recurrent bouts of canker sores are sensitive to gliadin. This protein is a component of gluten, which is found in all forms of wheat (including durum, and semolina), rye, oats, barley, and related grain hybrids such as kamut and triticale. When someone who is sensitive to gliadin consumes these grains, the intestine releases massive quantities of an immune protein called immunoglobulin A (IgA). This immune protein is ordinarily the body's first line of defense against disease-causing microorganisms that enter through the skin and mucosal surfaces. The immune system mistakenly binds IgA to cells in the lining of the mouth and treats them as if they had become infected.[2]

The immune disturbance that causes canker sores also interferes with normal absorption of nutrients. Many people who have canker sores are deficient in the B vitamins pyridoxine, riboflavin, or thiamine.[3] Iron deficiency is also a common problem.[4] Food *allergies,* however, are mediated by a different set of immunoglobulins than those involved in gliadin sensitivity and are not usually a contributing factor in canker sores.

TREATMENT SUMMARY

DIET

○ Avoid gluten.

NUTRITIONAL SUPPLEMENTS

○ Any complete B-complex multivitamin, daily.

HERBS

○ Aloe: gel applied to sores, several times a day.

○ Chamomile: tea, sipped slowly, several times a day.

○ Deglycyrrhizinated licorice (DGL): chewable tablets, several times a day.

See Part Three if you take prescription medication.

UNDERSTANDING THE HEALING PROCESS

The first step in treating canker sores is to stop the inflammatory process. Try to avoid *all* foods made with wheat or any other grain containing gluten. Sources of hidden gluten include caramel, gum, hydrolyzed plant protein (HPP), hydrolyzed vegetable protein (HVP), malt, maltodextrin, modified food starch, mono- and diglycerides, natural flavoring, soy sauce, texturized vegetable protein (TVP), and vinegar. Spelt, a wheatlike grain, has a different kind of gluten and is a good alternative to wheat for many people with canker sores (although not for people with celiac disease). At least one study found that people with canker sores usually benefit from a gluten-free diet even if they have no evidence of other changes usually associated with gluten sensitivity (see CELIAC DISEASE).[5]

B vitamins are frequently recommended for canker sores. Daily doses of 300 milligrams of vitamin B_1 (thiamine), 20 milligrams of vitamin B_2 (riboflavin), and 150 milligrams of vitamin B_6 (pyridoxine) have been found to give some people relief.[6] There is virtually no downside to using B vitamins. They are inexpensive and they do not cause side effects (although riboflavin may impart an orange color to the urine). Unfortunately, they are helpful only about 30 percent of the time. The people who are most likely to benefit from vitamin B supplementation are those who take the diuretic furosemide (Lasix) and heavy drinkers of coffee and tea.

Other vitamins and minerals have been used successfully to treat canker sores, but at risk of side effects. One study found that a daily dosage of 150 milligrams of zinc reduced recurrences of canker sores by 50–100 percent,[7] but the likely mode of action was reducing the immune system's production of neutrophils. This reduces the formation of canker sores but also reduces the immune system's ability to respond to bacteria and viruses. Iron deficiency has been found in about 15 percent of people with canker sores, but supplementation with iron when it is not needed can aggravate the rare,

but potentially deadly, iron storage disease hemachromatosis. Never take iron supplements unless you have had a blood test indicating that you are deficient in iron.

Herbal treatment is a better bet. Aloe gel stimulates the formation of a protective layer over mouth sores. One study found that aloe was more effective than the conventional treatment Orabase Plain.[8] Allergies to aloe are very rare. Taken internally in large doses, however, aloe is a laxative. Use only enough to cover the sore.

Chamomile teas soothe soreness in the mouth. They won't help, however, if they are prepared with *boiling* water. *Hot* water releases the volatile oil containing anti-inflammatory chamazulene, while boiling water causes it to evaporate. Chamazulene quenches free radicals that enable the formation of inflammatory leukotrienes,[9] and another compound in the essential oil serves as an antihistamine.[10] Allergic reactions to chamomile are rare but possible. Most European regulatory boards advise that chamomile should not be used during pregnancy.

Deglycyrrhizinated licorice (DGL) contains the anti-inflammatory chemicals found in licorice without glycyrrhizin, a chemical that can cause water retention, swelling, high blood pressure, and irregular heart rhythms. It is important to chew DGL tablets rather than swallowing them whole, since mixing DGL with saliva is required to release the healing agents. At least one study has found that a mixture of DGL and water applied to the inside of the mouth can shorten the healing time for canker sores, with complete healing typically occurring on the third day.[11]

CONCEPTS FOR COPING WITH CANKER SORES

○ Most toothpastes contain sodium lauryl sulfate (SLS), a foaming agent also found in shampoo and in "foaming bubble" floor and tile cleaners. Widely circulated stories that SLS can cause cancer are false, but there is good evidence that SLS aggravates canker sores. A Norwegian study reported in 1996 found that most canker sores were avoided just by using a toothpaste not containing SLS for 3 months,[12] although a British study in 1999 failed to confirm the results.[13] The difference between the results of the two studies could be as simple as differences in rinsing: 96 percent of SLS in toothpaste can be removed from the mouth with a 2-minute rinse.[14] Try rinsing more thoroughly after every brushing. If that doesn't help, try an SLS-free toothpaste such as CloSys II or Enamel Saver for 3 months to see if it helps.

○ Avoid foods and drinks that will irritate the sore. These include abrasive foods, such as potato chips and pretzels, and acidic foods, such as orange juice and vinegar.

○ Take care not to irritate the sore with your toothbrush or eating utensils.

○ Irritating caused by braces, rough fillings, or poorly fitted dentures can aggravate canker sores. Ask your dentist about adjustments if canker sores are a recurrent problem.

○ Antibiotic mouthwashes containing tetracycline are not appropriate for canker sores. The problem is not caused by infection, so an antibiotic will not help. Moreover, overuse of tetracycline can cause a yeast infection called thrush in adults and discolor teeth in children. An analgesic product containing benzocaine (Anbesol, Num-Zit, or Zilactin-B), on the other hand, will relieve pain but will not speed healing.

○ The medical literature reports at least one case in which a person with canker sores later developed a much more serious condition, celiac disease, after eating a normal diet for several years.[15] Some physicians suggest that anyone who has had canker sores should be tested for gliadin sensitivity, a measure of especially potent antibodies to the proteins in gluten. A blood test is not necessary; saliva testing is now available. For information, ask your physician to contact Great Smokies Diagnostic Laboratory in Asheville, North Carolina, 1-800-252-9303.

Capillary Fragility
See **Bruises**.

Car Sickness
See **Motion Sickness**.

Cardiac Arrhythmia
See **Irregular Heartbeat**.

Cardiomyopathy

SYMPTOM SUMMARY
○ Difficulty breathing after light exertion
○ Easily fatigued
○ Swollen ankles
○ Swollen abdomen

UNDERSTANDING THE DISEASE PROCESS

Cardiomyopathy is a condition of damage to the heart muscle. The most common form of cardiomyopathy is dilated congestive cardiomyopathy, in which the heart muscle has been damaged by coronary artery disease or heart attack. Diabetics are especially at risk for this form of cardiomyopathy. Dilated congestive cardiomyopathy can also occur after infection or exposure to certain toxins, as a side of effect of chemotherapy, and during pregnancy. Another form of cardiomyopathy, commonly referred to as "enlarged heart," is a hereditary condition.

According to the eminent cardiologist Demetrio Sodi-Pallares, a common feature of all forms of cardiomyopathy at a cellular level is an overwhelming influx of sodium.[1] When sodium goes in, calcium goes out. Without an adequate supply of calcium, the heart cell does not respond to electrical impulses to make it beat, unless there is destruction of its cholesterol lining. Electrons released during the destruction of the cell membrane change the electrical balance of the cell so that it can continue to beat. Only continuing degradation of the cell membrane enables the cell to function as part of the heart.

As the heart cell is being "burned" on the outside, it loses its ability to produce energy inside. Sodium is required for transporting glucose into cells. When salt builds up inside a cell, the accumulation of positively charged ions of sodium in the heart cell repels (like charges repelling each other) both additional sodium ions and the glucose they transport. The cell's glycogen supplies go down while its concentration of potentially toxic lactic acid goes up.

Finally, sick heart cells become swollen. When sodium goes in the cell, water follows. A peculiarity of cardiomyopathy is that as heart tissue is destroyed, the heart gets bigger. Cardiomyopathy causes an enlarged, energy-deprived, "water-logged" heart that beats less and less efficiently and eventually dies unless chemical and electrical balances can be restored.

TREATMENT SUMMARY

DIET

○ *Eliminate* added salt from your diet.

NUTRITIONAL SUPPLEMENTS

○ Coenzyme Q_{10}: 150–300 milligrams daily.

○ L-carnitine: 300 milligrams 3 times a day.

Diabetics can especially benefit from:

○ Pantethine: 300 milligrams 3 times a day.

HERBS

Most important:

○ Hawthorn in any one of the following forms, 3 times a day:

- Solid extract (standardized to contain 1.8 percent vitexin-4'-rhamnoside): 100–250 milligrams.
- Leaf and flowers as a tea: 1–2 teaspoons (3–5 grams).
- Fluid extract: 1–2 milliliters ($1/2$–1 teaspoon).

People with cardiomyopathy frequently also benefit from:

○ Arjuna (*Terminalia arjuna*): extract, as directed by dispensing herbalist.

○ Pushkarmoola (*Inula racemosa*): extract, as directed by dispensing herbalist.

See Part Three if you take prescription medication.

UNDERSTANDING THE HEALING PROCESS

Cardiomyopathy is a life-threatening condition for which a doctor's care is required. However, diet can work wonders. Additionally, there are several supplements that are generally helpful in dilated congestive cardiomyopathy. Consult your cardiologist before beginning supplemental therapy, and never stop taking a prescribed medication without your cardiologist's approval.

As this book is being written, 10,000 patients are involved in clinical trials of sodium-restricted diets in the treatment of cardiomyopathy throughout Latin America. The results of removing sodium from the diet in treating cardiomyopathy are sometimes dramatic. In as little as 2 weeks, the heart can return to its normal size and function—simply by removing the burden of sodium from ingested salt.

A truly salt-free diet is not easy. It is mandatory to eliminate all sources of excess sodium, including:

- All drugs containing sodium, such as Alka-Seltzer and aspirin.
- Anchovies, canned salmon, sardines, and shellfish in general.
- Any "fizzy" drink not specifically labeled as low-sodium.
- Any kind of salted, grilled meat, salted soup, or consommé.
- Bacon, ham, sausages, and all cured meats, pork or otherwise.
- Beer, carbonated beverages sweetened with sugar or aspartame, and mineral water.
- Beets, celery, and spinach.
- Breakfast cereals, bread, biscuits, pancakes, and waffles.
- Cheeses and other processed dairy products.
- Chocolate.
- Dried fruit and nuts.
- Peanuts, whether salted or not.
- Popcorn.
- Prepared foods of all types, especially salad dressings.

It is not unusual for patients to get very good results from sodium restriction—and to be told by their doctors that only medication can make cardiomyopathy better, so they go off their salt-restricted diets. Symptoms invariably return. It is important to let your doctor know you are attempting a rigorous salt-exclusion diet so dosages of your medications can be adjusted downward as you recover, but don't allow your doctor's skepticism to discourage you from this very important step in self-care.

Several supplements are also helpful in complementary care of cardiomyopathy. Coenzyme Q_{10} (CoQ$_{10}$) is synthesized by every cell in the body to capture electrons released as the mitochondria release the energy by combining sugar with oxygen. A solid, waxlike substance, CoQ$_{10}$ is made by the same chemical process that makes cholesterol, and, like cholesterol, CoQ$_{10}$ is especially abundant in the healthy heart. Since the heart muscle makes and uses energy 24 hours a day, it needs a large quantity of CoQ_{10}. Heart tissue biopsies of people with various heart diseases show a deficiency of CoQ_{10} of 50–75 percent of what is normal.[2] This effect is most severe at the point when circulation is restored to the heart muscle following a heart attack.[3]

As people age, the heart makes less CoQ_{10}. Certain cholesterol-lowering drugs also reduce the heart's supply of this vital enzyme. Replacing CoQ_{10} is important in treating angina.

In one study, 12 patients with restricted circulation were given 150 milligrams of CoQ_{10} daily for 4 weeks. Taking CoQ_{10} reduced the average frequency of angina attacks by 53 percent. CoQ_{10} treatment also allowed the angina patients to last longer on a treadmill before experiencing chest pain or abnormal EKGs.[4]

Even heart patients with severe cardiomyopathy benefit from CoQ_{10}. A Danish study found that treatment with the supplement for 12 weeks increased the output of the heart at rest and during exercise.[5] The supplement is similarly useful in treating hereditary hypertrophic cardiomyopathy, more commonly known as "enlarged heart." Doctors at the Langsjoen Clinic in Tyler, Texas, found that giving patients 200 milligrams of CoQ_{10} for 3 months reduced the thickness of the septum dividing the heart muscle by an average of 24 percent and the thickness of the posterior wall by 26 percent.[6]

There are very few precautions to take in the use of CoQ_{10}. The medical literature contains one report of CoQ_{10} decreasing the effectiveness of warfarin (Coumadin). It may improve sugar control in some cases of diabetes. If you are diabetic, check your blood sugars regularly when you take CoQ_{10}. Black pepper increases bloodstream levels of CoQ_{10}; seasoning your food with pepper would be helpful when you take CoQ_{10}.

L-carnitine also increases the heart's energy supply. L-carnitine carries fatty acids into the mitochondria, where they can be used for fuel. Most of the body's supply of L-carnitine is made in the kidneys and the liver. Stresses on these organs (such as diabetes or chronic alcohol abuse) diminish the supply of L-carnitine for the heart. When the heart has an inadequate oxygen supply, it quickly uses up its supply of L-carnitine and is then less able to produce energy.

Administering massive doses of L-carnitine, 2,000 milligrams of L-carnitine for every 100 pounds (45 kilograms) of body weight, after a heart attack has been shown to reduce heart damage.[7] A Japanese study found that taking 900 milligrams of L-carnitine daily allowed heart patients to last 2.4 minutes longer in their stress tests. An Italian study in which men with angina were given 1,000 milligrams of L-carnitine daily found they not only could last longer under stress, but could also work harder, as measured by a bicycle ergometer.[8] Approximately 1 in 30 people will experience nausea, heartburn, or gas when taking L-carnitine, but it is generally very free of side effects. People with seizure disorders, however, should consult with their physicians before taking this supplement.

Pantethine is a B-vitamin derivative that helps transport useful fatty acids into cells. It lowers total cholesterol, LDL, and triglycerides, and raises HDL without interfering with the production of L-carnitine. In one study involving diabetics, taking 600 milligrams of pantethine daily lowered triglyceride levels by 37 percent.[9] Generally, pantethine lowers total cholesterol by 15–25 percent and triglycerides by 25–40 percent. Taking much more than 600 milligrams per day can increase your susceptibility to sunburn, especially if you take the blood pressure medication lisinopril (Prinivil or Zestril).

Herbs used to treat cardiomyopathy open circulation. Hawthorn is both extraordinarily safe and extraordinarily effective in treating various forms of heart disease. This herb contains a variety of flavonoids. Some increase blood flow through the coronary arteries. Some increase left ventricular pressure, making each heartbeat stronger. Some accelerate the heart rate—and some decelerate it.[10] But the most important property of hawthorn is its ability to protect the heart from the effects of oxygen deprivation.

Heart cells, like many other tissues, are able to adapt to oxygen deprivation. They shift their energy production from pathways requiring the use of oxygen to pathways requiring the use of fatty acids. However, when their oxygen supply is restored, as it is when an angina attack ends, they are sometimes damaged and sometimes destroyed.

At the end of an attack of angina induced by the failure of the heart muscle to pump blood, the neutrophils of the immune system release a compound known as human neutrophil elastase (HNE), allowing the arteries to stretch back to a more normal size. The process of relaxing the artery, however, releases massive quantities of free radicals that disrupt the cholesterol coats of heart cells and interfere with the action of L-carnitine. At least one of the flavonoid compounds in hawthorn counteracts HNE.[11]

Hawthorn has several other beneficial effects. Animal studies have found that hawthorn stimulates the liver to use LDL cholesterol to make bile salts, cholesterol salts that are flushed out of the liver into the stool.[12] Other studies with laboratory animals have found that the hawthorn compound monoacetyl-vitexin rhamnoside relaxes the linings of the arteries, permitting greater blood flow, through a complicated chemical process.[13] And at least one animal study suggests that hawthorn can prevent irreversible tissue damage during heart attack.[14]

There are very few precautions for the use of hawthorn. It is almost completely nontoxic. Like many other natural treatments for angina, however, it can cause diarrhea the first few days you take it.

Arjuna has been used in Ayurvedic medicine for over 2,500 years as a "cardiac tonic." Ayurvedic physicians offer it as arjunatvagadi (arjuna in water), pardhadyaristam (grapes and arjuna fermented and boiled), arjunaghrtam (arjuna paste), and arjunatvak (arjuna powder). Animal experiments have shown that arjuna slows and strengthens the heartbeat and protects the heart from tissue destruction during oxygen deprivation. In a study of the use of the herb in treating mild angina, patients given the herb were found to have greater endurance in treadmill tests, without the complication of lowered blood pressure. Over a period of 3 months, 66 percent of stable angina patients and 20 percent of unstable angina patients showed improved EKGs.[15] Follow-up studies at the same clinic found that arjuna is also useful in treating cardiomyopathy caused by heart attack. Treatment with the herb reduced left ventricular mass by an average of 12 percent in 3 months.[16]

Arjuna is usually dispensed by a practitioner of Ayurvedic medicine. There have been no reports of side effects from arjuna products given by herbalists or physicians trained in Ayurveda. Dosage varies with the individual preparation.

Pushkarmoola is another Ayurvedic herb that grows in the foothills of the northwestern Himalayas. Traditional South Asian medicine uses pushkarmoola in the treatment of angina with shortness of breath. A small-scale study in India found that pushkarmoola was more effective than nitroglycerin in effecting favorable EKG changes (elevation of the S-T segment) and in relieving chest pain.[17] And a study involving 200 patients found that combining pushkarmoola with the traditional Indian herb guggul (*Commiphora mukkul*) in treatment for 6 months relieved shortness of breath in 60 percent of angina patients who had shortness of breath as a symptom at the beginning of the study. One in four patients experienced a complete remission of pain and showed a normal EKG by the end of 6 months of treatment.[18]

Like arjuna, pushkarmoola is also available from practitioners of Ayurveda. There are no reports of side effects from pushkarmoola products given by herbalists or physicians trained in Ayurveda.

CONCEPTS FOR COPING WITH CARDIOMYOPATHY

○ Following your diet plan can have unexpected results. If you are especially diligent in avoiding salt, your cardiologist may have to lower your dosage of digoxin.

○ If you have been taking St. John's wort for depression before being treated for cardiomyopathy, do not stop taking the herb abruptly. Your cardiologist will probably need to adjust several medications, including digoxin, when you stop taking the herb.[19] Always tell your doctor about any herbal supplements you take.

○ Immigrants from China sometimes suffer from Keshan disease, a form of cardiomyopathy related to selenium deficiency. Known only among people who have eaten a "one-sided diet," a limited variety of local foods in certain areas of northeastern China and Taiwan, this condition usually results from an inability of the heart to respond to viral infection after many years of eating foods grown in soils that lack selenium.[20] In rare cases, people with an inability to absorb selenium can also develop the disease.[21] Although taking a modest amount of supplemental selenium (100 micrograms a day) might help prevent disease in people who have recently immigrated from areas where it is common, once Keshan cardiomyopathy occurs it cannot be treated with selenium supplementation alone.

Cardiovascular Disease
See **Aneurysm; Angina; Cardiomyopathy; Congestive Heart Failure; High Cholesterol; High Triglyercides; Hypertension; Intermittent Claudication; Irregular Heartbeat; Peripheral Vascular Disease; Raynaud's Phenomenon.**

Carpal Tunnel Syndrome

SYMPTOM SUMMARY

○ Difficulty bringing the thumb across the palm to touch other fingers

○ Impaired fine finger movements

○ Numbness or tingling of the palm

○ Numbness or tingling of the thumb and adjacent fingers

○ Weak grip

○ Wrist pain in one or both hands

○ Tapping over the median nerve causes numbness

UNDERSTANDING THE DISEASE PROCESS

Carpal tunnel syndrome (CTS) is a painful compression of the median nerve. On its path to the hand, the median passes through an opening in the wrist known as the carpal tunnel. The ligaments and tendons inside the tunnel may be compressed by repetitive motion of the hand, causing the tunnel walls to close in. As the opening for the nerve narrows, it compresses. This causes numbness and tingling in the thumb, index finger, middle finger, and part of the ring finger. The pain of CTS keeps people awake at night and makes it difficult to pick up small objects.

There is disagreement among physicians as to whether most cases of CTS are job related. CTS in people under the age of 40 and affecting the dominant hand is much more likely to be associated with an anatomic variation in the structure of the hand.[1] There is some evidence that people with CTS suffer an abnormality in the formation of collagen in which the production of collagen is unusually sensitive to vitamin C.[2] That is, vitamin C, unless complemented by vitamin B₆, stimulates the production of defective collagen. Long-term treatment with growth hormone sometimes causes CTS,[3] and the condition is a common complication of any condition causing swelling, such as PMS or pregnancy, as well as acromegaly, diabetes, fungal infection, high blood pressure, hypothyroidism, kidney failure, multiple myeloma, obesity, and tuberculosis. The occupational groups most likely to develop CTS are artists, assembly workers, athletes, computer programmers, model makers, musicians, short order cooks, sign language communicators, and typists.

TREATMENT SUMMARY

NUTRITIONAL SUPPLEMENTS

○ Vitamin B₆: 200 milligrams daily.

○ Do *not* take supplemental vitamin C unless you also take vitamin B₆.

For pain relief, select from:

○ Bromelain: 250–500 milligrams 3 times a day.

○ Devil's claw: 405–520 milligrams up to 8 times a day.

○ Feverfew: 70–100 milligrams of dried extract daily.

○ Ginger (fresh): 2 tablespoons included in vegetable dishes, fruit salad, or used to make a tea.

○ Willow bark: 1 teaspoon in a cup of hot water or tea, as desired.

If you take steroid injections:

○ Glycyrrhizin: 250–500 milligrams daily for up to 6 weeks at a time.

See Part Three if you take prescription medication.

UNDERSTANDING THE HEALING PROCESS

The only nutritional supplement with a known effect on the disease process of CTS is vitamin B₆. This vitamin has little effect on the function of the hand, but is useful in relieving pain.[4] The *balance* between vitamin B₆ and vitamin C in the bloodstream may be more important in CTS. In a study of 441 adults with CTS, higher ratios of vitamin C to vitamin B₆ (such as might occur when taking supplemental vitamin C without vitamin B₆) were associated with the severity of pain and the frequency of pain, tingling, and waking up at night.[5]

Most of the studies involving vitamin B₆ used a dosage of 200 milligrams daily. This dosage is too much for pregnant women and nursing mothers, who should limit intake to 100 milligrams per day. There have been a very few cases in which taking 100–200 milligrams of vitamin B₆ a day aggravated existing nerve damage. Therefore, diabetics also should use no more than 100 milligrams per day if they have sensory neuropathy, that is, nerve damage to the hands and feet. Men who use sildenafil citrate (Viagra) should avoid high doses of this vitamin.

Vitamin B₆ requirements are affected by many medications. The use of oral contraceptives increases vitamin B$_6$ requirements. The vitamin is depleted during treatment with carbamazepine for bipolar disorder; cycloserine or ethionamide for tuberculosis; hydralazine for high blood pressure; penicillamine for arthritis, Wilson's disease, and certain skin conditions; and phenelzine for cocaine addiction, eating disorders, headaches, and panic attacks. If you take any of these prescription drugs and have carpal tunnel syndrome, you should take supplemental vitamin B$_6$. On the other hand, if you take levodopa for Parkinson's disease, theophylline for asthma, or phenytoin or valproic acid for seizures, you should not take vitamin B$_6$ supplements, since the vitamin can deactivate these medications. Regardless of the medications you take, if you experience abdominal pain, loss of appetite, nausea, vomiting, breast pain, or unexplained sensitivity to sun, discontinue use of the vitamin.

Several other supplements help relieve pain. Bromelain can start relieving pain and swelling almost as soon as you start taking it, provided you take it in an enteric-coated form (unavailable in the United States).[6] For those of us who have to take uncoated bromelain tablets, it is best to experiment with the smallest dose and increase by 250 milligrams a day until the highest recommended dose is reached. It may be necessary to take the highest recommended dose of uncoated bromelain for a week before obtaining relief.

Allergies to bromelain are very rare but not unheard of. Allergic reactions to this supplement are most likely to occur in people who are already allergic to pineapple, papaya, wheat flour, rye flour, or birch pollen. There has never been a report of an anaphylactic reaction to bromelain. There have been isolated reports of heavy periods, nausea, vomiting, and hives when bromelain is taken in very large overdoses (2,000 milligrams and higher).

Devil's claw relieves carpal tunnel pain, but only if it is taken in an enteric-coated form that protects its analgesic compounds from being digested in the stomach. Do not use devil's claw with NSAIDs such as aspirin and Tylenol, and avoid it entirely if you have duodenal or gastric ulcers.

Clinical trials with women who have arthritis found that taking 70–86 milligrams of feverfew every day for 6 weeks increased grip strength. There are a few reports of it helping people with carpal tunnel syndrome increase grip strength, although this application is not scientifically established. Like other herbs to relieve pain, feverfew can cause stomach irritation. Do not use it with NSAIDs and avoid feverfew if you have ulcers.

Two tablespoons of fresh ginger every day is likely to relieve pain and swelling even when pain relievers are discontinued, but the effect takes 1–3 months.

Willow bark is a natural substitute for aspirin. It contains salicin, a less potent pain reliever than the salicylates found in aspirin but one that does not generally cause bleeding or stomach irritation. Do not use willow bark during pregnancy, if you have tinnitus (ringing in the ears), or if you are allergic to aspirin. Do not give willow bark or aspirin to children who have colds or flu.

If you are taking injections of steroids to relieve pain, a licorice derivative called glycyrrhizin can help make them more effective. It increases the half-life of cortisol and other steroids, making them work longer to undo the damage done to your joints.[7] The downside of using glycyrrhizin for this purpose is that it *will* increase any side effects you experience from cortisone. When you take both glycyrrhizin and any corticosteroid drug, you are more likely to experience weight gain, puffiness, and elevated blood pressure. Do not take glycyrrhizin for more than 6 weeks at a time. Preferably, use it during your peak allergy season. Do not take glycyrrhizin if you have high blood pressure. DGL is another licorice derivative that does not aggravate side effects of steroid treatment, but it will not help carpal tunnel syndrome.

CONCEPTS FOR COPING WITH CARPAL TUNNEL SYNDROME

○ During an acute attack of CTS, a cold pack can reduce inflammation by constricting blood vessels and bringing swelling down. A flexible gel pack available from pharmacies, a plastic bag filled with ice, or even a package of frozen vegetables can be placed against your wrist for 10 minutes at a time to stop pain. Wrapping the cold pack in a towel can minimize discomfort to your skin.

○ Gentle exercise can relieve pain and prevent further injury to your carpal tunnel. Here are some examples:

- Lift your arms above your head and rotate them inward and outward.

- Wrap a rubber band around the fingers of one hand, from your thumb to your pinkie. Spread your fingers, hold to a count of 5, and then release.

- Hold one end of an elastic exercise band in your clenched fist, palm facing up, with the other end held under your foot. Slowly flex your wrist against the resistance provided by the elastic band. Repeat 10 times. Then grip the band in your fist with your palm facing down and do the same thing.

- Flex your wrists while holding a very light dumbbell, first palm up, then palm down.

- Extend your arms in front of you and circle your hands at the wrists, making circles first in one direction, then in the other.

- Use a spring-style or foam hand exerciser to strengthen your hand and wrists, following instructions provided for the product.

❍ Acupressure can also relieve swelling and numbness of carpal tunnel syndrome. To perform acupressure, take off your watch, if any, and begin with your right arm. With the thumb of your left hand, press the point two thumb widths above the center of the crease of your wrist on the inside of your right forearm. With the index finger of your left hand, press the point two thumb widths above the center of the crease of your wrist on the outside of your right forearm. Apply pressure to both points at the same time. Repeat the process using the thumb and index finger of your right hand to apply acupressure to your left arm.

Move up the outside of your arm (toward your elbow) a distance twice the width of your thumb and down the inside of your arm (toward your fingertips) to the middle of the crease of your wrist and then to the middle of your palm. As before, apply pressure to both sides simultaneously.

A dull ache after pressing acupressure points for 30 to 60 seconds is normal, but a sharp pain is a signal to stop. If there is a knot in a muscle at an acupressure point, it should dissipate after your have applied pressure for 30 seconds. If it does not, try acupressure on that arm again another day.

❍ No scientific study has explained how magnets work in CTS. The latest research finds that magnets *do* relieve pain, but so did a nonmagnetic wrap used as a placebo. It is possible that a study with more participants would find that magnets work better than weights strapped to the point of greatest pain in the wrist, but it is also possible that weight, rather than magnetism, is the way magnets relieve pain.[8] However magnets work, many people find that they help. The best results are obtained from button-sized magnets with strengths of 250–500 gauss or more. Magnets are placed positive side down at the same points used for acupressure. You can also purchase a wristband with the magnets already arranged and attached.

❍ Avoid high humidity and underheated rooms. CTS is often aggravated by damp, cool conditions.

❍ Split keyboards allow the user to hold the hands at a more natural angle. Keyless keyboards are another option.

❍ Sit up straight. When typing, keep wrists straight, with forearms horizontal and at a 90° angle to upper arms. Elbows should be hanging by the sides in a relaxed position.

❍ Try wearing a professionally fitted splint for several days (and nights, during sleep) to see if symptoms are reduced.

❍ Chiropractic care for CTS usually consists of exercise, chiropractic manipulation, and massage. Although chiropractic is not as effective in relieving pain as surgery, it is as effective as medically directed treatments and causes fewer side effects.[9]

Cat Scratch Fever

SYMPTOM SUMMARY

❍ Swelling at the site of a cat scratch resembling an insect bite, followed 2 weeks later by swelling of the lymph glands in the neck and under the arms

❍ Brucellosis, lymphoma, and tuberculosis cause very similar symptoms

UNDERSTANDING THE DISEASE PROCESS

Cat scratch fever, as its name suggests, is an infection spread to people by scratches from cats. Also known as bartonellosis, benign lymphoreticulosis, or cat scratch disease, cat scratch fever is caused by the bacterium *Bartonella henselae.* The bacterium is spread from cat to cat by fleas; kittens are more likely to become infected than adult cats. Most cats do not become ill when they contract *Bartonella,* although they may be temporarily out of sorts and more likely to scratch and bite. The Centers for Disease Control estimate that up to 60 percent of cats are infected with *Bartonella* in the southeastern United States, but only 4–7 percent of cats in colder climates are infected.

Children exposed to cat scratch fever show no symptoms for up to 2 weeks, but later develop swollen lymph glands and possibly tonsillitis. Children and adults with compromised immune systems, such as AIDS and cancer patients, are more at risk and can develop serious complications.

TREATMENT SUMMARY

O Do *not* give vitamin D to children with cat scratch fever.

UNDERSTANDING THE HEALING PROCESS

Cat scratch fever usually goes away without treatment. The only nutritional precaution during recovery is not to give children supplemental vitamin D, since giving vitamin D to children with active *Bartonella* infections can cause excessive of release of calcium into the bloodstream.[1]

CONCEPTS FOR COPING WITH CAT SCRATCH FEVER

O Declawing cats does not prevent cat scratch fever, since infection can occur without a cat scratch. Putting a cat down after an incident of cat scratch fever is also not necessary, since it is very rare for more than one member of a household to contract the disease. Possibly infected cats, however, should be separated from people with immune deficiencies.

Cataracts

SYMPTOM SUMMARY

O Cloudy or milky spot in the lens of the eye (pupil appears white instead of black)

O Filmy, foggy, fuzzy, or cloudy vision

O Changes in the way you see colors

O Double vision

O Halos around lights

O Impaired vision at night, especially around bright lights

O Need for frequent changes in eyeglasses

UNDERSTANDING THE DISEASE PROCESS

A senile cataract causes slow and painless loss of vision by clouding the lens of the eye. Senile cataracts are associated with aging, and supportive measures different from those for congenital cataracts (occurring at birth) and diabetic cataracts (associated with high blood sugars). Senile cataracts are the leading cause of loss of sight in most industrialized countries, and every year over 1 million operations to remove cataracts are performed in the United States alone.[1] This is nearly 500,000 more operations than the next nine most frequent types of surgery combined.[2]

Often the first hint of a developing cataract is when objects held close appear blurry. This kind of blurriness is not unlike farsightedness, except it can occur in only one eye. As the cataract progresses, it can cause glare and changes in color perception. Someone who has a cataract near the center of the lens may become nearsighted. Someone who has a cataract at the back of the lens may see double or see halos around bright lights. Ophthalmologists determine the size and location of cataracts with a red light, which makes white cataracts look black against the background of the lens.

The formation of senile cataracts is due to the cumulative effect of the same kinds of stresses that cause farsightedness. The cells at the equator of the eye have to grow especially rapidly by virtue of their position. This makes them especially susceptible to various kinds of environmental injuries. Over a period of several decades, smoking,[3] failure to protect the eyes from the ultraviolet rays of bright sunlight,[4] and antioxidant deficiencies cause tiny points of protein in the lens to coagulate. These microscopic opacities spread like the points of a star, growing toward the center of the lens, and slowly merging into larger areas of cloudiness that eventually interfere with sight.

For reasons that are not fully understood, the process of cataract formation is accelerated in people who have more than 22 percent body fat and in people whose body fat is concentrated in the abdomen rather than the hips.[5] Steroids and gout medications increase the risk of developing cataracts. Exposure to heavy metals accelerates the oxidative process that causes cataracts. Iron, nickel,[6] cadmium, copper, and lead are all found in cataract tissue. Cadmium exposure is especially dangerous for smokers.[7] Diabetes, galactosemia, hypothyroidism, hyperparathyroidism, neurofibromatosis, toxoplasmosis, and excessive consumption of vitamin D also contribute to cataracts.[8] Frequent diarrhea can cause electrolyte disturbances that cause cataracts.[9] Agricultural workers, Vietnam veterans, and drug-enforcement agents who use the herbicide paraquat are at increased risk for cataracts.[10] Sometimes a single exposure to radiation can cause the condition. The medical literature reports a case of a cataract that arose in an X-ray technician 20 years after exposure to radium irradiation while carrying radium needles in his pocket.[11] The most frequent and most preventable contributing factor to cataract formation, however, is vitamin deficiency.

TREATMENT SUMMARY

DIET

❍ Avoid butter, margarine, and salt.

❍ Include dark green, yellow, or orange fruits or vegetables in your daily diet.

NUTRITIONAL SUPPLEMENTS

❍ Lutein: 5 milligrams per day.

❍ Mixed carotenoids: 50,000 IU per day.

❍ Selenium: 400 micrograms per day.

❍ Vitamin C: 1,000 milligrams 3 times a day.

❍ Vitamin E: 600–800 IU per day.

HERBS

❍ Bilberry: 40–80 milligrams of 25 percent anthocyanidin extract, 3 times a day.

UNDERSTANDING THE HEALING PROCESS

The primary objective of nutritional supplementation for preventing cataracts is providing the eye with the nutrients it needs to make the antioxidant glutathione. When glutathione levels fall below a certain critical level, the proteins of the lens are no longer protected from ultraviolet radiation. They can begin to cross-link into the pointed star pattern that eventually forms a cataract. The lens also permanently loses its ability to pump sodium and potassium in and out of its cells. This interferes with the production of energy in the cells and leaves the lens vulnerable to swelling and inflammation.[12] Moreover, the lens temporarily loses its ability to detoxify free radicals of hydrogen peroxide.[13]

The key nutrients the eye needs to maintain its supply of glutathione are vitamins C and E. Simply taking vitamins C and E greatly reduces the risk of cataracts. One research team found that taking 400 IU of vitamin E alone reduces the risk of developing cataracts by 56 percent.[14] Taking just vitamin C or vitamin C in combination with vitamin E reduces the risk of cataracts by 70 percent.[15] Even just taking a multivitamin may reduce the risk of cataracts by 30 percent.[16] If you cannot afford any other nutritional supplements for your eye health, be sure to take at least a multivitamin tablet or vitamins C and E.

Strictly speaking, the benefits of taking vitamin C may only show up over the long term. In the Nurses' Health Study, a 10-year study of 50,283 women aged 45–67, taking supplemental vitamin C for a period of 10 years or greater was associated with a 77 percent lower incidence of early lens opacities and an 83 percent lower incidence of moderate lens opacities. In this study, no significant protection was noted from vitamin C supplementation for less than 10 years.[17]

Also, vitamin E may be more useful in preventing some kinds of cataracts than others. The Vitamin E and Cataract Prevention Study (VECAT) is a 4-year, prospective, randomized, controlled trial of vitamin E versus placebo for cataract prevention that is still in progress as this book is being written. Preliminary data from its examination of 1,111 participants aged 55–80 has found a strong relationship between vitamin E and the prevention of cortical cataracts (cataracts that cause distorted color perception and trouble driving at night) but not for nuclear cataracts (cataracts that cause nearsightedness).[18]

Selenium is an important cofactor of vitamins C and E. People who have cataracts have lower levels of selenium than people who do not.[19]

Beyond taking vitamins C and E, the next area for easy change is diet. Several epidemiological studies have found dietary links to increased or decreased risk of cataract. An Italian hospital study examined the dietary preferences of patients who had cataract surgery. Patients who ate the greatest quantities of meat, spinach, cheese, cruciferous vegetables, tomatoes, peppers, citrus fruits, and melon were the least likely to have cataract surgery. Patients who had consumed the greatest amounts of butter, total fat, salt, and oil (except olive oil) were the most likely to have cataract surgery.[20] The Nurses' Health Study found that regular consumption of spinach and kale was moderately protective for cataracts in women.[21] The Health Professionals Follow-Up Study, involving 36,644 male healthcare professionals, found that spinach and broccoli decreased risk of cataract in men.[22]

Lutein and zeaxanthin protect the lens against damage from ultraviolet light.[23] The Health Professionals Follow-Up Study found a 19 percent reduction in the rate of cataracts among men who consumed foods with the greatest amounts of these two carotenoids.[24] Among 77,466 women in the Nurses' Health Study, those who consumed the greatest amounts of lutein and zeaxanthin had a 22 percent decreased risk of cataract extraction compared with those who consumed the least.[25]

Riboflavin seems to protect the lens against nuclear cataracts (cataracts that cause nearsightedness as their first symptom). A clinical trial in Linxian, China, involving 23,249 participants found that the combination of riboflavin and niacin reduced the rate of nuclear cataracts among people aged 65–74 by 44 percent, provided the supplement was taken for 5–6 years.[26]

While nutritional supplements are useful in *preventing* cataracts, the herb bilberry may be useful in *stopping the progression* of cataracts. In a study of 50 patients with senile cataracts, a combination of bilberry and vitamin E for 4 months stopped the progression of cataracts in 24 out of 25 patients in the treatment group, compared to 19 out of 25 patients who did not received the combination.[27]

While the antioxidant supplements that fight cataracts are largely free of side effects, there are some precautions to be observed in their use. Selenium is better absorbed if it is not taken at the same time as vitamin C. Vitamin C taken in the form of vitamin C with bioflavonoids can interfere with the liver's ability to process statin drugs for controlling cholesterol, calcium channel blockers for hypertension such as nifedipine (Procardia), or cyclosporine for preventing transplant rejection. Vitamin E should be used with caution by those who take blood thinners such as Coumadin or Plavix.

CONCEPTS FOR COPING WITH CATARACTS

○ If you drink alcohol, drink in moderation. One study found that one drink of beverage alcohol (a free-radical scavenger for hydroxyl radicals), wine, beer, or spirits every day was associated with more than a 50 percent reduction in the rate of cataracts.[28] Another study found that drinking no alcohol at all, or drinking more than 2 drinks a day, however, was associated with a 100 percent increase in the rate of cataracts.[29]

○ Riboflavin (vitamin B_2) and niacin (vitamin B_3) are important factors in the development of cataracts when they are deficient.[30] Because of food-manufacturing practices, in North America, Australia, and New Zealand, deficiencies in these vitamins are only likely when they are depleted by interactions with prescription drugs; diet is more likely to be a factor in the United Kingdom and Ireland. If you are over 55 you should take 3 milligrams of riboflavin and 40 milligrams of niacin every day if you take any of the following prescription drugs:

- Antidepressants such as amitriptyline (Elavil) or imipramine (Tofranil)
- Chemotherapy with doxyrubicin (Adriamycin)
- Cholesterol-lowering medications such as:
  - Atorvastatin (Lipitor)
  - Cholestyramine or colestipol (LoCholest or Questran)
  - Lovastatin (Mevacor)
  - Pravastatin (Pravachol)
  - Simvastatin (Zocor)
- Metoclopramide (Mexalon or Reglan) for nausea and vomiting
- Oral contraceptives for any purpose

○ You should also take supplemental riboflavin and niacin if you are over 55 and you take Cholestin (red yeast rice), or if you regularly use psyllium fiber products such as Metamucil.

Celiac Disease

SYMPTOM SUMMARY

In infants and children:

○ Blood in stool

○ Bulging tummy in thin child

○ Clay-colored or floating stools

○ Decreased appetite

○ Diarrhea

- ○ Failure to thrive
- ○ Foul-smelling stools
- ○ Irritability
- ○ Slow development
- ○ Slow growth, wasting of the muscles in arms and legs
- ○ Vomiting
- ○ Weight loss

In adults:

- ○ Bloating, abdominal distension
- ○ Bone pain
- ○ Breathlessness due to anemia
- ○ Depression
- ○ Diarrhea
- ○ Discoloration of tooth enamel
- ○ Fatigue
- ○ Gas
- ○ Floating stools
- ○ Irritability
- ○ Muscle cramps
- ○ Nosebleeds
- ○ Seizures
- ○ Swelling throughout the body
- ○ Tingling or numbness in the legs (due to nerve damage caused by vitamin B deficiency)
- ○ Vomiting

UNDERSTANDING THE DISEASE PROCESS

Celiac disease, also known as sprue, is a digestive disease that damages the small intestine and interferes with the absorption of nutrients from food. The underlying cause of celiac disease is a hypersensitivity to gluten, a protein found in all forms of wheat (including durum, semolina, and spelt), rye, oats, barley, and related grain hybrids such as kamut and triticale. When someone who is sensitive to gluten consumes foods made from these grains, the intestine releases massive quantities of an immune protein called immunoglobulin A (IgA). This immune protein is ordinarily the body's first line of defense against disease-causing microorganisms that enter through the skin and mucosal surfaces. In celiac disease, IgA accumulates in the small pockets or villi that line the small intestine and treats them as if they had become infected.

The villi are especially important for absorbing essential fatty acids and fat-soluble vitamins. When they are attacked by the immune system, fat and the fat-soluble vitamins D and K fail to be absorbed and remain in the stool. This results in bulky, foul-smelling, frothy, greasy stools and diarrhea as well as serious nutritional deficiencies of vitamins and essential fatty acids. The resulting nutritional shortfalls may cause abdominal swelling, depression, fatigue, weight loss, and pain in the bones, joints, and/or muscles, as well as unusual markings on the nails and canker sores.

TREATMENT SUMMARY

DIET

○ Avoid *all* foods made with wheat or any other grain containing gluten. Sources of hidden gluten include caramel, gum, hydrolyzed plant protein (HPP), hydrolyzed vegetable protein (HVP), malt, maltodextrin, modified food starch, mono- and diglycerides, natural flavoring, soy sauce, texturized vegetable protein (TVP), and vinegar. Spelt, a wheatlike grain, has no gluten and is a good alternative to wheat in a variety of foods.

NUTRITIONAL SUPPLEMENTS

For additional relief of symptoms:

○ Selenium: 200 micrograms daily.

○ Vitamin E: 1,000 IU daily.

To prevent deficiencies:

○ Vitamin A: 5,000 IU daily. Women who are or who may become pregnant must take care not to exceed this dose.

○ Vitamin B: any complete vitamin B supplement containing both folic acid and vitamin B_{12}.

○ Vitamin D: 100–200 IU daily.

○ Vitamin K: 5 milligrams every other week, especially if taking antibiotics.

UNDERSTANDING THE HEALING PROCESS

A gluten-free diet is the key to controlling celiac disease. Most medical authorities note that about 10 percent of people with the disease do not respond even to rigorous elimination of gluten products from the diet. Eliminating milk and eggs can help most people in this group.

Vitamin B_{12} deficiency is not uncommon in people who have celiac disease.[1] It is important to provide folic acid to balance vitamin B_{12}, so a complete vitamin B supplement is recommended.

There is no direct evidence that selenium and vitamin E relieve symptoms of celiac disease. However, both vitamins protect an antioxidant enzyme known as glutathione peroxidase, which is known to be deficient in the condition. Clinical trials confirm that supplementation with these two vitamins corrects glutathione peroxidase deficiency in 6–8 weeks and levels continue to increase for at least 5 months; however, there is no immediate effect on symptoms of the disease.[2] Vitamins A, D, and K should be taken in low doses to prevent deficiency.

Children with celiac disease who do not strictly adhere to a gluten-free diet are at special risk for selenium deficiency.[3] Giving children over the age of three 100 micrograms of selenium once a week and including selenium-rich vegetables in the diet (such as broccoli and green onion) are enough to prevent deficiency.

CONCEPTS FOR COPING WITH CELIAC DISEASE

❍ If a gluten-free diet causes constipation, try drinking more water, increasing servings of fruits and vegetables and other remedies listed in under CONSTIPATION.

❍ The medical literature reports at least one case in which a person with canker sores later developed celiac disease after eating a normal diet for several years.[4] Some physicians suggest that anyone who has had canker sores should be tested for gliadin sensitivity, a measure of especially potent antibodies to the proteins in gluten. A blood test is not necessary; saliva testing is now available. For information, ask your physician to contact Great Smokies Diagnostic Laboratory in Asheville, North Carolina, 1-800-252-9303.

❍ About 1 in 30 cases of female infertility is attributable to untreated celiac disease.[5] A test for gliadin antibodies (as described above) should be performed in the process of diagnosing women's infertility. For reasons that are not fully understood, celiac parents are more likely to have girls than boys.[6]

❍ Women with celiac disease who become pregnant should take at least 400 micrograms of folic acid daily.

Absorption of folic acid is reduced by celiac disease, and deficiency in the vitamin can lead to birth defects.

❍ Iron-deficiency anemia caused by celiac disease is most effectively treated by a gluten-free diet rather than by taking iron supplements. Anemia usually resolves itself after 6–12 months of strict adherence to diet.[7]

❍ Non-food products such as lipstick, medications in pill form, and toothpaste may contain gluten. Health and beauty aids that are not ingested in normal use may be accidentally ingested when fingers come in contact with the mouth. In some cases, skin contact with gluten is enough to cause a reaction.

❍ "Starch" in the United States is usually corn starch, which is safe for people who have celiac disease. "Starch" in Europe, however, is usually wheat starch, which will cause a skin reaction.

❍ Many people with celiac disease buy bread machines to take advantage of the many gluten-free bread mixes available on the market. If you are buying a bread machine, keep in mind that gluten-free bread mixes are very heavy and not every bread maker can process them. Brands of bread makers that process gluten-free dough include the Black & Decker All-in-One (Model B1500-04), all Wellbilt machines, and the very expensive Zojirushi BBCCS-15.

❍ Be careful not to take any brand of vitamin E extracted from wheat. The formulation of vitamin E made by A. R. Grace & Company is safe for people with celiac disease, but the capsules themselves are made with beef gelatin and are neither halal nor kosher.

❍ Avoid fried foods, especially in fast-food restaurants. French fries are usually cooked in the same oil used to prepare breaded foods.

❍ If you drink alcohol, avoid beer (including rice beer, which contains malt), bourbon, gin, rye, and whiskey. Most vodkas do not cause a problem, and rum, sake, tequila, and wine are generally safe.

❍ Osteoporosis is a very rare complication of celiac disease. Osteomalacia causing multiple fractures, however, is more common with the condition. For additional information, see OSTEOMALACIA.

Celiac Sprue
See **Celiac Disease**.

Cellulite

SYMPTOM SUMMARY

❍ "Orange peel" texture to the skin with bulging, pitting, and deformation when pressed

❍ Tenderness of skin when pinched, pressed, or massaged

❍ Feeling of tightness in skin at rest

❍ Primarily affects the skin of the buttocks, hips, and thighs, but also may appear on the lower abdomen, nape of the neck, and upper arms

❍ More obvious when standing up than when lying down

UNDERSTANDING THE DISEASE PROCESS

Cellulite, not to be confused with cellulitis, is a condition that gives the skin a bumpy texture. It is most prevalent in the skin of the buttocks, hips, and thighs. The medical term for cellulite is *adiposis dermatosa*. As its technical name suggests, cellulite is a condition in which fat-cell chambers in the subcutaneous layer underlying the skin become enlarged, and the connective tissue holding them in place weakens. This gives the skin above the subcutaneous layer a dimpled appearance.

The subcutaneous layer of the skin on the thighs of both sexes consists of three layers of fat. Two sheets of connective tissue separate them. In men, the top layer of fat cells is crisscrossed by connective tissues that anchor it in place. The corium, the connective tissue separating subcutaneous tissues from the outermost layer of skin, is thick and protective.

In women, the top layer of fat cells consists of standing fat-cell chambers, which are separated by arching dividing walls. These walls extend alongside the fat chambers down to the corium. The corium is thin and more easily deformed.

These anatomical differences are the reason cellulite is seen almost exclusively in women. The differences in skin flexibility can be illustrated by a pinch test. Pinched skin in men easily returns to its original contours. Pinching the skin and subcutaneous tissue of the thighs of women results in the "mattress phenomenon." The skin forms bulges and pits. Pinching the skin and subcutaneous tissue of the thighs of men forms folds and furrows but not bulges and pits.[1]

While cellulite occurs in the fat layers of the skin, it is the result of displaced fluid rather than accumulated fat. Skin that is prone to cellulite has high concentrations of glycosaminoglycans, protein molecules that attract water.[2] Overproduction of glycosaminoglycans slows the flow of fluids through the skin. It increases pressure in the tiny blood vessels that oxygenate and bring nutrients to it. The constant high blood pressure localized in the skin leads to a buildup of a fibrous net that holds the standing fat chambers in place.[3] Then, when the skin is deformed, the dermis containing the fat chambers cannot move with the dermis between the fat chambers. This gives a dimpled orange peel or mattress texture to the epidermis above. As the condition progresses, the mattress phenomenon is permanent, distorting the skin whether or not it is moved or stretched.

TREATMENT SUMMARY

DIET

❍ If overweight, incorporate walking into any weight loss plan. Lose weight slowly, lowering consumption by no more than 250–300 calories per day.

NUTRITIONAL SUPPLEMENTS

❍ Rutin: 500 milligrams twice daily.

❍ Vitamin C: 1,000 milligrams daily.

❍ Vitamin E: 400 IU daily.

HERBS

❍ Bladderwrack, cola, and escin in cholesterol creams, applied to skin twice daily.

❍ Gotu kola (*Centella asiatica*) extract taken orally, 30 milligrams 3 times per day.

See Part Three if you take prescription medication.

In addition to any supplement program:

EXERCISE

❍ Walk at a pace raising the pulse to 50–60 percent of maximum for 45 minutes at least 3 times a week. This is important whether or not you are overweight.

UNDERSTANDING THE HEALING PROCESS

Women who have the financial means often consider surgery for cellulite, but effective surgical options for the condition are very limited. Since the cellulite is not merely the result of an accumulation of fat, liposuction will not reduce cellulite and sometimes may make it appear worse. Some plastic surgeons harvest fat from the abdomen and flank to fill in depressions. However, the results of fat injections are not always permanent, and the act of harvesting fat can cause complications if the fat is cut too close to the skin.

A "cellulite lift," designed to replace the "buttocks lift," was reported by the American Society for Aesthetic Plastic Surgery in 1990. This procedure requires an incision around the entire abdominal area, removing excess skin and pulling the skin up over the flank, thigh, and buttocks. Cellulite becomes less noticeable, but the procedure leaves an extensive scar.

A technique called subcision offers a relatively uncomplicated surgical treatment for advanced cellulite. In this procedure, the surgeon bruises the skin, breaks the septa that hold fat chambers in place, and then applies compression to maintain circulation to the area of the bruise. There is no scarring and there are relatively few reported complications, but the patient must wear compression stockings for 15 days, and relatively few surgeons are skilled in the procedure.[4]

Most women who suffer cellulite opt for nonsurgical treatment. The most recent research is promising. In July 2001 the French affiliate of Johnson & Johnson announced results of a double-blind, placebo-controlled study that found that a cream containing butcher's broom, caffeine, and retinol (a chemical relative of Retin-A), both relieved "orange peel" appearance of skin and improved circulation between the standing fat chambers of the skin.[5] This research is the first positive answer to the critics of cellulite therapy who previously could claim that no research backed the use of fat-dissolving compounds, such as those found in cola, in the treatment of cellulite.

While there are no "spot-reducing" diets that will shrink fat deposits causing cellulite, recent science has a great deal to say about the *causes* of fat deposits in the thighs of women. Researchers at the University of Pittsburgh School of Medicine have found that fatty-tissue distribution in the thighs is correlated to insulin resistance and not necessarily to total body weight.[6] That is, women who conscientiously manage their diets may have to endure cellulite regardless of their maintaining healthy body weight. The fat accumulated under conditions of insulin resistance is primarily between the muscles rather than under the skin. This fat does not accumulate in the standing fat-cell chambers, but affects the overall size of the thighs and pressure on the skin.

Reducing insulin resistance and shrinking fat deposits in thighs requires exercise. In the University of Pittsburgh study, none of the subjects exercised. They improved insulin resistance and lost weight by a reduced-calorie diet designed to take off 33 pounds (15 kilograms) in 12 weeks. Most of the fat lost in the thighs came from between the muscles rather than under the skin. Weight loss by calorie restriction, therefore, would have a minimal effect on cellulite.

On the other hand, a study of weight loss by a combination of dieting and exercise at the University of Maryland found that approximately equal percentages of fat were lost from between the muscles and underneath the skin of the thighs.[7] The University of Maryland study used an easier diet; participants in the test reduced calorie intake by 250–300 calories per day to lose approximately 15 pounds (7 kilograms) over 6 months. This approach had a much more significant effect on cellulite.

The combination of rutin, vitamin C, and vitamin E has not been clinically tested as a treatment for cellulite, but has been demonstrated to improve venous tone, venous capacity, and fibrinolytic balance. That is, it helps blood vessels contain fluids, increases the amount of blood that can flow through them, and helps break down fibers that interfere with circulation.[8] All of these effects are useful in the treatment of cellulite. Given the general health benefits of these supplements, they can be recommended for any person who has cellulite, although they may not have a direct and immediate effect on the condition.

Do not take rutin without vitamin C. Although rutin protects vitamin C from oxidation, it also slows the rate at which vitamin C is absorbed by cells. Rutin will interfere with the action of quinolone antibiotics (not to be confused with the anabolic steroid quinolone). Check Part Three before taking rutin if you are on any prescription antibiotic.

Bladderwrack (*Fucus vesiculosus*) is seaweed that has been used to treat obesity since the 1600s. It has a high content of iodine that may be absorbed through the skin and stimulate thyroid function, aiding in weight loss, although this common assumption has not been proven by scientific study. It softens, soothes, and tones the skin, and is incorporated into many cosmetics.

Cola is a rich source of caffeine. It is widely regarded to be lipolytic, or fat destroying. The first scientific evidence of its efficacy in the treatment of cellulite was reported in 2001.[9]

Escin (aescin) is an extract of horse chestnut seeds. It reduces the activity of enzymes that breakdown mucuslike complex sugars known as glycoacalyx in the walls of capillaries. This keeps fluid from escaping the blood vessel and moving into the surrounding tissue.[10] Since fluid accumulation is the pathological force creating cellulite, escin is helpful in controlling the condition. Escin has been clinically demonstrated to treat varicose veins, often seen with cellulite.[11]

Gotu kola acts in a way that complements other herbs commonly used in the treatment of cellulite. It stimulates the production of glycosaminoglycans, the building blocks for collagen, from which connective tissues are formed.[12] It increases the oxygen supply delivered through the capillaries.[13] Effects from using gotu kola are not immediate. Clinical studies show that it takes 2–3 weeks for the body to accumulate the maximum level of asiatic acid, gotu kola's principal active chemical constituent, although some changes occur on the cellular level in as little as 48–72 hours.[14]

None of these herbs is recommended for internal use by pregnant women. There is no risk, however, to using topical creams containing these herbs as directed on the label during pregnancy or nursing. Future products containing caffeine, ruscogenin (butcher's broom), and retinol are very likely to be helpful in treating cellulite and to carry a minimal risk for expectant mothers.

CONCEPTS FOR COPING WITH CELLULITE

Generations of women have used massage as a primary treatment for cellulite. *Endermologie* is a European technique that utilizes a suction roller device that is reported to break apart fat deposits that have been compartmentalized in the skin. This restores skin to a less dimpled appearance.

The reviews of Endermologie in the medical literature have been negative, although an explanation of the differences between anecdotal experience and clinical experience has recently surfaced. In 1997, physicians at the Bowman Gray School of Medicine at Wake Forest University published a report that massage was unlikely to have an effect on cellulite in less than 2 months.[15] British researchers then reported that only 10 of 35 women in their study reported improvement of skin appearance after 3 months of Endermologie.[16]

The latest explanation of the difference between individual reports of success with Endermologie and the relative lack of success in clinical trials comes from a study conducted at Vanderbilt University, by researchers choosing the unenviable task of massaging Yucatan pigs. A device similar to the Endermologie machine was confirmed to break up fat deposits and the fibrous growths holding them in place. Differences in success of treatment were accounted for not by variations in suction generated by the machine but by differences in the operators' technique. The physicians stated, "The actual force measured with each particular maneuver varied between different operators but not with different suction settings, suggesting that the technique of administering the treatments is the primary factor in creating the force within the tissue. This leads to the conclusion that deep mechanical massage is highly dependent on the individual operator of the device."[17]

Experiences with Endermologie confirm that massage is useful in treating cellulite. The watchword for success in home treatment is "harder." Deep tissue manipulation is essential to break up the standing fat chambers that cause dimpling of the skin. Massage that is as vigorous as possible within the limits of comfort and safety is required.

Cellulitis

SYMPTOM SUMMARY

○ Rash
- Appears suddenly; spreads rapidly
- Sharp borders
- Tight, stretched appearance to the skin
- Pain and tenderness in the affected area
- Thin red line along a vein leading away from the area of infection to the heart
- Warmth over the area of infection or general fever

○ Other signs of infection, such as:
- Chills, shaking
- Fatigue
- Muscle aches
- Nausea and vomiting
- Stiff joints
- Sweating

UNDERSTANDING THE DISEASE PROCESS

Cellulitis literally means inflammation of cells. It is most common on the face, especially around the eyes and behind the ears or on the lower legs, but it can also occur on other parts of the body. This inflammation is usually caused by infection with staph or strep bacteria that have entered the body through tiny cracks in the skin, or through a wound that is intentionally kept open, such as a catheter.

This skin infection is most common in people with poor circulation in their hands or feet and in diabetics. It can be a recurring problem in women who have had lymph nodes removed to treat breast cancer. It is a potentially life-threatening complication in HIV.

TREATMENT SUMMARY

NUTRITIONAL SUPPLEMENTS

○ Bioflavonoids: 1,000 milligrams per day.

○ Thymus extract: 500 milligrams of crude polypeptides daily.

○ Vitamin A: 5,000 IU per day.

○ Vitamin C: 500 milligrams 3–4 times a day.

○ Zinc picolinate: 30 milligrams per day.

HERBS

○ Echinacea: 150–300 milligrams of solid extract (3.5% echinacosides) 3 times a day, or dried root, freeze-dried plant, juice, fluid extract, or tincture as recommended on the label.

○ Goldenseal: as recommended on the label.

UNDERSTANDING THE HEALING PROCESS

The most recent understanding of how antibiotics work in treating cellulitis would surprise many patients who take them—as well as many doctors who prescribe them. Antibiotics in the class including erythromycin (macrolide antibiotics) act not by reducing infection, since reinfection reestablishes the bacteria almost as quickly as the antibiotics kill them, but by reducing inflammation. Antibiotics reduce inflammation by killing immune cells, specifically neutrophils, by simultaneously reducing the vigor of the immune response and the vigor of bacteria. Both of these actions limit damage to the skin. Macrolide antibiotics are effective in 60–80 percent of cases.[1] The natural treatments recommended here also relieve inflammation, but not at the expense of immune function.

Although there are no studies that directly confirm the usefulness of thymus extracts in treating cellulitis, there is considerable evidence that thymus extracts correct low immune function. In particular, research has shown that thymus extract normalizes the ratio of T-helper cells to T suppressor cells, maintaining a healthy immune response that neither destroys healthy tissue nor allows infectious microorganisms to flourish.[2]

Relatively low doses of vitamin A are sufficient to prevent "burnout" due to stress on the immune output of the thymus.[3] Vitamin A also enhances antibody response, increases the rate at which macrophages destroy bacteria, and stimulates natural killer cells.[4]

Vitamin C levels are quickly depleted during the stress of an infection.[5] In combination with bioflavonoids, it helps increase the stability of the ground substance, the "glue" between the skin and the tissues below it.[6]

Zinc is an important cofactor for vitamin A. When zinc is deficient, the immune system's ability to produce white blood cells in response to infection is reduced, thymic hormone levels are lower, the immune response in the skin is especially reduced, and phagocytosis, the process in which bacteria are engulfed and digested, is slowed. When zinc is deficient, all of these processes can be corrected by taking zinc supplements.[7]

A quick method for detecting zinc deficiency is a taste test. Powder a tablet of any zinc-based supplement or cold medication and mix with $1/4$ cup (50 milliliters) of water. Slosh the mixture in the mouth. People who notice no taste at all or who notice a "dry," "mineral," or "sweet" taste are likely to be zinc deficient. Anyone who notices a definite strong and unpleasant taste that intensifies over time is not likely to be zinc deficient.

Zinc picolinate is the most readily absorbed form of zinc. Do not take more than 50 milligrams of any zinc supplement daily. In rare cases, excessive intake of zinc depletes copper to cause anemia, that is, a deficiency of red blood cells, and neutropenia, a serious deficiency of white blood cells.

Echinacea relieves inflammation as effectively as antibiotics do, but instead of blunting the body's immune response, it enhances it. This herb is especially useful in stimulating phagocytosis. A study of oral administration of an *Echinacea purpurea* root extract (30 drops 3 times a day) to healthy men for 5 days resulted in a 120 percent increase in phagocytosis.[8] In laboratory tests, caffeic acid and echinacoside, two important chemical constituents of the herb, have been found to have specific antibacterial action against *Staphylococcus aureus.*[9]

Used on a short-term basis for cellulitis, echinacea should have no side effects. However, it is important to note that it is not recommended to prevent the disease.

Goldenseal contains berberine. This alkaloid kills *Helicobacter pylori,* a bacterium implicated in ulcers and chronic gastritis as well as chronic sinusitis.[10] One study of 275 patients with peptic ulcers found that sinusitis and hives were more common among those who tested positive for *Helicobacter pylori.* Treatment of the bacterial infection not only relieved ulcers but reduced sinusitis symptoms.[11]

CONCEPTS FOR COPING WITH CELLULITIS

❍ Keep the area of skin affected by cellulitis elevated, higher than the level of the heart. This reduces swelling.

❍ Apply hot, wet compresses to relieve pain. You can make a hot compress by soaking a clean towel in 2 cups of hot water to which you have added a teaspoon of powdered barberry, coptis, or goldenseal. These herbs contain berberine, which stops the multiplication of infectious bacteria. (Do not take these herbs internally in these dosages to treat skin infections.) Apply the hot towel (as hot you can stand it) to the affected skin. When the compress has cooled to body temperature, reheat the towel and reapply. Be sure to dry your skin after you have finished using the compress and to launder towels used for this purpose separately from other towels used by the family.

❍ Avoid external friction, such as that caused by tight-fitting clothes.

❍ Never squeeze or lance an area of skin infected with cellulitis yourself, especially if it is located on the face.

❍ Change your washcloth every time you wash, and change sheets and towels daily.

❍ Wash your hands frequently, especially after changing a dressing or applying ointment.

❍ If you take antibiotics, also take 1 or 2 capsules of *acidophilus* or *Lactobacillus* every day. These probiotics help restore the friendly bacteria in your intestine that are destroyed by antibiotic treatment.

❍ Flulike symptoms when you have a skin infection are a possible symptom of sepsis. See a physician immediately if you feel like you are coming down with the flu when you have cellulitis, particularly if the area of infection gets redder or hotter.

❍ Homeopathic physicians frequently treat cellulitis with Schuessler cell salts, particularly calcarea sulphurica (Calc Sulf) and silicea (silica). Homeopathic preparations should never be the sole treatment of this disease.

Cerebral Palsy

SYMPTOM SUMMARY

❍ Delayed development of sitting, crawling, reaching, and walking skills

❍ Difficulty feeding

❍ Hearing problems

❍ Joint contractions

❍ Limited range of motion

❍ Mental retardation

❍ Muscle contractions

❍ Peg Teeth

❍ Seizures

❍ Spasticity

❍ Speech difficulties

❍ Vision problems

UNDERSTANDING THE DISEASE PROCESS

Cerebral palsy comprises a group of chronic disorders impairing control of movement. They usually appear in the first few years of life and generally do not worsen over time. Cerebral palsy affects 2–3 of every 1,000 school-aged children.[1] At one time it was believed that cerebral palsy was the result of medical complications occurring around the time of delivery. However, there is growing evidence that the majority of cases are caused by exposure to toxins before birth or structural abnormalities of the central nervous system.[2] Symptoms of cerebral palsy include difficulty maintaining balance or walking, difficulty with fine motor tasks (such as writing or using scissors), and involuntary movements. The symptoms differ from person to person and may change over time. Some people with cerebral palsy are also affected by other medical disorders, including seizures or mental impairment, but cerebral palsy does not always cause profound disability.

Early signs of cerebral palsy usually appear before 3 years of age. Infants with cerebral palsy are frequently slow to reach developmental milestones such as learning to roll over, sit, crawl, smile, or walk. Cerebral palsy may be congenital or acquired after birth. Several of the causes of cerebral palsy, such as Rh incompatibility and rubella (German measles), are preventable with good prenatal care. Others, such as head injury and jaundice, are preventable during delivery and after birth. Cerebral palsy is not a progressive condition, so if there are new impairments, the problem may be something other than cerebral palsy.

There is no standard medical therapy for cerebral palsy. Special braces can compensate for muscle imbalance. Drugs and nutritional interventions can control seizures and muscle spasms. Counseling, mechanical aids to overcome physical disability, and physical, occupational, speech, and behavioral therapy add to quality of life. Cerebral palsy cannot be cured, but many people with cerebral palsy can enjoy near-normal lives if their neurological problems are properly managed.

TREATMENT SUMMARY

DIET

O Ensure adequate calorie intake.

NUTRITIONAL SUPPLEMENTS

O Boron: 3 milligrams twice a week for children; 3 milligrams per day for adults.

O Calcium: 250–300 milligrams a day for children, 800–1,150 milligrams a day for adults.

O Vitamin D: 200 IU per day for children; 400 IU per day for adults.

O Magnesium: 200 milligrams per day for children; 400–800 milligrams per day for adults.

UNDERSTANDING THE HEALING PROCESS

In the treatment of cerebral palsy, natural methods are complementary rather than alternative. That is, they enhance quality of life and complement standard medical interventions, but cannot replace them. On the other hand, small measures of self-help sometimes yield substantial improvements in day-to-day life experience.

Since many children with cerebral palsy have diffi-

culty eating, deficiencies in macronutrients (carbohydrates, proteins, and fats) is a common problem. Knowing how much to feed a child with cerebral palsy is complicated by the fact that the weight of the child is not necessarily a good measure of how much food the child needs for basal metabolism. Muscles that are inactive require relatively few calories, while muscles that are reactivated after physical therapy require more calories.[3] Impedance analysis, a painless procedure often offered at no cost at diet centers and health food stores can give an accurate estimate of the child's calorie needs.

Boron, calcium, magnesium, and vitamin D all help prevent fractures. Most of the studies of boron focused on the nutritional needs of women after menopause or adults with osteoporosis, but the research suggests that boron supplementation increases bloodstream concentrations of 25-hydroxycholecalciferol, a chemical related to vitamin D that helps bones use calcium and phosphate.[4] There is also very preliminary evidence that supplemental boron improves the function of the central nervous system.[5]

All but 2 out of 52 scientific studies have found that taking calcium helps prevent bone fractures. Calcium citrate is better absorbed than other forms, and all forms of calcium are best absorbed when taken in doses of less than 500 milligrams with food. H_2 blockers for heartburn (cimetidine, famotidine, mizatidine, or risendronate) block absorption of calcium and increase the need for supplemental calcium.

Scientists at the Loyola Medical Center in Chicago are investigating magnesium as a means of protecting nerve tissue in newborns to prevent cerebral palsy.[6] Magnesium's use in preventing fractures is better accepted. Be very careful not to exceed recommended doses, since magnesium supplements taken in overdose have the same result as taking milk of magnesia: loose stools. Don't take magnesium supplements with meals including foods rich in oxalic acid (beans, rhubarb, spinach, or sweet potatoes) or phytic acid (matzo, nuts, and soy), since these foods interfere with the absorption of magnesium.

Vitamin D's role in preventing fractures is still not fully understood, although the weight of the scientific evidence supports its use as a supplement for this purpose. There are also some indications it may help prevent seizures in children and young people who have cerebral palsy. Vitamin D may also stimulate muscle activity.[7] Vitamin D supplements are especially useful for people with cerebral palsy who take phenytoin (Dilantin) for seizures.

CONCEPTS FOR COPING WITH CEREBRAL PALSY

❍ Hippotherapy is physical rehabilitation accomplished by riding a horse. Because horseback riding gently and rhythmically moves the rider's body in a manner similar to a human gait, riders with physical disabilities often show improvement in flexibility, balance, and muscle strength. Used in Germany as a standard therapy for cerebral palsy since the 1960s, hippotherapy is only beginning to be studied in an organized fashion in the United States. A preliminary study at Therapeutic Riding of Tucson (Arizona) found that 8 weeks of horseback riding gave children with cerebral palsy a longer stride and a slower pace when walking. All five of the children in the group were found to expend more energy while walking, indicating greater muscular coordination and greater muscle involvement. Additionally, the five children in the preliminary study all showed higher scores on the Walking, Running, and Jumping dimension of the Gross Motor Function Measure (GMFM).[8]

❍ Hyperbaric oxygen therapy (HBOT) involves delivering 100 percent oxygen to body tissues under pressure, the equivalent of going 8–24 feet (3–8 meters) below sea level, in a special chamber. HBOT has become popular worldwide, but scientific research into its use is relatively recent. Most of the research into treating cerebral palsy has been conducted at the Hôpital Sainte-Justine at Jewish General Hospital in Montreal. Doctors at the Hôpital Sainte-Justine found that 25 children given 20-hour-long treatments at a pressure of 1.75 atmospheres developed finer hand-eye coordination and reduced spasticity.[9] Researchers at the Hôpital Sainte-Justine treated 111 children with either HBOT or slightly pressurized air. Both groups improved in speech, attention, memory, and functional skills, although the number of improvements did not predict the amount of treatment. That is, fewer treatments over the same period of time worked just as well.[10]

Adverse effects are not unheard of during HBOT. Ear problems are relatively common. Gas buildup in the stomach, occurring while the child is in the chamber, has to be released when the child is brought back to normal atmospheric pressure; there can be nausea, vomiting, and heartburn. In one poorly supervised treatment, a

child with cerebral palsy even developed a case of the bends. All of these complications, however, can be avoided by competent professional supervision of the therapy.

Cerebrovascular Accident
See **Stroke**.

Cervical Cancer, Preventing
See **Abnormal Pap Smears**.

Cervical Dysplasia
See **Abnormal Pap Smears**.

Chagas Disease

SYMPTOM SUMMARY
Acute phase:
❍ Swelling and peeling at the site of an insect bite
❍ Swelling of one eye for 30–60 days
❍ Fever
❍ Racing pulse
❍ Rash, lasting only a few days, without itching
❍ Fatigue
❍ Swollen lymph nodes

Chronic phase:
❍ Difficulty swallowing, need to drink water to swallow food
❍ Megacolon (severe constipation lasting a few days to a few months at a time)
❍ Hiccups
❍ Difficulty breathing after light exertion
❍ Rapid heartbeat
❍ Easily fatigued
❍ Swollen ankles
❍ Swollen abdomen

UNDERSTANDING THE DISEASE PROCESS

Chagas disease, or American trypanosomiasis, is an infection caused by *Trypanosoma cruzi,* a parasite related to the microorganism that causes sleeping sickness. It is spread by several families of blood-sucking insects. A major health problem in South America, Chagas disease infects over 18 million people in Latin America and as many as 675,000 people in the United States.

Trypanosoma cruzi spends its life cycle in one of two forms. Before the parasite enters the human body, it has a sail-like tail and a microscopic "muscle" for propelling itself through the bloodstream. This form of *Trypanosoma* is known as a trypomastigote. The trypomastigote settles inside a human cell and becomes an amastigote. As an amastigote, it loses its "muscle" and produces as many as 500 copies of itself. Amastigotes then convert back into trypomastigotes, breaking out of the cell and destroying it, reentering the bloodstream to repeat the cycle of destruction.

The rapid reproduction of the parasite creates cellular debris that swells the lymph glands and causes a characteristic swelling of one eye. Eventually the immune system can limit the numbers of *Trypanosoma* in circulation, but cannot get rid of the infection. For a period of many years, the body and the infection are at a standoff, but at some point, the weakened immune system creates white blood cells that mistakenly attack the human tissues rather than *Trypanosoma*. Massive destruction of the heart and nervous system occurs, along with severe inflammation of the esophagus. University of Georgia professor Rick Tarleton states that because scientists fear that a vaccine could produce similar reactions, a vaccine or chemotherapy for Chagas disease is only a remote possibility.

TREATMENT SUMMARY

NUTRITIONAL SUPPLEMENTS

O Zinc picolinate: 30 milligrams per day.

HERBS

O Cat's claw: tincture, 1 dropperful taken in a cup of water with 1 teaspoon of lemon juice, 2–3 times daily.

O Lapacho (Pau d'arco): standardized lapachol extract, 1–2 teaspoons daily.

O Avoid inositol and thymus extract.

UNDERSTANDING THE HEALING PROCESS

Despite the fact that 10 percent of the population of the Americas has been exposed to Chagas disease, medical treatment of the condition is in a relatively early stage of development. The only medication known to kill the parasite, benznidazole (sold under the trade names Radanil, Ragonil, and Rochagan) is not commercially available in the United States and Canada.

Laboratory experiments with animals have found that *Trypanosoma cruzi* grows 50 times more abundantly in zinc-deficient blood than in blood with normal concentrations of zinc.[1] Although clinical trials have never been conducted in humans, it is very likely that correcting zinc deficiency can increase resistance to Chagas disease.

A simple way to find out if you are zinc deficienct is to chew a zinc tablet. If there is no unpleasant taste, you are probably zinc deficient. If there is an objectionable metallic taste, you are probably not zinc deficient.

Zinc picolinate is the most readily absorbed form of zinc. Do not take more than 50 milligrams of any zinc supplement daily. In rare cases, excessive intake of zinc depletes copper and causes anemia, a deficiency of red blood cells, and neutropenia, a serious deficiency of white blood cells.[2]

Recent laboratory studies have found that *Trypanosoma cruzi* only causes damage to tissues when the body produces an inflammatory hormone known as interleukin-6 (IL-6).[3] A traditional South American herbal remedy for the condition, cat's claw, neutralizes IL-6.[4] This preliminary finding may eventually explain anecdotal reports of the usefulness of the herb in treating Chagas disease.

Tropical herb expert Leslie Taylor advises using tinctures rather than solid forms for most applications of cat's claw. Active tannins in the tinctures are released in the presence of citric acid, easily provided by lemon juice. If you use a brand of cat's claw made with vinegar, you do not need to add lemon juice. There is one report of an adverse reaction to cat's claw in lupus (although the authenticity of the product as cat's claw was not confirmed). As a precaution, do not use cat's claw if you have lupus or rheumatoid arthritis.

Lapacho is a source of lapachol, which at least in test-tube studies interferes with the trypomastigote's ability to move through the bloodstream.[5] There are anecdotal reports of the herb's ability to cure Chagas disease in animals and people, although clinical trials have not yet been conducted.

It is important to use only lapacho products that have been standardized for anthraquinones. While the earliest research suggested that progressive purification of lapacho reduces its antimicrobial properties, unscrupulous exporters sometimes use waste products—especially sawdust—in "natural" lapacho tinctures. If you prefer to use a natural product, buy from a reliable source such as Rainforest Market. More information is available from their website at www.rain-tree.com.

Avoid inositol supplements if you have Chagas disease. Almost all the molecules on the surface of the microorganism are synthesized with inositol.[6] The human immune system recognizes Chagas disease through a specialized group of T cells (white blood cells) known as CD8+ cells. Thymus extracts encourage the immune system to create a competing subset of immune cells, the CD4+ cells, and should be avoided in Chagas disease.

CONCEPTS FOR COPING WITH CHAGAS DISEASE

❍ Feeling faint or feeling a racing heartbeat after swallowing or clearing the throat is a sign that the heart has been affected by Chagas disease.[7] If you have ever been exposed to Chagas disease and experience this symptom, seek medical care as soon as possible.

❍ Temporary residents of areas of the world where Chagas disease is endemic (including the southwestern United States) can greatly reduce their risk of exposure to Chagas disease simply by avoiding domestic chickens. The insects that carry Chagas disease prefer chicken over human or dog blood and are not known to infect cats.

Chicken Pox

SYMPTOM SUMMARY

❍ Aches and fever, *followed 24 hours later by*
- Skin rash on back, chest, scalp, and shoulders
- Severe itching
- Blisters on eye, rectum, and/or vagina
- Crusting of rash in 2–4 days
- Darkening of crusts
- Scabs falling off in 9–13 days

UNDERSTANDING THE DISEASE PROCESS

Chicken pox is a painful infection of the skin caused by the *Varicella zoster* virus, the same virus that causes shingles. It begins with aches and fever that are followed about 24 hours later by blisters on the top half of the body. The blisters burst and crust over, causing an intense itch. The crust turns a dark brown and falls off, usually within 2 weeks of the beginning of the illness. Scarring is possible on the cheeks and around the eyes.

Widespread vaccination has made chicken pox a relatively rare condition, but antibiotic resistance has made complications of chicken pox more serious.[1] Scratching to relieve the itch of chicken pox creates tiny lesions that allow staph and strep bacteria to enter the body. These bacteria can cause abscesses of the skin, cellulitis, and bacterial pneumonia, among other complications. The viral infection itself can cause arthritis, ataxia (loss of coordination), and purple marks on the skin known as thrombocytopenia. Fortunately, only about 1 person in 1,000 has to be hospitalized for complications of chicken pox.[2]

TREATMENT SUMMARY

NUTRITIONAL SUPPLEMENTS:

❍ Bromelain *or* papain *or* chymotrypsin: as recommended on the product label, taken with a glass of water. Be sure to use an enteric-coated form.

❍ Vitamin B complex: 100 milligrams daily.

❍ Vitamin E: 100 IU per day for children (up to 800 IU per day for adults).

UNDERSTANDING THE HEALING PROCESS

There is some scientific evidence that the burning itch of *Varicella* infections can be relieved by proteolytic enzymes, the chemicals that help digest the proteins in food. The two richest plant sources of these enzymes are pineapple and papaya, which produce bromelain and papain, respectively. The proteolytic enzymes in these fruits have long been recognized for their use as "natural tenderizers" for meat. The body itself produces chymotrypsin, which is extracted from the pancreases of various animals.

Proteolytic enzymes were compared to the standard antiviral drug acyclovir (Zovirax) in a double-blind study involving 192 people. The participants in the test were given either the natural enzymes or the drug and evaluated on the seventh and fourteenth days of the study. Both groups had similar pain relief, although reddening of the skin was reduced more by acyclovir.[3] Similar results were found in a study involving 90 people.[4]

Proteolytic enzymes can be broken down by stomach acid. For this reason, most brands are "enteric-coated," covered with cellulose so that the tablet does not dissolve until it reaches the intestine. Make sure the brand you use is coated. Chymotrypsin is usually a pork product, so vegetarians and other persons who do not eat pork may prefer bromelain or papain. Holding the pill in the mouth can dissolve soft tissues, so always take proteolytic enzymes with water.

Digestive enzymes are safe for almost everyone. However, enteric-coated pancreatic enzymes given to children with cystic fibrosis have been known to cause a serious complication known as fibrosing colonopathy, probably due to an interaction between the enzymes and the coating of the tablet.[5] Frequent use of proteolytic enzymes can cause pale or pungent stools, and occasionally allergic reactions, such as sneezing, wheezing, or tearing. Hypersensitivity reactions to the enzyme preparations are usually caused by allergies to the pineapple, papaya, or pork from which the product was derived.

For 50 years, physicians have been reporting that vitamin B_{12}[6] and vitamin E[7] help relieve the pain of shingles. While no systematic studies have confirmed that these vitamins help relieve pain in chicken pox, it is likely that it will help.

CONCEPTS FOR COPING WITH CHICKEN POX

○ Never give aspirin to anyone who has chicken pox. The use of aspirin during any viral illness, but especially during chicken pox, can cause Reye's syndrome, a condition of serious inflammation in the brain and liver. It is also important not to give anyone with chicken pox foods containing chemicals similar to aspirin, including curry powder, dill, licorice, oregano, paprika, peppermint, prunes, raisins, turmeric, cakes made from mixes, chewing gum, or soft drinks. Early signs of Reye's syndrome are uncontrollable vomiting accompanied by combative behavior. Reye's syndrome is most common in children but can strike at any age. If persistent vomiting occurs during or up to 2 weeks after a chicken pox infection, see a doctor immediately.

○ Relieve itching with *cool* water by soaking or using compresses. Adding a cup of baking soda to bath water

may also be helpful. At night, treat the rash with calamine lotion or witch hazel cream to stop itching.

○ Doctors sometimes treat chicken pox in teenagers with the antiviral drug acyclovir (Zovirax), because chicken pox can sometimes cause serious complications in that age group. Acyclovir is also used as a supportive treatment of chicken pox in people whose immune systems are compromised by AIDS, antirejection drugs for transplants, chemotherapy, leukemia, or lymphoma. If you take the prescription medication acyclovir, you should also take 5–10 drops of essential oil of cloves in a small amount of water daily to increase the antiviral effectiveness of the drug.

○ There are a number of homeopathic remedies for chicken pox. Usually it is best to start with a single dose of the lowest strength (6C, 6X, or 12C) of the remedy matching the symptoms to be treated, and then wait for a response. If there is an improvement in symptoms, let the remedy continue to work until there is no more improvement, then take another dose. If there is no improvement, try a different potency (30X or 30C). Sometimes homeopathic medicines work for a few minutes, and sometimes they work for an entire day before another dose is needed.

• Antimonium tartaricum is a remedy for symptoms of early infection, before blisters have broken. Children who benefit from this remedy feel irritable, nauseous, and feverish. Later in the illness, this remedy relieves chest congestion and cough. This remedy may be indicated when eruptions are large and slow to emerge.

• Antimonium crudum is recommended for a child who usually is irritable and may object to being touched or looked at. The eruptions are sore, and touching them may bring on shooting pains.

• Apis mellifica is a remedy for pink and puffy blisters that itch a lot and hurt when touched.

• Belladonna is a remedy for eyes that are sensitive to light or for a pounding headache. This remedy relieves throbbing pain.

• Bryonia is a remedy for dry cough and dry mouth that are only relieved with cold drinks. Homeopathic physicians also use bryonia to treat persistent fever.

• Mercurius solubilis is a remedy for swollen lymph glands, bad breath, and body odor. Children who benefit from this preparation are sensitive to drafts and changes in temperature and feel worse at night.

• Pulsatilla is a remedy for the emotional toll of chicken pox. It is more effective when thirst is not a symptom.

• Rhus toxicodendron is a useful treatment when scratching has made itching worse. It also relieves sticky eyes and stiff muscles.

• Sulfur is a treatment for severe itch that causes loss of sleep at night.

• Urtica urens relieves stinging and burning sensations, especially if exposure to heat makes them worse.

Chinese Restaurant Syndrome

See **MSG Sensitivity**.

Chlamydia

SYMPTOM SUMMARY

In men:

❍ Pus or watery discharge from the penis

❍ Burning during urination or defecation

❍ Discharge from the penis or rectum

❍ Swollen or painful testicles

❍ Usually causes no symptoms at all

In women:

❍ Bleeding between menstrual periods

❍ Vaginal bleeding after intercourse

❍ Painful intercourse

❍ Vaginal discharge

❍ Burning during urination

❍ Urge to urinate more often than usual

❍ Abdominal pain

❍ Inflammation of the cervix with a yellow discharge that has a foul odor

❍ Often causes no symptoms at all

In babies exposed to chlamydia during delivery:

❍ Chlamydial conjunctivitis (eye infection)

❍ Chlamydial pneumonia

UNDERSTANDING THE DISEASE PROCESS

Chlamydia is the most common sexually transmitted disease in the United States. The Centers for Disease Control estimate that approximately 1 in 500 teenage males and 1 in 50 teenage females will contract the disease in any given year. Overall, about 5 percent of the United States population has been infected with chlamydia. It is 4 times as common as gonorrhea, 6 times as common as herpes, and 30 times as common as syphilis. It is most common in men and women under 25. The persons most at risk for chlamydia are those who have multiple sex partners or whose sex partners have multiple sex partners, people who don't use condoms, people with a history of sexually transmitted diseases, and sexually abused children.

Chlamydia is often referred to as the "silent epidemic" because one-half of men and three-quarters of women with the infection have no symptoms immediately after infection, although they can transmit the disease. In women, the most likely symptom is a yellow discharge with a foul odor.[1] In men, symptoms are indistinguishable from those of gonorrhea (see GONORRHEA). Symptoms, if they occur, begin 1–3 weeks following exposure.

Over time, chlamydia can cause serious complication. In women, chlamydia results in 250,000–500,000 cases of pelvic inflammatory disease (PID) every year in the United States. PID can scar and block the fallopian tubes, raising the risk of ectopic pregnancy, a potentially deadly pregnancy outside the uterus (see PELVIC INFLAMMATORY DISEASE). In men, chlamydia can cause alterations in the balance of the immune system that result in Reiter's syndrome: burning urination, followed by the formation of hard crust on the penis, followed by ulcers in the mouth and throat, inflammation of the eyes, and crippling arthritis.[2] Infants exposed to chlamydia can develop chlamydial pneumonia, which is very difficult to treat.

TREATMENT SUMMARY

NUTRITIONAL SUPPLEMENTS

❍ Acidophilus: 1,000 milligrams daily while taking erythromycin.

❍ Thymus extract: 500 milligrams of crude polypeptides daily.

❍ Vitamin A: 5,000 IU per day.

○ Vitamin E: 400 IU per day.

○ Zinc picolinate: 30 milligrams per day.

○ Do not take vitamin C while you are on antibiotics.

HERBS

○ Echinacea: 150–300 milligrams of solid extract (3.5% echinacosides) 3 times a day, or dried root, freeze-dried plant, juice, fluid extract, or tincture, as recommended on the label.

○ Goldenseal: as recommended on the label.

UNDERSTANDING THE HEALING PROCESS

The physician's first line of treatment for chlamydia is antibiotics. Adults usually receive a single dose of azithromycin or a week's worth of doxycycline. Pregnant women and children are usually given erythromycin. Antibiotics are most effective when the infection is least active. There is a 90–95 percent cure rate for people who test positive for the chlamydia infection but do not show symptoms. When there is active inflammation, studies have found cure rates as low as 0 percent for ciprofloxacin (Cipro) and averaging about 80 percent for other antibiotics. In chlamydia's current state of antibiotic resistance, azithromycin is extremely effective, especially for men.[3]

Since antibiotics can cure the disease in as little as a week, they are preferable to purely "natural" treatment. And since chlamydia causes up to 50 percent of cases of a potentially dangerous infection in women known as acute salpingitis, the speed of antibiotics is usually preferable to slower-acting natural treatments. Many supplements, however, are helpful in bringing the cure rate to almost 100 percent.

Acidophilus supplements have an important role in preventing recurrences of chlamydia, especially in women.[4] Vaginal colonies of these friendly bacteria prevent reinfection with chlamydia by secreting hydrogen peroxide. The specific strain *Lactobacillus acidophilus* NAS produces the greatest amount of hydrogen peroxide and also binds to the lining of the vagina more effectively than other forms of the supplement.

Women benefit from using *acidophilus* as a vaginal suppository. Men should take 1–2 capsules a day during antibiotic treatment. Side effects from *acidophilus* supplements are rare, but there can be belching, burping, or flatulence during the first 2–3 days they are taken.

There are no studies that directly confirm the usefulness of thymus extracts in treating chlamydia, but there is considerable evidence that thymus extracts correct low immune function. In particular, research has shown that thymus extract normalizes the ratio of T-helper cells to T suppressor cells, maintaining a healthy immune response that neither destroys healthy tissue nor allows infectious microorganisms to flourish.[5]

Relatively low doses of vitamin A are sufficient to prevent "burnout" due to stress on the immune output of the thymus.[6] Vitamin A also enhances antibody response, increases the rate at which macrophages destroy bacteria, and stimulates natural killer cells.[7] This dosage is extremely unlikely to cause side effects, and has never been associated with birth defects. Nonetheless, women who are or who could become pregnant should strictly limit their intake of supplemental vitamin A to 5,000 IU per day or less.

Some recent research suggests that vitamin E can help healthy tissues contain chlamydia infection and keep it from spreading. Chlamydia bacteria do not injur the cells in which they multiply. However, they release chemicals that cause an accelerated life cycle in healthy cells surrounding the cells they infect, killing them and providing an easy pathway for the spread of infection. Test-tube studies find that treating cells with vitamins C and E prevents this process.[8]

Taking 400 IU of vitamin E daily is unlikely to cause any problems. Be sure to avoid overdosing vitamin E, however, especially if you take aspirin or any prescription medication for thinning the blood, such as clopidogrel (Plavix) or warfarin (Coumadin). *If you are not on antibiotics,* it is also helpful to take 2,000–3,000 milligrams of vitamin C daily.

Zinc is an important cofactor for vitamin A. When zinc is deficient, the immune system's ability to produce white blood cells in response to infection is reduced, thymic hormone levels are lower, and the immune response in the linings of the urethra (in both men and women) and the cervix is especially reduced. Phagocytosis, the process in which bacteria are engulfed and digested, is slowed. All of these processes can be corrected by taking zinc supplements.[9]

A quick method for detecting zinc deficiency is a taste test. Powder a tablet of any zinc-based supplement or cold medication and mix with $\frac{1}{4}$ cup (50 milliliters) of water. Slosh the mixture in the mouth. People who notice no taste at all or who notice a "dry," "mineral," or "sweet" taste are likely to be zinc deficient. Anyone who notices a definite strong and unpleasant taste that intensifies over time is not likely to be zinc deficient.

Zinc picolinate is the most readily absorbed form of zinc. Do not take more than 50 milligrams of any zinc supplement daily. In rare cases, excessive intake of zinc depletes copper and causes anemia, a deficiency of red blood cells, and neutropenia, a serious deficiency of white blood cells.

Since echinacea is used to relieve inflammation, not everyone who has a chlamydia infection needs it. Men and women with urethritis and women with cervicitis, however, obtain relief of pain and swelling by taking the herb. One study found that a teaspoon of *Echinacea purpurea* juice is as effective in relieving pain and swelling as 100 milligrams of cortisone. Echinacea also enhances the immune system's response to bacterial infections. It is especially useful in stimulating phagocytosis, the process by which white blood cells surround and digest infectious bacteria. A study of oral administration of an *Echinacea purpurea* root extract (30 drops 3 times per day) to healthy men for 5 days resulted in a 120 percent increase in phagocytosis.[10]

Women who are trying to get pregnant should avoid *Echinacea purpurea*. It contains caffeoyl esters that can interfere with the action of hyaluronidase, an enzyme essential to the release of unfertilized eggs into the fallopian tube.[11]

There is laboratory evidence that *Echinacea angustifolia* contains chemicals that deactivate CYP3A4. This is a liver enzyme that breaks down a wide range of medications, including anabolic steroids, the chemotherapy drug methotrexate used in treating cancer and lupus, astemizole (Hismanal) for allergies, nifedipine (Adalat) and captopril (Capoten) for high blood pressure, and sildenafil (Viagra) for impotence, as well as many others. *Echinacea angustifolia* might help maintain levels of these drugs in the bloodstream and make them more effective, or it might also cause them to accumulate to levels at which they cause side effects. Switch to a brand of echinacea that does not contain *Echinacea angustifolia* if you experience unexpected side effects while taking any of these drugs.[12]

The use of echinacea by people who have HIV or AIDS has been a controversial topic among practitioners of natural healing. Echinacea stimulates immune function, but it also slightly increases production of T cells.[13] These are the immune cells attacked by HIV. When there are more T cells, the virus has more cells to infect. This gives the virus more opportunities to mutate into a drug-resistant form. The authoritative reference work *The Complete German Commission E Monographs* counsels against the use of echinacea for treating colds in people who have HIV or autoimmune diseases such as multiple sclerosis. Later communications between the senior editor of the *Monographs* and the German Food and Drug Administration revealed that the warning in the reference book was based on theoretical speculation rather than on practical experience.[14] Still, as a precaution, people with HIV should use echinacea only on a short-term basis, no more than a month at a time.

The combination of echinacea and goldenseal is especially useful in treating conditions that involve drainage. A study reported in 1999 that the combination of the two herbs stimulates the production of the immunoglobulins IgG and IgM, infection fighters that "remember" specific infections.[15] Goldenseal contains the general antibacterial compound berberine. This alkaloid kills a wide range of bacteria, including those in the same family as *Chlamydia.*

People's Pharmacy authors Joe and Teresa Graedon warn that goldenseal reportedly limits the effectiveness of the anticoagulants heparin and warfarin (Coumadin). Do not take goldenseal with these medications. Avoid supplements containing vitamin B$_6$ or L-histidine if you take goldenseal, since they can interfere with goldenseal's antibacterial action.

Although it may seem to defy nutritional common sense, people taking antibiotics for chlamydia infections should avoid vitamin C. Just as vitamin C gives people immunity to infections, it also gives chlamydia bacteria immunity to antibiotics.[16]

CONCEPTS FOR COPING WITH CHLAMYDIA

○ To avoid reinfection, it is necessary to identify and treat possibly infected sex partners. Abstinence from intercourse is essential until treatment is complete.

○ In addition to vitamin C, several other nutritional supplements should be avoided while you take antibiotics for chlamydia. Magnesium supplements interfere with the absorption of doxycycline, minocycline, and tetracycline. Quercetin and rutin can interfere with the body's absorption of ofloxacin. St. John's wort may make your skin more sensitive to sun if you take tetracycline.

○ Women who have chlamydia can benefit from douching with a solution of 2 tablespoons of Betadine (povidone iodine) in 1 quart (1 liter) of water once daily for a week. Betadine kills chlamydia on the lining of the vagina.[17] It is important *not* to use a traditional herbal remedy for cervicitis (a tampon soaked in 1 tablespoon goldenseal tincture, 1 tablespoon tea tree oil, and 1 tablespoon thuja oil for several hours, inserted, and left for 24 hours). This combination of herbs can cause irritation of the lining of the cervix that can help the chlamydia infection become established in deeper layers.

○ Any woman who thinks that she or her partner has chlamydia should tell her doctor immediately. This is especially important for pregnant women.

○ Women who take the Pill are slightly more at risk for contracting chlamydia than women who use other forms of contraception or no contraception at all. The high progesterone content in the most popular brands of oral contraceptives stimulates growth in the lining of the cervix, giving chlamydia more tissue to infect.

Cholelithiasis
See **Gallstones**.

Chondromalacia
See **Knee Pain**.

Chronic Abacterial Prostatitis
See **Prostatitis**.

Chronic Bacterial Prostatitis
See **Prostatitis**.

Chronic Bronchitis
See **Bronchitis, Chronic**.

Chronic Fatigue Syndrome (CFS)

SYMPTOM SUMMARY

Main symptom:

○ Fatigue:
- Lasting at least 6 months
- Not relieved by bed rest
- Severe enough to restrict activity
- Worst fatigue the individual has ever experienced

Other symptoms:

○ Fatigue lasting 24 hours or more develops after an amount of exercise that normally would be tolerated

○ Mild fever, under 101°F (38.8°C)

○ Muscle aches

○ Muscle weakness not explained by any other disorder

○ Nervous system symptoms:
- "Fuzzy" thinking
- Depression
- Headaches different from previous headaches in intensity, onset, or type
- Increased sensitivity of eyes to light (photophobia)
- Lapses of memory
- Short attention span

○ Sleep disturbances, either sleeping too much or sleeping too little

○ Sore throat

○ Tender lymph nodes in armpit or neck

UNDERSTANDING THE DISEASE PROCESS

Chronic fatigue syndrome (CFS) is a condition of persistent cycles of fatigue and recovery accompanied by numerous, variable symptoms affecting many body systems. CFS is a relatively common disorder, particularly in women. It is diagnosed in 522 women and 291 men per 100,000 people.[1] In addition to the characteristic persistent fatigue, CFS often causes cognitive dysfunction, gastrointestinal (GI) disturbance, headache, joint pain, and visual disturbances. It also can cause a sensation of pricking, tingling, or creeping on the skin that has no objective cause. This is referred to in the medical literature as paresthesia.

CFS damages the central nervous system. There may be reduced circulation and oxygenation of brain tissue,[2] or even tiny holes in the brain itself.[3] CFS damages the nerves that control the sense of balance[4] and those that coordinate walking.[5] It increases the production of the immune system's "attack chemicals" to dangerous levels, including interferon alpha, transforming growth factor beta,[6] interleukin-4, interleukin-6, interleukin-1 alpha,[7] and tumor necrosis factor alpha (TNF-alpha).[8]

Gluten sensitivity (celiac disease) can present the same symptoms as CFS, that is, neurological symptoms without causing digestive upset. Since this is a diagnosis that is often missed, it is worth the money and effort to take a simple saliva test for sensitivity to gluten and gliadin before accepting a diagnosis of CFS. (For further information, see CELIAC DISEASE.)

TREATMENT SUMMARY

DIET

○ Avoid alcohol.

○ Eat organically produced fruits and vegetables.

○ Try eliminating dairy and wheat from your diet.

NUTRITIONAL SUPPLEMENTS

○ Alpha-lipoic acid: 100 milligrams daily.

○ Coenzyme Q_{10}: 100 milligrams daily (especially important during respiratory infections).

○ Magnesium: 200–300 milligrams 3 times daily.

○ N-acetyl cysteine (NAC): 400 milligrams daily.

○ Selenium: 200 micrograms daily.

○ Vitamin C: 500–1,000 milligrams 3 times daily.

○ Vitamin E: 200–400 IU daily.

HERBS

○ Licorice (not DGL) : solid extract, 250–500 milligrams daily.

○ Siberian ginseng (eleutherococcus):

- 10–20 milliliters (2–3 tablespoons) of fluid extract, *or*

- 100–200 milligrams of 1% eleutheroside E extract, *or*

- 2–4 grams (1 tablespoon) of dried root, used in teas daily.

See Part Three if you take prescription medication.

UNDERSTANDING THE HEALING PROCESS

The aim of nutritional therapy for CFS is to stop a vicious cycle of oxidation and tissue damage to muscles and nerves. For reasons that have not been clearly elucidated, CFS causes a tremendous increase in the muscle and nerve production of the potent free-radical generator peroxynitrite. This chemical targets the mitochondria, the energy centers of muscle cells. It deactivates the mitochondrial enzymes succinic dehydrogenase and cis-aconitase so that muscle cells cannot make energy. Glucose byproducts that ordinarily would be transformed into the energy compound ATP are eliminated as waste in the urine.

At the same time, peroxynitrite causes oxidative damage to the cholesterol coats of nerve cells and also to their DNA. The nerve cells produce a chemical cocoon to protect them from mechanical damage by generating inflammatory hormones known as cytokines. These cytokines, however, release the chemical nitric oxide, which combines with another free-radical generator, superoxide, to form peroxynitrite, perpetuating the condition.[9] Antioxidant therapy breaks the cycle. Dietary changes keep the cycle from starting up again.

Avoid alcohol. Like people who suffer Gulf War syndrome or multiple chemical sensitivity, a majority of people who have CFS cannot tolerate alcohol.[10] That is, drinking alcohol may cause them to sweat, break out in hives or a rash, experience a sudden, intense headache, or pass out. Researchers at the University of Texas at San Antonio Medical School believe that a supersensitivity to alcohol, caffeine, food, or medication that begins with the onset of symptoms of CFS indicates exposure to environmental toxins.[11] Alternatively, it may indicate that symptoms are really due to celiac disease.

Eat organic. People with CFS frequently have elevated bloodstream levels of chlorinated hydrocarbon pesticides compared to normal control subjects. Some pesticides, such as 1,1-dichloro-2,2-bis(P-chlorophenyl)ethene (DDE), accumulate in the fatty outer layers of healthy nerve cells.

They make the cell membrane permeable to inflammatory agents, and they also deactivate useful proteins.[12] DDE, in particular, can easily cross the blood-brain barrier to affect neurological activity. When polychlorinated hydrocarbons accumulate in nerve tissue, natural resistance to chemical exposure is lost and food allergies become more frequent.[13]

Try eliminating dairy and wheat from your diet. Many people who suffer chronic fatigue have food intolerance, a condition differing from food allergy in that it activates the cytokine system, creating the specific chemicals that cause muscle and nerve damage in CFS. In an Australian study, 90 percent of CFS patients who eliminated wheat, milk, benzoates, nitrites, nitrates, and food colorings and other additives from their diet reported improvement in the severity of fatigue, fever, sore throat, muscle pain, headache, joint pain, and cognitive dysfunction. The elimination diet also resulted in a marked improvement in irritable bowel symptoms (alternating constipation and diarrhea, bloating, feeling of incomplete defecation) among all the participants in the study.[14]

Alpha-lipoic acid, N-acetyl cysteine (NAC), and selenium increase the body's supply of glutathione,[15] a vital antioxidant that protects nerve cells against additional lesions. NAC provides cysteine for glutathione synthesis, and alpha-lipoic acid is believed to increase intracellular glutathione levels by reducing the more abundant compound cystine to cysteine, bypassing the need for converting cystine to cysteine inside already-weakened cells.[16]

The glutathione that these supplements help the body produce is neuroprotective and may play a role in preventing additional nerve lesions.[17] Alpha-lipoic acid by itself also protects nerve cells. It binds nitric oxide and peroxynitrite so that they cannot interfere with the energy machinery in the mitochondria of muscle cells. Coenzyme Q_{10} has similar neuroprotective qualities and likewise has the ability to improve mitochondrial function.[18]

Vitamin E is another important antioxidant. The purpose of taking supplemental vitamin C and magnesium is to conserve vitamin E. Magnesium deficiency can interfere with the body's ability to make glutathione.[19]

The risk of side effects from taking this combination of supplements is minimal, but real. Alpha-lipoic acid can lower blood sugar levels, and should be used with caution by people who have either diabetes or hypo-glycemia. Smokers who have had bronchitis for 2 years or less should not take NAC unless they are quitting. There is some evidence that NAC may activate eosinophils, the white blood cells that may cause the progression of smoker's cough to chronic obstructive pulmonary disease.[20] NAC may cause headaches if taken with sildenafil (Viagra), and in rare cases can cause cysteine-crystal kidney stones. Diabetics who also have CF may find that taking NAC causes false readings in urine tests for ketones.

Selenium is better absorbed if it is not taken at the same time as vitamin C. Vitamin C taken in the form of vitamin C with bioflavonoids can interfere with the liver's ability to process statin drugs for controlling cholesterol, calcium channel blockers such as nifedipine (Procardia) for hypertension, or cyclosporine for preventing transplant rejection. Vitamin E should be used with caution by those who take blood thinners such as warfarin (Coumadin) or clopidogrel (Plavix).

Herbs such as licorice and Siberian ginseng complement antioxidant therapy. Unlike antioxidants that work on a molecular level, these herbs work on a whole-body level. About 95 percent of people who have CFS also have unusually low blood pressure. Oxygenated blood does not reach the brain, and depression results. Glycyrrhizin, a chemical found in licorice, causes sodium to flow out of cells into the bloodstream. To keep the concentration of sodium in the blood constant, the kidneys have to release less fluid, and blood pressure goes up. (Licorice products labeled DGL, or deglycyrrhizinated licorice, will not have this effect.) The value of licorice in treating CFS has been confirmed in a very preliminary study involving a single patient.[21]

While the primary immune imbalance in CFS involves the cytokines and the inflammatory reactions they produce, CFS also causes a deficiency in NK (natural killer) cells. These white blood cells are especially important in fighting viral infections; in fact, CFS was once known as low natural killer cell syndrome (LNKCS). At least in studies involving healthy volunteers, Siberian ginseng increases the numbers and activity of NK cells and greatly increases resistance to colds and flu.[22]

Do not use deglycyrrhizinated licorice (DGL) in the treatment of chronic fatigue syndrome. The chemical glycyrrhizin is essential in chronic fatigue treatment. The drawback to using glycyrrhizin is that it *will* increase any side effects you experience from prescription steroid treatments. When you take both glycyrrhizin and any corticosteroid drug, you are more likely to experience weight gain, puffiness, and elevated blood pressure. Do not take glycyrrhizin for more than 6 weeks at a time. Since glycyrrhizin relieves chronic fatigue by raising blood pressure, do not take glycyrrhizin if you already have high blood pressure.

Do not use Siberian ginseng if you take testosterone. The herb can cause testosterone to build up in the bloodstream to undesirably high levels.

CONCEPTS FOR COPING WITH CHRONIC FATIGUE SYNDROME

❍ If you choose to take the prescription medication acyclovir (Zovirax), you should also take 5–10 drops of essential oil of cloves in a small amount of water daily to increase the antiviral effectiveness of the drug.

❍ In the unlikely event you have days when you are capable of vigorous exercise, you should avoid it. Exercising to the point of being out of breath increases the production of free radicals that activate the peroxynitrite cycle that causes nerve and muscle cell damage in CFS.

Chronic Nonbacterial Prostatitis
See **Prostatitis**.

Chronic Obstructive Pulmonary Disease
See **Bronchitis, Chronic; Emphysema**.

Chronic Thromboangitis
See **Peripheral Vascular Disease**.

Chronic Venous Insufficiency
See **Varicose Veins**.

Circulatory Disease
See **Aneurysm; Angina; Cardiomyopathy; Congestive Heart Failure; High Cholesterol; High Triglyercides; Hypertension; Irregular Heartbeat; Peripheral Vascular Disease; Raynaud's Phenomenon**.

Cirrhosis of the Liver

SYMPTOM SUMMARY

Common symptoms:

❍ Appearance of small "spider veins" under the skin

❍ Bleeding hemorrhoids

❍ Confusion

❍ Erectile dysfunction

❍ Jaundice (yellowing of the skin)

❍ Loss of interest in sex

❍ Nausea

❍ Vomiting

❍ Vomiting blood

❍ Weakness

❍ Weight loss

Less frequent symptoms:

❍ Abdominal pain

❍ Bleeding gums

❍ Breast enlargement in men

❍ Clay-colored or pale stools

❍ Decreased volume of urine

❍ Fever

❍ Flatulence, gas

❍ Nosebleed

UNDERSTANDING THE DISEASE PROCESS

Cirrhosis is a condition of severe tissue damage in the liver. In the United States, the most common cause of cirrhosis is chronic alcoholism. Generally, about 15 percent of men who drink at least 80 grams of alcohol (the equivalent of 6 beers, 4 glasses of wine, or 6 shots of liquor) per day and women who drink at least 40 grams of alcohol (3 beers, 2 glasses of wine, or 3 shots of liquor) every day for 10–20 years develop cirrhosis. Cirrhosis may also result from hepatitis B, C, or D, cystic fibrosis, brucellosis, toxoplasmosis, the parasitic infection schistosomiasis, the iron-storage abnormality hemochromatosis, the copper-storage condition known as Wilson's disease, or toxic exposure to arsenic, oral contraceptives, certain kinds of mushrooms, or the herb colt's foot. One of the most insidious features of alcoholic cirrhosis of the liver is that the disease itself changes metabolic pathways in the liver so that alcohol has less and less effect on the central nervous system, so more and more is drunk with ever-increasing damage to liver tissue.[1]

Cirrhosis causes the liver to shrink in size and become distorted in shape. Bands of fibers surround liver cells and cut off circulation. Eventually large areas of tissue are surrounded by scar tissue and form nodules. In severe cases, cirrhosis can lead to liver failure and death. Cirrhosis may also occur in the bile ducts connecting the liver and gallbladder. The cause of this form of cirrhosis, primary biliary cirrhosis, is not known.

TREATMENT SUMMARY

NUTRITIONAL SUPPLEMENTS

O Phosphatidylcholine (lecithin): 900–1,000 milligrams per day.

O Selenium: 100 micrograms per day.

O S-adenosyl-L-methione (SAM-e): 1,600 milligrams per day.

O Taurine (for cramps): 3 grams daily.

HERBS

O Milk thistle, preferably as a silymarin phytosome: 420–600 milligrams per day.

O *Shakuyaku-kanzo-to* (for leg cramps): as directed on label.

See Part Three if you take prescription medication.

UNDERSTANDING THE HEALING PROCESS

Alcohol poisons liver tissue. For people with cirrhosis of the liver, the single most important step in self-care is to stop drinking. It is necessary to avoid all types of alcohol, including beer, wine, cocktails, and champagne. Alcohol adds calories to your diet and decreases your appetite, leaving less room for the protein your liver needs for healing. The combination of alcohol and acetaminophen (a pain reliever found in Tylenol and many over-the-counter cold medications) is especially damaging to the liver.

The use of phosphatidylcholine, also known as lecithin, in the treatment of cirrhosis is backed by long-term studies of alcohol-indulgent baboons. Heavy-drinking baboons given soy-derived phosphatidylcholine did not develop cirrhosis even after 8 years of heavy alcohol consumption, equivalent to 50 percent of their total calories.[2] Researchers believe that lecithin protects the liver by encouraging the breakdown of collagen in fibrous tissue.

Problems with phosphatidylcholine supplements are extremely rare. The supplement can cause diarrhea, nausea, or increased salivation. People with absorption problems, especially those with cystic fibrosis, should avoid phosphatidylcholine.

A number of studies support the use of SAM-e in the treatment of cirrhosis. A double-blind clinical trial found that 1,200 milligrams of SAM-e per day for 2 years decreased the overall death rate and the need for liver transplantation with alcoholic cirrhosis of the liver.[3] Later trials have found that doses as low as 180 milligrams per day may be helpful, especially for persons in earlier stages of cirrhosis.[4] The most important benefit of SAM-e in alcoholic cirrhosis is that it regulates the biochemical pathways so that alcohol has a greater effect on the central nervous system, and less has to be drunk for its drug effect.[5] SAM-e also acts in part by protecting the liver's supply of vitamin E,[6] so best results are likely to be obtained when there are adequate supplies of the vitamin.

Only the most preliminary clinical study supports the use of selenium in treating cirrhosis of the liver, but these laboratory experiments suggest that it could be very important. Selenium participates in a series of biochemical steps that make liver cells insensitive to tumor necrosis factor, a hormone the immune system ordinarily uses to destroy tumors that also destroys healthy tissues in the presence of alcohol. Cirrhosis patients with higher bloodstream concentrations of selenium have less severe liver damage.[7]

Relatively high doses of milk thistle, preferably taken

as a phytosome (the active ingredient silymarin chemically joined to phosphatidylcholine) reduce liver damage in alcoholic cirrhosis.[8] At molecular level, silibinin, one of the components of silymarin, prevents damage to the outer membranes of liver cells from free radicals of oxygen.[9] It helps liver cells use oxygen more efficiently, and assists in the formation of proteins.[10] Most important, it increases synthesis of proteins needed by the liver to repair itself.[11]

Milk thistle products are nontoxic, although they stimulate the production of bile, possibly making stools looser. Some people with cirrhosis may not benefit from taking silymarin. One study found that milk thistle is not helpful when there is a complication of cirrhosis known as portal hypertension.[12]

Muscle cramps are common in cirrhosis of the liver. A study sponsored by a Japanese herb manufacturer found that *shakuyaku-kanzo-to,* a traditional herbal formula containing peony root and licorice, stops leg cramps caused by cirrhosis. In the United States and Canada, *shakuyaku-kanzo-to* is sold under the following trade names:

- Peony and Licorice (Kanpo, Qualiherb)
- Peony and Licorice Combination (Blue Light, Brion, KPC, Ming Tong, Sheng Chang)
- Shao Yao Gan Cao Tang (most pharmacies associated with practitioners of Traditional Chinese Medicine)

Japanese physicians have also found that about 3 in 5 patients taking 3 grams of supplemental taurine daily experience relief from cramps.[13] Do not use taurine if you suffer congestive heart failure in addition to cirrhosis of the liver.

CONCEPTS FOR COPING WITH CIRRHOSIS OF THE LIVER

○ Ammonia is a normal byproduct of protein digestion. In advanced cirrhosis the liver is unable to remove ammonia from the blood. Ammonia can build up to levels that cause hepatic encephalopathy, a condition that can cause mental confusion, coma, or even death. A minority of people with hepatic encephalopathy can benefit from taking branched-chain amino acids (L-isoleucine, L-leucine, and L-valine). When there are adequate levels of B vitamins, the liver can use these amino acids to make proteins while producing a minimum of toxic ammonia. A German study published in the early 1980s reported that in 3 out of 4 cases, intravenous administration of branched-chain amino acids completely reversed hepatic encephalopathy.[14] More than 20 years of subsequent research has failed to prove that any single formula of branched-chain amino acids is best for treating cirrhosis, but there is general agreement among European physicians that amino acid supplements of this type are appropriate therapy.[15] Since taking too high a dose can cause serious side effects, only use branched-chain amino acids to treat cirrhosis after consultation with a nutritionally oriented physician.

○ A British study found that antioxidant supplementation can relieve the fatigue and chronic itching caused by biliary cirrhosis.[16] The British study used 100 milligrams of coenzyme Q_{10} plus a proprietary antioxidant formula sold in the United Kingdom as Bio-Antox (4 tablets per day). The Bio-Antox formula is equivalent to taking:

- Beta-carotene: 12 milligrams per day.
- S-adenosyl-L-methionine (SAM-e): 1,600 milligrams per day (a very high dose).
- Selenium: 300 micrograms per day.
- Vitamin C: 600 milligrams per day.
- Vitamin E: 800 IU per day.

People who have cirrhosis of the liver are unlikely to have conditions treated with medications that interact with these supplements. Mild gastrointestinal symptoms, such as diarrhea and nausea are possible the first 2–3 days while taking this combination. Since many people in the United States would find this dosage of SAM-e to be prohibitively expensive, it is best to start with a much lower dose, as little as 20 milligrams per day, and increase until benefits are noticed.

○ People with advanced cirrhosis are especially susceptible to internal bleeding. Natural medicine expert Steve Bratman advises his readers that oligomeric proanthocyanidins (OPCs) can help strengthen veins so that bleeding is less likely to occur. Grape seed extract, taken in a dosage of 50–100 milligrams per day, should help reduce internal bleeding without interfering with any medications people with cirrhosis of the liver are likely to take.

○ Practitioners of Traditional Chinese Medicine can prepare herbal treatments for ascites, typically containing the herb akebia (chocolate vine).

○ The severe abdominal swelling known as ascites is common in advanced cirrhosis. Disturbances of sodium metabolism cause both salt and fluid to build up in the body. Limiting salt intake is critically important in preventing ascites. To avoid ascites, eliminate:

- All drugs containing sodium, such as Alka-Seltzer and aspirin.
- Anchovies, canned salmon, sardines, and shellfish in general.
- Any "fizzy" drink not specifically labeled as low-sodium
- Any kind of salted, grilled meat, salted soup, or consommé.
- Bacon, ham, sausages, and all cured meats, pork or otherwise.
- Beer, carbonated beverages sweetened with sugar or aspartame, and mineral water.
- Beets, celery, and spinach.
- Breakfast cereals, bread, biscuits, pancakes, and waffles.
- Cheeses and other processed dairy products.
- Chocolate.
- Dried fruit and nuts.
- Peanuts, whether salted or not.
- Popcorn.
- Prepared foods of all types, especially salad dressings.

Cleft Lip and Cleft Palate

SYMPTOM SUMMARY

○ Cleft lip:
- Separation of the two sides of the lip prior to birth

○ Cleft palate:
- Opening in the roof of the mouth in which the two sides of the palate did not join together as the unborn baby was developing

○ Cleft lip and cleft palate can occur on either or both sides of the mouth.

UNDERSTANDING THE DISEASE PROCESS

Cleft lip and cleft palate are among the most common birth defects in the United States. According to the American Cleft Palate-Craniofacial Association, 1 of every 700 newborns is affected by cleft lip and/or cleft palate. Cleft lip and cleft palate are thought to be caused by a combination of genetic factors and nutritional deficiencies operating during the first trimester of pregnancy.

TREATMENT SUMMARY

NUTRITIONAL SUPPLEMENTS

○ Any complete vitamin B supplement containing at least 400 micrograms of folic acid, daily.

UNDERSTANDING THE PREVENTION PROCESS

Nutritional therapy alone may not prevent cleft lip and cleft palate. However, a recent study suggests that one of the most important factors causing these birth defects is a shortage of vitamin B_2 and folic acid, especially in women who have chronic diseases affecting vitamin absorption, such as celiac disease, Crohn's disease, cystic fibrosis, or dermatitis herpetiformis.[1] Some experts recommend that all women should take vitamin B supplements as long as they might become pregnant.

Climacteric
See Hot Flashes; Osteoporosis.

Cluster Headaches

SYMPTOM SUMMARY

○ "Clusters" of headaches, attacks generally lasting 6–8 weeks, causing 2–10 headaches a day, each headache usually lasting between 30 minutes and 2 hours

○ Horner's syndrome before attack
- Drooping of one eyelid
- Dilation of pupil on one side of face

○ Headaches commence 5–10 minutes after Horner's syndrome
- Intense pain on one side of the face
- Begins and stops rapidly

> - Worst in the eyes, nose, and cheek of the affected side of the face
> - Nasal congestion and tearing on the affected side of the face
> - Unlike migraine, no special need for dark or quiet
>
> ❍ Escalating number and intensity of headaches during first half of cluster, gradually becoming fewer and less intense as the cycle ends
>   - Attacks usually occur at same time of night or day
>   - Attacks in the same cluster usually affect the same side of the face, although attacks in the next cluster may affect the other side of the face

UNDERSTANDING THE DISEASE PROCESS

Cluster headaches (CH) are intensely painful headaches affecting one side of the face that occur in groups over a period of time, followed by weeks, months, or years of remission. Unlike migraine headaches, cluster headaches are more common in men than women. The pain of CH is described as "knifelike" rather than throbbing.

Attacks of cluster headaches may be triggered by stress, relaxation, extreme temperatures, glare, hay fever, or sexual activity. Also unlike migraine, cluster headaches are not usually triggered by specific foods. Some doctors note that there is a typical "cluster headache face": leonine features, spider veins radiating from the nose, broad chin, and vertical creases of the forehead. Sufferers of CH are frequently tall and rugged looking.[1]

TREATMENT SUMMARY

NUTRITIONAL SUPPLEMENTS

❍ Melatonin: 1–3 milligrams, 60–90 minutes before bedtime. Do not take melatonin during the day.

See Part Three if you take prescription medication.

UNDERSTANDING THE HEALING PROCESS

The current scientific thinking about CH is that they are a disorder of circadian rhythm, a disturbance of the body clock regulated by melatonin.[2] Supplemental melatonin usually helps, but it is most useful for people whose clusters occur at least a few weeks apart.[3] People

with chronic CH, cycles only a few days apart, may not benefit from melatonin.

CONCEPTS FOR COPING WITH CLUSTER HEADACHES

❍ Medical diagnosis of CH is important, since lung cancer and cancers of the nose and throat cause similar symptoms.

❍ Oxygen therapy is standard treatment for CH. Several clinical trials have confirmed that 15 minutes under an oxygen mask reduces the pain of headaches for most people. However, 1 in 4 people will experience a new headache when oxygen is removed.[4] Sufferers of chronic CH sometimes get better results with hyperbaric oxygen therapy.

❍ A nineteenth-century remedy for CH was to take a "snuff" of powdered cayenne pepper up the nose. Pharmaceutical companies are testing a prescription drug made from capsaicin, the active ingredient of cayenne pepper, called Civamide. Early tests have found that Civamide, like red pepper, causes irritation and sneezing. However, it reduces the frequency of cluster headaches by an average of over 50 percent.[5] Civamide will probably be released to the market in 2003 or 2004.

Cognitive Decline
See **Memory Loss**.

Cold Sores

SYMPTOM SUMMARY

❍ Itching, burning, and tingling about 2 days before blisters occur

❍ Small blisters on the lips, mouth, or gums
  - Appearing on red, raised, and painful skin
  - Crusting after several days
  - Filled with clear yellow fluid

❍ Yellow crusts fall off to reveal healed skin

❍ Possible fever

❍ Small blisters sometimes merge to form a single large blister

UNDERSTANDING THE DISEASE PROCESS

Cold sores (also known as fever blisters or herpes labialis) are a very common infection of the lips and mouth. The virus responsible for cold sores, *Herpes simplex* or HSV-1, can be transmitted in saliva during kissing or passed from one person to another by infected eating and drinking utensils, razors, toothbrushes, and towels. The easy transmission of the virus makes infection with herpesviruses extremely common. Epidemiologists agree that 90 percent of the population of the United States is infected with the virus before age 20.[1]

The first time you are exposed to the herpes simplex virus, sores may or may not develop. If the infection is going to cause your lips to break out, the cold sore will be felt 10–20 days after exposure. Whether nor not the first infection causes a sore, the virus usually remains in the nerve tissues of the face. Later triggering events cause additional bouts of sores. Usually the sores are less severe as time goes on.

Cold sores are a good measure of emotional stress, since emotional stress debilitates the immune system so that it cannot "remember" the virus that causes cold sores to keep it from multiplying.[2] Combined with stress, a later triggering event, such as some other kind of viral infection, sunburn, windburn, menstruation, or dental work reactivates the herpes simplex virus and causes another outbreak of sores.

TREATMENT SUMMARY

To prevent recurrences of cold sores:

DIET

❍ Avoid foods that contain high concentrations of the amino acid arginine, especially almonds, chocolate, Jell-O, and peanuts.

❍ Eat foods that contain high concentrations of the amino acid lysine, including most vegetables, chicken, fish, and turkey.

NUTRITIONAL SUPPLEMENTS

❍ L-Lysine: 1,000 milligrams 3 times a day. Pregnant women and nursing mothers should avoid lysine supplements.

To treat cold sore once they occur:

NUTRITIONAL SUPPLEMENTS

❍ Zinc oxide/glycine creams: applied at the first sign of inflammation.

HERBS

❍ Copaiba oil: applied to inflamed skin for fast relief of pain.

❍ Eleutherococcus (Siberian ginseng): 2,000 milligrams daily. Since this herb increases testorsterone, men with male-pattern baldness, benign prostatic hypertrophy, or prostate cancer should avoid it. Both men and women with acne should avoid Siberian ginseng.

❍ Kudzu Decoction (Ge Gen Tang or kakkon-to): as directed on label, daily.

❍ Any one of the following herbal creams:

• Licorice (glycyrrhetinic acid) cream, twice daily.

• Melissa cream, twice daily.

• Tea tree oil cream, applied to the lips 2–3 times daily.

See Part Three if you take prescription medication.

UNDERSTANDING THE HEALING PROCESS

Acyclovir (Zovirax) is the prescription drug of choice for treating cold sores, but it is expensive and it does not work for everyone. Moreover, the herpesvirus can become resistant to Zovirax and similar drugs so that these treatments eventually do not work. Only 5 percent of the strains of herpesvirus that cause cold sores do not respond to antiviral treatment at all, but these strains are most likely to occur in the people who need treatment the most, that is, babies born with herpes infections, people with AIDS or HIV, organ transplant recipients, and people taking chemotherapy.[3] Scientists believe that, eventually, all existing drug treatments for herpes will have to be replaced as the virus evolves.[4] Natural remedies, however, work nearly as well as Zovirax and do not run the risk of creating resistant strains of the herpesvirus.

Eat foods rich in the amino acid lysine, and avoid foods rich in the amino acid arginine to prevent herpes infections. The presence of arginine has been long believed to be a "trigger" for the virus to replicate itself.[5] Lysine has a chemical structure that is similar to that of arginine. It competes with and blocks arginine from entering the nerve tissues that harbor the herpesvirus between outbreaks.[6] Lysine more recently has been found to be essential to "coding" the virus so that it is recognized and destroyed by antibodies.[7] Lysine works slowly, however, so it is only useful in preventing cold sores, not in treating them.

A study published in 1979 suggests that zinc supplements in relatively high doses may be useful in controlling recurrent outbreaks of herpes.[8] However, the scientific evidence for the use of creams containing zinc and glycine to control the pain and inflammation caused by cold sores is stronger. A test sponsored by the Alterra Corporation found that applying zinc-based creams at the first sign of inflammation reduced the duration of cold sores by an average of a day and a half. Subjects treated with the zinc oxide/glycine cream also experienced reduction in overall severity of signs and symptoms, particularly blistering, soreness, itching, and tingling.[9]

Copaiba resin acts by reducing the permeability of capillary walls to histamine, the chemical responsible for painful swelling. The volatile oil of the herb is antimicrobial, and prevents secondary infections in eczema and psoriasis as well as herpes.[10]

Eleutherococcus, more commonly known as Russian or Siberian ginseng, has shown promise for the treatment of herpes. A 6-month double-blind trial of 93 men and women with recurrent herpes infections found that treatment with the herb eleutherococcus (2 grams daily) reduced the frequency of infections by almost 50 percent.[11]

The ancient Chinese herbalist Zhang Zhong-jing devised Kudzu Decoction as a means of treating diseases poetically described as "a bird that strains . . . to fly." Researchers in Japan recognized the metaphor as descriptive of herpes infection. Most viral infections, such as colds, are eliminated by the immune system in a few days or perhaps a few weeks. The herpesvirus, however, can remain in nerve tissues for many years without causing symptoms. It is activated when the body's overall resistance is weakened. The weakened immune system's only effective response to the infection is to destroy infected cells. The resulting cascade of inflammation and tissue damage can cause serious complications, and even result in death in infants and adults who are infected with both herpes and HIV.

Researchers at Toyama University in Japan studied the use of Kudzu Decoction as a herpes treatment. Their research found that the formula neither kills the virus directly nor activates the body's immune system. Instead, Kudzu Decoction blocks the tissue-damaging effects of the reactivated virus. In this way, the traditional Chinese herbal formula treats the disease without creating a worse condition in its place.[12]

Kudzu Decoction is nontoxic and safe for use in treating cold sores in children aged 6 and up. Over-the-counter brands of this formula available in the United States and Canada include:

○ Ge Gen Tang (Chinese Classics, Golden Flower Chinese Herbs, Honso , Kan Traditionals, Lotus Classics, ProBotanixx, Qualiherb, Sun Ten)

○ Kakkon-to (Tsumura)

○ Kakkonto Formula 026 (Kampo Institute)

○ Kampo4Cold/Flu Pueraria Formula (Honso)

○ Kudzu Releasing Formula (Kan Traditionals)

○ Pueraria Combination (Lotus Classics, Qualiherb, Sun Ten)

○ Pueraria Formula (Golden Flower Chinese Herbs)

○ Pueraria Plus Formula (Chinese Classics)

○ Shu Jin 1 (ProBotanixx)

Scientists at the University of Texas Medical Branch in Galveston have found that the primary antiviral chemical in licorice, 20 beta-carboxy-11-oxo-30-norolean-12-en-3 beta-yl-2-O-beta-D-glucopyranuronosyl-alpha-D-glucopyranosiduronic acid, more conveniently referred to as glycyrrhizin, protects the lips from opportunistic herpes infection. That is, this chemical prevents the spread of herpes by contact with infected eating utensils or glasses, or by kissing.[13] The latest research has found that glycyrrhizin stops the herpesvirus from "jumping the gap" between the nerve cells, in which it rests between outbreaks, and adjacent cells that carry it to the skin of the lips.[14] Clinical studies have found that licorice creams reduce the pain and healing time associated with cold sores and genital herpes. When used as a cream, licorice does not interact with prescription medications and does not cause side effects.

The latest double-blind, placebo-controlled clinical study in Germany found that melissa (also known as lemon balm) creams relieve the most intense pain of herpes inflammation, occurring on the second day of the outbreak. Melissa reduces total recovery time by an average of one day. It has a rapid effect on itching, tingling, burning, stabbing, swelling, tightening of the skin, and redness. The mechanism of action of the balm mint extract rules out the development of resistance of the herpesvirus. The German scientists conducting the study note that there is an indication that the intervals between the periods with herpes might be prolonged with mint balm cream treatment.[15]

Australian researchers have found that creams containing tea tree oil can reduce the time it takes cold sores to heal from average of 12 days to an average of 9 days. Patients in their study who took tea tree oil had lower concentrations of the virus in their saliva than patients who took Zovirax, meaning they were less likely to pass their infection to others. (This difference was not statistically significant.)[16]

CONCEPTS FOR COPING WITH COLD SORES

O If someone you know has a cold sore, don't kiss him or her and don't drink out of the same glass or use the same knife, fork, or spoon. Sharing towels, washcloths, or napkins is off-limits, too, because the virus may survive on the fabric.

O When you have cold sores, avoid acidic foods such as orange juice, lemons, and tomato sauce. They can irritate the sore.

O Sunburn on the lips reactivates the virus that causes cold sores. To avoid sunburn:

• In the summer, stay out of the sun especially between 10 A.M. and 3 P.M., when the sun's rays are strongest.

• Apply a lip moisturizer that contains sunscreen with an SPF value of 15 or greater.

• Exercise special care when boating or skiing. Sunlight reflected off the water or snow dramatically increases the potential for skin damage.

O Chapped, dry lips are also a risk factor for cold sores. To avoid chapped lips:

• Drink plenty of water. Adequate hydration helps regulate body temperature and prevents chapped lips in both winter and summer.

• Avoid extremely hot baths and showers.

• Apply moisturizer to your lips while they are still wet.

O Holding ice to the lip for 5–10 minutes relieves pain for 15–20 minutes.

O Bioflavonoids, propolis, and vitamins A, C, and E have all been found to play a role in preventing cold sores. They act too slowly, however, to be used in treating cold sores.

O A lip balm made of the herbs rhubarb (the aged root, not the fresh leaf) and sage is another effective herbal treatment for cold sores. A clinical study in Switzerland found that the rhubarb-sage combination cleared up cold sores as quickly as acyclovir (Zovirax), and was better for controlling pain, although acyclovir was better for controlling swelling. As this book is being written, this combination is only available from herbalists who make their own products and compounding pharmacists.

O There are a number of homeopathic remedies for cold sores. Usually it is best to start with a single dose of the lowest strength (6C, 6X, or 12C) of the remedy matching the symptoms to be treated, and then wait for a response. If there is an improvement in symptoms, let the remedy continue to work until there is no more improvement, then take another dose. If there is no improvement, try a different potency (30X or 30C). Sometimes homeopathic medicines work for a few minutes, and sometimes they work for an entire day before another dose is needed.

• Apis mellifica is a remedy for pink and puffy blisters that itch a lot and hurt when touched. If ice helps relieve some pain, apis mellifica should give complete relief. If cold sores do not feel better when ice is applied to them, apis mellifica may not help.

• Borax is also recommended for a tendency to be startled by loud noises and for fear of falling. Borax treats cold sores that cause a feeling of tightness in the lips.

• Dulcamara should be used when cold sores accompany a cold, particularly during chilly, rainy weather.

• Graphites are recommended for oozing, crusting cold sores.

• Natrum muriaticum is a remedy for cold sores that occur after sunburn.

• Rhus toxicodendron, taken at the first sign of an outbreak, relieves redness, pain, and itching.

Colds

SYMPTOM SUMMARY

○ Cough

○ Headache

○ Light fever, 102°F (38.8°C) or lower

○ Muscle aches

○ Nasal congestion

○ Runny nose

○ Sneezing

○ Sore throat

○ Tearing

UNDERSTANDING THE DISEASE PROCESS

At one time or another almost everyone catches a cold. The sneezing, tearing, runny nose, and scratchy throat of a cold are the immune system's response to infection with any one of hundreds of viruses. Virtually everything medicine knows about colds, however, concerns infection with the most common colds virus, rhinovirus.

Rhinoviral infection begins when the virus lands on the tear ducts or the nasal passages. Rhinoviruses can infect single cells or clusters of cells, more viruses being required to infect a cluster of cells than a single cell. Infection of individual cells does not cause symptoms, so it is usually necessary to be exposed to the virus for 120 hours or more during a 7-day period before "coming down with a cold."[1] For this reason, just being in the same room with someone who is sneezing or coughing without covering his or her mouth and nose, while socially objectionable, does not cause infection. The virus is usually transmitted by hand-to-hand contact. On the skin, the virus is harmless. Only when unwashed hands carrying the virus touch the eyes or nose does the virus have a chance to become infectious.

Once the virus has arrived at the tear ducts, it catches a ride on tears flowing backward through the duct. In the nose, the virus is transported backward through the beating action of the cilia, the fine hairs in the nose that capture dust and foreign particles. In either case, the colds virus is harmless until it reaches the back of the throat.

Once the rhinovirus has arrived at this area known as the posterior nasopharynx, it attaches either to LDL ("bad") cholesterol at the lining of a cell, or to the special adhesion molecules that glue the cells of the mucous lining to each other. The virus starts to multiply within the cells lining the nose and throat. One to two days later these cells begin to shed the virus through mucus and tears, making the infected person contagious. Just *after* the infected individual becomes capable of giving someone else a cold, the immune system sends neutrophils, lymphocytes, plasma cells, and eosinophils to inflame the nose and throat to trap the virus. These white blood cells kill the infected cells, and the nose and throat produce mucus to carry the dead cells, the white blood cells, and the virus out of the body.

How long you have to deal with the symptoms of a cold depends on the strength of your immune system. People with especially active immune systems can be infected with rhinovirus or other colds viruses and experience no symptoms at all. People whose immune systems produce large amounts of the hormone interleukin-2 (IL-2) produce less mucus and have fewer days with symptoms.

Stress makes colds worse. Both the production of mucus and the sneeze reflex are triggered by a signal from your brain that is made stronger by stress.[2] In one study of 394 volunteers, greater negative feelings predicted greater risk of catching a cold, no matter which virus the volunteers were exposed to.[3] Experiencing emotional stress just before being exposed to the virus is especially detrimental, and is associated with production of greater quantities of mucus.[4] Moderate drinkers are less likely to catch colds, while smokers are more likely.[5] People with a great deal of social contact can be presumed to be exposed to more colds viruses, but they are less likely to catch colds.[6]

Strictly speaking, there is no such thing as a "chest cold." Bronchial infections and pneumonia are caused by different microorganisms. However, catching a cold increases the risk of acquiring an infection of the lungs and bronchial passages, especially among infants,[7] young children,[8] older adults,[9] transplant recipients,[10] and people in nursing homes.[11] Catching a cold also makes an inner ear infection worse. Pressure in the nose and sinuses impairs drainage from the Eustachian tube and traps infection in the inner ear. The colds virus itself causes 32 percent of inner ear infections in children and 1–8 percent of inner ear infections in adults.[12] Most children who catch colds develop sinusitis, and 40 percent of sinus infections in adults are caused by rhinovirus.[13]

One in three hospitalizations for asthma[14] and 83 percent of cases of bacterial pneumonia in children with cystic fibrosis (CF) are triggered by colds.[15] And catching a cold increases the likelihood of spreading *Streptococcus,* the organism that causes strep throat, by 40 times.[16]

TREATMENT SUMMARY

At the first sign of symptoms, take (in order of importance):

○ *Zinc acetate or zinc gluconate:* lozenges, sucked, not swallowed whole, every 2 hours that you are awake.

○ *Echinacea purpurea:* juice (preferred), 20 drops every 2 hours that you are awake for the first day, then 3 times a day for 10 days.

○ Vitamin C: 2,000 milligrams a day.

For relief of symptoms:

HERBS

Choose a single form of the herb best suited to relieve the symptoms that bother you the most:

To relieve cough (antitussives):

○ Lobelia
  • Ointments: apply to the chest 2–3 times a day, *or*
  • Vinegar extract (acetract): No more than $1/2$ teaspoon 3 times a day. Take less if you experience nausea. Do not give to children.

○ Marshmallow
  • Tea: a rounded teaspoon of the herb in a cup of water as often as desired, *or*
  • Tincture: 1–3 teaspoons up to 4 times a day.

To treat sore throat (demulcents):

○ Elecampane
  • Tea: no more than $1/4$ teaspoon in a cup of water allowed to brew for 15 minutes, up to 3 times a day. *Strain before drinking.*

○ Ivy leaf (Hedera)
  • Extract: a dropperful by itself or in a small amount of water, 2–3 times a day.

○ Marshmallow
  • Tea: a rounded teaspoon of the herb in a cup of water as often as desired, *or*

  • Tincture: 1–3 teaspoons up to 4 times a day.

○ Plantain
  • Cough syrup: $1/2$ teaspoon 3 times a day, *or*
  • Tea: $1/4 - 1/2$ teaspoon of the herb brewed in hot water for 15 minutes.

○ Scutellaria (Chinese skullcap)
  • Fluid extract: $1/2 - 2$ teaspoons 1–3 times per day.

○ Slippery elm
  • Tea: 1 teaspoon in 1 cup of water as often as desired.

To break up phlegm (expectorants):

○ Anise
  • Aromatherapy: 10–20 drops of essential oil in a basin of hot water, vapors inhaled for several minutes once or twice a day. *Never drink essential oils of anise.*
  • Tea: bagged anise tea brewed in 1 cup of hot but not boiling water.

○ Horehound (also known as marrubio)
  • Cough lozenges containing horehound: as often as desired.
  • Tea (from the chopped herb available in hierberías): 1 teaspoon brewed in a cup of hot but not boiling water for 10 minutes, strained before drinking, 2–3 times a day.

○ Horseradish
  • Apply as a plaster once or twice a day.

○ Mullein
  • Tincture: $1/4 - 3/4$ teaspoon up to 4 times a day.

○ Mustard
  • Apply as poultice or plaster once or twice a day.

To stop coughing fits (spasmolytics):

○ Lobelia
  • Ointments: apply to the chest 2–3 times a day.
  • Vinegar extract (acetract): no more than $1/2$ teaspoon 3 times a day. Take less if you experience nausea. Do not give to children.

○ Thyme
  • Tea: $1/4 - 1/2$ teaspoon of the kitchen herb in 1 cup of hot water, 2–3 times daily.
  • Tincture: $1/3 - 1$ teaspoon, 2–3 times daily.

AROMATHERAPY

○ Add 5–10 drops of eucalyptus oil to the water in a vaporizer operated in your bedroom as your sleep.

To prevent colds, take:

○ Andrographis (Kan Jang): 200 milligrams daily.

○ Siberian ginseng (*Eleutherococcus*): 1 tablespoon of tincture or fluid extract daily, or eleuthero energy drinks as your diet allows.

See Part Three if you take prescription medication.

UNDERSTANDING THE HEALING PROCESS

An article published in the *Journal of the American Medical Association* in 1933 cynically stated that ". . . it is possible to convince the public that practically any preparation is of value for the prevention or treatment of colds."[17] The fact is, not every medication offered in the doctor's office—and not every supplement offered in the marketplace—helps everyone who has a cold, and products that relieve symptoms don't usually make your cold go away any faster. Doctors offer antibiotics to 60 percent of their patients with common colds, even though these drugs have no effect on the colds virus and only 2 percent of patients given antibiotics are helped by them.[18] Nose sprays do help cough and laryngitis, but they accomplish this by blunting a signal from the brain to produce mucus.[19] (The worse the aftertaste from using the spray, the more likely it is to help.) A similar effect can be accomplished just by taking a nap. The older antihistamines that cause drowsiness relieve sneezing and musus production in about half the people with colds who use them, but they also cause scratchy throat.[20] The newer non-sedating antihistamines do not help colds at all.[21]

If what the doctor can give doesn't help, what does? For starters, there is zinc. Zinc practically qualifies as a cure for the common cold. A recent medical study involving 218 volunteers found that using a nasal spray with zinc gluconate reduced the duration of a cold by a week. Colds lasted an average of 9 days among volunteers given a placebo and just 2 days among volunteers who started using zinc within 24 hours of their first symptoms.[22] The form and dosage of zinc are very important. Another study using a much lower (50 times smaller) dosage of zinc sulfate instead of zinc gluconate found no benefits at all.[23]

Zinc gluconate lozenges also stop colds. In a double-blind trial at the Cleveland Clinic Foundation, 100 people who were experiencing the early symptoms of a cold were given a lozenge that either contained 13.3 milligrams of zinc from zinc gluconate or was just a placebo. Participants took the lozenges every 2 hours while they were awake every day until their colds resolved. Taking the lozenges didn't help fever, muscle ache, scratchy throat, or sneezing, but it greatly helped headache, hoarseness, nasal drainage, sore throat, and coughing. Headache and hoarseness disappeared in 2 days (versus 3 days in the placebo group), nasal drainage in 4 days (versus 7 days), sore throat in just 1 day (versus 3 days), and coughing in 2.2 days (versus 4 day).[24] Lozenges made with zinc acetate also seem to be helpful.[25]

The catch with using zinc lozenges is that they have to taste bad to be good. Flavoring agents such as citric acid and tartaric acid stop zinc's action against the rhinovirus, although sweeteners such as mannitol and sorbitol (and other compounds with names ending in -ol) do not diminish zinc's effect. And even if the lozenge tastes bad, it won't help you if you swallow it. When you take zinc to fight a cold, you are not using it as a nutritional supplement. The zinc from a zinc lozenge has to enter your saliva, and the zinc-laden saliva has to remain in your mouth long enough to be transported to the back of your throat.

Echinacea can also stop a cold in its tracks, although not as dramatically as zinc. The best way to take echinacea to stop a cold is as a liquid extract or tincture (alcohol-free versions are available for children and for adults who are sensitive to alcohol), although other forms of echinacea also work. In a study reported in the *European Journal of Clinical Research,* 120 people were given either *Echinacea purpurea* juice (prepared by the German company that makes the American product Echinagard) or a placebo as soon as they started showing symptoms of a cold. The volunteers took 20 drops of echinacea or the placebo every 2 hours for 1 day, then 20 drops 3 times a day for a total of 10 days. Only 40 percent of those taking echinacea developed "real colds," compared to 60 percent of those taking the placebo. Among the volunteers who did develop colds, those taking echinacea started getting better in an average of 4 days compared to an average of 8 days for those who took the placebo.[26]

Other studies of echinacea have found similar results. The benefits of echinacea in treating colds seem to be greatest in people who have low T-cell counts,[27] such as people on chemotherapy or who use corticosteroids for lupus, multiple sclerosis, rheumatoid arthritis, or Sjögren's syndrome, or people with HIV or AIDS. Some people shouldn't use echinacea. Women who are trying to get pregnant should avoid *Echinacea purpurea.* It contains caffeoyl esters that can interfere the action of hyaluronidase, an enzyme essential to the release of unfertilized eggs into the fallopian tube.[28]

There is laboratory evidence that *Echinacea angustifolia* contains chemicals that deactivate CYP3A4. This is a liver enzyme that breaks down a wide range of medications, including anabolic steroids, the chemotherapy drug methotrexate used in treating cancer and lupus, astemizole (Hismanal) for allergies, nifedipine (Adalat) and captopril (Capoten) for high blood pressure, and sildenafil (Viagra) for impotence, as well as many others. *Echinacea angustifolia* might help maintain levels of these drugs in the bloodstream and make them more effective, or it might also cause them to accumulate to levels at which they cause side effects. Switch to a brand of echinacea that does not contain *Echinacea angustifolia* if you experience unexpected side effects while taking any of these drugs.[29]

Echinacea stimulates immune function, but it also slightly increases production of T cells.[30] These are the immune cells attacked by HIV. When there are more T cells, the virus has more cells to infect. This gives the virus more opportunities to mutate into a drug-resistant form. The authoritative reference work *The Complete German Commission E Monographs* counsels against the use of echinacea for treating colds in people who have HIV or autoimmune diseases such as multiple sclerosis. Later communications between the senior editor of the *Monographs* and the German Food and Drug Administration revealed that the warning in the reference book was based on theoretical speculation rather than practical experience.[31] Still, as a precaution, people with HIV should only use echinacea for *treating* colds rather than preventing them.

Vitamin C is the best-known natural treatment for colds. Dozens of scientific studies have found that vitamin C reduces the severity and duration of colds, but the results are usually not dramatic. A meta-analysis statistically combining the results of 21 studies found that taking any dosage of vitamin C beyond the RDA reduces the length of a cold by about 23 percent (about 2 days).[32] Higher doses of vitamin C, that is, up to 2,000 milligrams a day, get better results, especially in children. However, there is no scientific evidence that taking massive amounts of vitamin C (10,000 milligrams a day or more) provides any added benefit. In fact, taking vitamin C just at the beginning of symptoms seems to work as well as taking it throughout the course of a cold. [33]

People who take vitamin C need to disregard the adage "Starve a fever, feed a cold," at least with regard to carbohydrates. Vitamin C is most effective in an alkaline environment. Diets high in carbohydrates and refined sugars produce acidity, so if you are going to take vitamin C, your best results will come if you also restrict sugars and refined carbohydrates.[34] Very few people experience any side effects taking a dosage of 2,000 milligrams a day, although diarrhea or gas are possible. Take vitamin C with caution if you take certain prescription drugs. Vitamin C taken in the form of vitamin C with bioflavonoids can interfere with the liver's ability to process statin drugs for controlling cholesterol, calcium channel blockers such as nifedipine (Procardia) for hypertension, or cyclosporine for preventing transplant rejection.

There are a number of herbs that help relieve bronchitis. The best way to use them is to treat the symptoms that are the most bothersome to you. Anise and the related herb, star anise, contain an antimicrobial chemical, anethole.[35] The essential oil is especially deadly to molds and yeast infections.[36] Since anise stimulates production of secretions, it should be used to treat dry coughs rather than mucus-producing coughs.

Elecampane mostly consists of the sugar inulin (not to be confused with insulin), the same carbohydrate found in Jerusalem artichokes. The inulin in elecampane coats and soothes the throat. The herb also contains small amounts of volatile oils that act as counterirritants, desensitizing the throat to pain.

It is important not to use too much elecampane. The volatile oils in the herb can irritate the mouth and the bowel. There has been a single report in the medical literature of a potentially life-threatening allergic reaction to foods containing the same carbohydrates as elecampane. This experience has been cited as a reason not to use elecampane, but this allergy was to inulin, possibly to Jerusalem artichokes, rather than to any herb. There is no evidence whatsoever that the man who experienced a severe allergic reaction after eating foods containing inulin took any herb, including elecampane.[37] Nonetheless, if you are allergic to Jerusalem artichokes, do not take elecampane. There is also a report in the medical literature of a severe allergic reaction to Inutest, a highly refined form of inulin used to measure kidney function. Although this report also has been cited as a reason not to use elecampane, Inutest is not made from elecampane, and the allergic reaction to Inutest occurred after it was *injected* into a sensitive patient.[38]

Horehound, also known as marrubio, is a traditional remedy for bronchitis in the southwestern United States and Mexico. It is also widely used in the Arab world. Unlike over-the-counter remedies for bronchitis, it lowers blood pressure.[39] It also relieves the pain of sore throat.[40] Complications from using horehound are rare, but since it is a bitter and bitters stimulate production of stomach acids, people with gastroesophageal reflux disease (GERD), chronic heartburn, or peptic ulcers should use the herb in moderation.

Horseradish and mustard contain volatile oils that have antibacterial properties. They also open bronchial passages. While both herbs can be taken internally, they are more typically used in plasters and poultices.

Ivy leaf, also known as Hedera, is a common remedy for bronchitis in the Azores. Researchers have identified at least six chemicals in ivy leaf that stop bronchial spasms.[41] These compounds are not water soluble so the herb must be taken as an extract, although it can be mixed with water to make the extract easier to swallow. Ivy leaf is used to stop "coughing fits" caused by phlegmy coughs rather than dry coughs. Some samples of the herb can contain very small amounts of a nausea-inducing chemical known as emetine, so the herb should not be used by pregnant women or small children.

Lobelia contains the phlegm-dissolving plant chemical lobeline. This chemical acts on the same centers in the brain as nicotine, giving somewhat of the same sense of satisfaction as smoking.[42] Unlike nicotine, this plant chemical makes breathing deeper and stronger. It also stimulates the flow of blood to the heart by activating nerves in the carotid sinus.[43] In overdose, however, it can also activate the vagus nerve, which has roughly the same effect as a punch in the stomach. Too much lobeline, and too much lobelia, can cause nausea and vomiting.

Lobelia makes the brain less sensitive to amphetamines,[44] so it should not be taken by anyone who takes amphetamine or dextroamphetamine (Adderall), methamphetamine (Desoxyn), methylphenidate (Ritalin), or pemoine (Cylert). There is a widely held misconception that lobelia is toxic, but a systematic search of the medical literature failed to find any reports of lobelia poisoning.[45] Ear infections make it more likely that lobelia will cause stomach upset.

According to *The Complete German Commission E Monographs,* marshmallow contains healing sugars that line and soothe the throat and stop dry cough.[46] Marshmallow teas are more effective at stopping coughs than marshmallow cough drops or tinctures.[47] Marshmallow does not interact with medications, but it is nearly pure sugar and should be used with caution by people who have diabetes.

Mullein contains chemicals that kill bacteria and stop pain.[48] Taken at the same time as a flu treatment such as amatadine (Symmetrel), it greatly increases the probability that the flu treatment will work.[49] The combination of mullein and zanamivir (Relenza) has not yet been tested. Mullein does not generally cause any side effects, although some people may be allergic to it.

Plantain is both soothing and astringent. It contains both mucilages, slimy complex carbohydrates that coat the throat, and tannins, the same chemicals that are found in tea and that tighten the lining of the throat. One of its chemical components is aucubin, a chemical that locks itself to the proteins in the lining of the throat[50] and possibly forms a protective barrier against protection. Another of its components is a pectin, a sugar closely related to the pectin used in making jams and jellies, that in its purified form is as potent a stimulator of the immune system as gamma globulin.[51] Plantain is more useful in helping phlegm come up rather than in relieving dry cough. There are no interactions of plantain with prescription drugs, although it should not be taken at the same time as prescription drugs because it can interfere with their absorption.

Scutellaria is one of Traditional Chinese Medicine's most important herbs for treating respiratory infections. It contains a variety of anti-inflammatory chemicals that are antioxidant in some situations, protecting red blood cells, and prooxidant in others, activating the immune process.[52] It contains several chemicals that are effective in treating bronchitis secondary to infection with respiratory syncitial virus (RSV).[53] That is, unlike most other herbs and medications, scutellaria is antiviral rather than only antibacterial.

Slippery elm makes the lining of the throat "slippery" and reduces inflammation from eating and drinking. The complex carbohydrates in slippery elm are completely digestible and the product is wholly nontoxic. Teas can be made with 1/2–2 teaspoons of the bark depending on personal preferences. Slippery elm is also found in many herbal cough lozenges.

Thyme releases an essential oil known as thymol, which travels through the bloodstream to be exhaled through the lungs. Of all the herbs studied in the treatment of bronchitis, thyme has the longest half-life, lasting in the body for up to 20 hours.[54] There are reports that the essential oil of thyme, combined with essential oils of cinnamon, cloves, lavender, and mint, may reduce repeated infections in people who have bronchitis. The most common use of thyme, however, is treating coughing spasms in children.

Never take the essential oil of thyme by mouth. The essential oil should only be used in aromatherapy. The chopped herb can be used in teas. There are also commercially available fluid extracts and tinctures of thyme that are safe for use with either children or adults. In Europe, thyme is frequently combined with an extract made from a carnivorous plant, the sundew, to make cough drops such as Ricola.

Not to be neglected in taking care of a cold is aromatherapy. Although the concept of aromatherapy sounds exotic to many people, it is actually very basic: if you use a vaporizer, you use aromatherapy. Eucalyptus oil is a standard ingredient in cough drops and in oils added to humidifiers and vaporizers. While it does not increase breathing capacity, a study of 246 people with chronic bronchitis found that eucalyptus oils stop the worsening of cough that commonly occurs in the winter (in wet climates where heaters are used) or summer (in desert climates).[55]

Other essential oils can also be helpful in the vaporizer, or breathed in during a steaming bath. Chamomile, elderberry, and lemon balm relieve pain. Yarrow stops inflammation in the nose and throat.

While zinc, echinacea, and vitamin C are very useful in treating colds, other supplements are more useful for preventing colds. Unquestionably the best-documented herb for preventing colds is *Eleutherococcus,* also known as Siberian ginseng. This herb is not fully appreciated in the United States in part because the majority of the hundreds of research studies on its use in preventing winter illnesses were published in Russian.

Siberian ginseng is *not* the same plant as Chinese ginseng.

Clinical trials in the old Soviet Union enlisted the entire populations of cities in Siberia to test Siberian ginseng as a preventative for colds and flu. The largest of these studies found that taking Siberian ginseng for 8–10 weeks before the beginning of the cold and flu season reduced the incidence of these diseases by more than 95 percent.[56] As translator of the Soviet study, however, I must note that it was supervised, published, and publicized by a Soviet government agency responsible for exporting herbs. Studies conducted without such blatant commercial interest have found that Siberian ginseng stimulates the production of both B and T cells to boost immune power.[57] The noted natural health expert Dr. Michael Murray writes that Siberian ginseng prevents colds caused by exposure to cold, allergens, and, especially, emotional stress.[58]

Siberian ginseng has the interesting side effect of improving color vision, especially the ability to distinguish red and green.[59] It also increases the production of testosterone in men. A number of professional athletes use Siberian ginseng to prevent colds, and all of them are completely bald. Men who have prostate problems and women who have polycystic ovarian syndrome should avoid the herb.

Anothe herb that has been documented to prevent colds is "Indian echinacea," the South Asian herb andrographis. This herb was credited with saving India from the worldwide flu epidemic of 1919,[60] and has become a popular remedy for colds in Europe. A Chilean study enlisted 107 student volunteers, all 18 years old, to participate in a 3-month trial that used a dried extract of andrographis to prevent colds. Fifty-four of the students took two 100-milligram doses daily (a very low dose), and 53 were given a placebo. All the participants in the study were examined for symptoms of colds by a physician once a week for 12 weeks. At the end of the 3-month test period, only 16 students who used andrographis had had colds, compared to 33 of the placebo-group participants. Even a very low dose of andrographis reduced the risk of catching a cold by 50 percent.[61]

Although it is not as good for treating colds as echinacea, andrographis is known to be helpful for treating earache, sleeplessness, nasal drainage, and sore throat.[62] If you start taking andrographis after symptoms have already begun, you will probably not get results for 3–4 days. Much higher doses, 1,000–1,200 milligrams daily, are required for treating colds than for preventing colds.

Some people should not take andrographis. Some components of the herb stimulate gallbladder contraction, which can cause potentially severe pain in people who have gallstones. Extremely high doses of the herb, far more than anyone is likely to take, may cause infertility in men. One study found that male lab rats given the equivalent of 100 times a normal dose in humans experienced testicular atrophy,[63] although a follow-up study failed to confirm this side effect.

There is very little scientific evidence that taking vitamin C can prevent colds. One exception may be the sniffles that athletes get after a competition. For preventing colds after physical exhaustion, taking 500–1,000 milligrams of vitamin C a day is sufficient. To get protective benefits, you should start taking vitamin C at least 3 weeks before your athletic event. Vitamin E (200 IU per day) taken with vitamin C increases the benefit of vitamin C.[64]

There are many other natural products that are useful in treating colds. Bromelain, taken in doses of 500–750 milligrams 3 times a day between meals, helps break up sticky mucus. Do not take bromelain if you are allergic to pineapple. Fenugreek and thyme also help break up mucus.

Many people find that cat's claw stops the symptoms of a cold. If you take cat's claw, taking a teaspoon of lemon juice with the cat's claw tincture or drinking an orange juice chaser after taking the cat's claw capsule releases tannins that are especially useful in treating colds. A Native American remedy, osha, is helpful for relieving earache.

Several Asian herbal formulas have specific applications in treating colds.

❍ Kudzu Formula relieves colds with tension in the shoulders or the back of the neck. Brand names in the United States include:

- Ge Gen Tang (Chinese Classics, Golden Flower Chinese Herbs, Honso, Kan Traditionals, Lotus Classics, ProBotanixx, Qualiherb, Sun Ten)
- Kakkon-to (Tsumura)
- Kakkonto Formula 026 (Kampo Institute)
- Kampo4Cold/Flu Pueraria Formula (Honso)
- Kudzu Releasing Formula (Kan Traditionals)

- Pueraria Combination (Lotus Classics, Qualiherb, Sun Ten)
- Pueraria Formula (Golden Flower Chinese Herbs)
- Pueraria Plus Formula (Chinese Classics)
- Shu Jin 1 (ProBotanixx)

❍ Decoction to Construct the Middle or *ogi-kenchu-to,* offers relief of especially severe allergic symptoms in people who also have eczema or chronic digestive problems such as irritable bowel syndrome or peptic ulcer disease. Brand names of this formula in the United States include:

- Astragalus Formula (Golden Flower)
- Huang Qi Jian Zhong Tang (Lotus Classics, Qualiherb, Sun Ten)
- Ogi-kenchu-to (Honso, Tsumura).

CONCEPTS FOR COPING WITH COLDS

❍ Never give a child with a viral infection aspirin or foods containing chemicals similar to aspirin, including curry powder, dill, licorice, oregano, paprika, peppermint, prunes, raisins, turmeric, cakes made from mixes, chewing gum, or soft drinks. Reye's syndrome, a devastating illness involving pressure on the brain, can be triggered by consuming salicylates while recovering from viral infection.

❍ Acupressure applied to the webbing between the thumb and index finger relieves sinus pain and congestion.

❍ There are a number of homeopathic remedies for colds. Usually it is best to start with a single dose of the lowest strength (6C, 6X, or 12C) of the remedy matching the symptoms to be treated, and then wait for a response. If there is an improvement in symptoms, let the remedy continue to work until there is no more improvement, then take another dose. If there is no improvement, try a different potency (30X or 30C). Sometimes homeopathic medicines work for a few minutes, and sometimes they work for an entire day before another dose is needed.

- Aconitum napellus is recommended when symptoms come on suddenly, especially after a stressful or traumatic experience. Symptoms relieved by this homeopathic formula include scratchy throat, choking cough, tightness across the chest, and dry, stuffy nose.
- Alium cepa is recommended for runny nose with a

clear discharge, watery eyes, burning eyes, and sneezing.

• Arsenicum album is recommended for people who have frequent colds and sore throat. It is most effective when symptoms are worse at night and when thick, burning mucus is present.

• Baryta carbonica is recommended for people who catch colds easily after getting chilled. It treats runny nose, swollen lips, swollen tonsils, and adenoids.

• Belladonna is recommended when a cold comes on suddenly with flushed face and restlessness. Belladonna relieves "dried out" sinuses and earache.

• Dulcamara is recommended for colds that occur in chilly, wet weather. It is also helpful for allergies.

• Euphrasia relieves red eyes and frequent sneezing with a clear discharge. Helpful when symptoms interrupt sleep and when the person feels better after eating.

• Ferrum phosphoricum is said to stop a cold from developing if taken immediately after symptoms are first noticed. This remedy is used to relieve hacking cough after a cold has set in.

• Gelsemium treats fatigue, headache, fever, and chills. It is especially recommended when the person with the cold feels shaky. Gelsemium treats colds that occur in hot weather.

• Kali bichromicum helps break up thick, stringy mucus in the nose and throat.

• Mercurius solubilis treats colds in people who wake up sweaty. It also treats bad breath, swollen lymph nodes, and earache.

• Natrum muriaticum treats colds with a white (not clear) discharge, sneezing that is worse early in the morning, and chapped lips.

• Nux vomica treats stuffy head and runny nose.

• Phosphorus keeps colds from going to the chest, and is useful when one nostril is blocked and the other clear. Phosphorus is recommended for people who tend to get nosebleeds.

• Pulsatilla helps when the nose is stopped-up when indoors and runny when outdoors. It treats colds causing thick green or yellow mucus that are worse in the evening.

• Rhus toxicodendron treats colds that begin with stiffness and body aches before sneezing, tearing, cough, and sore throat occur.

Colic

SYMPTOM SUMMARY

In babies:

❍ Sudden outburst of excessive crying at about the same time every day

❍ Irritability

❍ Apparent abdominal pain demonstrated by bringing knees up to the stomach

UNDERSTANDING THE DISEASE PROCESS

Some babies cry more than others—some a lot more. Colic is a condition of early infancy characterized by loud crying, apparent abdominal pain, and irritability. Crying spells caused by colic usually last for 3–4 hours at a time. Colic typically starts 10 days to 3 weeks after birth and stops by the baby's fourth month. Babies who have colic usually start crying about the same time each day, but some infants may cry almost constantly.

Colic is more common in first-born children than in later children.[1] Breastfeeding seems to decrease the risk of colic in very young infants but to increase the risk of colic in older infants. One clinical study involving 89 breastfed and formula-fed infants found that at 2 weeks of age, 43 percent of formula-fed infants cried more than 3 hours a day but only 16 percent of breastfed infants cried more than 3 hours a day. At 6 weeks, however, the percentages were nearly reversed, 12 percent of formula-fed infants crying more than 3 hours a day versus 31 percent of breastfed infants.[2] Mothers who are older and better educated are more likely to seek medical care for colic.[3]

The causes of colic are not well known. It is not caused by hunger, pain, or too much gas. It may be due to air swallowed when the baby sucks on fingers or toes or the bottle, or it could be due to overfeeding the baby either cow's milk or breast milk. Colic is sometimes linked to an allergy to cow's milk. Some recent research suggests colic may be due to reflux esophagitis, a condition in which acid backs up from the stomach to the throat.

TREATMENT SUMMARY

Treatments that do not help:

❍ Simethicone (My Baby Gas Relief Drops, Digel, Gas-X, Mylanta).

Treatments that help, but involve serious medical risk:

○ Dicyclomine drugs (Bemote or Di-Spaz).

Treatments that help:

○ Carminative herbs (used as described in "Understanding the Healing Process").

○ Whey-based formulas (Neocate).

See the Drugs Interaction Guide if you take prescription drugs.

UNDERSTANDING THE HEALING PROCESS

For generations, parents of colicky babies have picked them up, talked to them, carried them around, offered them pacifiers, and given them a quiet place to rest. Clinical studies have not found that one method of calming the baby is better than another, but that any kind of reassurance helps.[4] Being careful to change diapers, placing the baby near the mother, and either putting the baby down to sleep or stimulating the baby with play was found in one study to be twice as effective as dietary changes alone.[5] On the other hand, while increasing specific parental interventions for colic helps, it does not lead to drastic improvement. One study found that colicky babies held for 4½ hours every day cried 5 minutes a day less than babies held for 2½ hours a day.[6] Balanced parental attention is best.

Clinical study suggests that the most commonly prescribed medication for colic, simethicone (My Baby Gas Relief Drops, Digel, Gas-X, Mylanta) does not help the condition. In one clinical trial, twice as many infants improved after taking no medication at all (the placebo) as did after taking simethicone.[7] Drugs that act on the baby's nervous system, such as dicyclomine (Bemote or Di-Spaz), do relieve colic[8] but make the baby very sensitive to hot weather and can also cause constipation.

Sugar water, low-lactose milk, and soy milk help relieve colic in some babies but not in others. The smell of soy milk may be a problem for some infants. Most babies prefer the smell of cow's milk or whey. A recent study in the Netherlands found that a whey-based formula reduced crying by an average of an hour a day.[9] Since whey-based formulas such as Nestlé-Carnation Good Start smell better and cost less, they are a useful treatment for colic. It is only necessary to give formula for *one* feeding a day. Other feedings can be breast milk or cow's milk. Results usually take about a week. Babies who tend to spit up may do better on amino-acid-based formulas such as Neocate.

An even less expensive treatment for colic is the use of carminative herbs. Chamomile teas have been used for centuries to treat colic. A clinical study found that giving babies ½ c (125 milliliters) of a calming tea made with chamomile, fennel, lemon balm, licorice, and vervain during crying spells, up to 3 times a day, was more effective than a placebo.[10] Teas made with cinnamon, fumitory, garden angelica (*Angelica archangelica*), and hyssop may also be helpful. Giving peppermint to infants should be avoided, since the burning action of the essential oil can cause spitting up or choking. The easiest way to use these herbs is to use herbal tea bags, available in health food stores and some food markets. Be sure to let the tea cool to room temperature before giving it to the infant.

European mothers sometimes make an herbal remedy for colic from caraway seeds. Mix a tablespoon (15 grams) of caraway seed with 1 cup (240 milliliters) of hot water and allow to stand for 10 minutes. Add ½ cup (120 milliliters) of glycerin, and store the resulting mixture in the refrigerator. Give the baby ½ teaspoon of the mixture every time crying starts.

CONCEPTS FOR COPING WITH COLIC

○ Feed the baby when he or she cries rather than on a fixed schedule. Babies' bodies do not have the same mechanisms to regulate energy as adults, so a baby's cry may be caused by low blood sugar. If feeding does not help, then try other measures.

○ Mothers who breastfeed colicky babies should avoid foods that may cause allergies in the child, especially cow's milk.

○ Chiropractic "finger massage," done by a professional, sometimes relieves colic in as little as 1 treatment,[11] and usually in 2 or 3 treatments.

○ Smoking during pregnancy increases the risk the newborn will have colic.[12]

○ There are a number of homeopathic remedies for colic. Usually it is best to start with a single dose of the lowest strength (6C, 6X, or 12C) of the remedy matching the symptoms to be treated, and then wait for a response. If there is an improvement in symptoms, let the remedy continue to work until there is no more improvement, then take another dose. If there is no improvement, try a different potency (30X or 30C). Sometimes homeopathic medicines work for a few minutes, and sometimes they work for an entire day before another dose is needed.

- Belladonna is a weaker version of the same active ingredient found in dicyclomine (Bemote or Di-Spaz). This treatment is recommended for babies who cry more, rather than less, when they are picked up.

- Chamomilla is recommended for babies who want constantly to be picked up or carried.

- Colocynthis is given to babies who cry when being carried on someone's arm or who cry when they roll over onto their stomachs.

- Dioscorea is given to babies who get relief from colic by bending backward.

- Magnesia phosphorica treats babies who get relief from the application of warmth.

- Nux vomica (the homeopathic preparation, not the emetic used to treat poisoning) is given to breast-fed babies who experience colic after the mother drinks coffee or soft drinks or eats chocolate.

Colitis

See **Inflammatory Bowel Disease; Irritable Bowel Syndrome.**

Colorectal Cancer

SYMPTOM SUMMARY

○ Most colorectal cancers do not cause symptoms. Blood in the stool that can only be measured by a simple medical test is often the only warning sign.

Some colorectal cancers will also cause:

○ Constipation or diarrhea lasting 2 weeks or more

○ Darker stools

○ *Dark* (not bright red) blood *in* (not on) the stool, or *bright red* blood (not dark) *on* (not in) the stool

○ Anemia that cannot be otherwise explained

○ Fatigue

○ Lower abdominal pain and tenderness

○ Narrow stools

○ Weight loss for no apparent reason

○ Lump in the anus

○ Bloating and gas

UNDERSTANDING THE DISEASE PROCESS

Colorectal cancer is a malignancy of the mucosal cells that line the inner wall of the colon and rectum. According to the Colon Cancer Alliance, colorectal cancer is the third most commonly diagnosed cancer in the United States, after breast cancer in women and prostate cancer in men. Approximately 1 in 18 people in the United States will develop colorectal cancer at some point in their lifetimes.

Colorectal cancer is most common in populations that tend to be lactose-intolerant, especially African-Americans. In the United States, African-Americans are 10 percent more likely than the general population to develop colorectal cancer and 30 percent more likely to die of the disease. Colorectal cancer usually strikes after the age of 60, but it can occur even in adults under 30 if there are genetic factors increasing risk of the disease.[1]

Risk factors for colorectal cancer include a history of colorectal polyps, personal or family history of cancer, ulcerative colitis, and Crohn's disease. Colorectal cancers developing near the rectum sometimes cause the stool to be *coated* with bright red blood. These cancers usually cause a steady pain that may be likened to sawing with a dull knife. Cancers developing on the right side of the colon can cause iron-deficiency anemia. These cancers also cause generalized abdominal pain and bleeding of brick-red blood. Cancers developing on the left side of the colon cause dark blood to be *mixed* with the stool due to colon obstruction; powerful straining is necessary to complete a bowel movement.

TREATMENT SUMMARY

DIET

○ Eat foods that are rich in available calcium, such as broccoli, Brussels sprouts, kale, mustard greens, turnips, and cold-water fish, as well as dairy products. If you eat dairy products, substitute *acidophilus*-enriched yogurt for milk as often as possible.

❍ Limit consumption of protein by eating at least 1 meat-free meal per day.

❍ Drink at least 8 glasses of water a day.

NUTRITIONAL SUPPLEMENTS

❍ Any multivitamin containing folic acid, daily.

UNDERSTANDING THE HEALING PROCESS

Preventing colon cancer is not so much a matter of what you eat as what you don't eat. High-calorie consumption, without regard to weight, increases the risk of colorectal cancer. Overweight, without regard to calorie consumption, increases the risk of benign colon polyps that can later become cancerous.[2] Increasing consumption of fiber can help prevent the development of colon cancer in people who eat a high-fat diet, but is not protective for people who eat a low-fat diet. Similarly, alpha- and beta-carotene and vitamin C protect against colorectal cancer in a high-fat diet but not in a low-fat diet.[3] For this reason, controlling weight and reducing intake of fat are more important than eating more fiber or taking specific nutritional supplements.

It also helps to exercise. A Taiwanese study found that men (but not women) who were physically active during their leisure time were much less likely to develop colon cancer. A study of over 75,000 people in Norway found that exercise reduces the risk of colon cancer in men, but added that high blood sugars and insulin resistance (which are associated with lack of exercise but can be treated without exercise) raised the risk of colon cancer in women.[4] A more recent study at the University of Utah reported that sedentary men, but not sedentary women, were more likely to develop a mutation causing inoperable colon cancer. In women, overweight, regardless of physical activity, predicted mutations leading to inoperable colon cancer.[5]

In addition to weight control, general dietary changes and general nutritional supplements can greatly reduce your risk of getting this form of cancer. The latest reports tell us that calcium is important in reducing the risk of colorectal cancer. The Harvard School of Public Health tracked 87,998 women in the Nurses' Health Study and 47,344 men in the Health Professionals Follow-up Study for 16 years. Men who consumed the most calcium (more than 1,250 milligrams per day) were 42 percent less likely than men who consumed the least calcium (less than 500 milligrams per day) to develop inoperable colorectal cancer. Women who consumed the most calcium were 27 percent less likely than women who consumed the least calcium to develop colon inoperable cancer. Calcium consumption also seemed to reduce the risk of developing operable colorectal cancers in women, although the findings were inconclusive. It did not have a similar benefit regarding the risk of operable colorectal cancers in men. The research team noted that 700 milligrams of calcium per day conferred almost as much cancer protection as 1,250 milligrams of calcium per day.[6]

Calcium acts by protecting the lining of the colon from potentially toxic reactions caused by red meat. The cancer risk of red meat is derived not from the fat in red meat but the blood.[7] The blood proteins in red meat release irritants that in turn trigger the multiplication of cells in the lining of the colon.[8] The release of trypsin to digest other proteins in red meat also inflames the lining of the colon.[9] The more colon cells are irritated, the more they multiply. The more cells multiply, the greater the chances of cancer-causing mutation.

At the present stage of scientific understanding, it appears the best way to get calcium is to drink milk. Finnish scientists have found that calcium and vitamin D by themselves do not necessarily lower the risk of colorectal cancer, and the consumption of large quantities of fermented milk products (such as cheese and butter) even increases the risk of colorectal cancer.[10] Yogurt, however, lowers the risk of colorectal cancer. Laboratory studies with white rats find that *acidophilus* and inulin (a carbohydrate abundant in Jerusalem artichokes, not to be confused with insulin) reduce the rate at which colon tumors form after exposure to carcinogenic chemicals.[11]

Calcium by itself, however, has no direct effect on the health of the colon. Calcium stops the proliferation of colorectal cancer cells only in the presence of vitamin D. Scientists at St. Luke's-Roosevelt Hospital in New York City have found that the greater the concentration of activated vitamin D in the colon, the fewer the actively multiplying cancer cells.[12] This finding explains the observation that the risk of dying from colorectal cancer is greatest in parts of the world that receive the least sunlight.[13] For this reason, getting regular sun—without burning—or taking 400–800 IU of vitamin D daily should help reduce the risk of colorectal cancer. For most people in North America and Europe, reducing fat consumption, increasing calcium consumption, helping calcium stay in the body by eating less red meat, and getting regular sun exposure greatly reduce the risk of colorectal cancer.

But what about colorectal cancer protection for people who don't eat a Western diet? A preliminary study in Taiwan of 163 colorectal cancer patients and 163 patients who did not have colon cancer suggests that drinking water is even more protective than drinking milk. Men who drank 8 glasses of water or more every day were 92 percent less likely to develop colon cancer than men who drank 5 glasses of water per day or fewer. Women who drank 8 glasses of water or more every day were 71 percent less likely to develop colon cancer than women who drank 5 glasses of water per day or fewer.[14] Drinking green tea may also help. Laboratory studies have found that green tea polyphenols alter the biochemical process that creates inflammatory hormones in the intestine, and may reduce the risk of colorectal cancer.[15]

The antioxidant selenium has long been considered cancer protective for the colon. For reasons that are not yet understood, selenium in foods, such as broccoli, offers greater cancer protection than selenium supplements.[16]

While few individual supplements have a proven role in preventing colorectal cancer, a study of over 88,000 women suggests that taking at least 400 micrograms of folic acid daily can reduce colorectal cancer risk by nearly 50 percent for women who drink alcohol.[17] Men and women who have ulcerative colitis and who take sulfasalazine (Azulfidine) should take supplements containing folic acid to prevent deficiency.

CONCEPTS FOR COPING WITH COLORECTAL CANCER

O Many people make the mistake of attributing rectal bleeding to anal fissures or hemorrhoids. Rectal bleeding can be caused by many factors, including cancer. Polyps and cancers do not bleed all the time, so an occurrence of rectal bleeding may be the first sign of colorectal cancer. Always have a medical evaluation to rule out colorectal cancer when you notice dark blood in stool.

O Taking a *baby* aspirin a day may reduce the risk of developing colon cancer. An adult aspirin taken daily has a much lower benefit. Japanese scientists have found that aspirin alters gene expression in several strains of colon cancer, including one kind of colon cancer resistant to conventional medical treatment.[18]

O If you have been told you have colon polyps, consider treatment with Traditional Chinese Medicine in addition to standard medical care. Magnolol, a chemical component of the Chinese herbs hou pou and magnolia that is found in many (but not all) Chinese and Japanese herbal formulas, stops the development of colorectal cancer cells just as they are duplicating their DNA to divide themselves into two. Freezing the growth process at just this point gives the cancer-protective gene p21 maximum opportunity to identify and repair the genetic damage that causes cancer. Taiwanese scientists have found that magnolol interacts with p21 both in the test tube and in the bodies of colorectal cancer patients.[19]

Common Cold
See **Colds**.

Condyloma
See **Genital Warts**.

Congestion, Nasal
See **Stuffy Nose**.

Congestive Heart Failure

SYMPTOM SUMMARY
O Cough

O Decreased production of urine

O Difficulty concentrating

O Difficulty sleeping

O Dizziness

O Fatigue

O Nausea

O Need to urinate at night

O Protruding neck veins

○ Rapid or irregular pulse

○ Shortness of breath after lying down

○ Shortness of breath, especially after exertion

○ Swelling in abdomen

○ Swelling of feet and ankles

○ Vomiting

○ Weight gain not related to excessive consumption of food or change in exercise habits

UNDERSTANDING THE DISEASE PROCESS

Congestive heart failure occurs when the heart is unable to pump enough blood to meet the body's circulatory needs. Symptoms of congestive heart failure vary, depending on whether the left or right chambers of the heart are damaged. When the damage is on the left side of the heart, blood backs up in the lungs making breathing difficult. The kidneys are unable to process fluids, and there is sudden weight gain. When the right chamber of the heart is damaged, there is accumulation of blood and other fluids in the feet and ankles and bloating of the abdomen, accompanied by extreme fatigue.

TREATMENT SUMMARY

DIET

○ *Eliminate* added salt from your diet.

NUTRITIONAL SUPPLEMENTS

○ Coenzyme Q_{10}: 150–300 milligrams daily.

○ L-carnitine: 500 milligrams 3 times a day.

○ Magnesium aspartate or magnesium citrate: 200–400 milligrams 3 times a day.

HERBS

Most important:

○ Hawthorn, any one of the following forms, 3 times a day:

• Solid extract (standardized to contain 1.8% vitexin-4'-rhamnoside): 100–250 milligrams.

• Leaf and flowers as a tea: 1–2 teaspoons (3–5 grams).

• Fluid extract: 1–2 milliliters ($^1/_2$–1 teaspoon).

People with damage from heart attack frequently also benefit from:

○ Arjuna (*Terminalia arjuna*): extract, as directed by dispensing herbalist.

○ Pushkarmoola (*Inula racemosa*): extract, as directed by dispensing herbalist.

See Part Three if you take prescription medication.

UNDERSTANDING THE HEALING PROCESS

Congestive heart failure is a life-threatening condition for which a doctor's care is required. However, diet can work wonders. Additionally, there are several supplements that are generally helpful in congestive heart failure caused by an underlying damage to the heart muscle, or cardiomyopathy. Consult your cardiologist before beginning supplemental therapy, and never stop taking a prescribed medication without your cardiologist's approval.

As this book is being written, 10,000 patients are involved in clinical trials of sodium-restricted diets in the treatment of cardiomyopathy and congestive heart failure throughout Latin America. The results of removing sodium from the diet in treating heart failure are sometimes dramatic. In as little as 2 weeks, the heart can return to its normal size and function—simply by removing the burden of sodium for ingested salt.

A truly salt-free diet is not easy. It is mandatory to eliminate all sources of excess sodium, including:

○ All drugs containing sodium, such as Alka-Seltzer and aspirin.

○ Anchovies, canned salmon, sardines, and shellfish in general.

○ Any "fizzy" drink not specifically labeled as low-sodium.

○ Any kind of salted, grilled meat, salted soup or consommé.

○ Bacon, ham, sausages, and all cured meats, pork or otherwise.

○ Beer, carbonated beverages sweetened with sugar or aspartame, and mineral water.

○ Beets, celery, and spinach.

○ Breakfast cereals, bread, biscuits, pancakes, and waffles.

○ Cheeses and other processed dairy products.

○ Chocolate.

○ Dried fruit and nuts.

○ Peanuts, whether salted or not.

○ Popcorn.

○ Prepared foods of all types, especially salad dressings.

It is not unusual for patients to get very good results from sodium restriction—and to be told by their doctors that only medication can make congestive heart failure better, so they go off their diets. Symptoms invariably return. It is important to let your doctor know you are attempting a rigorous salt-exclusion diet so dosages of your medications, *especially digoxin (Lanoxin)*, can be adjusted downward as you recover, but don't allow your doctor's skepticism to discourage you from this very important step in self-care.

Several supplements are also helpful in complementary care of the heart damage causing congestive heart failure. Coenzyme Q_{10} (CoQ_{10}) is synthesized by every cell in the body to capture electrons released as the mitochondria release the energy by combining sugar with oxygen. A solid, waxlike substance, CoQ_{10} is made by the same chemical process that makes cholesterol, and, like cholesterol, CoQ_{10} is especially abundant in the healthy heart. Since the heart muscle makes and uses energy 24 hours a day, it needs a large quantity of CoQ_{10}. Heart tissue biopsies of people with various heart diseases show a deficiency of CoQ_{10} of 50–75 percent of what is normal.[1] This effect is most severe at the point when circulation is restored to the heart muscle following a heart attack.[2]

As people age, the heart makes less CoQ_{10}. Certain cholesterol-lowering drugs also reduce the heart's supply of this vital enzyme. Replacing CoQ_{10} is important in treating heart disease of all kinds.

In one study, 12 patients with restricted circulation were given 150 milligrams of CoQ_{10} daily for 4 weeks. Taking CoQ_{10} reduced the average frequency of heart pain by 53 percent. CoQ_{10} treatment also allowed the angina patients to last longer on a treadmill before experiencing chest pain or abnormal EKGs.[3]

Even heart patients with severe heart damage benefit from CoQ_{10}. A Danish study found that treatment with the supplement for 12 weeks increased the output of the heart at rest and during exercise.[4] The supplement is similarly useful in treating hereditary hypertrophic cardiomyopathy, more commonly known as "enlarged heart." Doctors at the Langsjoen Clinic in Tyler, Texas found that giving patients 200 milligrams of CoQ_{10} for 3 months reduced the thickness of the septum dividing the heart muscle by an average of 24 percent and the thickness of the posterior wall by 26 percent.[5]

There are very few precautions to take in the use of CoQ_{10}. The medical literature contains one report of CoQ_{10} decreasing the effectiveness of warfarin (Coumadin). It may improve sugar control in some cases of diabetes. If you are diabetic, check your blood sugars regularly when you take CoQ_{10}. Black pepper increases bloodstream levels of CoQ_{10}; seasoning your food with pepper would be helpful when you take CoQ_{10}.

L-carnitine also increases the heart's energy supply. L-carnitine carries fatty acids into the mitochondria, where they can be used for fuel. Most of the body's supply of L-carnitine is made in the kidneys and the liver. Stresses on these organs (such as diabetes or chronic alcohol abuse) diminish the supply of L-carnitine for the heart. When the heart has an inadequate oxygen supply, it quickly uses up its supply of L-carnitine and is then less able to produce energy.

Administering massive doses of L-carnitine, 2,000 milligrams of L-carnitine for every 100 pounds (45 kilograms) of body weight, after a heart attack has been shown to reduce heart damage.[6] A Japanese study found that taking 900 milligrams of L-carnitine daily allowed heart patients to last 2.4 minutes longer in their stress tests. An Italian study in which men with angina were given 1,000 milligrams of L-carnitine daily found they not only could last longer under stress, but could also work harder, as measured by a bicycle ergometer.[7] Approximately 1 in 30 people will experience nausea, heartburn, or gas when taking L-carnitine, but it is generally very free of side effects. People with seizure disorders, however, should consult with their physicians before taking this supplement.

Magnesium is especially important for replacing the magnesium eliminated through the urine when congestive heart failure is treated with furosemide (Lasix).[8] Taking supplemental magnesium for 3–4 weeks helps reestablish normal heart rhythm and reduces the risk of sudden death.[9] Be sure to take no more than the recommended dosage, since overdosing magnesium can cause diarrhea.

Herbs used to treat congestive heart failure open circulation. Hawthorn is both extraordinarily safe and extraordinarily effective in treating various forms of heart disease, as was finally recognized by the American

Heart Association in an article printed in its journal in May 2002.[10] This herb contains a variety of flavonoids. Some increase blood flow through the coronary arteries. Some increase left ventricular pressure, making each heartbeat stronger. Some accelerate the heart rate—and some decelerate it.[11] But the most important property of hawthorn is its ability to protect the heart from the effects of oxygen deprivation.

Heart cells, like many other tissues, are able to adapt to oxygen deprivation. They shift their energy production from pathways requiring the use of oxygen to pathways requiring the use of fatty acids. However, when their oxygen supply is restored they are sometimes damaged and sometimes destroyed.

When heart pain is induced by the failure of the heart muscle to pump blood, the neutrophils of the immune system release a compound known as human neutrophil elastase (HNE), allowing the arteries to stretch back to a more normal size. The process of relaxing the artery, however, releases massive quantities of free radicals that disrupt the cholesterol coats of heart cells and interfere with the action of L-carnitine. At least one of the flavonoid compounds in hawthorn counteracts HNE.[12]

Hawthorn has several other beneficial effects. Animal studies have found that hawthorn stimulates the liver to use LDL cholesterol to make bile salts, cholesterol salts that are flushed out of the liver into the stool.[13] Other studies with laboratory animals have found that the hawthorn compound monoacetyl-vitexin rhamnoside relaxes the linings of the arteries, permitting greater blood flow, through a complicated chemical process.[14] And at least one animal study suggests that hawthorn can prevent irreversible tissue damage during heart attack.[15]

There are very few precautions for the use of hawthorn. It is almost completely nontoxic. Like many other natural treatments for angina, however, it can cause diarrhea the first few days you take it.

Arjuna has been used in Ayurvedic medicine for over 2,500 years as a "cardiac tonic." Ayurvedic physicians offer it as arjunatvagadi (arjuna in water), pardhadyaristam (grapes and arjuna fermented and boiled), arjunaghrtam (arjuna paste), and arjunatvak (arjuna powder). Animal experiments have shown that arjuna slows and strengthens the heartbeat and protects the heart from tissue destruction during oxygen deprivation. In a study of the use of the herb in treating mild heart pain, patients given the herb were found to have greater endurance in treadmill tests, without the complication of lowered blood pressure.[16] Follow-up studies at the same clinic found that arjuna is also useful in treating cardiomyopathy caused by heart attack. Treatment with the herb reduced left ventricular mass by an average of 12 percent in 3 months.[17]

Arjuna is usually dispensed by a practitioner of Ayurvedic medicine. There have been no reports of side effects from arjuna products given by herbalists or physicians trained in Ayurveda. Dosage varies with the individual preparation.

Pushkarmoola is another Ayurvedic herb that grows in the foothills of the northwestern Himalayas. Traditional South Asian medicine uses pushkarmoola in the treatment of angina with shortness of breath. A small-scale study in India found that pushkarmoola was more effective than nitroglycerin in effecting favorable EKG changes (elevation of the S-T segment) and in relieving chest pain.[18] And a study involving 200 patients found that combining pushkarmoola with the traditional Indian herb guggul (*Commiphora mukkul*) in treatment for 6 months relieved shortness of breath in 60 percent of angina patients who had shortness of breath as a symptom at the beginning of the study. One in four patients experienced a complete remission from pain and showed a normal EKG by the end of 6 months of treatment.[19]

Like arjuna, pushkarmoola is also available from practitioners of Ayurveda. There are no reports of side effects from pushkarmoola products given by herbalists or physicians trained in Ayurveda.

CONCEPTS FOR COPING WITH CONGESTIVE HEART FAILURE

❍ Following your diet plan can have unexpected results. If you are especially diligent in avoiding salt, your cardiologist may have to lower your dosage of digoxin.

❍ The diuretic drug furosemide (Lasix) can cause burning of the feet that is often mistaken for athlete's foot. A few days of taking any complete B-vitamin supplement will correct this side effect of the medication.

❍ If you have been taking St. John's wort for depression before being treated for cardiomyopathy, do not stop taking the herb abruptly. Your cardiologist will probably need to adjust several medications, including digoxin, when you stop taking the herb.[20] Always tell your doctor about any herbal supplements you take.

Conjunctivitis (Pinkeye)

SYMPTOM SUMMARY

○ Blurred vision

○ Crusts that form on the eyelid overnight

○ Eye pain

○ Gritty feeling or itching in the eyes

○ Red eyes

○ Sensitivity to light

○ Tearing

UNDERSTANDING THE DISEASE PROCESS

The conjunctiva is the thin mucous membrane on the underside of the eyelid. It is reflected onto the sclera or "white" of the eye. When the conjunctiva is infected, the resulting inflammation makes the sclera appear red or pink, hence the condition's name, pinkeye. Conjunctivitis is most commonly a viral infection, but the condition may also be caused by allergy, exposure to chemicals or smoke, or bacterial infection. When conjunctivitis is caused by bacterial infection, there may be a green or yellow discharge.

TREATMENT SUMMARY

NUTRITIONAL SUPPLEMENTS

○ Bioflavonoids: 1,000 milligrams per day.

○ Thymus extract: 500 milligrams of crude polypeptides daily.

○ Vitamin A: 5,000 IU per day.

○ Vitamin C: 500 milligrams 3–4 times a day.

○ Vitamin E: 400 IU per day for the first 2 months.

○ Zinc picolinate: 30 milligrams per day.

HERBS

○ Echinacea: 150–300 milligrams of solid extract (3.5% echinacosides) 3 times a day, or dried root, freeze-dried plant, juice, fluid extract, or tincture, as recommended on the label.

○ Goldenseal: capsules, as recommended on the label.

○ Herbal compresses and poultices made with barberry, calendula, chamomile, goldenseal, or Oregon grape root.

See Part Three if you take prescription medication.

UNDERSTANDING THE HEALING PROCESS

Common conjunctivitis does not require treatment, but conjunctivitis due to herpes requires urgent medical attention. If redness and swelling of the eyelids does not go away in 2–3 days, consider the possibility that it is caused by an allergy or a bacterial infection.

Bioflavonoids are especially important to eye health. They help stabilize the connective tissues supporting the eyelids[1] and strengthen the microscopic blood vessels serving the eyes.[2]

There are no studies that directly confirm the usefulness of thymus extract in treating conjunctivitis, but there is considerable evidence that thymus extract corrects low immune function. In particular, research has shown that thymus extract normalizes the ratio of T-helper cells to T suppressor cells, maintaining a healthy immune response that neither destroys healthy tissue nor allows infectious microorganisms to flourish.[3]

A German study of 41 people with chronic conjunctivitis published in the 1970s reported that people who have the condition tend to have relatively low bloodstream concentrations of vitamin A, as well as difficulty adjusting to changes in light.[4] This study does not prove that taking supplemental vitamin A reduces the risk of the inflammation, but other studies suggest that taking the vitamin will at least reduce the risk of spreading the infection.

Relatively low doses of vitamin A are sufficient to prevent "burnout" due to stress on the immune output of the thymus.[5] Vitamin A also enhances antibody response, increases the rate at which macrophages destroy bacteria, and stimulates natural killer cells.[6]

Vitamin C levels are quickly depleted during the stress of an infection.[7] In combination with bioflavonoids, it helps increase the stability of the collagen matrix of the connective tissues, the "glue" between the inner layer of the eyelid and the tissues supporting it.[8]

Zinc is an important cofactor for vitamin A. When zinc is deficient, the immune system's ability to produce white blood cells in response to infection is reduced, thymic hormone levels are lower, and the immune response in the lining of the eyelids is especially reduced. Phagocytosis, the process in which bacteria are engulfed and digested, is slowed. All of these processes can be corrected by taking zinc supplements.[9]

Echinacea relieves inflammation. One study found that a teaspoon of *Echinacea purpurea* juice is as effective in relieving pain and swelling as 100 milligrams of cortisone.[10] Echinacea also enhances the immune system's response to bacterial infections. It is especially useful in stimulating phagocytosis, the process by which white blood cells surround and digest infectious bacteria. A study of oral administration of an *Echinacea purpurea* root extract (30 drops 3 times per day) to healthy men for 5 days resulted in a 120 percent increase in phagocytosis.[11] Taking echinacea may help prevent secondary infections with bacteria.

Women who are trying to get pregnant should avoid *Echinacea purpurea.* It contains caffeoyl esters that can interfere with the action of hyaluronidase, an enzyme essential to the release of unfertilized eggs into the fallopian tube.[12]

The combination of echinacea and goldenseal is especially useful in treating conditions that involve drainage. A study reported in 1999 that the combination of the two herbs stimulates the production of the immunoglobulins IgG and IgM, infection fighters that "remember" specific infections.[13] Goldenseal contains general antibacterial compound berberine. This alkaloid kills a wide range of bacteria, including those in the same family as *Chlamydia,* which can cause conjunctivitis.

Traditionally, herbal teas have been applied to the eyelids as compresses or poultices. However, if absolute sterility is not ensured, further infection is possible. Potentially useful herbs include barberry, calendula, chamomile, goldenseal, and Oregon grape root. It is important to make the herbal tea with *boiling* water that is allowed to cool before making the compress, and to use a clean cloth. Sterile solutions of these herbs, and eyedrops with the herb eyebright, are commercially available.

CONCEPTS FOR COPING WITH CONJUNCTIVITIS

To prevent recurrence or spread of conjunctivitis:

○ Change pillowcases every 2–3 days.

○ Do not share eye cosmetics. Replace eye cosmetics frequently.

○ Do not share handkerchiefs or towels.

○ Keep hands away from the eyes.

○ Sterilize contact lenses.

○ Wash hands frequently.

Other helpful practices:

○ Apply a warm compress to the affected area several times a day. The viruses that cause conjunctivitis do not grow well under conditions of excessive heat.

○ The Mexican folk remedy for conjunctivitis, the chopped root of the madeira vine, available at *hierberías* in the Southwest, is being studied as a treatment for viral infections of the eye at the Pharmaceutical Institute of the University of Bonn in Germany. Herbalists have used it for generations in treating the pain and inflammation of conjunctivitis.

○ There are a number of homeopathic remedies for colds. Usually it is best to start with a single dose of the lowest strength (6C, 6X, or 12C) of the remedy matching the symptoms to be treated, and then wait for a response. If there is an improvement in symptoms, let the remedy continue to work until there is no more improvement, then take another dose. If there is no improvement, try a different potency (30X or 30C). Sometimes homeopathic medicines work for a few minutes, and sometimes they work for an entire day before another dose is needed.

• Apis mellifica is the homeopathic remedy for swollen, tearing eyes that are puffy and pink. There may be burning pain, and the eyelids may be stuck together.

• Argentum nitricum (homeopathic silver nitrate) is used to treat conjunctivitis that is worst in the corners of the eyes and that causes a yellow discharge.

• Hepar sulphuris calcareum relieves eyes that feel swollen or bruised, or eyes that feel like they are being drawn back into the head. People who are sensitive to the cold may benefit from this remedy.

• Mercurius solubilis dissolves a green discharge irritating the eyelids.

• Pulsatilla relieves eye inflammation or conjunctivitis accompanying a cold.

• Sulfur soothes itchy eyes, especially if they are bloodshot.

Constipation

SYMPTOM SUMMARY

○ Any unusual decrease in the frequency
of bowel movements or uncomfortable
hardening of the stool

UNDERSTANDING THE DISEASE PROCESS

Constipation is a condition in which the bowels move less frequently than expected or stools become hard, pelletlike, and difficult to pass. Constipation causes a number of subjective discomforts. These include straining, a feeling of fullness in the lower abdomen, and a sense of incomplete evacuation.

There is a wide variation in normal bowel habits, but most people move their bowels anywhere from 3 times a day to 3 times a week. Any frequency that is less than "normal" for you is considered constipation. Studies in the United States and the United Kingdom suggest that between 10 and 18 percent of otherwise healthy adults report frequent straining upon defecation, and about 4 percent have fewer than three bowel movements per week. Constipation is more common among women than men, and occurs in about 20 percent of people over age 65.[1]

Hard stools are formed when waste matter passes through the colon slowly. Soft stools are formed when waste matter passes through the colon quickly. The slow passage of stool through the colon is usually caused by failure to eat enough fiber or drink enough water. Constipation may also be a side effect of taking iron supplements, including narcotic pain relievers such as hydrocodone (Vicodin), calcium channel blockers for high blood pressure, such as amlopidine (Norvasc), diltiazem (Cardizem), nifedipine (Adalet, Procardia), and verapamil (Calan, Isoptin, Verelan), and antidepressants, such as fluvoxamine (Luvox), paroxetine (Paxil), fluoxetine (Prozac), and sertraline (Zoloft).

Constipation in and of itself is not usually regarded as a serious condition, but it may be a symptom of a serious condition, such as Chagas' disease, a complication of diabetes slowing the passage through the digestive tract known as gastroparesis, hypothyroidism, irritable bowel syndrome, or nerve damage caused by Lou Gehrig's disease, multiple sclerosis, Parkinson's disease, or spinal cord injury.

About 1 in 20 cases of constipation is caused by an outlet obstruction to defecation, also called an evacuation disorder. Constant use of stimulant laxatives over a period of years can cause the nerves controlling the colon to become dependent on them. When the laxative is discontinued, the muscles lining the colon do not respond to ordinary signals to propel stool forward but do respond to signals to hold stool in, and constipation results. Obstruction to defecation can also be caused by a pelvic floor disorder. This condition causes an inability to completely empty the rectum, so that there is a need to extract stool with a finger to complete bowel movement. Doctors usually diagnose pelvic floor disorders by having the patient strain to expel the index finger during a digital rectal exam. Motion of the puborectalis muscle backward during the digital rectal exam indicates that a lack of muscle coordination is causing constipation.

Physicians often look down on constipation as a concern of the elderly and the excessively self-involved, but constipation is an important risk factor for many other diseases. Slow transit of waste matter through the colon gives pathogenic bacteria a chance to reassemble the estrogen and testosterone broken down in the liver and excreted with bile. These reconstituted hormones reenter circulation and stimulate abnormal growth in the breasts in women and the prostate in men. At least one study suggests that chronic constipation is an important risk factor in colon cancer, finding that middle-aged adults who are constipated enough "to have to take something" once a month are twice as likely to develop the disease as those who never take laxatives, whereas middle-aged adults who are constipated enough to take laxatives once a week are 4 times as likely to develop the disease.[2]

TREATMENT SUMMARY
DIET

○ Gradually increase the amount of fiber in your diet so that you eat 5–9 servings of fruit and vegetables every day. Raw fruits and vegetables are preferable. Almonds, dried beans and peas, raw root vegetables (carrots, jicama, radishes, and turnip roots), dried pumpkin and sunflower seeds, whole-grain breads, oranges, apricots, prunes, and unpeeled apples are especially good sources of soluble fiber.

○ Avoid sugar.

O Drink 8 or more glasses of water every day.

O Avoid large, heavy meals. Eating smaller portions more often reduces the amount of food that has to pass through the colon at any one time.

O Avoid milk, wheat products, and beef.

NUTRITIONAL SUPPLEMENTS

O Fiber: 1–2 tablespoons of insoluble fiber (psyllium) or soluble fiber (orange pulp), taken with a glass of water daily. Do not take fiber at the same time you take nutritional supplements or medications.

O *Lactobacillus:* 1–2 billion live organisms (1–2 capsules), daily.

HERBS

Most effective choices:

O Ayurvedic and Chinese herbal remedies.

Additional herbs for relief of constipation on an occasional basis:

O Aloe, buckthorn, cascara sagrada, frangula, rhubarb, or senna (Senekot and related products): as directed on label, for up to 2 weeks.

O Dandelion: 20 drops of tincture in $1/4$ cup (60 milliliters) of water up to 3 times a day, may be used indefinitely.

O Ginger: 1 teaspoon (2–3 grams) made into a tea in 1 cup (240 milliliters) of hot water, 2–3 times a day, indefinitely.

O Hibiscus: Red Zinger tea, as desired.

O Kelp: eaten as a vegetable, as desired.

O Milk thistle: silymarin phytosomes, 120–240 milligrams per day, indefinitely.

See Part Three if you take prescription medication.

UNDERSTANDING THE HEALING PROCESS

The first thing that comes to mind for most people seeking to remedy constipation is bran. Bran makes larger stools that pass through the gut more quickly, [3] but there are complications in using bran effectively. Bran accelerates the passage of other kinds of food through the colon, but slows down the passage of food through the stomach.[4] The longer food stays in the stomach, the greater the likelihood of acid reflux, belching, burping,

or heartburn. Coarse bran is more useful in relieving constipation than fine bran, but it is also more likely to cause heartburn.[5] Once bran reaches the colon, it is the last food eliminated. If you eat bran for breakfast and skip lunch, the bran you eat will probably be eliminated in your next bowel movement. If you eat bran for breakfast and then eat an early lunch, bran does not get a chance to leave the colon and can cause swelling, bloating, and gas.[6]

Another popular food for relieving constipation is prunes. It is difficult to imagine how hundreds of millions of people around the world who eat prunes to encourage regularity could be wrong, so there is not a single scientific study validating their use in treating constipation. Scientists speculate that prunes stimulate bowel movements through a mechanism similar to milk of magnesia: their high content of the sugar sorbitol draws fluid into the colon and makes the stool softer and more watery. Prunes have another scientifically demonstrated nutritional value: they are a rich source of potassium, which is beneficial to cardiovascular health, and an important source of boron, which plays a role in the prevention of osteoporosis.[7] And no one can argue that they do not relieve constipation.

Most treatment plans for constipation include increased consumption of prepared fiber. Fiber is the part of plant food that is not digested. It adds bulk to the stools by absorbing water. There are two types of fiber, soluble and insoluble. Soluble fiber dissolves in water and is found in oat bran, barley, peas, beans, and citrus fruits. Insoluble fiber does not dissolve in water and is found in wheat bran and some vegetables. Fiber increases the transit time of stool through the colon and decrease the pressures within the colon.

Avoiding sugars also helps relieve constipation. Eating sugar raises blood sugars. When blood sugars are high, the central nervous system signals the digestive tract to absorb sugars more slowly.[8] This slows down the passage of food through the digestive tract, giving gas time to accumulate, and maximizes the amount of time irritating food allergens are in contact with the intestinal wall. Some naturopathic physicians speculate that sugar consumption is the most important contributing factor to spasmodic constipation in most cases in the United States.[9]

People who have frequent constipation can avoid the urge to pass gas by cutting down on saturated fats. Fat in any form (animal or vegetable) is a strong stimulus for colonic contractions after a meal. This in turn creates an urge to have a bowel movement, but bowel movement is difficult or impossible because the stool is hard. Gas, however, escapes. Many foods contain fat, especially meats of all kinds, poultry skin, whole milk, cream, cheese, butter, vegetable oil, margarine, shortening, avocados, and whipped toppings.

Maintaining the colon's supply of the friendly bacterium *Lactobacillus* is a helpful adjunct to treatments. Herbal stimulant laxatives such as aloe, buckthorn, cascara sagrada, frangula, rhubarb root, and senna contain complex sugars that have to be broken down by *Lactobacillus* before they can stimulate movement of the muscles lining the colon. *Lactobacillus* also breaks down fatty acids into forms that draw more water into the colon, softening the stool and making bowel movement easier.

Several herbal formulas from Chinese and Ayurvedic medicine are gentle, effective, and highly recommended in the treatment of constipation. These combinations are safe for long-term use, but should become unnecessary as dietary changes are made. Da Cheng Qi Tang, also known as Major Order the Chi Combination or Major Order the Qi Combination, is a gentle version of an herbal stimulant laxative. It relieves constipation in which it is necessary to strain to pass large, hard stools. This formula also relieves flatulence. This herbal formula is made by Honso, KPC Herbs, Lotus Classics, Qualiherb, and Sun Ten.

Gui Zhi Jia Shao Yao Tang, also known as Cinnamon and Peony Combination, relieves constipation in which pellets of loose stool are passed. It is also used to treat heartburn, stomach pain, and menstrual problems. This herbal formula is also made by KPC Herbs, Lotus Classics, Qualiherb, and Sun Ten.

Triphala is an ancient Indian remedy for constipation available from practitioners of Ayurvedic medicine. It is recommended when odor is a special problem.

The stimulant laxative herbs aloe, buckthorn, cascara sagrada, frangula, rhubarb root, and senna should not be used on a regular basis except by people who take opioid pain relievers such as hydrocodone (Vicodin). These herbs contain rhein anthrones, which are broken down by intestinal bacteria into forms that keep the large intestine from transporting water and minerals into the bloodstream. They also stimulate nerves that control the muscles that propel stool through the colon and deaden nerves that control the muscles that hold back stool. Over time, the nervous system of the colon can become dependent on the anthrones, so that severe constipation results when the herb is discontinued, except in people who use opioid pain relievers on an ongoing basis. Do not take stimulant laxatives for more than 2 weeks in any month unless your doctor directs you otherwise.

Numerous herbal products relieve symptoms of constipation and can be taken indefinitely. Dandelion tincture (20 drops in $1/4$ cup of water, 3 times a day on an empty stomach) and dandelion greens (eaten in salads as desired) stimulate the liver to secrete bile. This emulsifies fats in the colon and reduces the odor of stools. Ginger tea, made with a teaspoon of either fresh or dry ginger in the herbal or regular tea of your choice, relieves stomach cramps accompanying constipation. Hibiscus, the herb in Red Zinger tea (drunk no more than 3 times a day to avoid causing runny bowels), draws water into the intestine, softening the stool. Milk thistle (120–360 milligrams daily, preferably as phytosomes) also stimulates the production of bile by the liver, and is especially useful in relieving constipation in people who have cirrhosis of the liver or chronic hepatitis.

CONCEPTS FOR COPING WITH CONSTIPATION

○ If you have heart disease, use softening agents rather than bulking agents. This will help you avoid straining during bowel movements and consequently straining your heart.

○ Even if you are busy or embarrassed, make a trip to the bathroom whenever you feel like you might have a bowel movement.

○ Taking 15–20 minutes without distraction to use the bathroom every morning encourages regularity.

○ The most important thing you can do for an elderly person suffering chronic constipation is to provide dignity and privacy. Inaccessible toilets, inappropriate types of toilets, and reliance on other people for assistance contribute toward the development of constipation in the elderly.

○ Never take a bulking laxative at the same time as you take another nutritional supplement, herb, or prescription medication. The fibers in bulking laxatives will block absorption of supplements or medications.

○ If you don't exercise at all, chances are even a very modest level of activity, such as walking around the block, will help relieve constipation.[10] On the other hand, if you already exercise, chances are exercising more will not relieve constipation. Researchers at the University of California at Irvine studied the effects of having eight patients with chronic constipation increase their daily exercise from 3 kilometers (1.8 miles) to a 5 kilometers (3.0 miles) on a stationary bicycle. While there was improvement in the number and consistency of bowel movements and the amount of straining required, the improvement was very slight.[11]

○ If you must use a stimulant laxative, use aloe *juice* (not aloe latex) instead of other stimulant herbs such as senna (Senakot), buckthorn, cascara sagrada, or rhurbarb root. Aloe juice draws less water into the colon and is less likely to cause gas or cramping.[12] Aloe latex, also known as aloe bitters, acts faster than senna and the other herbal stimulant laxatives but also more likely to cause gas and cramping.

○ Toilet training commonly causes constipation. According to the medical literature, one in five toddlers becomes constipated for at least a month when learning to use the toilet.[13] Many parents find that children are more willing to use the toilet to urinate than to relieve their bowels. It is usually best to wait until your toddler expresses an interest in using the potty for both toilet functions before taking him or her out of underpants. To help you child begin a life time of healthy bowel habits, never scold or punish for failure to use the toilet, and do not refer to bowel movements as "nasty," "dirty," or "stinky."

○ Pelvic floor disorders are difficulty to treat with dietary modification or laxatives, but they sometimes respond to acupuncture or biofeedback.

○ Constipation alternating with diarrhea is a sign of irritable bowel syndrome (see IRRITABLE BOWEL SYNDROME). See your physician promptly if constipation symptoms include:

- Sudden constipation with abdominal cramps, and an inability to pass gas or stool. This is a medical emergency.
- Very thin, pencil-like stools.
- Dark, dried blood in stools.
- Abdominal pain and bloating

- Unexplained weight loss

○ There are a number of homeopathic remedies for constipation. Usually it is best to start with a single dose of the lowest strength (6C, 6X, or 12C) of the remedy matching the symptoms to be treated, and then wait for a response. If there is an improvement in symptoms, let the remedy continue to work until there is no more improvement, then take another dose. If there is no improvement, try a different potency (30X or 30C). Sometimes homeopathic medicines work for a few minutes, and sometimes they work for an entire day before another dose is needed.

- Bryonia relieves constipation causing large stools that are hard to expel.
- Calcarea sulphurica relieves stools that are at first hard, then sticky, then liquid.
- Causticum relieves straining during the release of long, stringy stools that may be coated with mucus.
- Graphites relieves perianal pain following straining at small "pills" of stool.
- Lycopodium relieves constipation accompanied by bloating and gas.
- Nux vomica is recommended when constipation is accompanied by sensitivity to cold, headaches, and painful tightness in the rectum.
- Sepia relieves a feeling of incomplete defecation.
- Silicea (silica) treats constipation marked by stools that start to come out but then go back in.
- Sulfur relieves highly odorous flatulence accompanied by dry stools.

Contact Dermatitis
See **Eczema**.

Convulsions
See **Epilepsy**.

Copper Overload
See **Wilson's Disease**.

Coronary Artery Disease/ Coronary Heart Disease

See **Aneurysm; Angina; Cardiomyopathy; Congestive Heart Failure; High Cholesterol; High Triglycerides; Hypertension; Irregular Heartbeat; Peripheral Vascular Disease; Raynaud's Phenomenon**.

Cough, Smoker's

SYMPTOM SUMMARY

- Dry cough, usually worst in the morning
- Frequent colds
- Headaches
- Reddish face, palms, or mucous membranes inside the mouth and nose
- Shortness of breath aggravated by altitude, exertion, or mild activity
- Vision abnormalities
- Wheezing

UNDERSTANDING THE DISEASE PROCESS

Smoker's cough is the well-known early morning cough of smokers. The peculiarity of smoker's cough is that it occurs when smoker's haven't been smoking, not when they have.

Normally, cilia, tiny hairlike formations lining the airways, beat in a rhythmic fashion to sweep harmful materials out of the lungs. Cigarette smoke contains chemicals that poison the cilia, causing some of the poison to remain in the lungs. When a smoker sleeps, some cilia recover and try to eliminate smoke that has remained in the lungs. After waking up, the smoker coughs because the lungs are trying to clear away the poisons that built up the previous day.

Over time, the cilia of smokers' lungs become accustomed to having to work twice as hard every morning. The fibers of the nerves activating them become supersensitive to the allergy-inducing chemical histamine.[1] They become hyperresponsive to dust, mites, allergens, and ozone so that even when the smoker doesn't smoke, he or she has smoker's cough.

Smokers who have smoker's cough are more likely to develop serious chronic lung conditions than smokers who don't.[2] Although there is some disagreement among medical studies, smoker's cough seems to be a bigger risk factor for smokers who have allergies.[3] The presence of eosinophils, the white blood cells most present at sites of allergic reactions and parasitic infections, predicts the progression of smoker's cough to conditions that cause chronic phlegm, such as bronchitis, emphysema, and pneumonia.[4]

TREATMENT SUMMARY

DIET

- Don't go on a low-fat, high-carbohydrate diet, but also avoid egg yolks, beef, and fried foods. Eat 2–3 servings of cold-water fish weekly.

NUTRITIONAL SUPPLEMENTS

- EPA and DHA (not to be confused with DHEA): 540 and 360 milligrams per day, respectively, or 1 tablespoon of flaxseed oil daily.
- N-acetyl cysteine (NAC): 400 milligrams a day.

UNDERSTANDING THE HEALING PROCESS

The obvious treatment for smoker's cough is to quit smoking. Most smokers are free of symptoms within 3 months of quitting smoking. In the meantime, there are several natural treatments that help.

Low-fat, high-carbohydrate diets are not advisable for people who have smoker's cough. High carbohydrate consumption increases the body's consumption of carbon dioxide. Several studies indicate that people with smoker's cough have difficulty eliminating carbon dioxide,[5,6] and a high-carbohydrate diet places additional stress on the lungs.

On the other hand, certain kinds of fats should be avoided. The biochemical process that makes the cilia supersensitive to allergens is made possible by the chemical thromboxane.[7] The body's production of thromboxane is greater when the diet includes egg yolks, beef tallow (often used in cooking fast-food French fries), and fried foods, and less when the diet includes fish oils. A study of 8,006 male smokers in Hawaii found that those who ate two or more servings of fish per week lost lung capacity at less than half the rate of those who did not eat the fish. The protective effect of fish oils was greatest for the smokers who smoked the most.[8] Another study published in *The New England Journal of Medicine* suggests that smokers are protected from the development of bronchitis, emphysema, and pneumonia when their diets include n-3 polyunsaturated fatty acids from any source.[9] EPA, DHA, and flaxseed oil are good sources of n-3 polyunsaturated fatty acids.

N-acetyl cysteine (NAC), used on a short-term basis, helps prevent especially bad attacks of smoker's cough *as you quit smoking.* Because NAC stimulates the action of eosinophils, it cannot be recommended for smokers who do not quit.

CONCEPTS FOR COPING WITH SMOKER'S COUGH

○ Eucalyptus oil is a standard ingredient in cough drops and in oils added to humidifiers and vaporizers. While it does not increase breathing capacity, a study of 246 people with chronic bronchitis found that eucalyptus oils stop the worsening of cough that commonly occurs in the winter (in wet climates where heaters are used) or summer (in desert climates).[10]

Cradle Cap
See **Seborrheic Dermatitis**.

Crescent Cell Anemia
See **Sickle-Cell Anemia**.

Crohn's Disease
See **Inflammatory Bowel Disease (IBD)**.

Croup

SYMPTOM SUMMARY

○ Barking cough

○ Hoarseness

○ Crowing sound when breathing is difficult

UNDERSTANDING THE DISEASE PROCESS

Croup is an infection that causes the windpipe (trachea) and voice box (larynx) to swell. It is usually part of a cold. Most commonly affecting children, croup causes fever, hoarseness, and a barking, hacking cough. Symptoms usually last 5–6 days.

TREATMENT SUMMARY

○ Follow the treatments recommended for colds. (See COLDS.)

UNDERSTANDING THE HEALING PROCESS

Croups are generally treated the same way as colds, although cough syrups are seldom helpful. If your child has mild difficulty breathing (stridor), try having him or her breathe moist air. This is called mist treatment.

1. Have your child breathe through a warm, wet washcloth placed over the nose and mouth. Do not hold the washcloth against the face, and remove it immediately if breathing difficulty worsens.

2. Run hot water in your shower or tub enclosure with the door closed. Once the shower or tub enclosure has become steamy or has fogged up, sit with your child in the room for about 10 minutes.

CONCEPTS FOR COPING WITH CROUP

○ See a doctor immediately, night or day, if the child's skin or lips turn blue or if the child starts drooling.

Cuts and Scrapes

SYMPTOM SUMMARY

○ Obvious open break in the skin caused by an identifiable physical injury

UNDERSTANDING THE DISEASE PROCESS

Any physical injury that results in an opening or break of the skin creates a wound. The immune system "cleans up" injured or infected tissue by a series of hormonal reactions that cause painful throbbing, redness, and swelling of surrounding tissues.

TREATMENT SUMMARY

SUPPLEMENTS

○ Vitamin C: 1,000 milligrams daily.

HERBS

○ Aloe: apply to wounds daily until healed.

○ Forskolin (a standardized extract of coleus): 5–10 milligrams 3 times daily.

○ Gotu kola (*Centella asiatica*): 60–120 milligrams of asiaticides daily. Should not be used by women who are trying to become pregnant.

○ Sangre de grado: apply to the skin immediately after injury to form a "second skin" and prevent infection.

UNDERSTANDING THE HEALING PROCESS

The most important thing to remember in treating wounds is to wash your hands before treating the wound. Wash the wound thoroughly with mild soap and water; then apply antibiotic and herbal ointments and a clean bandage.

The latest research on the use of vitamin C in the treatment of wounds has found that it keeps the basal layers of skin from contracting when the upper layers are injured. This allows regrowth of skin with a minimum of scarring.[1] A series of experiments with animals found that supplementation with relatively high dosages of vitamin C increases the strength of skin growing over the wound and accelerates closure.[2]

Aloe is anti-inflammatory, moisturizing, and emollient. It contains a number of antioxidant compounds that promote skin growth, including vitamins C and E and zinc. Unlike hydrocortisone creams used to relieve inflammation, aloe encourages skin-healing while relieving pain. Wounds treated with aloe vera gel heal as much as 3 days faster than burns and cuts treated with unmedicated dressings or with chemical antiseptic gels.[3]

In late 2001 researchers at the University of Nebraska Medical Center reported laboratory studies showing that forskolin prevented the action of a chemical-signaling system by which inflammatory hormones shut down fibroblasts, the cells that generate the extracellular connective tissue matrix.[4] Keeping fibroblasts at the site of the wound encourages the production of collagen and connective tissues across the region of damaged skin.

Gotu kola helps to prevent scarring. Keloids and hypertrophic scars, such as those caused by surgery, result from an extended period of inflammation which may go on for months or years without resolution. During this inflammatory phase, large numbers of swollen bundles of collagen are intermingled with cellular debris. This stage continues until sufficient numbers of fibroblasts are recruited in the wound to create well-defined collagen fibers. A clinical study found that 22 out of 27 patients' scars resolved with several months use of gotu kola.[5] The herb is especially effective when taken *before* surgery to prevent scarring.

The unprocessed resin of sangre de grado stimulates the production of collagen in wounds. This accelerates the formation of a protective crust over the wound.[6]

CONCEPTS FOR COPING WITH CUTS AND SCRAPES

○ If you have not had a tetanus shot in the last 5 years, you probably should get one. Consult your healthcare provider.

○ People who have diabetes or other conditions causing circulatory problems should check for infection in any cut or scrape as it heals, even if it seems minor.

○ Clinical studies show that antibiotic treatment does not prevent infection, but if the cuts and scrapes are extensive or if there is potential damage to hands and fingers, preventive antibiotic treatment is usually a good idea.[7] If you take antibiotics, take 1 or 2 capsules of *acidophilus* or *Lactobacillus* daily. This helps maintain the production of vitamin K in the intestine.

Cyclic Mastalgia
See **Premenstrual Syndrome (PMS)**.

Cyclothymia
See **Bipolar Disorder (Manic Depression)**.

Cyst, Breast
See **Fibrocystic Breast Disease**.

Cystic Fibrosis

SYMPTOM SUMMARY

○ No meconium stool (dark, greenish mass of bile, mucus, and stool) discharged in first 24 hours of life

○ Clubbing of fingers or toes

○ Coughing and wheezing

○ Delayed growth, slow weight gain

○ Diarrhea

○ Easily fatigued

○ Floating, foul-smelling stools that are pale or clay-colored

UNDERSTANDING THE DISEASE PROCESS

Cystic fibrosis (CF) is a devastating disease affecting the lungs, the digestive tract, the endocrine glands, and the reproductive system. There are at least 500 genetic mutations associated with this disease that can ultimately include arthritis, chronic obstructive pulmonary disease, diabetes, fibrosis of the liver, and gallstones.[1]

Like many other hereditary diseases, CF is autosomal recessive, that is, an individual must inherit genes that cause CF from both parents. In premodern times, inheriting *one* gene for CF actually conferred an advantage. People who carry only one CF gene, that is, about 1 in every 25 people, are more resistant to diarrhea and food-borne infections.[2] They may also be less likely to contract tuberculosis, more resistant to the flu, and less likely to suffer asthma during childhood and early adulthood.[3] Resistance to all of these diseases is conferred by decreased secretion, and the decreased secretion caused by having a single gene for CF does not appreciably interfere with normal life. Decreased secretion caused by having two genes for CF is a challenge to life itself.

In CF, the cells in the mucosal linings of the lungs and the digestive tract fail to secrete chloride ions, that is, they fail to release the chloride from sodium chloride. Since kidneys keep a nearly perfect balance of sodium and chloride ions throughout the body, there is no flow of fluids to the mucosal linings, which have the "right" balance of sodium and chloride without additional fluid.

The basis of this defect is an inability of the cells to respond to the chemical cyclic adenosine monophosphate (cAMP). This substance acts as a "second messenger" for dozens of hormonal processes. When a hormone comes in contact with the outer membrane of a cell, cAMP is released to carry a message to the organelles within the cell to perform desired functions. The cAMP system is a second messenger for anti-inflammatory hormones, both those manufactured by the body itself and those provided by medication. When this system does not work, the cells lining the lungs and digestive organs are essentially dry and irritated. Dehydrated mucus clogged with the byproducts of inflammation clogs airways and the secretory passages of the liver, pancreas, and gallbladder.

In the digestive system, this failure of fluid control affects the secretion of bile. This fluid is essential for emulsifying fats in the intestine so they can be absorbed into the hepatic portal vein for transport to the liver. When bile is not secreted, dietary fat remains in the intestine. In children with CF, the growing body does not receive enough calories, and fat is lost in large, bulky, frequent, floating, malodorous, fat-laden stools. The loss of energy normally provided by fats is compounded by additional energy expenditures (required by constant respiratory infections), frequent fevers, tissue breakdown (accelerated by the use of steroid inhalers), and an increase in effort just to breathe.[4]

The primary destructive effect of CF, however, is on the lungs. The destruction of airways by inflammation and their constant clogging with mucus is the cause of 90 percent of deaths from CF.[5]

Controlling respiratory infections is another ongoing challenge. Virtually every CF patient eventually has a respiratory infection with the bacterium *Pseudomonas aeruginosa*. This infectious agent thrives in moist environments: sinks, bathtubs, whirlpools, humidifiers, and swimming pools.[6] It is an extremely virulent infection. It releases proteases that "fool" white blood cells into ignoring chemical signals of the infection's presence. It emits a polysaccharide coat that protects against the chemical grappling hooks of white blood cells when they do detect the germ. And it frequently mutates into forms that resist antibiotics.[7] Both infectious bacteria and the immune system cells that control them release proteolytic enzymes, dissolving the collagen connections that give airways their shape.

As children with CF reach adulthood, the disease

affects mucous membranes throughout the body. In 98 percent of men with the disease, the various ducts that carry sperm from the testes, the epididymis, the seminal vesicles, and the vas deferens, are nonfunctional. In women, the Fallopian tubes may be blocked by mucus, and the vagina is inadequately lubricated. In both sexes there may be both osteoporosis and an overgrowth of bone called hypertrophic osteoarthropathy. Throughout life, there is an added risk of heat stroke, salt depletion, excessive activity of the sweat glands, and retinal hemorrhage.

TREATMENT SUMMARY

DIET

○ As surprising as it may seem, a diet in which 50 percent of calories or more is derived from plant seed oils is beneficial in CF.

NUTRITIONAL SUPPLEMENTS

○ Beta-carotene: children should be given the smallest dosage available, usually 3 milligrams or 5,000 IU, *once a week*. Adults may take up to 3 milligrams a day.

○ Coenzyme Q$_{10}$ (Ubiquinone): 60–100 milligrams daily, especially during respiratory infections.

○ Lecithin (for adults only): 1,200 milligrams every other day.

○ N-acetyl cysteine (NAC): 200 milligrams a day for children weighing less than 30 kilograms (66 pounds): 400 milligrams a day for larger children and adults.

○ Taurine: in children, 30 milligrams for each kilogram of body weight per day (150 milligrams for every 10 pounds of body weight per day). In adults, 500 milligrams 3 times a day.

○ Vitamin E: 200 IU a day for children; 800 IU a day for adults.

○ Vitamin K: 5 milligrams every other week if taking antibiotics.

UNDERSTANDING THE HEALING PROCESS

Conventional medical treatment is a must in CF. Complementary therapies simply are not adequate to control the disease. However, many nutritional interventions make meaningful contributions to the ongoing management of the condition. Their impact on the course of the disease is so significant that quality care in CF may be the ultimate in complementary healing, requiring both conventional medicine and "alternatives" for ongoing quality of life.

Unlike most conditions, CF requires high-energy diets. Fats, especially those from plant seed oils, are best in CF. Gamma-linolenic acid is especially important for children who are seriously underweight.[8] To help children gain weight, allow them to consume up to 3,000 calories a day but emphasize healthy oils such as fish oils, hempseed oil, olive oils, and safflower oils rather than animal fats. Do not attempt to increase calorie consumption by adding sugars.

Beta-carotene is a fat-soluble vitamin that is typically deficient in people who have CF. Very small doses of beta-carotene, as little as 850 IU per day, are enough to bring bloodstream levels up to normal in children.[9] Since the smallest dosage of beta-carotene on the market in the United States is 5,000 IU or 3 milligrams, giving beta-carotene once a week is adequate for children. There are no scientifically demonstrated benefits to children in taking the vitamin more frequently. Adults may benefit from as much as 5,000 IU or 3 milligrams of beta-carotene daily.

Animal studies have shown that coenzyme Q$_{10}$ greatly increases survival time after infection with *Pseudomonas aeruginosa.* It increases the activity of the bacteria-eating cells known as macrophages, and spares antioxidant vitamin E, reducing inflammation.[10] Although no scientific studies as yet confirm the use of CoQ$_{10}$ in treating CF in humans, there are numerous anecdotal reports that it helps.

Lecithin (also known as phosphatidylcholine) accelerates the conversion of cholesterol into forms that can be transported in the bloodstream.[11] Cholesterol is an essential component of the lining of every cell in the body. It is involved in the transport of other essential fatty acids. In cells affected by CF, membranes are recycled so frequently that their supply of cholesterol is depleted.[12] Supplemental lecithin helps the body provide cholesterol to the cells that need it. Since lecithin sometimes causes digestive upset, it is not recommended for children.

N-acetyl cysteine (NAC) is an amino acid derivative that can break the chemical bonds that make mucus sticky. A study involving 10 chronic lung disease patients and 10 healthy controls found that it increases the activity of white blood cells.[13] A study involving 52 CF patients found that using NAC for 3 months greatly increased lung capacity, especially in cases of *Pseudo-*

monas infection. NAC may cause headaches if taken with sildenafil (Viagra), and in rare cases can cause cysteine-crystal kidney stones. Diabetics who also have CF may find that taking NAC causes false readings in urine tests for ketones.

Taurine is an amino acid that latches on to bile salts to carry them away from the liver. Once the bile salts reach the intestine, taurine helps them attach to essential fatty acids to be reabsorbed into the body. This keeps nutritional fats from being excreted in stool. In one study, 92 percent of children given 30 milligrams of taurine for every kilogram of their body each day had fewer incidents of steatorrhea (floating, foul-smelling, and pale or clay-colored stools) and better reabsorption of bile salts.[14] Another study suggests that taurine supplementation increases absorption in the segment of the intestines known as the ileum, where 80 percent of bile acids reenter the bloodstream.[15]

Vitamin E is transported into the body by attachment to LDL cholesterol. Since people with CF have difficulty absorbing cholesterol from food, they tend to be deficient in vitamin E even if there are adequate levels of the vitamin in their diet.[16] Vitamin K is synthesized by bacteria in the intestine, so vitamin K levels go down during antibiotic treatment. However, taking vitamin K supplements as infrequently as every other week is usually sufficient.[17]

There are theoretical rationales for taking glutathione, L-carnitine, medium-chain triglycerides (MCTs), oligomeric proanthocyanidins (OPCs, Pycnogenols), and ursodeoxycholic acid (UDCA) in CF. They are unlikely to cause harm. However, since laboratory evidence for their use is scant and no clinical studies confirm them, they are not recommended here.

CONCEPTS FOR COPING WITH CYSTIC FIBROSIS

O Use pancreatic enzymes with caution. Although pancreatic enzyme replacement therapy (PERT) stops foul-smelling diarrhea and relieves abdominal pain, overuse of these enzymes can cause irreversible narrowing of the colon.

O If your doctor prescribes intravenous antibiotics, ask if aerosols are available. Intravenous (IV) administration of the newer antibiotic tobramycin (Tobradex), in particular, increases the risk of damage to the nerves in the middle ear and the kidneys. Aerosol tobramycin is

better absorbed in the lung tissues that need it and less likely to lead to antibiotic resistance.[18]

O Growth hormone treatment, although very expensive, improves breathing function in children with CF by increasing the size of the muscles of the diaphragm.[19] Nutritional supplements claiming to duplicate the effects of growth hormone, however, are unlikely to help and may even hurt. Gamma-oryzanol, for instance, increases muscle mass but lowers the body's secretion of growth hormone, and has an unknown effect on children with CF.

O Intensive exercise—under professional supervision—can lead to increased breathing capacity, higher body weight, and greater resistance to fatigue in just a few weeks.[20] A key concern before entering any supervised exercise program is making sure there is minimal danger of being exposed to respiratory infections. If an infection-free environment cannot be arranged, simply moving to a location 500–3,000 feet (150–1,000 meters) high in elevation and continuing modest exercise has some of the same benefits.

Cystitis

SYMPTOM SUMMARY

O Burning pain when urinating

O Increased frequency of urination

O Having to get up to urinate at night

O Cloudy, foul-smelling, or dark urine

O Lower abdominal pain

UNDERSTANDING THE DISEASE PROCESS

Cystitis, an infection-induced condition of inflammation in the urinary tract usually caused by *E. coli,* is the cause of 11 million visits to doctors every year in the United States alone.[1] Cystitis is one of the most common infections among women. Between 10 and 20 percent of women have at least one episode of bladder infection every year, and between 2 and 4 percent of women at any time are infected with the bacteria that cause bladder infections and do not know it. Between the ages of 20 and 50, cystitis is roughly 50 times more common in women than men, but the infection is common in baby boys and men over age 65. Cystitis is also relatively common among gay men.[2]

Urine is free of bacteria when it leaves the kidneys. Infectious bacteria can migrate upward through the urethra to the bladder (or, in rare instances, enter the urinary tract from the bloodstream). Bacteria are introduced into the urinary canal from fecal contamination or, in women, vaginal secretions.

Most bacteria that manage to enter the urethra are simply flushed away by the constant flow of urine. As women pass through menopause, however, hormonal changes tend to weaken the ligaments surrounding the urethral canal so that the free flow of urine is blocked. Pregnancy also places pressure on the urinary canal. In both situations, bacteria have greater opportunity to accumulate and grow hyphae, "hooks" that anchor them in the lining of the urinary canal. Both men and women with uncontrolled diabetes are especially susceptible to cystitis, since the high sugar content of their urine gives bacteria food on which to grow. Sexual intercourse and mechanical injury are other risk factors.

TREATMENT SUMMARY

DIET

○ Drink at least 8 glasses of water a day.

○ Drink 1 cup of unsweetened cranberry or blueberry juice beverages (usually containing 25% juice) every 8 hours.

○ Avoid sugar and alcoholic beverages.

HERBS

○ Echinacea: 150–300 milligrams of solid extract (3.5% echinacosides) 3 times a day, or dried root, freeze-dried plant, juice, fluid extract, or tincture, as recommended on the label.

○ Goldenseal:

• Dried root (or as tea): 1–2 grams 3 times a day, or

• Freeze-dried root: 500–1,000 milligrams 3 times a day, or

• Tincture (1:5): 4–6 milliliters (1–1.5 teaspoons) 3 times a day, or

• Fluid extract (1:1): 0.5-2.0 milliliters ($\frac{1}{4}$–$\frac{1}{2}$ tsp) 3 times a day, or

• Powdered solid extract (8% alkaloid): 250–500 milligrams 3 times a day.

○ Uva Ursi (see notes on use below):

• Dried leaves or as a tea: 1.5–4.0 grams (1–2 teaspoons) 3 times a day, or

• Freeze-dried leaves: 500–1,000 milligrams 3 times a day, or

• Tincture (1:5): 4–6 milliliters (1–1.5 teaspoons) 3 times a day, or

• Fluid extract (1:1): 1.0 milliliters ($\frac{1}{4}$–$\frac{1}{2}$ teaspoons) 3 times a day, or

• Powdered solid extract (10% arbutin): 250–500 milligrams 3 times a day.

Do not take uva ursi for more than 2 weeks at a time, or more often than 5 times a year.

See Part Three if you take prescription medication.

UNDERSTANDING THE HEALING PROCESS

Adequate hydration is fundamental to controlling bladder infections. Drinking 8 glasses of water ensures a regular flow of urine that keeps bacteria from accumulating in the urinary tract. Drinking sugary soft drinks and eating sweets, however, counteracts the beneficial effects of drinking water. Clinical study has shown that people who consume 100 grams of white sugar—the equivalent of a 44-ounce soft drink or a couple of slices of cake—have impaired immune responses to bacterial infection for at least 5 hours.[3] Drinking alcohol is also detrimental.

Cranberry juice was once thought to fight urinary tract infection by making the urine too acidic for bacterial growth, but later studies suggest that its mode of action is keeping *E. coli* from "taking root" in the urinary canal.[4] The most recent research found that drinking cranberry juice keeps 80 percent of antibiotic-treatable bacteria and 79 percent of antibiotic-resistant bacteria from adhering to the lining of the urethra. The effect begins 2 hours after cranberry juice is drunk and lasts 8 hours.[5] Blueberry and lingonberry juices are also effective.

Don't give cranberry juice to infants. The medical literature reports a case of cranberry juice intoxication in a 4-month-old baby given 180 milliliters (approximately $\frac{3}{4}$ cup) of cranberry juice. The baby developed diarrhea severe enough to cause dehydration. The cranberry juice acidified not only the urine but the child's entire system. The child recovered after being put on a lactose-free formula.[6]

Echinacea, goldenseal, or uva ursi taken by itself is of limited value in treating bladder infections, but all three herbs taken together make a potent infection-fighting combo. Echinacea relieves inflammation. One study found that a teaspoon of *Echinacea purpurea* juice is as effective in relieving pain and swelling as 100 milligrams of cortisone. Echinacea also enhances the immune system's response to bacterial infections. It is especially useful in stimulating phagocytosis, the process by which white blood cells surround and digest infectious bacteria. A study of oral administration of an *Echinacea purpurea* root extract (30 drops 3 times per day) to healthy men for 5 days resulted in a 120 percent increase in phagocytosis.[7] Similar effects are likely in women.

Goldenseal protects against *E. coli, Klebsiella, Proteus, Pseudomonas,* and staph infections, 5 of the 6 major causes of cystitis, accounting for nearly 98 percent of cases of the disease.[8] The combination of echinacea and goldenseal is especially useful in treating conditions that involve drainage. A 1999 study reported that the combination of the two herbs stimulates the production of the immunoglobulins IgG and IgM, infection fighters that "remember" specific infections.[9] Uva ursi offers added protection against *E. coli* and *Proteus,* but is only effective against *Proteus* if the urine is alkaline. The urine is made alkaline by avoiding sugars, fatty meats, alcohol, and *vitamin C supplements.* Taking vitamin C will make uva ursi ineffective against *Proteus.* Taking calcium, on the other hand, will help.

Women who are trying to get pregnant should avoid *Echinacea purpurea.* It contains caffeoyl esters that can interfere with the action of hyaluronidase, an enzyme essential to the release of unfertilized eggs into the fallopian tube.[10]

There is laboratory evidence that *Echinacea angustifolia* contains chemicals that deactivate CYP3A4. This is a liver enzyme that breaks down a wide range of medications, including anabolic steroids, the chemotherapy drug methotrexate used in treating cancer and lupus, astemizole (Hismanal) for allergies, nifedipine (Adalat) and captopril (Capoten) for high blood pressure, and sildenafil (Viagra) for impotence, as well as many others. *Echinacea angustifolia* might help maintain levels of these drugs in the bloodstream and make them more effective, or it might also cause them to accumulate to levels at which they cause side effects. Switch to a brand of echinacea that does not contain *Echinacea angustifolia* if you experience unexpected side effects while taking any of these drugs.[11]

Avoid all forms of echinacea if you are taking cocktail treatments for HIV. Echinacea stimulates immune function, but it also slightly increases production of T cells.[12] These are the immune cells attacked by HIV. When there are more T cells, the virus has more cells to infect. This gives the virus more opportunities to mutate into a drug-resistant form. This effect also makes echinacea inadvisable in autoimmune conditions, such as lupus, rheumatoid arthritis, and Sjögren's syndrome.

People's Pharmacy authors Joe and Teresa Graedon warn that goldenseal reportedly limits the effectiveness of the anticoagulants heparin and warfarin (Coumadin). Do not take goldenseal with these medications. Avoid supplements containing vitamin B_6 or L-histidine if you take goldenseal, since they can interfere with goldenseal's antibacterial action.

Never take uva ursi for more than 2 weeks at a time, and do not take the herb more than 5 times a year. Nausea, vomiting, and diarrhea may occur with prolonged use. Pregnant women and people with liver or kidney disease should not take uva ursi.

Many other herbs, including asparagus, birch leaf, buchu, couch grass, epimedium, and horseradish oil are commonly used to treat urinary tract infections, with varying degrees of success. Japanese medicine has considerable experience in using Polyporus Formula to treat urinary tract infections. Tsumura & Company confirms that approximately two-thirds of female patients who have a combination of symptoms modern Japanese doctors call "urethral syndrome"— painful urination and/or a sense of retained urine—find relief when taking this formula. About 6 percent of patients experience some degree of stomach upset when first taking the formula, but this side effect is not so great that they choose to discontinue the herbs. In the United States, Polyporus Formula is available under the following trade names:

○ Chorei-to (Tsumura)

○ Polyporus Combination (Lotus Classics, Sun Ten)

○ Zhu Ling Tang (Lotus Classics, Sun Ten)

CONCEPTS FOR COPING WITH CYSTITIS

○ During toilet training, girls should be taught to wipe away rather toward the vagina to prevent urinary tract infections.

○ Unprotected intercourse during the menstrual period increases the risk of infection for both partners. The endometrium both offers the woman protection against disease and hosts any gonorrheal bacteria that previously infected her; it is this layer that is sloughed off during menstruation.

○ The use of oral contraceptives (the Pill) reduces a woman's risk of infection with the bacteria that cause cystitis. Estrogens cause the cervix to secrete a thicker protective mucus, and diminish blood flow during the period.[13] On the other hand, use of the Pill increases a woman's risk of becoming infected with the sexually transmitted disease *Chlamydia,* especially during the second half of her period. The progesterone in the pill causes the cervix to grow tissues in such a way that a tissue layer favored by *Chlamydia* is more exposed.[14]

○ Urinate after sexual intercourse. Women who tend to develop bladder infections after intercourse should wash their labia and urethra with a strong tea of goldenseal (2 teaspoons/cup) both before and after sex.

○ Cystitis is sometimes interstitial, caused not by infection but by slow degeneration of the lining of the bladder or by pelvic adhesions interfering with the normal flexibility of the bladder. In these cases, gotu kola in a dosage of 30 milligrams, 3 times a day, may be helpful. Women who are pregnant should not take gotu kola.

○ If you take antibiotics, you should also take bromelain. In a Japanese study in the early 1970s, people with urinary tract infections received antibiotics plus either bromelain or a placebo. Infections cleared up in all the participants receiving bromelain but in only 46 percent of participants receiving just antibiotics.[15] Bromelain increases the body's absorption of antibiotics and enhances their bactericidal power.

○ Avoid iron supplements. Most bacteria "seek out" iron-bearing proteins such as transferrin by attaching themselves to the lining of the urethra.[16] They compete with their host for iron supplies. Deprived of iron, bacteria cannot cause urethral inflammation.[17]

○ Homeopathy offers many remedies for cystitis. Usually it is best to start with a single dose of the lowest strength (6C, 6X, or 12C) of the remedy matching the symptoms to be treated, and then wait for a response. If there is an improvement in symptoms, let the remedy continue to work until there is no more improvement, then take another dose. If there is no improvement, try a different potency (30X or 30C). Sometimes homeopathic medicines work for a few minutes, and sometimes they work for an entire day before another dose is needed.

• Aconitum napellus is among the most warming remedies, appropriate if urination is difficult after the person has been out in the cold. It is also used when bashful bladder is a problem.

• Apis mellifica, a homeopathic preparation of bee sting venom, is used to relieve burning and stinging sensations accompanying urination, especially if urination is strained. Homeopathic physicians sometimes recommend it when heat makes symptoms worse and cold relieves them.

• Belladonna relieves irritable bladder when only small amounts of dark urine are passed.

• Berberis vulgaris treats twinges of stabbing or cutting pain, or a sensation of burning that extends to the opening of the urthra. It is appropriate when the urge to urinate is worst when walking.

• Borax is a homeopathic remedy frequently recommended for children. It is most helpful for adults who also have motion sickness.

• Cantharis relieves a scalding sensation when only a few drops of urine can be passed. There may be a constant sensation of urinary urgency.

• Chimaphila umbellate treats urinary inflammation in people who have to strain to urinate.

• Clematis relieves dribbling, especially if there is a tingling sensation after urination.

• Equisetum (horsetail) treats cystitis when there is a feeling of fullness in the bladder that is worse immediately after urination.

• Lycopodium stops the urge to go to the bathroom at night. It is most useful when there is copious urination.

• Sepia treats "leaking." This remedy is especially helpful for women who have pelvic adhesions.

• Staphysagria is the remedy of choice for urinary tract infections in women that develop them after sexual intercourse. There may be a sensation that a drop of urine is stuck or rolling in the urethra, or a constant burning. This remedy is also used to treat people who are confined to bed or who have recently had catheters removed.

Dandruff

SYMPTOM SUMMARY

○ Dry or oily flakes of skin

○ No itching

○ Worse in winter

○ Dandruff may be accompanied by other symptoms of seborrheic dermatitis, including:

- Erythema (abnormal redness caused by capillary congestion) and scaly eruptions on the scalp and neck
- Intertrigo (chafing) on the groin and neck

UNDERSTANDING THE DISEASE PROCESS

Dandruff, flakes of skin falling from the scalp, is one of the most common of all skin conditions. Associated with seborrheic dermatitis, dandruff is a chronic inflammation of the upper layers of the skin. While the term dandruff only refers to scales of skin falling from the scalp, the underlying problem can cause flaking skin on the face and neck and chafing elsewhere on the body. Dandruff may be dry or oily, or both. Dandruff scales may be yellowish, and they may coalesce to form large patches with distinct borders.

Skin that produces dandruff is especially vulnerable to the yeast *Pityrosporum ovale,* but scientists have uncovered no single cause of the condition. Nutrient deficiencies, stress, and hormones are all likely factors in the disease, along with yeast infection. The observation that about 40 percent of AIDS patients suffer dandruff and seborrheic dermatitis,[1] however, suggests that yeast infection is the single most important factor in the condition.

TREATMENT SUMMARY

DIET

○ Avoid excessive protein intake (more than 6 servings of protein foods daily). Eat 3 ounces of cold-water fish 3 times weekly, *or*

○ Flaxseed or hempseed oil: 1 tablespoon per day.

NUTRITIONAL SUPPLEMENTS

○ Biotin: 3 milligrams 2 times a day.

○ Folic acid: 4–5 milligrams per day.

○ Vitamin B complex: 100 milligrams daily.

○ Zinc picolinate: 25 milligrams per day while taking folic acid.

HERBS

○ Aloe: apply any *Aloe vera* gel liberally once a day.

○ Dandelion (*Taraxacum officinale*): any of the following three forms and dosages, 3 times a day:

- Dried extract (4:1): 250–500 milligrams.
- Dried root: 4 grams.
- Fluid extract (1:1): 4–8 milliliters.

○ *Kami-shoyo-san:* take the dosage recommended on the label of any of the following products, which are based on this Kampo formula.

- Bupleurum & Peony Formula (Lotus Classics, Qualiherb, Sun Ten)
- Free and Easy Wanderer Plus (Golden Flower)
- Jia Wei Xiao Yao San (Lotus Classics, Qualiherb, Sun Ten)
- Kami-shoyo-san (Tsumura)
- Kampo4WomenMindEase (Honso)

OTHER NATURAL TREATMENTS

○ Honey: crude honey diluted with a small amount of warm water, left on the scalp for 3 hours at a time.

○ Pyridoxine ointment (50 milligrams of pyridoxine per gram of ointment in a water-soluble base, prepared by a pharmacy): apply to the scalp after shampooing and drying.

○ Bay oil, lavender oil, and sandalwood oil: mix 6–10 drops of any or all of these oils with a $1/2$ cup sesame oil, then apply the warm oil mixture to the scalp with a cotton swab. Allow the oils to soak into the scalp for at least 30 minutes before shampooing.

See Part Three if you take prescription medication.

UNDERSTANDING THE HEALING PROCESS

Dandruff is a condition in which the skin craves moisture. Applying a moisturizing oil of any kind, whether medicated or not, usually helps the condition.[2] It is particularly important not to attempt to "dry out" oily dandruff. Drying the scalp with overfrequent shampooing only tightens the skin and makes the natural elimination of sebum and dead skin cells more difficult. Dry skin ages more quickly.

Many medications cause dandruff as a side effect. These include dopamine for Parkinson's disease; hydralazine for congestive heart failure and high blood pressure; isoniazid (INH) for tuberculosis; penicillamine for kidney stones, rheumatoid arthritis, and Wilson's disease; and oral contraceptives.

There is a long-held belief in naturopathic medicine that excessive protein consumption, especially of fatty meats and eggs, aggravates skin conditions. It is possible that incomplete digestion of proteins or poor intestinal absorption of protein breakdown products results in elevated levels of certain amino acids in the bowels. Bacteria in the bowel metabolize these amino acids into cadaverine, putrescine, and spermidine. These compounds enter the bloodstream and remove a biochemical "brake" on skin-cell growth.[3] Multiplying unchecked, affected skin cells coalesce into rashes and produce oily, yellow flakes.

While this theory is unproved in the case of dandruff, limiting the consumption of fatty meats and eggs is of general benefit to health. Supplementing the diet with cold-water fish 3 times a week or taking a tablespoon of flaxseed or hempseed oil daily counteracts another effect of excessive protein consumption, the inflammatory arachidonic acid cascade.[4]

Dandruff in infants is greatly influenced by supplementation with biotin. A large part of the body's supply of this vitamin is produced by bacteria in the colon, which have not had a chance to be established in very young children. Supplemental biotin given to infants or taken by nursing mothers is effective against the related condition cradle cap (see SEBORRHEIC DERMATITIS).[5] In adults, however, biotin by itself is of no value in treating the condition.

Adults are more responsive to vitamin B supplements. Experimentally induced vitamin B_2 (riboflavin) deficiency produces drying and flaking of the skin.[6] Supplementation with vitamin B_{12} (cyanocobalamin) is helpful in oily dandruff, although oral vitamin B_{12} supplements do not relieve drying and flaking. (Injections of vitamin B_{12}, available from your doctor, may be helpful.)

Folic acid supplementation is helpful for oily dandruff. It is of little value in preventing dry dandruff.[7] Since folic acid may interfere with the absorption of zinc, take 25 milligrams of zinc picolinate daily while taking folic acid.

The gel from the leaves of the aloe (Aloe vera) plant is a proven remedy for skin damage of all kinds. In a 1999 study, 44 adults with seborrheic dermatitis, a skin condition that causes dandruff as well as other symptoms, applied either an aloe ointment or a placebo cream to affected areas twice daily for 4–6 weeks. A majority of those who used aloe reported that their symptoms improved significantly (62 percent versus 25 percent in the placebo group). Researchers determined that those using aloe had a significant decrease in scaliness, itching, and number of affected areas.[8]

Dandelion is a rich source of choline, an important nutrient for the liver and an important cofactor for vitamin B_{12}.

The traditional Japanese herbal remedy kami-shoyo-san is frequently recommended for women who experience dandruff or seborrhea after menopause. Traditional East Asian medicine teaches that the formula is best suited for women who experience fatigue, painful tension of the shoulder and neck muscles, anxiety, insomnia, constipation, and/or missed or scanty periods.

In the treatment of dandruff, honey is an ointment rather than a food. Honey has antifungal, antibacterial, and antioxidant properties. A study of the use of honey in the treatment of seborrheic dermatitis conducted in the United Arab Emirates involved 30 patients with chronic lesions on the scalp, face, and chest. Twenty patients were males and ten were females. All the participants in the study suffered severe dandruff, itching, and hair loss, as well as scaling and dry white plaques with crusts and fissures.

Half of the patients were asked to rub diluted crude honey (90 percent honey diluted in 10 percent warm water) on their scalps every other day. The honey was left for 3 hours before gentle rinsing with warm water. Patients were followed for 4 weeks. They were examined daily for itching, scaling, hair loss, and lesions. All of the patients who used honey showed a significant response. Itching was relieved and scaling disappeared within 1 week. Skin lesions were healed and disappeared completely within 2 weeks. In addition, patients who used honey reported reversal of hair loss.

After the end of the 4-week test period, all of the patients were instructed to use honey for 6 months. Fifteen complied. None of the patients who continued to use honey relapsed, while 12 out of 15 patients who did not continue using honey experienced a return of the lesions 2–4 months after stopping treatment.[9]

Treatment with pyridoxine (vitamin B_6) creams is helpful in treating seborrhea that causes greasy scales on the face or oily dandruff. In one study, all patients with these symptoms who took a pyridoxine cream cleared completely within 10 days.[10]

CONCEPTS FOR COPING WITH DANDRUFF

❍ Effective antidandruff shampoos contain selenium sulfide, menthol, or salicylic acid. If they become ineffective, switch to a zinc pyrithione shampoo such as Sebulon or Zencon.

Degenerative Arthritis
See **Osteoarthritis**.

Degenerative Joint Disease
See **Osteoarthritis**.

Dementia
See **Alzheimer's Disease**.

Dengue Fever

SYMPTOM SUMMARY

❍ "Saddleback" rash beginning on the torso and spreading to the face, arms, and legs 3–4 days after beginning of fever

❍ Joint pain

❍ Loss of appetite

❍ Nausea

❍ Severe headache

❍ Sudden, high fever

❍ Vomiting

❍ In a small number of cases, dengue fever can cause hemorrhagic shock, a medical emergency.

UNDERSTANDING THE DISEASE PROCESS

Dengue (pronounced Den-geh) fever is a mosquito-borne viral infection once almost wiped out but now resurgent in the tropics throughout the world. Dengue fever is not unknown in the United States. In 3 of the last 20 years there have been outbreaks in southern Texas. The Centers for Disease Control believe that all of southern Texas and the southeastern United States where the mosquito *Anopheles aegypti* is found are at risk.

The joint pain caused by dengue is so severe that in Texas the disease is nicknamed "break bone fever." Other symptoms of dengue include a characteristic "saddleback" rash beginning on the trunk of the body and spreading to the face, arms, and legs, as well as loss of appetite, nausea, vomiting, and high fever. Symptoms begin about a week after being bitten by an infected mosquito and usually last about a week.

TREATMENT SUMMARY

HERBS

❍ Goat's rue: Use tincture in dosage recommended by manufacturer.

Herbs are not adequate for treatment of hemorrhagic shock. Consult a physician immediately if shortness or breath or loss of consciousness occurs.

UNDERSTANDING THE HEALING PROCESS

Medical science has no cure or treatment for dengue fever. Unless shock occurs, doctors can only offer pain relievers, usually acetaminophen (Tylenol), and recommend lots of fluid. A traditional Mexican herbal remedy for dengue, however, may be helpful.

Scientists at the Autonomous University of Mexico in Mexico City have found that extracts of the Mexican goat's rue plants *Tephrosia madrensis, Tephrosia viridiflora,* and *Tephrosia crassifolia* slow the multiplication of the dengue virus under laboratory conditions.[1] Mexican *curanderos* treat dengue with a goat's rue tea, but tinctures of the herb should prove equally effective.

Goat's rue increases perspiration. Be sure to drink 8–10 glasses of water a day when taking this herb. It also can stimulate milk production in women. Do not rely on goat's rue for treatment of hemorrhagic shock.

CONCEPTS FOR COPING WITH DENGUE FEVER

❍ Prevention is the best treatment for dengue. When

traveling in the tropics, be sure to apply insect repellant when traveling through urban areas where water is allowed to stand—even cup-sized pools of water are enough for infection-bearing mosquitoes to multiply. The species of mosquito that carries dengue prefers to bite during the day, and frequents shaded or cool areas. Dengue is most common at elevations below 4,500 feet (1,500 meters).

Depigmentation

See **Vitiligo**.

Depression

SYMPTOM SUMMARY

A depressive episode is diagnosed if 5 or more of these following symptoms last most of the day, nearly every day, for a period of 2 weeks or longer.

○ Change in appetite and/or unintended weight loss or gain

○ Chronic fatigue

○ Chronic pain or other persistent bodily symptoms that are not caused by physical illness or injury

○ Difficulty concentrating and making decisions, as well as memory loss

○ Feelings of guilt, helplessness, hopelessness, or worthlessness

○ Lasting anxious, empty, or sad mood

○ Loss of interest in activities once enjoyed, including sex

○ Restlessness or irritability

○ Sleeping too much, or not enough

○ Thoughts of death or suicide, or suicide attempts

UNDERSTANDING THE DISEASE PROCESS

Depression is one of the most common illnesses worldwide. In the United States, 1 in 8 women and 1 in 12 men receives treatment for a depressive episode at some point in his or her lifetime.[1] Depression is even more common in other countries. For instance, 1 in 5 people in Lebanon experiences major depression.[2]

For many years, medicine has focused on "major depression," a combination of 5 or more symptoms lasting most of the day every day for 2 weeks or longer. This is the definition of clinical depression given in the authoritative *Diagnostic and Statistical Manual of Psychiatric Disorders* (*DSM-IV*). Researchers and physicians have come to realize, however, that even "subclinical" depression can have a profound impact on patients' lives and since the introduction of drugs such as Prozac, treatment of milder cases of depression has come in vogue. Mild to moderate depression is also amenable to self-care with diet, exercise, supplements, and herbs.

Causes of depression. Scholars for centuries attributed depression to supernatural causes, or, not unlike modern times, to parents. Hippocrates hypothesized that the alignment of the planets caused the spleen to secrete black bile, which then darkened the mood and caused melancholia. The Chinese physician Zhu Qi Shi stated, "Inherited causes of depression are due to one of the parents being too old or to exhaustion or disease at the time of conception." The great Arab physician Ishaq Ibn Imran also attributed depression to prenatal influences, specifically to the damage of semen during the act of intercourse from which the child was conceived. In *Anatomy of Melancholy* (1621), the English scholar Robert Burton stated that melancholic people are "born to melancholic parents."

In the late nineteenth century, supernatural theories of depression were replaced with psychological ones. The Viennese psychoanalyst Sigmund Freud offered a theory that depression begins with an early traumatic separation from a significant object of attachment. This loss predisposes the individual to depression, which is triggered by adult losses thought to revive the early traumatic loss. For 50 years psychological theories of depression predominated and the mode of treatment, for the few who could afford it, was the psychoanalyst's couch. The largely serendipitous discovery of drug treatments for depression, however, launched a movement to try to understand depression in biological terms.

In the 1960s, researchers in Europe and the United States proposed the biogenic amine hypothesis of depression. This "biopsychological" view holds that depression is the result of deficiencies of the neurotransmitters norepinephrine and serotonin in the brain. The proponents of this view held that deficiencies in these brain chemicals was genetically determined, thus, psychoanalytic approaches to the disease were invalid.[3] However, the antidepressant medications developed to compensate for deficiencies in norepinephrine and serotonin are ineffective about 40 percent of the time, so a more complex causality of the condition was called for.

The most recent scientific research concerning the nature of depression suggests both the psychoanalytic theories and biopsychological theories of the disease are partially correct. Traumatic events literally change the biochemistry of the brain through their effects on corticotrophin releasing factor, or CRF. Under conditions of stress, the hypothalamus of the brain produces CRF to signal the adrenal glands to release stress hormones. These hormones, including norepinephrine and epinephrine (adrenaline) stimulate the release of energy supplies from the liver and enable a fight-or-flight response to dangerous conditions. When there is a long period of emotional stress, the hypothalamus eventually becomes insensitive to stress and quits producing the energizing hormones.

Scientists have found indications of hormonal changes in laboratory animals for decades, but only recently have been able to show that these kinds of changes occur in humans. A study published in 2000 was the first to document hormonal changes indicating hypothalamic "burnout" have been found in major depression among women with a history of childhood abuse.[4] Laboratory studies with human volunteers have found that people with major depression have a blunted hormonal response to stimulation compared to people who are not depressed.[5] Scientists believe that prolonged distress physically changes the neurons in the brain so that the brain is less responsive to sensory input from the outside world.[6]

TREATMENT SUMMARY

DIET

○ Avoid both alcohol and stimulants, including caffeine and nicotine. Be aware that carbohydrate cravings are the body's signal that bloodstream concentrations of the amino acid that is needed to make the mood regulating hormone serotonin are low.

SUPPLEMENTS

○ High-potency multivitamins and minerals.

○ 5-HTP: 100–200 milligrams 3 times a day.

○ Fish oil: 5,000 milligrams per day.

○ Vitamin B_{12} and folic acid: 800 micrograms of each, daily.

If your budget permits:

○ SAM-e: take 200 milligrams twice daily for 2 days; 400 milligrams twice daily for a week; 400 milligrams 3 times a day for the next 10 days; after 20 days, take the full dosage of 400 milligrams 4 times a day.

HERBS

○ St. John's wort: 300 milligrams of an extract containing 0.3 percent hypericin, 3 times a day.

○ If anxiety is also a problem, take 70 milligrams of a kava extract standardized for kavalactones, 3 times a day (see ANXIETY).

Persons over the age of 50 who have not responded to Luvox, Paxil, Prozac, or Zoloft should take:

○ Ginkgo biloba: 80 milligrams of an extract containing 24% ginkgo flavonglycosides taken 3 times a day *in addition to* prescription antidepressants.

See Part Three if you take prescription medication.

UNDERSTANDING THE HEALING PROCESS

Sixty years ago, the preferred treatment for major depression was shock therapy, a technique that is frequently compared to rebooting a computer. Shock therapy reliably brought people out of major depression, but the technique was applied indiscriminately so that it was even banned in some cities. Shock therapy is now reserved for cases that do not respond to any other treatment.

In the 1960s shock therapy was replaced by drug therapy with a group of compounds known as tricyclic antidepressants, so-called because of their chemical structures that contain three benzene rings. The usefulness of these drugs in treating depression was discovered by accident. An investigator looking for a drug to quiet agitated psychotic patients noticed that the drug imipramine did not calm agitation, but had a profound lifting effect on severe depression.

The tricyclic antidepressants quickly replaced shock therapy (and are still in use today), but they have their own limitations. They cause sleepiness, lightheadedness, dry mouth, and blurred vision. People who use them have difficulty concentrating and thinking. They do not cause an elevation of mood in people who do not need them, but after 2–3 weeks of continuous use they begin to lift the mood of people with depression. They act on the brain by keeping the hormones norepinephrine and serotonin in the gaps between neurons, available to help transmit nerve impulses. Since norepinephrine is a "stress hormone," the drugs sometimes have the side effect of overstimulating the heart.

The next drugs to come in to common use for the treatment of depression were the monoamine oxidase inhibitors (MAOIs), which are still in use today. Monoamine oxidase is a hormone found in the liver and in nerve tissues that breaks down norepinephrine and serotonin. Inhibiting monoamine oxidase keeps norepinephrine and serotonin available for transmission of nerve impulses in the brain. Like the tricyclic antidepressants, MAOIs begin to lift depression after 2–3 weeks of continuous use. Also like tricyclic antidepressants, these drugs sometimes overstimulate the heart, raising diastolic blood pressure (the "bottom" number). They can induce both overexcitement and fatigue, sometimes concurrently.

The 1990s brought the widespread use of selective serotonin reuptake inhibitors (SSRIs) such as Luvox, Paxil, Prozac, and Zoloft. Like the tricyclic antidepressants, SSRIs keep nerve cells from reabsorbing serotonin, keeping the hormone in the gaps between neurons and thereby facilitating the transmission of messages in the brain. Unlike tricyclic antidepressants, SSRIs does not affect the reabsorption of norepinephrine, and so using them does not cause fatigue. Unfortunately, SSRIs have their own side effects, including loss of interest in or ability to perform sexual intercourse, nausea, vomiting, nightmares, and lucid dreams.

Diet, exercise, nutritional supplements, and herbs are free of these side effects. They have real, scientifically verified benefits on mild to moderate depression. Mixing medications with natural therapies, however, should be done with caution. Never stop taking a prescribed antidepressant in favor of a supplement without seeking your physician's advice. Abruptly quitting some prescription drugs can bring about a sudden return of symptoms before the supplement has a chance to work.

Alcohol is the world's first choice among depressants. The common misconception that alcohol is a stimulant is derived from a misunderstanding of the effects of small doses of alcohol. At first, alcohol depresses inhibitory control mechanisms that regulate excitatory neural synapses. Confidence abounds, the personality becomes expansive and vivacious, but then uncontrolled mood swings and emotional outbursts ensue. The consequences of actions performed under the influence of alcohol are frequently negative, and contribute to a situation in which depression is a natural response.

Caffeine is the world's first choice among stimulants. Overuse of caffeine, however, causes depression. One study found that among healthy college students, moderate and high coffee users scored higher on a depression scale (and had lower GPAs) than students who drank relatively little coffee.[7] Two studies have found that people experiencing major depression tend to consume high amounts of caffeine, the equivalent of 6 or more cups of coffee a day.[8,9] Another two studies positively correlate caffeine intake with the degree of mental illness in psychiatric patients.[10,11]

Although caffeine is bad for depression, the combination of caffeine and sugar is worse. In one study, 7 of 16 depressed patients became symptom-free simply by giving up caffeine and sugar.[12] In another study, 23 participants responding to an advertisement requesting test subjects "who feel depressed and don't know why, often feel tired even though they sleep a lot, are very moody, and generally seem to feel bad most of the time" were put on a coffee- and sugar-free diet for 1 week. They were then given either a capsule containing caffeine and a sugar-sweetened drink or a capsule containing cellulose and a drink sweetened with aspartame. About half of the test subjects who were given caffeine and Kool-Aid became depressed.[13]

Nicotine, like alcohol, caffeine, and sugar, is commonly considered a stimulant. In the short term, nicotine *is* a stimulant, triggering the release of norepinephrine and epinephrine (adrenaline) throughout the body, and heightening the sensitivity of sensory receptors throughout the body. In the long run, however, nicotine causes desensitization of the brain to norepinephrine in much the same manner as chronic stress.

The extraordinary complexity of the brain suggests that a deficiency in any nutrient may contribute to depression. For this reason, high-potency multivitamin and mineral supplements are a good idea for anyone dealing with the condition.

5-HTP (5-hydroxytryptophan) is an up-and-coming

nutritional supplement for the treatment of depression. This supplement is a source of the amino acid tryptophan in a form that readily enters the brain. The brain turns tryptophan into the mood regulator serotonin.

A clinical study involving 60 people with mild to moderate depression compared 5-HTP against Luvox (fluvoxamine), an antidepressant in the same family as Prozac. The study found that 5-HTP was slightly more effective than the prescription drug. More important, while Luvox caused the full range of side effects usually associated with SSRIs, 5-HTP only caused mild stomach upset in a few of the people who took it.[14]

5-HTP is a relatively safe supplement, but some people should avoid it. The most common side effects from 5-HTP are heartburn, nausea, and various kinds of stomach upset including, bloating, flatulence, and stomach rumbles. This complication is due to the fact that the digestive tract makes its own serotonin, which may be overabundant until it adjusts to the supplemental supply. About 2 in 5 people who use the supplement experience these effects during the first 2 weeks of using it. To avoid this complication, begin by taking a 50-milligram dose once or twice a day, gradually building up to a 100-milligram dose after 3 or 4 weeks.

There are no reports of adverse effects on the central nervous system from taking even high doses of 5-HTP. Theoretically, however, large doses of 5-HTP taken with the migraine medications naratriptan (Amerge), rizatriptan (Maxalt), sumatriptan (Imitrex), or zolmitriptan (Zomig), or any prescription medications for depression could cause "serotonin syndrome." In this rare condition of excess serotonin there may be agitation, confusion, heightened physical reflexes, racing pulse, and excessive sweating leading to hypertension, coma, and death. This condition has never been observed from supplementation with 5-HTP, but as a precaution, avoid using 5-HTP if you take any prescription drugs for depression or migraine. Persons who have angina, uncontrolled high blood pressure, a rare form of migraine known as Prinzmetal's angina, or who have had a heart attack should also avoid 5-HTP.

There are reports that combining 5-HTP with the Parkinson's disease drug carbidopa can cause symptoms similar to those of the skin disease scleroderma (see SCLERODERMA for symptoms).[15,16] 5-HTP probably should not be combined with conventional antidepressants.

Omega-3 fatty acids are known to be depleted in the red blood cells of persons with major depression.[17]

Tests are under way at Massachusetts General Hospital to determine the effective dosage of fish oil, a rich source of these essential fatty acids, in the treatment of depression. Fish oil is generally regarded as safe when taken in usual doses, although some people experience fishy burps. Large doses such as those recommended for bipolar disorder can cause loose stools. Fish oil counteracts clotting factors in the blood, and should be used only under a doctor's supervision by people who take Coumadin, heparin, or other blood thinners.

Drugs in the same class as Luvox, Paxil, Prozac, and Zoloft seem to work better when the body has adequate supplies of folic acid, which is frequently deficient in persons who have depression. A 10-week double-blind placebo-controlled trial of folic acid in 127 individuals with severe major depression being treated with Prozac found that women who took Prozac with the vitamin supplement got better faster than those who took Prozac alone. It is possible that the 500-microgram dose of the vitamin used in the study was not enough to produce a beneficial effect in men.[18]

Vitamin B_{12} supplementation is necessary when supplementing with folic acid, which is frequently deficient in persons who have depression. Vitamin B_{12} also works in tandem with SAM-e.

S-adenosyl-L-methionine (SAM-e) is effective but expensive. A full dosage of this supplement can cost $200 a month. The clinical studies of the supplement have compared it to tricyclic antidepressants, the most recent study finding it to be as effective in relieving mild depression as imipramine (Tofranil).[19] Occasionally people improve while taking as little as 20 milligrams of SAM-e a day, but scientists believe that the 200-milligram doses offered as an "affordable" supplement are too small to be effective. Effective treatment of depression with SAM-e requires a dosage of 1,600 milligrams a day. Start with a small dose and gradually increase over a period of 3 weeks to avoid stomach upset.

SAM-e may interfere with the Parkinson's disease drug L-dopa. Taking both SAM-e and prescription antidepressants may cause excessive production of serotonin, leading to anxiety, elevated blood pressure, and mania.[20] Do not combine SAM-e with L-dopa or prescription antidepressants except under the supervision of a physician who knows you are taking SAM-e.

St. John's wort is an extraordinarily well-researched herb. Nearly 180 studies document the efficacy of St. John's wort in treating anxiety, anorexia, depression,

St. John's Wort Study Misinterpreted, Says Herbal Science Group

The American public may be receiving misleading information about the effectiveness of the popular herbal dietary supplement St. John's wort, says the nonprofit American Botanical Council. ABC and some of its scientific advisors noted that a new clinical study being released to the media is being misinterpreted.

The long-awaited government-sponsored study on the effectiveness of the popular herb is being published this Wednesday, April 10 (2002) in the *Journal of the American Medical Association*. The study, conducted by researchers at Duke University and 11 other medical centers in the U.S., concludes that neither St. John's wort nor the drug sertraline showed any measurable benefit in patients with more *severe* forms of depression. Although the study was conducted in patients with moderate to *severe* depression, the herb has been tested and used mainly in patients with less severe forms of depression.

The study conducted from December 1998 to June 2000 included 340 moderate to severely depressed patients that were randomly assigned to three groups. Over an eight-week period, one group received a dose between 900–1500 milligrams of a leading brand of St. John's wort extract, one group took the antidepressant drug sertraline (50–100 mg), popularly know by its trade name Zoloft, and the third group took a placebo, a sugar or dummy pill. Patients who responded to treatment continued to receive their assigned treatment for an additional 18 weeks. Curiously, fewer of the patients in both the herb and the drug groups responded to the treatments than did those in the placebo group.

According to Jerry Cott, Ph.D., former Chief of the Psychopharmacology Research Program, at the National Institute of Mental Health, the NIH designed this trial to include a standard anti-depression drug (sertraline) as "an active comparator" to document the sensitivity of the trial, that is, the ability of this trial to detect an actual treatment effect. "The fact that the sertraline was not effective in the primary measures of depres-

sion demonstrates (according to the NIH's own design protocol) that this trial lacked assay sensitivity and should not be considered a successful study." Dr. Cott was involved in the original design of the trial when he worked for the NIMH.

He added that "this study does not invalidate the use of SJW in clinical depression. There are still many well-controlled trials supporting the use of St. John's wort in mild to moderate depression, and additional studies with more appropriate patient populations are in progress."

In Dr. Cott's estimation, this study could be considered "neutral," one that simply fails to show effectiveness of either treatment rather than proving the test drug doesn't work. "This result is not uncommon in pharmaceutical industry-sponsored studies, though normally they are not published. The study simply lacked the sensitivity to detect a difference." Dr. Cott is an expert on the effects of herbs and conventional drugs on mental disorders, including depression. He also formerly worked at the Food and Drug Administration where he evaluated clinical studies on new antidepressant drugs. (More information available at jerrycott.com.)

Dr. Steven Bratman, a physician-author in Fort Collins, Colorado agrees. "The conclusion of the study is taken too far. Both treatments have been found effective in the majority of clinical trials. This study, while not supporting the use of St. John's wort, doesn't discredit it either."

Dr. Bratman, co-author of the *Natural Pharmacy: Clinical Evaluation of Medicinal Herbs*, explained the intricacies of the interpretation of clinical studies of this type. "In many studies of antidepressants, perhaps as many as one-third, the tested drug doesn't do any better than placebo. The cause is probably a combination of the high placebo effect often seen in studies testing antidepressants and the relative coarseness and subjectivity of the type of rating scales that must be used to evaluate severity of depression." Dr. Bratman explained that these rating scales are by their very nature less precise than biomedical tests, such as those that measure cholesterol levels. "In consequence, it is quite easy for a truly effective anti-depressant, such as sertraline, to fail to prove efficacy in a given double-blind, placebo-controlled trial. The problem is not the treatment itself, but in the difficulties of studying such treatments."

Because this study included sertraline, a drug that previously has been shown effective, the inescapable conclusion is that details of the patient group and the methods by which the ratings were determined were such that this study could not discern the effectiveness of a known effective treatment. This also applies to St. John's wort (which has also been shown effective in many studies) as it does to sertraline.

Bratman took issue with the authors of the study when they used a secondary outcome measure to conclude that sertraline was more effective than placebo and therefore better than St. John's wort. According to the standard rules of interpreting clinical studies, one should take only the primary outcome measures as meaningful, he explained. On those measures, neither sertraline nor St. John's wort was effective. Digging into secondary measures is widely accepted as being inappropriate, he added.

Thus, when the authors conclude that St. John's wort is ineffective for moderate depression and shouldn't be used, noted Bratman, "it would be equally valid to say that sertraline is ineffective for moderate depression, and shouldn't be used," he added. "However, we know that this is not the case; looking at the body of published research as whole, both sertraline and St. John's wort *are* effective."

"Herbs should be tested according to a reasonable expectation of their previously documented benefits," said Mark Blumenthal, founder and executive director of the nonprofit American Botanical Council. He referred to 10 previous studies on St. John's wort extract where the herb preparation was compared directly with pharmaceutical antidepressants for treatment of mild to moderate depression. These studies indicated a comparable efficacy with St. John's wort and the conventional drugs.

He also noted, "In Germany many physicians use St. John's wort as a first-line remedy for mild to moderate depression; if it doesn't work, then they can always put the patient on more powerful, pharmaceutical anti-depressants."

Blumenthal added, "It is important for the NIH to continue conducting clinical trials on many popular herbal dietary supplements. This adds to the growing body of scientific information on their safety and efficacy. This process is a constructive contribution to the maturation of the herbal movement. At the same time, however, it is equally important that the results of these studies are accurately interpreted and communicated to the public. Unfortunately, it appears that some aspects of this first NIH-funded study are not being properly characterized." He also noted that the full text of the study is not available prior to this Wednesday, so it is not possible to adequately evaluate all the details.

The study was funded with $4 million from the National Institutes of Health's National Center for Complementary and Alternative Medicine. It was the first clinical trial established by the NIH to test the efficacy of herbal remedies. St. John's wort was chosen because at the time the study was designed and funded in 1996, St. John's wort had begun to significantly increase in popularity in the U.S. This new awareness was based on media reports of a meta-analysis (statistical review of clinical trials) of 23 European clinical trials that showed that St. John's wort was safe and effective in treating mild to moderate forms of depression.

Last April, another U.S.-based multi-center clinical trial on St. John's wort also failed to show any activity for the herb, again in more severely depressed patients. The placebo-controlled study was criticized for targeting patients that were too chronically and severely depressed and thus not consistent with the profile of patients normally included in clinical trials. It was also criticized for not including an active control, like the drug sertraline (Zoloft, produced by Pfizer, the funder of the study), to determine the level of response by the patients. Both trials used the leading German St. John's wort extract (known in Germany as Jarsin 300, made by Lichwter Pharma of Berlin, and sold in the U.S. as Kira by Lichtwer Pharma USA).

St. John's wort, also known by its scientific name *Hypericum perforatum*, is a traditional European herb that has drawn significant attention for its ability to help elevate mood in mild or moderately depressed people. At least 22 controlled clinical trials have been published in European medical journals suggesting that St. John's wort extract is a safe and effective remedy for mild to moderate depression. An estimated 131 million doses of St. John's wort were prescribed by psychiatrists in Germany in 1999, according to German sources.

The American Botanical Council is the nation's leading nonprofit organization addressing research and educational issues regarding herbs and medicinal plants. The 13-year-old organization occupies a 2.5 acre site in Austin, Texas where it publishes *HerbalGram*, a peer-reviewed journal on herbal medicine, and will publish a forthcoming book and continuing education course for healthcare professionals, *The ABC Clinical Guide to Herbs*, containing an extensive monograph on the safety and efficacy of St. John's wort. Information contact: ABC at P.O. Box 144345, Austin, TX 78714–4345, ph: 512-926-4900, fax: 512-926-2345. Website: www.herbalgram.org.

1. The study referred to in this release is Davidson, J.R.T., et al., "Effect of *Hypericum perforatum* (St. John's Wort) in major depressive disorder: A randomized controlled trial," *Journal of the American Medical Association*, 287, 1807–1814 (2002).

2. The previous United States study referred to in this release that found no response by St. John's wort is Shelton, R.C., et al., "Effectiveness of St John's Wort in major depression: A randomized controlled trial," *Journal of the American Medical Association*, 285(15), 1978–1986 (2001).

3. A comprehensive monograph on St. John's wort from ABC's forthcoming book *The ABC Clinical Guide to Herbs*, including summaries of 23 clinical trials and 122 references, can be viewed on the ABC website, www.herbalgram.org.

This April 9, 2002 press release is reprinted with permission of the American Botanical Council.

The American Botanical Council (ABC) is a membership-driven, nonprofit educational organization providing the public with accurate, science-based information on medicinal plants and phytomedicines. For more information about ABC or specific herbs, please visit www.herbalgram.org.

and sleep disturbances. In the European Union, St. John's wort is a prescription antidepressant prescribed by doctors and paid for by health insurance.

Various clinical studies have compared St. John's wort against the tricyclic antidepressants Elavil (amitriptyline) and Tofranil (imipramine) and against the SSRIs Paxil (fluoxetine) and Zoloft (sertraline). Clinical studies repeatedly find that St. John's wort is as effective as mainstream antidepressant drugs but with fewer side effects and a lower cost.

A psychiatric clinic in Darmstadt, Germany conducted a double-blind comparison trial of St. John's wort and Elavil. The 135 depressed patients were given either the herb or the prescription medication for 6 weeks. At the end of the trial, patients who had been taking St. John's wort had an average score on the Hamilton Depression Rating Scale of 8.8, compared to an average score of 10.7 for the patients treated with Elavil (that is, the patients taking St. John's wort were less depressed). The St. John's wort had fewer and milder side effects.[21]

A randomized, double-blind clinical comparison trial of St. John's wort and Tofranil conducted by the Remotiv-Imipramine Study Group in Germany involved 324 outpatients with mild to moderate depression at 40 outpatient clinics. After 6 weeks of treatment with either St. John's wort or Tofranil, the average score on the Hamilton Depression Rating Scale was 12.00 for patients taking St. John's wort and 12.75 for patients taking Tofranil. Adverse events such as agitation, anxiety, dizziness, retching, tiredness, and erectile dysfunction occurred in 63 percent of patients taking Tofranil, but only in 39 percent of participants taking St. John's wort. The most important difference between St. John's wort and Tofranil, however, was the patient's experience of anxiety while in treatment. The mean score on the anxiety-somatization subscale of the Hamilton measurement system was 3.79 in the St. John's wort group and 4.26 in the Tofranil group. Patients who took St. John's wort were significantly less likely to experience anxiety than patients who took Tofranil.[22]

Another German study compared St. John's wort to Prozac. Researchers enrolled 240 mildly to moderately depressed individuals into a randomized, double-blind, parallel-group comparison in which 114 patients received Prozac and 126 patients received St. John's wort. After 6 weeks of treatment, the mean Hamilton Depression Rating Scale decreased to 11.54 in the group taking

St. John's wort and 12.20 in the group taking Prozac. Eight percent of patients taking St. John's wort experienced adverse reactions, compared to 23 percent of patients on Prozac. The researchers concluded that St. John's wort and Prozac were equally effective in treating mild to moderate depression but that St. John's wort was a safer choice.[23]

A double-blind clinical study at St. John's Episcopal Hospital in Far Rockaway, New York tested the comparative benefits of St. John's wort and Zoloft. Thirty outpatients were given a low dose of either St. John's wort or Zoloft for a week, and then a standard dose of either St. John's wort or Zoloft for 6 weeks. A clinical response defined as a 50 percent reduction in scores on the Hamilton Depression Rating Scale was noted in 47 percent of patients receiving St. John's wort and 40 percent of patients receiving Zoloft. The difference between the two drugs was too small to say with statistical confidence which was more effective.[24]

Exactly how St. John's wort works is not known. The most recent research suggests that hyperforin, a chemical in the herb, modifies the expression of genes in parts of the brain that are physically changed by stress, specifically the hippocampus, locus coeruleus, and striatum.[25] These parts of the brain respond to adrenaline released in states of stress, excitement, and joy; restoring them to normal function may counteract other processes that cause depression.

Although the clinical evidence for St. John's wort is impressive, critics of herbal medicine correctly point out that it will not reliably treat severe depression. A well-publicized study published in the *Journal of the American Medical Association* in 2001 reported that only 24 percent of severely depressed patients given a relatively high dose of St. John's wort (1,200 milligrams of hypericin per day) went into remission during an 8-week trial, compared to 19 percent of patients who were given a placebo.[26] A similar controversy arose after reports of a clinical study in 2002. However, the news reports did not clarify that a response rate of less than 50 percent is typical for aggressive drug treatment of major depression, nor did the news reports compare side effects of standard medical treatments for major depression with side effects of St. John's wort. Nonetheless, anytime there is a risk of suicide, reliance on St. John's wort is inappropriate.

Do not take St. John's wort unless you have been off prescription antidepressants for at least 4 weeks. Prescription antidepressants linger in the bloodstream for a long time, and there have been several reports of "serotonin syndrome" (anxiety, elevated blood pressure, and mania) occurring when St. John's wort and medications such as Prozac are taken together.[27] Natural medicine specialist Dr. Steve Bratman notes that the antimigraine drug sumatriptan (Imitrex) and the pain-killing drug tramadol (Ultram) also raise serotonin levels and might interact similarly with the herb. St. John's wort may make the skin more sensitive to sun, especially if you also take oral contraceptives, sulfa drugs, tetracycline, the blood pressure medication lisinopril (Prinivil or Zestril), or the arthritis drug piroxicam (Feldene).

Most important, St. John's wort may reduce the effectiveness of chemotherapy drugs[28]—clozapine (Clozaril) or olanzapine (Zyprexa) for schizophrenia, cyclosporine (Neoral, Sandimmune, SangCya) for organ transplants,[29] digoxin (Lanoxin) for heart disease,[30] oral contraceptives, protease inhibitors for HIV,[31] theophylline (Theo-Dur) for asthma,[32] and warfarin (Coumadin)[33] used as a blood thinner. If you are taking St. John's wort and one of these medications at the same time, and then stop taking the herb, blood levels of the drug may rise. Increasing bloodstream concentrations of the drug may be dangerous in some circumstances.

Some research suggests that ginkgo helps the brain respond to the mood regulator serotonin. A study published in 1994 reported that older lab rats given ginkgo extracts grew addition serotonin receptor sites on brain cells. Ginkgo did not have this effect on younger animals.[34]

A clinical study then sought to determine whether giving ginkgo to older adults helped them respond to SSRIs such as Prozac. Forty patients between the ages of 51 and 78 who had depression that had not responded to Prozac were given either 80 milligrams of ginkgo extract 3 times a day or a placebo. By the end of the fourth week of the study, the average score of the ginkgo-treated patients on the Hamilton Depression Rating Scale had fallen from 14 to 7. In contrast, patients given a placebo had only dropped from 14 to 13.[35]

Ginkgo slightly thins the blood. For this reason, it should not be taken by people who take a daily aspirin or who are on blood thinners such as Coumadin or warfarin.

CONCEPTS FOR COPING WITH DEPRESSION

People with depression not only have trouble finding motivation to exercise, but the condition also has a direct effect on muscle tone. Sports physiologists have found that people with major depression have weaker biceps and hamstrings, but successful treatment with antidepressants improves muscle tone even without exercise.[36] Exercise itself, however, lifts mood.

In December 2001 researchers at University of Washington reported a study of 112 women aged 19–78 in a study of the effects of exercise and vitamin supplementation on mild to moderate depression. Women in the intervention group were instructed to take a brisk 20-minute outdoor walk at a target heart rate of 60 percent of maximum heart rate, to increase light exposure throughout the day, and to take a specific vitamin regimen. Women in the control group were not told to exercise and were given a placebo vitamin pill. The women in the study were otherwise in good health and took no other drugs or supplements for depression.

Pre- and post-intervention assessment utilized five measures of mood: Center for Epidemiology Studies Depression Scale, Profile of Mood States, Depression-Happiness Scale, Rosenberg Self-Esteem Scale, and the General Well-Being Schedule. The women in the intervention group improved on all five scales. Two-thirds of the women in the intervention group felt so much better by exercising that they participated in 100 percent of scheduled exercise sessions. The authors suggested that the type of intervention may provide an effective, easily managed therapy for mildly to moderately depressed women who prefer a self-directed approach or who have difficulties with the cost or side effects of medication or psychotherapy.[37]

Dermatitis Herpetiformis

SYMPTOM SUMMARY

○ Chronic skin eruption of itching lesions, papules, and vesicles in clusters resembling hives

○ Most common on the back, back of the neck, buttocks, elbows, knees, and scalp

UNDERSTANDING THE DISEASE PROCESS

Dermatitis herpetiformis is a disease that causes intense itching with a skin inflammation resembling hives. Patients often have no sign of the original lesions by the time they go to the doctor, because the itching is so intense and the original areas of skin inflammation are covered by raw abrasions and crusts induced by scratching. Itching frequently has a burning or stinging component. The onset of burning and stinging reliably predicts the eruption of whelps on the skin 12–24 hours later.

The underlying cause of dermatitis herpetiformis is a hypersensitivity to gliadin. This protein is a component of gluten, which is found in all forms of wheat (including durum, semolina, and spelt), rye, oats, barley and related grain hybrids such as kamut and triticale. When someone who is sensitive to gliadin consumes these grains, the intestine releases massive quantities of an immune protein called immunoglobulin A (IgA). IgA is ordinarily the body's first line of defense against disease-causing microorganisms that enter through the skin and mucosal surfaces.

In dermatitis herpetiformis, IgA binds to cells in the skin and treats them as if they had become infected. The body continues to secrete IgA, constantly inflaming the skin, until the affected individual stops eating foods containing gliadin or until the immune system becomes incapacitated. The benefits of changing diet, however, take several months.

Dermatitis herpetiformis is usually diagnosed by skin biopsy but there is a less painful alternative. Your doctor can order a test for gluten sensitivity that measures gluten antibodies in saliva. For information, ask your physician to contact Great Smokies Diagnostic Laboratory in Asheville, North Carolina, 1-800-252-9303.

TREATMENT SUMMARY

DIET

○ Avoid *all* foods made with wheat or any other grain containing gluten. Sources of hidden gluten include caramel, gum, hydrolyzed plant protein (HPP), hydrolyzed vegetable protein (HVP), malt, maltodextrin, modified food starch, monoglycerides, diglycerides, natural flavoring, soy sauce, texturized vegetable protein (TVP), and vinegar.

NUTRITIONAL SUPPLEMENTS

○ PABA (para-aminobenzoic acid):

• Three 500-milligram extended-release tablets taken with food, 3 times daily, *or*

• Aminobenzoate of potassium powder, one 2-gram packet taken with food, 3 times daily.

For no longer than 3 months:

○ Selenium: 200 micrograms daily.

○ Vitamin E: 1,000 IU daily.

UNDERSTANDING THE HEALING PROCESS

Since healing dermatitis herpetiformis with diet takes several months, many people with the condition opt to be treated with the antibiotic dapsone. This drug relieves symptoms in 24–48 hours, but anyone who takes more than 100 milligrams of the drug per day develops anemia. Other side effects may include damage to the bone marrow and liver, headache, and depression. Since the rash returns very quickly when the antibiotic is discontinued, the typical treatment strategy with dapsone and other agents for dermatitis herpetiformis is to find the lowest dosage possible while controlling symptoms, so that side effects diminish over time. As a British expert on the disease, Dr. Lionel Fry, notes, "Since side effects tend to occur early in treatment, patients may only have to attend hospital every six months once established on drug treatment."

Although natural healing of dermatitis herpetiformis requires discipline, it is free of side effects. Many sufferers of this form of dermatitis will choose the middle ground between medical and natural treatment, taking prescription drugs in the short term to control symptoms while waiting for diet to control the underlying disease.

A gluten-free diet is key to healing dermatitis herpetiformis. A 25-year study of dermatitis herpetiformis in the United Kingdom found that about a third of patients experience complete remission of symptoms simply by removing wheat and other gluten products from the diet. Virtually all of the remaining two-thirds of patients achieved partial relief of symptoms by partial adherence to the diet.[1] People with this condition who follow a gluten-free diet are also at much lower risk for developing lipomas, tumors of fatty tissue just beneath the skin.[2]

Most medical authorities note that about 10 percent of people with the disease do not respond even to rigorous elimination of gluten products from the diet. Eliminating milk and eggs can help most of the dermatitis herpetiformis sufferers in this group. An enzyme-linked immunosorbent assay (ELISA) of dermatitis herpetiformis patients has found that about 75 percent have serum antibodies reactive against gliadin, cow's milk, or the albumin protein in eggs.[3] Completely eliminating milk and eggs followed by carefully reintroducing them in small amounts several months later is a good test of the potential efficacy of permanently eliminating them from the diet.[4] Some milk- and egg-sensitive dermatitis patients will be able to tolerate small amounts of these foods if they strictly adhere to the gluten-free diet.

A single study in the 1950s found that treating dermatitis herpetiformis with very large dosages of PABA (9,000–24,000 milligrams per day) controlled symptoms for as long as 30 months. Symptoms of the disease rapidly recurred when PABA supplementation was stopped.[5] There is no evidence that taking as much as 24 grams (24,000 milligrams) of PABA daily causes any *serious* side effects. However, to provide a margin of safety, naturopathic physicians usually recommend taking no more than 6 grams (6,000 milligrams) of the supplement daily for no more than 3 months. Always take PABA with a full glass of water to avoid the nausea and vomiting that sometimes comes with taking high dosages of the supplement.

There is no direct evidence that selenium and vitamin E relieve symptoms of dermatitis herpetiformis. However, both vitamins protect an antioxidant enzyme known as glutathione peroxidase, which is known to be deficient in dermatitis herpetiformis. Clinical trials confirm that supplementation with these two vitamins corrects glutathione peroxidase deficiency in 6–8 weeks, and levels continue to increase for at least 5 months, however, there is no immediate effect on symptoms of the disease.[6,7]

CONCEPTS FOR COPING WITH DERMATITIS HERPETIFORMIS

○ If a gluten-free diet causes constipation, try drinking more water, increasing servings of fruits and vegetables, and following other remedies listed under CONSTIPATION.

○ Non-food products such as lipstick, medications in pill form, and toothpaste may contain gluten. Health and beauty aids that are not ingested in normal use may be accidentally ingested when fingers come in contact with the mouth. In some cases, skin contact with a gluten is enough to cause a reaction.

○ "Starch" in the United States is usually corn starch, which is safe for people who have dermatitis herpetiformis. "Starch" in Europe, however, is usually wheat starch, which will cause a skin reaction.

○ Many people with dermatitis herpetiformis buy bread machines to take advantage of the many gluten-free bread mixes available on the market. If you are buying a bread machine, keep in mind that gluten-free bread mixes are very heavy and not every bread maker can process them. Brands of bread makers that process gluten-free dough include the Black & Decker All-in-One (Model B1500–04), all Wellbilt machines (sold at Sears), and the very expensive Zojirushi BBCCS-15.

○ Be careful not to take any brand of vitamin E extracted from wheat. The formulation of vitamin E made by A. R. Grace & Company is safe for people with dermatitis herpetiformis, but the capsules themselves are made with beef gelatin and are neither halal nor kosher.

○ Avoid fried foods, especially in fast-food restaurants. French fries are usually cooked in the same oil used to prepare breaded foods.

○ If you drink alcohol, avoid beer (including rice beer, which contains malt), bourbon, gin, rye, and whiskey. Most vodkas do not cause a problem, and rum, sake, tequila, and wine are generally safe.

Dermographism
See **Hives**.

Diabetes

SYMPTOM SUMMARY

Type 1 Diabetes:

○ Increased thirst

○ Increased urination

○ Weight loss despite increased appetite

○ Nausea

○ Vomiting

○ Fatigue

Type 2 Diabetes:

○ Increased thirst

○ Increased appetite

○ Increased urination

○ Wounds that are slow to heal

○ Erectile dysfunction in men

○ Blurred vision

UNDERSTANDING THE DISEASE PROCESS

Diabetes (more technically, diabetes mellitus, literally "sugar diabetes") is a failure of the proper metabolism of sugar. Diabetes causes glucose to remain in the bloodstream rather than to be transported inside cells where it can be used as a source of energy. In full-blown diabetes, cells may be starved for energy and forced to burn fat and protein for fuel. The byproducts of protein breakdown accumulate with sugar in the bloodstream and increase the urgency of both urination and thirst. Even before the disease is fully developed, there can be blurred vision and slow healing of cuts, scrapes, and infections.

There are two major types of diabetes mellitus. Type 1 diabetes involves a complete or nearly complete failure of the cells in the pancreas to produce insulin. This form of diabetes usually strikes in childhood or early adulthood, although in rare cases older adults can develop type 1 diabetes after viral infections or as a complication of treatment for cancer or HIV. Children and young adults who develop type 1 diabetes carry genes that predispose them to the disease, but only about 40 percent of the carriers of these genes actually develop the disease. At one time researchers believed that the actual development of the disease involved an allergy to cow's milk or exposure to immune factors in the breast milk of diabetic mothers, but the current thinking is that viral infections, especially viral diarrhea, trigger the disease.[1] To the extent type 1 diabetes can be "caught" from breast milk from a diabetic mother, it can be prevented if the mother takes insulin to control blood sugars.[2]

Type 1 diabetes comes on suddenly. It typically is diagnosed in an emergency room. This form of diabetes must be treated with insulin. No existing therapy, conventional or alternative, can replace the need for taking 3–5 injections of insulin each and every day. Natural treatments for type 1 diabetes, however, can help the body use insulin more efficiently and help prevent complications.

Type 2 diabetes does not always require insulin injections, but this form of the disease is more insidious. Type 2 diabetes is sometimes only diagnosed after it causes a serious complication, such as loss of sight or ulceration of a foot or leg. Like type 1 diabetes, type 2 diabetes has both a genetic component and an environmental trigger. Some people are born with a genetic defect—actually a genetic characteristic that confers greater likelihood of survival between conception and birth—that causes every cell in their bodies to react to insulin in an unusual way. The outer membrane of every cell in the body holds proteins that act as a lock for which insulin is the key. These receptors grasp insulin and take it inside the cell. In people who are prone to type 2 diabetes, cells reduce the number of receptor sites for insulin if the amount of insulin in the bloodstream increases. That is, if the body makes more insulin, cells change so that they are less, rather than more, able to respond to it.

When people with this genetic characteristic gain weight or become physically inactive, a vicious cycle sets in. Increased body fat, especially over the abdomen, physically blocks the flow of blood to the fat cells that ordinarily store and convert sugar. Since glucose cannot reach fatty tissues, it remains in the bloodstream. The pancreas senses the additional sugar and makes more insulin. The additional insulin, however, causes fat cells to lose insulin receptor sites. Both sugar and insulin stay in the bloodstream, and cells lose still more insulin receptor sites, so the pancreas produces still more insulin.

Even when people have a genetic tendency toward type 2 diabetes and become overweight, however, diabetes is not necessarily inevitable. Vigorous daily exercise maintains circulation. If increased circulatory health keeps the blood flowing, the fat cells that use insulin to "catch" circulating glucose and turn it into fat can keep blood sugar levels normal. Alternatively, expanded muscle mass, also from exercise, enables muscle cells to use more glucose and also keep bloodstream glucose levels low.

But when overweight people with a hereditary tendency toward diabetes become inactive, diabetes results. Even while cells all over the body are losing their ability to respond to insulin, fat cells undergo changes that make them accumulate fat more readily and release them more slowly, compounding poor circulation caused by lack of exercise. As fat cells become "stuffed" with triglycerides, even if sugar reaches them, they cannot process it. Gaining weight becomes easier. The muscle cells are forced to do more and more of the work of keeping blood sugar levels normal, even while their own insulin resistance eventually forces them to use fats and their own proteins for fuel.[3]

The metabolic disruption caused by diabetes affects every cell of the body, but especially the eyes and nervous system. Unlike other tissues, the eyes, the brain, and the nerves do not have to rely on insulin transporters as their only way to receive glucose fuel. When blood sugars are high, glucose pours into these tissues faster than the tissues can use it, and toxic waste products build up. For this reason, especially in type 2 diabetes, the first obvious symptoms are usually psychological. Excess sugar "revs up" the brain so that many untreated type 2 diabetics appear slightly manic, with racing thoughts, racing speech, and a "go-go mind with a so-so body." Having too little energy for too much to do is a good time to see a doctor to make sure you do not have diabetes.

TREATMENT SUMMARY

This summary only recommends products that lower blood sugars by increasing insulin sensitivity. For lists of supplements useful in controlling specific problems, see individual entries for diabetic complications. (See FOOT ULCERS; GASTROPARESIS; NEUROPATHY; RETINOPATHY, DIABETIC).

NUTRITIONAL SUPPLEMENTS

(chosen with the help of a qualified healthcare practitioner)

❍ Alpha-lipoic acid: 200 milligrams daily.

❍ Biotin: 9–16 milligrams daily.

❍ Chromium (from brewer's yeast): 1,000 micrograms daily.

❍ Niacin (a cofactor for chromium): at least 20 milligrams but no more than 100 milligrams, daily.

❍ Vitamin C: up to 3,000 milligrams daily (higher amounts can raise blood sugars).

❍ Vitamin E: 800–1,000 IU daily.

See Part Three if you take prescription medication.

UNDERSTANDING THE HEALING PROCESS

The first difficult truth about healing a diabetic body is that you cannot control the disease if you do not know what your blood sugars are. After you have pricked your fingers (or your arms) thousands or tens of thousands of times, placed a drop of blood on a slide, and read your glucose level on a glucometer, you may have a fairly accurate sense of normal blood sugars. If your sugars are dangerously low or dangerously high, however, even this experience may not be enough. Blood sugar measurement—even after the introduction of the Gluco

Watch, which still requires skin pricks—is an absolute essential of diabetes management.

Fortunately, not all diabetics have to draw drops of blood to measure blood sugars every day, and modern lances are relatively less painful than those that existed even in 1995. If you have been told you have type 2 diabetes, you do not take insulin, and your blood sugars are *consistently* below 120 mg/dl (6.5 mM), you may only need to test your blood sugars one day a week. If you take Humalog or N insulin before meals, you may need to test your blood sugars every time you eat and when you get up in the morning. Ultrathin lancets reduce the pain of skin pricks and ultrasensitive glucometers reduce the amount of blood needed for a test, literally the size of a drop on the tip of a pin. Measuring and recording blood sugars is utterly essential to diabetic care.

The second difficult truth about healing a diabetic body is that, even if you have type 2 diabetes, if you do not manage your "honeymoon period" wisely you will probably have to take insulin injections. Insulin is made by the beta cells of the pancreas. When high blood sugars first set in, the beta cells attempt to compensate by making more and more insulin. Unfortunately, the body uses insulin 30 times more efficiently in transporting fats than in transporting sugars. You literally gain more while eating less. The underlying circulatory problems become worse and worse, and at some point, the beta cells in the pancreas burn themselves out. When 80 percent of the beta cells have been destroyed, you will need to start injecting insulin, and it is likely you will need insulin for the rest of your life. Most type 2 diabetics have a grace period of about 5 years before they effectively become type 1 diabetics if they do not rigorously control blood sugars and exercise.

The most difficult truth about healing a diabetic body is many medications, other than insulin, hurt as much as they help. The sulfonylureas, a group of drugs including acetohexamide (Dymelor), chlorpropamide (Diabinese), glimepiride (Amaryl), glipizide (Glucotrol), glyburide (DiaBeta, Glynase Prestab, Micronase), tolazamide (Tolinase), and tolbutamide (Orinase), lower blood sugars by stimulating the pancreas to produce insulin. This prevents diabetic complications, but accelerates the burnout of the insulin-producing beta cells.

The current craze in the medical treatment of diabetes, the thiazolidinedione drugs pioglitazone (Actos) and rosiglitazone (Avandia), have an even more insidious side effect. These drugs make insulin receptors more sensitive to insulin. Some recent research suggests they counteract a protein called resistin, which makes cells resistant to insulin.[4] These two effects enable fat and muscle cells to take sugar out of the bloodstream, lowering blood sugars. It also makes fat cells 30 times more efficient in taking fat out of the bloodstream, lowering triglycerides and cholesterol. Even worse, these drugs activate a gene, peroxisome proliferator-activated receptor gamma (PPAR-gamma), that causes fat cells to multiply, while they are becoming more efficient at storing fat. The short-term effect is weight gain without changing diet or exercise. Gains of 20 pounds (9–10 kilograms) are common. Gains of 100 pounds (45 kilograms), *without eating more or exercising less,* have been known to occur. No one knows whether the long-term effects of weight gain will eventually cancel out the short-term benefits of reducing blood sugar levels.

In all the bad news about diabetes, there is some good news. There are at least two basic diets that will help you control your blood sugars, although neither of them is a diet recommended by the American Diabetes Association. One approach is to essentially eliminate carbohydrates with an eating plan similar to the well-known Atkins diet. In this diet, all sweets (including "sugar-free" candies), desserts, pastries, rice, pasta, bread, crackers, fruit, fruit juices, creamers, *nonfat* yogurt, and cottage cheese are excluded, as are beets, carrots, corn, and potatoes. This leaves other vegetables, meat, fish, poultry, seafood, eggs, tofu, cheese, butter, whole-milk yogurt, and cream. Two kinds of crackers have a limited carbohydrate content and are permitted: Scandinavian crisp break and bran crisps. There are no occasions on which small amounts of sugar, desserts, or other concentrated carbohydrates are permitted.

While this approach is draconian, it is the easiest way for diabetics who cannot or do not exercise to maintain low blood sugars. Almost all diabetics (including those who take insulin) will have unacceptably high blood sugars (over 200 mg/dl or 11 mM) for at least 90 minutes after eating even one serving of carbohydrate. This severe carbohydrate-restricted diet prevents high blood sugars by eliminating the carbohydrates the digestive tract uses to make them. Since blood sugars are kept low, the high protein content of the diet does not damage the kidneys—although combining high protein with a high-sugar diet certainly does damage the kidneys. Since cholesterol receptors in the liver are not clogged by glucose, it does not raise cholesterol or triglycerides. Be warned, however, that getting off this high-protein, high-fat diet with a daily sweet or a favorite high-carbohydrate comfort food *will* cause elevated cholesterol and triglycerides and could eventually cause kidney damage.

Another way to maintain low blood sugars is with almost the reverse diet (but still no desserts). A diet that is high in unrefined carbohydrates, such as those found in whole grains, fruits, and vegetables, and low in both protein and fat keeps blood sugars low *in diabetics who exercise*. All vegetables and fruits, even celery sticks and spinach, contain carbohydrates that are eventually turned into glucose and which could eventually raise blood sugars. The carbohydrates in these foods, however, are released slowly, and sugar will not build up in the bloodstream if they are exercised away. That is, sugar will not build up in the bloodstream if fatty acids from eggs, meat, butter, cheese, margarine, and other fatty foods do not compete with glucose to use insulin to enter fat cells. If you eat both fruits and vegetables *and* meats and other fatty foods, or if you eat sugary foods on either diet, you gain no relative benefit; the only way you can lower your blood sugars is to eat less of everything—that is, the ADA diet. On the commonly prescribed ADA diet, you are permitted small portions of sweets (for example, a 1" slice, or 50 grams, of cake), but these foods *will* raise your blood sugars unless you exercise vigorously 90–120 minutes after eating them, not sooner, and not later. Eating a dessert today and exercising tomorrow does not help you maintain blood sugar control.

There are over 1,300 herbs and nutritional supplements that help lower blood sugars. The reason very few supplements are recommended here is that the overwhelming majority of them lower blood sugars by stimulating the pancreas to produce more insulin. Just like the sulfonylurea drugs, these natural products help control blood sugars and temporarily help prevent complications, but they accelerate the process that leads to insulin dependence. Other natural products lower blood sugars but aggravate common diabetic complications, such as gastroparesis. A few natural products lower blood sugars without increasing the production of insulin and are helpful in both type 1 and type 2 diabetes.

Alpha-lipoic acid reduces the concentration of a blood sugar byproduct known as fructosamine.[5] This chemical attaches to proteins and is a contributing factor in diabetic kidney disease. The supplement also stops the process of robbing fat cells of their sensitivity to insulin during the earlier stages of diabetes.[6] Laboratory experiments with animals have found that alpha-lipoic acid lowers blood pressure[7] and helps muscle tissues absorb glucose from the bloodstream,[8] although it is of limited benefit once insulin sensitivity has been established through exercise.[9] Alpha-lipoic acid does not interfere with medications commonly prescribed for diabetes, and can be taken in dosages of up 1,200 milligrams per day without side effects.

One of the more benign ways drugs such as Actos and Avandia lower blood sugars is by helping the body conserve its supplies of the B vitamin biotin.[10] Biotin protects beta cells in the pancreas from some of the detrimental effects of high blood sugars.[11] It may also slow the rate at which the liver releases stored sugars from glycogen,[12] and laboratory studies suggest it helps prevent neuropathy and retinopathy. Biotin works with alpha-lipoic acid to prevent the release of sugar from the liver.[13]

L-carnitine may help prevent the transmission of immune factors leading to diabetes from mother to child in breast milk.[14] (The mother takes the supplement.)

Diabetes seems to cause the body to excrete needed chromium into the urine.[15] Experiments with animals have found that supplemental chromium is especially helpful when blood sugars are especially high, so high that the body has begun to break down proteins inside cells because it cannot use insulin to transport glucose into cells. These experiments have also shown that chromium helps insulin resistance and high blood sugars caused by stress.[16]

Chromium that is derived from brewer's yeast is more beneficial than inorganic chromium.[17] Only about two out of three diabetic humans, however, benefits from taking chromium, and the supplement may prevent the production of harmful byproducts from blood sugars rather than lowering blood sugars in a way that will be noticed in blood tests.[18] The key to successful use of chromium may be making sure that the body has an adequate supply of its cofactor niacin. At least one study found that taking chromium by itself had no discernible benefit on diabetes, but taking both chromium and niacin lowered fasting blood sugars by 7 percent and reduced overall blood sugars (the total amount of glucose in the bloodstream over a 28-day period) by 15 percent—an enormous benefit.[19] Since high dosages of niacin can cause increased sensitivity to sunlight and sunburn and aggravate hot flashes or rosacea, be sure not to take more than 100 milligrams per day.

Vitamins C and E taken together help prevent injuries to muscles during exercise.[20] Vitamin E is important in preventing common diabetic complications, including atherosclerosis and neuropathy. Recent research suggests that melatonin taken in addition to vitamin E may be helpful in preventing kidney disease.[21]

Several other nutritional supplements may be helpful in some cases of diabetes. One group of clinical researchers concluded that "magnesium deficiency results in impaired insulin secretion while magnesium replacement restores insulin secretion."[22] However, magnesium cannot stimulate insulin secretion in beta cells that have been destroyed by high blood sugars, so it will not improve control over type 1 or advanced type 2 diabetes. If you have heart disease, however, magnesium is highly recommended (see ANGINA, CARDIOMYOPATHY, CONGESTIVE HEART FAILURE).

Vanadium in the form of vanadyl sulfate (50 micrograms 2 times a day) improves response to insulin in overweight, but not normal weight, diabetics.[23] Since it works by making the liver more responsive to insulin, it should be avoided by diabetics who have cirrhosis, fatty liver, or hepatitis. Milk thistle (a relatively high dose of 600 milligrams per day), however, can help relieve high blood sugars in diabetes caused by alcoholic cirrhosis of the liver.

CONCEPTS FOR COPING WITH DIABETES

○ Use glucose rather than orange juice or soft drinks to treat hypoglycemia caused by too much insulin, too much medication, or too much exercise. Glucose gel (available in tubes sold in pharmacies) can be smeared inside the mouth of a person who has passed out from low blood sugars. For a person weighing 200 pounds (90 kilograms), 15 grams of glucose, the equivalent of a tube of glucose gel or a roll of glucose tablets, is enough to raise blood sugars from the danger zone to a level supporting consciousness. Orange juice or a sugar-sweetened soft drink can be used to raise blood sugars but they do not act as quickly as glucose, and they cannot be given to someone who is unconscious.

○ Not everyone who has diabetes benefits from exercise. Generally, if your blood sugars are over 250 milligram/decilitre (13 mM), exercise will cause them to go up, not down. You need to establish basic control over your blood sugars

with diet, nutritional supplementation, and appropriate medication before beginning any exercise program.

○ Long periods of gentle exercise burn fat. Short periods of vigorous exercise trigger stress hormones that cause the liver to release more sugar than a diabetic's body can absorb. To lower blood sugars through exercise you need to exercise at your maximum capacity for at least 10–15 minutes, long enough for the body to burn the excess sugar. Once the sugar released from glycogen in the liver is used, exercise that is fast enough to make you mildly out of breath uses sugar 34 times faster than exercise that does not require heavy breathing. Since vigorous exercise can aggravate many complications of diabetes, it is essential that you stabilize your blood sugars and obtain a doctor's approval before starting heavy exercise. Since vigorous exercise can lower blood sugars very quickly, it is important that you exercise in a gym where trainers are aware of your condition and capable of giving you emergency glucose if your blood sugars fall too low.

○ Severe restriction of protein in the diet does not stop the progression of kidney disease,[24] although it may be necessary once kidney disease has occurred. It can, however, result in malnutrition.

Diabetic Complications
See **Foot Ulcers; Gastroparesis; Neuropathy; Retinopathy, Diabetic.**

Diaper Rash

SYMPTOM SUMMARY

○ Redness and irritation without crusting or skin flakes on regions of skin enclosed by a diaper

○ "Lucky Luke" pattern resembling the outline of a gun holster in babies who do not yet turn over

UNDERSTANDING THE DISEASE PROCESS

Diaper rash, for which the medical term is diaper dermatitis, is the most common skin disorder of infants in the United States. The National Ambulatory Medical Care Survey tracked 8.2 million visits to pediatricians for diaper rash during the 8 years the study was conducted.[1] While diaper rash is sometimes just an inflammatory reaction to the ammonia in urine retained by a wet diaper, persistent diaper rash is usually an overgrowth of *Candida albicans*.[2] This yeast normally inhabits healthy skin, but the conditions of warmth and moisture afforded by wet diapers give it opportunity to form an "overgrowth" on otherwise healthy skin.

The culprit in severe diaper rash is usually antibiotic treatment. Candida normally has to compete with other bacteria, such as *Peptostreptococcus* species, *Propionibacterium acnes, Staphylococcus epidermidis,* and others, for scarce resources on the skin. When competing bacteria are killed by antibiotics, *Candida* flourishes and causes diaper rash. A study of the effects of amoxicillin therapy on skin flora in infants found that during the first 3 days of antibiotic therapy counts of *Peptostreptococcus* species, *Propionibacterium acnes,* and *Staphylococcus epidermidis,* on the skin fell precipitously, while the density of yeast infection increased 14-fold. In the study, about 1 in 6 infants on amoxicillin developed diaper rash, the overgrowth of yeast continuing for about 2 weeks after the antibiotic was discontinued.[3]

When a baby is taken to the pediatrician for diaper rash, the pediatrician almost always prescribes an antifungal ointment such as betamethasone dipropionate, clotrimazole, nystatin, or triamcinolone. As a general rule, the stronger the treatment, the greater the risk of side effects. Betamethasone is a particularly potent steroid that can induce allergic reactions, which can only be diagnosed by the failure of diaper rash to heal. Betamethasone combined with clotrimazole is prescribed in 6 percent of visits to the pediatrician for diaper rash despite the fact that the manufacturer warns that it is not suitable for use in infants, specifically not suitable for diaper dermatitis.[4] Nystatin, an antifungal agent, and triamcinolone, a steroid, are provided together in prescription creams. Prolonged use of steroids retards development.

TREATMENT SUMMARY

DIET

❍ Nursing mothers should avoid cow's milk, eggs, and peanuts, and to a lesser extent, citrus fruit, while the baby has diaper's rash.

NUTRITIONAL SUPPLEMENTS

❍ *Acidophilus:* $1/8$–$1/4$ teaspoon applied to affected skin once daily after changing.

HERBS

❍ Simicort (licorice) cream, used topically.

UNDERSTANDING THE HEALING PROCESS

The key to controlling diaper rash is keeping the infant dry. Studies at the Kimberly-Clark Corporation have found that breathable diapers reduce the incidence of diaper rash by 38–50 percent. Candida colonies were two-thirds smaller when skin was covered by a breathable diaper.[6] Water-absorbent hydrogels are much more effective than petroleum jelly in relieving irritation in diaper rash and related conditions affecting adults.[7] Hydrogels, usually treated with zinc oxide, come in sheets that can be placed between the diaper and affected skin.

Babies who have persistent diaper rash may be reacting to allergens consumed by their mothers. In this case, mothers should try eliminating common food allergens, especially cow's milk, eggs, and peanuts, to see if there is improvement in the child.[8] Be careful with soy milk supplements for children. At least one study has found that infants with skin outbreaks tend to have allergies to soy.[9] If it is necessary to give formula to the baby, try formulas that are based on purified amino acids.

Probiotics such as *acidophilus* compete with *Candida* for nutrients available on the skin. Applying the probiotic directly to the skin avoids the possible complication of diarrhea if given in formula.

Simicort contains a medically useful form of licorice that keeps useful hormones from breaking down. One of the components of licorice, glycyrrhetinic acid, potentiates the effects of the natural anti-inflammatory hormone cortisol by inhibiting the enzyme 11-beta-hydroxysteroid dehydrogenase, which converts cortisol to an inactive form.[10]

CONCEPTS FOR COPING WITH DIAPER RASH

❍ Do not use Simicort with a prescription medication. Simicort increases the skin's retention of steroids made by the body itself as well as those provided by the medication with unpredictable effects.

❍ Use breathable diapers. Tight diapers or plastic bandages greatly increase the amount of the medication the baby's body absorbs.

❍ Boric acid, once a widely recommended home remedy, is not suitable for diaper rash. Even diluted boric acid washes have been known to cause diarrhea, kidney damage, and, ironically, dermatitis, in infants.

Diarrhea

SYMPTOM SUMMARY

○ Loose bowel movements

○ Frequent stools

○ Watery stools

UNDERSTANDING THE DISEASE PROCESS

Diarrhea is the passage of an increased amount of stool, usually with 3 or more bowel movements per day, or with excessively watery and unformed stools. Diarrhea may be accompanied by abdominal pain, cramping, fever, loss of appetite, and bloody or foul-smelling stools. Severe diarrhea, especially in the very young and very old, diabetics, and people who take medications for seizures, may require medical management.

Acute diarrhea is usually caused by infection, but certain foods and food additives can also trigger the condition. Sugars that are slowly absorbed, such as fructose and sorbitol, linger in the intestine and absorb water. If fructose or sorbitol consumption is the cause of diarrhea, stools will be frequent and runny but cramps, fever, and other symptoms are unlikely. Taking too much vitamin C or magnesium can cause diarrhea, as can allergies to specific foods, especially milk.

TREATMENT SUMMARY

NUTRITIONAL SUPPLEMENTS

For children's diarrhea:

○ Carob powder: $1/2$ ounce (15 grams), or approximately 2 tablespoons, mixed with applesauce or fruit for flavor.

To prevent traveler's diarrhea:

○ *Saccharomyces boulardii* (Sb): 150–500 milligrams 4 times per day, starting 3 days before travel.

To prevent recurrences of food poisoning:

○ Probiotics (*acidophilus, Bifidobacterium, Lactobacillus,* and/or *Streptococcus thermophilus*): as directed on the product label.

HERBS

For diarrhea caused by food poisoning or associated with intestinal parasites:

○ Goldenseal, barberry, coptis, or Oregon grape root: as directed on label.

For general diarrhea, traveler's diarrhea, and diarrhea caused by HIV and AIDS:

○ Sangre de grado: 125 milligrams, 4 times per day.

For cramping:

○ Chamomile: tea (made from tea bags), as desired.

For burning and irritation:

○ Slippery elm: 1 teaspoon of powdered herb in 1 cup (240 milliliters) of warm water, as often as desired.

For general diarrhea:

○ Dried (not fresh) bilberries, bilberry leaves, blackberry leaves, cranesbill, oak bark, or raspberry leaves: tea made with 1 heaping teaspoon of the herb in hot water, strained before drinking, as desired.

See Part Three if you take prescription medication.

UNDERSTANDING THE HEALING PROCESS

Mild diarrhea is often the body's way of ridding itself of food poisoning. Anything that keeps bacterial toxins inside the digestive tract prolongs other symptoms, such as cramping, fever, and abdominal pain. Taking medicines such as attapulgite (Kaopectate), bismuth subsalicylate (Pepto-Bismol), diphenoxylate (Lomotil, Lonox, Motofen), or opiates (codeine, paregoric) *before traveling* to prevent traveler's diarrhea can have the same adverse effect. When diarrhea is severe or continuous, treatment is required. A number of natural products have specific applications in treating different causes of the disease.

Carob is a gentle astringent that prevents the flow of fluids into the intestine and stops runny diarrhea. It is a traditional diarrhea treatment for children,[1] although it can also be used by adults.

A form of brewer's yeast known as *Saccharomyces boulardii* (Sb) can prevent traveler's diarrhea. It interferes with the toxic action of one of the most common causes of food poisoning, *Clostridium* bacteria,[2] and also stops diarrhea caused by other food bacteria[3] or the use of antibiotics.[4] Sb has also been found to stop diarrhea caused by ulcerative colitis and Crohn's disease.[5]

Other bacteria are especially useful in preventing recurrences of food poisoning. Diarrhea flushes both toxins and protective bacteria out of the intestine. Microorganisms that compete with and destroy the bacteria that cause diarrhea are replenished by probiotics such as *acidophilus, Bifidobacterium, Lactobacillus,* and *Streptococcus thermophilus.* [6]

Sb is a safe supplement, but there have been four cases of fungal infection after taking the supplement—all of them through contamination of a catheter after urination or defecation of the microorganism. There is one report of meningitis caused by *Bifidobacterium* in an infant. There have been a few cases of fungal infection after taking *Lactobacillus,* all of them in conjunction with an underlying health condition, that is, cancer, diabetes, or recent surgery.

Goldenseal, barberry, coptis, and Oregon grape root contain berberine, a potent antibacterial that can be used to control diarrhea caused by food poisoning. Berberine does not stop diarrhea immediately. The body still has to expel the toxins created by the food-borne bacteria even after the bacterial infection is controlled. Scientific study has found that berberine kills the organism that causes cholera, and stops *E. coli* bacteria from attaching themselves to the lining of the intestine. It also slows the growth of the microorganisms that cause giardiasis and leishmaniasis, tropic waterborne infections that frequently cause persistent diarrhea.[7]

The content of berberine in different formulations of these herbs varies from brand to brand, so it is necessary to follow label directions. An appropriate dosage of any herb that contains berberine is enough of the herb to provide 400 milligrams of berberine a day. In overdose, berberine can cause constipation, heartburn, shortness of breath, and flulike symptoms. Pregnant women should not take berberine, because it can stimulate uterine contractions. Infants should not be given herbs that contain berberine by mouth, because it can cause jaundice. Coptis powders in diapers are acceptable.

The latex of the rainforest herb sangre de grado has been clinically demonstrated to treat general diarrhea, traveler's diarrhea, and diarrhea caused by HIV and AIDS. Except in HIV and AIDS, 125 milligrams taken 4 times a day is enough and larger amounts do not offer additional relief. In HIV and AIDS, 500–700 milligrams of the herb taken 4 times a day is needed to control loose stools. This rainforest herb is especially useful in controlling diarrhea caused by eating meat contaminated with *E. coli.*[8]

Dried bilberries, bilberry leaves,[9] blackberry leaves, cranesbill, oak bark,[10] and raspberry leaves[11] all contain tannins that stop the leakage of fluids into the intestine and gradually "dry up" runny diarrhea. (Never use *fresh* bilberries to treat diarrhea; they may make diarrhea worse.) Chamomile teas made with hot (not boiling) water release an essential oil that stops cramping.[12]

Slippery elm bark contains an abundance of complex carbohydrates. Taken by mouth, this herb triggers a reflex causing the stomach to produce large quantities of mucus to coat and protect the entire digestive tract.[13] This dilutes the mucus reaching the skin around the anus and reduces irritation. Since slippery elm bark is a food as well as an herb, it is completely nontoxic.

CONCEPTS FOR COPING WITH DIARRHEA

❍ At least one clinical study has found that acupuncture is nearly twice as effective as antibiotics in treating diarrhea in infants.[14] *Gently* rubbing the Zu San Li point, the site most commonly used for acupuncture treatment of diarrhea, found at the front of the leg just below the knee, may also help.

❍ If you frequently experience diarrhea after drinking milk or eating dairy products, you may be lactose intolerant. Lactaid is an over-the-counter product that may reduce diarrhea caused by eating or drinking dairy foods and other products containing milk sugars, including convenience foods and medications. It treats an enzyme deficiency for milk sugar rather than an allergy to milk. To determine if Lactaid may be helpful to you, eat a normal breakfast and include a large, 12-ounce glass of milk of any kind. Over the next 6 hours, keep track of any discomfort you may have (if you experience any kind of severe reaction, consult a physician). The next day, prepare an identical breakfast with another 12-ounce glass of milk. Swallow a Lactaid tablet with your first sip of milk. If your symptoms are not as bad on the second day, Lactaid may be beneficial for you.

❍ Colostrum (from cows immunized for rotavirus) has been shown to treat diarrhea in children infected with rotavirus.[15] Colostrum (from cows exposed to the disease bacteria) has successfully treated diarrhea caused by *Clostridium, Crytosporidium, E. coli,* and *Helicobacter.* Commerically available colostrum, however, is not likely to have the same effect. For infants with viral diarrhea, probiotics or synbiotics containing *Bifidobacterium bifidus* and *Streptococcus thermophilus* are more likely to be helpful.[16] For infants and small children with other forms of infectious diarrhea, nine clinical studies confirm that *Lactobacillus* is both safe and effective.[17]

❍ An extraordinarily large number of South American herbs treat diarrhea, including abuta, acerola, ageratum, amargo, amor seco, bold, cajueiro, calumba, carapia, carqueja, chanca piedra, chuchuhuasi, copaiba, epazote, fedegosa, gervão, graviola, guacatong, guajava, guaraná, guava, iporuru, jatoba, mango, marcuja, mullaca, mutamba, papay, pedra huma-caa, periwinkle, picao preto, simaruba, tayuya, tiririca, tumeric, and vassourinha. Several of these herbs, especially simaruba, are useful in treating difficult cases of diarrhea contracted during travel to the tropics, such as amoebic dysentery. For more information on how to use these herbs, and for supplies of hard-to-get tropical herbs, see www.rain-tree.com or contact Raintree Nutrition in Austin, Texas.

❍ There are a number of homeopathic remedies for diarrhea. Usually it is best to start with a single dose of the lowest strength (6C, 6X, or 12C) of the remedy matching the symptoms to be treated, and then wait for a response. If there is an improvement in symptoms, let the remedy continue to work until there is no more improvement, then take another dose. If there is no improvement, try a different potency (30X or 30C). Sometimes homeopathic medicines work for a few minutes, and sometimes they work for an entire day before another dose is needed.

• Argentum nitricum, or homeopathic silver nitrate, treats diarrhea associated with nervous tension, such as a school exam or giving a speech. It is also recommended for diarrhea accompanied by bloating and flatulence, or occurring after eating too much sugar.

• Arsenicum album is recommended for diarrhea accompanied by a burning sensation in the digestive tract. Simultaneous diarrhea and vomiting is treated with this remedy, as is food poisoning.

• Bryonia treats diarrhea accompanying the flu, especially diarrhea that is worse in the morning.

• Chamomilla treats abdominal cramping and gas with hot, green, runny diarrhea.

• Colocynthis treats diarrhea that follows sharp abdominal pain that is relieved by bending over at the waist. Do not use homeopathy to treat abdominal pain that is not accompanied by diarrhea. Seek medical attention if abdominal pain is not quickly relieved by passing stool.

• Ipecacuanha is a homeopathic preparation of ipecac, the medication used to treat certain kinds of poisoning by inducing vomiting. In homeopathic doses, ipecac stops vomiting as well as diarrhea accompanying it.

• Phosphorus relieves continuous diarrhea accompanied by thirst.

• Podophyllum treats diarrhea with rumbling stomach and abdominal gurgling. Homeopaths recommend it for stomach upset occurring in hot weather and for diarrhea that is worse in the morning.

• Pulsatilla treats diarrhea following consumption of fatty foods.

• Sulfur stops hot, burning, urgent diarrhea, especially in people who have hemorrhoids.

Digestive Problems
See **Bloating; Flatulence; Heartburn; Peptic Ulcer Disease.**

Diphtheria

SYMPTOM SUMMARY

❍ Thick, gray, and attached membrane over the tonsils and throat

❍ Fever

❍ Sore throat

❍ Swollen lymph nodes

❍ Sometimes only causes ulcers on the skin

After recovery:

❍ Hoarseness

❍ Infection of heart muscle

❍ Membranes obstructing airways

UNDERSTANDING THE DISEASE PROCESS

Diphtheria is a bacterial disease that can infect the throat (respiratory diphtheria) or the skin (cutaneous diphtheria). A common childhood disease before World War II, mandatory vaccination has made the condition very rare in the United States and most developed nations today. In 1993 and 1994, there was a serious outbreak of diphtheria in countries of the former Soviet Union, with more than 50,000 cases reported. There also have been a few very isolated cases in the United States, most recently among some Northern Plains Indian populations.

The bacterium that causes diphtheria is spread from person to person by contact with microscopic droplets of saliva and mucus suspended in the air after uncovered coughs and sneezes. In its early stages, diphtheria can be mistaken for a bad sore throat. As the disease progresses, it releases a toxin that causes a fuzzy gray membrane to cover the tonsils and throat. This membrane interferes with breathing. In severe cases, children who have diphtheria can have trouble with both breathing and swallowing and have rapid heartbeat, slurred speech, and pale or bluish skin from oxygen deprivation.

Diphtheria is seldom life-threatening, although it can cause serious complications. Although medically treated diphtheria almost never results in death, the mortality rate among unvaccinated children is 10 times higher than among children who have had their DPT shots.

TREATMENT SUMMARY

To increase the effectiveness of DPT vaccination:

❍ Vitamin A: 25,000 IU administered once, at the same time as the vaccination.

To lower the risk of cardiac complications:

❍ L-carnitine: 100 milligrams twice a day for 5 days.

See Part Three if you take prescription medication.

UNDERSTANDING THE HEALING PROCESS

Modern complementary healthcare in the United States has very little experience with diphtheria. It is known that giving a child 200 milligrams of L-carnitine for 5 days greatly reduces the risk of infection in the heart muscle,[1] and that giving an infant 25,000 IU of vitamin A at the same time as their DPT vaccination confers greater immunity to the disease.[2]

CONCEPTS FOR COPING WITH DIPHTHERIA

❍ In addition to L-carnitine, homeopathic physicians may be able to suggest effective treatments for child-

hood diphtheria. Tests sponsored by the US Army found that exposure to homeopathic doses of diphtheria toxin would be useful if diphtheria toxin were used in bioterrorism.[3] Before the introduction of antibiotics, homeopathic remedies offered the best treatment of diphtheria and significantly lowered rates of mortality and complications.[4]

Discoid Lupus Erythematosus
See **Lupus.**

Diverticulitis and Diverticulosis

SYMPTOM SUMMARY

❍ Abdominal cramps

❍ Bloating

❍ Constipation

❍ Fever and chills

❍ Nausea

UNDERSTANDING THE DISEASE PROCESS

In diverticular disease, portions of the colon form pouches. The development of these pouches is caused by diverticulosis. Inflammation of the pouches is called diverticulitis.

The pouches form as a result of straining to pass a hard, dry stool. Pressure from straining at stool causes the pouches to form at weak points in the wall of the colon. The pouches themselves do not necessarily cause any symptoms, but if fecal matter collects in them, they can become infected and inflamed.

Diverticulitis usually clears up on its on. Continued straining at stool can cause blood vessels in the pouches in the lining of the colon to break and bleed. If an abscess forms in the lining of the colon, however, feces and pus can flow into the pelvic or stomach area and cause a potentially life-threatening condition known as peritonitis. Bleeding or severe abdominal cramps are always indications of the need for immediate medical attention.

TREATMENT SUMMARY

DIET

○ Gradually increase the amount of fiber in your diet so that you eat 5–9 servings of fruit and vegetables every day. Raw fruits and vegetables are preferable. Almonds, dried beans and peas, raw root vegetables (carrots, jicama, radishes, and turnip roots), dried pumpkin and sunflower seeds, whole-grain breads, oranges, apricots, prunes, and unpeeled apples are especially good sources of soluble fiber.

○ Avoid sugar.

○ Drink 8 or more glasses of water every day.

○ Avoid large, heavy meals. Eating smaller portions more often reduces the amount of food that has to pass through the colon at any one time.

○ Avoid milk, wheat products, and beef.

NUTRITIONAL SUPPLEMENTS

○ Fiber: 1–2 tablespoons of insoluble (psyllium) or soluble (orange pulp) fiber taken with a glass of water, daily. Do not take fiber at the same time you take nutritional supplements or medications.

○ Glucomannan: 3–4 grams daily.

See Part Three if you take prescription medication.

UNDERSTANDING THE HEALING PROCESS

The most useful thing you can do to heal diverticulitis is to treat constipation. Drink more water. Eat more fiber. And if you take supplemental fiber, make sure it contains cellulose. A study of 43,881 American male healthcare professionals found that taking fiber with cellulose cut the risk of developing diverticular disease in half.[1]

Glucomannan is a water-soluble fiber extracted from the konjac root. It is also found in dates. Unlike other kinds of fiber, glucomannan is a laxative. That is, it both adds bulk to the stool and increases the urge to have a bowel movement. It also reduces the appetite, lowers LDL cholesterol, and encourages weight loss.

Clinical studies have found that only about 40 percent of people who take 2 grams of glucomannan a day have fewer attacks of diverticulitis,[2] but there are two things you can do to make glucomannan more effective. One is to increase the dose. Some studies have found that 3 grams is a more effective dosage for relieving constipation.[3] The other is to eat yogurt or to take probiotics such as *acidophilus* or *Lactobacillus*. Konjac fiber is broken down in the intestine by these friendly bacteria.[4]

Never take glucomannan just before going to bed. Always take this supplement with at least a glass of water. Taking glucomannan with too little water to chase it down can cause it to swell before it reaches the intestines. In a few cases, glucomannan has swollen and blocked the throat. Tablet forms of glucomannan should be avoided, since they tend to absorb water and swell in a single location in the intestine, possibly causing a blockage.

CONCEPTS FOR COPING WITH DIVERTICULAR DISEASE

○ Repeated attacks of diverticulitis, while extremely uncomfortable, are not usually associated with severe complications. A modern medical perspective on frequent attacks of the disease is that they should not be treated with surgery unless complications arise.[5]

○ Diverticulosis on the right side of the colon is unusually common in China. Among ethnic Chinese, the single strongest lifestyle factor in predicting diverticular disease is meat consumption. Chinese people who eat the most meat are nearly 25 times more likely to develop diverticular disease than Chinese people who eat the least meat. For reasons that are not yet understood, among Chinese people, vegetable or fruit consumption frequency, laxative use, supplemental fiber intake, smoking, and family history seem to have no relevance to diverticular disease.[6]

Down Syndrome

SYMPTOM SUMMARY

○ Flattened nose, protruding tongue, and upward-slanting eyes

○ Physical and mental developmental delays

UNDERSTANDING THE DISEASE PROCESS

Down syndrome is the most common birth defect, occurring in approximately 1 in 660 births. This well-known condition is caused by the presence of a third copy of chromosome 21, and usually, although not invariably, results in mental retardation and other problems.

TREATMENT SUMMARY

NUTRITIONAL SUPPLEMENTS

○ Acetyl-L-carnitine: up to 2,000 milligrams per day, initial dosage chosen in consultation with the child's physician.

See the Drug Interactions Guide if prescription medications are taken.

UNDERSTANDING THE HEALING PROCESS

Nutritional therapy cannot reverse Down syndrome, but supplementation with acetyl-L-carnitine during the first 5 years of life may greatly relieve learning disabilities. Carnitine is responsible for several chemical processes, including the metabolism of cholesterol in the linings of brain cells, the transfer of electrical signals between nerves, and protection against nerve tissue damage by free radicals of oxygen. Children with Down syndrome tend to have L-carnitine deficiencies during the first 5 years of life, gradually correcting themselves by age 13.[1] In an Italian study, Down syndrome children given acetyl-L-carnitine supplements for 90 days showed significant improvement in visual memory and attention.[2]

Children on seizure medications may need especially high doses of acetyl-L-carnitine, so the initial dosage is best chosen in consultation with the child's physician. Doctors usually recommend 100 milligrams per day for every kilogram (2.2 pounds) of the child's body weight, up to a maximum of 2,000 milligrams per day. It is important to use acetyl-L-carnitine, a chemically modified form of L-carnitine that is more readily absorbed by the brain.

CONCEPTS FOR COPING WITH DOWN SYNDROME

○ Children with Down Syndrome tend to have slow metabolisms and to burn fewer calories than children who do not have the condition. Children with Down

syndrome are as active as their peers *yet use fewer calories overall,* primarily because they use less energy when they are resting or sleeping. Down children have a natural tendency to be overweight. Since nutrient deficiency is possible when calories are restricted, parents of Down children should encourage physical exercise to help the child maintain normal weight.

Duchenne Muscular Dystrophy

SYMPTOM SUMMARY
○ Muscle weakness

UNDERSTANDING THE DISEASE PROCESS

Duchenne muscular dystrophy is one of the most common progressive childhood genetic disorders in the world, affecting approximately 1 in every 3,500 male newborns worldwide. Boys with Duchenne dystrophy develop difficulty walking and begin falling due to muscle weakness as toddlers, and by 8–10 years of age the muscle weakness has progressed to the point where most are wheelchair bound. By their late teens, most DMD children have succumbed to their disease, usually as victims of respiratory failure.

TREATMENT SUMMARY

NUTRITIONAL SUPPLEMENTS

○ Creatine*

○ Glutamine*

○ L-acetyl-carnitine*

*Do not use supplements in Duchenne muscular dystrophy without consulting a physician and/or pharmacist.

UNDERSTANDING THE HEALING PROCESS

As this book is being written in late 2002, the Cooperative International Neuromuscular Research Group is beginning clinical trials of combinations of the supplements creatine, glutamine, and L-acetyl-carnitine as an intervention in Duchenne muscular dystrophy. Experiments with animals used as a model of Duchenne dystrophy have found that creatine encourages regeneration of muscle tissue and improves energy metabolism within muscle cells.[1] Clinical studies have found that Duchenne dystrophy interferes with muscle cells' ability to absorb the "nonessential" amino acid glutamine, making it an "essential" amino acid in this condition.[2] Duchenne dystrophy also interferes with the body's use of L-carnitine,[3] essential for healthy heart function.

CONCEPTS FOR COPING WITH DUCHENNE MUSCULAR DYSTROPHY

○ Results of the supplementation trials for Duchenne dystrophy may not be available until 2005. For the latest information on the use of these nutritional aids, visit the website of the Muscular Dystrophy Association at www.mdausa.org.

Duhring's Disease

See **Dermatitis Herpetiformis**.

Duodenal Ulcer

See **Peptic Ulcer Disease**.

Dupuytren's Contracture

SYMPTOM SUMMARY

○ Small lump in the palm, usually in the crease of the hand closest to the ring and little fingers

○ As the disease progresses, the affected finger is drawn toward the palm

UNDERSTANDING THE DISEASE PROCESS

Dupuytren's contracture (named after a nineteenth-century French baron) is a condition caused by the cumulative thickening of muscle fibers in the palm. Biochemical changes cause the fibroblasts, cells that produce flexible collagen for the skin, to become myofibroblasts, cells that produce "tough" collagen for muscle. The misplaced collagen forms a small lump in the palm and eventually causes a finger or fingers to be drawn inward.

Dupuytren's contracture can involve one or both hands and eventually the toes, although it tends to appear after age 50 and develop slowly. It is not usually related to injury. The condition is more common in men than women, usually strikes people of northern European descent, and is associated with habits and diseases that cause chronic vitamin deficiencies, such as alcoholism, cigarette smoking, diabetes, or treatment with seizure medications.[1]

TREATMENT SUMMARY

NUTRITIONAL SUPPLEMENTS

○ Vitamin E: 800 IU daily.

HERBS

○ *Hochu-ekki-to* (Japanese herbal formula): as directed on the label.

UNDERSTANDING THE HEALING PROCESS

The current understanding of Dupuytren's contracture is that it is a disorder of collagen production resulting from misdirected biological signals. Abnormalities in the production of blood-clotting agents, among other factors, signal the tissues in the palm that they need to become "tougher." The immune system can slow the process by releasing a chemical known as interferon gamma, "interfering" with the production of unnecessary collagen.[2]

Vitamin E has a well-known effect on blood clotting, making the blood more slippery. Three British researchers in the 1950s tried treating Dupuytren's contracture with vitamin E alone. A dose corresponding to 667 IU a day for 10 months produced moderate improvements in contraction.[3] A dose corresponding to 444 IU a day for 3 months produced no changes.[4] Vitamin E should be regarded as helping rather than curing the condition, perhaps delaying the need for surgery.

Although Dupuytren's contracture is very rare in Japan, the Japanese herbal formula *hochu-ekki-to* has been used for centuries to treat similar conditions. According to traditional East Asian medicine, a condition such as Dupuytren's contracture results from a deficiency of *ki* (life force) in the "earth" organs, the spleen (digestive function) and stomach. When the person has become "ungrounded" from healthy habits regarding diet, exercise, or thought, the spleen and stomach lose their capacity to generate needed energies. Since these organs supply energy to the muscles and the flesh, deficiency in them makes the arms and legs flabby and weak or fibrous and lifeless. The masters of East Asian herbal medicine devised this formula nearly 1,000 years ago to correct this pattern.

The analogy of alcoholism and cigarette smoking to becoming "ungrounded" from healthy habits does not offer a theoretical scientific rationale for using the treatment. Laboratory study, however, does. Japanese studies have found that *hochu-ekki-to* stimulates the production of interferon gamma in the bone marrow, liver, and spleen in laboratory animals.[5] Since interferon gamma slows the biochemical changes that induce Dupuytren's contracture, it is possible that future studies will confirm a similar effect in humans.

Brands of *hochu-ekki-to* available in the United States include:

- Added Flavors Supplement the Center & Boost Qi (Blue Poppy Herbs)
- Arouse Vigor (Kan Herbals)
- Breaking Clouds (Three Treasures)
- Bu Zhong Yi Qi Tang (Asian Patents, Blue Poppy Herbs, Chinese Classics, Golden Flower Chinese Herbs, Health Concerns, Kan Herbals, Lotus Classics, ProBotanixx, Qualiherb, Sun Ten, Three Treasures)
- Central Chi Tea (Asian Patents)
- Ginseng & Astragalus (Qualiherb)
- Ginseng & Astragalus Combination (Sun Ten)
- Ginseng & Astragalus Formula (Golden Flower Chinese Herbs)
- Hochuekkito Formula 017 (Kampo Institute)
- Raise Qi (Health Concerns)
- Tonify Qi & Ease the Muscles (Three Treasures)
- Yi Qi (Probotanixx)

CONCEPTS FOR COPING WITH DUPUYTREN'S CONTRACTURE

○ The general rule for surgery for Dupuytren's contracture is better sooner than later. The best results are obtained with early treatment.

Dyslexia

SYMPTOM SUMMARY

○ Difficulty determining the main idea of a written sentence

○ Difficulty learning to recognize written words

○ Difficulty rhyming

UNDERSTANDING THE DISEASE PROCESS

Dyslexia is an innate difficulty in mastering language. The condition results in an inability to recognize letters, numbers, and words rapidly; confusion between left and right; difficulty understanding spoken words; and, sometimes, poor muscular coordination. Dyslexia affects about 1 in 10 children in the United States, Canada, and the United Kingdom. About 1 in 25 children has dyslexia so severely that he or she cannot learn in an ordinary classroom setting. The condition is more common in boys than in girls.[1]

In dyslexia the left side of the brain is deprived of its advantages in processing verbal information. People with normal abilities to understand language tend to process concepts on the left side of the brain and to process images and feelings on the right side of the brain. People who have dyslexia do not have an advantage in verbal processing in the left brain.

Dyslexia also affects the eyes. In dyslexia, the eyes do not keep a focus on written words. Normally, the eye's magnocellular system moves the gaze in an orderly fashion across the printed page. If a letter or word is skipped, the muscles of the eye move its focus back to missing information. In dyslexics, the eyes may not be coordinated, or the magnocellular system may not work, so that letters appear to move or float out of sequence.[2]

TREATMENT SUMMARY

NUTRITIONAL SUPPLEMENTS

○ Docahexaenoic acid (DHA): 500 milligrams per day for children under 12; 1,000–2,000 milligrams daily for adults.

UNDERSTANDING THE HEALING PROCESS

Scientists believe that at least in adults, defects in the magnocellular system in the eyes is associated with a deficiency of essential fatty acids. The greater the deficiency, the worse the symptoms of dyslexia. Severe fatty acid deficiencies in adults with dyslexia manifest themselves not only as problems with reading and writing, but also with understanding spoken words.[3] Inherited metabolic defects in processing essential fatty acids seem to debilitate the eyes' magnocellular system, crippling their ability to process fast, changing information from the visual world.[4]

There are very strong indications that supplying the

body with more essential fatty acids can compensate for defects in the way it processes them. A scientific study has concluded that boys with better reading and math skills have higher bloodstream concentrations of DHA than boys with poorer reading and math skills,[5] and small-scale clinical studies have confirmed that taking DHA improves athletic skills[6] and night vision in children with dyslexia.[7]

As this book is being written, testing is underway in the United Kingdom to see if taking DHA has a direct and measurable effects on academic skills. The researchers plan to study 120 dyslexic English children who will be given either a fatty acid supplement or a placebo for a period of 6 months. Each child will be given a breath test for abnormalities in fatty acid metabolism before and after treatment, and standard measures of attention, visual perception, and motor control will be recorded. This will be the first good indication of whether DHA helps dyslexics in the classroom. It is already known that DHA helps dyslexics function better outside the classroom.

People who have hemophilia and people who take blood-thinning medications should not take DHA. Otherwise, adverse reactions to this supplement are very rare, although some people experience "fishy" breath and diarrhea when first taking it.

Dyslipidemia
See **High Cholesterol; High Triglycerides.**

Dysmenorrhea

SYMPTOM SUMMARY

○ Pain beginning 24 hours before and lasting 72 hours after menstruation

○ May be accompanied by:

- Backache
- Cramping
- Diarrhea
- Dizziness or fainting spells
- Headache
- Nausea and vomiting
- Pain radiating down to anterior thigh

UNDERSTANDING THE DISEASE PROCESS

Menstrual cramps are an extremely common condition. Approximately 2 in 5 women in the United States experiences menstrual cramps for 2–3 days every month, and 1 in 10 women has to take time away from regular daily activities because of menstrual pain.[1] Menstrual cramps may be caused by primary or secondary dysmenorrhea. Primary dysmenorrhea is the result of the accumulation of inflammatory hormones called prostaglandins during the menstrual cycle. Prostaglandins cause constriction of the blood vessels in the lining of the uterus and rhythmic contraction with the pulsing of blood. Most women are more sensitive to pain during the middle of their menstrual cycles and less sensitive to pain during their period, due to the action of estrogen. Women who suffer menstrual cramps may lack a sensitivity to estrogen causing them to lack pain protection during their period.[2]

Secondary dysmenorrhea combines the effects of excess prostaglandins with pain from endometriosis or uterine injury. Primary dysmennorhea usually begins in the late teens or early 20s. Secondary dysmenorrhea usually first occurs when a menstrual cycle occurs without ovulation, that is, its underlying cause is uterine injury but it does not occur until a woman starts using the Pill. It is important to distinguish dysmenorrhea from appendicitis, ectopic pregnancy, endometriosis, ovarian cysts, ovarian torsion, and pelvic inflammatory disease. Pain that regularly occurs shortly before to shortly after the period is most likely to be dysmenorrhea.

TREATMENT SUMMARY

DIET

○ Avoid fatty foods and sugar.

NUTRITIONAL SUPPLEMENTS

○ Calcium: at least 1,200 milligrams per day.

○ Fish oil: 5 grams per day (optional).

HERBS

○ *Toki-shakuyaku-san* (Japanese herbal remedy), fennel seed oil, black cohosh, blue cohosh, and corydalis.

UNDERSTANDING THE HEALING PROCESS

Bestselling diet author Dr. Barry Sears suggests that the formation of inflammatory prostaglandins can be controlled by a "zone diet," especially with fish oil supplements. There is some research confirming that limiting simple sugars and consuming essential fatty acids on a regular basis could be useful in preventing menstrual cramps.

Calcium is a simple and effective treatment for menstrual cramps. Researchers at Columbia University found that taking 1,200 milligrams of calcium daily reduced reported menstrual cramps by 48 percent in a group of 500 women, although the full effects of calcium supplementation took 2–3 months.[3] Earlier studies by some of the same researchers found that calcium also relieves water retention and depression.[4] Since calcium is useful in preventing or treating many other conditions, almost every woman can benefit from calcium supplements. The Columbia University researchers used calcium carbonate, although there are numerous anecdotal reports that calcium citrate (the form of calcium recommended for preventing osteoporosis) also reduces cramping.

The herbal remedy with the clearest scientific explanation for treating menstrual cramps is the Japanese herbal remedy known as *toki-shakuyaku-san.* Laboratory studies in Japan have confirmed that this mixture of dong quai and peony stops the production of the prostaglandins that cause the blood vessels in the uterus to cramp. The formula is widely available in the United States and Canada under several trade names:

- Dang Gui & Peony (Qualiherb)
- Kampo4Women MenopauEase (Honso)
- Tangkuei & Peony Formula (Lotus Classics)
- Tang-Kuei and Peony Formula (Golden Flower Chinese Herbs, Sun Ten)
- Toki-shakuyaku-san (Honso, Tsumura)

Another herb that has a clear scientific backing for use in treating menstrual cramps is fennel seed oil. Research at the University of Tehran has found that it stops uterine contractions that cause cramping and pain, although it does not improve circulation within the uterus.[5]

Always dilute fennel seed oil in water or a tea. Drunk without dilution, fennel seed oil can cause heartburn or gas, although in a tea it stops heartburn or gas. Fennel seed teas, while effective, work more slowly.

Other herbs are somewhat less reliably useful for treating menstrual pain. Both black cohosh and the unrelated blue cohosh are traditional remedies for men-

strual cramping. Neither herb should be used during pregnancy. Corydalis contains tetrahydropalmatine, a potent analgesic and sedative. It is better to use buffered, standardized herbal formulas containing corydalis rather than the herb itself. A widely available preparation of corydalis is the Chinese herbal remedy An Zhong San, which combines corydalis and fennel. An Zhong San relieves menstrual cramping along with a variety of "abdominal" symptoms, such as bloating, diarrhea, and gastritis. Common brand names of An Zhong San in the United States and Canada include:

- An Zhong San (KPC Herbs, Lotus Classics, Qualiherb, Sun Ten)
- Anchu-san (Honso, Tsumura)
- Cardamon & Fennel (Qualiherb)
- Cardamon & Fennel Formula (Sun Ten)
- Fennel & Galanga Formula (KPC Herbs, Lotus Classics)

Avoid herbal formulas that combine corydalis with California poppy since they may increase, rather than decrease, uterine contractions.

The remedy for menstrual pain in Native American herbal medicine is the aptly named crampbark, also known as viburnum. This herb relieves severe cramps that are associated with nausea, vomiting, and sweaty chills. Use crampbark tinctures as directed on the label. Traditional healers in the United States also often recommend tinctures of false unicorn root or vervain. Both herbs have a long history of successful use, although neither has been verified through scientific study.

CONCEPTS FOR COPING WITH MENSTRUAL CRAMPS

❏ Teenaged girls with menstrual cramps may benefit from taking vitamin E.[6] Start 400 IU of vitamin E 2 days before the period and continue for 5 days.

❏ B vitamins are useful in treating many aspects of PMS, but they do not relieve menstrual cramps.

❏ Secondhand tobacco smoke increases the rate of menstrual cramps, as does exposure to dirt, dust, toxic chemicals, and noise. A study of women in China by the Harvard School of Public Health found that exposure to just 3 cigarettes a day may increase a woman's probability of experiencing menstrual cramps in any given month by up to 800 percent.[7]

○ Many chiropractors apply high-velocity, low-amplitude (HVLA) treatments to the lower back to treat menstrual cramps. Chiropractic manipulation is thought to minimize back pain that is felt in the abdomen even though it originates in the spine. It is also thought to increase blood supply to the uterus so that blood vessels in the uterus do not constrict as severely. A review of the research literature has found that 3 out of 4 clinical trials find a small benefit in chiropractic manipulation, although a simple back rub is also effective.[8]

○ Women who suffer social or personal loss are more likely to experience menstrual pain. Having access to a social support network reduces menstrual pain.[9]

○ Acupuncture may be helpful in treating menstrual cramps. A Chinese study found that 42 out of 49 women treated with acupuncture were free of pain for 3 consecutive months.[10]

○ There are a number of homeopathic remedies for menstrual cramps. Usually it is best to start with a single dose of the lowest strength (6C, 6X, or 12C) of the remedy matching the symptoms to be treated, and then wait for a response. If there is an improvement in symptoms, let the remedy continue to work until there is no more improvement, then take another dose. If there is no improvement, try a different potency (30X or 30C). Sometimes homeopathic medicines work for a few minutes, and sometimes they work for an entire day before another dose is needed.

• Belladonna is recommended when the menstrual period comes early and brings a flow of bright, red blood. Menstrual cramps may be accompanied by a sensation of heat. The woman who most benefits from homeopathic belladonna has symptoms that would be caused by an overdose of the herb belladonna, pounding or throbbing sensations, racing pulse, and eyes that are sensitive to light.

• Bovista treats menstrual cramps that occur with fluid retention, weight gain, and puffiness. Women who have diarrhea at their periods are especially likely to benefit from this remedy.

• Caulophyllum treats menstrual cramps in women who have irregular periods. Pain radiating to the lower back and legs and flare-ups of arthritis are strong indications for this remedy.

• Cimicifuga is a homeopathic preparation of black cohosh most suitable for women who experience shooting pains in the neck or back, or acne or other skin outbreaks during their period.

• Cocculus treats menstrual cramps accompanied by insomnia. The woman most likely to benefit from this remedy may experience a "hollow" feeling in the lower abdomen along with nausea and/or vomiting.

• Colocynthis is recommended when menstrual cramps are worsened by personal loss or emotional upset. Homeopathic physicians often recommend this remedy when menstrual pain is relieved by leaning forward or bending over.

• Lachesis is used when cramping is worst just before the period and is relieved when the menstrual flow starts. Discomfort when wearing belts or necklaces is another indication for this remedy.

• Lilllium tigrinum is recommended for women who tend to enforce household rules with severity during their period. The physical symptoms it treats include a feeling that the uterus is falling, and discomfort that is relieved by crossing the legs at the knees.

• Magnesia phosphorica treats menstrual pain accompanying a dark discharge containing mucus. The period may start too early, and there may be special sensitivity to cold or painful stimulation of the skin.

• Nux vomica relieves pain that is worst just above the tailbone. Strong reaction to overindulgence in food or alcohol is another indication for this remedy.

• Pulsatilla, also known as silverweed, is most frequently recommended to girls who have just started their periods. Clotting in the discharge, sensitivity to heat, and irritability are also indications for pulsatilla.

• Sepia is used when the period comes late. It is also helpful when symptoms are relieved by a warm bath or moist heat.

• Veratrum album treats heavy periods causing cramps. Discomfort treated by this remedy is worst during cold weather and at night.

E. coli Infection

SYMPTOM SUMMARY

○ Diarrhea and/or fever after eating unwashed vegetables or undercooked beef

UNDERSTANDING THE DISEASE PROCESS

E. coli is an infectious bacterium that enters food through contamination with human or animal fecal waste. Infection with *E. coli* often leads to bloody diarrhea, and occasionally to kidney failure. The Centers for Disease Control estimate that 73,000 people are infected with *E. coli* every year. Approximately 1 in 1,000 cases ends in kidney failure and death.

By far the most common contaminated food is hamburger meat. Person-to-person contact in families and child care centers is also an important mode of transmission. Infection may occur after drinking raw milk and after swimming in or drinking sewage-contaminated water.

TREATMENT SUMMARY

NUTRITIONAL SUPPLEMENTS

❍ *Lactobacillus:* 1 or 2 capsules, 2–3 times a week on an ongoing basis.

UNDERSTANDING THE HEALING PROCESS

The best defense against *E. coli* is *Lactobacillus,* the healthy bacteria that normally reside in the human intestine. Lactobacilli secrete enzymes that interfere with *E. coli*'s ability to use simple sugars, and other chemicals that keep *E. coli* from "rooting" in the intestinal wall.[1]

Lactobacillus has to be in the intestine before *E. coli,* otherwise the secretions of the two competing strains of bacteria can cause diarrhea. The best approach is to eat yogurt or to take 1 or 2 capsules of *Lactobacillus* concentrate on a daily basis.

CONCEPTS FOR COPING WITH *E. COLI*

❍ Most people infected with *E. coli* recover without antibiotics or other specific medical treatment in 5–10 days. There is no scientific evidence that antibiotics improve the course of disease, and it is even thought that treatment with some antibiotics may precipitate kidney complications. Antidiarrheal agents, such as loperamide (Imodium), "lock in" *E. coli* infection and should also be avoided.

❍ To avoid *E. coli* infection:

• Cook hamburger and ground beef thoroughly. Ground meats can turn brown before disease-causing bacteria are killed, so use a digital instant-read meat thermometer to ensure the thickest part of the patty has been heated to at least 160°F. If you do not use a meat thermometer, avoid eating ground meat that is still pink. If you are served a rare hamburger in a restaurant, return the meat and ask that it be reheated and placed on a fresh bun with fresh condiments.

• In the kitchen, keep raw meat separate from ready-to-eat foods. Wash utensils, counters, plates, and hands with hot, soapy water after they touch raw meat.

• Avoid unpasteurized milk and juices, as well as alfalfa sprouts.

• Be sure to wash fruits and vegetables, especially if they are to be eaten raw.

• Avoid swallowing lake or pool water while swimming.

• Make sure children (or adults) with diarrhea wash their hands thoroughly in warm, soapy water after using the bathroom. Anyone with diarrhea should avoid swimming in a public pool, sharing a bath or shower, and preparing food for others.

• Keep fingernails trimmed. Dr. Michael Doyle and his team at the University of Georgia put hamburger contaminated with *E. coli* under the nails of volunteers. The subjects then washed their hands thoroughly, and the researchers measured how much bacteria was left. They found that volunteers who used nail brushes had the fewest bacteria. However, if the volunteers had long fingernails, even nail brushes weren't effective for cleaning contamination from the hands.

❍ See also DIARRHEA.

Ear Infections

SYMPTOM SUMMARY

❍ Moderate to severe pain in the ears

❍ Difficulty hearing

❍ Difficulty sleeping

❍ Fluid draining from the ear

❍ Loss of balance

❍ Runny nose

UNDERSTANDING THE DISEASE PROCESS

Otitis media, or infection of the middle ear, is the most common illness in children under the age of 15. Depending on the study, epidemiologists estimate that between 84 and 93 percent of all children in the United States have at least one ear infection. The frequency of ear infections is highest in those aged 2 years or younger, and it sharply declines in children older than 6 years.[1]

Ear infections tend to become chronic because of the anatomy of the ear. The immune system isolates infections by causing inflammation. The cells lining the narrow Eustachian canal absorb nitrogen from the air in the canal. The middle ear develops a negative pressure that traps both the infection and the inflammation to cause an ongoing problem.

Researchers once thought that abnormalities of the Eustachian tube could be caused by either allergy or infection, and there is little disagreement that foreign objects stuck in the ear can block the canal. The latest thinking, however, is that the abnormality of the ear canal leading to symptoms results from a reaction of the lining to infectious bacteria rather than from an allergic reaction. Multiple scientific studies have revealed that the same infectious bacteria are present in the ear even when the child also suffers allergies, whether the symptoms are short-term or chronic.[2]

Various factors increase the risk of repeated ear infections. Allergies, while not causing ear infections, aggravate them. Airplane travel and swimming can trap air in the ear. For reasons scientists do not understand, Native Americans, especially Eskimos and children of the Navajo Nation, tend to get more frequent and more severe ear infections. The risk of ear infection is not increased by passive exposure to cigarette smoke (at least smoke from the kinds of cigarettes available in the United States), although the children of mothers who smoked while they were pregnant are slightly more likely to develop otitis media.[3]

Children who have repeated ear infections tend to lose their ability to hear high pitches.[4] Loss of hearing may occur even when symptoms are mild or unnoticed.

TREATMENT SUMMARY

NUTRITIONAL SUPPLEMENTS

○ Lemon- or cherry-flavored cod liver oil: 1 teaspoon daily for children under 3; 2 teaspoons daily for children aged 3–6; 1 tablespoon daily for children over the age of 6 and adults.

○ Any age-appropriate multivitamin and mineral supplement *containing selenium,* daily.

HERBS

○ Echinacea: as directed on the label.

UNDERSTANDING THE HEALING PROCESS

Parents with a holistic orientation to healthcare tend to give their children a wide range of products to fight ear infections. While many traditional remedies have some value, only two are of exceptional value in treating otitis media. The best evidence supports the use of one of the oldest remedies, cod liver oil.

Researchers at The New York Eye and Ear Infirmary at Columbia University gave children aged 6 months to 5 years 1 teaspoon of lemon-flavored cod liver oil (containing both EPA and vitamin A) and $1/2$ tablet of a selenium-containing children's chewable multivitamin and mineral tablet per day. At the end of the study, children who receive the supplement were up to 25 percent less likely to be put on antibiotics for ear infections.[5] Finding a brand of cod liver without an offensive taste may be problematic, but the supplement itself causes very few side effects.

The mainstay of herbal therapy for otitis media is echinacea. Surprisingly, no scientific study has ever considered whether echinacea is specifically useful for ear infections, although a study is underway at the University of Arizona. Echinacea is the best herb for ear infections because it is both an anti-inflammatory, opening the Eustachian canal, and an immune stimulant. Children are unlikely to be on any medications that interact with echinacea, although children with HIV should only be given echinacea for 2 weeks at a time.

CONCEPTS FOR COPING WITH EAR INFECTIONS

○ Children who are breastfed tend to have fewer ear infections, although breastfeeding is not a guarantee against the disease. Breast milk contains a form of iron that stops of the growth of one of the kinds of bacteria that causes middle ear infections, *Haemophilus influenzae.*[6]

❍ If your child is treated with ciprofloxacin (Cipro), avoid sprouts, buckwheat, and supplements containing copper, magnesium, quercetin, or rutin. These foods and supplements interfere with the action of the drug. On the other hand, giving the antibiotic with pineapple juice increases its absorption into the child's bloodstream.

❍ Ear drops with garlic, mullein, and/or St. John's wort do relieve pain and inflammation, but the oil can obscure the doctor's view of the middle ear. Do not give your child ear drops the morning before he or she goes to the doctor.

❍ Don't give a baby who has an ear infection a bottle when he or she is lying on his or her back. In this position the baby can aspirate milk up the nose and into the ear canal, feeding bacteria and prolonging the infection. Healthy children can be given a bottle when they are in a supine position, but they should be picked up after feeding to make sure any milk that has been sucked up their noses drains back down the throat.[7]

❍ If you choose to use cough syrups, be sure only to use brands that are both sugar- and alcohol-free. Since cough syrups are taken without brushing the teeth and are formulated to coat the throat (and the teeth), sugar in cough syrups is a major cause of cavities in children who have ear infections.

❍ Chewing gum can prevent ear infections. The sweetener xylitol slows the growth of the *Pneumococcus* bacteria that cause ear infections by interfering with their ability to attach to lining of the ear canal. Finnish researchers found that giving children 10 pieces of xylitol-sweetened gum a day reduced the rate of ear infections by 40 percent, with no side effects (although the researchers noted that xylitol lozenges caused stomach upset in roughly 1 in 10 children).[8] One important consideration in the use of xylitol to control ear infections is that children must chew the gum when they are well, not only when they are sick. Starting the gum once an ear infection has developed does not help.[9] Another consideration is that the gum must be used several times a day, not just once. If the xylitol is not used constantly, bacteria have an opportunity to take hold.

❍ There have been two clinical studies of homeopathy as a treatment method for childhood ear infections. In a Swiss study children were given an individualized homeopathic remedy for pain. If the first remedy did not relieve pain within 6 hours, they were given a second homeopathic remedy matched to their personality type and particular symptoms. Pain control was achieved for 33 percent of children within 6 hours and another 39 percent of children within 12 hours. Children given placebo remedies were not as likely to experience relief of pain.[10] A study at the University of Washington also found that children given homeopathic treatment were 10–20 percent more likely to recover than children given no treatment at all.[11]

❍ The best way to treat a child with homeopathy is to select an appropriate remedy, wait 6 hours, and if necessary, try a second appropriate homeopathic remedy. Common remedies for otitis media include:

• Aconitum napellus treats throbbing pain when the child is fearful or restless.

• Belladonna is used when the child has fever and a flushed face, and especially when the right ear is most affected.

• Chamomilla is recommended when the child suffers "spells" of intense pain and throws tantrums.

• Ferrum phosphoricum is used when symptoms have just started, or when fatigue is marked.

• Hepar sulphuris calcareum is used when there is drainage, and especially when the child is sensitive to drafts.

• Pulsatilla treats ear problems that follow a cold or are accompanied by stuffy nose.

Ears, Ringing
See **Tinnitus**.

Eating Disorders
See **Anorexia; Bulimia**.

Eclampsia
See **Preeclampsia and Eclampsia**.

Eczema

SYMPTOM SUMMARY

○ Flare-ups and remissions of inflammation

○ Itching and scratching

○ Symptoms last longer than 6 weeks

○ Patches of irritation, exudation, and scaling

○ Personal or family history of asthma, food allergies, or hay fever

○ Worst in the folds of skin where the limbs bend

UNDERSTANDING THE DISEASE PROCESS

Eczema is the manifestation of an allergic state in the skin. Seventy percent of people who have eczema also have asthma, food allergies, and/or hay fever. Eighty percent of people who have eczema have elevated levels of immunoglobulin E (IgE) antibodies. In any kind of allergic attack, these immunoglobulins cause mast cells to break open and spill histamine, which in turn dissolves healthy skin cells as if they had been infected or injured.

Eczema tends to affect different parts of the body at different ages. Infants with eczema typically have weeping inflamed patches and crusted plaques on the face, neck, and groin. Children and adolescents are more likely to have eczema in the folds of skin where the limbs bend.

About half of children who have eczema spontaneously recover when they reach adulthood. Adults who have the disease usually have localized inflammation, such as hand eczema or lichen simplex chronicus, crusty inflammation on the ankles or backs of the feet.

Crusted and weeping lesions are especially at risk for infection with *Staphylococcus aureus*. Physicians typically treat eczema with antihistamines first, followed by topical steroids in more severe cases.

TREATMENT SUMMARY

DIET

○ Children and adults should consume 1 serving of cold-water fish 3 times a week. Infants should be breast-fed rather than given cow's milk or soy.

NUTRITIONAL SUPPLEMENTS

○ EPA and DHA (not to be confused with DHEA): 540 and 360 milligrams per day, respectively, or 1 tablespoon of flaxseed oil daily.

○ Evening primrose oil (EPO): 3,000 milligrams per day.

○ Prebiotics and probiotics: as directed on product label.

○ Quercetin: 400 milligrams 3 times a day, before meals.

○ Vitamin A: 50,000 IU per day. Women who are or who may become pregnant should strictly limit their intake of vitamin A to 5,000 IU per day or less.

○ Vitamin E: 400 IU per day.

○ Zinc picolinate: 50 milligrams per day until symptoms subside, then 30 milligrams per day.

HERBS

○ Burdock (*Arctium lappa*) or Dandelion (*Taraxacum officinale*): 500 milligrams solid extract capsules, 3 times per day.

○ Coleus forskolii: 50 milligrams of 18% forskolin extract, 3 times per day.

○ Licorice: 250–500 milligrams of solid extract (4:1) capsules, 3 times per day.

Other useful treatments:

○ Simicort or other cream containing glycyrrhetinic acid, or cream containing chamomile or witch hazel, or zinc oxide cream, daily. Do not apply zinc oxide creams to "oozing" skin.

UNDERSTANDING THE HEALING PROCESS

As early as the 1930s, scientists recognized that infants who have eczema suffer a deficiency of essential fatty acids.[2] Much more recently, scientists proved that errors in the body's metabolism of essential fatty acids causes eczema rather that the other way around.[3] The discovery of the causes of eczema, however, is a good example of how double-blind studies can be used to bias an investigation toward the investigators' favorite product, in this case, steroids.

In the 1920s researchers noticed that scaly conditions of the skin resulted from deficiencies of essential fatty acids.[4] Limited by the research techniques of their time, researchers began treating eczema with the sources of essential fatty acids known to them, lard, cod liver oil, corn oil, and linseed oil. While these products are not good sources of the omega-3 fatty acids used today, they are excellent sources of the n-6 fatty acid linolenic acid, from which the skin can produce its own omega-3 fatty acids.

The problem with using these products in treatment was that enormous quantities of lard or corn oil had to be consumed to have an effect on eczema. In most cases 100–120 grams (approximately a cup of corn oil or lard, yielding 10 or 12 grams of the therapeutic linoleic acid) needed to be eaten every day. While consuming these large quantities of fatty oils may have had other health effects, it did treat eczema, and became a standard treatment for the disease by the 1940s.[5]

In the late 1940s a new product for treating skin inflammation came on the scene, steroids. These drugs became widely popular on the basis of publicity of a double-blind, placebo-controlled clinical trial that found, despite the experience of hundreds of thousands of people, essential fatty acids could not control eczema. This 1954 study enlisted 27 children with eczema and treated them with boric acid and coal tar—at that time alternatives to treatment with corn oil—or 0.27 grams of linoleic acid. The experiment was blinded so that the clinician did not know which children were receiving which treatment. Since the amount of linoleic acid given the children was less than 3 percent of a therapeutic dose, the children in the linoleic acid group did not get better, whereas the children given boric acid and coal tar improved. In a second experiment, all the children were given boric acid and coal tar, but some of the children were also given a very small dose of linoleic acid. The children given linoleic acid did no better than the children who were given boric acid and coal tar.[6]

The results of the study were widely publicized as scientific proof that treating eczema with essential fatty acids did not work. Since the study had been conducted with the "new" double-blind approach, its findings were reported as unassailable. Fast-acting steroid creams then quickly became the treatment of choice for atopic skin conditions.

Research into the nutritional treatment of eczema was stalled for over 30 years. However, since that time, newer scientific research has confirmed that deficiencies of essential fatty acids cause scaliness, redness, weeping, and inflammation. Fatty acid deficiency increases the rate at which skin cells multiply,[7] makes them more permeable to water,[8] induces the formation of abnormal keratinocytes, and accelerates the production of natural steroid hormones in the skin.[9]

Corn oil and lard, of course, would still be effective in the treatment of eczema, but research has determined that the fatty acids that have the greatest influence on the health of the skin are n-3 fatty acids, which the body makes from n-6 fatty acids. People who have eczema have a deficiency in the enzymes needed to convert n-6 fatty acids to n-3 fatty acids. In turn, the deficiency of n-3 fatty acids leads to a deficiency of the hormonal "brake" on the process of inflammation, prostaglandin E_1 (PGE_1), and a shortage of the control chemical for the immune system, cyclic adenosine monophosphate (cAMP). When these two chemicals are deficient in the skin, the immune system runs amok, destroying healthy skin cells and stimulating their rapid replacement.

Fish oils are rich sources of polyunsaturated n-3 fatty acids, which the body does not produce in sufficient quantities in eczema. Dietary supplementation with fish oils causes these desirable fatty acids to be incorporated into the linings of skin cells, protecting them from attack by neutrophils, tissue-destructive cells of the immune system.[10] Studies have found that breastfeeding offers infants significant protection against eczema, as well as against allergies in general.[11] Babies who are breastfed but still develop eczema typically are showing a reaction to allergens consumed by their mothers. In this case, mothers should try eliminating common food allergens, especially cow's milk, eggs, and peanuts, to see if there is improvement in the child.[12] Be careful with soy milk supplements for children. At least one study has found that infants with eczema tend to have allergies to soy.[13] If it is necessary to give the baby formula, try formulas that are based on purified amino acids.

Only about 1 in 40 children and adults who has eczema also has an allergy to cow's milk.[14] About 1 in 20 children with eczema has an allergy to hamburger meat and other beef products,[15] although well-done burgers are less likely to cause a reaction than rare ones.[16]

Prebiotics are indigestible food ingredients that selectively stimulate the growth and activity of friendly bacteria in the colon. Probiotics are live microorganisms that benefit the body by improving the balance of intestinal microflora. Prebiotics and probiotics are often packaged together, for example, *acidophilus* with pectin maximizes the effectiveness of the probiotic.

Breastfed infants of nursing mothers given *Lactobacillus* GG had significantly improved eczema, compared with infants not exposed to this probiotic. In a

Finnish study, infants given a combination of *acidophilus* and *Lactobacillus* in a supplement containing whey protein showed less extensive and less severe eczema and faster development than a control group.[17] Probiotics act on eczema by suppressing an autoimmune response over a period of 4–8 weeks. *Lactobacillus* bacteria have been identified with changes in immune sensitivity, although both *acidophilus* and *Lactobacillus* bacteria have a beneficial effect on the disease in very young children.[18]

Probiotics may prevent the development not only of eczema but also of asthma and hay fever in toddlers who are considered at high risk for atopic disease, that is, children of parents who have at least one close relative who has these conditions. In another double-blind, placebo-controlled clinical study in Finland, children who were given *Lactobacillus* for 6 months were half as likely to develop eczema by age 2 as children who were not.[19]

There is no direct evidence that probiotics can help adults who have eczema, but they are likely to help. Since there are so many different products containing friendly bacteria on the market, specific dosing recommendations cannot be given here. Follow recommended dosages listed on the product label. Probiotics occasionally cause flatulence. If this occurs, lower the dose.

In the early 1980s nutritionally oriented physicians recognized that if the underlying metabolic problem in childhood and adult eczema is a failure to convert linoleic acid to gamma-linolenic acid (GLA), supplementing with GLA should help. British studies found that giving 2, 4, or 6 grams of evening primrose oil (EPO) daily to adults with eczema corrected their fatty acid profiles measured by blood tests.[20] Japanese studies found that giving the same dosages to children with eczema produced the same desirable results.[21] Other studies found that taking EPO for a month lowered the levels of the stress hormones epinephrine and norepinephrine in the skin,[22] and reduced roughness of inflamed skin.[23] Placebo-controlled studies found that EPO is beneficial when rubbed into the skin[24] (although the expense of EPO makes this inadvisable for most patients), relieves hyperactivity associated with eczema,[25] and relieves exacerbations of eczema associated with PMS.[26]

Two double-blind, placebo-controlled studies reported negative results in treating eczema with EPO. In one study, the authors found that GLA levels went up in patients who were treated with EPO and in patients who were not, suggesting that the EPO and the placebo were switched.[27] In another study, the authors created a novel scoring system to show that EPO failed to relieve symptoms, although a standard scoring system would have indicated that it did. They also failed to report that improvements in the placebo group were rapidly reversed, whereas improvements in the EPO group persisted.[28,29]

Quercetin was once known as "vitamin P," an essential cofactor for vitamin C. Quercetin stops the biological signals that tell mast cells to release histamine, the inflammatory agent in allergic reactions.[30] It also short-circuits a series of biochemical steps necessary for the formation of leukotrienes, slow-acting agents of allergic inflammation.[31] Quercetin interacts with a number of medications. It increases the toxicity of the cancer chemotherapy drug Platinol (cisplatin), the antirejection drug cyclosporine (Neoral, Sandimunne) given to transplant patients, and the high blood pressure medication nifedipine (Procardia). Quercetin competes for receptor sites and decreases the effectiveness of quinolone antibiotics, which include:

- ciprofloxacin (Cipro, Baycip, Cetraxal, Ciflox, Cifran, Ciplox, Cyprobay, Quintor)
- enoxacin (Penetrex)
- gatifloxacin (Tequin)
- gemifloxacin (a relatively new drug)
- grepafloxacin (Raxar)
- levofloxacin (Levaquin)
- lomefloxacin (Maxaquin)
- moxifloxacin (Avelox)
- norfloxacin (Amicrobin, Anquin, Baccidal, Barazan, Biofloxin, Floxenor, Fulgram, Janacin, Lexinor, Norofin, Noroxin, Norxacin, Orixacin, Oroflox, Urinox, Zoroxin)
- ofloxacin (Floxin)
- sparfloxacin (Zagam)
- temafloxacin (Omniflox)
- trovafloxacin (Trovan)

Vitamin A lowers the production of the inflammatory IgE, which is overabundant in eczematous skin. Vitamin A's effects are most noticeable when inflammation is minimal. That is, severe eczema is considerably less responsive to vitamin A treatment.[32]

There is some recent laboratory evidence that vitamin E could be formulated in a way to prevent delayed hypersensitivity reactions, such as those that cause eczema.[33] Clinical testing of vitamin E in the treatment of eczema, however, has been disappointing. Adults given 600 IU of vitamin E with or without 600 micrograms of selenium daily for 12 weeks failed to improve in a British study reported in 1989.[34] Nonetheless, vitamin E is useful as a cofactor for vitamin A. In laboratory studies with animals, the amount of vitamin A in the bloodstream stays low regardless of intake until vitamin E levels are normal. Vitamin E supplementation is useful even if vitamin A is not taken, since it complements the vitamin A available from the diet.

Both hair[35] and blood[36] analyses find lower levels of zinc in children who have eczema than in healthy children. On the other hand, hair and blood analysis shows that copper and the blood protein that binds it are higher in children who have eczema than in healthy children. These findings support the frequent recommendation of zinc supplementation as a treatment for childhood eczema. Similar findings have not, however, been found in the most recent study of adults with eczema.[37] That is, the data do not support the idea that adults with eczema are zinc deficient. However, there is some evidence that zinc supplementation can bring about a balance between the actions of antibodies and white blood cells, which is important in eczema.[38] For this reason, there *may* be some benefit for *temporary* high-dose supplementation with zinc for eczema in adults who are zinc deficient, discontinued when symptoms improve. Maintenance supplementation with zinc is useful since zinc, like vitamin E, is a cofactor for vitamin A.

A quick method for detecting zinc deficiency is a taste test. Powder a tablet of any zinc-based supplement or cold medication and mix with 1/4 cup (50 milliliters) of water. Slosh the mixture in the mouth. People who notice no taste at all or who notice a "dry," "mineral," or "sweet" taste are likely to be zinc deficient. Anyone who notices a definite strong and unpleasant taste that intensifies over time is not likely to be zinc deficient.

Burdock is a rich source of inulin, which activates the alternate complement pathway (ACP),[39] a secondary means of immune defense against bacterial infection. The ACP is especially important to eczema patients, since constant scratching leaves the skin at risk for infection with *Staphylococcus aureus.* Over 90 percent of people with eczema develop staph infections at some point during the disease.[40]

Dandelion is also a useful source of inulin. If capsulated burdock or dandelion is unavailable, take 2–8 grams of dried root, 1–2 teaspoons of fluid extract, or 1–2 teaspoons of fresh juice of either herb daily.

There is laboratory evidence that forkskolin, the primary active chemical constituent of coleus, is highly antiallergenic.[41] Forskolin stimulates the production of greater quantities of cyclic adenosine monophosphate (cAMP). This substance acts as a "second messenger" for dozens of hormonal processes. When a hormone comes in contact with the outer membrane of a cell, cAMP is released to carry a message to the organelles within the cell to perform desired functions. The cAMP system is a second messenger for anti-inflammatory hormones, both those manufactured by the body itself and those provided by medication. Forskolin is especially helpful when used with steroids to control inflammation.

While coleus helps the body form second messengers for hormones, licorice keeps useful hormones from breaking down. One of the components of licorice, glycyrrhetinic acid, potentiates the effects of hydrocortisone creams by inhibiting the enzyme 11-beta-hydroxysteroid dehydrogenase, which converts hydrocortisone to an inactive form.[42] Glycyrrhetinic acid conserves both the hormones produced by the body and those provided by medication. In one clinical study, 93 percent of eczema patients demonstrated improvement while being treating with glycyrrhetinic acid alone, indicating the conservation of body-made hormones, compared to 83 percent of patients using cortisone.[43] Licorice may be taken internally, most conveniently in capsule form (do not use DGL to treat eczema) or in a cream such as Simicort.

Chamomile, also known by its botanical name *Matricaria,* is widely used in Europe to treat both psoriasis and eczema. When chamomile is treated with hot water, it releases chamazulene, a potent antioxidant that absorbs free radicals needed for an allergic response.[44] Chamazulene also inhibits the formation of inflammatory leukotrienes.[45] The essential oil, which has to be extracted by a different process, stops the release of histamine by mast cells, further blunting any allergic reactions in the skin.[46]

A double-blind, placebo-controlled clinical test of the use of witch hazel creams in the treatment of eczema showed that witch hazel was less effective than hydrocortisone, but offered a significant anti-inflammatory effect without the side effects of prednisone.[47]

Zinc oxide gels hydrate the skin.[48] They will exacerbate weeping eczema, but are suitable for dry skin.

CONCEPTS FOR COPING WITH ECZEMA

Important steps in self-care:

○ Avoid allergens whenever possible.

○ Avoid excessive washing of the skin. Washing the skin too often dries it out.

○ Avoid scratching when you itch. If you must relieve the itch, gently rubbing with the flat of your hand is less likely to do damage.

○ Avoid wool and polyester clothing. Wool scratches. Polyester traps oils on the skin. Rubber and elastic may also be irritating.

○ Ease dry skin by applying a damp cloth to the skin. The cloth traps humid air and allows moisture to build up in the skin from within.

○ Take quick showers instead of long baths. The natural moisturizing agent of the skin, sodium PCA, can leach out, especially in alkaline water. Chlorinated swimming pools are more acidic than bath water and less damaging to the skin, but swims should also be brief.

○ Use hypoallergenic laundry detergents. Add vinegar to the rinse cycle to remove laundry soap.

○ Use the cream or ointment your doctor recommends on a regular basis, and as a soap substitute, to keep the skin supple and to prevent drying.

○ Wear gloves to avoid exposure to chemicals and strong detergents. Vinegar, lemon, and baking soda are friendly cleansers.

○ Try to shampoo the hair no more often than twice a week. Shampoo damage to the skin can be treated by application of a small amount of jojoba oil.

○ Keep infants in a dust-free environment, preferably in rooms without carpets or drapes. At least one study found that infants with eczema tended to have allergies to dust mites, which burrow into the skin.

○ There have been no scientific studies of the use of homeopathy for the treatment of eczema, but a number of traditional treatments are available for various combinations of symptoms and personality types. Remedies include:

• Antimonium crudum, for children who crave sour foods such as pickles.

• Arsenicum album, for people who are neat and orderly and who tend to scratch a lot.

• Arum triphyllum, for outbreaks on the lower face, especially around the mouth.

• Calendula, for outbreaks that tend to get infected.

• Graphites, for eczema on sun-damaged or wrinkled skin.

• Mezereum, for outbreaks that then crust over, especially in people who have sensitive stomachs.

• Petroleum, for cracked skin.

• Rhus toxicodendron, for outbreaks that are especially inflamed, red, or swollen.

• Sulfur, for outbreaks that are aggravated by bathing or showering in warm or hot water.

Edema

See **Bruises; Congestive Heart Failure; Preeclampsia and Eclampsia; Varicose Veins.**

Elevated Blood Pressure

See **Hypertension.**

Emphysema

SYMPTOM SUMMARY

○ Bluish discoloration of the skin (caused by lack of oxygen)

○ Chronic cough

○ Chronic shortness of breath, especially on exertion

○ Wheezing

In later stages of the disease:

○ Anxiety

○ Bulging eyes

○ Clubbed fingers or toes

○ Dizziness

○ Fatigue

- Flared nostrils
- Impotence
- Inability to concentrate
- Insomnia, tired upon waking
- Morning headaches
- Swollen ankles, feet, and legs
- Temporary cessation of breathing
- Unplanned weight loss
- Vision abnormalities
- Volatile temper

UNDERSTANDING THE DISEASE PROCESS

Emphysema is a condition in which alveoli (air sacs) of the lungs become hyperextended and cannot return to their normal volume. These larger air sacs lose "suction" as tiny holes form, and the lungs lose their ability to take in oxygen and let out carbon dioxide. The underlying cause of these tissue changes is an imbalance of two kinds of protein enzymes. One type of enzyme, called protease, normally clean up dead or injured cells. Another type of enzyme, called antiprotease, prevents unintended damage when the lungs are inflamed. Over a period of years, the chemicals in cigarette smoke and certain gases and viral infections upset the balance of proteases and antiproteases so that the "elastic" in the air sacs is destroyed.

TREATMENT SUMMARY

DIET

- Don't go on a low-fat, high-carbohydrate diet, but also avoid egg yolks, beef, and fried foods. Eat 2–3 servings of cold-water fish weekly.

NUTRITIONAL SUPPLEMENTS

- EPA and DHA (not to be confused with DHEA): 540 and 360 milligrams per day, respectively, or 1 tablespoon of flaxseed oil daily.

- N-acetyl cysteine (NAC): 400 milligrams a day if you do not smoke.

AROMATHERAPY

- Add 5–10 drops of eucalyptus oil to the water in a vaporizer operated in your bedroom as your sleep.

UNDERSTANDING THE HEALING PROCESS

Neither mainstream medicine nor natural medicine offers a cure for emphysema. Quitting smoking, however, greatly reduces the severity of symptoms. Medical examination of the 29,133 participants of the Alpha-Tocopherol Beta-Carotene Cancer Prevention Study found that quitting smoking reduced the number of days the lungs formed phlegm by 84 percent and the number of coughs by 78 percent.[1] Clearly, the most important step in the care of emphysema is to quit smoking. Additionally, several natural interventions make living with emphysema easier.

People with emphysema need to stay away from low-fat, high-carbohydrate diets. High carbohydrate consumption increases the body's consumption of carbon dioxide. Several studies indicate that people with chronic obstructive pulmonary disease have difficulty eliminating carbon dioxide,[2,3] and a high-carbohydrate diet places additional stress on the lungs.

On the other hand, certain kinds of fats should be avoided. The biochemical process that makes the lungs sensitive to allergens is made possible by the chemical thromboxane.[4] The body's production of thromboxane is greater when the diet includes egg yolks, beef tallow (often used in cooking fast-food French fries), and fried foods, and less when the diet includes fish oils. A study of 8,006 male smokers in Hawaii found that those who ate 2 or more servings of fish per week were found to lose lung capacity at less than half the rate of those who did not. The protective effect of fish oils was greatest for the smokers who smoked the most.[5] Another study published in the prestigious *New England Journal of Medicine* suggests that smokers are protected from the development of bronchitis, emphysema, and pneumonia when their diets include n-3 polyunsaturated fatty acids from any source.[6] EPA, DHA, and flaxseed oil are good sources of n-3 polyunsaturated fatty acids.

N-acetyl cysteine (NAC) is an amino acid derivative that can break the chemical bonds that make mucus sticky. A study involving 10 chronic lung disease patients and 10 healthy controls found that NAC increases the activity of infection-fighting white blood cells.[7] A total of 8 double-blind, placebo-controlled scientific studies concur that regular use of NAC can significantly reduce the frequency of severe attacks of bronchitis.[8]

Not everyone with emphysema should take NAC. Smokers with emphysema should not take NAC unless they are quitting. There is some evidence that NAC may activate eosinophils, the white blood cells that may cause the progression of smoker's cough to chronic obstructive pulmonary disease.[9] NAC may cause headaches if taken with sildenafil (Viagra), and in rare cases can cause cysteine-crystal kidney stones. Diabetics who also have cystic fibrosis may find that taking NAC causes false readings in urine tests for ketones.

Eucalyptus oil is a standard ingredient in cough drops and in oils added to humidifiers and vaporizers. While it does not increase breathing capacity, a study of 246 people with chronic bronchitis found that eucalyptus oils stopped the worsening of cough that commonly occurs in the winter (in wet climates where heaters are used) or summer (in desert climates).[10]

People who have emphysema are frequently deficient in antioxidant vitamins such as vitamin A, vitamin C, vitamin E, coenzyme Q_{10}, and beta-carotene. It would seem logical that taking supplemental antioxidants would help emphysema, but this is not necessarily the case. There is considerable evidence that consuming *low* doses of these antioxidants *in the form of fruits and vegetables* helps in various kinds of chronic obstructive pulmonary disease, including emphysema, even among elderly long-term smokers,[11] whereas taking specific supplements (notably beta-carotene and vitamin C) does not.[12]

Many people are unaware that free radicals are not solely harmful, but they are involved in many defense reactions of the cells. High levels of antioxidants may disturb these reactions with unpredictable and unexpected consequences. Therefore, if you take antioxidants, take the smallest possible dose. Better yet, get your antioxidants from the most available and most balanced natural sources, fruits and vegetables.

CONCEPTS FOR COPING WITH EMPHYSEMA

❍ Ask your doctor about getting vaccinated against flu and pneumonia.

❍ Avoid exposure to colds and influenza at home or in public, and avoid respiratory irritants such as secondhand smoke, dust, and other air pollutants.

❍ Avoid tight belts, bras, and girdles.

❍ If you must use a vacuum cleaner, be sure it has a disposable dust bag. Use extreme caution not to break the bag when discarding it.

❍ When cooking, always use your exhaust fan, or make sure there is good ventilation.

❍ If you do drive and gas up your car yourself, try to get upwind from the pump so that you do not gas yourself as well as the car.

❍ If walking is difficult for you, a urinal by the bedside can be extremely helpful. There are urinal containers made especially for women.

❍ If being constantly short of breath makes daily activities difficult, try these energy-saving shortcuts:

• Don't engage in physical activities until an hour or more after eating. Digestion draws blood, with its oxygen, away from muscles leaving them less able to cope with extra demands. This is the very same reason that children are taught not to go swimming right after meals.

• If you feel breathless, use pursed-lip breathing.

• Making a bed is one of the most demanding of household tasks. If you must do it yourself, try making half the bed while you are still in it. Pull the top sheet and blanket up on one side and smooth them out. Exit from the unmade side, which is then easy to finish.

• If you find taking a shower or bath demanding, try taking a shower or bath while sitting on a bath stool. A terrycloth robe will eliminate the effort of drying; just blot.

• If you must go up and down stairs and cannot afford a mechanical chair lift (they are very expensive), have a table or chair at the top of the stairs on which you can lean or sit.

Endometriosis

SYMPTOM SUMMARY

❍ Heavy or long periods

❍ Inability to become pregnant

❍ Pain before and during menstrual period

❍ Pain during sexual intercourse

❍ Painful urination or bowel movements

❍ Pelvic inflammation or tenderness

❍ Rectal bleeding during menstrual period

❍ Spotting before menstrual period

UNDERSTANDING THE DISEASE PROCESS

Endometriosis is a chronic condition in which the endometrium, the inner lining of the uterus that is shed each month during menses, passes inward rather than outward. Clear, black, or red cysts and adhesions become implanted within the pelvic cavity, and light brown cysts may accumulate in the ovaries. The accumulation of uterine tissue inside the pelvis causes pain and bleeding just before and during the menstrual period. Epidemiologists estimate that 10–15 percent of all women of child-bearing age suffer endometrosis, and that the condition is a factor in 50 percent of all cases of women's infertility.[1]

Retrograde menstruation occurs in 90 percent of women, but causes endometriosis only 10–20 percent of the time. Researchers believe that uterine tissue that is not removed during menstruation creates cysts only in the absence of an enzyme (17-beta-hydroxysteroid dehydrogenase type 2) to convert an especially potent form of estrogen, 17-beta-estradiol, into a more gently effective hormone, estrone.[2] The 17-beta-estradiol form of estrogen strongly stimulates the growth of uterine tissue during the first 14 days of the menstrual cycle. It also stimulates the growth of misplaced uterine tissue in the pelvis. The growth of all forms of uterine tissue is stopped by progesterone.

TREATMENT SUMMARY

NUTRITIONAL SUPPLEMENTS

❍ Fish oil: 3 grams daily.

UNDERSTANDING THE HEALING PROCESS

Since endometrial cysts grow in the presence of estrogen and shrink when they are deprived of estrogen, all of the standard medical treatments for the condition involve decreasing estrogen levels. Depriving a woman's body of estrogen, of course, has serious side effects. The drugs danazol and medroxyprogesterone acetate stop ovulation and ensure infertility. Mifepristone (RU-486), recently introduced for the treatment of endometriosis, stops the period altogether and can cause abortion. The hormone progesterone acts as a natural "brake" on the growth of the uterus after the first half of the menstrual cycle, and leads to the sloughing off of the endometrium during menstruation. Therapeutic progesterone, however, can stop menstruation but may or may not stop ovulation.[3] In the face of these problems, even physicians recognize the need for alternative methods of treatment.

Natural therapy for endometriosis focuses on limiting inflammation rather than limiting estrogen. The best-researched supplement for this purpose is fish oil. There is solid clinical evidence that taking fish oil relieves menstrual pain.[4] There is no evidence that fish oil will cause endometrial tissue to shrink, but it is certain that it will not interfere with the normal action of estrogen.

It may be necessary to take fish oil through 2 menstrual cycles to notice any benefit. Some women may experience mild diarrhea or "fishy burps" when first taking the supplement. These can be avoided by using pharmaceutical-grade fish oil, or by substituting DHA from microalgae. Avoiding fried foods and sugar will enhance the effect of the supplement.

CONCEPTS FOR COPING WITH ENDOMETRIOSIS

❍ There is epidemiological evidence that women who consume 7 cups of coffee a day or more are twice as likely to develop endometriosis as women who consume 3 cups of coffee a day or less.[5] There is no conclusive clinical evidence that reducing coffee consumption or switching to decaf causes a medically measurable reduction in symptoms, but many women find that drinking less coffee helps.

❍ The most frequently prescribed medication for endometriosis, danazol (Danocrine), can cause deepening of the voice and other "masculine" side effects. Reversing the side effects requires discontinuing the drug, but side effects can usually be avoided by women who exercise regularly.[6]

❍ The traditional herbal remedy for endometriosis is vitex, usually combined with dandelion, motherwort, and/or prickly ash. Like fish oil, vitex reduces pain but probably has no effect on endometrial tissue itself. Vitex has not been clinically tested.

❍ The traditional Chinese herbal treatment for endometriosis, Dan Gui Shao Yao San, a combination of dong quai, peony, atractylodis, alisma, angelica, ligusticum root, and poria mushroom has been clinically tested in Japan and found to relieve endometrial pain.[7] Safe and reliable formulations of Dan Gui Shao Yao San are available in the United States and Canada under the following brand names:

- Dang Gui & Peony (Qualiherb)
- Kampo4Women MenopauEase (Honso)
- Tangkuei & Peony Formula (Lotus Classics)
- Tang-Kuei and Peony Formula (Golden Flower Chinese Herbs, Sun Ten)
- Toki-shakuyaku-san (Honso, Tsumura)

Enteritis, Regional
See **Inflammatory Bowel Disease (IBD)**.

Epididymitis

SYMPTOM SUMMARY

- Blood in semen
- Discharge from urethra (opening at the end of the penis)
- Enlarged testicles
- Fever
- Pain in the groin
- Painful intercourse or ejaculation
- Painful swelling of the scrotum
- Painful urination
- Tender, swollen groin on affected side
- Tender, swollen testicle on affected side

UNDERSTANDING THE DISEASE PROCESS

Epididymitis is an inflammation of the epididymis, the C-shaped structure surrounding each testicle. The epididymis contains a twisting tubule in which the sperm mature before they travel to the vas deferens and spermatic cord, eventually reaching the ejaculatory canal. During their stay in the epididymis, sperm acquire the ability to "swim" in the cervical passage after intercourse. Sperm are tightly packed in the tubes and held in place by mucuslike proteins so that only a relative few are released in each ejaculation.

The tight twists and turns of the vessels controlling the outflow of sperm intensify inflammation in the testicles. As inflammation spreads up the vas deferens, an external ring that functions as a "valve" for sperm keeps the duct itself from swelling. This increases the pressure inside the testicles, which may double in size. The lymph canals also swell. Pain radiates out the vas deferens, and can become flank pain. Usually only one testicle is affected. There is sometimes a slight fever.

Older men and athletes may develop "chemical epididymitis." In this syndrome, vigorous exercise or straining on a full bladder causes "retrograde urination." The epididymis becomes inflamed by the overflow of sterile urine.[1]

Especially in men under 35, most cases of epididymitis are caused by infection. About 20 percent on men who get mumps develop, epididymo-orchitis, swollen testicles specifically linked to the swelling of the lymph glands caused by mumps. Epididymitis can also be caused by tuberculosis, and in older men who are not sexually active, epididymitis is usually from an *Enterobacteriacea* or *Pseudomonas* infection. But the overwhelming majority cases of epididymitis in younger men involve sexually transmitted microorganisms, typically *Chlamydia* in heterosexual men[2] and *E. coli* in homosexual men.[3] Both of these microorganisms can produce symptoms as serious as those caused by gonorrhea. Generally, *Chlamydia* causes heavy discharge and pain above the testicles, while *E. coli* causes less discharge, swollen testicles, and redness.

Testicular aches and pains are not usually a cause for alarm; however, *sudden onset of severe testicular pain is a medical emergency.* Testicular torsion, that is, twisting of blood vessels serving the testes, must be surgically treated in 6 hours or less to be assured of recovery. If a young man complains of abdominal pain, the scrotum should always be carefully examined because abdominal pain often precedes testicular pain in testicular torsion. The table on the following page summarizes the differences between epididymitis, which is not a medical emergency, and testicular torsion.

TREATMENT SUMMARY

NUTRITIONAL SUPPLEMENTS

- Bioflavonoids: 1,000 milligrams per day.
- Thymus extract: 500 milligrams of crude polypeptides daily.
- Vitamin A: 5,000 IU per day.
- Vitamin C: 500 milligrams 3–4 times a day.
- Zinc picolinate: 30 milligrams per day.

DISTINCTIONS BETWEEN EPIDIDYMITIS AND TESTICULAR TORSION

	Epididymitis	Testicular Torsion
Placement of testicles	Normal	Elevated, seem to be drawn up
Prehn's sign (lifting the testicles)—should only be done by physician if pain is severe	Relieves pain	Does not relieve pain
Pyuria (pus in the urine)	Common	Unusual
Skin	Adheres to the testes	Loose

HERBS

In all cases:

❍ Bromelain: 250 milligrams 4 times a day between meals and at night before bedtime.

In cases associated with bacterial infection:

❍ Echinacea: 150–300 milligrams of solid extract (3.5% echinacosides) 3 times a day, or dried root, freeze-dried plant, juice, fluid extract, or tincture, as recommended on the label.

❍ Goldenseal: as recommended on the label.

See Part Three if you take prescription medication.

UNDERSTANDING THE HEALING PROCESS

The healing process for epididymitis is very straightforward and the pain of epididymitis is highly motivating for sensible self-care. Bed rest and ice packs applied to the testicles are recommended for the first 48 hours after the diagnosis of symptoms. (Other sources of testicular pain have potentially devastating consequences; therefore, self-diagnosis is not recommended.) After the initial pain has subsided, wearing an athletic supporter will be helpful. It is important to empty the bladder before engaging in any strenuous physical activity.

Most cases of epididymitis are treated with antibiotics. The supplements recommended here will relieve inflammation and accelerate the healing process. It is important not to stop taking antibiotics before taking the entire prescription, since early termination of antibiotic treatment leaves only the most virulent bacteria behind to establish chronic infection.

Although there are no studies that directly confirm the usefulness of thymus extract in treating epididymitis, there is considerable evidence that thymus extract corrects low immune function. In particular, research has shown that thymus extract normalizes the ratio of helper T cells to suppressor T cells, maintaining a healthy immune response that neither destroys healthy tissue nor allows infectious microorganisms to flourish.[4]

Relatively low doses of vitamin A are sufficient to prevent "burnout" due to stress on the immune output of the thymus.[5] Vitamin A also enhances antibody response, increases the rate at which macrophages destroy bacteria, and stimulates natural killer cells.[6]

Vitamin C levels are quickly depleted during the stress of an infection.[7] In combination with bioflavonoids, it helps increase the stability of the ground substance, the "glue" between the epididymis and the tissues around it.[8]

Zinc is an important cofactor for vitamin A. When zinc is deficient, the immune system's ability to produce white blood cells in response to infection is reduced, thymic hormone levels are lower, the immune response in the skin is especially reduced, and phagocytosis, the process in which bacteria are engulfed and digested, is slowed. When zinc is deficient, all of these processes can be corrected by taking zinc supplements.[9]

A quick method for detecting zinc deficiency is a taste test. Powder a tablet of any zinc-based supplement or cold medication and mix with $1/4$ cup (50 milliliters) of water. Slosh the mixture in the mouth. People who notice no taste at all or who notice a "dry," "mineral," or "sweet" taste are likely to be zinc deficient. Anyone who notices a definite strong and unpleasant taste that intensifies over time is not likely to be zinc deficient.

Zinc picolinate is the most readily absorbed form of zinc. Do not take more than 50 milligrams of any zinc supplement daily. In rare cases, excessive intake of zinc depletes copper to cause anemia, that is, a deficiency of red blood cells, and neutropenia, a serious deficiency of white blood cells.

Bromelain serves as an all-purpose inflammation treatment. Bromelain stops the production of kinins and prostaglandins that cause inflammation, and accelerates recovery time. It increases the effectiveness of antibacterial herbs by increasing the permeability of the barrier between the bloodstream and the testes.[10]

Echinacea relieves inflammation. One study found that a teaspoon of *Echinacea purpurea* juice is as effective in relieving pain and swelling as 100 milligrams of cortisone.[11] Echinacea also enhances the immune system's response to bacterial infections. It is especially useful in stimulating phagocytosis, the process by which white blood cells surround and digest infectious bacteria. A study of oral administration of an *Echinacea purpurea* root extract (30 drops 3 times per day) to healthy men for 5 days resulted in a 120 percent increase in phagocytosis.[12]

Women who are trying to get pregnant should avoid *Echinacea purpurea*. It contains caffeoyl esters that can interfere with the action of hyaluronidase, an enzyme essential to the release of unfertilized eggs into the fallopian tube.[13]

There is laboratory evidence that *Echinacea angustifolia* contains chemicals that deactivate CYP3A4. This is a liver enzyme that breaks down a wide range of medications, including anabolic steroids, the chemotherapy drug methotrexate used in treating cancer and lupus, astemizole (Hismanal) for allergies, nifedipine (Adalat) and captopril (Capoten) for high blood pressure, and sildenafil (Viagra) for impotence, as well as many others. *Echinacea angustifolia* might help maintain levels of these drugs in the bloodstream and make them more effective, or it might also cause them to accumulate to levels at which they cause side effects. Switch to a brand of echinacea that does not contain *Echinacea angustifolia* if you experience unexpected side effects while taking any of these drugs.[14]

Avoid all forms of echinacea if you have HIV. Echinacea stimulates immune function, but it also slightly increases production of T cells.[15] These are the immune cells attacked by HIV. When there are more T cells, the virus has more cells to infect. This gives it more opportunities to mutate into a drug-resistant form. This effect also makes echinacea inadvisable in autoimmune conditions, such as lupus, rheumatoid arthritis, and Sjögren's syndrome.

The combination of echinacea and goldenseal is especially useful in treating conditions that involve drainage. A study reported in 1999 that the combination of the two herbs stimulates the production of the immunoglobulins IgG and IgM, infection fighters that "remember" specific infections.[16] Goldenseal contains the general antibacterial compound berberine. This alkaloid kills a wide range of bacteria, including those in the same family as *Chlamydia*.

People's Pharmacy authors Joe and Teresa Graedon

warn that goldenseal reportedly limits the effectiveness of the anticoagulants heparin and warfarin (Coumadin). Do not take goldenseal with these medications. Avoid supplements containing vitamin B_6 or L-histidine if you take goldenseal, since they can interfere with goldenseal's antibacterial action.

CONCEPTS FOR COPING WITH EPIDIDYMITIS

○ Epididymitis can also affect women. Women who suspect they may have been exposed to *Chlamydia* or *E. coli* through sexual intercourse but do not yet have symptoms may benefit from the Chinese herb epimedium, a traditional East Asian treatment for venereal infections. It stimulates the production of urine so that *Chlamydia* or *E. coli* bacteria cannot lodge in the lining of the urethra. It is also directly antibacterial against *Chlamydia* and *Neisseria gonorrhea*, stimulating macrophages from the immune system to engulf and digest the bacteria.[17]

Epilepsy

SYMPTOM SUMMARY

○ Seizures:
- Tonic (stiffening of the body, dilation of the pupils)
- Clonic (sudden muscle jerks)
- Atonic (loss of muscle tone and/or consciousness)

UNDERSTANDING THE DISEASE PROCESS

Epilepsy is a condition of repeated seizures caused by abnormal electrical discharges from cells in the brain. Epilepsy is not a single disease; it is a group of disorders, often in the cerebral cortex. The various forms of epilepsy may be secondary to an identifiable brain abnormality or neurological disorder, or are they may be "idiopathic," lacking a clear cause.

TREATMENT SUMMARY

NUTRITIONAL SUPPLEMENTS

○ Vitamin E: 400 IU per day (same dosage for children and adults).

UNDERSTANDING THE HEALING PROCESS

Epilepsy can be difficult to manage with drugs. Considerable recent research has been devoted to managing the condition in adults as well as children by ketogenic diet, a nearly all-fat diet that forces the brain to subsist on ketone bodies rather than sugars. Up to 60 percent of epileptics who go on the diet have a 50 percent reduction in seizures for at least a few months.[1] The requirements of the diet are exacting and require professional guidance. Additional information about the diet is available from your neurologist or from www.neuro.jhmi.edu/Epilepsy/keto.html, the John's Hopkins Epilepsy Center, or from Charlie Foundation To Help Cure Pediatric Epilepsy, 1223 Wilshire Blvd #815, Santa Monica, CA 90403-5406 or 1-800-367-5386.

Nutritional treatments for epilepsy are problematic, because of the delicate balances required to avoid seizures. Antioxidants such as vitamin E are thought to prevent the "kindling" of epileptic seizures and also to protect brain cells from damage during seizures. A study at the Hospital for Sick Children in Toronto found that 400 IU of vitamin E a day in addition to regular seizure medication resulted in significant reduction of seizures in 10 of 12 cases of childhood epilepsy.[2] Unfortunately, clinical trials of vitamin E in treating epilepsy in adults have yielded inconsistent results, but, unlike many other supplements, vitamin E is not known to cause any adverse effects.

CONCEPTS FOR COPING WITH EPILEPSY

❍ Avoid blackcurrant and evening primrose oil. There are reports that these supplements can aggravate temporal lobe seizures (seizures characterized by changes in sensation and personality). Laboratory studies with animals suggest fish oil should be helpful in preventing seizures, but there have been no clinical trials of the use of fish oil in treating epilepsy conducted with human volunteers.

❍ Bloodstream concentrations of antiseizure medications must be maintained within a narrow range to be effective. Excessive perspiration or excessive consumption of fluid can alter medication levels and trigger a seizure. Avoid drinking more than 1 or 2 glasses of water (or the equivalent) in any 2-hour period, but be sure to replace lost fluids when you are perspiring heavily.

❍ If you take valproic acid (Depakene, Depakote) for seizures, you are at special risk for liver damage and you should have liver enzyme levels (ALT and AST) periodically checked. If taking the drug is beginning to elevate liver enzymes, take 120 milligrams of silymarin (milk thistle) extract 3 times a day to counteract liver damage.

❍ Seizure medications interact with many herbs and nutritional supplements. See Part Three for further information.

Erectile Dysfunction

SYMPTOM SUMMARY

❍ Inability to achieve or maintain sufficiently firm erection for intercourse

UNDERSTANDING THE DISEASE PROCESS

Erectile dysfunction, or ED, is the modern medical term for the inability to achieve or maintain a sufficiently hard erection for sexual intercourse. Although at least 15 different medical conditions can cause ED, the greater physiological mystery is not why erections are sometimes difficult to achieve but why erections do not occur all the time. In healthy men, specialized hormone docking sites called alpha-adrenergic receptors are almost always occupied by the stress hormone epinephrine. This hormone tells the nerves that they should keep the circulation of blood into the penis at a minimum so that it remains flaccid. The nerves locking blood out of the penis are part of the sympathetic nervous system, the part of the nervous system activated by emotional and physical stress.

The power of the sympathetic nerves controlling the penis can only be overcome by strong signals delivered by the other half of the nervous system, the parasympathetic nerves. Touching the penis or other erogenous zones—as well as certain sights, sounds, smells, or thoughts—triggers the parasympathetic nerves to signal the blood vessels to open and an erection to form. The sympathetic nervous system can be activated by will or fear, however, so that the erection is lost.

It is possible to compare an erection to filling a tire with air. Achieving an erect tire requires air forced into the tire under pressure. It takes an intact "tire" without a hole to maintain the air and allow it to expand. A defect in either the flow or air into the tire or in the lining of the tire will cause it to "go flat."

When ED occurs as a side effect of prescription medication, symptoms usually occur rapidly. ED caused by various kinds of circulatory problems, however, usually develops slowly with little loss of sexual desire. ED accompanying cirrhosis of the liver or heart disease may also involve loss of sexual desire.

TREATMENT SUMMARY

HERBS

O Yohimbe: try a dose of 5 milligrams. If you experience enhanced erectile function, then *skip a day* and take 5 milligrams every other day (or less frequently). If you do not experience better erections, wait 2 days and try taking two 5-milligram doses in the same day. Some men need 50 milligrams of yohimbe in 5 doses on the day they have sex. Do not take yohimbe every day. Always take 1 or preferably 2 days off the herb for maximum effect.

NUTRITIONAL SUPPLEMENTS

For diabetic men:

O Alpha-lipoic acid: 400 milligrams twice a day for 4 months, then 100 milligrams 3 times a day thereafter.

UNDERSTANDING THE HEALING PROCESS

When ED is due to medication, the simplest course of action is to ask your doctor to prescribe a different drug. Among the types of drugs frequently interfering with men's sexual function are blood pressure medications, diuretics, cholesterol medications, chemotherapy, epilepsy medications, drugs for HIV, and steroids. Alcohol, amphetamines, Ecstasy, and marijuana also can contribute to ED.

Until the late 1990s, most of the commonly available medications for ED were taken by injection into the penis, a definite detriment to spontaneous lovemaking. Vacuum pumps to enlarge the penis are difficult to operate, and an implanted balloon requires surgery most men are reluctant even to consider. The introduction of Viagra (sildenafil) in 1998, however, revolutionized the medication treatment of ED.

Viagra acts on the simple principle that the penis must be filled with blood before an erection can occur. The drug stimulates the production of nitric oxide (NO) in the nerves that line the arteries emptying into the penis, dilating them and allowing the flow of blood.

The drawbacks to using Viagra are that it is expensive and seldom covered by insurance, and it does not always work. Many men find yohimbe to be an effective alternative. Yohimbe is an herbal medication made of the bark of an African tree (*Corynanthe yohimbe,* also referred to as *Pausinystalia yohimbe*). One of the components of yohimbe, yohimbine, was the only medication approved by the FDA for the treatment of impotence before the advent of Viagra. The rainforest herbs igpepo, pamprana, quebracho, and rauwolfia are also natural sources of yohimbine.

Yohimbe is the best-known natural treatment for ED and the nearest natural equivalent to Viagra. Its primary active chemical constituent, yohimbine, is similar to Viagra in that it treats impotence regardless of cause. Also like Viagra, yohimbine acts by stimulating the flow of blood into the penis. Yohimbine unlocks norepinephrine (a chemical similar to adrenaline) bound to alpha-adrenergic receptors on the nerves controlling blood flow to the organ. This forces blood into the penis and makes an erection possible. The norepinephrine released from the alpha-adrenergic nerves is absorbed by non-adrenergic, non-cholinergic nerves. This action performs the same function as Viagra, generating the formation of nitric oxide and increasing blood flow into the penis. The plant chemical also stimulates cholinergic nerves that encourage the production of more NO, relaxing smooth muscles that trap blood inside the penis and make the erection sustainable.[1]

Unlike Viagra, yohimbe has a wide range of effects on the central nervous system stimulating interest in sex. When taken in doses of up to 30 milligrams, yohimbe is an antidepressant. It stimulates the production of the reward chemical dopamine in the brain, changing brain chemistry so that it is easier to give your sexual partner your fullest attention. Unlike medications for ED that also change the brain's dopamine system, such as bromocriptine (Parlodel), the effectiveness of yohimbe and yohimbine does not diminish over time.

Understanding how yohimbe works is important to using it successfully. In men who take yohimbe every day, the body readjusts its production of norepinephrine so that this stress hormone is always bound to alpha-adrenergic receptors. Only when yohimbe "takes the nervous system by surprise" does it have a beneficial effect on erection. This is why some clinical studies in which men were given a single high dose of yohimbe every day did not find it to be effective,[2] but others in which men took roughly the same amount of the herb in 6 tablets, rather than 1, found it to be highly effective.[3]

Standardized extracts of yohimbe or prescription yohimbine are your best sources of the chemical. In the mid-1990s, chemical analysis of over-the-counter yohimbe bark products found that not a single brand contained even 10 percent yohimbe bark, some containing no yohimbe or yohimbine at all.[4] To find a dosage that is effective for you, start with a single 5-milligram dose and see if there is any improvement in erectile capacity when you engage in sexual activity. Then skip a day, increasing the dosage up to 50 milligrams to find an effective level.

Yohimbe may be taken with Viagra, but should *never* be taken with the antidepressant trazodone (Deseryl, Trialodine). This combination can cause priapism, a painful erection that has to be surgically deflated to prevent permanent tissue damage to the penis. Yohimbe also should not be combined with butyl nitrite ("poppers"). It is ineffective when taken with some drugs used to increase sexual desire, such as bromocriptine or selegiline (deprenyl, Jumex). The blood pressure medication clonidine is an antidote to yohimbine, and makes yohimbe completely ineffective.

Many men find it difficult to sleep for 18 to 24 hours after taking either the herb yohimbe or the prescription medication yohimbine. Tranquilizers and herbal sleep aids such as kava-kava will not help insomnia caused by yohimbe.

Diabetic men may especially benefit from taking alpha-lipoic acid. Up to 70 percent of men with diabetes develop ED within 5 years of diagnosis with diabetes. Constant exposure to high blood sugars causes glycosylation, a kind of biochemical caramelizing, of nerve fibers in the linings of the arteries serving the penis. The arteries become unable to produce the nitric oxide needed to open the flow of blood for an erection, even when stimulated by drugs such as Viagra.[5]

Alpha-lipoic acid reverses glycosylation. German physicians recommend taking 800 milligrams of encapsulated alpha-lipoic acid for 3 months, and 100 milligrams 3 times a day thereafter.[6] Up to 1,800 milligrams of alpha-lipoic acid a day may be helpful during the first 3 weeks, but since very high doses of the supplement can lower blood sugars unpredictably, you should not take this large a dose without consulting your physician. The first effects of alpha-lipoic may be the restoration of sensation, rather than erection, but erections will return

in time with the use of the supplement, provided blood sugars are carefully regulated. (See also NEUROPATHY.)

L-arginine is frequently recommended for ED, and may increase the effectiveness of Viagra, since it provides the chemicals from which NO is made. Clinical studies of L-arginine have used relatively small doses, no more than 3,000 milligrams per day,[7,8] and using more than 5,000 milligrams of L-arginine may make ED worse. The herbs damiana, ginseng, and muira puama are also frequently recommended for ED, but their effects are unpredictable and they do not help the majority of men who take them.

CONCEPTS FOR COPING WITH ERECTILE DYSFUNCTION

❍ If you have ED, you should not take any saw palmetto for prostate problems. Saw palmetto keeps testosterone from stimulating both prostate enlargement and normal penile functions. Take pygeum instead.

❍ Cocaine, amphetamine, and methamphetamine all lead to a strong shrinkage of the male genitals. These drugs liberate adrenaline from nerve endings throughout the body and cause increased excitement and sexual desire. However, they also produce massive amounts of norepinephrine that binds to alpha-adrenergic receptors in the nerves of the penis, blocking the flow of blood to the organ and making erection difficult or impossible. The street drug Ecstasy has a similar effect, but through a different physiological process. Using yohimbe or Viagra with these drugs keeps them from inducing ED, but having sex under conditions of impaired judgment increases the risk of pregnancy, STDs, and HIV.

❍ While there are no scientific studies confirming the use of homeopathy in the treatment of ED, homeopathic remedies are entirely safe and frequently effective. The best way to use homeopathy is to choose an appropriate remedy (or consult a homeopathic physician for an appropriate remedy), and to take the remedy for 30 days. If there is no improvement in erections in a month, discontinue the remedy.

- Agnus castus is recommended when there is a cold sensation in the penis, frequent urination, and disturbed sleep. Homeopathic physicians often recommend this remedy for men who develop ED after many years of frequent sexual activity or, in some cases, excessive masturbation. The homeopathic literature suggests that agnus castus is appropriate for men who are anxious about disease conditions or who have problems with inattention or memory loss.

• Argentum nitricum treats ED occurring after intercourse is initiated. Men who need this remedy usually have cravings for sweets and salt, and may be described as volatile or artistic.

• Caladium remedies the complete absence of erection despite sexual excitement. Men who benefit from this remedy may have nocturnal emissions without dreams.

• Causticum treats ED occurring with incontinence, especially loss of urine when coughing, laughing, or sneezing, or prostate problems. Homeopathic theory associates this remedy with the need to check things, such as returning home in the middle of a trip to make sure the appliances are turned off, checking bank balances several times a day, and so on.

• Lycopodium treats ED in men who are sexually inexperienced or lacking in self-confidence. Homeopathy teaches that this remedy is appropriate for men who have problems with bloating and flatulence or who have the need for rest or sleep late in the day.

• Selenium metallicum is given to men who develop ED after a serious illness. Loss of body hair or eyebrows is a sign that homeopathic selenium is an appropriate remedy.

• Staphysagria treats ED in men who suffer embarrassment in a sexual context. Homeopathic doctors typically offer this remedy to men from religious backgrounds with strong prohibitions on sexual activity.

Eye Concerns

See **Blepharitis; Cataracts; Conjunctivitis; Glaucoma, Chronic; Macular Degeneration; Night Vision, Impaired; Retinitis Pigmentosa; Retinopathy of Prematurity; Retinopathy, Diabetic.**

Eyelids, Sticky

See **Blepharitis.**

Facial Nerve Palsy/ Facial Paralysis
See **Bell's Palsy**.

Fatigue, Chronic
See **Chronic Fatigue Syndrome (CFS)**.

Fatty Liver
See **High Triglycerides**.

Female Infertility

SYMPTOM SUMMARY

○ Failure to conceive after 1 year of unprotected intercourse

UNDERSTANDING THE DISEASE PROCESS

Infertility in women can be secondary to a host of treatable diseases, most notably endometriosis, hypothyroidism, and polycystic ovarian disease. The most common direct cause of women's infertility is periodic anovulation, that is, the failure of the ovaries to release an egg prior to the menstrual period. Neither medical nor natural interventions are likely to produce immediate results, but a variety of methods can be used together to enhance the likelihood of becoming pregnant. The following interventions are most likely to help women who experience scanty flow during their period, indicating failure to ovulate. When symptoms include acne, facial hair, sensitivity to cold, heavy periods, or complete absence of periods, other treatable conditions should be considered (see AMENORRHEA, ENDOMETRIOSIS, HYPOTHYROIDISM, PELVIC INFLAMMATORY DISEASE).

TREATMENT SUMMARY

NUTRITIONAL SUPPLEMENTS

○ Take any multivitamin containing vitamin E, daily.

○ Avoid quercetin.

HERBS

❍ Vitex: 35–40 milligrams once a day, discontinued when pregnancy occurs.

See Part Three if you take prescription medication.

UNDERSTANDING THE HEALING PROCESS

Generally speaking, women trying to become pregnant should avoid alcohol, caffeine, and smoking. Scientific studies of the role of alcohol in female infertility present conflicting results, but it appears that drinking during the third week of the menstrual cycle (2 weeks after menstruation) reduces a woman's chance of becoming pregnant.[1] Drinking during early pregnancy, of course, has detrimental effects on the baby. Caffeine does not have a detrimental effect on the development of the unborn child,[2] and is not likely to have an effect on fertility unless there is endometriosis, in which case it greatly reduces chances of conception. Some chemicals in tobacco smoke actually increase fertility, but the overall effect of smoking is to lower progesterone levels and decrease the thickening of the lining of the uterus during the first half of the menstrual cycle, decreasing chances of implantation of a fertilized egg.[3]

Various vitamin deficiencies have been associated with reduced fertility, but the amounts needed to compensate for them are small. A multivitamin tablet taken daily enhances fertility, one study finding that it reduced the time required to become pregnant by about 5 percent, but it also slightly increases the likelihood of having twins or triplets.[4] Vitamin E seems to be most important to fertility. Folic acid is important to the baby's normal development.

Vitex is frequently recommended for women's infertility. The German Commission E stated that vitex is useful for increasing the volume of the corpus luteum, that is, it compensates for scanty periods. In a German study, 67 women in their 20s and 30s who had scanty periods or no periods at all took vitex once daily for 3 months. Thirty-eight became pregnant during the trial.[5] Men must not take vitex, and women should discontinue the herb when they become pregnant. There is a slightly increased risk of multiple births from taking the herb.

Women trying to become pregnant must be careful not to take supplemental quercetin, a plant flavonoid found in onions and grapefruit that blocks the action of the enzyme hyaluronidase. This enzyme breaks down hyaluronic acid, which forms a protective sticky coat around the egg and must be broken down for the egg to be released.

CONCEPTS FOR COPING WITH FEMALE INFERTILITY

❍ Prolonged foreplay may decrease the likelihood that a woman will get pregnant from that act of sexual intercourse. Magnetic resonance imaging studies show that during sexual arousal without intercourse the uterus rises and the anterior vaginal wall lengthens, increasing the distance the sperm must travel to the egg. Variations to the missionary position may be preferable for couples seeking conception, since the penis assumes a boomerang shape when the man is on top.[6]

❍ Women who are 20 percent underweight or overweight are less likely to conceive. Weight gain or weight loss programs may be helpful.

❍ Women who are contemplating pregnancy should take folic acid, 1 tablet a day (400 milligrams). This will decrease the risk of neural tube defects such as spina bifida (a hole in the spine), anencephaly (absent brain), and hydrocephaly (water in the brain). Folic acid is also present in foods such as spinach, green beans, fortified cornflakes, and oranges.

❍ Natural family planning can be used to increase or decrease chances of conception, although strong commitment from both partners is necessary for the method to be successful. A woman's fertility is greatest:

- When there is an appearance of clear, thin, elastic, and watery (like egg white) cervical mucus for 4 days. This mucus appears shortly before and shortly after the egg is released.

- When body temperature rises approximately 1°F (0.5°C) for approximately 2 days. A woman's body temperature rises just after the egg is released. It is necessary to take temperatures at the same time every day (preferably while still in bed in the morning) with an especially sensitive thermometer available from drugstores. Body temperature remains elevated until the next period starts.

- At the time of ovulation. Not every woman ovulates on the fourteenth day of her menstrual cycle. Keeping track of body temperature will give a good measure of when in the cycle ovulation occurs.

Fetal Alcohol Syndrome

SYMPTOM SUMMARY

○ Shortened eyelids

○ Thin upper lip

○ Crest in the upper lip

○ Flattened nose

○ Low birth weight

○ Slow development

UNDERSTANDING THE DISEASE PROCESS

Fetal alcohol syndrome (FAS) is a collection of symptoms caused by a mother's use of alcohol during pregnancy. Problems with learning, attention, memory, and problem solving are common, along with poor coordination, impulsiveness, and speech and hearing impairment. Learning problems may persist throughout life.

TREATMENT SUMMARY

NUTRITIONAL SUPPLEMENTS

During pregnancy, the mother should take:

○ Vitamin A: not more than 5,000 IU per day.

○ Zinc picolinate: 15 milligrams per day.

UNDERSTANDING THE HEALING PROCESS

The most important thing to be understood about FAS is that there is no safe time and no safe form of alcohol for an expectant mother to drink. Once the child is born, FAS cannot be corrected through nutritional means. Women who have drank before they found out they were pregnant *may* be able to limit damage to the unborn child through nutritional supplementation.

Although the use of vitamin A during pregnancy is associated with rare instances of birth defects, these usually result from taking 300,000 IU or more in a single dose during the first few weeks of pregnancy. Scientists believe that a mother's drinking alters the developing child's ability to use vitamin A, and that supplemental vitamin A *in limited doses may* compensate.[1]

Zinc deficiency in the mother leads to low birth weight in the child. Taking more zinc than is needed to correct deficiency has no special benefit for the child.[2] A dose of 15 milligrams per day during pregnancy is sufficient.

CONCEPTS FOR PREVENTING FETAL ALCOHOL SYNDROME

○ Any woman who could become pregnant should take folic acid, 1 tablet a day (400 milligrams). This will decrease the risk of neural tube defects such as spina bifida (a hole in the spine), anencephaly (absent brain), and hydrocephaly (water in the brain). Folic acid is also present in foods such as spinach, green beans, fortified cornflake, and oranges.

Fever Blisters
See **Cold Sores**.

Fibrocystic Breast Disease

SYMPTOM SUMMARY

○ Premenstrual breast pain or tenderness localized in cysts

○ Usually affects both breasts

UNDERSTANDING THE DISEASE PROCESS

Fibrocystic breast disease, or fibroadenomas of the breast, are tender cysts in women's breasts that become especially inflamed and painful several days before and during the menstrual period. The cause of fibrocystic breast disease is unknown. Approximately 10 percent of fibroadenomas disappear each year, and most stop growing after they are approximately 1 inch (2–3 centimeters) in size. About 2 in 5 women experience fibrocystic breast disease between the ages of 20 and 45.

Cysts in the breasts may calcify after menopause. Cysts grow rapidly in the presence of estrogen, and may be aggravated during pregnancy or by estrogen replacement therapy. Having fibrocystic breast disease roughly doubles a woman's risk of developing breast cancer, but 4 out of 5 women with the condition do *not* develop cancer.[1]

TREATMENT SUMMARY

DIET

○ Avoid chocolate, coffee, guaraná, maté, and tea.

○ Drink at least 8 glasses of water every day.

○ Eat high-fiber foods at every meal.

○ Eat yogurt or take 1–2 capsules of *Lactobacillus acidophilus* every day.

NUTRITIONAL SUPPLEMENTS

○ Wobenzym: as directed on the label.

○ Vitamin B complex: 10 times the RDA.

○ Beta-carotene: 50,000–300,000 IU daily.

○ Evening primrose or flaxseed oil: 1 tablespoon daily.

○ Vitamin B_6: 25–50 milligrams 3 times daily.

○ Vitamin C: 500 milligrams 3 times daily.

○ Vitamin E: 400–800 IU of D-alpha tocopherol daily.

○ Zinc: 15 milligrams daily.

See Part Three if you take prescription medication.

UNDERSTANDING THE HEALING PROCESS

Maintaining low estrogen levels is important to minimize the pain of fibrocystic breast disease. The liver breaks down excess estrogen and releases estrogen byproducts into the bile that is carried to the intestine. However, if the bile salts carrying estrogen stay in the intestine too long, they can be reabsorbed. Fiber and fluid keep estrogen from being reabsorbed. Women who have bowel movements every day are over 80 percent less likely to develop fibrocystic breast disease than women who have bowel movements only every other day.[2]

Regularity is not the only factor in keeping estrogen reabsorption to a minimum. Some microorganisms living in the intestine can reassemble estrogen byproducts into active estrogen that causes inflammation of the breast. Taking 1–2 capsules of *Lactobacillus* or eating yogurt with active cultures every day provides beneficial bacteria that keep these microorganisms at bay.

Caffeine (the active ingredient in coffee, guaraná, maté, and black tea), theobromine (the pleasure chemical in chocolate), and theophylline (an important active chemical in both black and green tea) interfere with a "second messenger" system in the breast that essentially tells breast cells to stop responding to the effects of estrogen during the menstrual period. Women have differing levels of sensitivity to these chemicals, but one study found that 75 percent of women who reduce their consumption of coffee, chocolate, colas, and tea and 98 percent of women who eliminate consumption of these beverages experience less breast pain.[3] Some research

suggests that the threshold level for aggravating breast pain in most women is about 2 cups of coffee or 4 cans of soda daily. Researchers have also found that drinking coffee reduces testosterone, a hormone related to maintenance of sexual desire.[4]

The best scientific evidence for any nutritional supplement for treating fibrocystic breast disease supports the use of enzyme therapy. A German clinical study of the enzyme preparation Wobenzym reported that *all* women receiving the enzyme reported improvement, more than benefited from medically directed hormone therapy.[5] Adverse reactions to Wobenzym have never been reported.

Dozens of scientific studies over 40 years come to no conclusions as to the real benefit of vitamins and minerals in treating fibrocystic breast disease. Different women seem to respond to vitamins in different ways. The best approach is to begin with a full range of supplements for 3 months and to gradually eliminate supplements one by one to see if improvement is sustained.

CONCEPTS FOR COPING WITH FIBROCYSTIC BREAST DISEASE

○ Fibrocystic breast pain can be reduced by a well-fitted brassiere or sometimes by going braless. Changing the brassiere can give immediate relief, and is the first step in controlling fibrocystic breast pain.

○ Many women report that eating soy foods and taking soy isoflavones reduces cyclical breast pain.

○ The best supplement for hard-to-treat fibrocystic breast disease is vitamin A in high doses. Women whose breast pain did not respond to elimination of caffeine or to ordinary painkillers were given 150,000 IU of vitamin A a day in a study at the University of Montreal. Eighty percent of the women tested had beneficial results with vitamin A and a dramatic reduction in the level of pain. Forty percent of the women had at least a 50 percent decrease in the size of their breast lumps. The reduction in breast pain persisted 8 months after the women in the study quit taking vitamin A.[6] This dosage of vitamin A, however, could have toxic effects on an unborn child during the first trimester of pregnancy, and some women will experience headaches. Do not take high doses of vitamin A unless you cannot become pregnant. Women who are or who may become pregnant should strictly limit their intake of vitamin A to 5,000 IU per day or less. Many experts recommend provitamin A, beta-carotene, as a substitute for vitamin A on the basis of the University of Montreal study, but no study has confirmed the benefit of treating breast cysts with beta-carotene.

Fibroids

SYMPTOM SUMMARY

○ Heavy bleeding during menstruation

○ Abdominal pain similar to menstrual cramps

○ Urge to urinate when lying down, especially at night

○ Dyspareunia, pain during sexual intercourse

○ Constipation

○ Larger fibroids may form palpable hard lumps in the lower abdomen

○ In severe cases, the contour of the uterus may resemble that of pregnancy

○ Many women with fibroids have no symptoms

○ If menstrual bleeding is severe enough to cause anemia, there may also be shortness of breath, pale skin, headaches, and ringing in the ears.

UNDERSTANDING THE DISEASE PROCESS

A uterine fibroid, known in medicine as a leiomyoma or simply as a myoma, is a noncancerous growth of muscle and connective tissue in the uterus. The size of a fibroid ranges from the head of a pin to a large melon, individual tumors sometimes weighing as much as 20 pounds (9 kilograms). Uterine fibroids are the most common tumor of the female reproductive organs. Some studies estimate that up to 80 percent of women between the ages of 30 and 50 have uterine fibroids, although only 25 percent of women experience symptoms. In the United States, African-American women are especially likely to suffer fibroids, and they tend to have more numerous fibroids causing pain and anemia.

Uterine fibroids can do serious damage to fertility. Fibroids can block the cervix so that sperm cannot reach the uterus. They can block the fallopian tubes so that the egg cannot reach the uterus. They can distort the endometrium so that a fertilized egg cannot attach itself and begin growth. When pregnancy is achieved, small fibroids are enough to increase the risk of miscarriage.

Fibroids pressing against the urinary canal elevate the risk of urinary tract infections, and any fibroid can cause pain.

The growth of fibroids is fueled by estrogen. Fibroids often first appear during pregnancy, when a woman's body produces enormous quantities of estrogen, and disappear during menopause, when estrogen production is greatly decreased. The hormone progesterone also plays a role in the growth of fibroids. These two hormones together keep the fibroid alive and protect it from natural processes that would cause it to shrink and die.

The risk factors for fibroids are high estrogen levels, such as the use of high-estrogen oral contraceptives, use of estrogen replacement therapy, or overweight. Poor circulation does not accelerate the formation of fibroids, but it can make existing fibroids intensely painful. Women who have high blood pressure, especially women who begin taking high blood pressure medication before age 35, are especially likely to suffer painful fibroids. Other risk factors include history of pelvic inflammatory disease or chlamydia, infections caused by a poorly fitted IUD, and regular use of feminine hygiene products containing talcum powder.[1]

TREATMENT SUMMARY

DIET

○ Avoid beef and ham, emphasize green vegetables and fruit.

HERBS

○ Black cohosh: 250–500 milligrams 3 times a day.

See Part Three if you take prescription medication.

UNDERSTANDING THE HEALING PROCESS

Research into the interrelationship of diet and fibroids is limited, but Italian investigators found that women with uterine myomas reported more frequent consumption of beef, other red meat, and ham and less frequent consumption of green vegetables, fruit, and fish. The study of 1,557 women found that eating more beef roughly doubled the risk of having fibroids, whereas eating more green vegetables cut the risk of fibroids in half.[2]

No herb is more useful in treating fibroids than black cohosh. This widely used women's herb contains chemicals that keep estrogen from stimulating the proliferation of cells,[3] stopping the growth of fibroid tissue. Laboratory studies specifically confirm that black cohosh, unlike so many other hormone-related products, absolutely does not stimulate the growth of cancerous cells.[4] Unlike medications for uterine fibroids, black cohosh does not block the *beneficial* actions of estrogen.

Three classes of compounds in black cohosh bind to receptor sites in the reproductive tract, the brain, and other organs that otherwise would receive estrogen. This reduces overall estrogen activity when estrogen levels are high. Other compounds in black cohosh compounds block the formation of luteinizing hormone (LH), which stimulates a surge of estrogen production in the first 14 days of the menstrual period. This stimulates estrogen production when estrogen levels are low. The dual action of the herb allows it to stabilize the body's estrogen usage.[5]

Taking more than 3,000 milligrams of black cohosh a day may cause abdominal pain, nausea, headaches, and dizziness. Women who are pregnant or breastfeeding should not use black cohosh.

The Female Reproductive System

The uterus or womb is a pear-shaped organ between the bladder and the lower intestine. It consists of two parts, the body and the cervix.

The cervix is the lower third of the uterus. It has a canal opening into the vagina known as the os, which carries menstrual blood out of the uterus.

The upper two-thirds, or body, of the uterus is lined with the endometrium, a thick inner layer rich in blood vessels. During pregnancy estrogen stimulates the endometrium to expand to support the growing fetus. When a woman of reproductive age is not pregnant, the endometrium grows and is slouged off through the monthly period of menstruation.

At the sides of the body of the uterus are two fallopian tubes, conduits through which the ovaries release the egg. Within the ovaries are 200,000 to 400,000 follicles, cellular sacs containing the materials needed for the egg to mature.

CONCEPTS FOR COPING WITH UTERINE FIBROIDS

○ Women who take the estrogen-sequestering drug leuprolide (Lupron) for uterine fibroids are at risk for bone loss. Taking supplemental ipriflavone can reduce the risk of bone loss and also keep LDL cholesterol levels down during treatment with this drug.[6]

○ Uterine fibroids become cancerous in approximately 1 out of 10,000 cases. Uterine fibroids do not increase your risk for uterine or any form of cancer.

○ Many women use herbal products containing dioscorea, or wild yam, to treat problems in menopause. Some dioscorea creams contain progesterone that is not declared on the label, and which activate fibroids. Use either dioscorea tincture or creams that are clearly identified as not containing synthetic progesterone.

○ Surgical adhesions are a frequent complication of hysterectomy for fibroids. For further information, see PELVIC ADHESIONS.

Filiariasis
See **Lymphedema**.

Flatulence

SYMPTOM SUMMARY
○ Abdominal bloating

○ Excessive release of gas (more than 20 times a day)

UNDERSTANDING THE DISEASE PROCESS

Flatus or flatulence is air or gas in the intestine that is released through the rectum. Everyone passes gas. Flatus is a normal byproduct of eating. Approximately 17 milliliters of air, a little more than a tablespoon, goes down with every bite of food or swallow of water. This gas builds up to a volume between a pint and half a gallon ($1/2$–2 liters) and has to be released 6–20 times a day. Approximately 99.999 percent of the volume of flatus is odor-free. However, very small traces of the sulfur-containing gases hydrogen sulfide, dimethyl sulfide, and methanethiol are sufficient to cause intense odor.

Inflammation of the intestinal wall may cause sudden release of large amounts of flatus. Excess gas may be released from carbonated beverages or formed in the large intestine as the result of bacterial action on undigested food. Approximately 30 percent of the population of the United States—including 50 percent of Hispanics, 80 percent of African-Americans, and 90 percent of Asian Americans—lacks an enzyme needed to digest milk sugars. Even healthy people cannot digest large quantities of fructose sugars from fruit or the complex polysaccharides found in beans, broccoli, cabbage, cauliflower, or Brussels sprouts.

Flatulence is usually not a serious medical problem. Flatulence, accompanying severe steady pain in the upper abdomen or yellowing of the skin or eyes, however, requires urgent medical attention.

TREATMENT SUMMARY

DIET

○ Cinnamon, dandelion greens, the Mexican herb epizote (used to prepare *frijoles* or bean dishes), fennel seeds, or flaxseed *powders* (not whole flaxseeds) can be used in recipes to reduce gas formation.

○ Keep a flatulographic record to identify offending foods. Write down a list of the foods you eat and note whether you pass gas after eating them. A diary of what you eat with notes of excessive flatulence will help you identify the foods you need to avoid. Common offenders are apples, apricots, bagels, baked beans, barley, beets, black-eyed peas, bog beans, bran, breakfast cereals, broccoli, Brussels sprouts, cabbage, cauliflower, chickpeas, chili, corn, cucumbers, dairy products (in people who are lactose intolerant), eggs, eggplant, fava beans, leeks, lentils, lettuce, lima beans, nuts, oat flour, onions, pasta, peanut butter, peanuts, peas, peppers, pinto beans, pistachios, popcorn, prunes, raisins, sesame seeds, soybeans, soy milk, tofu, whole wheat flour, and whole-grain breads. The no-calorie sweeteners sorbitol and xylitol may also cause gas.

HERBS

Take any one of the following herbs.

○ Angelica (European angelica or *Angelica archangelica*):
  • Essential oil, 10 drops in $1/4$ cup of water after meals, *or*
  • Fluid extract, $1/2$–1 teaspoon after meals.

○ Aniseed:
  • Tea made with 1 teaspoon of crushed seed or 1 tea bag in 1 cup of hot water steeped 10–15 minutes, up to 3 times a day after meals.

○ Caraway:
  • Oil, 1–2 drops in $1/4$ cup of water or on a sugar cube taken after meals.

○ Chamomile:
  • Tea made with 1 teaspoon of crushed herb or 1 tea bag in 1 cup of hot water steeped 10–15 minutes, up to 4 times a day, after or between meals.

○ Fennel:
  • Tea made with 1 teaspoon of crushed seed or 1 tea bag in 1 cup hot water steeped 10–15 minutes, up to 3 times a day after or between meals.
  • Fennel-seed candies after meals.

○ Ginger:
  • Capsules (400–500 milligrams), 1 before meals, *or*
  • Chewable tablets (67.5 milligrams), one after each meal, *or*
  • Ginger juice with other fruit juices, as desired.

○ Lavender:
  • Prepare an infusion from 1 teaspoon of chopped herb drawn in $2/3$ cup of hot water for 10 minutes, strained before drinking, *or*
  • Place 1–4 drops of lavender oil on a sugar cube and eat the cube.

○ Peppermint:
  • Tea made with 1 teaspoon of peppermint or 1 tea bag in $2/3$ cup of hot water allowed to steep in a closed container for 10 minutes.

It is also possible to prepare a homemade peppermint liqueur by leaving 8 ounces of peppermint leaves in a bottle of vodka for 10 days, shaking the bottle every 2–3 days. Strain the mixture before storage. Take $1/2$–1 teaspoon of the liqueur between meals.

See Part Three if you take prescription medication.

UNDERSTANDING THE HEALING PROCESS

There are two basic approaches to controlling flatulence: avoid offending foods, or calm the digestive tract to minimize the release of gas. The herbal treatments presented here minimize the release of gas.

Angelica is an appropriate remedy for people who do not care for herbal teas. It stimulates the production of gastric juices and helps the digestion of meats and fatty foods. It also prevents spasmodic flatulence.

Using angelica several times a day *plus* taking oral contraceptives, sulfa drugs, tetracycline, the blood pressure medication lisinopril (Prinivil or Zestril), or the arthritis drug piroxicam (Feldene) could increase the risk of sunburn. Do not use angelica if you take any of these drugs.

Aniseed is a traditional remedy for flatulence, as well as for bronchitis, colds, coughs, fevers, and sore throat. It is an ingredient in paregoric, an opium mixture once given to colicky babies. It is particularly useful in controlling spasmodic flatulence. It acts by increasing secretions in the digestive tract that encourage passing gas in smaller, unnoticed quantities.[1] Foods prepared with aniseed, such as aniseed cookies and ouzo, have the same effect as the herb, but would have to be consumed in quantity to control flatulence.

Many recipes from the Caucasus, the Near East, the Himalayas, Mongolia, and Morocco include caraway oil to prevent flatulence from gassy foods. It relieves bloating, cramps, and nervous stomach. In folk medicine caraway oil is used to induce menstruation, so it should be avoided by women who have heavy periods.

Chamomile has been used for centuries to treat flatulence. When chamomile is placed in hot water, it releases chamazulene. This chemical stops the release of free radicals involved in food allergy reactions.[2] The essential oil blocks the release of histamine, protecting the digestive tract from irritation.[3]

Essential oils are lost by boiling or evaporation, so it is important to brew chamomile teas with hot, but not boiling, water and in a teapot or other closed container. Allergic reactions to chamomile are rare but possible. Most European regulatory boards advise that chamomile should not be used during pregnancy.

Fennel promotes the passage of food through the intestines while stopping muscle spasms that allow the escape of gas.

Never take pure fennel *oil* by mouth. It can cause acid stomach and intestinal irritation. In women, daily consumption of fennel seed may increase estrogen levels. Women who have estrogen-sensitive disorders (such as fibroids or fibrocystic breast disease) should not take fennel on a regular basis.

Ginger counteracts biochemical changes that occur after eating high-fat meals. Specifically, it deactivates Platelet Activating Factor (PAF), a hormonal agent of gastrointestinal inflammation.[4] It increases the rate at which food passes through the intestines, reducing the amount of bacterial fermentation in the gut.[5]

Ginger inhibits the body's synthesis of the stress hormone thromboxane, one of the chemical triggers for the formation of a thrombus, or blood clot.[6] For this reason, it should not be taken by people who suffer anemia or sickle-cell anemia or who have low levels of blood-clotting factors due to liver disease. It also should be avoided by people who take blood thinners, such as aspirin, clopidogrel (Plavix), ticlopidine HCl (Ticlid), or warfarin (Coumadin). Taking these medications with ginger could result in unexpected bleeding. Ginger also increases the absorption of barbiturates, increasing sleepiness.

Lavender encourages the secretion of bile from the gallbladder, making it easier to digest fats. People who have gallstones should avoid the herb, since it increases flow through the bile duct.

Lavender is also mildly sedating. In laboratory studies with animals, the essential oils of lavender counter the anxiety-inducing effects of caffeine.[7] This property makes the herb especially useful for people whose flatulence is worse under conditions of emotional duress or after drinking coffee.

Peppermint is probably the world's most widely used remedy for bloating and gas. It is especially helpful for flatulence associated with a "nervous stomach." The essential oil slows the rate at which the intestines contract to expel both stool and gas, making emissions smaller, less noisy, and less frequent.[8]

Peppermint stimulates the release of bile, so it should be avoided by people who have gallstones, gallbladder inflammation, or severe liver damage. Anyone who has an allergy to menthol should also avoid peppermint.

CONCEPTS FOR COPING WITH FLATULENCE

○ Eat slowly to avoid swallowing air.

○ Don't drink carbonated beverages or any beverages through a straw. This will reduce the amount of air getting into your stomach.

○ Avoid chewing gums sweetened with sorbitol or xylitol. These sweeteners contain complex carbohydrates that are not absorbed through the lining of the intestine. Instead, they remain in the gut where they are fermented by intestinal bacteria. The action of chewing gum also causes the swallowing air, increasing the volume of gas.

○ The Flatulence Filter, a portable seat cushion containing activated charcoal, traps disagreeable odors. Tests at the Minneapolis Veterans Affairs Medical Center found that it traps over 90 percent of the sulfur gases that cause the stink of flatulence, including hydrogen sulfide, methanethiol, and dimethyl sulfide.[9] The cushion is available for purchase by calling UltraTech Products at 1–800–316–8668 (outside the United States, 1–410–631–4776) or by writing UltraTech Products, Inc., 11191 Westheimer #123, Houston, Texas 77042.

○ If you find flatulence to be a problem while taking a psyllium-based laxative such as Metamucil, switch to a soluble-fiber laxative such as Citrucel.

○ Angostura bitters are made from gentian, an herb that is so bitter that it induces a gastric reflex to release digestive juices. People who can stand the taste find that taking the bitters greatly reduces bloating and gas after eating meat and fatty foods. People who have gallstones should avoid Angostura and other kinds of bitters, because all bitters stimulate the flow of bile.

○ Contrary to common belief, drinking beer does not cause gas. Hops, in fact, relieves stress-related digestive problems, although they are more effective taken as an herb than in beer.

○ The herb marrubio (horehound), found in the southwestern United States, is a bitter that also relieves gas caused by eating fatty foods. Marrubio is traditionally taken as a tea, made by steeping 1 teaspoon of the chopped herb in 1 cup of hot water in a closed vessel for 10 minutes. The tea is strained before it is drunk.

○ The methane and oxygen in flatus make it somewhat flammable. Setting flatus on fire has actually occurred, with serious injury to the emitter of the gas.

○ If you experience severe flatulence after traveling abroad, you may have a persistent infection known as giardiasis. See GIARDIASIS for further information.

○ Pepto-Bismol helps control odor, although it does not necessarily stop the release of gas. Bismuth subsalicy-late, the "pink" in Pepto-Bismol, reduces odor by taking hydrogen sulfide out of the flatus. Hydrogen sulfide is the chemical responsible for rotten egg smell. Do not take Pepto-Bismol if you are sensitive to aspirin or NSAIDs such as Indocin (indomethacin), Motrin (ibuprofen), or Orudis (ketoprofen). Do not take Pepto-Bismol every day, since the bismuth in the product could build up to toxic levels.

○ Activated charcoal is advisable for people who cannot take Pepto-Bismol. Like Pepto-Bismol, activated charcoal does not reduce the volume of gas,[10] but traps obnoxious odors. It is important not to take activated charcoal with prescription medications, especially acetaminophen, the antiseizure medications Depakene and Depakote (valproic acid), Dilantin (phenytoin), and Tegretol (carbamazepine), the heart medications Lanoxin (digoxin) and Lasix (furosemide), most pain relievers for arthritis, and the antibiotic tetracycline. For more information and a free sample, write to Requa, Inc., Dept. P, P. O. Box 4008 Greenwich, CT 06830.

○ Bean-O is an over-the-counter product that may reduce flatulence caused by eating fiber-rich foods such as beans, bran, and broccoli. The product is an enzyme, alpha-galactosidase, which helps break down the complex sugars found in gassy foods into simple sugars that the body can comfortably digest. These additional sugars add 2 to 6 percent to total calories of carbohydrate foods. Bean-O has no effect on proteins or gluten. Despite these drawbacks, many people find Bean-O to be the answer for persistent gas problems. There is also a version for pets called CurTail. For additional information and/or a free sample, call toll-free 1–800–257–8650 between 8:30 A.M. and 5:30 P.M. EST.

○ Lactaid is an over-the-counter product that may reduce flatulence caused by eating or drinking dairy foods and other products containing milk sugars, including convenience foods and medications. It treats an enzyme deficiency for milk sugar rather than an allergy to milk. To determine if Lactaid may be helpful to you, eat a normal breakfast and include a large, 12-ounce glass of milk of any kind. Over the next 6 hours, keep track of any discomfort you may have (if you experience any kind of severe reaction, consult a physician). The next day, prepare an identical breakfast with another 12-ounce glass of milk. Swallow a Lactaid tablet with your first sip of milk. If your symptoms are not as bad on the second day, Lactaid may be helpful.

Flu

SYMPTOM SUMMARY

○ Chills

○ Dry cough

○ Fatigue

○ Fever up to 104°F (40°C)

○ Muscle aches

○ Nausea

○ Runny or stuffy nose

○ Sneezing

○ Sore throat

○ Vomiting

○ Most common in winter months (November to April in the northern hemisphere, June to October in the Southern hemisphere)

○ Onset of symptoms is usually sudden and intense

UNDERSTANDING THE DISEASE PROCESS

Influenza, commonly referred to as the flu, is a disease caused by the influenza virus. It causes many of the same symptoms as a cold, but comes on more quickly and is more severe. Every year, millions of people catch the flu. According to the Centers for Disease Control, between 10 and 20 percent of the entire population of the United States gets the flu each year. An average of 114,000 people per year have to be admitted to the hospital, and 20,000 people per year die of the flu, making it a leading cause of death, especially among small children, people over 65, and people with cancer, HIV, or other diseases causing a compromised immune system. In nursing homes, 60 out of 100 patients can be affected, with up to 30 fatalities. A person over age 65 is at risk because the immune system is weakened and, over the years, "forgets" it has been exposed to influenza.

There are three types of influenza viruses, influenza A, B, and C. Influenza A is typically spread from person to person (although a particularly deadly strain of influenza A was spread from chickens to people in Hong Kong in 1997), but influenza B and C can be spread from human to human or from animals to humans. Influenza A infections are the most common, while influenza B infections are the most deadly. Influenza C causes a very mild illness that does not cause epidemics.

The flu virus is spread when an infected person coughs, spits, speaks, or sneezes and sends virus particles in the air to be inhaled by other people. Less often, the flu is spread when sputum or mucus of an infected person lands on a doorknob or other surface and is then touched by another person who then touches his or he nose or mouth. To cause infection, the spherical influenza virus must insert protein spikes called hemagglutinin into the linings of red blood cells. Once it has entered the cells, the virus multiplies in the linings of the nose and throat for 3–7 days before causing symptoms, but it can be transmitted from person to person just a few hours after infection. An infected person sheds and spreads the virus for about a week, although people with weakened immune systems (people with cancer, HIV, or taking immunosuppressant drugs after transplant) are infectious for up to 2–3 weeks.

The influenza virus is constantly mutating so every epidemic is caused by a different strain of the infection. The immune system seldom gets a chance to use its "memory" to fight the flu, so that it is possible for people to get the flu many times during their lifetimes. Vaccination and/or other measures are necessary every year to avoid getting the flu.

TREATMENT SUMMARY

NUTRITIONAL SUPPLEMENTS

For general prevention:

○ Selenium: 100 micrograms per day, beginning at least 3 months before flu season.

○ If you get the flu every year, have a test for iron deficiency.

As soon as you know you have been exposed to the flu:

○ Vitamin C: take 1,000 milligrams every hour for 6 hours, then 1,000 milligrams 3 times per day until symptoms subside.

○ Vitamin E: 400–1,000 IU daily.

HERBS

For general prevention:

○ Ginseng: extract, as directed on the label, beginning 4 weeks before vaccination and continuing throughout flu season.

As soon as you know you have been exposed to the flu:

○ *Echinacea purpurea:* juice (preferred), 20 drops every 2 hours you are awake for the first day, then 3 times a day for 10 days.

○ Elderberry (*Sambucus*): beginning in October and continuing through March, 1–2 teaspoons of extract daily for children, 2–4 teaspoons of extract daily for adults.

See Part Three if you take prescription medication.

UNDERSTANDING THE HEALING PROCESS

Tens of millions of people take flu shots to prevent the flu. The problem with relying on flu shots is that they are not always effective. Flu vaccines have to be made months before flu season. This requires epidemiologists to make a best guess as to which strain of the flu virus will cause the next year's epidemic. If the scientists' prediction of the strain is correct, influenza vaccinations will prevent infection in 70–90 percent of healthy people under 65. They are only 30–60 percent effective in the elderly and for people who have chronic diseases.

There are several natural products that help prevent catching the flu. Selenium can more than double the immune system's response to vaccines and infection, but selenium deficiency takes at least 100 days to correct.[1] For this reason, it is important to begin taking selenium in late summer to help prevent the flu. If you do catch the flu, having an adequate supply of selenium in your body greatly reduces the risk of developing pneumonia.[2]

Iron is necessary for the immune system's response to the flu virus.[3] People who catch the flu every year should have a blood test for iron deficiency, and if (and only if) iron levels are low, take iron supplements.

Testing the well-known herbal formula Ginsana, scientists at the University of Milan found that taking ginseng every day beginning a month before getting a flu shot and for 3 months thereafter reduces the incidence of both colds and flu by two-thirds. Ginsana increased antibody levels by more than 50 percent and nearly doubled the number of natural killer (NK) cells by the eighth week of the study. There were very few adverse reactions to the herb, primarily insomnia.

Megadoses of vitamin C, preferably started before symptoms appear, greatly reduce the severity of the flu. A study of 462 students aged 18–32 found that symptoms of colds and flu were reduced up to 85 percent by high-dose vitamin C treatment.[4] Some people will experience loose bowels on the first day of vitamin C treatment, but this is a transient side effect. Since the body can become dependent on high levels of vitamin C, it is important only to take doses of 3,000 milligrams per day when you know you have been exposed to the flu. Vitamin E is an important cofactor for vitamin C, and animal studies show that vitamin E lowers the likelihood of developing pneumonia.[5]

Echinacea is the most frequently used herb for treating the flu, but it is not necessarily the first choice for treating the flu. In a study reported in the *European Journal of Clinical Research,* 120 people were given either *Echinacea purpurea* juice (prepared by the German company that makes the American product Echinagard) or a placebo as soon as they started showing symptoms of a cold or flu. The volunteers took 20 drops of echinacea or the placebo every 2 hours for 1 day, then 20 drops 3 times a day for a total of 10 days. Only 40 percent of those taking echinacea developed "real colds" or flu, compared to 60 percent of those taking the placebo. Among the volunteers who did develop colds or flu, those taking echinacea started getting better in an average of 4 days compared to an average of 8 days for those who took the placebo.[6]

Other studies of echinacea have found similar results. The benefits of echinacea in treating colds and flu seem to be greatest in people who have low T-cell counts,[7] such as people on chemotherapy or who use corticosteroids for lupus, multiple sclerosis, rheumatoid arthritis, or Sjögren's syndrome, or people with HIV or AIDS. Some people shouldn't use echinacea. Women who are trying to get pregnant should avoid *Echinacea purpurea.* It contains caffeoyl esters that can interfere with the action of hyaluronidase, an enzyme essential to the release of unfertilized eggs into the fallopian tube.[8]

There is laboratory evidence that *Echinacea angustifolia* contains chemicals that deactivate CYP3A4. This is a liver enzyme that breaks down a wide range of medications, including anabolic steroids, the chemotherapy drug methotrexate used in treating cancer and lupus, astemizole (Hismanal) for allergies, nifedipine (Adalat) and captopril (Capoten) for high blood pressure, and sildenafil (Viagra) for impotence, as well as many others. *Echinacea angustifolia* might help maintain levels of these drugs in the bloodstream and make them more effective, or it might also cause them to accumulate to levels at which they cause side effects. Switch to a brand of echinacea that does not contain *Echinacea angustifolia* if you experience unexpected side effects while taking any of these drugs.[9]

Echinacea stimulates immune function, but it also slightly increases production of T cells.[10] These are the immune cells attacked by HIV. When there are more T cells, the virus has more cells to infect. This gives it more opportunities to mutate into a drug-resistant form. The authoritative reference work *The Complete German Commission E Monographs* counsels against the use of echinacea for treating colds and flu in people who have HIV or autoimmune diseases such as multiple sclerosis. Later communications between the senior editor of the *Monographs* and the German Food and Drug Administration revealed that the warning in the reference book was based on theoretical speculation rather than practical experience.[11] Still, as a precaution, people with HIV should only use echinacea for *treating* the flu rather than preventing it.

Elderberry does not pose these problems. In fact, it is recommended for people who have HIV, people on chemotherapy, and people with other serious immune problems.[12] More important, it has a very specific effect on the influenza virus.

Dr. Madeleine Mumcuoglu discovered that elderberry contains a protein that prevents hemagglutinin, the "spikes" of the flu virus, from attaching to cells. This action effectively confines the flu virus and limits the duration of symptoms. Clinical studies at Hebrew University in Jerusalem have found taking elderberry extract reduces the duration of flu symptoms from an average of 6 days to 2–3 days.[13] Elderberry is effective against both influenza A and influenza B. An added advantage to the use of elderberry is its record of safety. There are no known adverse reactions to the use of the herb, although the possibility of an individual allergic reaction can never be discounted. Children may respond best to an elderberry formula made with glycerin rather alcohol or sugar syrup.

Wild indigo, also known as baptisia, is sometimes recommended for treatment of flu. It is best used in combination with echinacea. The two herbs taken together have a greater immunostimulant effect than either separately.

Osha, like elderberry, is effective against both A and B strains of the flu. It is most often taken as a tea.

CONCEPTS FOR COPING WITH INFLUENZA

○ While vomiting, diarrhea, and being "sick to your stomach" can sometimes be related to the flu—particularly in children—these problems are rarely the main symptoms of influenza. Influenza is primarily a respiratory disease, and gastrointestinal symptoms usually point to another cause.

○ The herb mullein contains chemicals that kill bacteria and stop pain.[14] Taken at the same time as a flu treatment such as amatadine (Symmetrel), it greatly increases the probability that the flu treatment will work.[15] The combination of mullein and zanamivir (Relenza) has not yet been tested. Mullein does not generally cause any side effects, although some people may be allergic to it.

○ N-acetyl cysteine (NAC) helps relieve flu symptoms in people who have chronic bronchitis, cystic fibrosis, emphysema, tuberculosis, or other chronic obstructive pulmonary diseases. Take 600 milligrams 3 times a day for up to 10 days.

○ There are a number of homeopathic remedies for the flu. Usually it is best to start with a single dose of the lowest strength (6C, 6X, or 12C) of the remedy matching the symptoms to be treated, and then wait for a response. If there is an improvement in symptoms, let the remedy continue to work until there is no more improvement, then take another dose. If there is no improvement, try a different potency (30X or 30C). Sometimes homeopathic medicines work for a few minutes, and sometimes they work for an entire day before another dose is needed.

• Aconitum napellus relieves sudden and severe symptoms of flu that come with anxiety, palpitations, racing pulse, constricted pupils, fever, and severe thirst. Most homeopathic physicians recommend this remedy for symptoms beginning after exposure to cold or wind.

• Apis mellifica relieves pain that begins with swollen tonsils and sore throat and spreads to the eyes and ears. Unlike aconitum, apis is used when there is little thirst.

• Arsenicum album relieves a bundle of symptoms including diarrhea, nausea, vomiting, runny nose, and sneezing fits. The head may feel feverish while the rest of the body is cold.

• Belladonna, like aconitum, relieves sudden, severe symptoms, but belladonna is more appropriate for "red" symptoms (red face, rashes, fever, and red and inflamed sore throat). There may be alternating fever and chills, or the hands and feet may feel cold while the rest of the body feels feverish.

• Bryonia is recommended for people who become emotionally out of sorts and when the worst symptom of flu is muscle pain. This remedy may also be appropriate when stomach pain is a prominent symptom.

• Eupatorium perforliatum, the homeopathic preparation of the herb boneset, relieves "aches in the bones," especially in the legs and lower back. Chills may be felt in the legs and back, pain in the eyes, and a heavy sensation in the head.

• Ferrum phosphoricum is most appropriate when prominent symptoms are dry and hard cough, strong thirst, vomiting after eating, fever, headache, and rosy cheeks. This remedy is usually recommended during the early stages of the flu.

• Gelsemium treats headache that is worse at the back of the head, with drooping eyes and all-over achiness. Symptoms successfully treated with gelsemium become worse over a period of several days.

• Nux vomica is best used when abdominal cramps and nausea are the primary symptoms. There may also be oversensitivity to light and sound and extreme sensitivity to drafts and chills despite high fever.

• Phosphorus is recommended when flu causes flushes in the face. The person most responsive to this treatment is likely to feel anxious and in need of reassurance.

• Rhus toxicodendron treats symptoms relieved by taking hot baths, especially bone and muscle aches. Bloating, a red tongue, a slight cough, and stiffness are other symptoms.

• Sulfur is recommended for people who take a long time to get over symptoms. People who respond well to this treatment tend to have low fever, reddened tongue and throat, and experience a burning sensation when coughing or sneezing.

Fluid Retention
See **Bruises; Congestive Heart Failure; Preeclampsia and Eclampsia; Varicose Veins**.

Folliculitis
See **Abscesses of the Skin**.

Folling's Disease
See **Phenylketonuria (PKU)**.

Foot Odor

SYMPTOM SUMMARY

○ Abnormal, offensive odor of the feet not necessarily associated with perspiration

UNDERSTANDING THE DISEASE PROCESS

Foot odor is seldom a topic of polite conversation, even though many people suffer from this embarrassing and at times frustrating problem. Foot odor is a problem especially for active people whose feet sweat a lot. Fortunately, foot odor can usually be controlled with simple measures.

Intense and disagreeable foot or body odor, also known as bromhidrosis, is an abnormality of the secretory glands of the skin. The secretory glands of the skin are divided into two types, eccrine and apocrine. Eccrine glands are distributed over the entire skin surface. They are primarily involved in regulating body temperature by producing sweat. Apocrine glands have a limited distribution, involving the feet, skin around the reproductive organs, and breasts. They have no role in regulating body temperature but are responsible for the release of pheromones, chemical attractants and repellents that have a role in social interaction.

Excessive foot or body odor usually involves the apocrine glands. Various species of *Corynebacterium* bacteria colonize in the apocrine glands and feed on fatty acids. Intense body odor is due to the odor of the rancid fatty acid byproducts the bacteria produce. Sweat released by the eccrine glands softens the skin and encourages the release of the offending fatty acid byproducts, and spreads the odor across the body with the flow of sweat.[1]

Smelly feet are the most common manifestation of bromhidrosis. The condition is most common in young adults, and is only rarely seen in persons over the age of 40. Foot odor associated with excessive sweating is generally seen only in children. Persistent body odor that is resistant to personal hygiene is a relatively rare condition.

While body odor is usually only unpleasant, certain kinds of body odors indicate serious underlying conditions. Fish-odor syndrome, in which the body exudes the odor of rotting fish, results from the failure of the liver to process L-carnitine. There is an excessive excretion of the chemical trimethylamine in urine, sweat, and breath. Persons with this condition may experience tachycardia (fast heart rate) and severe high blood pressure after eating cheese (which contains tyramine) and after using nasal sprays containing epinephrine. The syndrome is associated with various psychological reactions, including social isolation, clinical depression, and attempted suicide. This condition can result from an inherited genetic abnormality or from overdosing the supplement L-carnitine.

A body odor like nail polish is a sign of ketoacidosis, a complication of uncontrolled diabetes. Diabetics suffering ketoacidosis usually experience dehydration that is not relieved by drinking water, visual disturbances, and severe mood swings. Ketoacidosis in and of itself does not usually cause death, but requires urgent medical care to prevent serious complications.

TREATMENT SUMMARY

HERBS

○ Tea tree oil, in emollient form (8% tea tree oil) or tea tree solution (40%), rubbed into the feet daily.

UNDERSTANDING THE HEALING PROCESS

"Wash and dry" is primary care for foot odor. It is important both to remove *Corynebacterium* bacteria from the skin and to deprive them of an environment conducive to their growth and spread. Other helpful practices include:

Washing:

○ Wash briskly with antibacterial soap, including between the toes.

○ Dry the skin between the toes with a hair dryer.

Footwear:

○ Allow shoes to air out for at least 24 hours after use.

○ Wear absorbent socks and change them frequently.

○ Wear shoes that "breathe."

Over-the-counter products:

○ Antiperspirants can decrease moisture.

○ Tea tree oil usually controls *Corynebacterium* overgrowths after 2–3 weeks of daily application.[2] If tea tree oil is not adequate to control foot odor, see your healthcare provider for an evaluation of special circumstances.

Foot Ulcers
(Diabetic Complication)

SYMPTOM SUMMARY

○ Openings of the skin on the soles of the feet that fail to heal

○ Signs that feet are at risk for ulceration:

  • Bunions

  • Claw toes

  • Hammer toes

  • Mallet toes

  • Feet widening and flattening with age

UNDERSTANDING THE DISEASE PROCESS

Wounds to the feet that will not heal are a common complication of advanced diabetes. The National Institute of Diabetes and Digestive and Kidney Diseases (NIDDKD) estimates that 15 percent of all people with diabetes eventually have a foot ulcer, and 6 out of every 1,000 people with diabetes have an amputation. Foot ulcers are most common in diabetics who have neuropathy (see NEUROPATHY).

Suffering a permanent loss of sensation similar to numbness in the lips after getting a shot of anesthetic in the dentist's office, diabetics with advanced neuropathy lose the ability to distinguish sharp and dull pain in their feet. Minor cuts and scrapes can go unnoticed and untreated and develop into potentially serious bacterial infections. The healing process in the foot is further impeded by poor circulation in the capillaries of the skin. These microscopic blood vessels become clogged and cannot be opened by surgical means. The combination of these two processes makes diabetic feet especially vulnerable to slow-to-heal wounds and hard-to-treat infections.

TREATMENT SUMMARY

NUTRITIONAL SUPPLEMENTS

❍ Magnesium aspartate or magnesium citrate: 200–400 milligrams 3 times a day.

❍ Selenium: 400 micrograms per day.

❍ Vitamin C: 1,000 milligrams 3 times a day.

❍ Vitamin E: 600–800 IU per day.

See Part Three if you take prescription medication.

UNDERSTANDING THE HEALING PROCESS

Scientific investigation into the use of nutritional supplements in preventing and treating diabetic foot ulcers is very recent and very limited. Physicians at the Hospital General in Durango, Mexico have noted that nearly 95 percent of their diabetic patients who have foot ulcers are deficient in magnesium. Low magnesium levels are associated with a nearly 300 percent increase in the risk of developing foot ulcers in type 2 diabetes.[1] Whether magnesium supplementation would lower the risk of developing foot ulcers has not been scientifically established, but the benefits of magnesium in controlling cardiac arrhythmias and congestive heart failure, which are common in type 2 diabetics, make taking magnesium a sensible choice.

Magnesium is the primary element in milk of magnesia, and magnesium supplements can cause diarrhea. Usually the effect is short-term and takes places the first 2 or 3 days the supplement is taken. In heart patients, supplemental magnesium can interfere with the body's ability to absorb quinolone antibiotics that may be used in the treatment of foot ulcers, including:

❍ ciprofloxacin (Cipro, Baycip, Cetraxal, Ciflox, Cifran, Ciplox, Cyprobay, Quintor)

- enoxacin (Penetrex)
- gatifloxacin (Tequin)
- gemifloxacin (a relatively new drug)
- grepafloxacin (Raxar)
- levofloxacin (Levaquin)
- lomefloxacin (Maxaquin)
- moxifloxacin (Avelox)

- norfloxacin (amicrobin, anquin, baccidal, barazan, biofloxin, floxenor, fulgram, janacin, lex, Amicrobin, Anquin, Baccidal, Barazan, Biofloxin, Floxenor, Fulgram, Janacin, Lexinor, Norofin, Norxacin, Orixacin, Oroflox, Urinox, Zoroxin)
- ofloxacin (Floxin)
- sparfloxacin (Zagam)
- temafloxacin (Omniflox)
- trovafloxacin (Trovan)

Magnesium supplements can also interfere with the absorption of tetracycline. You should not use magnesium supplements if you have myasthenia gravis. They may exacerbate muscle weakness and precipitate a myasthenic crisis.

Laboratory evidence suggests that the failure of foot ulcers to heal may be related to a deficiency of the antioxidant glutathione.[2] Key nutrients for maintaining the body's supply of glutathione are selenium and vitamins C and E. Like magnesium, these supplements have not been conclusively demonstrated to help heal foot ulcers, but their general benefit to health justifies taking them.

CONCEPTS FOR COPING WITH DIABETIC FOOT ULCERS

To prevent foot problems from developing, people with diabetes should follow these rules for foot care:

❍ Check your feet and toes daily for any cuts, sores, bruises, bumps, or infections. Use a mirror if necessary. If you are visually impaired, ask a spouse, family member, or friend to inspect your feet daily.

❍ When you wash your feet, use warm (not hot) water and a mild soap. Test the water temperature with your wrist before putting your feet in the water. Doctors do not advise soaking your feet for long periods, since you may lose protective calluses. Dry your feet carefully with a soft towel, especially between the toes. Washing the feet every day is best.

❍ Cover your feet (except for the skin between the toes) with cold cream, a lotion containing lanolin, or petroleum jelly before putting on shoes and socks. Diabetes makes the feet sweat less than normal. Using a moisturizer helps prevent dry, cracked skin.

❍ Wear shoes that fit your feet well and allow your toes

to move. After years of neuropathy, the feet are likely to become wider and flatter. Most diabetes clinics can refer you to stores that carry shoes for diabetics, or, if needed, to a pedorthist, a specialist who can provide you with corrective shoes or inserts. Always choose shoes that have:

- Firm heels for support and stability
- Plenty of room for the toes
- Removable insoles for flexible fit
- Rocker soles, designed to reduce pressure on the ball of the foot

❍ Break in new shoes gradually, wearing them for only an hour at a time at first.

❍ Open-toe sandals especially designed for diabetics, such as Ambulator Conform Sandals, are available to accommodate claw toes, hammer toes, mallet toes, and bunions, all relatively common problems in diabetic feet. Orthotic insoles provide additional protection for patients with ball-of-foot pain. Anti-Shox Gel Sox are designed to cushion and protect the foot in the areas most susceptible to pain. The unique gel decreases friction against the foot for immediate comfort. Comfort n' Care Seamfree Socks allow blood to circulate evenly across the foot, and are made of a fabric that wicks moisture away from the skin.

❍ Ask your doctor to check your feet at every visit. Call your doctor if you notice that a sore is not healing well.

❍ Avoid sitting with your legs crossed. Crossing your legs can reduce the flow of blood to the feet.

❍ Cut your toenails straight across. Be careful not to leave any sharp corners that could cut the next toe.

❍ Examine your shoes before putting them on to make sure they have no tears, sharp edges, or objects in them that might injure your feet.

❍ If your feet are cold at night wear socks. Do not use heating pads or hot water bottles, since burns may not be felt.

❍ Never go barefoot, especially outdoors. Always wear shoes; sock alone do not protect the feet from cuts and punctures.

❍ Test the water temperature with your elbow before stepping into a bath.

❍ Use an emery board or pumice stone to file away dead skin, but do not remove calluses. Do not try to cut off any growths yourself, and do not use wart remover on your feet.

❍ Wear thick, soft socks and avoid wearing slippery socks, mended socks, or socks with seams.

Forgetfulness
See **Memory Loss**.

Fragile Capillaries
See **Bruises**.

Frostbite

SYMPTOM SUMMARY

❍ Clumsiness

❍ Coldness and stiffness

❍ Pain, throbbing, burning, or electrical sensations upon rewarming

❍ Stinging, burning, numbness

❍ Most commonly affects hands and feet, although ears and nose are also susceptible to frostbite. Deeper tissues are injured in severe cases.

❍ Cracked nails as frostbite heals

UNDERSTANDING THE DISEASE PROCESS

Frostbite is frozen skin, a condition that is worse when the skin is dehydrated. People from warm climates, African-Americans, and Arabs tend to get especially severe frostbite when exposed to severe cold.[1] After recovery from frostbite, the injured area is especially sensitive to cold.

TREATMENT SUMMARY

DIET

❍ Drink at least 3 quarts (3 liters) of water daily when exposed to cold.

HERBS

❍ Aloe: applied with Trental to severe frostbite.

O Ginkgo: 70–80 milligrams 3 times a day when cold weather starts.

See Part Three if you take prescription medication.

UNDERSTANDING THE HEALING PROCESS

Adequate hydration increases circulation and lowers the risk of frostbite. Taking ginkgo on a regular basis starting at the beginning of winter also reduces the risk of frostbite. A French expedition to the Himalayas found that mountaineers who took ginkgo had warmer skin, fingers, and toes than mountaineers who did not.[2] If you do get frostbite and are treated with Trental, discontinue ginkgo.

CONCEPTS FOR COPING WITH FROSTBITE

O When you observe frostbite, come indoors immediately. Remove all wet clothing. Immerse chilled body parts in warm—never hot—water until sensation returns, or if water is not available, cover frozen areas with a blanket. The best way to warm tissues is in a whirlpool at 106–108°F (42–44°C). Thawing usually takes 20–60 minutes. When the skin is thawed, it regains a rosy color.

O Do not test water with a frostbitten hand. If your hands are frostbitten, you will not be able to sense excessive heat and could be burned. Have someone else check water temperature if your hands have frostbite.

O Never use direct heat on frozen tissue.

O Do not thaw skin that is at risk for refreezing, for instance, if you are still in an unheated car or cabin.

O Do not rub snow on frostbitten skin. Any massage of the area can cause further injury.

O Rewarming is accompanied by a burning sensation. Blisters usually form as the skin thaws.

O It is better to walk to shelter with frozen feet than to attempt rewarming at the scene. However, walking on frostbitten feet may cause tissue chipping or fractures.

O Doctors will usually debride (surgically remove) clear blisters to reduce injury from inflammation. Blue or black blisters are left intact to prevent bleeding.

O For first aid, apply a loose dressing over the skin. Soaking the dressing in aloe helps. The combination of aloe and Trental (pentoxifylline) is better for healing than either alone.

Fungal Infection
See **Athlete's Foot**; **Ringworm**.

Galactorrhea

SYMPTOM SUMMARY

O Nipple discharge

- Clear or milky fluid, not discolored

- May involve one or both breasts

- Occurs only when pressure is applied to the breast

O Possible breast tenderness or breast lump

O Possible cracking or redness of the skin surrounding the nipple

UNDERSTANDING THE DISEASE PROCESS

Lactation, or the production of breast milk, is a normal condition in women occurring after delivery of a baby. Galactorrhea is the untimely production of breast milk. Many women who have had a baby can express a small amount of breast milk up to years after childbirth. Secretion of breast milk at other times, however, is a relatively rare condition usually signaling a hormonal imbalance.

The production of breast milk is controlled by the hormone prolactin, which is secreted by the pituitary gland in the brain. In about 30 percent of cases, galactorrhea in women is associated with a tumor of the pituitary gland. When excessive milk production is associated with a pituitary tumor, there will also be skipped menstrual periods and measurably high prolactin levels in the bloodstream. Prolactin levels can also be elevated when there are tumors in the ovaries (in women) or testicles (in men). When galactorrhea is due to a hormonal imbalance, both breasts are involved.

Milk production from one breast, especially after menopause, is in rare cases a sign of breast cancer. When breast cancer is a cause, however, the expressed milk is usually discolored. More often galactorrhea involving a single breast is associated with a benign tumor.

Many medications cause galactorrhea as a side effect. These include oral contraceptives, antidepressants, tranquilizers, heroin, morphine, and some medications for high blood pressure. Galactorrhea can also occur after using the herbs anise, blessed thistle, fennel, fenugreek, milk thistle, or silymarin. Release of breast milk by women is not uncommon during sexual stimulation. Scratchy blouses or poorly fitted bras can aggravate the condition.

Galactorrhea is more likely to be a nuisance than a serious medical condition. Women should consult a doctor promptly, however, if unexpected milk production occurs with skipped menstrual periods, headaches, trouble seeing, loss of interest in sex, acne, or growth of hair on the chest or chin. There are no established natural health practices for men with this condition. Men with galactorrhea should consult an endocrinologist.

TREATMENT SUMMARY

Do not take any treatment for galactorrhea unless you know you are not pregnant.

HERBS

For women only:

❍ Vitex (chasteberry): 80–100 milligrams of dry extract (two 40-milligram tablets or one 100-milligram tablet) daily.

See Part Three if you take prescription medication.

UNDERSTANDING THE HEALING PROCESS

Often misunderstood as *increasing* milk production, vitex, also known as chasteberry, has been used for centuries for *decreasing* unwanted milk production. The fruits of the chasteberry tree contain iridoids and flavonoids that mimic human sex hormones.[1] They have a special influence on the pituitary gland's manufacturing of prolactin, modulating the brain's production of the reward chemical dopamine in such a way that prolactin production is decreased, especially during times of stress.[2] They also bind to endorphin receptors in the brain, lowering the sensation of stress.[3] Over 50 percent of women who use vitex will also experience fewer unpleasant symptoms during their premenstrual period.[4]

While vitex is the best natural treatment for galactorrhea, there are a number of precautions for its use. It may be necessary to take this herb for up to 3 months, or 3 menstrual cycles, to get results. Women who use vitex should also use contraception. While the herb does not cause birth defects, in rare instances it appears to induce multiple ovulations resulting in twins and triplets.[5] Although women who have galactorrhea are not likely to be on estrogen replacement therapy (ERT), the herb should not be combined with ERT (Premarin, Premphase, Prempr, Provera), since it can potentially slow the rate at which the liver removes estrogen from circulation. Men trying to become fathers should not take vitex, since laboratory experiments with dogs indicate that it interferes with sperm production.[6] Most important, vitex should not be taken with the commonly prescribed medication for galactorrhea, bromocriptine (Parlodel), since the combination can cause unpredictable effects on anxiety and mood.

CONCEPTS FOR COPING WITH GALACTORRHEA

❍ Avoid stimulating your breasts.

❍ Avoid touching your nipples or having your nipples touched during sexual activity.

❍ Don't do breast self-exams more than once a month.

❍ Unexpected milk production is a symptom of several health conditions.

• In women who are not pregnant, missing a period plus galactorrhea is frequently a sign of hypothyroidism. There will also be fatigue, dry skin, sensitivity to cold weather, and unintentional weight gain. Restoring normal levels of thyroid hormone stops galactorrhea.

• Unexpected milk production in both breasts with headache, blurred vision, and loss of peripheral vision can be a sign of a pituitary tumor. If you experience these symptoms, see a physician.

• Reddish breast milk produced by one breast can be a sign of a breast tumor. See a physician for breast cancer testing.

• An outbreak of acne or growth of hair on the chest or chin with galactorrhea is a symptom requiring urgent medical attention. This combination of symptoms can result from ovarian cysts or ovarian cancer in a relatively early, treatable stage.

Gallbladder Attack
See **Gallstones**.

Gallstones

SYMPTOM SUMMARY

○ Abdominal pain

- Occurs within minutes of eating
- In the upper-middle or upper-right quadrant of the abdomen
- May radiate to the right shoulder blade or to the back
- Sharp, cramping, or dull
- Worse after a high-fat meal

○ Clay-colored stools

○ Flatulence

○ Heartburn

○ Bloating

○ In severe cases, yellow or green coloration of the skin—*an indication that medical attention is urgently needed*

UNDERSTANDING THE DISEASE PROCESS

Gallstones are crystalline precipitates of fats and minerals normally flushed out from the liver with yellow-green fluid known as bile through the gallbladder. Every year over 1 million people in the United States alone are diagnosed with gallstones, and over 300,000 cholecystectomies (surgical removals of the gallbladder) are performed. Some studies estimate that 8 percent of men and 20 percent of women in the United States have gallstones.[1]

A gallstone forms when the bile becomes supersaturated with cholesterol, calcium, the pigment bilirubin, or a combination of all three. Since cholesterol is a fat, it cannot be carried through the watery fluid of the bile unless it is joined to a carrier, lecithin. If cholesterol is overabundant, if lecithin is in shortage, or if the liver fails to produce enough bile to flush it downward to the gut, cholesterol tends to accumulate and form stones in the gallbladder. Stones grow very slowly, usually about a tenth of an inch (2 millimeters) in diameter a year, and cannot be felt until they have been forming in the gallbladder for 8–10 years. Calcium and bilirubin almost always collect with the cholesterol during the formation of the stone.

Women are 2 to 4 times more likely than men to develop gallstones. Estrogen suppresses the formation of bile salts that attract and carry cholesterol out of the gallbladder. Both pregnancy and the use of the contraceptive Pill raise estrogen levels and increase the risk of developing gallstones.

TREATMENT SUMMARY

DIET

○ Avoid sugar and consume moderate amounts of fat in your diet.

○ When dieting, take 3,000–5,000 milligrams of pharmaceutical-grade fish oil daily.

○ Avoid gallstone-attack triggers such as pork, onions, and eggs.

NUTRITIONAL SUPPLEMENTS

○ Water-soluble fiber: at least 5,000 milligrams per day.

UNDERSTANDING THE HEALING PROCESS

Since cholesterol is the principle component of gallstones, lowering cholesterol is the key to preventing the formation of gallstones. Bloodstream cholesterol levels, however, are not related to the risk of gallstones—in fact, some studies have found that lower levels of cholesterol in the blood[2] and taking cholesterol-lowering medications[3] are associated with *increased* risk of gallstones. The important cholesterol level for gallstones is not the amount of cholesterol in the blood but the amount of cholesterol in the bile. Cholesterol concentrations in the bile are not related to the amount of either LDL or HDL in the blood, but rather to the concentration of triglycerides.[4]

When the diet is rich in refined sugars or the kind of fructose found in corn syrup, the liver is forced to store energy in the form of triglycerides. Long-chain triglycerides are absorbed by fat cells and contribute to weight gain. Medium-chain triglycerides (MCTs), sometimes referred to as "the lean fats," can be used by the liver itself for energy. When so many MCTs are created that they spill over into the bile, however, they compete with cholesterol for carriers and leave some cholesterol behind. This increases the rate at which gallstones are formed.[5]

Crash diets, especially those that are very low in fat and high in carbohydrates, increase the formation of MCTs and sometimes trigger gallstone attacks. The solution, however, is not to eat more fat. Essential fatty acids from fish oil counteract the negative effects of dieting. Fish oils reduce the cholesterol content of the bile and, based on the results of the single clinical study of their use, prevent gallstones in women dieters. Physicians at the Médica Sur Clinic in Mexico City gave women fish oil, ursodeoxycholic acid, or a placebo while they strictly observed a 1,200-calorie-a-day reducing diet. At the end of 6 weeks, cholesterol nucleation time, a measure of how easily stones can form from cholesterol, had been lowered significantly in the women who had been taking fish oil but not in the women who had received ursodeoxycholic acid or a placebo.[6]

The other supplement that is always useful in treating gallstones is fiber. Wheat bran has been reported to reduce the relative amount of cholesterol in bile of a small group of people whose bile contained excessive cholesterol (a risk factor for gallstone formation).[7] The same effect has been reported in people who already have gallstones.[8] Any kind of fiber should be taken with plenty of fluid.

Several other supplements can be helpful but should be used with caution. Chenodeoxycholic acid and ursodeoxycholic acid dissolve stones about 30 percent of the time, but they have to be taken for several years, usually cause diarrhea, and can cause liver damage. Theoretically, supplemental lecithin (phosphatidylcholine) should help stop the formation of gallstones, since the geometry of the cholesterol molecule requires 50 bile salt carriers without lecithin and only 7 bile salt carriers with lecithin. No clinical study, however, has found that lecithin used by itself relieves gallstones. Silymarin (milk thistle) stimulates the production of bile and can help flush small stones painlessly—or flush large stones painfully. Peppermint oil may slowly dissolve stones, but it can also cause heartburn.

CONCEPTS FOR COPING WITH GALLSTONES

O An olive oil "liver flush" is a very popular remedy for gallstones. Typically, 1 cup of unrefined olive oil is taken with the juice of 2 lemons every morning for several days. Many people pass huge "stones" while on the flush. However, what is mistaken for stones is a soapy mixture of calcium, olive oil, and lemon juice produced in the intestine itself rather than in the liver.

A "liver flush" probably does more harm than good. Oleic acid, the main component of olive oil, increases the development of gallstones in laboratory animals by increasing the cholesterol content of bile. Moreover, consumption of a large quantity of any kind of oil causes contraction of the gallbladder and increases the likelihood of a stone blocking the bile duct.

O Postmenopausal estrogen replacement therapy consisting of estrogen plus progestin increases a woman's risk of needing gallbladder surgery by about 40 percent.[9]

O MCTs taken to enhance athletic performance will not increase the risk of gallstones, provided they are used just before workouts and are not taken on rest days.

O Sunbathing increases the risk of gallstones in fair-skinned people. Scientists theorize that the exposure to sunlight increases the production of pigments in the skin that have to be processed by the liver. Pigment byproducts form a platform on which stones can form in the bile. One survey found that a "positive attitude toward sunbathing" was associated with a 2,560 percent increase in risk of gallstones.[10]

O Exercise prevents gallstones. Studies of 60,290 women and 45,813 men by the Harvard School of Public Health found that:

• Men who watch more than 40 hours of television a week have up to 7 times greater risk of developing gallstones than men who watch 6 hours of television per week or less.[11]

• Women who spend more than 60 hours sitting at work, driving, reading, or watching television have up to 4 times greater risk of developing gallstones compared to women who spend less than 6 hours a week in sedentary pursuits.[12]

O Vitamin C is sometimes recommended for gallstones, but it is beneficial only in the long run. Vitamin C only changes cholesterol nucleation time, a measure of how fast cholesterol turns into stones in the gallbladder.[13] Taking vitamin C will not affect existing gallstones.

O Drinking coffee seems to increase the risk of gallstones in women but protect against gallstones in men. The Ulm Gallstone Study, conducted in Germany in 1994 and 1995, found that the men and women who drank the most coffee had a slightly (8 percent) higher risk of getting gallstones.[14] In contrast, American researchers studying men found that those who drank 2 or 3 cups of regular coffee every day had a 40 percent lower risk of developing gallstones and men who drank

4 or more cups of regular coffee every day had 45 percent lower risk of developing gallstones. Decaffeinated coffee did not lower risk; only regular coffee was protective.[15] Drinking coffee with cream, which is the rule in Germany, may cancel out the protective effect.

○ Constipation was once thought to be a cause of gallstones, but recent research fails to confirm this idea. Nutritionists at the Harvard School of Public Health surveyed 79,829 women and found that those who had only two bowel movements a week were actually somewhat less likely to develop gallstones than those who had more than one bowel movement a day. The use of laxatives was related to a lower risk of gallstones, although not in a meaningful way; women who used laxatives once a month had a 16 percent lower risk of gallstones, while women who used laxatives once a day had a 12 percent lower risk.[16]

○ Men who drink can lower their risk of gallstones by drinking less but drinking more frequently. Men consuming 1–2 alcoholic drinks 5–7 days per week have lower rates of gallstones compared both to men who never drink and to men who drink heavily once or twice a week.[17]

○ Homeopathy can be used to relieve the symptoms of gallstones but is not a substitute for necessary medical care. Usually it is best to start with a single dose of the lowest strength (6C, 6X, or 12C) of the remedy matching the symptoms to be treated, and then wait for a response. If there is an improvement in symptoms, let the remedy continue to work until there is no more improvement, then take another dose. If there is no improvement, try a different potency (30X or 30C). Sometimes homeopathic medicines work for a few minutes, and sometimes they work for an entire day before another dose is needed.

• Berberis vulgaris treats sharp twinges of pain radiating outward from the gallbladder to the groin and the pelvic bone and up the back. Pain is worse when standing up, or when moving from seated to standing position.

• Calcarea carbonica treats gallbladder in people who have a "sweet tooth." It is also helpful when pains extend to the chest and are made worse from leaning forward.

• Chelidonium majus is often recommended for pain extending to the back, right shoulder, and shoulder blade. Pain is worse when riding in a car or plane. There may be a sensation of "belt tightening," as if a tight string or rope were pulled across the abdomen.

• Colocynthis treats pain relieved by doubling over or by putting hard pressure on the abdomen. Persons who are responsive to this remedy tend to have gallbladder attacks after emotionally upsetting events.

• Dioscorea is indicated for pain that is relieved by leaning backward or sitting in a recliner, but not by lying down.

• Lycopodium is recommended when gallstones are accompanied by gassiness or bloating. People who respond well to this remedy typically enjoy sweetened coffee or tea and tend to tire in the late afternoon and evening.

• Nux vomica treats stitching pains that travel upward, nausea, and cramps.

• Podophyllum is appropriate when there is constipation with clay-colored stools that are dry and hard to pass and may alternate with watery diarrhea.

Gardnerella
See **Vaginosis**.

Gastritis

SYMPTOM SUMMARY
○ Abdominal cramps

○ Dark stools

○ Hiccups

○ Loss of appetite

○ Nausea

○ Vomiting

○ Vomiting blood or "coffee grounds" (flakes of dried blood)

UNDERSTANDING THE DISEASE PROCESS

Gastritis is a condition of inflammation of the lining of the stomach. The most common cause of gastritis is infection with *Helicobacter pylori,* a bacterium adapted to life in the highly acidic environment of the stomach. In the United States, about 35 percent of the population is infected with the bacterium, although improvements in water quality in the latter half of the twentieth century have brought the rate of new infections down to about 1 percent per year. In the rest of the world, especially where drinking water is not germ-free, more than 50 percent of the population has the infection. People of British and Scandinavian descent and people of African descent are especially like to suffer infectious gastritis, while people of southern European and Middle Eastern descent often have a hereditary immunity to the disease. Infection with *H. pylori* substantially increases the risk of developing a cancer of the stomach known as MALT lymphoma. The lifetime risk of gastric cancer among people infected with *H. pylori* is between 1 and 3 percent.[1]

Gastritis is also common in people who take aspirin or acetaminophen (Tylenol) on a regular basis to control arthritic pain, and in alcoholics. It is a common side effect of chemotherapy. Whatever the cause, constant inflammation of the stomach lining over a period of years can lead to the development of peptic ulcers or, paradoxically, an inability of the stomach to produce the acid needed to digest food (see HYPOCHLORHYDRIA). In severe cases, the inability of the stomach to extract vitamin B_{12} leads to the vitamin-deficiency disease pernicious anemia (see ANEMIA, PERNICIOUS AND MEGALOBLASTIC).

TREATMENT SUMMARY

DIET

❍ Vegetables in the cabbage family, especially raw cabbage juice, greatly relieve ulcer pain and accelerate healing by stimulating the production of mucus. They are not recommended, however, for gastritis sufferers who also have irritable bowel syndrome, who benefit from glutamine supplements instead.

❍ When inflammation flares up, eat bananas that have not ripened so much that they are soft.

NUTRITIONAL SUPPLEMENTS

❍ Bismuth subcitrate: 240 milligrams twice daily before lunch and dinner.

❍ Gamma-oryzanol: 300–600 milligrams daily.

❍ *Lactobacillus* (especially during the first week of any antibiotic treatment): 1–2 billion live organisms daily.

❍ Vitamin C: 5,000 milligrams taken in 4 doses (1 dose of 2,000 milligrams, then 3 doses of 1,000 milligrams

each) every day for 1 month, followed by at least 500 milligrams a day.

See Part Three if you take prescription medication.

UNDERSTANDING THE HEALING PROCESS

Many people with chronic gastritis find that vegetables in the cabbage family and bananas that are slightly less than ripe are the best food when stomach pain flares up. Cabbage, broccoli, cauliflower, and kale contain flavonoids that reduce the stomach's production of acid in response to stress through a biochemical mechanism similar to that activated by drugs like Zantac.[1] The beta-carotene in these vegetables may help keep gastritis from becoming chronic.[2] In at least two animal studies, the dried extract of green banana stopped the formation of ulcers by stimulating the growth of protective mucosal cells in the lining of the stomach.[3,4]

Bismuth subcitrate is an especially safe form of the active ingredient of Pepto-Bismol. Children should take bismuth subcitrate rather than bismuth subsalicylate (Pepto-Bismol), since bismuth subsalicylate can mask Reye's syndrome, a potentially dangerous complication of colds and flu. Bismuth subcitrate is available from compounding pharmacists, who can be located through the International Academy of Compounding Pharmacists, 1–800–927–4227.

Gamma-oryzanol is a chemical found in rice bran oil that is closely related to antioxidants in the Vitamin E family. It reduces the secretion of stomach acid.[5] A Japanese study found that all participants who had erosive gastritis experienced relief of symptoms after taking gamma-oryzanol for 2 weeks. However, some people taking as much as 600 milligrams of gamma-oryzanol for 6 months may experience dry mouth, flushing, headaches, and daytime sleepiness.[6] If this occurs, reduce the dosage.

Lactobacillus is extremely helpful during the first week of any antibiotic treatment for *H. pylori*. A study at the Catholic University in Rome followed 120 people given a standard therapy for *H. pylori* consisting of 3 antibiotics—clarithromycin, pantoprazole, and tinidazole—for 1 week. Sixty participants were given *Lactobacillus* supplements for 2 weeks, and 60 were given a placebo. The antibiotics caused bloating, diarrhea, and taste disturbances in both groups, but these unpleasant effects were greatly reduced in the group given *Lactobacillus*.[7]

However, *Lactobacillus* not only counteracts the side effects of antibiotics, it is itself a natural antibiotic, as well as an anti-inflammatory. Thirty patients followed in an 8-week study at Tokai University School of Medicine in Japan were found to have lowered levels of *H. pylori* and reduced inflammation after treatment with *Lactobacillus* alone.[8] The Japanese study used yogurt, eaten in quantities as desired but eaten every day, as the source of the friendly bacteria.

Vitamin C is useful when gastritis is caused by *H. pylori* infection. In one clinical study in which 51 ulcer patients were given 5,000 milligrams of vitamin C a day (divided into 4 doses), 30 percent were free of infection by the end of 1 month.[9] It has not been scientifically determined that taking this relatively high dose of vitamin C for more than a month will do additional good. It is important to drink 8 glasses of water a day when taking this much vitamin C. A few people will experience diarrhea when taking 5,000 milligrams of the vitamin a day; do not take this much vitamin C if you have a history of kidney stones.

In the long run, vitamin C is probably extremely important in the prevention of stomach cancer. The concentration of vitamin C in gastric juice is lower in people who have *H. pylori* infections that in those who do not.[10] This is probably due to the bacterium's destruction of tissues in the lining of the stomach that secrete vitamin C.[11] When *H. pylori* are eliminated, vitamin C levels go up. Since vitamin C prevents the conversion of dietary nitrites into carcinogenic nitrosamines, vitamin C is probably important in protecting against carcinomas of the stomach.[12]

CONCEPTS FOR COPING WITH GASTRITIS

○ The amino acids arginine, cysteine, and glutamine sometimes relieve gastritis caused by taking aspirin or similar pain relievers.

○ Demulcent herbs, such as bladderwrack, marshmallow, and slippery elm relieve inflammation by coating the lining of the stomach. Taken as warm teas, they do not interfere with any medications.

Gastroesophageal Reflux Disease (GERD)

See **Heartburn.**

Gastrointestinal Indigestion

See **Bloating; Flatulence; Heartburn.**

Gastroparesis
(Diabetic Complication)

SYMPTOM SUMMARY

○ Bloating

○ Belching

○ Feeling full after eating only a few bites of food

○ Nagging dull pain in the upper abdomen

○ Heartburn that is not helped by antacids

○ Alternating constipation and diarrhea (diarrhea that is worse at night)

○ Loss of appetite

○ Nausea and vomiting

UNDERSTANDING THE DISEASE PROCESS

Gastroparesis (gas-tro-par-EES-is) is a complication causing a paresis, or paralysis, of the digestive tract resulting in delayed emptying of the stomach into the intestines. Affecting 30–50 percent of all people with diabetes, this form of nerve damage occurs after a prolonged period of poor blood sugar control, usually 5–10 years. High blood sugars may cause damage to the nerves controlling the movement of food through the digestive tract, without observable symptoms. Only about half of diabetics who have the nerve damage associated with gastroparesis ever experience bloating, constipation, diarrhea, loss of appetite, nausea, or vomiting as a result, and the experience of these symptoms may not be constant in the other half.[1]

The way diabetes causes gastroparesis is by damaging the stomach's "pacemaker." The stomach has two parts. The upper portion is called the fundus, where swallowed food and liquid collect. The antrum, the lower portion, is where food is churned back and forth until it is broken into small fragments and then squirted out into the duodenum, the first part of the small intestine.

The same electrical wave that causes the muscles in the heart to contract causes the muscles lining the stomach to contract and move food from the fundus to the antrum, then from the antrum to the intestines. The normal rate of contraction is about 3 times a minute, much slower than the heart, but enough for the process of digestion. Gastroparesis occurs when the rate of the electrical wave slows and the stomach contracts less frequently. In gastroparesis, the food rests in the stomach relying on acid and digestive enzymes to break it down and gravity to carry it to the intestines.

TREATMENT SUMMARY

NUTRITIONAL SUPPLEMENTS

○ Bromelain with papain or bromelain with trypsin: 1 tablet 30 minutes before each meal.

Before fatty meals add:

○ Pancreatin: 1 tablet (1,000,000 USP), 30 minutes before eating.

See Part Three if you take prescription medication.

UNDERSTANDING THE HEALING PROCESS

Bromelain is a protein-dissolving enzyme found in the pineapple. When it is taken with another digestive enzyme, usually papain or trypsin, it accelerates the digestion of solid food in the stomach and speeds the digestive process. Older research suggests that it may activate the "pacemaker" controlling both the stomach and heart.[2] Pancreatin helps with the digestion of animal fats.[3]

CONCEPTS FOR COPING WITH GASTROPARESIS

○ High-fat foods, including vegetable oils, cause a delay in emptying the stomach and should be avoided in gastroparesis. High-fiber foods, including cabbage and broccoli, tend to stay in the stomach and should be avoided when symptoms are particularly severe. Liquid foods pass through the stomach faster than solid foods, and eating 4–6 small meals rather than 2 or 3 large meals also helps.

○ Amitriptyline (Elavil), the antidepressant drug commonly prescribed for diabetic neuropathy, can make gastroparesis worse. Be sure to take digestive enzymes before meals if you also take Elavil.

○ Avoid energy drinks containing the South American herbs guaraná or yerba maté (also known just as maté). These herbs contribute to weight loss as advertised, but do so by delaying the rate at which food passes through the stomach.[4]

○ Clinical studies have confirmed that acupuncture stimulates the production of the enzymes gastrin and motilin in diabetic patients with gastroparesis. These enzymes stimulate the movement of food and liquids through the digestive tract and compensate for nerve damage.

Genital Herpes
See **Herpes**.

Genital Warts

SYMPTOM SUMMARY

○ Abnormal vaginal bleeding (not associated with a menstrual period) after sexual intercourse

○ Genital sores

○ Increased dampness or moisture in the area of growths

○ Increased vaginal discharge

○ Itching of the penis, scrotum, or anal or vulvar areas

○ Raised wartlike tumors on the genitals

○ Cauliflowerlike growths around the anus or female genitalia

UNDERSTANDING THE DISEASE PROCESS

Genital warts, also known as condyloma acuminatum, are the result of infection with the human papillomavirus (HPV). Genital warts are among the most common sexually transmitted diseases in the United States. According to the American Social Health Association, approximately 5.5 million new cases of sexually transmitted HPV infections are reported every year. At least 20 million Americans are already infected.

Anogenital warts develop on the skin and mucosal

surfaces of the external sex organs and around the anus. In circumcised men, sexually transmitted warts most commonly occur on the shaft of the penis. Perianal warts are more common in homosexual men but may develop in heterosexual men as well. In women, genital warts usually first appear on the labia, and spread to other parts of the vulva and to the vagina and cervix. The complications of genital warts include itching and occasional bleeding. Large masses of genital warts may cause mechanical problems, such as obstruction of the birth canal. Anxiety, depression, and embarrassment are common psychological reactions to the condition.

HPV is spread by skin-to-skin contact. Like many other venereal diseases, genital warts frequently produce no outward symptoms. The incubation period for HPV disease is typically 3–4 months, and may take 1–2 years. HPV infection begins in the basement membrane of the skin, and spreads upward as skin cells migrate to the surface. The virus affects the skin so that all the layers of skin except the basement membrane grow at an accelerated rate. The pile-up of keratin produces long fingers of skin tissue. When the DNA of the virus becomes fully integrated with the DNA of the cell, it can become cancerous.

TREATMENT SUMMARY

NUTRITIONAL SUPPLEMENTS

○ Beta-carotene: 200,000 IU per day.

○ Folic acid: 2.5 milligrams per day.

○ Pyridoxine (Vitamin B$_6$): 50 milligrams 3 times per day.

○ Selenium: 400 micrograms per day.

○ Vitamin A: 50,000 IU per day. Women who are or who may become pregnant should strictly limit their intake of vitamin A to 5,000 IU per day or less.

○ Vitamin B$_{12}$: 1 milligram per day.

○ Vitamin C: 1,000 milligrams per day.

○ Vitamin E: 800 IU per day.

○ Zinc picolinate: 30 milligrams per day.

UNDERSTANDING THE HEALING PROCESS

Medical treatment of genital warts consists of several unpleasant treatment options. Condyloma are removed by application of liquid nitrogen; burning with electricity, surgical excision, or laser ablation; or the application of 5-fluorouracil (5-FU), a chemical more typically used in chemotherapy for cancer. All of these approaches are painful. None of these approaches guarantees warts will not reappear.

It is unusual for genital warts to resolve without these treatments. When they do, it is the result of cell-mediated immunity, that is, the activation of white blood cells to engulf and digest HPV-infected skin cells. Since recurrence of genital warts is more likely to result from reactivation of existing infection than new infection,[1] attention to nutritional factors is important to make recurrence less likely. Attention to nutrition is also important for persons who have only been exposed to HPV. A study of college women in the late 1980s found that 11.4 percent carried antibodies to human papillomavirus while only 2 percent had genital warts, suggesting that many were unaware they had been infected with the disease.[2]

Most of the research regarding nutrition and HPV has focused on preventing the progression of HPV infection of the cervix to cervical cancer. Findings in these studies point to nutritional interactions that are likely, although not proven, to help prevent progression of infection in both men and women infected with the virus.

Beta-carotene is especially important for women who have been exposed to HPV. One study found that women who develop cervical dysplasia have an average of two-thirds as much beta-carotene in their bloodstreams (13.9 micrograms per deciliter compared to 21.3 micrograms per deciliter) as healthy women.[3] Carotenes enhance the activity of the immune system in both men and women,[4] and ensure the normal adhesion of skin cells to each other.[5] Since genital warts are a result of skin cells "coming loose" from the basement membrane, beta-carotene may protect against their formation.

Folic acid uptake into the cervix may be deficient even when folic acid levels in the bloodstream are normal.[6] Folic acid and vitamin B$_{12}$ together are necessary for normal responses of white blood cells to viral challenges,[7] although they may not have a direct bearing on the progression of HPV infection.[8]

Many of the older drugs for seizure disorders interfere with the body's ability to absorb folic acid. These include carbamazepine, fosphenytoin, phenytoin, phenobarbital, and valproic acid. Folic acid is also depleted by NSAIDs, such as ibuprofen, indomethacin, naproxen, and sulindac, and by sulfa drugs, cholestyramine and colestipol for lowering cholesterol and colchicine for treating gout. If you take any of these medications and have genital warts, you should take supplemental folic acid. Avoid overdosing, since *high* levels of folic acid can interfere with the body's metabolism of many of these drugs.

Pyridoxine (vitamin B$_6$) deficiency is associated with decreased antibody production.[9] Serum levels of pyridoxine are 33 percent lower in women in whom HPV progresses to cervical cancer than in healthy women.[10]

The use of oral contraceptives increases pyridoxine requirements. The vitamin is depleted during treatment with carbamazepine for bipolar disorder; cycloserine or ethionamide for tuberculosis; hydralazine for high blood pressure; penicillamine for arthritis, Wilson's disease, and certain skin conditions; phenelzine for cocaine addiction, eating disorders, headaches, and panic attacks; and valproic acid for seizure disorders. If you take any of these prescription drugs and have genital warts, you should take supplemental pyridoxine. On the other hand, if you take levodopa for Parkinson's disease, theophylline for asthma, or valproic acid for seizures, you should not take pyridoxine supplements, since the vitamin interferes with the body's use of these medications.

Selenium is an important cofactor for vitamin E. It is theorized that men and women who develop genital warts have low levels of the antioxidant glutathione peroxidase, which normalizes with vitamin E and selenium treatment. Glutathione peroxidase puts a break on inflammation reactions throughout the body, especially in the skin. Selenium intake and selenium levels in the bloodstream are both inversely proportional to the risk of developing all kinds of cancer of the skin.[11]

Vitamins A, C, and E encourage the multiplication of healthy cells but prevent the multiplication of HPV-infected cells, at least in the test tube. The strongest effect is observed from vitamin E,[12] but all three vitamins should be taken together since they increase each other's availability to cells. Studies at the Northern Ireland Centre for Diet and Health report that supplementing with vitamin C increases the amount of available vitamin E in the bloodstream by about 10 percent. The studies also report that supplementing with vitamin E increases the amount of available vitamin C in the bloodstream by about 60 percent.[13] Vitamin E is an important cofactor for vitamin A. In laboratory studies with animals, the amount of vitamin A in the bloodstream stays low regardless of intake until vitamin E levels are normal. Vitamin E supplementation is useful even if vitamin A is not taken, since it complements the vitamin A available from the diet.[14]

Inadequate vitamin C intake is a risk factor for the progression of HPV infection to cervical carcinoma.[15] Vitamin C supplementation is especially needed when the diet is high in sugar. Glucose and vitamin C compete for sites on the membrane from which to enter cells.[16] Vitamin E supplementation boosts the immune system's response to viral infections and activates helper T cells.[17]

A study of 206 women found an inverse relationship between zinc levels in the bloodstream and the progression of HPV to cancer.[18] No studies have examined the use of zinc in treating HPV infection in men, but adequate levels of zinc are likely to prevent secondary infection of bruised or crumbled warts in both sexes.

Supplementation with zinc is indicated for persons who have a zinc deficiency. A quick method for detecting zinc deficiency is a taste test. Powder a tablet of any zinc-based supplement or cold medication and mix with $1/4$ cup (50 milliliters) of water. Slosh the mixture in the mouth. People who notice no taste at all or who notice a "dry," "mineral," or "sweet" taste are likely to be zinc deficient. Anyone who notices a definite strong and unpleasant taste that intensifies over time is not likely to be zinc deficient.

CONCEPTS FOR COPING WITH GENITAL WARTS

O Smoking increases the probability genital warts will become cancerous. Cancers of the anus, penis, and vulva frequently begin as genital warts.[19]

GERD
See **Heartburn**.

Gestational Hypertension
See **Hypertension**.

Giardiasis

SYMPTOM SUMMARY

○ Greasy, mushy, and intensely malodorous stools

○ Diarrhea alternating with constipation

○ Abdominal cramps

○ Nausea

○ Loss of appetite

○ Heartburn

○ Sulfurous belching ("purple burps")

○ Symptoms usually come on slowly, but some people may have several days of explosive diarrhea shortly after contracting the infection

UNDERSTANDING THE DISEASE PROCESS

Giardiasis, caused by the intestinal parasite *Giardia,* is one of the most common causes of diarrhea in the world. Epidemiologists estimate that up to 65 percent of children in day care contract giardiasis, and the condition is a common complaint among backpackers in the Rocky Mountains of the United States and throughout the developing world.[1]

Swallowing just 10 to 25 microscopic cysts of the parasite is enough to cause *Giardia* infection in the upper bowel. Once the infection is established, it tends to persist. Most people with giardiasis lose at least 10 pounds (4.5 kilograms). Dehydration from the condition is potentially dangerous in small children.

TREATMENT SUMMARY

HERBS

○ Barberry, coptis, goldenseal, or Oregon grape root: used only under the supervision of an experienced herbalist.

UNDERSTANDING THE HEALING PROCESS

Untreated, giardiasis lasts for weeks. Treated with medication, giardiasis still lasts for weeks. The most effective medication for giardiasis, quinacrine (Atabrine), is not available in the United States. American physicians usu-

ally prescribe metronidazole (Flagyl), which has to be used over a period of about 2 months. This drug causes dizziness and headaches and leaves a metallic taste in the mouth. If taken with alcohol, it causes severe nausea and vomiting. If taken with garlic, it potentially can cause bruising or bleeding.

The herbal alternatives to Flagyl are the herbs containing berberine—barberry, coptis, goldenseal, and Oregon grape root. Clinical studies conducted in India confirm that berberine controls giardiasis after about 2 weeks; however, the required dose of the berberine-containing herb is about 200 milligrams per day in adults and 50–100 milligrams per day in children.[2] This dosage is enough to elevate blood pressure and cause hot flashes and headaches, so it is important to enlist the help of an experienced herbalist before attempting herbal treatment of this condition. You should not take B vitamins when using any of these herbs to control *Giardia*; vitamin B_6 gives the infection resistance to berberine.

CONCEPTS FOR COPING WITH GIARDIASIS

○ Whenever any member of a household, including an infant, contracts giardiasis, it is especially important to wash hands before feeding the baby and after changing diapers. In a day-care setting, transmission of giardiasis is reduced by using diapers that can contain stool and urine. Diapers should have waterproof outer covers or the children should be dressed in plastic pants.

○ Bleach kills *Giardia* in warm water, but not in cold water.

○ Hikers should boil water or use adequate chlorination or filters before drinking water from streams, especially when hiking through the Four Corners area of the southwestern United States.

○ Giardiasis can be spread through sexual contact; oral-genital or oral-anal contact spreads the disease.

○ Children who have asymptomatic giardiasis (that is, no diarrhea, heartburn, or burps) may nonetheless have difficulty digesting milk products.[3] Other protein sources may be helpful for children recovering from the disease. Children recovering from giardiasis may be deficient in copper, iron, and zinc.[4] A daily multivitamin and mineral supplement is enough to correct deficiency.

○ See also DIARRHEA.

Gilbert's Syndrome

SYMPTOM SUMMARY

○ Mild yellowing of the skin and the whites of the eyes (jaundice)

○ Abdominal pain in the upper right quadrant

○ Fatigue

○ Nausea

○ Usually does not turn the urine dark brown (which would a sign of a more serious condition)

UNDERSTANDING THE DISEASE PROCESS

Gilbert's syndrome is a common, inherited disorder that affects the liver's ability to process the greenish brown pigments in bile called bilirubin. The resulting buildup of bilirubin in the bloodstream can lead to yellowing of the skin (jaundice) but the liver itself remains normal. Affecting 3–7 percent of the population, Gilbert's syndrome is more common in men than in women and usually is first noticed in late adolescence or early adulthood after a bout of the flu or a period of fasting.

The symptoms of Gilbert's syndrome are most likely to recur after an infection or while dieting to lose weight. They can also occur after the consumption of ordinary substances that activate certain detoxification pathways in the liver, specifically those in which the liver combines glucuronic acid with the toxin to neutralize it. The liver uses its glucuronidation pathways to detoxify aspirin, menthol (the aromatic compound in peppermint), vanillin (artificial vanilla), and benzoates used as food preservatives. When someone with Gilbert's syndrome consumes these common substances, the liver is unable also to use the glucuronidation process to dispose of bile.

TREATMENT SUMMARY

NUTRITIONAL SUPPLEMENTS

○ S-adenosyl-L-methionine (SAM-e): 200 milligrams, twice a day.

UNDERSTANDING THE HEALING PROCESS

Glucuronidation is accomplished by the enzyme UDP-glucuronyl transferase. This enzyme is activated by d-limonene, a chemical found in orange and lemon zest, caraway oil, and dill seed. Simply eating foods with d-limonene or taking s-adenosyl-L-methionine (SAM-e) extends the liver's supply of the enzyme sufficiently to allow it to process bilirubin. When bilirubin is eliminated by the liver, symptoms cease.[1,2]

CONCEPTS FOR COPING WITH GILBERT'S SYNDROME

○ Including citrus zest, caraway oil, and dill weed oil (available at gourmet food shops) in your diet will help relieve symptoms.

Gingivitis

SYMPTOM SUMMARY

○ Inflammation of the gums (also known as gingival) with redness and swelling

○ Blood appears on the toothbrush even after gentle brushing of the teeth

○ Gums appear bright red or reddish purple

○ Gums appear shiny

○ Gums bleed easily

○ Gums are tender when touched

○ Mouth sores

UNDERSTANDING THE DISEASE PROCESS

Gingivitis is a condition of chronic irritation of the gums. Gingivitis is caused by long-term deposits of plaque, the sticky material that develops on the exposed surfaces of the teeth, consisting of blood, food debris, and mucus. The toxins produced by the bacteria in plaque cause the gums to become infected, shiny, swollen, and tender.

The cause of gingivitis can be as simple as overly vigorous brushing. Misaligned teeth, ill-fitting bridges, crowns, and dentures, and sharp edges of fillings can also cause gum irritation. Bacterial growth in the gums is enhanced in a number of health conditions, including uncontrolled diabetes, collagen disease, leukemia, anemia, vitamin deficiency states, and pregnancy. Bacteria grow unchecked in the absence of regular brushing and flossing. Gingivitis becomes increasingly common with increasing age. In the United States, the rate of all kinds of periodontal disease is 15 percent at age 10, 38 percent at age 20, 46 percent at age 35, and 54 percent at age 50. Men have a greater tendency to gingivitis than women.[1]

Gingivitis is the early stage of a more serious condition, periodontitis. In this more serious condition, hardened plaque, or tartar, pries the gum away from the teeth and the bony structures that support the teeth. Tooth loss usually follows.

TREATMENT SUMMARY

DIET

○ Avoid sugar.

○ Drink black *tea* (without sugar) as often as desired.

NUTRITIONAL SUPPLEMENTS

○ Quercetin: 500 milligrams 3 times a day.

○ Selenium: 400 micrograms per day.

○ Vitamin A: 15,000 IU per day. Women who are or who may become pregnant should strictly limit their intake of vitamin A to 5,000 IU per day or less.

○ Vitamin C: 1,000 milligrams 3 times a day with meals.

○ Vitamin E: 400 IU per day.

○ Zinc picolinate: 30 milligrams a day.

○ Folic acid: 2 milligrams (five 0.4-milligram tablets) a day should be taken by pregnant women and women who take oral contraceptives, and anyone who takes phenytoin (Dilantin) for seizures or methotrexate for cancer, psoriasis, or rheumatoid arthritis.

HERBS

○ Chamomile tea can be used as a soothing beverage or even as a mouthwash.

See Part Three if you take prescription medication.

UNDERSTANDING THE HEALING PROCESS

The objectives in healing gingivitis include decreasing inflammation, increasing immune resistance, decreasing the time the gums take to heal, and enhancing the integrity of the membranes lining the gums. The recommendations in the treatment summary are discussed as they contribute to these objectives.

Sugar feeds the bacteria that cause plaque. It draws fluid out of the gums and interferes with their absorption of vitamin C. It also weakens immune resistance by interfering with the chemical signals that the gums send to the immune system to attract polymorphonuclear leukocytes, large white blood cells that are the first line of defense against excessive accumulations of bacteria. The effects of sugar on the gums are most severe in people with chronic diseases that already depress the activity of polymorphonuclear leukocytes, such as diabetes, Crohn's disease, Down syndrome, Chediak-Higashi syndrome, and juvenile periodontitis.[a]

In much of East Asia even today, green tea is used as a toothpaste. Green and black teas contain two chemical compounds, (-)-epigallocatechin gallate and (-)-epicatechin gallate, which together prevent the transfer of sugar from the saliva to bacteria.[3] Deprived of sugar, bacteria do not grow and cannot cause inflammation.

Quercetin, a chemical found in green tea, onions, red wine, and St. John's wort, belongs to a family of compounds that stabilize collagen in the gums by preventing the release of histamine. Quercetin may be especially valuable for treating gingivitis in people who have food allergies.

Vitamin A stimulates the production of keratin, the protein that "toughens" the gums. It is also necessary for the production of collagen to heal wounds made by bacterial infection.[4] Vitamin A is especially important in treating gingivitis in people who have hepatitis C, Crohn's disease, ulcerative colitis, short bowel syndrome, pancreatic disease, cystic fibrosis, or Whipple's disease.

Side effects from accidental overdosing of vitamin A are rare, but they are significant. The first signs of vitamin A overdose are dry skin and chapped lips, especially in dry weather. Later signs of toxicity are headache, mood swings, and pain in muscles and joints. In massive doses, vitamin A can cause liver damage. In the first 3 months of pregnancy, it can cause birth defects. Women who are or who may become pregnant should strictly limit their intake of Vitamin A to 5,000 IU per day or less. Discontinue vitamin A at the first sign of toxicity.

Gum disease may be a sign of vitamin C deficiency. It is possible to take considerably more than the RDA of vitamin C and still be deficient, if the body has become accustomed to high doses. That is, someone who drinks large quantities of fruit juices and stops, or who takes high doses of vitamin C and stops, may become vitamin

C deficient even while eating a healthy diet. If gingivitis occurs, it is best to assume that there is a functional deficiency of the vitamin and take the supplement.

Vitamin E speeds up the healing of wounds. It is especially important if mercury amalgams are present. Mercury depletes the gums of the antioxidant enzymes catalase, glutathione peroxidase, and superoxide dismutase. At least in animal studies, this toxic effect of mercury is counteracted by vitamin E.[5] Selenium is an important cofactor for vitamin E.

Zinc is essential to dozens of enzymatic processes, including those that send a signal to polymorphonuclear leukocytes to fight bacterial infection. Zinc is also needed for the gums to make enzymes that slow down the process of tissue destruction initiated by endotoxins released by bacteria.[6] Gum disease is especially severe when there is a deficiency of zinc coupled with an excess of copper.[7]

While it is important to take zinc in treating gingivitis, it is equally important not to take too much. Except where otherwise directed, do not take more than 50 milligrams of any zinc supplement daily. In rare cases, excessive intake of zinc depletes copper to cause anemia, that is, a deficiency of red blood cells, and neutropenia, a serious deficiency of white blood cells.

Chamomile tea (and actually, teas made of several related plants, such as calendula, chrysanthemum, cosmos, and the flower but not the oil of safflower) contains triterpenes that stop inflammation.

CONCEPTS FOR COPING WITH GINGIVITIS

❍ To prevent gingivitis, floss daily. To treat gingivitis, floss after every meal and at bedtime.

❍ Regular cleanings by a dentist remove plaque that may develop even with diligent brushing and flossing. Most dentists recommend having the teeth cleaned once or twice a year, every 3 months if gingivitis is active.

❍ Don't bite your nails or pick your teeth. Both practices can damage tender gums.

❍ The active ingredient in Listerine mouthwash is thymol, a compound found in the herb thyme. Thymol is a potent antibacterial agent.

❍ Faulty fillings are a common cause of gingivitis. Overhanging margins accumulate plaque and offer a shelter for bacteria. Mercury amalgams deplete antioxidant enzymes in small areas of the gums, exposing the glycosaminoglycans and proteoglycans that make up the collagen matrix of the gums to bacterial attack.[8]

❍ The herb bloodroot is the source of mouthwashes and toothpastes labeled as containing benzophenanthridine alkaloids or sanguinarine. These compounds cause bacteria to "clump" so that they cannot form colonies on the gums. Some studies indicate they are not as effective in controlling plaque as the synthetic chemical chlorhexidine,[9] but alternating mouthwashes containing sanguinarine and mouthwashes that do not offers maximum benefit.

❍ Electric toothbrushes are recommended for persons who have problems with manual strength or dexterity.

❍ Consider using a tongue cleaner as a final step in oral hygiene. Cleaning the soft plaque from the back of the tongue removes most of the bacteria and other debris that are the primary source of plaque—and are frequently are the cause of halitosis. A tongue cleaner should have smooth, well-rounded cleaning edges. Unbreakable stainless steel is preferable to potentially breakable plastic. Avoid cleaners that have holes that can trap the plaque you are trying to remove.

Glaucoma, Chronic

SYMPTOM SUMMARY

❍ Blurred or foggy vision

❍ Chronic mild headaches

❍ Frequent changes of eyeglasses or contacts, none of which are satisfactory

❍ Inability to adjust the eyes to darkened rooms

❍ Seeing rainbow-colored halos around lights

Acute glaucoma, characterized by severe eye pain, cloudy vision with halos appearing around lights, red eyes, dilated pupils, and/or nausea and vomiting is a medical emergency. The use of scopolamine for motion sickness greatly increases the risk of an attack. Seek a doctor's attention immediately if you experience the symptoms of acute glaucoma.

UNDERSTANDING THE DISEASE PROCESS

Glaucoma is a condition of poor circulation within the eye. All types of glaucoma can cause damage to the optic nerve, resulting in tunnel vision or loss of sight. Glaucoma is the leading cause of blindness among African-Americans[1] and the second-most-common cause of blindness in the United States as a whole.[2] Risk factors other than being of African-American descent include diabetes, high blood pressure, migraine, nearsightedness, and the use of cholesterol-lowering medications and steroids.

The progress of glaucoma is insidious. There are usually no symptoms or only vague symptoms during the early stages of the disease. The only hint something is wrong may be difficulty parking a car into a parallel slot or missing words in reading, or difficulty adjusting to dim light. Once the optic nerve has begun to atrophy, peripheral vision is lost first. The tunnel of good vision grows smaller and smaller until blindness finally results.

The most common form of glaucoma is the so-called open-angle form of the disease. The lens is nourished by a watery fluid known as the aqueous humor, rather than by the bloodstream. This nourishing fluid is produced by the ciliary bodies at the edges of the lens. It has to flow around a 180°bend to reach the canal of Schlemm, a porous vein that transports essential nutrients and oxygen into the cornea. If this angle is closed, circulation to the cornea is cut off and intense pain and rapid destruction of the optic nerve results. If circulation is merely impeded as the angle remains open, the consequences are a lesser amount of pain and slow destruction of the optic nerve.

Changes in the structure of the collagen of the eye precede circulation problems. A filtration barrier keeps large particles from entering the aqueous humor. This barrier is composed of glycosaminoglycans (GAGs). In eyes affected by glaucoma, chondroitin sulfate builds up and hyaluronic acid is depleted in the filtration barrier.[3] This imbalance makes the filtration barrier inelastic and impermeable to fluids, with the result that the cornea

COMMONLY PRESCRIBED GLAUCOMA MEDICATIONS AND THEIR POTENTIAL SIDE EFFECTS

Category	Medication	Possible Side Effects
Nonselective Adrenergic Nerve Fiber Stimulants	Allergan (dipivefrin)	Frequent allergic reactions
Selective Adrenergic Nerve Fiber Stimulants	Apraclonidine	Frequent allergic reactions, racing pulse
	Alphagan (brimonidine)	Fewer allergic reactions, but causes dry mouth
Beta-blockers	Betimol (timolol hemihydrate) Betoptic (betaxolol HCl) Betagan (levobunolol HCl) Ocupress (carteolol HCl) Optipranolol (metipranolol) Timoptic-XE (timolol maleate)	Bronchial spasms, confusion, depression, erectile dysfunction, fatigue, hair loss, heart failure, and/or shortness of breath. Timolol lowers HDL ("good") cholesterol levels and raises total cholesterol levels in women 60 years and older.
Carbonic Anhydrase Inhibitors (without diuretics)	acetazolamide, Dichlorphenamide, Ethoxzolamine, Methazolamide	Anorexia, depression, electrolyte disturbances, fatigue, kidney stones, sensation of prickling, tingling, crawling skin
	Trusopt (dorzolamide)	No side effects (applied directly to the eye)
Cholinergic Nerve Fiber Stimulants	Carboptic (carbachol)	Detached retina, diarrhea, headache, frequent urination
	Pilagan, Pilocar (pilocarpine)	Bronchial spasms, high blood pressure, racing pulse
Cholinesterase Inhibitors	Demecarium, Echotihophate iodide, Isoflurophate, Neostigmine, Physostigmine	Increase cell division in the eye, raising the risk of cataract formation and detached retina
Carbonic Anhydrase Inhibitors (with diuretics)	Ak-Zol, Dazamide, Diamox, Diamox Sequels (acetylzolamide)	Potassium deficiencies causing fatigue or muscle weakness
Prostaglandin Analogs	Xalatan (latanoprost)	Darkens the iris

ceases to be well hydrated and pressure builds up behind the barrier.[4]

Russian scientists have found that ineffective antioxidant defense systems also contribute to the progress of glaucoma. Patients with advanced glaucoma were especially likely to have low levels of glutathione in both the aqueous humor and the bloodstream.[5] Patients with advanced glaucoma had on average twice the levels of oxidation of essential fatty acids in the vitreous humor inside the eye.[6]

While glaucoma is usually associated with elevated intraocular pressure (IOP), glaucoma is not the same as elevated IOP. Normal IOP ranges from 7–22 mg/Hg. Approximately 90 percent of people with IOPs greater than 22 mg/Hg never develop glaucoma, while some people with normal IOPs (especially migraine sufferers) nonetheless develop optic nerve injury.[7] People with elevated IOP who avoid the damage to the optic nerve do so because they maintain good circulation despite elevated pressure.

TREATMENT SUMMARY

NUTRITIONAL SUPPLEMENTS

❍ Alpha-lipoic acid: 75–150 milligrams daily.

❍ Bioflavonoids with rutin: 500–1,000 milligrams daily.

❍ Magnesium: 200 milligrams daily.

❍ Melatonin: 0.1–1.0 milligrams daily.

❍ Thiamine: 200–250 milligrams daily.

❍ Vitamin C: 50–250 milligrams for every pound of body weight (100–500 milligrams per kilogram) daily, taken in divided doses. Consult your physician or naturopath before beginning high-dose vitamin C therapy.

For glaucoma patients taking beta-blockers, such as Betimol (timolol hemihydrate), Betoptic (betaxolol HCl), Betagan (levobunolol HCl), Ocupress (carteolol HCl), Optipranolol (metipranolol), or Timoptic-XE (timolol maleate):

❍ Coenzyme Q_{10}: 30 milligrams per day.

See Part Three if you take prescription medication.

UNDERSTANDING THE HEALING PROCESS

In much of the world, surgery is the first line of treatment for glaucoma. British physicians, in particular, cite poor patient compliance with prescribed regimens of eye drops or oral medications and seek to avoid ongoing drug expense. Surgery is successful in lowering intraocular pressure in 80 percent of cases, but there is a risk of bleeding, and even successful surgery increases the risk of developing cataracts.

In the United States, because of the risks of surgery, most ophthalmologists treat glaucoma with medication first. With one exception, however, all of the commonly prescribed medications for glaucoma have serious side effects. (The medication that does not cause side effects, dorzolamide, must be applied as an ointment directly to the eye.) See the table "Commonly Prescribed Glaucoma Medications and Their Potential Side Effects."

Alpha-lipoic acid supplements raise the levels of glutathione, the important antioxidant in tears[8] and in red blood cells.[9] About half of people with glaucoma who take alpha-lipoic acid supplements for 1 month will experience better color perception.[10]

Bioflavonoids are helpful in a wide range of eye problems, including poor night vision, nearsightedness, and retinopathy. A small-scale study in Italy found that the bioflavonoids found in bilberry increase circulation in the retina in glaucoma patients, even after a single dose (equivalent to 800 milligrams of bilberry standardized extract).[11] The bioflavonoid rutin has been used to lower IOPs when patients are unresponsive to medication alone.[12]

Do not take rutin without vitamin C. Although rutin protects vitamin C from oxidation, it also slows the rate at which vitamin C is absorbed by cells. Rutin will interfere with action of quinolone antibiotics (not to be confused with the anabolic steroid quinolone). The antibiotics that may interact with rutin include:

• ciprofloxacin (Cipro, Baycip, Cetraxal, Ciflox, Cifran, Ciplox, Cyprobay, Quintor)

• enoxacin (Penetrex)

• gatifloxacin (Tequin)

• gemifloxacin (a relatively new drug).

• grepafloxacin (Raxar)

• levofloxacin (Levaquin)

• lomefloxacin (Maxaquin)

• moxifloxacin (Avelox)

• norfloxacin (Amicrobin, Anquin, Baccidal, Barazan, Biofloxin, Floxenor, Fulgram, Janacin, Lexinor, Norofin, Noroxin, Norxacin, Orixacin, Oroflox, Urinox, Zoroxin)

- ofloxacin (Floxin)
- sparfloxacin (Zagam)
- temafloxacin (Omniflox)
- trovafloxacin (Trovan)

Taking rutin, zinc, or magnesium together with the antibiotic will make the antibiotic less effective.

Magnesium is especially important for people with glaucoma who also suffer migraine or Raynaud's disease or who are unusually sensitive to the cold. A small-scale study at the University Eye Clinic in Basel, Switzerland found that giving glaucoma patients 121.5 milligrams of magnesium a day for 4 weeks improved peripheral vision and also improved peripheral circulation.[13]

IOP falls toward normal levels in the early morning when there are normal levels of melatonin, which is depleted by exposure to bright light and use of beta-blockers (such as Timoptic). One experiment found that melatonin corrects elevated IOP caused by exposure to bright light within an hour; the effect lasted for up to 4 hours.[14]

A comparison of 38 people with glaucoma to 12 healthy controls found that people with glaucoma tend to have deficient levels of thiamine despite adequate intake of the vitamin in their diets. Adequate supplies of thiamine are especially important for the health of the optic nerve.[15] Supplemental thiamine is especially important for people with glaucoma who take digoxin (Digox) or furosemide (Lasix) for congestive heart failure after a heart attack.

Vitamin B_{12} has no effect on IOP, but seems to prevent deterioration of the optic nerve. A trial involving glaucoma patients receiving a relatively high dosage of vitamin B_{12} for 5 years found no lowering of IOP, but no progression of loss of visual field.[16]

Very high doses of vitamin C can dramatically lower IOP. Vitamin C alone has been used to achieve normal eye pressures in some glaucoma patients who were unresponsive to acetazolamide or pilocarpine. In one study involving 25 patients, a single dose of 500 milligrams of vitamin C for every kilogram of body weight lowered IOP by an average of 16 mm/Hg in 4–5 hours. The effect was maintained for 8 hours.[17] Some glaucoma patients will respond to as little as 2,000 milligrams per day, but others will require as much as 35,000 milligrams to lower IOP.

There are several theoretical explanations for the effectiveness of vitamin C in lowering IOP. It is a well-known antioxidant. Laboratory tests have found that it stimulates the production of hyaluronic acid, which is deficient in glaucomatous eyes.[18] This makes the filtration barrier more elastic and helps fluid flow through the eye.

High dosages of vitamin C almost always cause diarrhea at first, although the effect usually goes away in 3–4 days and can be avoided entirely if vitamin C is administered by injection. High dosages can also cause kidney stones. Abruptly discontinuing a high daily dosage of vitamin C can lead to symptoms of vitamin C deficiency. Before starting any high-dosage regimen of vitamin C, consult with your physician to make sure it will not aggravate any other health conditions or interfere with medications.

Coenzyme Q_{10} reduces the side effects beta-blockers have on the cardiovascular system. It prevents reduction in the output of the heart and hastens the restoration of normal pulse rates after each dose of medication. A Japanese study of 16 patients found that taking coenzyme Q_{10} to relieve side effects of treatment with Timoptic (timolol) did not interfere with the medication's beneficial effects on glaucoma.[19]

Vanadium is an antagonist to chromium. Taking vanadium supplements may cause elevations of IOP tending to "stretch" the lens, making it difficult to focus. Chondroitin sulfate is a substitute for glucosamine sulfate, which makes the meshwork of the eye less elastic. Although there are no reports of elevated IOPs after administration of chondroitin, caution is advisable.

CONCEPTS FOR COPING WITH GLAUCOMA

○ Avoid supplements containing vanadium. If you take chondroitin, be sure to inform you ophthalmologist and have your eyes checked at least once every 6 months.

○ Avoid the use of corticosteroids (asthma inhalers, cortisone skin medications, etc.). They inhibit the synthesis of collagen needed for the vascular health of the eye.[20]

○ Everyone should have an eye exam including screening for glaucoma every 2 years after the age of 35. Screening at least once a year is recommended for persons who have a family history of glaucoma.

Gluten Sensitivity
See **Celiac Disease.**

Goiter

See **Hypothyroidism**.

Gonorrhea

SYMPTOM SUMMARY

In men:

❍ Discharge at the tip of the penis, may be clear or purulent (thick, yellowish, puslike)

❍ Dripping or "leaking" urine

❍ Increased urgency of urination

❍ Pain upon urination

❍ Red or swollen opening of the penis (urethra)

❍ Stained underwear

❍ Tender, swollen, or painful testicles

In women:

❍ Burning or painful urination

❍ Hesitation in starting the flow of urine

❍ Mouth sores

❍ Pain during sexual intercourse

❍ Sore throat

❍ Vaginal discharge

❍ Fever, abdominal pain, and tenderness of the pelvic region if the infection has spread to the Fallopian tubes

UNDERSTANDING THE DISEASE PROCESS

Gonorrhea is an infection caused by *Neisseria gonorrhea,* one of the most common infectious bacteria. There are almost 400,000 cases of gonorrhea reported each year to the Centers for Disease Control in the United States, and there are probably many more cases than go undiagnosed. As many as 90 percent of the sexual partners of an infected male will contract the disease.

Gonorrhea is easily transmitted through sexual intercourse, including anal and oral sex. A man has a 1 in 5 chance of contracting the disease through a single act of vaginal intercourse with an infected woman. Women have a slightly higher rate of infection than men.

In men, gonorrhea bacteria can infect the urethra, causing burning, painful urination and discharge; the throat, producing a severe sore throat; and the anus and rectum, producing a condition called proctitis. The microorganisms can spread from the urethra to other parts of the reproductive tract causing epididymitis (infection of the epididymis, a structure attached to the testicle), prostatitis (inflammation of the prostate gland), or periurethral abscess (collection of pus around the opening of the penis). If gonorrhea is untreated, it may lead to urethral stricture (a narrowing of the urethra interfering with the flow of urination), urinary tract infection, and ultimately even kidney failure. Anorectal gonorrhea is relatively common in gay men who have the condition, while up to 25 percent of gay men who have gonorrhea have a throat infection.

In women, gonorrhea can infect the vagina, causing vaginitis, an irritated vagina with drainage; the throat, producing a severe throat; and the anus and rectum, causing proctitis. Gonorrhea bacteria may spread through the cervix and uterus and into the Fallopian tubes, the tubes that carry the egg into the uterus. When gonorrhea reaches the Fallopian tubes, it is referred to as pelvic inflammatory disease (PID). Gonorrheal infection of the Fallopian tubes can have a devastating effect on women's fertility. A single episode of PID increases the risk of ectopic pregnancy by 600 percent. Two episodes of PID causes an average 13 percent loss of fertility. Three occurrences of PID reduce fertility by 70 percent.[1]

PID can spread beyond the Fallopian tubes into the peritoneal cavity, causing peritonitis, and, typically in adolescent girls, settle into a joint, causing gonococcal arthritis. Slightly fewer than 25 percent of women who develop gonorrhea have throat infection.

In rare instances, young children can contract gonorrhea without sexual intercourse. A newborn may acquire the infection during childbirth. Young girls may contract the disease through contact with a recently contaminated object, such as a damp cloth.

The symptoms of gonorrhea usually appear 2–5 days after sexual activity with an infected partner, although symptoms may not manifest for as long as 2 weeks. Men may be asymptomatic, so that they transmit the disease without knowing they have it.

TREATMENT SUMMARY

NUTRITIONAL SUPPLEMENTS

❍ Beta-carotene: 1,000,000 IU per day for the first 2 months.

○ Bioflavonoids: 1,000 milligrams per day.

○ Chlorophyll: 10 milligrams of a fat-soluble form 4 times per day for 1 month. Chlorophyll should not be taken orally before infection has been confirmed.

○ Thymus extract: 500 milligrams of crude polypeptides daily.

○ Vitamin A: 5,000 IU per day.

○ Vitamin C: 500 milligrams 3–4 times per day.

○ Vitamin E: 400 IU per day for the first 2 months.

○ Zinc picolinate: 30 milligrams per day.

HERBS

○ Bromelain: 250 milligrams 4 times a day between meals and at night before bedtime.

○ Comfrey: 500 milligrams of freeze-dried herb 3 times a day, or 30 drops of 1:1 fluid extract twice a day.

○ Echinacea: 150–300 milligrams of solid extract (3.5% echinacosides) 3 times a day, or dried root, freeze-dried plant, juice, fluid extract, or tincture, as recommended on the label.

○ Goldenseal: as recommended on the label.

For men or *women who have difficulty urinating:*

○ Polyporus Formula: as directed on the label. In Traditional Chinese Medicine, it is referred to as *zhu ling tang.* This product has several common brand names in the United States, including:

- Chorei-to (Tsumura)
- Polyporus Combination (Lotus Classics, Sun Ten)
- Zhu Ling Tang (Lotus Classics, Sun Ten)

UNDERSTANDING THE HEALING PROCESS

At one time, gonorrhea was easily treated with penicillin. Since the Vietnam War, many strains of gonorrhea found in the American population no longer respond to treatment with penicillin. The new standard of treatment is a battery of potent antibiotics, including:

○ Cefixime: 400 milligrams by mouth, 1 time.

○ Cefpodoxime proxetil: 200 milligrams by mouth, 1 time.

○ Ceftriaxone: 125 milligrams injected into a muscle, 1 time.

○ Cefuroxime (Axotal): 1,000 milligrams by mouth, 1 time.

○ Ciprofloxacin: 500 milligrams by mouth, 1 time.

○ Enoxacin: 400 milligrams by mouth, 1 time.

○ Erythromycin: 550 milligrams by mouth 4 times a day for 1 week.

○ Ofloxacin: 400 milligrams by mouth, 1 time.

○ Spectinomycin: 2,000 milligrams injected into a muscle, 1 time.

These nine antibiotics are thought necessary to control the multiple strains of gonorrhea that are now in general circulation. Some newer single-dose antibiotics are highly effective in treating uncomplicated gonorrhea. A study of gatifloxacin, for instance, found that a single dose eradicated urethral, rectal, and pharyngeal (throat) infections in 100 percent of men and 99 percent of women treated.[2] Gonorrhea in women, however, can be very difficult to treat. An older study found that 15 percent of women with gonorrheal PID failed to respond to antibiotic treatment.[3]

Although there are no studies that directly confirm the usefulness of thymus extract in treating gonorrhea, there is considerable evidence that thymus extract corrects low immune function. In particular, research has shown that thymus extract normalizes the ratio of T helper cells to T suppressor cells, maintaining a healthy immune response that neither destroys healthy tissue nor allows infectious microorganisms to flourish.[4]

Relatively low doses of vitamin A are sufficient to prevent "burnout" due to stress on the immune output of the thymus.[5] Vitamin A also enhances antibody response, increases the rate at which macrophages destroy bacteria, and stimulates natural killer cells.[6]

The related compound beta-carotene is especially important to the health of the ovary. When gonorrhea infects the ovary, beta-carotene helps limit cell damage caused by inflammation. Beta-carotene is also useful in limiting tissue damage in other organs in both men and women. It also enhances various immune functions such as antibody levels, the beneficial effects of interferon, and white blood cell activity.

To a limited extent, chlorophyll taken orally increases the iron supply available to the gonococcus before it "takes root" in the reproductive tract by stimulating the production of hemoglobin. For this reason, men and women who merely suspect they have been exposed to gonorrhea should avoid oral chlorophyll supplements and chlorophyll chewing gums. In women, a chlorophyll douche taken after suspected contact lowers the risk of infection. Chlorophyll breaks down carbon dioxide into oxygen and creates an environment unfavorable to the anaerobic gonorrhea bacteria.

After infection, orally administered chlorophyll is helpful to both sexes. It is theorized that it creates an oxygenated environment on the soft tissues lining the reproductive tract that is unfavorable for strong development of bacterial colonies.[7]

Vitamin C levels are quickly depleted during the stress of an infection.[8] In combination with bioflavonoids, it helps increase the stability of the collagen matrix of the connective tissues, the "glue" between the reproductive tract and the tissues around it.[9] Its anti-inflammatory activity helps prevent urethral stenosis in men and pelvic scarring in women.

Zinc is an important cofactor for vitamin A. When zinc is deficient, the immune system's ability to produce white blood cells in response to infection is reduced, thymic hormone levels are lower, the immune response in the skin is especially reduced, and phagocytosis, the process in which bacteria are engulfed and digested, is slowed. When zinc is deficient, all of these processes can be corrected by taking zinc supplements.[10]

A quick method for detecting zinc deficiency is a taste test. Powder a tablet of any zinc-based supplement or cold medication and mix with 1/4 cup (50 milliliters) of water. Slosh the mixture in the mouth. People who notice no taste at all or who notice a "dry," "mineral," or "sweet" taste are likely to be zinc deficient. Anyone who notices a definite strong and unpleasant taste that intensifies over time is not likely to be zinc deficient.

Zinc picolinate is the most readily absorbed form of zinc. Do not take more than 50 milligrams of any zinc supplement daily. In rare cases, excessive intake of zinc depletes copper to cause anemia, that is, a deficiency of red blood cells, and neutropenia, a serious deficiency of white blood cells.

Bromelain serves as an all-purpose inflammation treatment. Bromelain stops the production of kinins and prostaglandins that cause inflammation, and accelerates recovery time. It increases the effectiveness of antibacterial herbs by increasing the permeability of the barrier between the bloodstream and the reproductive organs.[11] Bromelain is especially useful in preventing adhesive scar tissue from forming in the ovaries in women and urethra in men.

Comfrey contains allantoin, a stimulant to cell regeneration. Allantoin also stops the infiltration of white blood cells into the linings of the reproductive organs, limiting inflammation.[12] It should not be used by women who are or who may become pregnant, or by nursing mothers. Never gather comfrey in the wild for personal use; the aerial parts of the plant are reliably nontoxic, but the other parts of the plant are highly toxic.

Echinacea relieves inflammation. One study found that a teaspoon of *Echinacea purpurea* juice is as effective in relieving pain and swelling as 100 milligrams of cortisone.[13] Echinacea also enhances the immune system's response to bacterial infections. It is especially useful in stimulating phagocytosis. A study of oral administration of an *Echinacea purpurea* root extract (30 drops 3 times per day) to healthy men for 5 days resulted in a 120 percent increase in phagocytosis.[14]

Women who are trying to get pregnant should avoid *Echinacea purpurea*. It contains caffeoyl esters that can interfere with the action of hyaluronidase, an enzyme essential to the release of unfertilized eggs into the fallopian tube.[15]

There is laboratory evidence that *Echinacea angustifolia* contains chemicals that deactivate CYP3A4. This is a liver enzyme that breaks down a wide range of medications, including anabolic steroids, the chemotherapy drug methotrexate used in treating cancer and lupus, astemizole (Hismanal) for allergies, nifedipine (Adalat) and captopril (Capoten) for high blood pressure, and sildenafil (Viagra) for impotence, as well as many others. *Echinacea angustifolia* might help maintain levels of these drugs in the bloodstream and make them more effective, or it might also cause them to accumulate to levels at which they cause side effects. Switch to a brand of echinacea that does not contain *Echinacea angustifolia* if you experience unexpected side effects while taking any of these drugs.[16]

Avoid *long-term* use of all forms of echinacea if you have HIV. Echinacea stimulates immune function, but it also slightly increases production of T cells.[17] These are the immune cells attacked by HIV. When there are more T cells, the virus has more cells to infect. This gives it more opportunities to mutate into a drug-resistant form. This effect also makes echinacea inadvisable in autoimmune conditions, such as lupus, rheumatoid arthritis, and Sjögren's syndrome.

The combination of echinacea and goldenseal is especially useful in treating conditions that involve drainage. A 1999 study reported that the combination of the two herbs stimulates the production of the immunoglobulins IgG and IgM, infection fighters that "remember" specific infections.[18] Goldenseal contains the general antibacterial compound berberine. This alkaloid kills a wide range of bacteria, including those in the same family as *Chlamydia.*

People's Pharmacy authors Joe and Teresa Graedon warn that goldenseal reportedly limits the effectiveness of the anticoagulants heparin and warfarin (Coumadin). Do not take goldenseal with these medications. Avoid supplements containing vitamin B_6 or L histidine if you take goldenseal, since they can interfere with goldenseal's antibacterial action.

Epimedium is a traditional East Asian treatment for venereal infections. It stimulates the production of urine so that *Chlamydia* or *E. coli* bacteria cannot lodge in the lining of the urethra. Japanese physicians report that epimedium stimulates muscle growth in the sphincter muscles. This helps the inguinal ring regulate pressure in the epididymis. It is also directly antibacterial against *Chlamydia* and *N. gonorrhea,* stimulating macrophages from the immune system to engulf and digest the bacteria.[19]

Japanese medicine has considerable experience in using Polyporus Formula to treat urinary tract infections. Tsumura & Company confirms that approximately two-thirds of female patients who have a combination of symptoms that modern Japanese doctors call "urethral syndrome," painful urination and/or a sense of retained urine, find relief when taking this formula. About 6 percent of patients experience some degree of stomach upset when first taking the formula, but this side effect is not so great that they choose to discontinue the treatments.

CONCEPTS FOR COPING WITH GONORRHEA

○ Avoid iron supplements. Gonorrhea bacteria "seek out" iron-bearing proteins such as transferrin in attaching themselves to the lining of the urethra.[20] They compete with their host for iron supplies. Deprived of iron, gonorrhea cannot cause inflammation.[21]

○ Survey data show that many adolescent males and young men who have gonorrhea are unwilling to use condoms and unwilling to have sex with a single partner.[22] These are the major risk factors for the disease.

○ In the United States, uncircumcised men contract gonorrhea at a rate approximately 60 percent higher than circumcised men.[23]

○ Women who have gonorrhea should avoid or cut down on smoking. A study of 197 women hospitalized for their first PID infection found that women who smoke were 1.7 times more likely to have PID than women who did not, regardless of the number of cigarettes smoked per day.[24] Another study found that women who smoked more than 10 cigarettes per day were more likely to develop PID than women who smoked fewer than 10 cigarettes per day.[25] The few studies touching on the issue of smoking and gonorrhea in men do not establish a relationship between smoking and the progress of the disease.

○ Unprotected intercourse during the menstrual period increases the risk of infection for both partners. The endometrium both offers the woman protection against disease and hosts any gonorrheal bacteria that previously infected her, and it is this layer that is sloughed off during menstruation.

○ Overfrequent use of douches is not recommended for women, since they disturb the protective bacteria that naturally reside in the vagina and cervix. A woman who believes she has been exposed to gonorrhea may benefit from a single douche with water-soluble chlorophyll solution. One study found that use of douches 3 or more times per month was associated with a 360 percent increase in risk for PID, although the high number may reflect repeated exposure to the infection.[26]

○ Homosexual men are more likely to be infected with gonorrhea and other microorganisms if they use douches or enemas before intercourse.[27]

○ The use of IUDs for contraception greatly increases a woman's risk of contracting gonorrhea. The surface of the IUD hosts colonies of infectious bacteria while the presence of the device reduces immune capacity.[28]

○ The use of oral contraceptives (the Pill) reduces a woman's risk of infection with gonorrhea. Estrogens cause the cervix to secrete a thicker protective mucus, and diminish blood flow during the period.[29] On the other hand, use of the Pill increases a woman's risk of becoming infected with *Chlamydia,* especially during the second half of her period. The progesterone in the pill causes the cervix to grow tissues in such a way that a tissue layer favored by *Chlamydia* is more exposed.[30]

Gout

SYMPTOM SUMMARY

○ Joint pain

- Begins suddenly, often described as "arthritis developing in one day"
- In one or more joints, most commonly in the big toe, ankle, or knee

○ Joint swelling and stiffness

○ Redness and warmth in the affected joint

○ Skin lump over the affected joint, may drain chalky material

○ Fever

UNDERSTANDING THE DISEASE PROCESS

Gout is a form of arthritis caused by a buildup of the metabolic byproducts of uric acid in joints. It causes sudden attacks of pain and tenderness in joints, usually the metarsophalangeal joint of the big toe, but sometimes in other joints, such as the ankles, hands, knees, and wrists. The first attack usually occurs at night. Joints rapidly become warm, red, and tender, and the skin over them often appears as if it had been infected. Untreated, pain and swelling usually continue for 3–10 days.

The pain of gout results from the accumulation of needlelike crystals of a salt of uric acid known as monosodium urate. These crystals accumulate in a joint and invade surrounding tissues during an acute attack. So much monosodium urate can accumulate in the synovial fluid in the joint that it takes on a chalky color. The immune system floods the joint with neutrophils to remove injured tissue. The influx of neutrophils compounds pain and swelling, and over the long term can destroy a joint.

Uric acid is formed from the breakdown of purines, one of the two classes of components of DNA, RNA, and ATP. The recycling of purines depends on the enzyme xanthine oxidase, which generates a potent free radical known as superoxide. Overconsumption of foods that are rich in purines can produce more uric acid than the xanthine oxidase system can process. Excessive consumption of alcohol, surgery or serious illness, or withdrawal from ACTH, steroid medications, or medications for the treatment of gout can disable the xanthine oxi-

dase system so that it cannot process normal levels of purines. Any of these imbalances can precipitate an attack.

Gout is most commonly a disease of men over the age of 50. Women only represent 5–17 percent of all cases of gout, and the condition is almost never seen in women before menopause except in women with a strong family history of the condition.[1]

TREATMENT SUMMARY

DIET

○ Eliminate foods high in purine from your diet, including anchovies, baker's and brewer's yeast, bouillon, brains, broth, caviar, consommé, dried beans and peas, goose, gravy, heart, herring, kidneys, liver, mackerel, meat extracts, partridge, sardines, scallops, shrimp, sweetbreads, and yeast extracts (such as Marmite and Vegemite). Curtail consumption of foods containing moderate amounts of purines, including asparagus, dried beans and legumes, fish, mushrooms, poultry, and spinach.

○ Lose weight by reducing calories rather than by vigorous exercise.

○ Drink at least 8 glasses of water daily to dilute the uric acid concentration of urine.

○ Avoid alcohol, especially beer. Heavy drinking is the most frequent trigger for gout attacks.

○ Eat cherries.

NUTRITIONAL SUPPLEMENTS

○ Take quercetin and bromelain if you cannot eat cherries.

○ Avoid trace mineral supplements containing molybdenum. Molybdenum surplus causes a condition very similar to gout.[2]

○ Avoid megadoses of vitamin C. They may increase the production of uric acid.

○ Avoid high doses (over 50 milligrams per day) of niacin. Niacin competes with uric acid for excretion into the urine.

○ Avoid iron supplements. Excess iron in the bloodstream can cause uric acids to form in joints.

See Part Three if you take prescription medication.

UNDERSTANDING THE HEALING PROCESS

The standard medical intervention for acute attacks of gout is colchicine. This potent anti-inflammatory drug was originally isolated from the autumn crocus. It is extremely effective at controlling inflammation. Up to 75 percent of patients show major improvement in symptoms within the first 8–12 hours of taking the drug. However, colchicine has serious side effects. It can cause bone marrow dysfunction, depression, hair loss, liver damage, respiratory problems, and seizures. Even worse, taking a dose of colchicine low enough to avoid these side effects doubles risk of death from heart failure attack. And the way to avoid increased risk of death from heart failure is to increase the dose of colchicine, increasing the risk of nonfatal side effects.[3] Moreover, colchicine is only an anti-inflammatory. It does nothing to prevent future attacks of gout.

A natural approach to treating gout aims to keep uric acid within normal levels. Considerable personal discipline is required to overcome the condition, but the combination of dietary changes and nutritional supplementation usually prevents further attacks.

The first step in controlling uric acid is reducing consumption of foods that contain purines, since these foods increase uric acid production. Alcohol must also be avoided, since alcohol impairs kidney function and accelerates the breakdown of purines into forms that become uric acid. It is also important to reduce consumption of refined carbohydrates and saturated fats, since these foods increase uric acid retention. High-protein diets must also be avoided, since the amino acids they provide displace uric acid in the cleansing apparatus of the kidneys and force it back into the bloodstream.

The next step in controlling uric acid is reducing insulin resistance, the inability of muscle cells to accept sugars. The simplest ways of reducing insulin resistance are vigorous exercise and weight loss. *Vigorous* exercise is not recommended for sufferers of gout since it may precipitate uric acid crystals in the kidneys. In some cases, a deficiency of the enzyme HGPRTase may cause excessive release of hypoxanthine in muscles being exercised.[4]

Limitations on exercise leave diet as the principal means of reducing insulin resistance in gout. A clinical study at the University of Witwatersrand in South Africa that enrolled 13 men with gout found that following a calorie-restricted diet for 4 months normalized uric acid levels in a majority of participants in the trial. The diet consisted of 1,600 calories a day, 40 percent derived from carbohydrate, 30 percent from protein, and 30 percent from fat; simple sugars were replaced with complex carbohydrates, and saturated fats were replaced with polyunsaturated fats. Participants lost an average of 15 pounds (7.7 kilograms), and the frequency of attacks was reduced from an average of 2 per month to 1 attack every other month.[5]

Very nearly the only food gout sufferers can eat as much as they want of is cherries. Consuming $1/2$ pound (250 grams) of fresh or canned cherries every day is widely recognized as lowering uric acid levels and preventing attacks of gout. Cherries, blueberries, and other dark and red-blue berries are rich sources of anthocyanidins and other flavonoids. These natural healing agents have the ability to cross-link the proteins in collagen, reinforcing the collagen matrix of cartilage and tendons. They also prevent the synthesis and release of histamine, leukotrienes, and prostaglandins, compounds that cause the intense pain of gout.

If you cannot eat cherries, try taking 125–250 milligrams of quercetin 3 times a day between meals. Quercetin also stops the synthesis and release of histamine, leukotrienes, and prostaglandins, and has some actions similar to the drug allopurinol.[6] Bromelain, taken in doses of 125–250 milligrams with quercetin 3 times a day, increases the body's absorption of quercetin and may break up uric acid crystal deposits. There is some evidence dandelion and stinging nettle may also break up uric acid deposits that cause gout, since they help dissolve uric acid kidney stones.

There are good theoretical rationales for taking eicosapentaenoic acid (EPA), folic acid, vitamin E, and the herb devil's claw. EPA limits the production of leukotrienes that cause tissue damage. Folic acid inhibits xanthine oxidase, the enzyme responsible for producing uric acid. Vitamin E also inhibits the production of leukotrienes and is an important antioxidant. Devil's claw relieves joint pain, but only if it is taken in an enteric-coated form that protects its analgesic compounds from being digested in the stomach. All of these products are likely to offer some relief from pain and swelling, but none has been comprehensively tested as a treatment for gout.

CONCEPTS FOR COPING WITH GOUT

○ Taking a baby aspirin a day can *increase* your risk of gout.[7] Taking several aspirin a day lowers risk of gout, but may be too much to protect against other conditions.

❍ Pseudogout, a condition of sudden, intense pain and swelling in joints caused by calcium crystals rather than uric acid crystals, affects 3 percent of the population by age 50, and 50 percent of the population by age 90, although it is occasionally seen in teenagers.[8] Dietary restriction is not necessary and will not help pseudogout, although anti-inflammatories such as devil's claw and willow bark will relieve pain.

❍ Naturopathic physicians Michael Murray and Joseph Pizzorno report that saturnine gout, that is, gout associated with lead poisoning is much more common than might be expected. Lead leached out of crystal decanters containing alcohol beverages or poorly glazed pottery containing acidic foods can be a major contributor to gout. (See LEAD EXPOSURE.)

❍ Recent studies have found that some commercial preparations of ginkgo contain colchicine,[9] although not at levels high enough to cause side effects. Whether ginkgo contains enough colchicine to affect gout is yet to be determined.

Granulomatous Ileocolitis

See **Inflammatory Bowel Disease (IBD)**.

Hair Loss, Male-Pattern

SYMPTOM SUMMARY

❍ *Gradual* loss of hair

- From the front hair line back in men
- Diffusely across the crown in women

UNDERSTANDING THE DISEASE PROCESS

Male-pattern hair loss, or androgenetic alopecia, is an extremely common condition in both men and women. In this form of hair loss, there is a gradual transition from large, thick pigmented hairs to thinner, shorter hairs and finally to short, wispy, nonpigmented vellus "fuzz" in the involved areas. The hair follicles are slowly reset to a permanent resting stage so that when hair falls out, it is not replaced.

TREATMENT SUMMARY

NUTRITIONAL SUPPLEMENTS

❍ Beta-sitosterol: 100 milligrams per day.

HERBS

❍ Saw palmetto: 400 milligrams per day.

UNDERSTANDING THE HEALING PROCESS

Many supplements are recommended for male-pattern hair loss, but none are proven. However, a very preliminary randomized, placebo-controlled study of a combination of saw palmetto and beta-sitosterol found that 6 out of 10 men with male-pattern baldness taking the two supplements stopped losing hair and began to grow new hair. Doses were relatively high: 400 milligrams a day of saw palmetto extract and 100 milligrams per day of beta-sitosterol. The combination may also be helpful for women suffering hormone-related hair loss.[1]

No side effects have been observed from the use of beta-sitosterol. Men who have erectile dysfunction should avoid saw palmetto.

CONCEPTS FOR COPING WITH MALE-PATTERN HAIR LOSS

❍ Male-pattern hair loss may be accelerated by other, correctable health conditions. Alopecia areata, which causes loss of patches of hair, can mimic male-pattern hair loss. Hypothyroidism and iron deficiencies also cause loss of hair. Never begin taking iron supplements until a blood test has confirmed iron deficiency. See also ALOPECIA AREATA.

Halitosis

SYMPTOM SUMMARY

Treatable halitosis presents:

❍ Bad breath, plus

- "Craters" between the teeth on the gums
- Foul taste in the mouth
- Grayish film on the gums
- Painful, red, and swollen gums
- Profuse bleeding from the gums in response to irritation or pressure

❍ Symptoms may appear very suddenly

UNDERSTANDING THE DISEASE PROCESS

Everyone occasionally has halitosis, also known as bad breath. Onions, garlic, and cheeses are frequent offenders. When the food is fully digested, the odor goes away.

Especially unpleasant bad breath not related to what you eat or drink, however, is usually caused by bacterial infection. Trench mouth, the most common form of bad breath caused by bacteria, can also cause a particularly painful form of gingivitis. Also known as acute necrotizing ulcerating gingivitis or Vincent's stomatitis, the term "trench mouth" is derived from a popular term for the condition when it was especially common among soldiers in trenches in World War I.

Trench mouth is essentially an overgrowth of bacteria that normally reside in the mouth. The mass of bacteria secretes toxic enzymes that dissolve the collagen of the gums and overwhelm the gums' ability to repair themselves. Trench mouth is almost never seen in people who have access to good oral hygiene. It is most common in men and in those aged 15–35.

TREATMENT SUMMARY

DIET

○ Avoid sugar.

○ Drink black or green tea without sugar as often as desired.

NUTRITIONAL SUPPLEMENTS

○ Quercetin: 500 milligrams 3 times a day.

○ Selenium: 400 micrograms per day.

○ Vitamin A: 15,000 IU per day. Women who are or who may become pregnant should strictly limit their intake of vitamin A to 5,000 IU per day or less.

○ Vitamin C: 1,000 milligrams 3 times a day with meals.

○ Vitamin E: 400 IU per day.

○ Zinc picolinate: 30 milligrams per day.

○ Folic acid: 2 milligrams (five 0.4-milligram tablets) a day should be taken by pregnant women and women who take oral contraceptives, and anyone who takes phenytoin (Dilantin) for seizures or methotrexate for cancer, psoriasis, or rheumatoid arthritis.

HERBS

○ Chamomile tea can be used as a soothing beverage or even as a mouthwash.

UNDERSTANDING THE HEALING PROCESS

When bad breath is caused by trench mouth, it is not only embarrassing, it is painful. If trench mouth is untreated or treatment is delayed, the infection can spread to the cheeks, lips, or jawbone. Bacterial infection can destroy these tissues. To treat trench mouth you need to decrease inflammation, increase immune resistance, and help the gums to heal.

Sugar feeds the bacteria that cause plaque. It draws fluid out of the gums and interferes with their absorption of vitamin C. It also weakens immune resistance by interfering with the chemical signals that the gums send to the immune system to attract polymorphonuclear leukocytes, large white blood cells that are the first line of defense against excessive accumulations of bacteria. The effects of sugar on the gums are most severe in people with chronic diseases that already depress the activity of polymorphonuclear leukocytes, such as diabetes, Crohn's disease, Down syndrome, Chediak-Higashi syndrome, and juvenile periodontitis.[1] Eliminating sugar is the most important thing you can do to stop bacterial bad breath.

In much of East Asia even today, green tea is used as a toothpaste. Green and black teas contain two chemical compounds, (-)-epigallocatechin gallate and (-)-epicatechin gallate, which together prevent the transfer of sugar from the saliva to bacteria.[2] Deprived of sugar, bacteria do not grow and cannot cause inflammation. Drinking tea deprives bacteria even of the sugars provided by starchy foods such as rice, potatoes, and bread.

Quercetin, a chemical found in green tea, onions, red wine, and St. John's wort, belongs to a family of compounds that stabilize collagen in the gums by preventing the release of histamine. Quercetin may be especially valuable for treating chronic bad breath in people who have food allergies.

Use quercetin with caution if you take certain prescription drugs. Quercetin increases the toxicity of the cancer chemotherapy drug Platinol (cisplatin), the antirejection drug cyclosporine (Neoral, Sandimunne) given to transplant patients, and the high blood pressure medication nifedipine (Procardia). It competes for receptor sites and decreases the effectiveness of quinolone antibiotics, which include:

• ciprofloxacin (Cipro, Baycip, Cetraxal, Ciflox, Cifran, Ciplox, Cyprobay, Quintor)

• enoxacin (Penetrex)

- gatifloxacin (Tequin)
- gemifloxacin (a relatively new drug)
- grepafloxacin (Raxar)
- levofloxacin (Levaquin)
- lomefloxacin (Maxaquin)
- moxifloxacin (Avelox)
- norfloxacin (Amicrobin, Anquin, Baccidal, Barazan, Biofloxin, Floxenor, Fulgram, Janacin, Lexinor, Norofin, Noroxin, Norxacin, Orixacin, Oroflox, Urinox, Zoroxin)
- ofloxacin (Floxin)
- sparfloxacin (Zagam)
- temafloxacin (Omniflox)
- trovafloxacin (Trovan)

Vitamin A stimulates the production of keratin, the protein that "toughens" the gums. It is also necessary for the production of collagen to heal wounds made by bacterial infection.[3] Vitamin A is especially important for controlling bad breath in people who have hepatitis C, Crohn's disease, ulcerative colitis, short bowel syndrome, pancreatic disease, cystic fibrosis, or Whipple's disease.

Side effects from accidental overdosing of vitamin A are rare, but they are significant—especially when liver disease is a contributing factor to bad breath. The first signs of vitamin A overdose are dry skin and chapped lips, especially in dry weather. Later signs of toxicity are headache, mood swings, and pain in muscles and joints. In massive doses, vitamin A can cause liver damage. In the first 3 months of pregnancy, it can cause birth defects. Women who are or who may become pregnant should strictly limit their intake of vitamin A to 5,000 IU per day or less. Discontinue vitamin A at the first sign of toxicity.

Bad breath with gum disease is almost always a sign of vitamin C deficiency. It is possible to take considerably more than the RDA of vitamin C and still be deficient, if the body has become accustomed to high doses. That is, someone who drinks large quantities of fruit juices and stops, or who takes high doses of vitamin C and stops, may become vitamin C deficient even while eating a healthy diet. If trench mouth occurs, it is best to assume that there is a functional deficiency of the vitamin and take the supplement.

Take vitamin C with caution if you also take certain prescription drugs. Vitamin C taken in the form of vitamin C with bioflavonoids can interfere with the liver's ability to process statin drugs for controlling cholesterol, calcium channel blockers for hypertension such as nifedipine (Procardia), or cyclosporine for preventing transplant rejection.

Vitamin E speeds up the healing of foul-smelling and infected gums. It is especially important if mercury amalgams are present. Mercury depletes the gums of the antioxidant enzymes catalase, glutathione peroxidase, and superoxide dismutase. At least in animal studies, this toxic effect of mercury is counteracted by vitamin E.[4] Selenium is an important cofactor for vitamin E.

The most noticeable side effect from taking too much selenium is bad breath, a garlicky smell. Do not take vitamin C and selenium at the same time, or the selenium will be poorly absorbed. Vitamin E should be used with caution by those who take blood thinners such as clopidogrel (Plavix) or warfarin (Coumadin).

Zinc is essential to dozens of enzymatic processes, including those that send a signal to polymorphonuclear leukocytes to fight bacterial infection. Zinc is also needed for the gums to make enzymes that slow down the process of tissue destruction initiated by endotoxins released by bacteria.[5] Gum disease is especially severe when there is a deficiency of zinc coupled with an excess of copper.[6]

While it is important to take zinc in treating trench mouth, it is equally important not to take too much. Except where otherwise directed, do not take more than 50 milligrams of any zinc supplement daily. In rare cases, excessive intake of zinc depletes copper to cause anemia, that is, a deficiency of red blood cells, and neutropenia, a serious deficiency of white blood cells.

Chamomile tea (and actually, teas made of several related plants, such as calendula, chrysanthemum, cosmos, and the flower but not the oil of safflower) contains triterpenes that stop inflammation. Allergic reactions to chamomile are rare, but the herb sometimes causes sniffles or stomach upset.

CONCEPTS FOR COPING WITH BAD BREATH CAUSED BY INFECTION

❍ Remove decayed gum tissue with a mouthwash of *diluted* hydrogen perioxide. Do not swallow.

❍ To prevent recurrences of trench mouth, floss after every meal and at bedtime.

❍ Regular cleanings by a dentist remove bacteria-laden plaque that may develop even with diligent brushing and flossing. Most dentists recommend having the teeth cleaned once or twice a year, every 3 months if trench mouth is a problem.

○ Don't bite your nails or pick your teeth. Both practices can damage tender gums.

○ The active ingredient in Listerine mouthwash is thymol, a compound found in the herb thyme. Thymol is a potent antibacterial agent.

○ Faulty fillings create a breeding ground for the bacteria that cause trench mouth. Overhanging margins accumulate plaque and offer a shelter for bacteria. Mercury amalgams deplete antioxidant enzymes in small areas of the gums, exposing the glycosaminoglycans and proteoglycans that make up the collagen matrix of the gums to bacterial attack.[7]

○ The herb bloodroot is the source of mouthwashes and toothpastes labeled as containing benzophenanthridine alkaloids or sanguinarine. These compounds cause bacteria to "clump" so that they cannot form colonies on the gums. Some studies indicate they are not as effective in controlling plaque as the synthetic chemical chlorhexidine,[8] but alternating mouthwashes containing sanguinarine and mouthwashes that do not offers maximum benefit.

○ If you smoke, stop.

○ Consider using a tongue cleaner as a final step in oral hygiene. Cleaning the soft plaque from the back of the tongue removes most of the bacteria and other debris that are the primary source of plaque—and frequently are the cause of halitosis. A tongue cleaner should have smooth, well-rounded cleaning edges. Unbreakable stainless steel is preferable to potentially breakable plastic. Avoid cleaners that have holes that can trap the plaque you are trying to remove.

○ Avoid trace mineral supplements containing molybdenum. Molybdenum is essential to the process of sulfoxidation, the metabolic step in which the sulfur found in foods such as garlic is metabolized. Molybdenum activates the enzyme sulfite oxidase. Bad breath is a more commonly recognized problem in countries in which the diet contains high amounts of molybdenum.

Hardening of the Arteries
See **Atherosclerosis.**

Hashimoto's Thyroiditis
See **Hypothyroidism.**

Hay Fever
See **Allergies.**

Headache
See **Cluster Headaches; Migraine; Tension Headaches.**

Hearing Problems
See **Acoustic Trauma; Tinnitus.**

Heart Problems
See **Angina; Atherosclerosis; Cardiomyopathy; Congestive Heart Failure; Irregular Heartbeat; Mitral Valve Prolapse.**

Heartburn

SYMPTOM SUMMARY

○ Uncomfortable burning or warmth in the chest 30–60 minutes after eating

○ Pain may radiate to arms, back, jaws, or throat

○ Pain is worse when lying down or bending over

○ Stomach acid can cause sore throat, hoarseness, or damage to the enamel of the teeth

○ You should seek emergency medical care if you experience:

- Throwing up blood or passing blood in your bowel movements
- Severe pain
- Difficulty swallowing
- Dehydration
- Unintentional weight loss

UNDERSTANDING THE DISEASE PROCESS

Heartburn is an uncomfortable burning or feeling of warmth in the chest that has nothing to with the heart. Food travels from the mouth to the acidic environment in the stomach through a narrow tube called the esophagus. At the base of the esophagus lies the lower esophageal sphincter (LES), which is essentially a valve to keep digested food and stomach acid from traveling back up the throat. When the LES does not close completely, the lower part of the esophagus can be burned by stomach acid and cause the sensation of heartburn.

About one in three people experiences heartburn occasionally; some people suffer heartburn after every meal. People who suffer from certain medical conditions may have an increased risk of heartburn. These conditions include diabetes, hiatal hernia, and autoimmune diseases such as Raynaud's phenomenon and scleroderma. Heartburn can also be aggravated by medications, especially aspirin, heart and blood pressure medications, and the asthma drug Theo-Dur (theophylline). Most of the time, however, heartburn is due to dietary indiscretion.

TREATMENT SUMMARY

DIET

❍ Avoid large meals.

HERBS

❍ Deglycyrrhizinated licorice (DGL): 2 tablets (500 milligrams) *chewed* and swallowed 15 minutes before meals and 1 hour before bedtime.

❍ Slippery elm: tea as desired.

UNDERSTANDING THE HEALING PROCESS

The conventional wisdom concerning heartburn is that certain foods relax the LES and allow stomach acid to come up. These foods are thought to include alcohol, caffeinated coffee and tea, chocolate, citrus fruits and juices, fatty foods, peppermint, peppers, and tomatoes. Strictly speaking, peppers do not cause heartburn; they only heighten the sensation of pain when it occurs and cause the pain to be felt sooner.[1] At least one study has found that the majority of people who have heartburn continue to experience symptoms even after eliminating other typical problem foods.[2] However, everyone with heartburn can benefit from eating small meals.

Scientists at the Cattedra di Gastroenterologia at the University of Milan devised a sophisticated experiment to make exact measurements of gastroesophageal reflux after a high-calorie, high-fat meal, a high-calorie, balanced meal, and a reduced-calorie, balanced meal in a group of heartburn sufferers. They found that the high-calorie meal with the least amount of fat actually caused the greatest amount of heartburn. The low-calorie meal caused less heartburn than either of the high-calorie meals.[3]

The explanation of these results is that stuffing your stomach forces food back into the esophagus. For most heartburn sufferers, eating less is more important than avoiding any particular food.

Two herbal remedies relieve heartburn. Deglycyrrhizinated licorice (DGL) is a form of licorice root that has been processed to remove glycyrrhizin, a chemical that can cause elevated blood pressure and water retention in some people. Two studies have found that DGL is as effective as drugs in the same family as Zantac in controlling ulcers,[4,5] although its use in treating heartburn is based on anecdotal experience. DGL must be chewed before it is swallowed to release anti-inflammatory compounds.

Slippery elm teas contain mucilages that coat and soothe the esophagus and stomach. They do not cause any kind of side effect and they do not interact with any medications, although they are not calorie-free.

CONCEPTS FOR COPING WITH HEARTBURN

❍ There is a long list of herbs used to treat indigestion that should not be used to treat heartburn. Bitters that stimulate the production of stomach acid should be avoided. These include absinthe, andrographis (used as a tea), Angostura bitters, barberry, bitter orange, blessed thistle, boldo, centaury, devil's claw (enteric-coated capsules for arthritis pain relief are OK), gentian, goldenseal, greater celandine, horehound, Oregon grape root, prickly ash, vervain, wormwood, yellow dock. People susceptible to heartburn should also avoid betaine HCl.

❍ Anything that puts pressure on the stomach aggravates heartburn: tight belts or constricting clothing, bending, lifting, obesity, or pregnancy.

❍ Avoid lying down for at least 3 hours after eating. If you suffer nighttime heartburn, elevate the head of your bed at least 6 inches (15 centimeters) by placing bricks under the bedposts. Do not prop up with pillows. This puts pressure on your stomach and makes heartburn worse.

Heavy Periods
(Menorrhagia)

SYMPTOM SUMMARY

○ Loss of more than 80 milliliters ($\frac{1}{3}$ cup) of blood during the menstrual period

○ Clots

○ Flooding

○ Need to change sanitary napkins during the night

UNDERSTANDING THE DISEASE CONDITION

Heavy periods, or menorrhagia, involve any loss of blood during the menstrual period that the woman finds excessive. Arbitrarily defined as a loss of more than 80 milliliters ($\frac{1}{3}$ cup) by the medical profession, heavy periods are defined differently by different women. One study found that 40 percent of women losing more than 80 milliliters of blood during their period regarded their periods as scanty, while 20 percent of women losing less than 20 milliliters regarded their periods as heavy.[1]

Heavy periods are not unusual after dilation and curettage and in women who use IUDs for birth control, women who have had ectopic pregnancies, or women who have uterine fibroids, endometriosis, pelvic inflammatory disease, severe liver disease, or myeloma. They also may be caused by thyroid deficiencies, or low levels of luteinizing hormone (LH), the hormone that stops the growth of blood vessels in the uterus in the middle of the menstrual cycle. About 1 percent of all women have a hereditary condition known as von Willebrand's disease, which also causes nosebleeds and bleeding gums.[2] Heavy periods have also been associated with deficiencies of essential fatty acids, iron, and vitamins A, C, E, and K.

TREATMENT SUMMARY

NUTRITIONAL SUPPLEMENTS

○ Bioflavonoids: 250 milligrams per day.

○ Chlorophyll: 25 milligrams per day.

○ Iron sulfate: 25 milligrams per day—only if blood tests show low ferritin levels.

○ Vitamin A: 25,000 IU per day. Women who are or who may become pregnant should strictly limit their intake of vitamin A to 5,000 IU per day or less.

○ Vitamin E: 200 IU per day.

HERBS

○ Shepherd's purse (*Capsella bursae pastoris*): 1 teaspoon in a cup of hot water brewed as a tea, 3 times a day.

UNDERSTANDING THE HEALING PROCESS

Heavy periods are usually not a sign of a more serious condition. Generally speaking, heavy periods that occur on a regular cycle can be treated with nutritional measures, while irregular periods usually indicate a deeper hormonal imbalance. Other signs a gynecologist's help is needed include bleeding after intercourse and bleeding between periods. When the possibility of other disease conditions has been eliminated, then it is possible to begin a nutritional and herbal program to which up to 92 percent of women with heavy periods respond.

Chlorophyll is a source of vitamin K, which helps the blood make clotting factors. It also makes iron more available to the lining of the uterus, which may indirectly reduce the tendency to bleed.

Vitamin A deficiencies are common in women who have menorrhagia. A South African study found that bringing vitamin levels up to normal alleviated heavy periods in 92 percent of patients.[3] The dosages recommended for heavy periods will not cause side effects, but women who are or who could become pregnant should not take more than 5,000 IU per day of vitamin A, since recommended dosages can cause birth defects if consumed during the first 3 months of pregnancy.

Vitamin C with bioflavonoids strengthens the linings of the capillaries serving the uterus. One study found that 14 out of 16 women taking vitamin C with bioflavonoids improved with treatment. Vitamin C may be especially helpful for women who have heavy periods who take the antidepressants paroxetine (Paxil) or fluvoxamine (Luvox).[4]

Vitamin E may be especially helpful for women with heavy periods who use IUDs. Taking as little vitamin E as 100 IU every other day can sometimes significantly improve symptoms in women who use IUDs.[5]

Heavy periods ordinarily do not result in enough blood loss to cause iron deficiency. However, at least one medical study suggests iron deficiency can cause heavy periods. Physicians writing in the *Journal of the American Medical Association* in the 1960s found that 75 percent of women given iron supplements had less menstrual blood loss, provided there were no other identifiable disease conditions contributing to the problem. Women who did not respond to iron supplements tended later to develop uterine fibroids and endometriosis.[6]

Before taking iron supplements, it is essential to determine that there is an iron deficiency—not every woman who has heavy periods is deficient in iron, and women who have the iron-storage disease hemochromatosis can be seriously harmed by taking iron supplements. Some women who need iron supplements prefer to remain anemic, since iron tablets can cause constipation, diarrhea, and/or especially foul-smelling flatulence.

Drinking orange juice with iron tablets helps the intestine absorb the iron. Do not take iron with supplements containing calcium, inositol hexaphosphate, magnesium, vanadium, or vitamin E, since taking the supplements together may interfere with absorption of one supplement or the other. Do not take iron supplements with antacids, or if you have a history of gastritis, gastrointestinal bleeding, or peptic ulcer disease. You also should not take iron with L-dopa, penicillamine, thyroxine, or most antibiotics, since iron can interfere with the absorption of these prescription drugs.

Herbs such as shepherd's purse stop heavy bleeding—as long as you continue to take them. Shepherd's purse has a high content of oxalic acid, which some scientists believe account for its ability to stop bleeding due to functional abnormalities in the uterus, such as fibroid tumors. Senecio, witch hazel, geranium, trillium, betel nut (*Areca catechu*), and blue cohosh also stop bleeding, but present safety concerns. Blue cohosh, in particular, can cause miscarriage or birth defects if taken in the first 3 months of pregnancy.

CONCEPTS FOR COPING WITH HEAVY PERIODS

❍ Medical studies have found that oral contraceptives reduce blood loss.[7] And IUDs increase menstrual bleeding, especially during the first 6 months of their use.[8]

❍ Several scientific studies have found that the number of pads used during each period is not a good measure of menstrual blood loss.

❍ Bleeding that is worst during the first 3 days of your period suggests a specific biochemical imbalance that can be corrected by reducing intake of beef, beef tallow (often used in cooking fast-food French fries), eggs, and deep-fried food, and by taking fish oils, DHA (not DHEA), or EPA on a regular basis.

❍ Homeopathic medicine offers a range of treatments for heavy periods. Usually it is best to start with a single dose of the lowest strength (6C, 6X, or 12C) of the remedy matching the symptoms to be treated, and then wait for a response. If there is an improvement in symptoms, let the remedy continue to work until there is no more improvement, then take another dose. If there is no improvement, try a different potency (30X or 30C). Sometimes homeopathic medicines work for a few minutes, and sometimes they work for an entire day before another dose is needed.

- Bovista is indicated when premenstrual diarrhea is also a symptom. Women who have problems with fluid retention may also benefit from this remedy.

- Calcarea carbonica is a styptic for periods that come early or are unusually long. There may be sugar cravings, breast pain, digestive upsets, or heavy sweating along with heavy periods.

- Caulophyllum is appropriate for women who also have pelvic inflammation, or whose arthritic symptoms are worst around their periods.

- Chamomilla is appropriate when heavy periods are accompanied by emotional tension.

- Cimicifuga is specified when there is headache or neck pain, or outbreaks of rashes.

- Kreosotum treats heavy periods accompanied by pelvic and abdominal skin irritation.

- Lachesis treats bloating and abdominal tension as well as hot flashes and headaches.

- Lillium tigrinum relieves a feeling of the uterus pushing out that is relieved by crossing the legs.

- Lycopodium treats late periods that cause heavy flow. It is also appropriate for women who become bulimic at the time of their periods.

- Nux vomica is appropriate when there is also constipation or a feeling of pain in the tailbone.

- Pulsatilla is typically given to girls who have just started their periods.

- Veratrum album is appropriate when cold drinks or air conditioning brings relief of premenstrual symptoms.

Hemorrhoids

SYMPTOM SUMMARY

○ Anal itch

○ Blood on toilet tissue

○ Bright red blood in stool (dark red blood indicates bleeding other than hemorrhoids)

○ Pain during bowel movements

○ Rectal bleeding, especially after bowel movements

UNDERSTANDING THE DISEASE PROCESS

Hemorrhoids are varicose veins in the anus and rectum that can ache and bleed. Hemorrhoids are very common. There are some estimates that 50 percent of people over 50 years of age and up to one-third of the total population of the United States has hemorrhoids to some degree.[1]

Hemorrhoids may be internal, within the rectal canal, or external, around the anus. The most common symptom of internal hemorrhoids is bright red blood covering the stool, on toilet paper, or in the toilet bowl. However, an internal hemorrhoid may protrude through the anus outside the body, becoming irritated and painful. This is known as a protruding hemorrhoid. The most common symptom of external hemorrhoids is painful swelling in the form of a hard lump around the anus that results when a blood clot forms. This is a thrombosed external hemorrhoid.

Hemorrhoids are a distortion of an arteriovenous network surrounding the anus and making bowel control possible. These vascular cushions extend into the rectal canal and prevent stool from escaping between bowel movements. Downward pressure during defecation presses them back against the walls of the rectum allowing stool to escape. Advancing age or aggravating conditions deteriorates the connecting fibers that anchor the cushions to the wall of the rectum, causing them to become congested, bleed, and prolapse, sometimes protruding outside the anus.

Scientists researching the causes of hemorrhoids have identified increasing age, chronic diarrhea, pregnancy, pelvic tumors, obesity, and prolonged sitting and straining as significant risk factors.[2] Curiously, constipation is not a significant cause of hemorrhoids; one study even showed that chronic diarrhea is 12 times more likely to cause hemorrhoids than chronic constipation.[3] Any condition that leads to chronic straining to keep the anal sphincter closed, especially diseases that cause chronic diarrhea (Crohn's disease, irritable bowel syndrome, ulcerative colitis, and others) greatly increases the risk of hemorrhoids.[4]

TREATMENT SUMMARY

DIET

○ *Gradually* increase the amount of fiber in your diet so that you eat 5–9 servings of fruit and vegetables every day. Raw fruits and vegetables are preferable. Almonds, dried beans and peas, raw root vegetables (carrots, jicama, radishes, and turnip roots), dried pumpkin and sunflower seeds, whole-grain breads, oranges, apricots, prunes, and unpeeled apples are especially good sources of soluble fiber.

○ Avoid sugar.

○ Drink 8 or more glasses of water every day.

○ Avoid large, heavy meals. Eating smaller portions more often reduces the size of bowel movements.

NUTRITIONAL SUPPLEMENTS

○ Citrus bioflavonoids containing diosmin and hesperidin: 500 milligrams twice a day.

○ Vitamin C: at least 1,000 milligrams a day.

○ Fiber: 1–2 tablespoons of insoluble fiber (psyllium) or soluble fiber (orange pulp) taken with a glass of water daily. Do not take fiber at the same time you take other nutritional supplements or medications.

HERBS

○ *Collinsonea* (stone) root: tincture, as directed on the label.

○ Dioscorea (Wild yam): 400 milligrams in capsule form daily.

○ Slippery elm bark: 1 teaspoon in 1 cup of water as often as desired.

○ Witch hazel creams (such as Venetone): applied to the anus 1–2 times daily.

○ Extracts of horse chestnut and red oak and essential oils of cypress and/or frankincense are also soothing.

UNDERSTANDING THE HEALING PROCESS

Conventional treatment for hemorrhoids consists of taking fiber, drinking more water, and using stool softeners, rectal suppositories containing anti-inflammatory steroids, topical preparations (Anusol, Preparation H, Hemorid), and medicated wipes (Tucks). Severe cases, especially when interior hemorrhoids prolapse or when they contain blood clots, may need to be treated surgically.

While these treatments relieve hemorrhoids, citrus bioflavonoids at least partially prevent flare-ups of hemorrhoids. A French researcher gave 120 hemorrhoid sufferers Daflon 500, a tablet containing a mixture of the citrus bioflavonoids diosmin and hesperidin, or a placebo for 2 months. During that time, 24 of the test participants taking bioflavonoids experienced at least one attack of hemorrhoids lasting an average of 2.6 days. Among test participants given a sugar pill, 42 experienced at least one attack of hemorrhoids lasting an average of 4.6 days. People taking bioflavonoids also reported lower levels of pain.[5] Clearly, this test did not show that bioflavonoids cure hemorrhoids, but they can reduce pain and accelerate healing. Other studies have found that citrus bioflavonoids begin to work in as little as 7 days,[6] and that they help stop bleeding after hemorrhoid surgery.[7]

Other bioflavonoids are also available to treat hemorrhoids, such as barley leaf extracts and Scotch broom, but they should be used with caution by anyone takes antibiotics or many other prescription medications (see QUERCETIN in Part Two). Horse chestnut, oligomeric proanthocyanidins (OPCs), and gotu kola do not pose as many potentially negative interactions with drugs and possess many healing properties relevant to treating hemorrhoids, but they are not as well documented as the citrus bioflavonoids diosmin and hesperidin.

If you take citrus bioflavonoids, be sure also to take vitamin C. Scientists are unsure of the interaction between citrus bioflavonoids and vitamin C. Citrus bioflavonoids and vitamin C were once thought to be synergistic, but some recent studies suggest that diosmin and hesperidin may actually interfere with the body's ability to absorb this vitamin. To be sure vitamin C requirements are met, take at least a small dose (500 milligrams) of vitamin C when taking citrus bioflavonoids.

Along with taking bioflavonoids, it is important to relieve constipation by taking fiber. Constipation does not cause hemorrhoids, but the pain and inflammation caused by hemorrhoids is greatly relieved by treating constipation. Since fiber and prunes don't give reliable results (see CONSTIPATION), most treatment plans for constipation include increased consumption of prepared fiber. Fiber is the part of plant food that is not digested. It adds bulk to the stools by absorbing water. There are two types of fiber, soluble and insoluble. Soluble fiber dissolves in water and is found in oat bran, barley, peas, beans, and citrus fruits. Insoluble fiber does not dissolve in water and is found in wheat bran and some vegetables. Fiber increases the transit time of stool through the colon and decrease the pressures within the colon.

Avoiding sugars also helps relieve constipation. Eating sugar raises blood sugar levels. When blood sugars are high, the central nervous system signals the digestive tract to absorb sugars more slowly.[8] This slows down the passage of food through the digestive tract, giving gas time to accumulate, and maximizes the amount of time irritating food allergens are in contact with the intestinal wall. Some naturopathic physicians speculate that sugar consumption is the most important contributing factor to most cases of spasmodic constipation in the United States.[9]

CONCEPTS FOR COPING WITH HEMORRHOIDS

❍ Many people benefit from daily sitz baths. As its name suggests, a sitz bath is a warm bath in which the patient sits, immersing the buttocks in warm water for up to 20 minutes at a time. Several herbs can be added to the bath water for added relief of anal fissures. Burnet, horsetail, and oak bark are anti-inflammatory. A dropper of valerian tincture is widely reported to relieve spasms. Essential oils of calendula, chamomile, or yarrow may be added to the bath to relieve inflammation.

❍ Homeopathy offers a number of remedies for hemorrhoids, chosen on the basis of individual characteristics. Usually it is best to start with a single dose of the lowest strength (6C, 6X, or 12C) of the remedy matching the symptoms to be treated, and then wait for a response. If there is an improvement in symptoms, let the remedy continue to work until there is no more improvement, then take another dose. If there is no improvement, try a different potency (30X or 30C). Sometimes homeopathic medicines work for a few minutes, sometimes they work for an entire day before another dose is needed.

- Aesculus hippocastanum treats sore, swollen, aching hemorrhoids accompanied by a painful sensation of a "bundle of sticks" in the rectum lasting for hours after bowel movement. This remedy is most successful for people who also have lower back pain and who are sore and achy, with a swollen feeling.

• Aloe relieves prolapsed hemorrhoids (hemorrhoids swollen and protruding out the anus). Diarrhea and flatulence are indicators for this remedy.

• Arnica, frequently used to treat sports injuries, is also used to treat hemorrhoids made worse by heavy lifting or athletic activity.

• Calcarea fluorica treats bleeding and itching hemorrhoids. Constipation and flatulence are indications for this remedy.

• Graphites treats burning hemorrhoids in people who are overweight, tend to have a ruddy complexion, and have a strong joie de vivre.

• Hamamelis is the homeopathic remedy for hemorrhoids that are made worse by sitting in a warm bath. Bleeding and soreness are other indications for this remedy.

• Ignatia treats hemorrhoids that are accompanied by stabbing pain. It is especially recommended when rectal prolapse follows bowel movements.

• Nux vomica relieves hemorrhoids accompanying chronic constipation. Food, alcohol, tobacco, or drug addictions are an indication for this remedy.

• Pulsatilla treats hemorrhoids occurring during pregnancy or that worsen around the menstrual period.

• Sulfur relieves hemorrhoids accompanied by flatulence with a strong, offensive odor.

Hepatic Encephalopathy
See **Cirrhosis of the Liver**.

Hepatitis A

SYMPTOM SUMMARY

2–6 weeks after exposure to the virus:

○ Headache

○ Loss of appetite

○ Low-grade fever

○ Muscle aches similar to the flu

○ Nausea

○ Vomiting

○ Urine may become dark after about 4 weeks, indicating an immune reaction in the liver

After dark urine appears:

○ Abdominal pain (in about half of cases)

○ Itch

○ Jaundice (yellowing of the skin), most notable in elderly persons with the disease, may be very slight in children

○ Joint pain

○ Pale stools

○ Rash on the legs

UNDERSTANDING THE DISEASE PROCESS

Hepatitis A is a relatively mild, and, in the twenty-first century in North America, relatively uncommon viral infection of the liver. For the most recent year for which statistics are available, the Centers for Disease Control report that there were approximately 32,000 diagnosed cases in the United States. The disease is most common among small children in day care, day-care workers, sewage workers, male homosexuals, and travelers returning from developing countries.

The hepatitis A virus (HAV) is spread by person-to-person contact, but people with HAV are infectious only after jaundice (yellowing of the skin) has developed. Symptoms usually occur 2–6 weeks after infection. The damage done by HAV infection is usually very mild, with symptoms caused by the immune system rather than by the virus itself. Symptoms usually dissipate in less than 3 months. Death from HAV occurs in only about 1 in 5,000 cases, almost all of these in the elderly.[1]

TREATMENT SUMMARY

NUTRITIONAL SUPPLEMENTS

○ Vitamin B: any complete vitamin B supplement, daily.

○ Vitamin C: at least 1,000 milligrams per day.

HERBS

○ Glycyrrhizin: as directed on the label.

UNDERSTANDING THE HEALING PROCESS

Care for hepatitis A mainly consists of watchful waiting.

The infection can deplete water-soluble vitamins, so it is important to replace vitamins B and C. Avoid high doses of vitamin C, since they may cause diarrhea. The licorice derivative glycyrrhizin is known to kill HAV in the test tube; it is safe for general use but should be avoided by people who take steroids or medications for high blood pressure.

CONCEPTS FOR COPING WITH HEPATITIS A

❍ Because the symptoms of hepatitis A are mediated by the immune system, "immune stimulant" supplements are not helpful. Many naturopaths recommend silymarin (milk thistle), but this herb should be avoided if there is diarrhea or heartburn.

❍ Hepatitis A is much more common in Mexico than in the United States. Be sure to drink and brush your teeth with purified water (*agua purificada*), and avoid raw fish (ceviche), raw fruits and vegetables, and fruit juices (*liquadas*) unless you know they have been prepared under sanitary conditions.

Hepatitis B

SYMPTOM SUMMARY

6 weeks to 6 months after exposure to the virus:

❍ Abdominal pain

❍ Clay-colored stools

❍ Cough

❍ Dark urine

❍ Fever

❍ Joint pain

❍ Rashes

❍ Sore throat

❍ Often no symptoms at all

Chronic infection:

❍ Appearance of characteristic purple blotches under the skin

❍ Bleeding hemorrhoids

❍ Confusion

❍ Erectile dysfunction in men

❍ Jaundice (yellowing of the skin)

❍ Loss of interest in sex

❍ Nausea

❍ Vomiting

❍ Vomiting blood

❍ Weakness

❍ Weight loss

Distinguished from other forms of viral hepatitis only by blood test

UNDERSTANDING THE DISEASE PROCESS

The hepatitis B virus (HBV) is a common infection of the liver. About 1 million people in the United States have chronic hepatitis B, and every year another 200,000 to 300,000 persons are exposed to the virus. At least 10,000 require hospitalization, and several hundred die of liver failure. People with HBV infection often develop chronic liver disease and have a 200-fold increased risk of liver cancer. Worldwide, over 300 million people carry this hepatitis virus. HBV was once thought to be transmitted exclusively by sexual contact and contaminated blood products, but scientists now know that the virus can be spread through contaminated food.[1]

TREATMENT SUMMARY

DIET

❍ Make breakfast your largest meal, to avoid nausea later in the day.

NUTRITIONAL SUPPLEMENTS

❍ Vitamin E: 1,000 IU daily.

HERBS

❍ *Sho-saiko-to* (if you are not taking interferon therapy): as directed on label.

UNDERSTANDING THE HEALING PROCESS

There is no specific medical therapy for the early, acute stages of hepatitis infection. It is important to eat a high-energy diet during this stage of the disease, although it is better to avoid animal protein should liver damage (indicated by blood test) occur. Eating more at breakfast can help you avoid nausea later in the day. Fortunately,

90 percent of people who go through acute HBV infection recover completely.[2]

Clinical studies have found that supplemental vitamin E slows the reproduction of HBV. It is of special benefit for people coming off treatment with interferon or Epivir.[3] People with HBV are unlikely to be prescribed aspirin, clopidogrel (Plavix), or warfarin (Coumadin), but people who have any form of chronic liver disease should not take vitamin E with these drugs or with ginkgo.

Other clinical studies of people with HBV have found that the Japanese herbal formula *sho-saiko-to* increases the immune system's production of interferon, a chemical that interferes with the reproduction of the virus.[4] The key drawback to the use of *sho-saiko-to* is that it can overstimulate the body's production of interferon when used in combination with interferon therapy. An autoimmune form of pneumonia can result. Do not use *sho-saiko-to* at any time during the months you take interferon therapy. *Sho-saiko-to* is available in the United States and Canada as:

- Liver Kampo (Honso)
- Minor Bupleurum Combination (Lotus Classics, Qualiherb, Sun Ten)
- Minor Bupleurum Formula (Chinese Classics, Golden Flower Chinese Herbs)
- Minor Bupleurum Formulation (Kan Traditionals)
- Sho-saiko-to (Honso, Tsumura)
- Xiuao Chai Hu Tang (Chinese Classics, Golden Flower Chinese Herbs, Herbal Times, Honso, Kan Traditionals, Lotus Classics, Qualiherb, Sun Ten)

CONCEPTS FOR COPING WITH HEPATITIS B

○ Silymarin, a group of chemicals in milk thistle, is very useful in treating cirrhosis but does not reduce symptoms of acute HBV.

○ A cut that is slow to stop bleeding is a sign of liver damage. If you experience any form of unusual bleeding, consult a physician.

○ HBV is not spread from mother to child by breast-feeding.

○ Taking Coenzyme Q_{10} increases the body's immune response to HBV vaccine. Swedish studies have found that taking 180 milligrams of CoQ_{10} daily for the 90 days during which the three hepatitis vaccine injections are being received increases the body's production of

antibodies by more than 50 percent in young people.[5] Studies at Tufts University in Boston found an even more striking effect in the elderly. Taking just 400 IU of vitamin E daily for 9 months produced a 600 percent increase in antibodies to hepatitis B.

○ The physician's first line of treatment for HBV is interferon (Intron A) Most patients develop flulike symptoms when treated with interferon; ask your doctor about timing your treatment later in the day, when side effects will be less severe, should this effect occur. About 15 percent of people treated with interferon develop severe depression, often with risk of suicide. There is no supplement that can reduce the side effects of interferon, but there are supplements that may make it more effective.

- Iron deficiency interferes with the action of interferon, but iron excess accelerates liver damage. Make sure your physician has measured serum ferritin and prescribed iron supplements, if necessary, before taking interferon. Do not take over-the-counter iron supplements, since unnecessary iron supplementation can make the underlying disease worse.

- There are preliminary indications that N-acetyl cysteine (NAC) and thymus extract will increase the effectiveness of interferon against hepatitis B. They will not stop the drug's side effects. If your doctor approves, take 400 milligrams of NAC daily and thymus extract as directed on the label. NAC may cause headaches if taken with sildenafil (Viagra), and in rare cases can cause cysteine-crystal kidney stones. Diabetics who also have CF may find that taking NAC causes false readings in urine tests for ketones.

○ When interferon fails, doctors may prescribe a drug more commonly used for AIDS, lamivudine (Epivir). This drug is much less likely to cause side effects, but there is a risk that the virus can become resistant to the drug when it is the sole medication. Taking a B-vitamin supplement containing riboflavin daily reduces the risk of a relatively rare side effect of the medication, lactic acidosis. Taking a vitamin E supplement is important when coming off the medication. Clinical trials at the Universita di Bologna in Italy found that patients finishing a course of Epivir who supplemented with vitamin E were far more likely to achieve normal liver enzyme (ALT) levels and negative tests for HBV-DNA if they took 1,000 IU of vitamin E daily during the 12 months after completing treatment with the drug.[7]

○ Also see CIRRHOSIS OF THE LIVER.

Hepatitis C

SYMPTOM SUMMARY

Usually no symptoms until disease is in an advanced stage

Common symptoms after condition has caused cirrhosis of the liver:

○ Appearance of small "spider veins" under the skin

○ Bleeding hemorrhoids

○ Confusion

○ Erectile dysfunction in men

○ Jaundice (yellowing of the skin)

○ Loss of interest in sex

○ Nausea

○ Vomiting

○ Vomiting blood

○ Weakness

○ Weight loss

Less frequent symptoms after development of cirrhosis:

○ Abdominal pain

○ Bleeding gums

○ Breast enlargement in men

○ Clay-colored or pale stools

○ Decreased volume of urine

○ Fever

○ Flatulence

○ Nosebleed

UNDERSTANDING THE DISEASE PROCESS

Nearly 4 million Americans are infected with the hepatitis C virus (HCV). Worldwide, nearly 170 million people have HCV. Infection due to HCV accounts for 20 percent of all cases of acute hepatitis, an estimated 30,000 new acute infections, and 8,000–10,000 deaths each year in the United States.[1]

Hepatitis C infections can live in the liver for years and even decades causing little damage. People with hepatitis C who continue to drink heavily are 27 times more likely to die of the disease than those who abstain from alcohol completely. Among people infected with the virus who avoid alcohol and drugs, only about 1 in 5 develops cirrhosis of the liver. Most of these unfortunate few share a common and treatable condition, insulin resistance.

Insulin resistance is an inability of the body to move sugar out of the bloodstream and into cells in response to the hormone insulin. The condition is usually associated with overweight, specifically with abdominal fat. Lowering fat in the diet and losing weight usually lessen insulin resistance.

In hepatitis C, insulin resistance causes a cascade of changes in the liver's need to process hormones and fat. Insulin in the skin and muscles ordinarily puts a brake on the action of hormone-sensitive lipase, the enzyme responsible for releasing fatty acids from fat cells. In insulin resistance, this hormone is no longer suppressed. Fat cells churn out free fatty acids that are ultimately stored in the liver. In addition, stress hormones, growth hormone, and the sugar-releasing compound glucagon are increased in response to increased levels of insulin. The liver is forced to recycle these hormones at the same time it deals with the stress of hepatitis C. And the fatty acids themselves stimulate the formation of fat in the liver. The result is an ever-increasing burden of fatty acids and hormones adding to the liver's stress.

TREATMENT SUMMARY

DIET

○ Reduce calorie consumption.

NUTRITIONAL SUPPLEMENTS

As soon as possible after diagnosis:

○ Alpha-lipoic acid: 200 milligrams daily.

○ Chromium (from brewer's yeast): 1,000 micrograms daily.

After diagnosis of cirrhosis:

○ Selenium: 100 micrograms per day.

HERBS

After diagnosis of cirrhosis:

○ Milk thistle, preferably as a silymarin phytosome: 420–600 milligrams per day.

○ *Shakuyaku-kanzo-to* (for leg cramps): as directed on label.

See Part Three if you take prescription medication.

UNDERSTANDING THE HEALING PROCESS

Australian researchers tested 19 people with chronic hepatitis C in a 90-day test of diet and exercise. Some participants had previously been treated with interferon and some had not, but all had some degree of fibrosis (leading to cirrhosis), steatosis (significant risk of developing diabetes), and inflammation (indicating tissue death). All 23 participants were significantly overweight and all had measurable insulin resistance.

The Australian test participants modified their diet by a simple rule: eat less. Average food consumption in the group was lowered from 2,740 to 1,620 calories per day (50 percent carbohydrate, 20 percent protein, and 30 percent fat), enough for most to lose 1 pound a week. Participants gradually increased exercise to 30 minutes a day. Participants engaged in aerobic exercise, such as a brisk walk, but did not do strength training.

The diet and exercise changes in this program were hardly rigorous, but the results were impressive. Serum ALT, a measure of liver tissue destruction, steadily decreased as the participants lost weight. Fatty liver, fibrosis, and inflammation improved in almost all the participants. Most important, in four of the participants, smooth muscle antibodies, the measure of damage to the liver by the immune system itself, completely disappeared.

The Australian research team believes that any man with a waist measure of more than 37 inches (94 centimeters) and any woman with a waist measurement of more than 32 inches (80 centimeters) can benefit from gentle changes in diet and exercise to lose weight. Massive weight loss is not necessary. Losing as little as 2.5 percent of one's total body weight is frequently enough to stop the progression of the disease.[2]

Weight loss, however, is only one tool in overcoming insulin resistance. Alpha-lipoic acid reduces the concentration of a blood sugar byproduct known as fructosamine. This sugar-coated protein modifies the action of immune cells so that they are more likely to attach to and attack liver tissue. This chemical attaches to proteins and is a contributing factor in diabetic kidney disease. The supplement also stops the process that robs fat cells of their sensitivity to insulin during the earlier stages of diabetes. Laboratory experiments with animals have found that alpha-lipoic acid lowers blood pressure and helps muscle tissues absorb glucose from the bloodstream, although it is of limited benefit once insulin sensitivity has been established through exercise. Alpha-lipoic acid can be taken in dosages of up to 1,200 milligrams per day without side effects, but 100 milligrams per day is sufficient.

Chromium relieves insulin resistance and high blood sugars caused by stress. Chromium that is derived from brewer's yeast is more beneficial than inorganic chromium. Take 1,000 micrograms a day. Chromium works even better when taken with its cofactor niacin, but since niacin can cause harmless changes in liver tissue that can be mistaken for liver cancer in CAT scans, people with hepatitis C should not take it.

Vanadium in the form of vanadyl sulfate is frequently recommended for insulin resistance in people who are overweight (although it is not as effective in people who are normal weight). Since it works by making the liver more responsive to insulin, however, it should be avoided by anyone who has cirrhosis, fatty liver, or any other complication of hepatitis C.

Several supplements help once cirrhosis of the liver is diagnosed. Only the most preliminary clinical study supports the use of selenium in treating advanced liver damage caused by hepatitis C, but these laboratory experiments suggest that it could be very important. Selenium participates in a series of biochemical steps that make liver cells insensitive to tumor necrosis factor, a hormone the immune system ordinarily uses to destroy tumors that also destroys healthy tissues in the presence of alcohol. Cirrhosis patients with higher bloodstream concentrations of selenium have less severe liver damage.[3]

Relatively high doses of milk thistle, preferably taken as a phytosome (the active ingredient, silymarin, chemically joined to phosphatidylcholine) reduce liver damage in alcoholic cirrhosis.[4] At molecular level, silibinin, one of the components of silymarin, prevents damage to the outer membranes of liver cells from free radicals of oxygen.[5] It helps liver cells use oxygen more efficiently, and assists in the formation of proteins.[6] Most important, it increases synthesis of proteins needed by the liver to repair itself.[7]

Milk thistle products are nontoxic, although they stimulate the production of bile, possibly making stools looser. Some people with cirrhosis may not benefit from taking silymarin. One study found that milk thistle is not helpful when there is a complication of cirrhosis known as portal hypertension.[8]

Muscle cramps are common in advanced hepatitis C. A study sponsored by a Japanese herb manufacturer found that *shakuyaku-kanzo-to,* a traditional herbal formula containing peony root and licorice, stops leg cramps caused by cirrhosis. In the United States and Canada, *shakuyaku-kanzo-to* is sold under the following trade names:

- Peony and Licorice (Kanpo, Qualiherb)
- Peony and Licorice Combination (Blue Light, Brion, KPC, Ming Tong, Sheng Chang)
- Shao Yao Gan Cao Tang (most pharmacies associated with practitioners of Traditional Chinese Medicine)

Japanese physicians have also found that about 3 in 5 patients taking 3 grams of supplemental taurine daily experience relief from cramps.[9] Do not use taurine if you suffer congestive heart failure in addition to cirrhosis of the liver. Do not use the Japanese herbal remedy *sho-saiko-to* if you have hepatitis C.

CONCEPTS FOR COPING WITH HEPATITIS C

○ Ammonia is a normal byproduct of protein digestion. In advanced hepatitis C the liver is unable to remove ammonia from the blood. Ammonia can build up to levels that cause hepatic encephalopathy, a condition that can cause mental confusion, coma, or even death. A minority of people with hepatic encephalopathy can benefit from taking branched-chain amino acids (L-isoleucine, L-leucine, and L-valine). When there are adequate levels of B vitamins, the liver can use these amino acids to make proteins while producing a minimum of toxic ammonia. A German study published in the early 1980s reported that in 3 out of 4 cases, intravenous administration of branched-chain amino acids completely reversed hepatic encephalopathy.[10] More than 20 years of subsequent research has failed to prove that any single formula of branched-chain amino acids is best for treating cirrhosis, but there is general agreement among European physicians that amino acid supplements of this type are appropriate therapy.[11] Since taking too high a dose can cause serious side effects, only use branched-chain amino acids to treat cirrhosis after consultation with a nutritionally oriented physician.

○ Practitioners of Traditional Chinese Medicine can prepare herbal treatments for ascites, typically containing the herb akebia (chocolate vine).

○ People who have cirrhosis of the liver are unlikely to have conditions treated with medications that interact with the supplements recommended here. However, a popular Japanese herbal remedy recommended for hepatitis B, *sho-saiko-to,* can cause deadly interstitial pneumonia when used by people undergoing treatment with interferon.

○ See also CIRRHOSIS OF THE LIVER.

Herniated Disk
See **Back Pain**.

Herpes

SYMPTOM SUMMARY

On first contact with the herpesvirus:

○ Fatigue

○ Fever

○ Loss of appetite

○ Muscle pain

Prior to outbreak:

○ Reddening of skin

○ Burning, itching, tingling, and pain

After the outbreak:

○ Eruption of blisters filled with clear, straw-colored fluid

○ Blisters break, forming painful ulcers that crust over in 7–14 days

○ Outbreaks may occur on genitals, anus, inner thigh, or mouth

○ Men develop painful urination if the lesion is near the opening of the urethra.

○ Women frequently develop painful urination and vaginal discharge.

Because the herpesvirus is transmitted through secretions from the oral or genital mucosa, common sites of infection in men include the shaft and head of the penis, the scrotum, inner thighs, and anus. Women are infected on the labia, vagina, cervix, anus, and inner thighs. The mouth can be a site of infection in both sexes.

UNDERSTANDING THE DISEASE PROCESS

Two viruses cause herpes, herpes simplex virus type 1 (HSV-1), and herpes simplex virus type 2 (HSV-2). HSV-1 is generally associated with cold sores. HSV-2 is generally associated with genital outbreaks. Since initial oral herpes infection, usually occurs in childhood, HSV-1 is not classified as a sexually transmitted disease.

The virus responsible for cold sores, HSV-1, can be transmitted in saliva either during kissing or by eating and drinking from contaminated utensils. HSV-1 can cause genital herpes through transmission during oral-genital sex. Thus, both strains of the virus may be transmitted by sexual contact. HSV-2 is transmitted by direct contact with oral or genital secretions.

Infection with the herpesvirus is extremely common. Epidemiologists agree that 90 percent of the population of the United States has been exposed to HSV-1 (oral herpes) and about 22 percent of the population has been exposed to HSV-2 (genital herpes). Most of the people who have been exposed to herpes are between the ages of 19 and 39.[1]

HSV-2 infection is more common in women than in men. Antibodies for the virus are found in 26 percent of women compared to 18 percent of men over the age of twelve. HSV-2 infection is more common in African-Americans than in Caucasians. Approximately 17 percent of Caucasian adults and 46 percent of African-American adults harbor HSV-2, but only 1 in 5 ever develops a medically diagnosed outbreak of the disease.

Some infectious disease experts believe the reason only 1 in 5 persons infected with HSV-2 ever receives appropriate medical care is that the disease is very often misdiagnosed. Individuals who consult a physician about the more common manifestations of genital herpes may be told that they have genital trauma, yeast or urinary tract infections, bladder dysfunction, hemorrhoids, or even flea bites. The reason for the frequent misdiagnosis of the disease is that it usually causes very mild symptoms. The differences between the most common symptoms of herpes and the classic symptoms of herpes described in medical books are summarized in the table "Symptoms of Genital Herpes" on the following page.

Treatment and care of mild cases of herpes is important. Research suggests that the virus can be transmitted even in the absence of clinical disease, so that a sexual partner without obvious genital herpes may still transmit the illness. Some experts believe that the spread of herpes by people who do not have active symptoms may actually contribute more to the spread of genital herpes than active sores.

Serious complications may be associated with herpes infection. The herpesvirus has been implicated in causing cancer of the cervix. The risk of cervical cancer increases when HSV is present in combination with

SYMPTOMS OF GENITAL HERPES			
Disease Type	Severity	Symptoms	Time to Healing
Typical Symptoms			
Typical (80 percent of cases)	Least severe of all manifestations	Burning, itching, and soreness of the genitals with little or no pain. Ulcers are not observed due to the small number, small size, or internal anal, cervical, rectal, urethral, or vulvar location.[2]	A few days
Classic Symptoms			
All outbreaks		**On mucous membranes:** ulcers without blisters or crusting **On skin:** Clusters of small painful blisters that ulcerate, crust, and heal.[3]	
First outbreak	Most severe pain and ulceration	Fever, headache, muscle pain, and painful urination. 80 percent of women have cervical inflammation. Ulcers form in about 10 days.	3 weeks
Recurrent outbreaks	Less severe manifestations of the disease	Burning, itching, tingling, and pain up to 48 hours before appearance of blisters. 20 to 40 percent of patients will not have warning signs before blisters develop.[4]	5 days

human papillomavirus (HPV), the virus responsible for genital warts. For pregnant women, the presence of either type of herpesvirus on the genitalia or in the birth canal is a threat to the infant. Subsequent infection to the newborn infant can lead to herpetic meningitis, herpetic viremia, chronic skin infection, and even death.

Herpes infection also poses a serious problem for people with AIDS, cancer patients undergoing chemotherapy or radiation therapy, or persons with asthma, rheumatoid arthritis, or skin conditions treated with steroids. These people may suffer infections of various organs including:

- Encephalitis—a very serious infection of the brain. If untreated, approximately 60–80 percent of those who contract this condition will progress to coma and death within a few days. Those who recover often suffer some impairment, ranging from mild neurological impairment to paralysis.

- Herpetic esophagitis—infection of the esophagus causing painful ulcers.

- Herpetic hepatitis—inflammation of the liver and eventual liver failure.

- Herpetic keratitis—herpes infection of the eye leading to scarring within the cornea and eventual blindness.

- Persistent infection of the mucous membranes and skin of the nose, mouth, and throat.

- Pneumonitis—infection of the lung causing a life-threatening pneumonia.

TREATMENT SUMMARY

DIET

❍ Avoid foods that contain high concentrations of the amino acid arginine, especially almonds, chocolate, Jell-O, and peanuts. Eat foods that contain high concentrations of the amino acid lysine, including most vegetables, chicken, fish, and turkey.

SUPPLEMENTS

❍ Bioflavonoids: 1,000 milligrams per day.

❍ L-lysine: 1,000 milligrams 3 times a day. Pregnant women and nursing mothers should avoid lysine supplements.

❍ Propolis: 650 milligrams 3 times a day.

❍ Thymus extract: 500 milligrams of crude polypeptides daily.

❍ Vitamin A: 50,000 IU daily. Women who are or who may become pregnant should strictly limit their intake of vitamin A to 5,000 IU per day or less.

❍ Vitamin C: 2,000 milligrams daily.

HERBS

❍ Copaiba oil: applied to inflamed skin for fast relief of pain.

❍ Eleutherococcus (Siberian ginseng): 2,000 milligrams daily. Since the herb stimulates testosterone production, men with incipient male-pattern baldness, benign prostatic hypertrophy, or prostate cancer should avoid it. Both men and women with acne should avoid this herb.

❍ Kudzu Decoction (Ge Gen Tang or *kakkon-to*): as directed on label, daily. Brands include:

- Ge Gen Tang (Chinese Classics, Golden Flower Chinese Herbs, Honso , Kan Traditionals, Lotus Classics, ProBotanixx, Qualiherb, Sun Ten)

- Kakkon-to (Tsumura)

- Kakkonto Formula 026 (Kampo Institute)

- Kampo4Cold/Flu Pueraria Formula (Honso)

- Kudzu Releasing Formula (Kan Traditionals)

- Pueraria Combination (Lotus Classics, Qualiherb, Sun Ten)

- Pueraria Formula (Golden Flower Chinese Herbs)

- Pueraria Plus Formula (Chinese Classics)

- Shu Jin 1 (ProBotanixx)

❍ Licorice (glycyrrhetinic acid) cream: apply twice daily.

❍ Melissa cream: apply twice daily.

For cold sores:

❍ Zinc/glycine cream: apply at the first sign of inflammation.

UNDERSTANDING THE HEALING PROCESS

Herpes has no cure. No one becomes immune to the disease after having it. Even when symptoms disappear, the virus can still be spread through intimate contact.

Condoms are the best protection against acquiring genital herpes from sexual activity. Latex condoms protect against the transmission of the virus. Lambskin and animal membrane condoms do not. The virus can penetrate them. The female condom has been tested and shown to successfully reduce transmission risk as well.

Individuals with genital herpes should avoid sexual

contact when active lesions are present. In addition, individuals with known genital herpes but without current clinical symptoms should inform their partners that they have the disease. This precaution allows both parties to use barrier protection to prevent the spread of the infection.

Eating foods rich in the amino acid lysine and avoiding foods rich in the amino acid arginine is of proven value in controlling herpes infections. The presence of arginine has long been believed to be a "trigger" for the virus to replicate itself.[5] Lysine has a chemical structure that is similar to that of arginine. It competes with and blocks arginine from entering the nerve tissues that harbor the herpesvirus between outbreaks.[6] Lysine more recently has been found to be essential in "coding" the virus so that it is recognized and destroyed by antibodies.[7]

In a study conducted in the mid-1980s, herpes patients were given lysine in a large dosage (3,000 milligrams per day) along with restriction of chocolate, gelatin, and nuts. After 6 months, herpes outbreaks were 25 percent less frequent among patients treated with lysine than in the placebo group.[8] Apparently a high dosage is necessary for successful treatment. A clinical test using a lower dosage of lysine (1,200 milligrams) failed to show that lysine supplementation helps control herpes outbreaks.[9]

Bioflavonoids, propolis, and vitamin C act synergistically to control herpes outbreaks. In a study in which women were given 3,000 milligrams of water-soluble bioflavonoids and 3,000 milligrams of vitamin C beginning at the onset of symptoms, blisters healed in an average of 4.4 days in the treatment group compared to 10 days in the placebo group.[10] In a study in Ukraine, women with cervical herpes were treated with either propolis or the commonly prescribed medication acyclovir. Women given propolis were twice as likely to have crusted rather than open lesions on the third day of treatment. They were slightly less than twice as likely to show complete healing of the outbreak on the tenth day. Moreover, only women in the propolis group showed improvement in yeast infections during the course of treatment.[11]

French studies have found that a chemical constituent of propolis, 3-methylbut-2-enyl caffeate, eliminates 99.9 percent of the herpesvirus under test tube conditions.[12] However, the antiviral effect of propolis is even greater when combined with bioflavonoid compounds.[13] The healing properties of propolis have not been confirmed for propolis taken orally rather than in creams, and the synergistic effect of these three supplements has not been confirmed in clinical studies, but the preliminary evidence is strong enough to merit their inclusion in any nutritional program for herpes.

Thymus extracts have been shown to prevent the frequency and severity of recurrent herpes outbreaks in persons with immune deficiency. Thymus extract appears to increase the production of antibodies in response to the virus, and to make natural killer cells more active.[14]

Next to using latex condoms, taking vitamin A may be one of the most considerate things you can do for your partner if you have genital herpes. A study of 273 women who had herpes at the University of Washington found that those who had high concentrations of vitamin A in the bloodstream were 15 times less likely to shed the herpesvirus, potentially infecting their partners, than women who suffered vitamin A deficiency. Only 2 percent of women with high levels of vitamin A were potentially infectious at the time of the test.[15] Although the tests were conducted on women who were also HIV positive and did not use oral contraception, and have not been repeated in a study including men, it is likely that vitamin A is extraordinarily useful in slowing the spread of herpesvirus.

A single study published in 1979 suggests that zinc supplements in relatively high doses may be useful in controlling recurrent outbreaks of herpes.[16] However, the scientific evidence for the use of creams containing zinc and glycine to control the pain and inflammation caused by cold sores is stronger. A test sponsored by the Alterra Corporation found that applying zinc-based creams at the first sign of inflammation reduced the duration of cold sores from an average of 6.5 days to 5 days. Subjects treated with the zinc oxide/glycine cream also experienced reduction in overall severity of signs and symptoms, particularly blistering, soreness, itching, and tingling.[17]

Copaiba resin acts by reducing the permeability of capillary walls to histamine, the chemical responsible for painful swelling. The volatile oil of the herb is antimicrobial, and prevents secondary infections in eczema and psoriasis as well as herpes.[18]

Eleutherococcus, more commonly known as Russian or Siberian ginseng, has shown promise for the treatment of herpes. A 6-month double-blind trial of 93 men and women with recurrent herpes infections found that treatment with the herb eleutherococcus (2 grams daily) reduced the frequency of infections by almost 50 percent.[19]

The ancient Chinese herbalist Zhang Zhong-jing devised Kudzu Decoction as a means of treating diseases poetically described as "a bird that strains . . . to fly." Researchers in Japan recognized the metaphor as descriptive of herpes infection. Most viral infections, such as colds, are eliminated by the immune system in a few days or perhaps a few weeks. The herpesvirus, however, can remain in nerve tissues for many years without causing symptoms. It is activated when the body's overall resistance is weakened. The weakened immune system's only effective response to the infection is to destroy infected cells. The resulting cascade of inflammation and tissue damage can cause serious complications, and even result in death in infants and adults who are infected with both herpes and HIV.

Researchers at Toyama University in Japan studied the use of Kudzu Decoction as a herpes treatment. Their research found that the formula neither kills the virus directly nor activates the body's immune system. Instead, Kudzu Decoction blocks the tissue-damaging effects of the reactivated virus. In this way, the traditional Chinese herbal formula treats the disease without creating a worse condition in its place.[20]

Scientists at the University of Texas Medical Branch in Galveston have found that the primary antiviral chemical in licorice, 20 beta-carboxy-11-oxo-30-norolean-12-en-3 beta-yl-2-O-beta-D-glucopyranuronosyl-alpha-D-glucopyranosiduronic acid, more conveniently referred to as glycyrrhizin, protects damaged skin from opportunistic herpes infection, that is, herpes that could be spread by contact with infected bandages or medical instruments.[21] The latest research has found that glycyrrhizin stops the herpesvirus from "jumping the gap" between the nerve cells, in which it rests between outbreaks, and adjacent cells that carry it to the skin.[22] Clinical studies have found that licorice creams reduce the pain and healing time associated with cold sores and genital herpes.

The latest double-blind, placebo-controlled clinical study in Germany found that melissa (also known as lemon balm) creams relieve the most intense pain of herpes inflammation, occurring on the second day of the outbreak. Melissa reduces total recovery time by an average of 1 day. It has a rapid effect on itching, tingling, burning, stabbing, swelling, tightening of the skin, and redness. The mechanism of action of the balm mint extract rules out the development of resistance of the herpesvirus. The German scientists conducting the study note that there is an indication that the intervals between the periods with herpes might be prolonged with mint balm cream treatment.[23]

CONCEPTS FOR COPING WITH HERPES

❍ Ice, applied 10 minutes on, 5 minutes off, relieves burning, itching, and pain prior to recurrent outbreaks.

❍ There is laboratory evidence that omega-3 fatty acids, pyruvate, and vitamin E applied in a topical formula help control outbreaks. These supplements are likely to help when taken orally.

Herpes Simplex
See Cold Sores.

Herpes Zoster
See Shingles.

Hiccups

SYMPTOM SUMMARY

❍ Eruption of air through the mouth from the stomach with a characteristic sound, usually occurring without warning and beyond conscious control

UNDERSTANDING THE DISEASE PROCESS

Hiccups, known in the medical literature as *singultus*, are sharp, unpredictable, recurring contractions of the diaphragm causing a sudden escape of air. Anatomically, a hiccup is the opposite of a belch. In a belch, the muscles of the abdomen are felt contracting in an upward stroke opening the top of the stomach just before the release of gas. In a hiccup, the muscles of the abdomen are felt contracting in a downward stroke closing the bottom of the stomach just after the release of gas. A belch is felt erupting and sometimes can be stopped. A hiccup comes on without warning and usually cannot be stopped.

Since hiccups stop the downward flow of food, some scientists believe they perform the same safety function as vomiting. Hiccups prevent the body from receiving tainted or excessive quantities of food.

The trigger for a hiccup is the stimulation of one of two nerves, either the phrenic nerve, which controls the diaphragm, or the vagus nerve, which connects to the brain and controls respiration, digestion, and the pulse rate. Anything that causes these nerves to be excessively stimulated, such as swallowing air while eating or talking too fast, drinking too much alcohol, smoking or secondhand smoke, eating hot, cold, or spicy foods, or overeating, can cause hiccups.

Hiccups occur in healthy people, but can also be a sign of disease. One research group found that 28 percent of hiccups cause the reflux of gastric acid.[1] Hiccups cause the acid reflux rather than the other way around.[2] Hiccups may also be caused by any respiratory disease that causes irritation of the vagus nerve, such as pneumonia, and by stroke causing injury to the "hiccup center" in the brain. Hiccups are one of many symptoms of pleural effusion of cancers, that is, the spread of cancer to the lungs, or acute pancreatitis. They may be a side effect of treatment with commonly prescribed drugs for epilepsy. And they are a common complication of ear infections or foreign bodies lodged against the eardrum.

TREATMENT SUMMARY

Treatments not requiring assistance:

❍ Hold your breath while bearing down with the abdominal muscles.

❍ Sprinkle a lemon wedge with Angostura bitters. Bite the lemon and swallow the bitters.

❍ Sprinkle a teaspoon of salt into a cup of warm water and drink.

❍ Breathe in and out of a *paper* bag.

❍ Stimulate the soft palate by rubbing it with a finger or cotton swab to the point of gagging for several minutes. Alternatively, stimulate the soft palate by allowing a teaspoon of sugar to dissolve at the base of the tongue or by drinking a glass of ice water.

Treatments requiring the assistance of others:

❍ Expose the hiccups sufferer to a sudden, low-pitched, loud, unexpected sound.

UNDERSTANDING THE HEALING PROCESS

Curing hiccups has been a concern of medicine for thousands of years. A passage in the *Dialogues* of the Greek philosopher Plato records, "When Pausainis came to pause, Aristodemus said that the turn of Aristophanes was next, but either he had eaten too much or from some other cause he had the hiccup, and was obliged to change with Eryximachus, the physician, who was reclining on the couch below him. 'Eryximachus,' he said, 'you ought either to stop my hiccup or to speak in my turn until I am better.' 'I will do both,' said Eryximachus, 'I will speak in your place and do you speak in mine; and while I am speaking, let me recommend that you hold your breath, and if this fails, gargle with a little water; and if the hiccup still continues, tickle your nose with something and sneeze, and if you sneeze once or twice, even the most violent hiccup is sure to go. In the meantime, I will take your turn and you shall take mine.' "

In the twenty-first century, friends continue to help each other control hiccups. Among the more colorful approaches to curing the malady are jumping out of a plane, drinking a glass of water while someone presses the ears closed, counting sheep (and its variation, counting people), tickling the rib cage, kissing, having someone deliver a swift punch to the abdomen (not recommended), swallowing a teaspoon of vinegar and sugar together in one gulp, eating pickled habañero peppers, and smoking marijuana, catnip, and/or fennel (also not recommended). Many traditional remedies for hiccups, however, have a scientific basis and some have even been scientifically tested.

Holding your breath while bearing down on the abdominal muscles opens the stomach slowly and allows gas to escape slowly, circumventing a hiccup. Attempting to imitate a belch will have the same effect.

Angostura bitters are made from the herb gentian, a plant so bitter that 1 part of gentian in 58,000 parts of water has a disagreeably bitter taste. Their intense bitter taste causes a reflex action by the vagus nerve to secrete fluids into the stomach, altering stomach pressure.

Hiccups sometimes result from hyponatremia, low sodium levels caused by a deficiency of salt in the diet. In the United States, low sodium levels are rare, but taking a pinch of salt in a cup of warm water sometimes helps.

Breathing in and out of a paper bag (never use plastic) increases the carbon dioxide (CO_2) content of inhaled air. Receptors in the blood vessels respond to changes in CO_2 levels by increasing the rate of respiration, interrupting the hiccups cycle.

Stimulating the soft palate activates a cranial nerve controlling the glottis, the "gate" through which hiccups pass. Rubbing the soft palate, letting a spoonful of sugar dissolve in the mouth, or drinking cold water shuts the gate.

Sudden, loud sounds are a favorite home remedy for hiccups. Research shows that sounds either of an intensity between 70 and 125 decibels, at least as loud as a lawn mower but not quite as loud as sitting in the front row at a rock concert, or in a low pitch, about 1,000 Hz, are the most likely to break a contraction cycle in the long muscles of the diaphragm that cause hiccups.[3]

Popping a paper bag into which a hiccups sufferer has been breathing in and out interrupts the hiccups cycle in two different ways. The loud, low sound stimulates a new rhythm in the diaphragm, and the sudden movement of air into the lungs resets the vagus nerve.[4]

CONCEPTS FOR COPING WITH HICCUPS

○ Massage of the smooth muscles over the carotid artery, *done by a massage professional,* frequently relieves hiccups. Do not attempt self-massage of the carotid artery, as syncope (fainting) may result.

High Blood Pressure
See **Hypertension.**

High Blood Sugar
See **Diabetes.**

High Cholesterol

SYMPTOM SUMMARY

Defined in terms of LDL cholesterol:

○ 190 mg/dl and fewer than 2 risk factors

○ 160 mg/dl and 2 or more risk factors

○ 130 mg/dl and evidence of heart disease

Risk factors:

○ Age/sex
  - Men older than 45 years
  - Women older than 55 years, or women who have hysterectomy and who are not on estrogen replacement therapy

○ Current cigarette smoking

○ Diabetes mellitus

○ Family history of premature coronary heart disease
  - Father, grandfather, or brother diagnosed before age 55
  - Mother, grandmother, or sister diagnosed before age 65

○ Hypertension—blood pressure greater than or equal to 140/90 mm Hg, or taking drugs for high blood pressure

○ Low HDL-C, below 35 mg/dl (subtract 1 risk factor if HDL-C is greater than 60 mg/dl)

UNDERSTANDING THE DISEASE PROCESS

High cholesterol, or polygenic hypercholesterolemia, is the most common health concern among North Americans over the age of 40. The American Heart Association defines high cholesterol in otherwise healthy people as a total cholesterol over 240 mg/dl or LDL cholesterol over 190 mg/dl. High cholesterol in people with prior evidence of heart disease, smoking, diabetes, or other risk factors is defined at lower levels.

The relationship between cholesterol levels and risk of heart disease is not straightforward. Cholesterol in and of itself is beneficial, rather than harmful, and all kinds of cholesterol are required throughout the body. Cholesterol is extracted from food to form cholymicrons, large globules of cholesterol and proteins to make the cholesterol soluble in the bloodstream. Cholymicrons carry cholesterol from the intestine to the liver, and triglycerides to the muscles for energy. After an extremely high-fat meal, the blood can be literally milky with cholymicrons, but their presence in the bloodstream is short-lived. Cholymicrons in and of themselves do not have a role in hardening of the arteries or heart disease.

The other forms of cholesterol are manufactured by

the liver. The largest particles of cholesterol have the lowest density. Attached to a protein to make it soluble, this cholesterol is known as very-low-density lipoprotein or VLDL. This form of cholesterol is especially important to athletes, as it transports energy stored from carbohydrate loading from the liver to the muscles. As VLDL downloads triglycerides to the muscles and to fat cells, it gradually shrinks down to a heavier cholesterol core of low-density lipoprotein, or LDL.

This form of cholesterol fuels the immune system. Monocytes, the white blood cells that surround and destroy the larger infectious microorganisms, such as bacteria, depend on LDL as their energy source. LDL plays an especially important role in protecting against respiratory infections. Not just the immune system, however, but the entire body requires LDL cholesterol. Cells throughout the body have LDL receptors that "dock" circulating LDL to extract the cholesterol essential to maintaining the cell wall, in effect a raincoat keeping the contents of the cell from dissolving into the bloodstream.

Eventually enough cholesterol has been extracted that the circulating fat is reduced to a small amount of cholesterol and a roughly equal amount of protein. This small and compact form of cholesterol is known as high-density lipoprotein, or HDL. This is the form of cholesterol that prevents hardening of the arteries. Particles of low-density lipoprotein, or LDL, cholesterol are larger and more likely to get caught in the lining of the artery. Particles of high-density lipoprotein, or HDL, are smaller and are less likely to get caught in the lining of the artery.

Simply getting stuck in the lining of an artery does not change cholesterol into an artery-clogging plaque. Only the smallest and oldest of the LDL particles, those most easily seeded with free radicals, are oxidized and initiate hardening of the arteries.[1] Cholesterol particles of varying sizes are normally passed through the linings of the arteries to feed underlying tissues. For cholesterol to form a plaque, it has to be damaged, either by oxygen or by free radicals, before it is eaten with food or after it is produced by the liver. To monocytes, the damaged cholesterol appears to be an infected cell. The damaged cholesterol triggers the release of chemical factors that cause the monocyte to adhere to the lining of the artery and transform itself into a macrophage, a cell that is capable of absorbing dozens of times its normal size in cholesterol and infected tissue. The macrophage, rather than the cholesterol itself, clogs the artery. The more HDL is present near the oxidized LDL, however, the less likely the macrophage is to attach itself and create a plaque.[2]

This complicated process explains why some people with normal cholesterol levels get cardiovascular disease and some people with elevated cholesterol levels do not. Enormous studies involving hundreds of thousands of people are frequently cited as proving the truism that there is no level of LDL cholesterol that should not be lowered, and the evidence does show that taking cholesterol lowering drugs lowers the risk of death. What the evidence does not show is that lowering cholesterol in and of itself lowers the risk of death. The studies show that how high your LDL cholesterol levels are when you begin taking medication predicts your risk of cardiovascular disease. How much you lower them with medication does not.

One such study, the Air Force/Texas Coronary Atherosclerosis Prevention Study (AFCAPS/TexCAPS) followed 6,605 men and women aged 45–73 for 5 years. Taking a standard 20- or 40-milligram-a-day dose of lovastatin (Mevacor) unquestionably lowered the risk of heart disease. People who did not take Mevacor had a 1 in 135 chance of heart attack or stroke in any given year, while people who took Mevacor had a 1 in 145 chance of heart attack or stroke in any given year. More interestingly, this study found that while changes in LDL levels did not predict heart disease, changes in the levels of the carrier proteins for LDL, apoAI and apoB, did.[3]

TREATMENT SUMMARY

DIET

○ Use olive oil in cooking as frequently as possible.

NUTRITIONAL SUPPLEMENTS

○ Vitamin E: 800 IU per day.

HERBS

○ Red yeast rice (Cholestin): as directed on label.

See Part Three if you take prescription medication.

UNDERSTANDING THE HEALING PROCESS

If changes in cholesterol levels cannot tell you whether your risk of heart disease is higher or lower, should you ignore cholesterol? No, but there are other blood tests that are now widely available that can give you and your doctor valuable treatment information. Lower levels of the lipoproteins apoAI and apoB are a good indication of improving cardiovascular health. And the value of cholesterol-lowering medications is not that they lower cholesterol, but that they stop the inflammation that attracts monocytes to the walls of arteries to build cholesterol plaques.

An astonishing range of naturally occurring substances lower cholesterol levels. These include fish oil,[4] flaxseed,[5] garlic,[6] hazelnuts,[7] macadamia nuts,[8] pistachio nuts,[9] oat bran,[10] psyllium powders typically used to treat constipation,[11] soy,[12] stanol ester margarines,[13] and yogurt,[14] among many others. An equally astonishing range of naturally occurring substances slow the oxidation of LDL cholesterol and the progress of atherosclerosis: cranberry extract,[15] the polyphenols in crème de cacao,[16] germanium (a component of computer chips),[17] hibiscus (the herb responsible for the tart taste of Red Zinger tea),[18] lycopene from tomatoes,[19] melatonin,[20] perilla leaf (used in making some kinds of sushi)[21], and even an oyster extract,[22] among many others. There is no reason you should not take any of these products you wish if you have high cholesterol. Only one natural supplement, however, is known both to lower cholesterol levels and reduce risk of cardiovascular disease. It is red yeast rice.

The use of red yeast rice in China was first documented in the Tang Dynasty in A.D. 800. It has been used to make rice wine, and as a food preservative for maintaining the color and taste of fish and meat. The medicinal properties of red yeast rice were described in detail in the ancient Chinese pharmacopoeia, *Ben Cao Gang Mu-Dan Shi Bu Yi,* published during the Ming Dynasty (A.D. 1368–1644).

Red yeast rice (Cholestin) contains a naturally occurring form of lovastatin (Mevacor), a commonly prescribed cholesterol-lowering medication. The first clinical study of red yeast rice was conducted in China. Physicians gave 324 people with high cholesterol (average total cholesterol, 230 mg/dL; average LDL, 130 mg/dl; average HDL, under 40 mg/dl) either red yeast rice or a placebo for 8 weeks. Total cholesterol dropped by 23 percent, LDL cholesterol by 31 percent, and triglycerides by 34 percent. Serum HDL levels increased by 20 percent.[23]

A second study gave 65 adults with high cholesterol either 2.4 grams of red yeast rice daily or a placebo. Participants in this study were asked to follow a diet of 30-percent fat, 10-percent saturated fat with no more than 300 milligrams of cholesterol daily. After 8 weeks, the participants in the study who had been given red yeast rice had an average 18-percent reduction in total cholesterol, 23-percent reduction in LDL cholesterol, and 16-percent reduction in triglycerides. In this study, there were no changes in HDL levels.[24]

Unlike lovastatin (Mevacor), red yeast rice (Cholestin) has never been known to cause serious side effects. Red yeast products have only caused headaches and stomach upset. Some precautions, however, are prudent. Like lovastatin, red yeast should be avoided by women who are or who may become pregnant, by nursing mothers, and by anyone with kidney or liver disease. It should not be taken with antibiotics, cyclosporine (a medication for preventing rejection of transplants), niacin, or protease inhibitors.

If you have been prescribed any of the statin drugs atorvastatin (Lipitor), lovastatin (Mevacor), pravastatin (Pravachol), or simvastatin (Zocor), ask your doctor about using red yeast rice. Treatment with this natural supplement costs significantly less than the prescription drug.

The Mediterranean diet is rich in olive oil. Many studies have found that the Mediterranean diet is associated with significant reductions in the risk of death from complications of atherosclerosis. The Lyon Diet Heart Study compared a diet rich in olive oil with a standard low-fat diet for patients with heart disease. Atherosclerosis patients on the Mediterranean diet showed a 76-percent reduction in angina, pulmonary embolism, heart attack, and stroke after 27 months of the study. This finding was considered so significant that the study was stopped so that all participants could add olive oil to their diets.[25] No clinical study has ever found any other diet to protect more against death from heart attack.[26]

Clinical studies suggest that only a few people who take vitamin E on a regular basis can expect their arteries to clear as a result. However, taking vitamin E may keep atherosclerosis from getting worse.[27] The very latest scientific speculation suggests that vitamin E may be extremely important in *preventing* atherosclerosis, since vitamin E is oxidized before LDL is oxidized, in effect protecting it from the physiological processes that cause the formation of atherosclerotic plaques. Vitamin E is more important in the earlier stages of atherosclerosis than in the later stages of the disease.[28]

Some studies suggest that 100–200 IU of vitamin E

per day may be as effective in treating atherosclerosis as the most widely sold dosage of the vitamin, 400–800 IU. However, since dosages for preventing atherosclerosis have not been determined, 800 IU is better for people who are currently in good health.

CONCEPTS FOR COPING WITH HIGH CHOLESTEROL

○ Any cholesterol reduction program is easier if you lose weight. Losing weight causes fat cells to produce more of a hormone known as adiponectin. As fat cells get smaller, this hormone makes it easier for fatty acids to leave the bloodstream for storage as body fat. While this makes losing weight harder, it makes lowering cholesterol easier.[29]

○ Coenzyme Q_{10} helps the heart operate more effectively when its oxygen supply is limited. This supplement is especially useful for persons who take statin drugs, such as atorvastatin (Lipitor), lovastatin (Mevacor), pravastatin (Pravachol), or simvastatin (Zocor). It is recommended for people who take red yeast (Cholestin), which is also a statin. Statins interfere with the body's ability to produce both coenzyme Q_{10} and cholesterol.

○ Low-fat diets are more likely to lower cholesterol in men than in women.[30] Many people find that reducing dietary cholesterol by eating less meat and fewer eggs does not lower their bloodstream cholesterol levels. Meta-analysis of 27 clinical studies has found that changing consumption of dietary fat only helps people with more than 2 risk factors, and that the total lowering of risk of mortality from *all* causes is only about 2 percent.[31] The greatest danger comes from a diet that is high in both carbohydrates and fat, leading to high levels of VLDL and cholesterol that literally cause the blood to become "cloudy." Non-diabetics can avoid this condition by dietary moderation; diabetics need to keep blood sugars low at all times. See DIABETES.

○ European, especially German, physicians frequently recommend garlic as a means of reducing the risk of atherosclerosis.[32] No fewer than 37 placebo-controlled clinical studies consistently find that using garlic for 1–3 months lowers total cholesterol levels by as much as 25 mg/dl (depending on the preparation of garlic used, 12–25 mg/dl in 3 months). However, no study has found that garlic helps lower cholesterol for as long as 6 months and no study has found that garlic prevents or cures atherosclerosis.[33] What may be much more important, however, is preliminary evidence that garlic stops the oxidation of LDL cholesterol.[34]

○ Hibiscus, a herb found in Red Zinger tea, stops the oxidation of LDL cholesterol. Two of the plant chemicals found in hibiscus are stronger antioxidants than vitamin E.[35]

○ Smokers benefit from taking vitamin C. A study at the University of California at Berkeley found that taking 500 milligrams of vitamin C a day greatly lowered the concentration of bloodstream levels of F(2)-isoprostane levels, an index of oxidant stress. A mixture an antioxidants including alpha-lipoic acid, vitamin E, and vitamin C also lowered levels of this dangerous prooxidant, but not as effectively as vitamin C alone.[36] Since vitamin E is important in fighting other factors influencing atherosclerosis,[37] smokers should take both vitamins C and E.

○ Very preliminary research indicates that transcendental meditation lowers blood pressure and reduces or reverses atherosclerosis. Since transcendental meditators also tend to give up red meat and quit smoking, it is not clear how much improvement in health is due to meditation itself.[38]

○ Untreated gum disease, especially when there are high cholesterol levels, increases the risk of atherosclerosis by 50 to 100 percent.[39]

○ Type 2 diabetics sometimes have the option of controlling their blood sugars with or without insulin. While there are many drawbacks to the use of insulin, insulin therapy tends to open arteries. In as little as 3 months, as much as 25 percent more blood can flow through arteries of type 2 diabetics who have begun insulin treatment.[40] This partially compensates for high cholesterol levels.

○ Taking more 1,000 milligrams of niacin a day, sometimes recommended for high cholesterol, can raise homocysteine levels. For this reason, niacin should not be taken for high cholesterol except under a doctor's supervision.

○ Very high cholesterol, levels of 300–4,000 mg/dl, is *not* helped by statin drugs or by red yeast rice. When cholesterol levels are this high, the main component of cholesterol is VLDL, which is not affected by these medications, although some physicians have found that an extremely low-sodium diet reduces very high cholesterol to levels close to normal in 4–6 weeks.[41] In the absence of sodium restriction, it is essential to lower triglyceride levels. (See HIGH TRIGLYCERIDES.)

O Scientists at the University of Iowa have been able to lower cholesterol levels in healthy volunteers by, of all things, hamburgers. A daily dose of ground beef fortified with 2,700 milligrams of phytosterols was found to lower total cholesterol by an average of 9 percent and LDL cholesterol by an average of 14 percent over a 4-week trial.[42] Hamburgers without the phytosterols do not have the same effect, although soy or tofu burgers do.

High Homocysteine

SYMPTOM SUMMARY

O Blood test measuring homocysteine level over 16 mmol/L

In extreme cases:

O Abdominal pain, nausea, or vomiting after meals

O Canker sores

O Fever without evidence of infection

O Darkened skin on the back of the fingers and toes

O Swollen, red, or shiny tongue

UNDERSTANDING THE DISEASE PROCESS

The amino acid homocysteine is a normal byproduct of the body's metabolism of another amino acid, methionine. When there is not enough folic acid, homocysteine tends to accumulate. Researchers disagree whether high levels of homocysteine cause heart disease in both men and women, but there is general agreement that high homocysteine is a risk factor for cardiovascular disease in women, independent of high cholesterol. At least one study has found that the combination of suppressed anger and high homocysteine levels predicts heart disease, although this effect is marked only in women who are above normal weight.[1] Increased homocysteine levels are a risk factor for the development of many other diseases, including Alzheimer's disease, Crohn's disease, embolism, diabetes, hypothyroidism, miscarriage, osteoporosis, and stroke.

The folic acid deficiency that leads to high homocysteine levels can result from any of a number of causes. Because folates are destroyed by prolonged exposure to heat, people that mostly eat food cooked in kettles of boiling water may be predisposed to folic acid deficiency. Folic acid deficiency is common in heavy drinkers, in people with liver or kidney disease, and in people treated with drugs that fight cancer or arthritis by depriving cells of folic acid, such as methotrexate. Folic acid deficiency can also occur as a result of vitamin B_{12} deficiency, the kidneys forced to eliminate folic acid when there is not enough vitamin B_{12} to prevent accumulation of methylene THFA.

TREATMENT SUMMARY

NUTRITIONAL SUPPLEMENTS

O Folic acid: 400–1,000 micrograms per day.

O Vitamin B_6: 10–50 milligrams per day.

O Vitamin B_{12}: 50–300 micrograms per day.

O Zinc picolinate: 15 milligrams per day.

UNDERSTANDING THE HEALING PROCESS

Since high homocysteine levels are due to a deficiency of the vitamin folic acid, correcting high homocysteine levels is simply a matter of replacing folic acid—along with the other B vitamins needed for its use. Zinc is also supplemented because zinc deficiency keeps the intestine from absorbing B vitamins.

Not every B vitamin lowers homocysteine. Taking more than 1,000 milligrams of niacin a day, sometimes recommended for high cholesterol, can raise homocysteine levels. For this reason, niacin should not be taken for high cholesterol except under a doctor's supervision. Doctors sometimes treat high homocysteine with betaine (trimethylglycine) or choline in very high doses, but this should not be attempted unless treatment with B vitamins is not successful.

CONCEPTS FOR COPING WITH HIGH HOMOCYSTEINE

O Homocysteine levels go up during dieting to lose weight. Taking supplemental folic acid while dieting may not only keep homocysteine levels down but may also increase the percentage of weight lost from fat rather than muscle tissue.[2]

High Triglycerides

SYMPTOM SUMMARY

Blood test indicating:

❍ Borderline high triglycerides: 150–199 mg/dL

❍ High triglycerides: 200–499 mg/dL

❍ Very high triglycerides: 500 mg/dL or higher

UNDERSTANDING THE DISEASE PROCESS

High triglycerides are a common diagnosis in the United States. Triglycerides are energy packets manufactured by the liver and delivered to the muscles by very-low-density lipoprotein (VLDL) cholesterol. Any condition that increases the production of VLDL cholesterol—such as overeating fatty or sugary foods—or decreases the use of triglycerides—such as a sedentary lifestyle—increases triglycerides.

Very high concentrations of triglycerides, in the range of 1,000–2,000 mg/dL or more, require so much cholesterol to carry them that the blood can take on a milky appearance. In a test tube allowed to stand, blood containing extremely large amounts of triglyceride eventually forms a creamy layer on top. Triglyceride levels this high can cause a variety of symptoms: skin outbreaks on the back, buttocks, and chest (caused by accumulation of VLDL cholesterol in the skin), yellow creases on the palms, and liver enlargement caused by fatty liver. Triglyceride levels over 4,000 mg/dL cause accumulation of cholesterol in the blood vessels of the eyes.

Lower levels of triglycerides also cause damage. Digesting high-fat meals releases massive quantities of free radicals in the process of attaching triglycerides to the cholesterol needed to transport them. These free radicals compete with the lining of blood vessels for antioxidants from vitamin E, and the flow of blood through the coronary arteries can be reduced by as much as 20 percent.[1]

As the waistline increases, triglycerides increase, especially in men. Generally speaking, men with a waistline in excess of 36 inches (90 centimeters) tend to have elevated triglycerides.[2] Men with excessive abdominal fat tend to use all of their fat-dissolving enzymes on that fat, and do not have enough enzymes left over to process the triglycerides and cholesterol in high-fat or high-sugar meals.[3] The effect is especially severe when high-fat meals containing over 2,000 calories of energy are consumed.

TREATMENT SUMMARY

NUTRITIONAL SUPPLEMENTS

❍ Fish oil: 10 grams (10,000 milligrams) daily.

❍ Vitamin E: 800 IU per day.

HERBS

❍ Garlic extract tablets: 900 milligrams daily.

See Part Three if you take prescription medication.

UNDERSTANDING THE HEALING PROCESS

If you have been told you have high triglycerides, the most important things you can do are to reduce your consumption of calories—especially from sweets—and to take vitamin E. Antioxidant vitamin E can reverse the shrinkage of coronary arteries caused by free radicals from the metabolism of triglycerides—in less than a day.[4]

Taking 10 grams of fish oil daily can drastically lower your triglyceride levels. Studies with animals suggest that fish oil can be especially helpful for diabetics.[5] Clinical studies confirm that fish oil lowers triglyceride levels in humans.

The omega-3 fatty acids that lower triglyceride levels are found in albacore, mackerel, salmon, and tuna, but it is necessary to eat about 1 pound of fatty fish a day to get enough to have a measurable effect. Most people will find that taking fish oil capsules is less expensive (and less caloric, the required amount of fish oil providing about 100 calories, and the required amount of fish providing at least 750 calories). Cod liver oil is less expensive and has a similar effect on triglyceride levels, but it contains high concentrations of vitamins A and D that can be toxic at levels high enough to lower triglycerides, especially for women. Flaxseed oil does not lower triglycerides.

If you take fish oil, you should also take garlic. In some cases, fish oil supplementation can raise LDL cholesterol levels. Taking garlic counteracts this side effect.

Some people notice bad breath after taking either fish oil or garlic extract. If this occurs, change brands. If you experience diarrhea or burping when first taking fish oil, lower the dosage to 1 capsule a day and increase by 1 capsule every day until you are taking the needed 10 grams.

CONCEPTS FOR COPING WITH HIGH TRIGLYCERIDES

○ High-carbohydrate diets (more than 60 percent of calories from carbohydrates) raise triglyceride levels, even if refined sugars are avoided.[6] It is not necessary to avoid dietary fat completely to lower triglyceride levels, only to eat fats and protein foods in moderation.

○ Reducing the fat content of the diet is a double-edged sword. If fat is reduced in the diet and there is resulting weight loss, especially around the waist, the body can more easily process triglycerides with the enzymes it has. If fat is reduced in the diet without weight loss, the body slows down the production of HDL (desirable) cholesterol to increase the production of VLDL (highly undesirable) cholesterol to transport triglycerides made from dietary sugars.

○ Doctors frequently treat high triglycerides with niacin. This B vitamin is very effective, but the levels of niacin needed to reduce triglyceride levels can cause a variety of undesirable side effects, most notably flushing and headaches. People with rosacea must completely avoid niacin.

○ Several medications can cause severely elevated triglyceride levels. These include estrogen replacement therapy without progesterone, Nolvadex (tamoxifen), Retin-A (tretinoin) for acne, birth control pills with high estrogen content, and high doses of beta-blockers or diuretics for high blood pressure.

HIV and AIDS

SYMPTOM SUMMARY

HIV infection:

○ Flulike symptoms occur in some people a few weeks after contracting the virus, otherwise, no symptoms

Initial symptoms of AIDS:

○ Frequent fevers and sweats

○ Lack of energy

○ Mouth, genital, or anal sores from herpes infections.

○ Persistent or frequent yeast infections

○ Persistent skin rashes or flaky skin

○ Short-term memory loss

○ Weight loss

Symptoms of advanced AIDS:

○ Abdominal cramps, nausea, vomiting

○ Confusion, forgetfulness

○ Cough

○ Difficult or painful swallowing

○ Extreme fatigue

○ Fever

○ Lack of coordination

○ Mental symptoms such as confusion and forgetfulness

○ Nausea, abdominal cramps, and vomiting

○ Persistent, severe diarrhea

○ Seizures

○ Severe headaches with neck stiffness

○ Vision loss

○ Weight loss

○ Coma

UNDERSTANDING THE DISEASE PROCESS

The human immunodeficiency virus, more commonly known as HIV, infects over 1.1 million people in the United States, and tens of millions more worldwide. Although a few people experience flulike symptoms immediately after they are infected with HIV, most people with HIV experience no symptoms until the disease has destroyed the majority of their primary infection-fighting cells, the CD4+ or helper T cells. The destruction to the immune system allows for infections of every organ system, causing a collection of symptoms known as acquired immunodeficiency syndrome, or AIDS. Multiple-drug cocktail therapy appears to greatly extend life, but there is currently no cure for AIDS.

TREATMENT SUMMARY

DIET

O Use supplemental nutrition drinks (such as Boost or Ensure) as often as possible.

NUTRITIONAL SUPPLEMENTS

O L-arginine: 20 grams per day.

O L-glutamine: 14 grams per day.

O L-leucine as HMB: 3 grams per day.

O Magnesium chloride (extended release): 500–600 milligrams daily.

O Melatonin: 20 milligrams, *taken in the evening.*

O Vitamin E: 200 IU per day.

Avoid or use with caution:

O Creatine.

O Ornithine alpha-ketoglutarate.

HERBS

O Cat's claw: tincture, 1 dropperful taken in a cup of water with 1 teaspoon of lemon juice, 2–3 times daily.

See Part Three if you take prescription medication.

UNDERSTANDING THE HEALING PROCESS

The mainstream medical therapy for HIV and AIDS is a drug "cocktail" of up to 30 tablets of up to 10 medications that must be taken in precise dosages, at precise times, and following other precise conditions, daily. Since upward of 200 vitamins, minerals, herbs, and other nutritional supplements have possible or proven supportive value in AIDS, the full range of constructive and destructive interactions between prescription medications and natural treatments is simply too great to describe here. Instead, this entry addresses treatment of the most common correctable cause of death in AIDS, wasting.[1] Treatments listed here are compatible with any program of medication or natural healing.

Far too often, wasting is considered only as an inevitable symptom of the end stages of AIDS rather than as a condition that affects the whole course of AIDS and that can be treated. Diligent attention to loss of appetite and weight in the early stages of AIDS can stop opportunistic infections, prevent suffering, and extend life. If wasting is ignored, however, there is a point of no return. In AIDS patients, death is usually imminent if one-third of body weight has been lost.[2]

Nothing in this book is intended to discourage you from seeking medical intervention to stop your body from wasting away. In AIDS, there are initial reports of good results from the anabolic steroids. Speakers at international AIDS conferences have reported that oxandrolone (Oxandrin) prevents wasting in women who have AIDS. Dr. Marc Hellerstein of the University of California at Berkeley reports that a medically administered combination of oxandrolone, testosterone, and exercise can enable recovery of 2 pounds (1 kilogram) of body mass a week in men in the earlier stages of AIDS. The FDA-approved marijuana derivative dronabinol has been found to increase weight in Alzheimer's patients[3] (although it can cause changes in mental state that are more severe than those induced by marijuana). Growth hormone, a very expensive therapy, can lead to weight gain in the elderly with other conditions.[4] The recommendations here can be used with medical therapies for wasting, or, if medical intervention is not available, in place of them.

High-protein dietary supplement drinks are a mainstay in treating wasting. The advantage of these drinks is that they are easily digested, conserving part of the 5–10 percent of total calories the body burns just to digest food. Various brands tend to be of equal value. However, if ornithine alpha-ketoglutarate (which lowers blood sugars as part of the process of stimulating the growth of muscle) is part of the supplementation plan, it is better to use a formula that prevents hypoglycemia, such as Glucerna.

The amino acid L-arginine stimulates the production of natural killer (NK) cells. In a clinical study of clinically stable men and women with AIDS who had viral loads below 10,000 copies/mL, taking 20 grams of arginine a day for 2 weeks increased the production of NK cells more than 50-fold. In this study, no participant experienced any side effects from the use of arginine.[5] One study found that the combination of arginine, glutamine, and a form of leucine known as beta-hydroxy-beta-methylbutyrate (HMB) helped AIDS patients regain weight at a rate of approximately 3/4 pound (300 grams) a week over an 8-week period.[6]

People who have Kaposi's sarcoma should not take amino acid supplements. Glutamine is the most abundant amino acid in the body. It helps maintain the immune system, it protects the lining of the gastrointestinal system, and it is critical to building healthy tissues. But it is also an essential element for cell division, and the cytokines that cause weight loss in AIDS are triggered by cell division.[7] It is also possible that glutamine supplements could stimulate the growth of Kaposi's sarcoma.

Magnesium is essential to the synthesis of fat, protein, and nucleic acids. Deficiencies of magnesium cause irregular heartbeats, muscle weakness, seizures, and loss of appetite. They may play a role in the production of the cytokines that cause weight loss in AIDS.[8]

The best form of magnesium for people with AIDS is a slow-release formulation of magnesium chloride. Magnesium is the active ingredient in the laxative milk of magnesia, so don't take magnesium supplements if diarrhea is a problem.

There have been reports in the medical literature for a number years that melatonin can prevent wasting. A study of 86 cancer patients in Italy found that giving 20 milligrams of melatonin every evening prevented weight loss without requiring additional consumption of food.[9] The same group of scientists also found that melatonin appeared to slow the process of angiogenesis, the growth of new blood vessels to supply solid tumors.[10] Melatonin may be helpful for AIDS-related cancers.

Melatonin supplements should not be taken by people who have melanoma. People who have seizures should also avoid melatonin. The only other significant precaution in the use of this supplement is that it must be taken in the evening, rather than during the day, to assist nighttime sleep.

Mexican clinics treating as many as 3,000 AIDS patients anecdotally report preventions of cachexia (wasting) after treatment with cat's claw. These results have not been scientifically documented, but recent research confirms that the herb inhibits production of the cytokines IL-6 and TNF-alpha.[11] This may be the mode of its healing action.

Tropical herb expert Leslie Taylor advises using tinctures rather than solid forms for most applications of cat's claw. Active tannins in the tinctures are released in the presence of citric acid, easily provided by lemon juice. If you use a brand of cat's claw made with vinegar, you do not need to add lemon juice. There is one report of an adverse reaction to cat's claw in lupus (although the authenticity of the product as cat's claw was not confirmed). As a precaution, do not use cat's claw in the treatment of cachexia associated with advanced lupus or rheumatoid arthritis.

There are some supplements that should be avoided by people who are experiencing wasting or who have diseases that cause wasting. It would seem logical to treat cachexia with creatine, since it is well known to stimulate muscle growth. In younger persons in the early stages of HIV, creatine supplementation might help. By the time muscle wasting has begun to occur, however, creatine will only add water weight.

Ornithine alpha-ketoglutarate (which is not the same as L-ornithine) stimulates the production of growth hormone by stimulating the production of arginine. One study has found it can stimulate appetite and weight gain in the elderly.[12] Part of its mode of action, however, is the production of insulin. Use of the amino acid can cause hypoglycemia, which is especially dangerous for people who have conditions of intellectual impairment, such as Alzheimer's disease or senile dementia.

CONCEPTS FOR COPING WITH HIV AND AIDS

○ For every 1°C (1.8°F) increase in body temperature, resting calorie consumption goes up 17 percent.[13] Early treatment of fevers is very important in stopping weight loss.

○ Use echinacea to *treat* infections rather than to *prevent* them. Echinacea stimulates immune function, but it also slightly increases production of T cells.[14] These are the immune cells attacked by HIV. When there are more T cells, the virus has more cells to infect. This gives the virus more opportunities to mutate into a drug-resistant form. The authoritative reference work *The Complete German Commission E Monographs* counsels against the use of echinacea for treating colds in people who have HIV or autoimmune diseases such as multiple sclerosis. Later communications between the senior editor of the *Monographs* and the German Food and Drug Administration revealed that the warning in the reference book was based on theoretical speculation rather than practical experience.[15] Still, as a precaution, people with HIV should only use echinacea for *treating* colds rather than preventing them.

○ There are numerous anecdotal reports on marked improvement of AIDS-related diarrhea after taking the South American herb sangre de grado. For more information or to buy the herb, visit www.rain-tree.com.

Hives

SYMPTOM SUMMARY

○ Itching

○ Swelling of the surface of the skin into red or skin-colored welts (wheals) with clearly defined edges

○ Sudden onset

○ Welts change shape, disappear, and reappear within minutes or hours

○ Welts turn white when touched

○ New welts develop when the skin is scratched

○ Welts enlarge, spread, or join together to form large flat, raised areas

More severe cases may be accompanied by:

○ Chills

○ Dizziness

○ Flushing

○ Headaches

○ Loss of consciousness

○ Muscle pain

○ Nausea

○ Racing pulse

○ Shortness of breath

○ Vomiting

○ Wheezing

Angiodema is a condition similar to hives, except the swelling is below the surface of the skin.

UNDERSTANDING THE DISEASE PROCESS

Hives, known in the medical literature as urticaria, are a localized itchy outbreak of the skin. In this essentially allergic reaction, the skin breaks out in bumps surrounded by elongated flares. These "hives" are referred to as wheals or welts. The welts tend to be pink, but they turn white when touched. Welts may coalesce into plaques covering substantial areas of skin.

Hives are intensely itchy. They may involve any area of the body from the scalp to the soles of the feet, and appear in crops of 24- to 72-hour duration. The most common sites for hives are the hands, feet, and face. Angioedema, a swelling below the skin caused by the same allergic mechanism, usually occurs around the eyes and in the lips. While hives usually go away without treatment, angioedema in the upper respiratory tract may be life threatening and requires immediate medical attention.

A survey of college students indicates that about 1 in 5 people has hives at some point in his or her life. Hives may occur at any age, but young adults in their twenties are the most frequently affected.[1] The precise causes of the condition vary from person to person. They are discussed by category below.

Aspirin sensitivity is observed in up to 67 percent of persons who have recurrent outbreaks of hives.[2] Aspirin alters the metabolism of free fatty acids so that it favors the production of leukotrienes. These are hormonal messengers that make the walls of blood vessels more permeable to histamine. Aspirin also makes the lining of the intestines more permeable to allergens, increasing the risk of reaction to common food allergens such as cheese, chocolate, eggs, milk, pineapple, shellfish, and strawberries. At least one study found that taking a single adult aspirin daily for 3 weeks desensitizes the immune system to aspirin and also to foods,[3] but the benefits vanish if aspirin is discontinued.

The newer and considerably more expensive COX-2 inhibitors, such as Celebrex and Vioxx, greatly reduce the risk of allergy. Celebrex induces a sensitivity reaction in 1 in 3 aspirin-sensitive hives sufferers, Vioxx in 1 in 30.[4]

Cholinergic urticaria is a heat reflex in which stimulation of the sweat glands by cholinergic nerve fibers results in pinpoint welts surrounded by reddened skin. The stress causing cholinergic urticaria may be passive overheating, such as in a warm bath or sauna, emotional stress, or physical exercise. The outbreaks in this form of the condition usually arise within 2 to 15 minutes after provocation. They last for up to an hour. The heat reflex may also cause headache, swelling around the eyes, tearing, and, occasionally, gastric upset or asthma.

Cold urticaria is a reaction of the skin to contact with cold air, objects, or water. When cold stimuli provoke hives, the welts are usually restricted to the area of exposure. They develop within a few seconds after the removal of the cold object and rewarming of the skin. The cold reflex is more pronounced during dieting, or when there are also multiple insect bites, parasitic infections, viral infections, or when penicillin is being used.

Cold urticaria is a common symptom of mononucleosis. In myeloma (muscle cancer), the development of a cold reflex reaction may precede the diagnosis of cancer by several years.

Dermographism is the appearance of hives when moderate pressure is applied to the skin. They may occur as a result of contact with watchbands, bracelets, garters, necklaces, bedding, or towels. Dermographic lesions usually start 1–2 minutes after contact and appear at first as redness. The color change is followed 1–3 minutes later by swelling and wheals. Dermographic hives usually resolve within 2–3 hours. This form of hives is most common in persons who are obese. It is frequently seen with diabetes, thyroid disorders, or yeast infections.

The most familiar cause of hives is food allergy. The most frequent offenders are chocolate, eggs, fresh fruit, legumes (especially peanuts), milk, and shellfish.

Two factors increase the risk of outbreaks of hives after eating allergenic foods. One is incomplete digestion. A study published in the 1940s reported that of 77 patients diagnosed with chronic hives, 65 failed to produce enough stomach acid to break down the proteins that cause allergies. Treatment with hydrochloric acid and a vitamin B complex relieved symptoms in most of the patients in the study.[5] Failure to secrete sufficient gastric acid is especially common in persons over the age of 60.[6] In older persons, it may be a major contributing factor in repeated outbreaks of hives after consuming allergenic foods.

Another contributing factor to recurrent food allergies is the permeability of the intestinal wall. This is the reason reactions to food are more severe when they are consumed after taking aspirin.[7] Aspirin irritates the lining, increasing its permeability and easing transport of allergens into the bloodstream. Alcohol, NSAIDs, and many food additives have a similar effect. Consuming any substance that irritates the lining of the digestive tract increases the severity of the food allergy that causes hives.

Food colorings, especially yellow dye #5 (tartrazine), can provoke hives in about 0.1 percent of the population.[8] Tartrazine is added to almost every food and even antihistamines, antibiotics, sedatives, and steroids. This yellow dye modifies fatty-acid metabolism in the same manner as aspirin and increases the susceptibility of the skin to allergic inflammation.

Food flavorings are a major factor in many cases of hives in children. A wide range of salicylic acid esters flavors cake mixes, chewing gum, puddings, and soft drinks. These chemical relatives of aspirin also occur naturally in curry powder, dill, licorice, oregano, paprika, peppermint, prunes, raisins, and turmeric. The average child consumes as much as 200 milligrams of salicylate per day.[9] This dosage approaches the amount of salicylate in children's aspirin. Other flavorings, including aspartame,[10] cinnamon, menthol, and vanilla[11] may produce urticaria in some individuals.

The food preservatives BHA (butylated hydroxyanisol) and BHT (butylated hydroxytoluene) provoke reactions in about 15 percent of individuals who have chronic hives.[12] As many as 44 percent of persons with chronic hives are allergic to benzoates, which occur in relatively high concentrations in fish and shrimp.[13] Sulfites, which are sprayed on fruits, vegetables, and shrimp to keep them fresh in countries outside the United States, aggravate a wide range of allergic conditions, including asthma and hives. Sulfites occur naturally in beer and wine.

About 1 in 10 people is allergic to penicillin, and about 1 in 4 of those allergic to penicillin will develop urticaria, angioedema, or anaphylaxis after taking it.[14] Penicillin is a common additive to livestock feeds. Hives and anaphylactic reactions have been traced to penicillin in frozen dinners,[15] milk,[16] and soft drinks.[17] Among patients with chronic hives *and* an allergy to penicillin, about half will improve on a dairy-free diet.[18]

TREATMENT SUMMARY

NUTRITIONAL SUPPLEMENTS

Taken on an ongoing basis for prevention:

○ Quercetin: 250 milligrams 20 minutes before meals.

○ Vitamin B$_{12}$: 100 micrograms per day.

Other useful treatments (used when hives break out):

○ Simicort or other cream containing glycyrrhetinic acid, cream containing chamomile, or zinc oxide cream, daily. Do not apply zinc oxide creams to "oozing" skin.

UNDERSTANDING THE HEALING PROCESS

The primary treatment of hives consists of avoiding the sources of skin reaction. Control of symptoms can be accomplished through the use of nonsedating histamines, such as astemizole (Hismanal), cetirizine (Zyrtec), and loratadine (Claritin), but at the expense of dry mouth, nose, and throat. The sedating histamines brompheniramine (Dimetapp), chlorpheniramine (Chlor-Trimeton), clemastine (Tavist-1), and diphenhydramine (Benadryl) also control symptoms, but, as their name suggests, induce drowsiness. Reducing the risk of future outbreaks can only be accomplished through nutritional supplementation.

Quercetin was once known as "vitamin P," an essential cofactor for vitamin C. Quercetin stops the biological signals that tell mast cells to release histamine, the inflammatory agent in allergic reactions.[19] It also short-circuits a series of biochemical steps necessary for the formation of leukotrienes, slow-acting agents of allergic inflammation.[20]

Quercetin interacts with a number of medications. It increases the toxicity of the cancer chemotherapy drug Platinol (cisplatin), the antirejection drug cyclosporine (Neoral, Sandimunne) given to transplant patients, and the high blood pressure medication nifedipine (Procardia). It competes for receptor sites and decreases the effectiveness of quinolone antibiotics, which include:

- ciprofloxacin (Cipro, Baycip, Cetraxal, Ciflox, Cifran, Ciplox, Cyprobay, Quintor)
- enoxacin (Penetrex)
- gatifloxacin (Tequin)
- gemifloxacin (a relatively new drug)
- grepafloxacin (Raxar)
- levofloxacin (Levaquin)
- lomefloxacin (Maxaquin)
- moxifloxacin (Avelox)
- norfloxacin (Amicrobin, Anquin, Baccidal, Barazan, Biofloxin, Floxenor, Fulgram, Janacin, Lexinor, Norofin, Noroxin, Norxacin, Orixacin, Oroflox, Urinox, Zoroxin)
- ofloxacin (Floxin)
- sparfloxacin (Zagam)
- temafloxacin (Omniflox)
- trovafloxacin (Trovan)

Vitamin B_{12} is especially useful in protecting against allergies to sulfites. In one study, 2,000 micrograms of vitamin B_{12} taken in a tablet that was allowed to dissolve under the tongue prevented reactions to sulfites in 17 of 18 sulfite-sensitive subjects.[21]

Chamomile, also known by its botanical name *Matricaria,* is widely used in Europe to treat various inflamma-tory skin conditions including hives. When chamomile is treated with hot water, it releases chamazulene, a potent antioxidant that absorbs free radicals needed for an allergic response.[22] Chamazulene also inhibits the formation of inflammatory leukotrienes.[23] The essential oil, which has to be extracted by a different process, stops the release of histamine by mast cells, further blunting any allergic reactions in the skin.[24]

Licorice keeps useful hormones from breaking down. One of the components of licorice, glycyrrhetinic acid, potentiates the effects of hydrocortisone creams by inhibiting the enzyme 11-beta-hydroxysteroid dehydrogenase, which converts hydrocortisone to an inactive form.[25]

Horton's Headache
See **Cluster Headaches**.

Hot Flashes

SYMPTOM SUMMARY

○ Sensation of rushing blood followed several minutes later by sensation of heat

○ Radiates from face to chest and upper body

○ May be accompanied by dizziness, headache, redness in the face, and profuse sweating

UNDERSTANDING THE DISEASE PROCESS

Hot flashes are a common discomfort during the years before menopause, the complete cessation of menstruation. Menstrual cycles shorten and become irregular for 2–7 years prior to entering a true menopausal state. Hot flashes are most common during this time. They also occur in women who enter a surgically induced menopause after removal of their ovaries.

Most women sense a hot flash is coming on several minutes before it actually occurs. The hot flash causes a sudden sensation of heat and warmth starting in the face and spreading to the chest and other parts of the upper body. The heat is wavelike, "flushed" through the body, lasting from several minutes to half an hour. The sensation of heat may be accompanied by headache, dizziness, redness, and profuse sweating. The frequency of hot flashes ranges from 1 or 2 an hour to 1 or 2 a week. They may be triggered by emotional stress, drinking hot liquids or alcoholic beverages, or by exposure to loud noises.

Hot flashes are most common in women between the ages of 40 and 56. They are considerably more common among African-American women than in other racial groups. A survey published in the *Journal of the American Medical Association* reported that, in the United States, 29 percent of white women and 53 percent of African-American women experience hot flashes during menopause.[1]

When hot flashes occur after the cessation of menstruation, it is assumed they are due to menopause. If there is any doubt whether the condition is menopause-related, a blood test for elevated follicle-stimulating hormone (FSH) will confirm that hot flashes are due to change of life. Diabetes, malaria, and diet can cause hot flashes that are easily distinguished from hot flashes during menopause by timing. In diabetes, eating hot peppers can cause sweating and a sensation of heat while eating or immediately after meals. The hot flashes caused by malaria are "tidal," that is they occur at approximately the same time every day, alternating with chills.

TREATMENT SUMMARY

NUTRITIONAL SUPPLEMENTS

❑ Soy isoflavones (daidzein plus genistein): 100 milligrams daily. Up to 400 milligrams per day may be helpful.

HERBS

❑ Black cohosh: 500–1,000 milligrams daily.

UNDERSTANDING THE HEALING PROCESS

The hormonal cause of hot flashes is reduced production of estrogen. There is no doubt that estrogen replacement therapy reduces the frequency and severity of hot flashes as well as insomnia and vaginal dryness during menopause, although it is not as helpful in older women.[2] However, there is also little doubt that estrogen replacement therapy increases a woman's risk of several potentially deadly diseases. The July 17, 2002 edition of the *Journal of the American Medical Association* published the results of a study that followed 16,608 women for an average of 5 years and found

that using estrogen replacement therapy increased the risk of breast cancer by 26 percent, stroke by 41 percent, and pulmonary embolism by more than 100 percent. However, it should be noted that the study also found lower numbers of colon and endometrial cancers that more than offset the increased numbers of cases of breast cancer.[3] Another recent study that followed 44,241 postmenopausal women for approximately 20 years concluded that estrogen use is associated with an increased risk of ovarian cancer. In this study, women who used estrogen alone for 10–19 years were twice as likely to develop ovarian cancer than women who did not use hormones during and after menopause. For women who used estrogen for 20 or more years, the risk of ovarian cancer increased to 3 times that of women who did not use postmenopausal hormones. The risk of ovarian cancer may be elevated for as long as 29 years after a woman quits using estrogen replacement therapy.[4] For these compelling reasons, many women seek alternatives to estrogen therapy.

Scientific research into herbal alternatives for estrogen treatment for hot flashes has produced puzzling findings, most commonly that both the herb and the placebo it was compared against relieved hot flashes equally well. Some researchers have found that women in their studies learned what herb was being tested and went out and bought it for use in addition to the placebo. Nonetheless, there is general agreement that women who have not had breast cancer benefit from the use of soy products and black cohosh, and, more important, that these products do not carry the risks associated with estrogen.

A study of 40 women given 100 milligrams of soy isoflavones daily for 4 months found considerable lowering of total and LDL cholesterol but no effect on HDL cholesterol or triglyceride levels, suggesting that soy does not harm the heart. This dosage of soy isoflavones also significantly relieved hot flashes.[5] (Taking as little as 40 milligrams of isoflavones a day lowered LDL cholesterol levels an average of 18 percent in women taking the supplement for 12 weeks, but did not relieve hot flashes.[6]) A study of 177 women suffering 5 or more hot flashes per day at the Advanced Care Center in New Jersey found that 100 milligrams of a combination of the soy isoflavones daidzein and genistein relieved hot flashes and had no effect on the uterus.[7]

Soy products do not offer relief as quickly as hormone replacement,[8] but the body of clinical research considered as a whole indicates that most women will experice relief from hot flashes by taking 100 milligrams of soy isoflavones (daidzein + genistein) daily. Soy foods are also helpful, but fermented soy foods such as miso and brewed soy sauce (labeled shoyu or tamari, although the latter is technically an inaccurate term) are best.

Black cohosh can be used with or without soy to relieve hot flashes. At least five studies have confirmed that black cohosh relieves symptoms of menopause, one study even finding it more effective than estrogen replacement therapy.[9] Since full effects of the herb are not experienced for up to 6 months, many women begin taking the herb several months before they plan to discontinue hormone replacement therapy.

A few women suffer stomach upset during the first 1–3 weeks of taking black cohosh. If stomach upset is a problem, consider treatment with *kami-shoyo-san,* described below.

CONCEPTS FOR COPING WITH HOT FLASHES

❍ Keep room temperatures low and wear layers of clothing that can be removed if you have a hot flash.

❍ Try deep breathing if a hot flash is coming on.

❍ Avoid spicy foods, especially hot peppers. The capsaicin in hot peppers activates a nerve pathway that causes profuse sweating from the face.

❍ Treating constipation with fiber may reduce hot flashes. A study in Finland found that taking 15 grams (3 heaping tablespoons) of fiber in the form of guar gum reduced both hot flashes and total cholesterol over a period of 3 months.[10]

❍ Treatment of hot flashes in women who have had breast cancer is problematic. Estrogen-sequestering drugs such as tamoxifen (Nolvadex) greatly increase the symptoms of menopause. Black cohosh,[11] soy beverages, and soy protein powders do not reliably help,[12] but soy isoflavones and fermented soy foods may be useful. Doctors in Japan often offer women experiencing side effects of Nolvadex a standardized herbal treatment called *kami-shoyo-san,* a combination of angelica, bupleurum, Cornelian cherry, ginger, licorice, mint, moutan, peony, poria mushroom, and white atractylodis root. A study of 13 women experiencing drug-induced meno-

pause at the Osaka City University Medical School in Japan found that all 13 obtained relief of hot flashes, insomnia, and mood swings when given this formula or a very similar combination of herbs. Augmented Rambling Powder (*kami-shoyo-san*) does not raise estrogen levels and does not diminish the effectiveness of Nolvadex against cancer.[13] In the United States and Canada, *kami-shoyo-san* is available under the following trade names:

- Bupleurum & Peony Formula (Lotus Classics, Qualiherb, Sun Ten)
- Free and Easy Wanderer Plus (Golden Flower)
- Jia Wei Xiao Yao San (Lotus Classics, Qualiherb, Sun Ten)
- Kami-shoyo-san (Tsumura)
- Kampo4WomenMindEase (Honso)

❍ The Oriental herb dong quai is popular in the treatment of menopausal symptoms. It contains a chemical that can stop the production of free radicals that cause a vein to dilate and "flush" just before a hot flash.[14] A clinical study at the Kaiser Permanente centers in California failed to find benefits from taking the herb for hot flashes, but this preliminary study focused on women with the highest levels of estrogen in their bodies.[15]

❍ Ginseng enhances energy, vitality, and sense of well-being—but does not relieve hot flashes.

❍ Clinical study of magnet therapy for menopausal symptoms in women treated for breast cancer has yielded puzzling results. Researchers at the School of Nursing at Vanderbilt University studying the use of magnets at six acupuncture points for relieving hot flashes found that placebo (fake) magnets were more effective than real magnets, but both real and fake magnets relieved symptoms.[16]

❍ If you choose to take hormone replacement therapy despite the risks, consider adding soy and black cohosh to your treatment program. A study by the University of California at San Francisco found that women using combination therapy reported greater improvement in vaginal dryness, libido, and mood than those using HRT alone.[17]

Housemaid's Knee
See **Knee Pain.**

Human Bites

SYMPTOM SUMMARY

○ Skin break with no bleeding, *or*

○ Puncture wound, *or*

○ Crushing injury

UNDERSTANDING THE DISEASE PROCESS

A human bite is a wound to flesh caught between the teeth of the upper jaw and the teeth of the lower jaw of a human. Human bites may be caused by an actual bite or by glancing some part of the body, such as the knuckles, against the teeth. Human bites frequently cause puncture wounds, which present a high risk of infection.

TREATMENT SUMMARY

Nutritional supplements and herbs do not substitute for first-aid care, described below.

NUTRITIONAL SUPPLEMENTS

○ Vitamin C: 1,000 milligrams daily.

HERBS

○ Aloe: apply to wounds daily until healed.

○ Forskolin (a standardized extract of coleus): 5–10 milligrams 3 times daily.

○ Gotu kola (*Centella asiatica*): 60–120 milligrams of asiaticides daily. Should not be used by women who are trying to become pregnant.

○ Sangre de grado: apply to the skin immediately after injury to form a protective crust (sometimes called a "second skin") and prevent infection.

FIRST AID FOR HUMAN BITES

○ Before treating the bite, wash your hands thoroughly with soap and water.

○ If the bite is not bleeding, wash it with running water for 3–5 minutes and then cover lightly with a clean dressing.

○ If the bite is bleeding actively, control the bleeding with direct pressure with a clean, dry cloth or by elevating the area of the bite to a level above the heart.

○ Never put a wound from a human bite in your own mouth.

○ To avoid being bitten, never put your hand near or in the mouth of someone who is having a seizure.

○ People who have diabetes or other conditions causing circulatory problems should consult a physician after any bite, even if it seems minor.

UNDERSTANDING THE HEALING PROCESS

The human mouth usually contains more infectious bacteria than an animal mouth. For this reason, attention from a healthcare practitioner after receiving a human bite is important. In addition to bacteria that cause infection, there is a risk of injury to tendons or joints when the bite extends below the skin.

Vitamin C accelerates healing. The latest research on the use of vitamin C in the treatment of wounds has found that it keeps the basal layers of skin from contracting when the upper layers are injured. This allows regrowth of skin with a minimum of scarring.[1] A series of laboratory experiments found that supplementation with relatively high dosages of vitamin C increases the strength of skin growing over the wound and accelerates closure.[2]

Aloe is anti-inflammatory, moisturizing, and emollient. It contains a number of antioxidant compounds promoting skin growth, including vitamins C and E and zinc. Unlike hydrocortisone creams used to relieve inflammation, aloe encourages skin healing while relieving pain. Wounds treated with aloe vera gel heal as much as 3 days faster than burns and cuts treated with unmedicated dressings or with chemical antiseptic gels.[3]

Forskolin stops a chemical signaling system by which inflammatory hormones shut down fibroblasts, the cells that generate the extracellular connective tissue matrix.[4] Keeping fibroblasts at the site of the wound encourages the production of collagen and connective tissues across the region of damaged skin.

Gotu kola helps to prevent scarring. Keloids and hypertrophic scars, such as those caused by surgery, result from an extended period of inflammation which may go on for months or years without resolution. During this inflammatory phase, large numbers of swollen bundles of collagen are intermingled with cellular debris. This stage continues until sufficient numbers of fibroblasts are recruited in the wound to create well-defined collagen fibers. A clinical study found that 22 out of 27 patients' scars resolved after several months of using gotu kola.[5] The unprocessed resin of sangre de grado stimulates the production of collagen in wounds. This accelerates the formation of a protective crust over the wound.[6]

Human Immunodeficiency Virus

See **HIV and AIDS**.

Huntington's Disease

SYMPTOM SUMMARY

- Behavioral changes:
  - Antisocial attitudes
  - Hallucinations, paranoia
  - Mood swings, irritability
  - Restlessness
- Unusual facial movements, grimaces
- Need to turn head to shift gaze
- Unsteady gait
- Progressive development of choreiform movements—may be slow and uncontrolled, or sudden, jerky movements of the arms, face, legs, or trunk
- Progressive dementia
  - Disorientation or confusion
  - Loss of intellectual skills such as spelling or math
  - Loss of judgment
  - Loss of memory
  - Unusual speech patterns
- Anxiety
- Difficulty swallowing

UNDERSTANDING THE DISEASE PROCESS

Huntington's disease (HD), results from genetically programmed degeneration of brain cells, called neurons, in certain areas of the brain. This degeneration causes uncontrolled movements, loss of intellectual faculties, and emotional disturbance. Huntington's disease was once known as Huntington's *chorea,* referring to choreiform movements, such as jerking movements of the arms, face, legs, or trunk.

HD is a familial disease. It is passed from parent to child through a mutation in the normal gene. Each child of an HD parent has a 50–50 chance of inheriting the HD gene. If a child does not inherit the HD gene, he or she will not develop the disease and cannot pass it to subsequent generations. A person who inherits the HD gene will sooner or later develop the disease. Whether one child inherits the gene has no bearing on whether others will or will not inherit the gene.

Some early symptoms of HD are mood swings, depression, irritability or trouble driving, learning new things, remembering a fact, or making a decision. As the disease progresses, concentration on intellectual tasks becomes increasingly difficult. The patient may have difficulty feeding himself or herself and swallowing. The rate of disease progression and the age of onset vary from person to person.

TREATMENT SUMMARY

DIET

- Avoid dietary sources of glutamate, including red meats, cheeses, and pureed tomatoes.

- Eliminate aspartame, hydrolyzed vegetable protein, and MSG from your diet.

NUTRITIONAL SUPPLEMENTS

- Coenzyme Q_{10}: 30 milligrams per day.

- Melatonin: 1 milligram daily, taken 2 hours before bedtime.

- Vitamin C: 5,000 milligrams daily taken in 4 doses (2,000 milligrams before breakfast, 1,000 milligrams before lunch and dinner, and at bedtime). Lower the dosage if stomach upset occurs.

- Vitamin E: 800 IU daily.

UNDERSTANDING THE HEALING PROCESS

The scientific understanding of the nutritional therapy of HD is in its very early stages. Recently, British researchers discovered an important part of the mechanism through which HD destroys brain tissues. Molecules of the huntingtin protein, a compound that ordinarily functions harmlessly in the cytoplasm, is damaged by free radicals so that it clumps and migrates to the nucleus of the cell, crippling its DNA. The "gates" releasing the free radicals that do this damage are activated by glutamate, a salt of the amino acid glutamine.[1] This discovery suggests that controlling either free radicals or glutamate might slow down the disease process. Research is very preliminary and effective dosages have not yet been established, but there is at least a chance that dietary restrictions and antioxidant supplements will help HD sufferers in the early stages of the disease.

Since the damage in HD is unleashed by the action of glutamate, eliminating glutamate from the diet should be the top priority of nutritional care. Monosodium glutamate, or MSG, should be completely eliminated from the diet. Hydrolyzed vegetable protein, a brown powder used to enhance the flavor of prepared soups and sauces is another source of concentrated glutamate that must be eliminated from the diet. Red meats, cheese, and pureed tomatoes are likewise concentrated sources of glutamate and should be avoided. The glutamate in whole tomatoes is bound in a way that it takes longer to digest and never reaches nerve tissue unless tomatoes are eaten in massive quantities.

It is also important to avoid aspartame (NutraSweet). Aspartame contains aspartate, which acts on nerve tissue in the same way as glutamate. Even though the amount of aspartate absorbed by the brain from a single soft drink is very small, its effects are cumulative, so NutraSweet must be eliminated from the diet.[2]

Physicians at Harvard Medical School treated a small number of HD patients with coenzyme Q_{10}. They found that the supplement increased the availability of oxygen in brain tissue.[3] The immediate goal of their research was to expand the basic understanding of the disease rather than to find nutritional treatments, so no conclusions on dosing or likely effects can be drawn from their study. However, CoQ_{10} is likely to be helpful in HD.

Preliminary research into the use of melatonin in HD has been conducted at the University of Texas Health Center in San Antonio. Melatonin crosses the blood-brain barrier easily into the brain, and is known to protect nerve tissue from free-radical damage. Melatonin stimulates a variety of antioxidant enzymes including superoxide dismutase, glutathione peroxidase, and glutathione reductase. Since superoxide dismutase production is defective in about 10 percent of people who have HD, melatonin may help compensate for the deficient enzyme.[4] Research at the Max-Planck Institute in Berlin has failed to find that melatonin "untangles" damaged nerve cells,[5] but it is possible that it is beneficial in the early stages of the disease. Melatonin is very unlikely to have a detrimental effect on HD. Clinical studies of the use of melatonin in treating HD, however, have not been conducted, and the dosage recommended here is merely a "best guess."

Vitamin C is an important cofactor for vitamin E, making it more available and increasing its concentrations in the bloodstream. Vitamin E, in turn, may be helpful in the early stages of HD. Scientists at the John's Hopkins University School of Medicine conducted a clinical trial in which 73 HD patients were given either vitamin E or a placebo. Vitamin E treatment had no statistically significant effects overall, but the authors noted that it may slow the progression of symptoms if taken in the early stages of the disease.[6]

CONCEPTS FOR COPING WITH HUNTINGTON'S DISEASE

O A genetic test, coupled with a complete medical history and neurological and laboratory tests, help physicians diagnose HD. Presymptomatic testing is available for individuals who are at risk for carrying the HD gene. In 1 to 3 percent of individuals with HD, no family history of HD can be found.

Hyperactivity
See **ADD/ADHD.**

Hypercholesterolemia
See **High Cholesterol.**

Hyperemesis Gravidarum
See **Morning Sickness.**

Hyperhomocysteinemia
See **High Homocysteine.**

Hyperlipidemia
See **High Cholesterol; High Triglycerides.**

Hypertension

SYMPTOM SUMMARY

- Headache
- Anxiety
- Blurred vision
- Chest pain beneath the breastbone
- Confusion
- Either pale skin or redness in the face and neck
- Fatigue
- Muscle twitches and tremors
- Nausea and vomiting
- Nosebleed
- Sensation of heartbeat
- Sweating
- Tinnitus (ringing or buzzing in the ears)
- Often causes no symptoms

Diagnostic Summary:

- Borderline high blood pressure: 120–160/90–94
- Mild high blood pressure: 140–160/95–104
- Moderate high blood pressure: 140–180/105–114
- Severe high blood pressure: 160+/115+

UNDERSTANDING THE DISEASE PROCESS

For most of us, our first experience with chronic illness is high blood pressure. Hypertension does not respect healthy lifestyles. Even people who maintain normal weight, exercise regularly, maintain healthy cholesterol levels, and eat a heart-healthy diet can be, and frequently are, diagnosed with the condition. Nine out of 10 Americans will develop hypertension by the age of 60, and 6 out of 10 eventually take high blood pressure medication.[1]

If blood pressure readings are consistently higher than 160/110, doctors usually insist on prescription medication. But when blood pressure is between 120 and 160 systolic (the pressure generated when the heartbeats) or between 80 and 94 diastolic (the pressure when the heart is at rest), the diagnosis is "borderline hypertension." This condition of slightly elevated blood pressure can be treated with medication just to lower the numbers, or it can be treated with nutrition to correct its underlying causes.

Borderline hypertension is usually "essential" or "primary," meaning it is not associated with an abnormality in a specific organ. Until a few years ago, the causes of essential hypertension eluded medical science, but recent research has revealed that this nearly universal health problem begins as with cholesterol—but not high cholesterol.

The human body produces two principal forms of cholesterol: bulky, low-density particles of cholesterol known as low-density lipoprotein, or LDL; and compact, high-density particles of cholesterol known as high-density lipoprotein, or HDL. LDL cholesterol is typically termed "bad" and HDL cholesterol is typically termed "good," but actually both forms are necessary for the body. The larger LDL particles serve as a food for some of the body's largest cells, the immune system's macrophages, the cells that surround and engulf foreign bodies and microorganisms (as well as LDL cholesterol itself). The smaller HDL cholesterol particles are used by every cell in the body to make their protective linings, serving as a "rain slicker" keeping their contents from dissolving in the watery bloodstream.

Under conditions of stress or poor nutrition, the larger surface of LDL is particularly vulnerable to attack by free radicals of oxygen. Without adequate levels of antioxidant free-radical quenchers such as vitamin E, LDL cholesterol combines with oxygen to form lyso-phosphatidylcholine, better known by its acronym LPC. This chemical, the primary component of artery-hardening oxycholesterol, thickens artery walls and encourages inflammation.

In people with normal blood pressure, oxycholesterol does not get a chance to damage arteries. A balanced immune system produces antibodies to LPC that keep it from accumulating in the linings of blood vessels. Antibodies to LPC perform the immune system's equivalent of a surgical strike, dissolving the oxidized cholesterol before it can form artery-clogging plaques. In people with borderline high blood pressure, however, the immune system fails to produce the antibodies that clean up LPC. Their immune systems are forced to use the immune system's equivalent of a battering ram, the macrophages. These "cholesterol gobblers" surround and engulf LPC but become stuck in the intima, the inner lining of the artery wall. The intima slowly thickens and squeezes the artery so that blood pressure slowly increases. It is important to understand that the immune deficiencies that cause borderline high blood pressure do not affect the immune system as a whole. Only the antibodies to oxidized cholesterol are out of balance.

TREATMENT SUMMARY

NUTRITIONAL SUPPLEMENTS

○ Sesamin: six 500-milligram sesamin capsules, or 3 tablespoons of sesame oil a day. If you cannot find sesamin or sesame, also helpful are blackcurrant, evening primrose, flaxseed (linseed), and/or pumpkinseed oils.

○ Fish oil: at least 3, but no more than 5, grams per day.

○ Vitamin E: 1,200 IU per day.

○ Vitamin C: 2,000 milligrams per day.

○ Folic acid: 10 milligrams per day.

○ L-arginine: at least 3, and up to 21, grams daily.

UNDERSTANDING THE HEALING PROCESS

Fortunately, it is possible to rebalance the immune system so that LDL does not accumulate as LPC. The surprising solution to the problem of oxidized cholesterol is fat, the essential fatty acids found in purified natural oils, such as sesamin in sesame oil and docosahexaenoic acid (DHA) found in fish oil. One of the newest additions to the supplement shelf, sesamin, stops the oxidation of LDL into the artery-clogging LPC. It also slows the production of the arterial inflammatory arachidonic acid,[2] a fat made in abundance from greasy foods and sugars. Sesamin also activates an enzyme that breaks down LPC into its harmless unsaturated form. Sesamin extracts are not yet widely available in the United States, but sesamin is found in sesame oil.

In general, sesamin acts on the same metabolic pathways as the better-known DHA. Fish oils containing DHA are a gentle way to lower blood pressure. A clinical study at the University of Florence in Italy studied men with borderline high blood pressure who took a little more than 3 grams of fish oil a day for 2 months. This DHA-rich supplement lowered systolic blood pressures by an average of 5 mm/Hg and diastolic pressures by an average of 6 mm/Hg. The benefits of taking fish oil

peaked at 4 months and slowly declined when the supplement was discontinued.[3]

While sesame and fish oils act in a similar way, many people will prefer sesame. The advantage of sesame is that it is vegetarian. Derived from the bottom of the food chain, sesame is far less likely to contain pesticides and environmental contaminants, even though modern manufacturing processes have greatly reduced the risk of toxic contamination of fish oil. Sesame also does not cause fish oil's occasional but highly objectionable side effects, diarrhea and fishy-smelling burps. Both sesamin and DHA from fish oil, however, are highly useful in stopping the progress of borderline hypertension.

Fish oil is especially helpful for people who also have diabetes, although the full effect of the supplement in diabetes does not occur until it has been taken for at least 6 months.[4] Taking more than 5 grams a day of either oil, moreover, may hurt more than it helps, providing a different fat for free radicals to attack, unless there is also regular supplementation with antioxidants such as vitamins C and E.[5]

Antioxidant deficiencies are a key cause of borderline high blood pressure, and antioxidant supplements lower borderline high blood pressure. In people with normal blood pressure or borderline high blood pressure, taking 1,200 IU of vitamin E every day for 2 months reduces the "stickiness" of macrophages on the lining of arteries.[6] This prevents macrophages from burrowing into the intima and causing hardening of the arteries resulting in elevation in blood pressure. Taking 2,000 milligrams of vitamin C for just 10 days has the same effect,[7] and taking the same dose of vitamin C for 4 weeks also relaxes arteries and lowers blood pressure.[8] Recent large-scale research has found that people who consume the least vitamin C have the highest blood pressures, and vice versa.[9]

In treating high blood pressure, it is important to take enough vitamin C and enough vitamin E. Some studies have found no benefit from taking only 400 IU of vitamin E[10] or only 1,000 milligrams of vitamin C a day (in the case of smokers).[11] It is also important to be sure to take *both* vitamins every day. Studies at the Northern Ireland Centre for Diet and Health have found that taking vitamin C increases the amount of available vitamin E in the bloodstream by about 10 percent. Taking vitamin E increases the amount of available vitamin C in the bloodstream by about 60 percent.[12]

Another important supplement for heart health in

general is folic acid. This B vitamin is very well known for its ability to lower bloodstream concentrations of homocysteine, an important risk factor in heart disease. It is less well known for its ability to enable blood vessels to stay flexible and keep blood pressure down after fatty meals.[13] For this benefit, most people need to take at least 10 milligrams of folic acid daily for at least 2 weeks, although people with especially high cholesterol levels may notice improvement in blood pressure while taking just 5 milligrams of folic acid a day.[14]

The amino acid L-arginine is also very useful in lowering blood pressure. Survey studies have found that women who consume more protein (about 25 percent of their total calories), and therefore more L-arginine, are significantly less likely to develop coronary heart disease.[15] High doses of supplemental L-arginine can produce dramatic increases in arterial blood flow. A clinical trial involving participants with high cholesterol levels found that taking 21 grams of L-arginine a day for 4 weeks increased blood flow by 3.9 percent.[16] Another clinical trial involving participants with confirmed coronary disease found that taking 21 grams of L-arginine a day for 4 weeks increased arterial blood flow by 4.7 percent.[17] These percentages sound like small improvements, but they correspond to a 6- to 8-point drop in blood pressure without side effects, comparable to a low dose of most prescription blood pressure medications.

Relatively high doses of L-arginine are best. Studies have found that taking as little as 3 grams of L-arginine daily can help, but results may take 6 months.[18] You should not take L-arginine if you have herpes.

These measures are usually curative in borderline high blood pressure, but they are only helpful in more severe cases. If you have blood pressure high enough that you have to take medication, see Concepts for Coping with Hypertension for additional information.

CONCEPTS FOR COPING WITH HYPERTENSION (BORDERLINE, MILD, MODERATE, AND SEVERE)

○ Allow time for supplements to work. Any prescription medication your doctor offers you will take several weeks to begin to work. The same is true of nutritional supplementation. If you have borderline hypertension, ask your doctor for time to make your supplement program work.

○ Take your blood pressure at least once a week, preferably at the same time of day and with the same monitor.

○ When only systolic (upper number) pressures are elevated, CoQ_{10} may be very helpful. A study by the Veterans Health Administration found that men with isolated systolic hypertension who took 60 milligrams of CoQ_{10} daily for 3 months had decreases in systolic pressure of 8–25 points without decreases in diastolic (lower number) pressures.[19] The advantage of CoQ_{10} over other treatments is that it avoids the complication of orthostatic hypotension, feeling faint (or actually passing out) when moving from a seated to a standing position, as could be caused by drugs that lower both systolic and diastolic pressures.

○ Drinking caffeinated coffee tends to lower diastolic pressures (the bottom number). Blood pressure elevation after drinking coffee is greatest 1 hour after consumption. The long-term effect on blood pressure of drinking 1 cup of caffeinated coffee a day is very small—considerably less than 1 mm/Hg—but drinking 5 or more cups of coffee a day increases the lifetime risk of developing high blood pressure.[20] One study found that people over 70 who drink 5 or more cups of regular coffee a day had their blood pressure lowered by 4/3 mm/Hg after 1 day of drinking decaf.[21]

○ Aromatherapy with ylang-ylang is widely reported to lower blood pressure.

○ Herbs used to treat high blood pressure tend to treat symptoms rather the underlying disease, but they can be very useful adjuncts to vitamin and essential fatty acid supplementation. Among the more helpful herbs are:

• Coleus, usually found as forskolin extract, lowers blood pressure while strengthening the heartbeat and lowering the pulse rate.

• Dong quai, usually used to treat complaints of menopause, increases the resting period between heartbeats and lowers blood pressure.

• Hawthorn increases circulation but typically lowers blood pressure.

• Oligomeric proanthocyanidins (OPCs), such as grape seed and pine bark extracts, protect against tissue damage caused by high blood pressure, especially in diabetics.

○ The natural sweetener stevia has been shown to lower blood pressure in laboratory experiments with animals.[22] Stevia also lowers blood sugars.

❍ Avoid table salt and salty foods, but also eat more fruits and vegetables. Sodium restriction alone is a very effective means of lowering blood pressure—provided salt and hidden sodium are almost completely eliminated from the diet. This means not only avoiding visible salt and salty foods, but even avoiding seemingly safe foods such as carrots, beets, celery, bread, and egg whites. Very few people can follow a truly sodium-restricted diet. An intermediate approach, however, was proven effective by the Dietary Approaches to Stop Hypertension (DASH) trial, a clinical study focusing on the special needs of women and African-Americans. The DASH trials found that slightly limiting salt consumption (by eliminating the use of table salt and by avoiding salty foods such as luncheon meats and pickles) combined with eating more fruits, vegetables, and low-fat dairy products lowered blood pressures an average of 11/5 mm/Hg in about 2 weeks.[23]

❍ No single food is a cure for hypertension, although some foods eaten in moderation are helpful. There is purely anecdotal evidence, for instance, that eating a substantial serving of celery (1/4 pound, or about 110 grams) every day begins to lower blood pressure after about a week. The effect in the single documented case was substantial, from an unhealthy 158/96 to a healthy 118/82 in just 7 days.[24] However, there are problems in using celery alone as a blood pressure treatment. No one knows if the effect wears off or becomes greater the more celery you eat. Celery contains furanocoumarins that cause the same side effect as prescription ACE inhibitors: sensitivity to sun and sunburn. People who take ACE inhibitors such as lisinopril (Prinivil, Zestril) for high blood pressure should avoid eating more than an ounce (30 grams) of celery a day.

❍ Garlic and onions are also helpful in lowering blood pressure. If you are concerned about bad breath, consider taking a garlic supplement such as Kwai. Recent research has found that taking 600 milligrams of Kwai garlic extract daily lowered systolic blood pressures (the upper number) 8–11 mm/Hg and diastolic blood pressures an average of 6 mm/Hg. More is not better—taking more than 600 milligrams of Kwai daily did not lower blood pressures further.[25]

❍ In addition to other measures, homeopathy may be useful in borderline hypertension. Your best measure of the effectiveness of any homeopathic remedy for hypertension is whether it makes you feel better; if it does, continue using it. Homeopathy is not an acceptable substitute for other treatments (natural or prescription) for this condition.

❍ Argentum nitricum is a remedy for "stage fright" or anticipatory stress causing high blood pressure and other symptoms. It also relieves diarrhea, dizziness, headache, and racing pulse. Those who benefit most from this remedy are people who have strong cravings for sugar and salt.

❍ Aurum metallicum is a treatment for high blood pressure associated with ongoing stress, especially in people who relieve stress with alcohol. An important indication for this preparation is symptoms becoming worse at night.

❍ Belladonna is the homeopathic remedy for symptoms caused by overdoses of the herb belladonna, redness in the face and neck, dilated pupils, throbbing headache, sensation of racing pulse so strong it can be felt not just in the heart but throughout the body. Another indication for this treatment is cold hands and feet.

❍ Calcarea carbonica relieves high blood pressure in people who tend to get cold and clammy. They are easily tired by exertion, but can also have a racing pulse when lying down. People who benefit from calcarea carbonic tend to like sweets and to have problems with weight control.

❍ Glonoinum is the homeopathic remedy for "being out of it," in addition to a pounding heartbeat, especially in hot weather or after drinking alcohol or taking drugs.

❍ Lachesis treats logorrhea, a tendency to spew out words while experiencing constriction in the chest. People who benefit from lachesis may become "purple" or "blue" with rage. Symptoms treated by this remedy are typically worse after sleeping.

❍ Natrum muriaticum treats high blood pressure in people who keep their emotions inside. A craving for salt and symptoms that get worse as the day progresses are other indications for this remedy.

❍ Nux vomica relieves high blood pressure in people who take offense easily. Constipation and hemorrhoids are also common in the personality type treated by this remedy, as are sugar cravings and a tendency to drink a lot of coffee.

❍ Phosphorus treats high blood pressure in people who tend to get "spacey" with redness in the face, nosebleed, or dizziness. Craving cold drinks and improvement after sleeping or eating are other indications for this remedy.

○ Plumbum, the homeopathic remedy made from minute amounts of lead, treats the symptoms caused by lead: degeneration of the nerves, hardening of the arteries, tics, twitches, and paralysis. Homeopaths also recommend plumbum for people who develop high blood pressure while "living in the fast lane," and then become fatigued or depressed when symptoms develop.

○ Sanguinaria treats high blood pressure occurring with "red" symptoms: red cheeks, red neck, heartburn, reddened skin from allergies, burning pains of the skin, sunburn, and migraine. Symptoms are usually worse on the right side of the body.

Hypertriglyceridemia

See **High Triglycerides**.

Hypochlorhydria

SYMPTOM SUMMARY

○ "Acne" consisting of dilated blood vessels in the face

○ Belching

○ Chronic intestinal parasites

○ Constipation, diarrhea, or indigestion

○ Cracked, peeling, or weak fingernails

○ Iron deficiency

○ Itching around the anus

○ Multiple food allergies

○ Sense of fullness after eating

○ Undigested food in stool

○ Yeast infections

UNDERSTANDING THE DISEASE PROCESS

In hypochlorhydria the stomach produces insufficient gastric acid. Although much more is written about conditions of excess stomach acid, deficient stomach acid also produces symptoms. In addition to the indications listed above, hypochlorhydria is a contributing factor in Addison's disease, asthma, celiac disease, dermatitis herpetiformis, diabetes, eczema, gallbladder disease, hepatitis, hives, hyperthyroidism, hypothyroidism, lupus, myasthenia gravis, osteoporosis, pernicious anemia, psoriasis, rheumatoid arthritis, rosacea, Sjögren's syndrome, and vitiligo.

The ability of the stomach to secrete gastric acid declines with age. It is also diminished by infection with *Helicobacter pylori,* the bacterium best known as the causative agent of peptic ulcers. Most people who are infected with *H. pylori* do not develop ulcers, but they may develop low-grade symptoms misidentified with other conditions. Low gastric acid production allows the bacterium to survive in the lining of the stomach. As it multiplies in the stomach, the production of stomach acid is further reduced, increasing opportunities for the growth of the bacterium. Ulceration may not occur, but subtle nutritional deficiencies resulting from insufficient acid to digest food cause a wide range of seemingly unrelated symptoms.

Doctors can diagnose hypochlorhydria with a test known as the Heidelberg gastric analysis, in which the patient is fitted with a waistband receiver to measure pH signals sent by telemetry in a capsule swallowed after drinking baking soda. A simpler diagnostic tool, however, is to try the remedies listed below and see if symptoms improve.

TREATMENT SUMMARY

NUTRITIONAL SUPPLEMENTS

○ Vitamin C: 500–1,000 milligrams 3 times a day.

○ Vitamin E: 400 IU daily.

HERBS

○ Deglycyrrhizinated licorice (DGL): 200–400 milligrams 3 times a day.

UNDERSTANDING THE HEALING PROCESS

Low levels of the antioxidant vitamins C and E encourage the colonization of the lining of the stomach by *H. pylori*.[1,2] They decrease the risk of ulcer formation, since the mechanism through which *H. pylori* damages the gastric mucous membrane is oxidation. They also protect the DNA of stomach cells, reducing the risk of stomach cancer.[3]

Deglycyrrhizinated licorice (DGL) contains flavonoid compounds that inhibit the growth of *H. pylori.* Licorice flavonoids stimulate the production of mucus to coat and protect the stomach. DGL also increases the life span of intestinal cells and improves blood flow to the intestinal lining.[4]

Bismuth compounds such as bismuth subsalicylate found in Pepto-Bismol coat the lining of the stomach and protect it from infection. Some research suggests that bismuth will best help people who have at least some symptoms of indigestion, that is, not just acne, perianal inflammation, or weak nails.[5] Bismuth subcitrate, a form of bismuth available from compounding pharmacists, is more effective at controlling the infection, although it is also more expensive. Bismuth subcitrate is available from compounding pharmacists, who can be located through the International Academy of Compounding Pharmacists, 1-800-927-4227.

CONCEPTS FOR COPING WITH HYPOCHLORHYDRIA

○ Always avoid antacids. Many people find symptoms of hypochlorhydria are relieved by bismuth subsalicylate (Pepto-Bismol).

Hypoglycemia

SYMPTOM SUMMARY

○ Anxiety

○ Confusion

○ Rapid pulse

○ Shakiness

○ Sweating

○ Weakness

○ In extreme cases, loss of consciousness, coma, or even death

UNDERSTANDING THE DISEASE PROCESS

Hypoglycemia is a state of low blood sugar. The condition can occur after skipping meals (fasting hypoglycemia) or it can be a reaction to overeating (reactive hypoglycemia), the result of the body's overproduction of insulin in response to a high-carbohydrate meal. Fast-

ing hypoglycemia can occur at any time of day, but reactive hypoglycemia typically occurs 2–4 hours after eating.

Reactive hypoglycemia is more common among women than men. This form of hypoglycemia never leads directly to coma and death, although loss of consciousness can contribute to serious or even fatal accidents. The majority of diabetics on insulin occasionally "overshoot" and experience low blood sugars. Taking too much insulin can in rare instances result in coma or death.

TREATMENT SUMMARY

DIET

○ Eat whole grains and fruits. Avoid refined sugar. Eat 4–6 smaller meals, rather than 1–2 larger meals, a day.

NUTRITIONAL SUPPLEMENTS

○ Chromium: 200 micrograms per day.

UNDERSTANDING THE HEALING PROCESS

Many people who think they have hypoglycemia do not in fact suffer from low blood sugars. A simple blood test involving putting a drop of blood on a test strip in a blood glucose meter can determine whether low blood sugar is the cause of symptoms. Readings below 45 mg/dl indicate reactive hypoglycemia. Diabetics should always test their blood sugars when they begin to feel sweaty, weak, or faint. Readings below 70 mg/dl within 2 hours of taking fast-acting (N or Humalog) insulin indicate a need for sugar.

Anyone who has reactive hypoglycemia should avoid sweets. The pancreas normally releases a surge of insulin as carbohydrates are being digested so that blood sugars are kept in the normal range. In reactive hypoglycemia, eating desserts or large servings of white bread, Irish potatoes, or rice can trigger the release of excessive amounts of insulin so that sugars fall below the normal range. When symptoms of hypoglycemia occur, the appropriate treatment is to take the kind of sugar the body needs, glucose, rather than orange juice, cola, or candy. A small amount of glucose can be readily absorbed and bring blood sugar levels back to normal. A larger amount of sucrose is required to give the body the sugar it needs immediately, and the excess can cause another, milder round of hypoglycemia a few hours after the first.

Fasting-acting glucose gels are available in tubes at pharmacies, and glucose tablets are also effective. Glucose is not as palatable as table sugar and few hypoglycemics will take glucose unless there is a real need. If glucose is not available, cola (not diet), juice, or candy will also bring blood sugars back to normal, but they do not act as quickly as glucose.

There is considerable anecdotal evidence to support the use of chromium in the treatment of hypoglycemia. Experiments have show that chromium makes muscle cells more sensitive to insulin resistance, so that they take sugar out of the bloodstream more rapidly, and the body is less likely to overproduce insulin as it attempts to lower blood sugars as food is digested. Chromium may be especially useful for hypoglycemics whose symptoms are worse during periods of emotional stress.[1]

Contrary to some recommendations, taking magnesium if you have hypoglycemia is not a good idea. Magnesium increases the body's production of insulin, and additional insulin aggravates reactive hypoglycemia.[2]

CONCEPTS FOR COPING WITH HYPOGLYCEMIA

○ Use glucose rather than orange juice or soft drinks to treat hypoglycemia caused by too much insulin, too much medication, or too much exercise. Glucose gel (available in tubes sold in pharmacies) can be smeared inside the mouth of a person who has passed out from low blood sugars. For a person weighing 200 pounds (90 kilograms), 15 grams of glucose, the equivalent a tube of glucose gel or a roll of glucose tablets, is enough to raise blood sugars from the danger zone to a level supporting consciousness. Orange juice or a sugar-sweetened soft drink can be used to raise blood sugars but they do not act as quickly as glucose, and they cannot be given to someone who is unconscious.

Hypothyroidism

SYMPTOM SUMMARY

○ Fatigue

○ Weakness

○ Pale skin

○ Swelling of the thyroid, or goiter

○ Sensitivity to cold

○ Weight gain

○ Arthritis

○ Brittle nails

○ carpal tunnel syndrome

○ Constipation

○ Depression

○ Easy bruising

○ High blood pressure

○ Hives

○ Numbness, especially in the fingers and toes

○ Snoring

In women:

○ Heavy periods

○ Galactorrhea

UNDERSTANDING THE DISEASE PROCESS

Hypothyroidism is a condition in which the thyroid gland fails to produce adequate levels of thyroid hormone. It is usually caused by disease within the thyroid gland itself, but in rare cases it can arise from disturbances in the hypothalamus and pituitary or result from a general resistance to thyroid hormone.

In the early stages, hypothyroidism often eludes diagnosis. The symptoms of hypothyroidism can affect almost any organ. They are nonspecific in their early stages and do not necessarily occur in any sequence. These symptoms may include brittle nails, thinning hair, joint pain, muscle pain, muscle cramps, pale skin, dry skin, headaches, and, in women, heavy periods. As the disease progresses, there may be hoarseness, swollen ankles, carpal tunnel syndrome, constipation, and/or shortness of breath. In advanced cases there is a lack of mental acuteness, loss of balance, and sleep apnea. In one study, 43 percent of people with hypothyroidism developed carpal tunnel syndrome and 46 percent suffered some degree of shrinking in the muscles.[1] About 25 percent of people who have hypothyroidism develop other immune-mediated diseases, such as chronic auto-immune hepatitis, lupus, pernicious anemia, Sjögren's syndrome, or vitiligo. High cholesterol is also common with the condition and contributes to increased risk of atherosclerosis. People with deficient thyroid hormone production who are also diabetic are at special risk of developing anemia.[2]

The most frequent cause of hypothyroidism is Hashimoto's disease or Hashimoto's thyroiditis, an attack on the thyroid by the immune system. In this condition, the immune system develops antibodies to thyroid peroxidase (TPO) and thyroglobulin (TG), both components of thyroid cells. Generally the onset is slow and results in progressive destruction of the thyroid gland. Ironically, the immune system's destruction of the thyroid leading to hypothyroidism may begin hyperthyroidism, in which the thyroid produces excessive quantities of thyroid hormones.

Destruction of the thyroid can also result from the iron-storage disease hemochromatosis, leukemia, sarcoidosis, thyroid cancer, or tuberculosis. It can occur in AIDS as a direct result of infection with *Pneumocystis carinii,* and it is not unusual as a side effect of treatment with various chemotherapy drugs, such as interferon, lithium, or the heart drug amiodarone. Extreme iodine deficiency, which is rare outside South Asia and a few isolated areas of Central Europe, is another possible cause.

Hypothyroidism caused by disease in the thyroid gland itself is sometimes accompanied by an enlargement of the gland known as goiter. This condition responds to dietary restrictions that are not necessary in all cases of hypothyroidism. (See Concepts for Coping with Hypothyroidism).

TREATMENT SUMMARY

NUTRITIONAL SUPPLEMENTS

❍ Use iodized salt daily, or eat bladderwrack or kelp, weekly.

❍ Selenium: 100 micrograms daily.

❍ Zinc picolinate: 15–30 milligrams daily.

❍ Avoid niacin.

HERBS

❍ Kidney Chi Pill from *The Golden Cabinet.*

UNDERSTANDING THE HEALING PROCESS

Since iodine is almost always available at adequate levels in the modern diet, iodine supplements and iodine-rich foods such as bladderwrack and kelp are of limited benefit *by themselves* in treating hypothyroidism. People whose thyroids have not been surgically or chemi-

cally destroyed may benefit from supplementation with selenium and zinc. Selenium deficiency lowers the activity of the antioxidant enzyme glutathione peroxidase activity in the thyroid gland, thus allowing hydrogen peroxide produced during thyroid hormone synthesis to destroy cells.[3] Selenium supplementation reverses this effect—but selenium without adequate amounts of iodine makes hypothyroidism worse. Do not take selenium unless you also use iodized salt on a daily basis or take an iodine supplement. Zinc is also required for normal function of the enzyme, but a minimum of supplementation, 15–30 milligrams per day, is sufficient.

People with hypothyroidism frequently develop high cholesterol and high homocysteine levels, but taking niacin to correct these problems is not advisable. In one case, thyroid hormone levels fell in two people who were taking niacin for high cholesterol so that one was diagnosed with hypothyroidism. When the niacin was discontinued for 1 month, thyroid hormone levels returned to normal.[4] Some recent research has even found that the basic rationale for taking niacin was faulty; studies of women with deficient thyroid function has found that their increased risk of heart disease is not related to unusually high homocysteine levels,[5] and that supplemental niacin has no special advantage in hypothyroidism.

People with minimal thyroid function (that is, people whose hypothyroidism did not result from medical removal of the thyroid) may benefit from treatment with the traditional Chinese herbal remedy Kidney Chi Pill from *The Golden Cabinet* (referring to a book of herbal formulas constituting a "golden" medicine cabinet, written in the third century A.D.). A Chinese clinical study found that people with hypothyroidism who took the herbs for 1 year experienced marked improvement of symptoms and increased bloodstream concentrations of thyroid hormones.[6] Traditional Chinese Medicine teaches that this formula is especially helpful in treating hypothyroidism complicated by urinary incontinence or copious urination.

Kidney Chi Pill from *The Golden Cabinet* is a combination of the herbs aconite, alisma, cinnamon, Cornelian cherry, dioscorea, moutan, poria mushroom, and rehmannia. It is is available in the United States and Canada under the following trade names:

- Dynamic Warrior (Jade Pharmacy)
- Essential Yang (Golden Flower Herbs)
- Jin Gui Shen Qi Wan (Blue Light)

Practitioners of Traditional Chinese Medicine can formulate an herbal tea equivalent to these patent medicines anywhere in the world.

CONCEPTS FOR COPING WITH HYPOTHYROIDISM

○ Taking large amounts of iodine supplements because you think you might have low thyroid function can have disastrous effects. Massive doses of supplemental iodine will overstimulate the thyroid so that the immune system is activated to attack the thyroid, causing the very condition iodine supplementation is intended to prevent. Eating large quantities of sea vegetables such as kelp can have a similar effect,[7] but not always. The most recent research in Japan found that antibodies to thyroid hormone and thyroid disease were no higher in regions where kelp is a primary food, such as in the Okinawan diet, due to the fact that Okinawan kelp is relatively low in iodine.[8]

○ Most people with hypothyroidism will need medically prescribed thyroid hormone replacements, primarily levothyroxine (Synthroid, Levothroid, Levoxyl). Natural therapies for hypothyroidism make it easier to live with the condition, but do not substitute for medication. Some doctors use desiccated thyroid, also called thyroid extract (for example, Armour Thyroid) as an alternative to synthetic thyroid hormones. Dessicated thyroid extract contains two biologically active hormones, thyroxine and triiodothyronine, whereas the most commonly prescribed thyroid-hormone preparations contain only thyroxine. One study showed that the combination of the two hormones contained in desiccated thyroid is more effective than thyroxine alone, especially in fighting depression and improving mental acuity and for women who have to take thyroid hormone replacement after surgery for thyroid cancer.[9] Dried thyroid products sold in health food stores have had most of the thyroid hormone removed and are not effective for people with hypothyroidism. Intact desiccated thyroid is available only by prescription.

○ A number of foods contain goitrogens, compounds that cause the formation of goiter by interfering with the normal synthesis of thyroid hormone. These foods include canola (rapeseed) oil, broccoli, raw Brussels sprouts (cooked Brussels sprouts do not have this effect), cabbage, kale, lima beans, sweet potatoes, soy (including soy sauce, tofu, and miso), tapioca, and pearl millet. Avoiding these foods helps prevent and slowly correct goiter.

○ When eating outside the United States, avoid hamburgers. Several outbreaks of thyrotoxicosis have been attributed to a practice, now banned in the United States, called "gullet trimming," in which meat in the neck region of slaughtered animals is ground into hamburger meats. Because thyroid glands are reddish in color and located in the neck, it was not unusual for gullet trimmers to get thyroid glands into hamburger or sausage meat. For anyone who has normal thyroid hormone levels (by virtue of having a healthy thyroid or through the use of medication), eating hamburger meat prepared in this way can get doses of thyroid hormone sufficient to cause sleeplessness, nervousness, headache, fatigue, excessive sweating, and weight loss.

IBD
See **Inflammatory Bowel Disease (IBD)**.

IBS
See **Irritable Bowel Syndrome (IBS)**.

Idopathic Endolymphatic Hydrops
See **Ménière's Disease**.

Ileitis
See **Inflammatory Bowel Disease (IBD)**.

Ileocolitis/Ileitis
See **Inflammatory Bowel Disease (IBD)**.

Impetigo
See **Boils and Carbuncles**.

Impotence

See **Erectile Dysfunction**.

Indigestion

See **Bloating; Flatulence; Heartburn; Hiccups**.

Infertility

See **Female Infertility; Male Infertility**.

Inflammatory Bowel Disease (IBD)

SYMPTOM SUMMARY

Crohn's Disease:

○ Abdominal tenderness, especially in the lower right side

○ Fatigue

○ Flatulence

○ Intermittent diarrhea

○ Loss of appetite

Ulcerative Colitis:

○ Abdominal cramps

○ Bloody diarrhea

○ Hemorrhoids

○ Perianal inflammation

○ Weight loss

UNDERSTANDING THE DISEASE PROCESS

Inflammatory bowel disease (IBD) commonly refers to ulcerative colitis and Crohn's disease, chronic conditions of inflammation of the lower gastrointestinal tract of unknown caused. Crohn's disease also is referred to as granulomatous ileocolitis, regional enteritis, or terminal ileitis.

In Crohn's disease, there are segments of inflammation involving not just the lining of the bowel but their supporting tissues. Over time, the intestine develops a cobblestone appearance, as ulcers form and heal in its various layers. The pockets of inflammation caused by Crohn's disease are usually isolated, in the colon (in 25 percent of patients), in the small intestine (in 30 percent of patients), or in the large intestine (in 40 percent of patients). Usually the rectum is not affected by Crohn's disease, but there can be inflammation of the mouth, tongue, esophagus, and stomach. Fistulas, secondary openings of the anus to the outside of the body, can occur.

In ulcerative colitis, inflammation usually begins in the rectum, spreads upward a certain distance, and abruptly stops. The small intestine, stomach, and mouth are never involved. The radiological image seen after a barium enema is more like a pipe than a series of cobblestones.

IBD is a disease most commonly seen in North America and Northern Europe, and it strikes 4 times as many Caucasians as members of other races. It is especially common among Ashkenazi Jews. IBD typically first appears in the late teens or 20s, although first cases are also clustered among people aged 55–65. Interestingly, smokers are much less likely to get IBD than former smokers or nonsmokers, and nicotine patches have been tried as a treatment for the condition.

TREATMENT SUMMARY

DIET

○ Avoid any prepared food product containing stabilizers, emulsifiers, or carrageenan.

NUTRITIONAL SUPPLEMENTS

○ Any multivitamin and mineral supplement: as directed on the label, daily.

○ Complete probiotic formula (preferably containing both *Lactobacillus acidophilus* and *Bifidobacteria*): 1–2 capsules daily.

○ Fish oil: 3–10 grams daily.

○ Vitamin E: 100–200 IU daily.

○ Vitamin K: 5 milligrams every other week.

HERBS

○ Slippery elm or Robert's Formula: as desired.

UNDERSTANDING THE HEALING PROCESS

When research scientists want to induce inflammatory

bowel disease in lab rats, they feed them carrageenan. This seaweed derivative is used as an emulsifier and stabilizer in almost every prepared food product containing milk, including ice cream, yogurt, coffee creamer, and cheese spreads. Carrageenan by itself (even in enormous quantities) does not cause intestinal inflammation in humans. However, when it is used as a food by the intestinal bacterium *Bacteroides vulgatus,* it creates a toxic chemical that accelerates the course of both Crohn's disease and ulcerative colitis.

This bacterium is especially abundant in the intestine when there is chronic inflammation. People with IBD should be careful to avoid any product containing carrageenan, and if eating prepared foods is unavoidable, take probiotics to provide bacteria to compete with *B. vulgatus.* Yogurt is an acceptable probiotic in IBD as long as it is not made with emulsifiers or stabilizers.

Some people with IBD have identifiable food allergies and do better when they eliminate offending food items from their diet. Some clinical trials have found that IBD patients do better when they completely eliminate gluten and dairy,[1] but others have found that IBD patients do better when they receive concentrated wheat and dairy proteins.[2] For this reason, it is premature to suppose that there is a connection between allergies and symptoms in all cases of IBD, and food allergies have to be considered on a purely individual basis. When there is a food allergy that aggravates symptoms of IBD, it is most likely to be tied to yeasts and molds used in making bread and cheese.[3] A majority of people with IBD, however, do not have food allergies. High-fiber foods, such as beans, fruit, and nuts, can irritate the colon but do not usually cause allergies.

Several supplements are generally helpful in IBD. Frequent bouts of diarrhea, loss of appetite, and side effects of medication interfere with the absorption of nutrients from food. People with IBD are especially prone to developing deficiencies of vitamins A, B_{12}, C, D, E, and K, folic acid, calcium, copper, magnesium, and selenium.[4] A daily multivitamin tablet with minerals is always indicated. People who have surgery for Crohn's disease are especially likely to develop vitamin D deficiency[5] and should consult with their physicians about taking a vitamin D supplement to avoid osteoporosis.

At least one clinical study has found that probiotic *Lactobacillus acidophilus* and *Bifidobacterium* greatly reduce the risk of recurrence of "pouchitis," an inflammatory condition that commonly occurs after surgery for IBD. Scientists at the University of Bologna in Italy reported that 3 out of 20 patients given probiotics suffered relapses of pouchitis over a 9-month period, whereas all 20 patients given a placebo suffered flare-ups of the condition.[6] The are no contraindications for the probiotics in IBD.

Fish oil is widely recommended for treatment of IBD, and the clinical data indicate it at least prolongs remission, although it does not prevent relapses of the disease.[7] If fishy-smelling burps are a problem, switch to evening primrose oil.

Deficiencies of vitamin E and vitamin K tend to occur at the same time, and at any given time about a third of people with IBD are deficient in these two vitamins.[8] Vitamin K is especially likely to be depleted during treatment with antibiotics. The doses needed to prevent deficiency are so small that they are highly unlikely to interfere with any prescription drugs. Zinc supplements are frequently recommended in IBS, but zinc levels are actually above normal when the disease is active, and very few IBS sufferers are deficient in zinc.[9]

Demulcent herbs, such as slippery elm, relieve inflammation by coating the lining of the colon and rectum. Taken as a warm tea, they do not interfere with any medications. Robert's Formula is a combination of baptisia (wild indigo), cabbage powder, *Echinacea angustifolia,* geranium, goldenseal, marshmallow root, and slippery elm. Available from naturopathic physicians and compounding pharmacists, Robert's Formula is both demulcent and anti-inflammatory.

CONCEPTS FOR COPING WITH INFLAMMATORY BOWEL DISEASE

O Some physicians recommend medium-chain triglycerides (MCTs) as a nutritional supplement for IBD patients. MCTs are easily absorbed through the intestine and readily converted to energy, but very little MCT is stored as fat.

Influenza
See **Flu.**

Injuries
See **Burns; Cuts and Scrapes; Sunburn.**

Insect, Spider, and Tick Bites

SYMPTOM SUMMARY

❍ Itchy bumps, grouped where the bites occur

❍ Intense itching due to allergic reaction

UNDERSTANDING THE DISEASE PROCESS

Insect bites are a fact of life throughout most of the United States and most of the world. East of the Mississippi River, biting flies, mosquitoes, and ticks account for most bites. In California and the arid Southwest, crawling scorpions and spiders are a greater problem.

Bites from insects and other creepy-crawlies are not merely a nuisance, they frequently transmit disease. Up to 90 percent of ticks in the northeastern United States carry Lyme disease. In parts of southern Texas, typhus is carried by possums and spread to house cats by fleas that then bite humans. Throughout much of the United States, fire ants swarm and sting in great numbers when their mounds are disturbed (although they do, however, feed on ticks). Rocky Mountain spotted fever, despite its name, is especially common in ticks in North Carolina. Mouse mites in New York City carry a disease related to chicken pox. Throughout much of the country, mosquitoes carry encephalitis and West Nile virus.

Insect-borne illness is an even bigger problem outside the United States. South American sand flies carry leishmaniasis and bartonellosis. Onchoceriasis, spread by black flies, is a major cause of blindness in Africa. Elephantiasis in Africa and East Asia is caused by filarial worms transmitted by mosquitoes.

Injury to the skin from an insect bite is usually minimal. Typically the skin inflammation results from an allergic reaction rather than the bite itself. Sometimes skin injury results from a toxin injected by the bite, such as the toxin of the brown recluse spider.

TREATMENT SUMMARY

❍ Apply any insect repellant containing DEET before going outdoors.

For relief of itch or inflammation:

❍ Simicort: as directed on label.

UNDERSTANDING THE HEALING PROCESS

Preventing insect bites is one area of health where natural is not better. Recent studies at the University of North Carolina at Chapel Hill have found that "natural" insect repellants containing citronella or other botanicals repel insects for an average of 20 minutes. Spray-on insect repellants containing DEET offer nearly complete protection for up to 5 hours. Wristbands soaked in insect repellant typically offer no protection at all.[1]

There is natural therapy once bites occur, however. For minor insect bites, apply Simicort, a cream made with licorice extract. One of the components of licorice, glycyrrhetinic acid, potentiates the effects of the natural anti-inflammatory hormone cortisol by inhibiting the enzyme 11-beta-hydroxysteroid dehydrogenase, which converts cortisol to an inactive form.[2]

CONCEPTS FOR COPING WITH INSECT, SPIDER, AND TICK BITES

❍ Accurate identification is essential when assessing the need for treatment for scorpion and spider bites. The only potentially lethal scorpion in the United States, found in Arizona and northern Mexico, is small, tan-to-buff in color, and has a blunt thorn on its tail. This scorpion may have "racing stripes." The black widow is a large, shiny black spider with what looks like a red hourglass on its abdomen. The brown recluse is a small brown spider with long legs and an "hourglass" or "violin case" pattern on its abdomen. Bites by desert scorpions require immediate medical attention. A bite by a black widow can cause intense abdominal pain, and also requires urgent medical care. If you are bitten by a brown recluse, put ice on the bite and seek emergency medical attention. Untreated brown recluse bites can cause extensive tissue damage that must be surgically treated.

❍ Bedbugs prefer to bite bats and birds, but after seasonal migrations of their preferred hosts, they wander into houses in search of alternate food sources. A sure sign of a bedbug bite is three bites in a row.

❍ The ticks that carry Lyme disease are small, brown, and pear-shaped, and have black legs. The ticks that carry Rocky Mountain spotted fever and tularemia have ornate mouth parts and a single glowing white spot in the middle of their backs. Remove an attached tick as soon as it is detected. Ticks usually bite in folds of skin or where creases in clothing stop their movement. To remove the tick, place *one end* of a pair of tweezers under the tick as close to the skin as possible and pull upward with steady pressure. Do not squeeze the tick, since this can force the contents of the tick's stomach into the bite and infect the wound. Do not use alcohol, turpentine, or a hot match to remove ticks, since these methods can cause the tick to vomit into the wound, transmitting the bacteria that cause Lyme disease. A plastic device known as a "tick nipper" is also effective.

Insomnia

SYMPTOM SUMMARY

- ○ Awakening at night
- ○ Difficulty falling asleep
- ○ Anxiety
- ○ Apathy
- ○ Daytime fatigue and drowsiness
- ○ Depression
- ○ Difficulty concentrating
- ○ Episodes of stopped breathing
- ○ Irritability
- ○ Loud snoring
- ○ Lower-leg movements during sleep
- ○ Memory problems
- ○ Sleep attacks during the day

UNDERSTANDING THE DISEASE PROCESS

Insomnia is the most common sleep disorder. It is a condition of difficulty in initiating or maintaining sleep, waking up too early in the morning, and/or the experience of nonrestorative sleep. Lost sleep is a major public health problem. Approximately 200,000 automobile crashes occur each year because of drivers' excessive sleepiness.[1] Daytime sleepiness has been implicated as the cause of several major catastrophes, such as the Three Mile Island meltdown, the erroneous launch of the *Challenger* space shuttle, and the grounding of the Exxon *Valdez* oil tanker.

Approximately one in three adult Americans suffers insomnia during the course of a year.[2] Insomnia is more common among women[3] and older people[4] and is

associated with lower incomes and lower educational levels.[5] Insomnia is associated with a higher risk for emotional problems,[6] decreased enjoyment of interpersonal relationships, and decreased perceived mood and wellness.[7] Insomnia causes impaired memory and concentration, decreased ability to accomplish daily tasks, and diminished capacity to solve problems.[8]

Despite the frequency and importance of the condition, most doctors place a low priority on treating it. In a Gallup poll conducted in 1995, only 1 in 20 people with insomnia ever received medical treatment for the condition.[9] In a recent survey of 222 hospitalized patients, investigators noted sleep complaints in half of these patients and diagnosable sleep disorders in 40 percent. However, none of the clinical charts made any mention of sleep.

TREATMENT SUMMARY

DIET

○ Avoid caffeine (coffee, tea, chocolate). Unless you are diabetic, be sure to consume a carbohydrate food 1–2 hours before bedtime.

SUPPLEMENTS

Taken 45 minutes to 1 hour before bedtime:

○ Niacin: 100 milligrams.

○ Magnesium: 250 milligrams.

○ 5-HTP or L-tryptophan: 100–300 milligrams.

○ Melatonin: 0.3 milligrams.

○ Vitamin B_6: 50 milligrams.

Take supplements with a glass of juice. Avoid protein foods for 2 hours before bedtime.

HERBS

Taken 45 minutes to 1 hour before bedtime:

○ Passionflower in any of the following forms:

- • Dried herb in tea: 4–8 grams.
- • Dry powdered extract containing 2.6 percent flavonoids: 300–400 milligrams.
- • Fluid extract: $1/2$–1 teaspoon.
- • Tincture: $1 1/2$–2 teaspoons.

○ Valerian in any of the following forms:

- • Dried root as a tea: 2–3 grams.

- Dry powdered extract containing 0.8 percent valerenic acid: 150–300 milligrams.
- Fluid extract: $1/2$–1 teaspoon.
- Tincture: $1^1/_2$–2 teaspoons.

○ *Avoid* ephedra, guaraná, and maté.

○ Women experiencing insomnia as a symptom of menopause and who do not take estrogen therapy may benefit from 200 milligrams of ginseng taken daily, in addition to other treatments.

○ Kava is appropriate if anxiety is an important contributing factor (see ANXIETY). Small-scale clinical studies suggest that kava may be a better choice than valerian for people who are troubled by vivid dreams, but passionflower and valerian may be better choices for people who have diseases affecting balance or causing dizziness.[10]

UNDERSTANDING THE HEALING PROCESS

While there is considerable variability in "normal" sleep, most adults are comfortable with 6–8 hours daily, taken in a single period.[11] Normal sleep consists of 4–6 cycles defined by electroencephalograph (EEG) in 2 categories: non-rapid eye movement (NREM) sleep and rapid eye movement (REM) sleep.

Stage 1 NREM sleep is a very light sleep, from which the sleeper can be readily aroused. In this stage the EEG shows mixed frequencies of low voltage. The majority of the night's sleep is spent in stage 2 of NREM sleep. This stage is recognized by steep spindles on the EEG. Stages 3 and 4 of NREM are referred to as delta sleep or slow-wave sleep.

In REM sleep, as its name suggests, there are episodes of rapid eye movement. During REM sleep, the muscles rest. Muscle tone goes flat.[12]

Getting enough sleep is essential for maintaining good health. Sleep is a restorative process that balances the autonomic nervous system (regulating breathing and digestion), the endocrine glands, and the immune system. In groups of people who suffer sleep disturbances due to various diseases, including alcohol dependence, depression, and HIV, losses of immune function coincide with loss of sleep.[13]

The link between sleep and the immune system is the hormone interleukin (IL)-6. This hormone is secreted by "germ-eating" macrophages in response to infectious challenge. It plays a key role in the processes that lead to the production, proliferation, and maturation of two other components of the immune system, the B and T cells. IL-6 concentrations are low during the daytime and high at night in healthy individuals. However, loss of sleep[14]—and snoring[15]—deplete the body's supply of IL-6. For this reason, sleep disturbances lower resistance to infectious disease,[16] increase the risk of cancer,[17] and accelerate the progression of inflammatory diseases such as rheumatoid arthritis.[18]

Getting a good night's sleep is important to weight control. Scientists at the University of Chicago found that young male volunteers who were restricted to 4 hours of sleep for 6 consecutive nights were significantly less tolerant of glucose.[19] This means their bodies had to produce more of the hormone insulin to move the same amount of glucose from the bloodstream into the muscle cells that use it. Insulin moves not only sugar but also fat, and fat cells have 300 times as many insulin receptors as muscle cells. In other words, the effect of increasing the amount of insulin in the bloodstream has 300 times as great an impact on fat storage as on muscle power.

For people over the age of 35, sleep deprivation works against weight control in a second way. Growth hormone deficiency is linked to increased obesity, loss of muscle mass, and reduced exercise capacity. The body regenerates growth hormone during sleep. How much growth hormone the body is capable of producing during sleep, however, depends on regular sleep.

The University of Chicago researchers also found that, during the daytime hours, the bloodstream concentration of growth hormone is about 2.1–2.2 picograms per milliliter. During sleep, the concentration of the hormone almost doubles in the first 30 minutes, to 4.0 picograms per milliliter, and soars to 5.7 picograms per milliliter about an hour after falling to sleep. After 2 hours, concentrations of growth hormone fall back to their daytime levels.

When the body is deprived of sleep, growth hormone levels are flat. The Chicago researchers measured growth hormone in volunteers who had been restricted to 4 hours of sleep for 6 nights. During the day, their growth levels were also 2.1–2.2 picograms per milliliter. During sleep, however, the hormone peaked at a concentration of only 3.8 picograms per milliliter.

While sleep deprivation depletes growth hormones, it increases stress hormones. The same study found that cortisol levels (which also increase during sleep) were 60 percent higher at night in sleep-deprived subjects.

Sleep deprivation even causes further sleep deprivation. The study at the University of Chicago also found that in healthy individuals, levels of the sleep-inducing hormone nearly triple 3$\frac{1}{2}$ hours after the onset of sleep. They fall to lower levels as the night progresses but are nearly twice as high at either the beginning or the end of sleep as they are during the day. In sleep-deprived individuals, melatonin levels are also higher during sleep, but only about half as high as otherwise would be expected.[20]

The clear conclusion of the scientific literature is that getting enough sleep is essential to a healthy immune system and weight control. The literature shows that the effects of insomnia go beyond mental fatigue even to cause muscle loss. Pharmaceutical approaches to treating insomnia restore sleep and help restore hormonal balance—with side effects. Diet, supplements, and herbs also restore sleep with a minimum of side effects.

The most basic treatment for insomnia is to avoid stimulants. These include sources of caffeine, such as coffee, tea, and chocolate, and stimulant herbs, such as ephedra, guaraná, and maté. It is also important to avoid hypoglycemia. Low blood sugar levels promote awakening by the release of stress hormones that release sugars stored in the liver. Low blood sugar levels are not a problem, of course, in diabetes.

The neurotransmitter serotonin is an initiator of sleep. It is especially important in slow-wave sleep, the sleep during which the body regenerates essential hormones. The brain manufactures serotonin from the amino acid L-tryptophan. This amino acid is best absorbed by the brain when blood sugars are relatively high. Since it has to compete with other amino acids for absorption into the brain, it should not be taken with meals, especially meals of high-protein foods.

Supplementation with L-tryptophan by itself produces modest benefits in the treatment of insomnia. A small-scale placebo-controlled clinical trial at the University of Manitoba found that a 2,400-milligram dose of L-tryptophan reduced the time needed to fall asleep an hour after it was taken. L-tryptophan is effective even if it is taken in the middle of the day, but the effect of the supplement wears off over time. A relatively high dose of the amino acid is needed if it is taken 2 hours before trying to go to sleep.[21]

Some researchers believe that 2,000 milligrams is the largest dose of L-tryptophan the body can use. Under conditions of stress, or when there is a vitamin B$_6$ deficiency, the body converts L-tryptophan into kynurenine,

a chemical compound that cannot be used by the brain.[22] It is possible that taking more than 1,200 milligrams of L-tryptophan per day is hazardous for persons who also take the MAO inhibitors phenelzine (Nardil) or tranylcypromine (Parnate). There have been reports of serotonin syndrome, a condition causing agitation, confusion, delirium, heavy sweating, racing pulse, and blood pressure fluctuations, in people who have taken both the prescription drug and L-tryptophan.[23] These problems can be avoided by the use of 5-HTP, an intermediate product of the conversion of L-tryptophan into serotonin.

5-HTP is readily absorbed by the brain even when blood sugars are low. It does not have to compete with other amino acids for transport into the brain, so it can be taken with meals. And unlike L-tryptophan, it cannot be shunted into the production of niacin or other proteins, although adequate magnesium levels are essential for its use. While 5-HTP is converted into serotonin, other important neurotransmitters become more abundant as a result of 5-HTP supplementation. These include dopamine, norepinephrine, and endorphins.[24]

A clinical study has found that 5-HTP increases REM sleep. Eight test participants were given 200 milligrams of 5-HTP at 9:15 P.M. and another 400 milligrams at 11:15 P.M. Taking the supplement increased the amount of time spent in restorative REM sleep from an average of 98 minutes to an average of 118 minutes. The researchers repeated the experiment without the 400-milligram dose, and found that it induced a lesser increase of REM sleep time.[25]

Melatonin is especially useful in treating insomnia in adults over 50. A study at the Massachusetts Institute of Technology found dosages of melatonin from 0.1 gram to 3 grams all improved sleep in insomniacs, although they had no effect on people who did not have insomnia. Melatonin has its greatest effect on the third and fourth hours of sleep. The MIT researchers found that the most effective dose was 0.3 grams. A 0.1-gram dose improved sleep but did not bring melatonin levels to normal. A 3-gram dose also improved sleep but could cause shakes and chills.[26]

Dutch researchers have tested melatonin in the treatment of insomnia in children aged 6–12. They found that a relatively high (5.0-milligram) dose for a week helped children fall asleep an average of half an hour earlier and to sleep as much as 1 hour longer each night. The only side effect noted was mild headache in 2 of the 33 children in the study, and only 1 of the 33 children in the study was not helped by the supplement. The researchers noted that 1 child developed a mild seizure disorder during the trial, but they did not believe that melatonin caused the condition.[27]

Passionflower consists of the dried flowering and fruiting top of a perennial climbing vine native to northeastern Mexico and Texas. It contains a number of flavonoid compounds, one of which, chrysin, acts on the same sites in the brain as the benzodiazepine drugs Librium and Valium,[28] but without causing daytime drowsiness.[29] Since passionflower is used in folk medicine as a stimulant to childbirth, pregnant women should not take it.

Valerian has been used as a sleep aid for over 1,000 years.[30] It contains valepotriates, valerenic acid, and other water-soluble chemicals that contribute to its sedative properties.

Valerian is a clinically effective source of GABA, a chemical that blocks extraneous nerve impulses in the brain.[31] A clinical trial with 128 volunteers given 400 milligrams of valerian extract at bedtime found that the herb improved sleep quality, decreased the time needed to fall asleep, and reduced the number of awakenings during the night.[32] A study in which participants were given 135 milligrams of a dry extract of valerian 3 times a day found that the herb improved slow-wave sleep and decreased the amount of time spent in stage 1 sleep.[33]

Valerian is generally a very safe herb, although there have been reports of withdrawal symptoms in persons who quit using it abruptly after taking higher-than-recommended dosages for a period of several years. Valerian has an additive effect when used with barbiturates or benzodiazepine tranquilizers. Do not use both the herb and these prescription medications.

A pilot study conducted by an herbal products company in Switzerland found that the combination of valerian and hops is also helpful in treating mild insomnia. Thirty patients were given a combination of 250 milligrams of valerian extract and 60 milligrams of hops extract. After 2 weeks of treatment, polysomnography showed a decline in sleep latency, that is, the time required to go to sleep, and also in the time required to wake up. More important, the combination of the two herbs increased slow-wave sleep, the period in which the body replenishes IL-6, growth hormone, and melatonin. There were no side effects from the herbal treatment.[34]

There are a number of studies that indicate that ginseng is effective in treating insomnia in both men and women. Since it is relatively expensive, however, it is recommended only for special cases. A Japanese clinical study, involving 12 postmenopausal women suffering emotional disturbance with menopause and 8 postmenopausal women without any symptoms of menopause, tested the efficacy of the herb as a treatment for insomnia. The scientists found that the ratio of the stress hormone cortisol to bloodstream concentrations of DHEA was significantly higher in women who suffered insomnia than in women who did not. Taking ginseng for 30 days lowered the cortisol/DHEA ratio in the women who had insomnia (although not to the levels of the women who did not have insomnia) and relieved depression, fatigue, and insomnia.[35]

Do not take ginseng if you are also taking estrogen replacement therapy (ERT). Animal studies indicate that the herb stimulates estrogen production by the ovaries,[36] and the combination of ERT and ginseng may be excessive.

CONCEPTS FOR COPING WITH INSOMNIA

❍ Get 20 minutes or more of aerobic exercise daily, in the morning or afternoon, not before bedtime.

❍ In addition to diet, supplements, and herbs, you may be able to induce sleep by progressive relaxation. After you have stretched out or curled up in bed into a position you find comfortable, flex your feet as tightly as you can and hold the tension as you count from 1–10. Release the tension for 2 or 3 seconds, take a breath, and then press your calves as firmly as you can against the mattress, again holding the tension as you count from 1–10. Release and repeat the process with your thighs, back, hands, and arms. Many people fall asleep before they use all their muscle groups.

❍ Speak with your prescribing physician about changing the dosage of beta-blockers, oral contraceptives, and thyroid hormones if you experience insomnia while taking any of these drugs. Avoid the use of marijuana.

❍ If you have trouble getting up in the morning, turn on bright lights. The transition from dim to bright light in the morning induces an immediate increase in bloodstream levels of the "wake-up" chemical cortisol.[37]

❍ If you take a nap, turn off the lights. Try to nap before noon. Napping in the dark and in the morning shifts the brain's production of melatonin so that you can get to sleep sooner at night, whereas napping in bright light and in the afternoon shifts the brain's production of melatonin so that you stay up longer at night.[38]

O Edginess when you have been deprived of sleep is natural, and the effect gets worse as the day progresses. Research at the University of Chicago has found that people who have a "sleep debt" after getting only 4 hours of sleep a night for 6 nights have higher levels of the stress hormone cortisol, especially in the early evening.[39]

O People over the age of 70 who have difficulty sleeping at night may benefit from exposure to bright light for 2 hours in the late morning and 2 hours in the middle of the afternoon every day. Studies at the Akita University School of Medicine in Japan have found that exposure to bright light for 4 hours a day increases the secretion of melatonin, reestablishes circadian rhythms, and relieves sleep disturbances.[40]

O Acupuncture of the ear and scalp sometimes produces immediate relief of insomnia. Acupuncture probably relieves insomnia by the same mechanisms through which it relieves pain.[41]

O A sleep-inducing effect from at least one homeopathic medication has been measured by electroencephalographs (EEGs) in laboratory experiments with rats, showing that its effect is not due to a placebo effect.[42] Among the many homeopathic medications for insomnia are:

- Aconitum napellus, when fear and agitation prevent falling asleep.
- Arsenicum album, for insomnia in people who are obsessed with detail.
- Calcarea carbonica, when insomnia is caused by joint pain.
- Cocculus, for jet lag.
- Coffea cruda, when either happy or disturbing thoughts keep the person awake.
- Ignatia, when insomnia follows grief or disappointment.
- Kali phosphoricum, for insomnia when dieting.
- Nux vomica, for insomnia after overindulgence in food, drink, or coffee.
- Silicea (silica), for sleepwalking.
- Sulfur, for itching, especially in hot weather.
- Zincum metallicum, for restless arms and legs.

Intermittent Claudication
See **Peripheral Vascular Disease.**

Intestinal Malabsorption
See **Celiac Disease; Cirrhosis of the Liver; Cystic Fibrosis; Inflammatory Bowel Disease; Pancreatitis.**

Irregular Heartbeat

SYMPTOM SUMMARY

No symptoms at all, or any or all of the following:

- Anxiety
- Dizziness
- Fainting
- Sensation of fluttering or pounding in the chest
- Unusual awareness of the heartbeat

UNDERSTANDING THE DISEASE PROCESS

Irregular heartbeat, or cardiac arrhythmia, is a disturbance of the heart rhythm. Irregularities in the way the heartbeats may be entirely benign, and, in fact, a lack of variability in the heart rate predicts increased risk of death from all causes in the elderly.[1] However, when the different parts of the heart do not beat in synchrony, changes in pressure in the heart can lead to insufficient circulation or heart attack.

TREATMENT SUMMARY

NUTRITIONAL SUPPLEMENTS

O Magnesium aspartate or magnesium citrate: 200–400 milligrams 3 times a day.

See Part Three if you take prescription medication.

UNDERSTANDING THE HEALING PROCESS

Magnesium is the most helpful supplement for all kinds of cardiac arrhythmias as deficiencies of magnesium are common in people who have arrhythmias.[2] A study at

St. George's Hospital School in London found that people who had had heart attacks and who were treated with furosemide (Lasix) had 24 percent fewer incidents of tachycardia (racing heartbeat) after taking magnesium for 6 weeks.[3] Later investigators commented that this change in EKGs suggested there would be significantly fewer cases of sudden death from all causes.[4]

Don't overdose magnesium. It is the primary element in milk of magnesia, and magnesium supplements can cause diarrhea. Usually the effect is short-term and takes places the first 2 or 3 days the supplement is taken. In heart patients, supplemental magnesium can interfere with the body's ability to absorb quinolone (such as Cipro).

Magnesium supplements can also interfere with the absorption of tetracycline. You should not use magnesium supplements if you have myasthenia gravis. They may exacerbate muscle weakness and precipitate a myasthenic crisis.

Essential fatty acids are frequently recommended for cardiac arrhythmias, especially since the publication of a paper entitled "Prevention of Fatal Cardiac Arrhythmias by Polyunsaturated Acids" in the *The American Journal of Clinical Nutrition*.[5] While there is no reason not to believe essential fatty acids will eventually be found to prevent cardiac arrhythmias in humans, the results reported in this paper were based only on tests with surgically prepared exercising dogs and test-tube cultures of heart cells taken from baby rats.

Copper is also sometimes recommended for treating irregular heartbeats. This recommendation is based on the experience of just three patients, and should be considered premature. Potassium supplementation was once important in treating cardiac arrhythmias, but nowadays relatively few people with arrhythmias benefit from supplemental potassium—because modern prescription drugs have been specifically designed to help the body retain potassium. If you take hydrochlorothiazide (the active ingredient in Dyazide, HCTZ, HydroDIURIL, Maxzide, and Moduretic) as your *only* heart medication, you can benefit by increasing your consumption of fruits and vegetables, valuable sources of potassium, and by taking a supplemental source of potassium such as Slo-K. Large-scale surveys have found that potassium deficiencies are associated with cardiac arrhythmias, and at least for people who take hydrochlorothiazide, supplemental potassium can prevent arrhythmias.[6]

However, potassium supplements must be avoided by people who take potassium-sparing diuretics (amiloride, sprionolactone, or triamterene) or ACE inhibitors for blood pressure (benazepril, captopril, enalapril, fosinopril, lisinopril, moexipril, perindopril, quinapril, ramipril, or trandolapril). The combination of potassium supplements with these medications can produce incapacitating or even deadly arrhythmias. If you do not know whether your blood pressure medication is one of these drugs, ask your pharmacist before taking any potassium supplement.

CONCEPTS FOR COPING WITH CARDIAC ARRHYTHMIAS

○ Avoid caffeine. Many people are not sensitive to it, but some people can experience irregular heartbeats after drinking just 1 cup.[7]

Irritable Bowel Syndrome (IBS)

SYMPTOM SUMMARY

General symptoms IBS shares with other intestinal diseases:

○ Alternating constipation and diarrhea

○ Painful bowel movements

○ Undigested food in stool

Specific symptoms that distinguish IBS from other intestinal diseases:

○ Abdominal bloating

○ Feelings of incomplete defecation

○ Looser stools with onset of pain

○ More frequent bowel movements at onset of pain

○ Passage of mucus from the rectum

○ Relief of abdominal pain by defecation

Related terms include irritable colon, non-ulcer dyspepsia (irritable bowel syndrome may occur simultaneously with ulcers), spastic bowel, and spastic colon.

UNDERSTANDING THE DISEASE PROCESS

Irritable bowel syndrome (IBS) is a condition of chronic intestinal discomfort. IBS sufferers may experience lower abdominal pain, bloating, constipation alternating with diarrhea or frequent diarrhea, gas, mucus, urgent bowel movement, and a feeling of incomplete evacuation after a bowel movement. The symptoms of IBS usually remain below the waist. However, the condition may also cause difficulty swallowing, a sensation of a lump in the throat, acid indigestion, nausea, and chest pain.

According to the International Foundation for Functional Gastrointestinal Disorders, IBS affects between 25 and 55 million people in the United States. It results in 2.5 to 3.5 million yearly visits to physicians, and it affects men and women of all ages and of all races. The prevalence of IBS in the general population of Western countries varies from 6–22 percent. IBS affects 14–24 percent of women and 5–19 percent of men. The prevalence is similar in Caucasians and African-Americans, but appears to be lower in Hispanics.

Many IBS sufferers report that their symptoms began with a major life event: a death, a divorce, incarceration, or a financial crisis. Some IBS sufferers develop the disease after abdominal surgery or a bout with another intestinal disease. Recurrences of IBS sometimes occur after consumption of a food to which the IBS sufferer is sensitive. But while a flare-up of IBS may occur in response to any of these stimuli, it can also occur for no apparent reason at all.

IBS is not a "psychosomatic" illness. While many IBS sufferers understandably develop social anxieties after they develop a disease causing frequent diarrhea and flatulence, most IBS sufferers have normal psychological profiles before they develop the disease.[1] On the other hand, attitudes definitely affect the course of the disease. IBS sufferers who conceal aggressive tendencies are less likely to improve when given antidepressants.[2] IBS sufferers who have dissociative tendencies, that is, who are in a state of denial about traumatic events in their lives, are also more likely to suffer longer and more severe symptoms.[3] And people who suffer dysthymia, an affective disorder characterized by chronic mildly depressed or irritable moods often accompanied by other symptoms (such as eating and sleeping disturbances, fatigue, and poor self-esteem), are 33 times more likely to have IBS than people who do not.[4] This statistic, however, does not reveal whether IBS causes dysthymia or

dysthymia causes IBS. A large number of IBS sufferers spent their childhood years in privileged or wealthy homes. Higher socioeconomic standing is frequently associated with excessive cleanliness, which has been found in dozens of studies to predispose children growing up in those homes to developing allergies. IBS is also associated with childhood use of antibiotics.[5]

Since the exact causes of the condition are unclear, IBS falls into a category of diseases physicians call functional. This description means that, while the bowel obviously does not function properly, there is no obvious cause. People who have IBS tend to have other functional diseases, including:

- Chronic fatigue syndrome (CFS)
- Dysmenorrhea
- Fibromylagia syndrome (FMS)
- Irritable bladder syndrome
- Irritable bowel syndrome (IBS)
- Migraine headaches
- Multiple chemical sensitivity syndrome (MCSS)
- Myofascial pain syndrome (MPS)
- Periodic limb movement (PLMS)
- Restless leg syndrome (RLS)
- Temporomandibular joint disorder (TMJ)
- Tension headaches

The reason individuals can experience a wide range of symptoms from several disorders is not clear, but a person who has the symptoms of one disease on the list is likely to have symptoms from several diseases on the list.

On the other hand, IBS can be distinguished from other intestinal diseases. IBS differs from celiac disease in that people with celiac disease experience marked intestinal symptoms such as diarrhea and gas upon the consumption of foods that contain gluten, such as products made from wheat, oats, rye, and barley. When celiac disease sufferers eliminate food containing gluten, the symptoms disappear. IBS also differs from Crohn's disease or ulcerative colitis. In IBS there is no trace of blood in the stool, and no history of fever or chills.

IBS is not life threatening. It does not lead to Crohn's disease or colon cancer. IBS is, however, serious. IBS greatly diminishes quality of life. People with IBS are more likely to miss work, more likely to be placed in the hospital, and more likely to endure uncomfortable and embarrassing diagnostic procedures. The symptoms of

IBS fluctuate over time, but even 5 years after the first episode, 35 percent of IBS sufferers will continue to have the disease.[6]

TREATMENT SUMMARY

DIET

❍ Avoid dairy products if you are lactose intolerant. Avoid gas-producing vegetables such as beans, broccoli, cabbage, and lentils, and limit alcohol to at most 1–2 drinks a day.

❍ Avoid excessive consumption of fats. Symptoms may be eased just by eating smaller portions and avoiding butter, fatty meats, fried foods, margarine, and salad dressings.

❍ Increase fiber but not by taking bran. Eat 5–9 servings of fruits and vegetables daily or take *water-soluble* fiber supplements to ensure adequate fiber intake. Eat just enough fiber so that you have soft, easily passed, and painless bowel movements.

❍ Avoid products containing refined sugar.

❍ Avoid foods to which you are allergic.

NUTRITIONAL SUPPLEMENTS

❍ *Lactobacillus:* 1–2 billion live organisms daily.

❍ Quercetin (for relief of diarrhea symptoms): 250 milligrams 20 minutes before meals.

HERBS

❍ Peppermint oil: enteric-coated capsules, 0.2–0.4 milliliters twice a day between meals.

❍ Robert's Formula: as directed by the compounding pharmacist.

UNDERSTANDING THE HEALING PROCESS

Medical treatment for IBS consists mainly of increased dietary fiber plus drugs that calm the muscles that cause bowel spasm. However, doctors sometimes overlook other causes of IBS symptoms that are much easier to treat.

A percentage of patients labeled as having IBS in fact have an inability to digest fructose (corn syrup or fruit sugar), lactose (milk sugar), or sorbitol, a common "no-calorie" sweetener.[7] Before beginning any program of treatment for IBS, whether traditional or holistic, it is extremely useful to verify that the problem is not a failure to digest these ubiquitous sweetening agents. Try excluding fructose, lactose, and sorbitol from your diet for at least a week before beginning a treatment program for IBS.

It is important to understand that specific foods can exacerbate IBS symptoms, but they are not the sole cause of typical IBS symptoms. To determine which foods trigger which symptoms, it is necessary to start with a very basic, bland diet and gradually add a new food each day recording any symptoms associated with that particular food.

It is important to avoid overconsumption of fats. Eating causes contractions of the colon. This in turn usually causes an urge to have a bowel movement within 30–60 minutes after a meal. In people with IBS, the urge may come sooner with cramps and diarrhea. The urgency of the response is often related to the number of calories and, especially, the amount of fat in a meal. Fat in any form (animal or vegetable) is a strong stimulus of colonic contractions after a meal. Many foods contain fat, especially meats of all kinds, poultry skin, whole milk, cream, cheese, butter, vegetable oil, margarine, shortening, avocados, and whipped toppings.

Most treatment plans for IBS include increased consumption of fiber. Fiber is the part of plant food that is not digested. It adds bulk to the stools by absorbing water. There are two types of fiber, soluble and insoluble. Soluble fiber dissolves in water and is found in oat bran, barley, peas, beans, and citrus fruits. Insoluble fiber does not dissolve in water and is found in wheat bran and some vegetables. Fiber increases the transit time of the colon and decreases the pressures within the colon.

While fiber is almost universally recommended for IBS, the scientific evidence that it helps any symptom other than constipation is equivocal. In theory, high-fiber diets keep the colon mildly distended, which may help to prevent spasms from developing. A double-blind, placebo-controlled study of 28 IBS patients for 6 months found that *bran* does not always result in lighter stools, and even when it does, improvement in the full range of symptoms of IBS is unrelated to the effects of bran.[8] Diarrhea does not improve in response to bran. Constipation does improve in response to bran, but only because the stools are larger and pass through the gut more quickly, not because there are more trips to the bathroom.[9]

The reason studies do not find consistent results for the use of bran as a source of fiber is that bran can cause food allergies that aggravate IBS. Water-soluble fiber is likely to give better results.

Eating sugar raises blood sugar levels. When blood sugars are high, the central nervous system signals the digestive tract to absorb sugars more slowly.[10] This slows down the passage of food through the digestive tract, giving gas time to accumulate, and maximizes the amount of time irritating food allergens are in contact with the intestinal wall. Some naturopathic physicians speculate that sugar consumption is the most important contributing factor to IBS in most cases in the United States.[11]

Food allergies contribute to IBS symptoms suggestive of vascular instability, such as excessive sweating, fatigue, headaches, hyperventilation, and palpitations or racing pulse. They are also usually the culprit when flatulence and gas is a major symptom.[12] One study found that two-thirds of IBS sufferers have at least one food allergy, and many have more than one food allergy.[13] The most common allergies of IBS patients are dairy products (40–44 percent) and grains (40–60 percent).[14]

Clinical tests in Sweden have found taking supplemental *Lactobacillus* (not *acidophilus*) rapidly reduces gas production. Benefits are noticed in as little as 2–3 days.[15]

Quercetin was once known as "vitamin P," an essential cofactor for vitamin C. It has pharmacological actions very similar to those of cromolyn sodium, a common prescription medication for IBS. Quercetin stops the biological signals that tell mast cells to release histamine, the inflammatory agent in allergic reactions.[16] It also short-circuits a series of biochemical steps necessary for the formation of leukotrienes, slow-acting agents of inflammation.[17]

Quercetin interacts with a number of medications. It increases the toxicity of the cancer chemotherapy drug Platinol (cisplatin), the antirejection drug cyclosporine (Neoral, Sandimunne) given to transplant patients, and the high blood pressure medication nifedipine (Procardia). It competes for receptor sites and decreases the effectiveness of quinolone antibiotics, which include:

- ciprofloxacin (Cipro, Baycip, Cetraxal, Ciflox, Cifran, Ciplox, Cyprobay, Quintor)
- enoxacin (Penetrex)
- gatifloxacin (Tequin)
- gemifloxacin (a relatively new drug)
- grepafloxacin (Raxar)
- levofloxacin (Levaquin)

- lomefloxacin (Maxaquin)
- moxifloxacin (Avelox)
- norfloxacin (Amicrobin, Anquin, Baccidal, Barazan, Biofloxin, Floxenor, Fulgram, Janacin, Lexinor, Norofin, Noroxin, Norxacin, Orixacin, Oroflox, Urinox, Zoroxin)
- ofloxacin (Floxin)
- sparfloxacin (Zagam)
- temafloxacin (Omniflox)
- trovafloxacin (Trovan)

Peppermint oil is the best known and most effective natural treatment for IBS. Especially outside the United States, the medical profession recognizes the value of peppermint oil in that menthol, the principal active ingredient in peppermint oil, is a standard pre-treatment for stopping muscle spasms before they start in lower gastrointestinal diagnostic procedures such as endoscopy.[18]

Peppermint oil acts by stopping the absorption of sugar in the upper intestine.[19] This action helps keep blood sugars lower, and stops a series of physiological reactions that otherwise would slow down the passage of food through the intestine. Peppermint reduces abdominal pain, abdominal bloating, flatulence, frequency of trips to the bathroom, and boborygmus, or stomach rumbles. Peppermint oil is especially helpful in reducing the pain of IBS in children. A clinical trial at the University of Missouri found that 75 percent of children with IBS given peppermint oil capsules received relief of pain within 2 weeks.[20] Research in Germany has found that combinations of peppermint, caraway, fennel, and/or wormwood oils are also effective.

It is important to use peppermint oil in enteric-coated capsules, and to swallow them without chewing. The coating on the capsule ensures that the peppermint oil is not released until it reaches the intestine, where it is needed. Pure peppermint oil can cause belching or heartburn.

Robert's Formula is a combination of cabbage powder, *Echinacea angustifolia,* geranium, goldenseal, marshmallow root, slippery elm, and wild indigo. It is an old-time favorite of naturopathic physicians for the treatment of IBS. Cabbage normalizes the secretion of stomach acid.[21] *Echinacea angustifolia* is strongly anti-inflammatory. Geranium has an astringent action that causes proteins in the lining of the intestines to cross-link, healing ulcers.[22] Goldenseal contains berberine, which is also found in barberry and coptis. This natural antiseptic inhibits the growth of many disease-causing bacteria, including *Helicobacter pylori*, which infects the stomach.[23] The complex polysaccharides in marshmallow root stimulate phagocytosis, the immune process in which cells called macrophages engulf and neutralize infectious microorganisms. Slippery elm reinforces the actions of all the other herbs with its own soothing mucilage. Wild indigo, also known as baptisia, contains compounds that fight digestive infections and greatly increase the immune-stimulant effect of echinacea.

Health food stores carry Robert's Formula under many different labels. Take only 1–2 teaspoons of the mixture with ½ cup of water daily, to avoid overdosing echinacea.

CONCEPTS FOR COPING WITH IRRITABLE BOWEL SYNDROME

○ The Chinese herbal preparation Fang Feng Tong Sheng Tang (known in English as Ledebouriella Decoction that Sagely Unblocks) received headlines when an article in the *Journal of the American Medical Association* confirmed that it helps control symptoms of IBS. Not reported in the media, or in the medical journal, was that this formula is most useful in treating symptoms when constipation, not diarrhea, is the principle symptom.

○ To reduce gas, avoid smoking, chewing gum, excessive liquid intake, and carbonated drinks.

○ Stimulant laxatives, including herbal stimulant laxatives such as buckthorn, cascara sagrada, rhubarb root, and senna, tend to harm the bowel when taken over a long period of time. The nerves controlling the propulsion of stool become dependent on the stimulant. If a laxative is needed, osmotic laxatives like lactulose and sorbitol are preferable over stimulant laxatives.

○ Heating pads, hot baths, or hot drinks help to slow abdominal spasms and provide relief from abdominal pain. For patients with severe pain, it is common to take antidepressants. These are used to block the transmission of pain from the gut to the brain. The antidepressants doctors give for this purpose are usually prescribed in very low dosages and are in a class of drugs that are relatively inexpensive, usually less than $10 (total cost) for a month's supply.

○ Many people with IBS have a history of physical trauma or sexual abuse. This makes them more sensitive to body movements. Therapies to relieve post-traumatic stress will also relieve IBS.

Jaundice
See **Hepatitis A**.

Jellyfish Stings

SYMPTOM SUMMARY

○ Raised, red, painful, itching rash, usually limited to the area of skin in contact with the jellyfish

○ Symptoms last for days to weeks

○ Sting to the eyes can cause severe inflammation, redness, swelling, and tearing; abrasions to the lens can do permanent damage to sight

○ In rare instances, headaches, vomiting, muscle spasms, fever, chills, or shock

UNDERSTANDING THE DISEASE PROCESS

More than 100 species of jellyfish sting humans, causing reactions ranging from a mild itch to sudden death. The Portuguese man-of-war lives in the warm waters of the eastern coast of North America. This enormous creature can have tentacles up to 100 feet (33 meters) long that continue to release venom up to 2 weeks after they are detached from the jellyfish's main body. "True jellyfish" are smaller and much less toxic, with the exception of the box jellyfish found in the waters off the northern and eastern coasts of Australia. Stings from the box jellyfish can cause shock and even death. Sea corals, sea urchins, and sea anemones also release similar toxins, but serious complications from them are rare.

The jellyfish's stinger is triggered by contact (or transfer of the jellyfish to fresh water), bursting out of the tentacle like a jack-in-the-box. The stinger of even a small jellyfish possesses a terrific force; the jellyfish stores venom under an internal pressure of 150 atmospheres and the stinger's load of venom is released with a force of 40,000 G.[1] A sharp, hollow tube delivers venom to the skin, usually causing a mild sting. One type of jellyfish, the thimble jellyfish, releases eggs that can lodge in swimwear. A rash develops on the skin under swimwear 24 hours after contact and usually lasts about 5 days. This reaction is known as sea bather's eruption.

TREATMENT SUMMARY

○ Follow first-aid procedures listed below.

○ Vinegar: apply to the bite.

UNDERSTANDING THE HEALING PROCESS

The first step in treating a jellyfish sting is to remove the person receiving the sting from the water. In Australia, a jellyfish sting requires immediate emergency medical attention. In North America, simple first-aid measures are usually adequate.

It is very important to rinse a jellyfish sting in salt water or not to rinse it at all. The jellyfish tentacle swells in the presence of fresh water and releases additional venom. Applying vinegar (or urine) to the wound deactivates stingers that have not yet discharged and reduces the toxicity of venom on the skin.

The next step of treatment is to remove the stinger. Use tweezers or forceps and wear protective gloves, taking care not to come in contact with the stinger. Once the stinger is removed, it is important to keep the area of the body that was stung still, so that venom is not circulated further into the skin.

When these first-aid measures are completed, the only thing to do is to take pain relievers and wait for improvement. Shortness of breath, vomiting, or severe pain require medical attention.

CONCEPTS FOR COPING WITH JELLYFISH STINGS

○ Wearing a Lycra wetsuit can prevent stings.

○ Do not dive, swim, or surf where large numbers of jellyfish have been reported.

○ Do not touch live corals without gloves.

○ Stings from sea anemones, sea cucumbers, and sea urchins are also treated with vinegar. Although they do not usually produce a sting, they may cause a bizarrely shaped, painless rash several days after exposure.[2] The rash usually heals over the course of a few weeks.

○ Any jellyfish sting to the eyes, mouth, or genitals requires medical attention in addition to immediate first aid. Do not attempt to remove a stinger from the eyes unless you are a medical professional.

Jet Lag

SYMPTOM SUMMARY

○ Constipation

○ Early awakening or insomnia

○ Fatigue

○ Headache, fuzzy thinking

○ Irritability

○ Reduced immunity

UNDERSTANDING THE DISEASE PROCESS

Jet lag is a condition of desynchronization of the biological clock regulating the body and the outside world. It is caused by drastic changes in the sleep-wake cycle. While jet lag is most commonly associated with travelers journeying east to west, artificial jet lag can be induced by working night shifts, working rotating shifts, or by staying up all night. Artificial jet lag is a special problem of physician-interns, management trainees for 24-hour businesses, soldiers under battle-alert conditions, and persons who live in disaster areas.

TREATMENT SUMMARY

SUPPLEMENTS

○ Melatonin: 3 milligrams, taken at your normal bedtime *on arrival* (if traveling) or *when you resume day shifts*. Do not take melatonin late at night after staying up late. Gradually reduce dosage to 1 milligram or less if you do not have trouble sleeping, discontinuing after 1 week.

UNDERSTANDING THE HEALING PROCESS

The Argonne jet-lag diet (see inset) has been used for over 20 years, but the evidence in support of it is largely anecdotal. Although many travelers (including the author of this book) can confirm from personal experience that it works, more travelers opt for melatonin and/or prescription drugs.

Melatonin has been clinically tested for treating jet lag. A 1986 study of 17 travelers flying from San Fran-

The Argonne National Laboratory Recommends a 3-Day Diet for Reducing Jet Lag

1. Determine what the breakfast time will be at the destination on the day of arrival. You will break your final fast (see below) at the destination breakfast time.

2. Alternate eating to a pattern of feast-fast-feast-fast 3 days before departure as follows:

   - Three days before departure, feast. Eat as much as you want of a high-protein breakfast and lunch and a high-carbohydrate dinner. No coffee except between 2 and 5 P.M.

   - Two days before departure, fast except for light meals of salads, light soups, fruits, and juices. No coffee except between 3 and 5 P.M.

   - The day before departure, feast again.

   - On the departure day, fast. Going west, you only need to fast half the day.

3. Breaking the Final Fast

   - Westbound: if you drink caffeinated beverages, take them the morning before departure.

   - Eastbound: take any caffeinated beverages between 6 and 11 P.M. If the flight is long enough, sleep until destination breakfast time. Wake up and feast, beginning with a high-protein breakfast.

   - Turn lights on. Stay awake and active.

At your travel destination:

   - Feast on high-protein breakfasts and lunches to stimulate the body's active cycle.

   - Suitable foods include steak, eggs, hamburgers, high-protein cereals, and green beans.

   - Feast on high-carbohydrate suppers to stimulate sleep. They include spaghetti and other pastas (but no meatballs), crepes (but no meat fillings), potatoes, other starchy vegetables, and sweet desserts.

Before your return home, repeat the process with special attention to fast days. Fast days help deplete the liver's store of carbohydrates and prepare the body's clock for resetting for the return trip. Suitable foods include fruit, light soups, broths, skimpy salads, unbuttered toast, or half pieces of bread. On these days, keep calories and carbohydrates to a minimum.

---

cisco to London (8 time zones away) found that the 8 subjects who took 5 milligrams of melatonin experienced essentially no symptoms while the 9 travelers given a placebo experienced noteworthy symptoms.[1] Most people sleep well with melatonin, and wake up the next morning with few symptoms of jet lag, although most will have some fatigue from the flight itself. More recently, the U.S. Army conducted studies in the use of melatonin in preventing jet lag in aviation personnel in rapid deployments overseas, and confirmed that melatonin greatly reduces sleep disturbance and increases proficiency in task performance. The U.S. Army study used a relatively high dosage of melatonin, 10 milligrams.[2] At least 10 other studies report similar results.

With melatonin and other drugs for reestablishing body rhythms, timing is critical. The pineal gland produces melatonin at night. Taking melatonin is a signal to the pineal gland that it is night, so taking melatonin during the day can induce artificial jet lag. Early clinical studies rejected melatonin as a sleep aid, noting that users were less alert, more sleepy, and had more sluggish reaction times, but these findings resulted from giving the supplement to the test subjects during the day.[3]

The prescription drug zolpidem (Ambien) is more effective than melatonin in controlling jet lag, but is more likely to produce side effects, including nausea, vomiting, and confusion.[4]

CONCEPTS FOR COPING WITH JET LAG

O Cocculus is the standard homeopathic remedy for jet lag.

Kanner's Syndrome
See Autism.

Kidney Stones

SYMPTOM SUMMARY

○ Excruciating, radiating pain originating in the flank or kidney

○ Nausea, vomiting, abdominal swelling

○ Chills, fever, and frequent urination when there is infection

UNDERSTANDING THE DISEASE PROCESS

Kidney stones are sharp and irregular precipitates of minerals from the urine. They pass down the slender tube leading from the kidney to the bladder, and from the bladder to the urethra, following the path urine uses to exit the body. Small stones may pass unnoticed, but larger stones cause excruciating pain.

Most kidney stones are composed of calcium and oxalic acid. These chemicals normally stay dissolved in the urine, but when urinary output is greatly reduced, when the urine loses its acidity, or when the chemicals are released into the urine in very large quantities, tiny crystals may precipitate out of the urine and begin to form stones. Sometimes infectious microorganisms such as *Proteus* serve as a framework for developing kidney stones. Calcium oxalate tends to precipitate out of the urine first. Small brown or black stones that look like seeds or berries form when the urine is slightly alkaline. Urine that is more alkaline causes calcium phosphate to crystallize along with calcium oxalate. Stones formed from these chemicals are lighter and tend to form "horns." Extremely alkaline urine forms crystals of magnesium ammonium phosphate, light brown stones with a painful "staghorn" well known to anyone who has suffered the condition. The urine can also form small, elliptical, translucent stones from uric acid, and stones with a "cut" appearance from cysteine.

Kidney stones are common. Up to 15 percent of men and 6 percent of all women will develop at least one stone, with recurrence in about half these people.[1] Medical science is only beginning to understand why some people develop stones and others do not. In the United States, women are more likely to develop stones if they have a history of high blood pressure, if they have not used calcium supplements, and if their diets are low in magnesium-rich foods such as beans, broccoli, nuts and seeds (especially peanuts), soy, and leafy green veg-

etables.[2] Women whose sisters develop kidney stones are more likely to develop kidney stones themselves if their urine is high in calcium and unusually alkaline.[3] Making urine more alkaline by using cranberry extract tablets is a risk factor for kidney stones in women.[4] Men are more likely to develop stones if they have uncontrolled high blood pressure.[5] Men whose brothers have kidney stones are more likely to develop kidney stones as they grow older and if their urine potassium levels are low or their urine calcium levels are high.[6] Children on extremely high-fat diets are at risk of kidney stones unless they consume adequate amounts of fluid.[7]

TREATMENT SUMMARY

DIET

○ Drink 8–10 glasses of water daily.

NUTRITIONAL SUPPLEMENTS

○ GLA (gamma-linolenic acid): up to 10 grams per day.

○ Inositol nicotinate: 4 grams (eight 500-milligram capsules) daily, or $1/2$ ounce of rice bran, daily.

○ Potassium-magnesium citrate: dosage should be chosen in consultation with a physician.

○ Vitamin B_6 (pyridoxine): 50 milligrams 3 times per day.

UNDERSTANDING THE HEALING PROCESS

The simplest yet most essential task in preventing kidney stones is drinking enough water. Adequate hydration helps ensure that the volume of urine will be enough to dissolve the minerals that can cause stones. Some other beverages are also helpful. Survey data collected by the Harvard School of Public Health shows that consuming 1 cup (240 milliliters) of coffee daily (regular or decaffeinated) reduces the risk of kidney stones by 10 percent, the same amount of tea by 14 percent, beer by 21 percent, and wine by 39 percent. (The data do not show that drinking large quantities of any of these beverages eliminates the risk of kidney stones). Juices tend to be harmful. The same survey also found that drinking a cup of apple juice daily increased the risk of developing kidney stones possibly by 75 percent, and drinking a cup of grapefruit juice daily increased the risk of kidney stones by as much as 85 percent.[8] While using cranberry juice tablets increases the risk of kidney stones in women, no study has found that cranberry juice itself increases the risk of kidney stones.

Since most stones are made of calcium, it would seem logical that reducing dietary calcium would reduce the risk of stones. Reducing consumption of calcium-rich foods does reduce the amount of calcium in the urine, but it increases the amount of the other component of most kidney stones, oxalate. Rather than reducing the risk of stones, a low-calcium diet nearly doubles the risk of recurrent kidney stones, at least in men.[9] Even taking calcium supplements, *in the form of calcium citrate*, does not increase the risk of kidney stones.[10]

Similarly, since most kidney stones contain oxalate, it would seem logical to limit consumption of foods that are high in oxalic acid, such as almonds, beet greens, bran, chocolate, rhubarb, spinach, strawberries, and tea. No study, however, has found that restricting consumption of these foods increases the risk of kidney stones, and some studies have found that consumption of leafy green vegetables, peanuts, and tea actually reduce the risk of kidney stones. The vitamin K in leafy green vegetables may be one reason vegetarians have a lower incidence of kidney stones.

Consumption of animal protein is likewise an accepted risk factor for kidney stones, but clinical testing has found that only about one-third of people who get kidney stones are adversely affected by a high-protein diet.[11] It seems sensible to avoid excessive consumption of meat, but severe protein restriction probably will not help.

The latest and most useful nutritional supplement for treating kidney stones is potassium-magnesium citrate. A 3-year study found that taking this supplement reduced the risk of recurrent kidney stones by a whopping 80 percent.[12] The initial dosage of the supplement, however, must be chosen in consultation with a physician. Supplements containing potassium have the potential to raise blood levels of potassium too high, primarily in people with impaired kidneys. Potassium supplements reduce the effectiveness of antibiotics (especially those used to treat bladder infections), aspirin, lithium, and oral diabetes medications. They can increase bloodstream concentrations of amphetamines, methamphetamines, and ephedrine to toxic levels. You must consult with a physician before taking potassium-magnesium citrate with any of these medications.

Other supplements that are not as helpful as potassium-magnesium citrate, are still beneficial. Inositol nicotinate, derived from rice bran, greatly reduces the rate at which calcium forms crystals in the urine.[13] It is likely that the inositol content in bran explains its long-known effectiveness in treating kidney stones.

There is a possibility that taking substantially more than the recommended dose of inositol could result in flushing, itching, dizziness, palpitations, and a "sugar rush." Inositol nicotinate has only recently been introduced to the market in the United States. However, in the 30 years it has been used in Europe, adverse reactions have been very rare. You may substitute $1/2$ ounce of rice bran for inositol if adverse symptoms occur.

Vitamin B_6 may reduce the risk of kidney stones in women. A study of 85,557 women by the Harvard School of Public Health found that women consuming the greatest amount of the vitamin had risk reduced by approximately one-third.[14] A study of 45,251 men by the Harvard School of Public Health found that consuming vitamin B_6 reduced risk of kidney stones by approximately 10 percent.[15] Since vitamin B_{12} is possibly linked to increased risk of kidney stones, it is best to use a B_6 supplement rather than a complete B vitamin.

A number of herbs are approved for the treatment of kidney stones in Germany, including asparagus, birch leaf, bishop's weed fruit, couch grass, goldenrod, horsetail, lovage, petasites, shiny restharrow, and stinging nettle (a combination of the leaf and root). These herbs increase urination and may be of some value in the long-term prevention of kidney stones and urinary tract infections. The herb khella is well known for its ability to relax the ureter and allow a stone to pass, but it has to be taken during an acute attack. Ruta graveolens (gravel root), peucedanum, leptotania, and hydrangea are similarly useful during an acute attack. Aloe latex (aloe taken by mouth in a capsule form) bind calcium and may prevent stones, but it also has a potent laxative effect.

CONCEPTS FOR COPING WITH KIDNEY STONES

○ Mineral water is helpful for people who have kidney stones. It reduces concentrations of both calcium oxalate and uric acid.[16]

○ Drink lemonade rather than orange juice. Some physicians recommend citrus juices for preventing kidney stones. As noted above, citrus juices are typically harmful. Drinking citrus juices acidifies the urine, making minerals more soluble, and increases levels of citrate, which keeps oxalate from combining with calcium.

However, it also increases production of oxalate, enough that the overall effect is to increase the production of calcium oxalate stones. The only citrus juice that may be helpful and has not been found to be harmful is lemon juice, which contains five times the content of citrate found in other citrus juices.

○ Women (and men) who have calcium oxalate stones (stones without "horns") are at special risk of developing osteoporosis if they consume a high-salt diet.[17]

○ If you take vitamin C, be sure to drink 8–10 glasses of water daily. While taking 1,500 milligrams of supplemental vitamin C daily substantially reduces the risk of kidney stones,[18] taking vitamin C while dehydrated can cause formation of kidney stones in just a few days.[19]

Knee Pain

SYMPTOM SUMMARY

○ Persistent pain, inflammation, and/or swelling in the knee

UNDERSTANDING THE DISEASE PROCESS

Knee pain is a common problem among runners and regular participants in sports that involve running. The kneecap (patella) moves up and down in a shallow groove at the lower end of the thigh bone (femur). It is connected on top to the quadriceps from the front of the upper leg. It is connected below to the lower leg bone, or tibia, by a narrow band of fibrous tissue known as the patellar tendon.

Regular running can cause the surface of the kneecap to become rough and irritated where it fits into a narrow groove of the thigh bone. Vigorous exercise or overweight can cause degeneration of the cartilage in the knee joint where the upper leg (femur) and lower leg bone (tibia) join. Either form of degeneration can cause chronic and sometimes intense knee pain. The condition of irritation of the undersurface of the kneecap is known as patellofemoral syndrome or chondromalacia.

TREATMENT SUMMARY

Take any one *of the following for relief of pain:*

NUTRITIONAL SUPPLEMENTS

○ SAM-e: 400 milligrams 3 times a day.

HERBS

○ Boswellic acids: 400 milligrams per day.

○ Capsaicin cream: apply to the knee daily. If you are sensitive to capsaicin, substitute diluted essential oils of peppermint, eucalyptus, rosemary, or wintergreen.

○ Devil's claw (as an alternative to aspirin or NSAIDs): 405–520 milligrams up to 8 times a day.

○ Willow bark (as an alternative to aspirin or NSAIDs): 1 teaspoon in a cup of hot water or tea, as desired.

○ Yucca (leaf): 2–4 grams (1–2 teaspoons) per day.

If you use aspirin or NSAIDs on a regular basis, take:

○ DGL (Deglycyrrhizinated licorice): chew and swallow 1–2 380-milligram tablets of DGL 20 minutes before meals, 3 times a day.

See Part Three if you take prescription medication.

Causes of Knee Pain

- Patellofemoral syndrome
- Blood disorders, such as sickle-cell anemia or hemophilia (very rare)
- Chronic infection, parasites (very rare)
- Irritation of the patellar tendon (jumper's knee)
- Osgood-Schlatter's disease ("growing pains," most common in teenagers)
- Rheumatoid arthritis
- Scar tissue

Knee pain is made worse by:

- Downhill running
- Flat feet
- Inadequate cushioning in footwear, pounding shocks absorbed during hiking, jogging, or running
- Knock knees
- Overweight
- Weak front and inner thigh muscles

UNDERSTANDING THE HEALING PROCESS

Treating knee pain is important for preserving the strength of the knee, especially in older adults.[1] Older persons with arthritis in the knee and younger persons with chondromalacia who do not treat knee pain can find they experience "slippage" or "giving way" of their knees during activities such as walking, stair climbing, or standing from a sitting position. The degeneration of the knee resulting from disuse after failure to treat knee pain can end recreational activity, interfere with work, or even cause a person to lose the ability to walk.[2]

A number of alternative healing techniques are clinically demonstrated to be effective in treating knee pain. Frequent exposure to cold (such as working in a cold storage room) increases knee pain,[3] but ice packs are universally recommended for treating injury and swelling to the knee. (Not everyone benefits from applying ice packs to the knee. Use other methods if applying ice increases rather than decreases pain.) Numerous reports confirm that transcutaneous electrical stimulation (TENS) relieves knee pain, but it is important to start at the lowest setting and gradually increase the voltage applied to the knee.

Clinical studies at Holcomb HealthCare Services in Nashville, Tennessee, and University of Texas Medical Branch in Galveston have found that magnets begin to reduce knee pain in as little as 1 hour and increase mobility and flexibility of the knee. In the University of Texas study, 2 participants reported that after 2 weeks of treatment with the magnets they could walk without using a cane. One participant in the UT study was able to resume running and surfing. Many participants noted decreased pain at night and less stiffness in the morning.[4] Thick magnets imbedded in ceramics or neodymium are more effective than thin magnets imbedded in plastic or rubber. Magnets that are strong enough to relieve pain sometimes cause mild tingling sensations. The best magnets are labeled as having a field of at least 300 gauss or 0.8–1.0 Tesla.

SAM-e, best known for treatment of depression, also relieves pain. Various studies have found SAM-e as good or better for pain relief as Advil, Motrin, Naprosyn, and Nuprin. A study involving 20,641 people with osteoarthritis of the finger, hip, knee, and spine found that SAM-e alone was as effective as their ordinary pain relievers.[5] Another study involving 734 subjects found that it was more effective than Naprosyn (naproxen sodium).

The advantage of SAM-e is that it very seldom causes side effects. In the longest-running study involving the supplement, various minor side effects occurred in 20 out of 97 patients from time to time during the first 18 months of the intervention. In the final 6 months of the study, however, no patients experienced any side effects from SAM-e. Patients received relief of morning stiffness, pain at rest, and pain on movement, and depression.[6]

Although herbal treatments for knee pain are not especially well documented, several herbs are likely to be helpful if used on an occasional basis. Animal studies show that boswellic acid extracts (produced from the Ayurvedic herb guggul) stop inflammation, increase glycosaminoglycan synthesis, and improve blood flow to joints.[7] When used at a dosage of 400 milligrams per day, there are no reported side effects from this product. The Ayurvedic formula Yogaraj Guggulu has the same effect.

Both boswellic acids and Yogaraj Guggulu alter the body's production of thyroid hormone, and should be avoided by people who have Graves' disease or hyperthyroidism. They also should be avoided by persons taking beta-blockers, especially propanolol (Inderal, Inderide), or calcium channel blockers, especially diltiazem (Cardizem), for high blood pressure, since either product can make these drugs less available to the body.[8]

Capsaicin, devil's claw, and willow bark offer pain relief. Capsaicin is the chemical that gives hot peppers their heat. As anyone who has cooked with chiles knows, capsaicin can cause burning, redness, and inflammation, especially to the eyes and mouth. The first time capsaicin cream is applied to the skin over a painful knee, it causes these symptoms, but the nerve fibers serving the back of the leg become insensitive to it—and to knee pain.[9]

Capsaicin works best when there is good circulation to the skin to which it is applied.[10] Do not apply capsaicin to your legs if you have diabetes, and never apply capsaicin to ulcerated skin. It is also important to keep capsaicin out of your nose and eyes. Allergic reactions to the herb are rare but are not unknown, and there have been cases of hypothermia in people who used capsaicin in an especially cold room. It is theoretically possible that capsaicin absorbed into the bloodstream could reduce the bioavailability of aspirin; if you use capsaicin, use pain relievers other than aspirin.

Devil's claw relieves knee pain, but only if it is taken in an enteric-coated form that protects its analgesic compounds from being digested in the stomach. Do not use devil's claw with NSAIDs such as aspirin and Tylenol and avoid it entirely if you have duodenal or gastric ulcers.

Willow bark is a natural substitute for aspirin. It contains a less potent pain reliever than the salicylates found in aspirin that does not generally cause bleeding or stomach irritation. Do not use willow bark during pregnancy, if you have tinnitus (ringing in the ears), or if you are allergic to aspirin. Do not give willow bark or aspirin to children who have colds or flu.

Natural health experts Dr. Michael Murray and Dr. Joseph Pizzorno suggest that yucca reduces inflammation in various forms of joint pain through a unique pathway, stopping the production of bacterial toxins in the intestines. They base their suggestion on the scientific observation that bacterial endotoxins stop proteoglycan synthesis, and that yucca contains natural soaps that break up the fat components of the bacterial endotoxins.[11] Although research has not yet confirmed their theory, many sufferers of osteoarthritis report that yucca seems to help if it is used over a period of several months.

CONCEPTS FOR COPING WITH KNEE PAIN

❍ A dull ache is not usually a problem, but a sharp pain in the knee requires that you rest it until the pain stops. Squatting and going down stairs are the most frequent causes of knee pain.

❍ Wearing a bandage around the knee can prevent swelling. Make sure the bandage is not so tight that it cuts off circulation. Your doctor may prescribe a brace or support to help keep the kneecap in the track or groove.

❍ Ice is frequently recommended for knee pain but it does not always help.

❍ Sports that are easy on the knees include walking, slow jogging, swimming (with a flutter kick), and cross-country skiing. Cycling on hills, baseball, hockey, and downhill skiing may cause problems for some people. Basketball, football, racquetball, running (especially sprints and running on hills), soccer, and squash frequently result in knee injuries.

❍ If you suffer chronic knee pain, you should not do full arc extension exercises, bending your leg to a 90-degree angle with a weight at the ankle. Older persons with knee pain should avoid knee exercises of any kind until a medical examination has confirmed osteoporosis and resulting bone loss are not a problem. With physician approval, useful knee exercises include:

• Hamstring stretch:

• *Sitting.* Sit on the floor. With your back straight, lean forward from the hip and reach down over your leg until you begin to feel your muscles stretch. Hold for 10 seconds and relax.

• *Standing.* Prop up the injured leg with the knee locked. Bend standing leg slightly. Place hands on lower thigh just above the knee. With your back straight, bend forward from the hip until you begin to feel a stretch under your thigh. Hold for 10 seconds and relax.

• Single quadriceps stretch:

• *Standing.* With your back straight, pull your foot back until you feel your thigh muscle gently stretch. Slowly and gently push down and back with your knee. Hold for 15 seconds and relax. Discontinue if you feel pain.

❍ Proteolytic enzymes relieve pain and swelling when taken after surgery. A double-blind, placebo-controlled trial of 80 individuals undergoing knee surgery found that treatment with mixed proteolytic enzymes after surgery significantly improved mobility and decreased swelling.[12] Take bromelain *or* papain *or* chymotrypsin, in dosages recommended on the product label, with a glass of water. Since proteolytic enzymes can reduce blood-clotting factors, they should not be taken *before* surgery.

Kwashiorkor

SYMPTOM SUMMARY

❍ Medical examination of the infant will detect an enlarged liver and low levels of albumin in the blood

❍ Fatigue, lethargy, and irritability, *followed by*

❍ "Chubby cheeks" or "sugar baby" appearance, occurring *with* swelling in the arms and legs without skin changes, *followed by*

❍ Thin arms and legs and enlarged belly, *followed by*

❍ Blistering with appearance of flaky paint across the child's body

UNDERSTANDING THE DISEASE PROCESS

Kwashiorkor is a disease of protein, fatty acid, and zinc deficiency in infants and young children. The term "kwashiorkor" comes from a Kwa language spoken along the coast of the African nation of Ghana and means "sad child." Children developing kwashiorkor may receive adequate or even excessive calories, but lack of other nutrients causes slow starvation. Failure to treat the condition eventually results in shock, coma, and death, but even infants who are successfully treated after the disease has progressed to the skin-blistering stage suffer permanent physical and mental deficits. Specific micronutrient deficiencies cause complications; vitamin A deficiency is a factor in pneumonia, and selenium deficiency can cause heart failure.[1]

Children in the United States, United Kingdom, Canada, Australia, and other developed nations are not immune to kwashiorkor. Hundreds of cases have been reported in the United States alone. While kwashiorkor can result from child abuse, it is more often the case that parents of babies with kwashiorkor are well educated and conscientious, providing the child with regular medical care. The condition most often occurs when parents replace mother's milk or formula with sugar water, rice, or rice cereal, usually to treat diarrhea or eczema, on the presumption that the child is allergic to cow's milk.[2] Well-meaning parents simply do not know to offer their child additional protein. Kwashiorkor also occasionally occurs in older children of less nutritionally astute parents who are allowed to subsist on chips and sodas.

TREATMENT

NUTRITIONAL SUPPLEMENTS

❍ Baby formula containing amino acids, essential fatty acids, and zinc as part of a balanced blend of micronutrients in every serving.

UNDERSTANDING THE HEALING PROCESS

If you believe your infant or small child may be malnourished, seek a doctor's advice. There are many causes of malnutrition that cannot be treated just by improving the child's diet.

Kwashiorkor is completely correctable if it is treated in the "chubby cheeks" stage, and intervention at any stage can result in a greatly improved future life for your child. Any formula containing at least 10 percent fat and 12 percent protein is adequate to correct symptoms. Improvement is usually noticeable in a week and recovery usually occurs in 6 weeks if treatment is begun early enough. Pregestimil and Ultracare are among the most frequently used brands of formula for feeding babies with protein deficiency.

CONCEPTS FOR COPING WITH KWASHIORKOR

❍ Breastfeeding is best for the baby, but if mother's milk is not available and you suspect your infant has milk allergies or gluten sensitivity, consider a balanced milk substitute such as Ultracare. Although it has a rice milk base, it contains essential fatty acids and micronutrients necessary for the child's normal growth. It only contains enough protein, however, to prevent, not treat, protein deficiency.

❍ Vegan diets for infants are possible, but require careful planning. During the first 6 months of life, mother's milk is essential. Soy milk should not be used as the primary beverage for the child until after the first birthday. Soy and other protein sources can be introduced at 7 or 8 months. Breastfed vegan infants may need supplements of vitamin B_{12} if the mother's diet is inadequate; older infants may need zinc supplements and reliable sources of iron and vitamins D and B_{12}.

❍ Kwashiorkor, being rare in the United States, is sometimes confused with other deficiency diseases, such as zinc deficiency (as in acrodermatitis enteropathica), fatty acid deficiency (caused by cystic fibrosis or intestinal inflammation), or biotin deficiency (caused by a hereditary condition in which the child lacks an enzyme). Giving a child with kwashiorkor supplements to treat these conditions will help, but symptoms will persist. When there is a question whether the condition could be kwashiorkor, giving all necessary nutrients is the best approach.

Lactation, Insufficient

SYMPTOM SUMMARY

❍ Failure of breastfed baby to gain weight on a biweekly basis

UNDERSTANDING THE DISEASE PROCESS

Insufficient lactation is a relatively uncommon condition in which a nursing mother is not able to produce enough milk to feed her baby. This usually occurs during the first 6 weeks after birth. Reduced milk supply may result from an insufficient number of feedings, limiting length of feedings, or improper positioning at the breast. It can also be related to premature delivery, diabetes,[1] or obesity.[2]

A small number of women who do not produce enough breast milk have an insufficient amount of milk-producing tissue, sometimes as a result of breast reduction. Some medications, such as antihistamines, birth control pills, and sedatives, decrease the milk supply. Excessive caffeine (over 5 cups of coffee a day), fatigue, and smoking may cause poor milk ejection reflex, the release of breast milk in response to the baby's suckle.

Babies may also play a part in insufficient feeding. A baby with a short or tight frenulum (the tissue anchoring the tongue to the floor of the mouth) may not be able to nurse properly until the frenulum stretches on its own over time.

Regular monitoring of the nursing infant's weight by a health professional is essential to ensure the child is adequately fed. In rare cases, dehydration and even death of the child has resulted from insufficient feeding.

TREATMENT SUMMARY

DIET

❍ Avoid fava beans, miso, and yogurt.

HERBS

❍ Cabbage leaves: hold fresh cabbage leaves (placing them in the brassiere or under a loosely taped strip of gauze) to the breast to relieve inflammation.

❍ Fennel: 100–600 milligrams of encapsulated herb, up to 3 times daily.

❍ Fenugreek: 2–4 610-milligram capsules daily.

❍ Milk thistle: 70–210 milligrams 3 times daily.

Do not take:

❍ Chaste tree fruit *(agnus castus)*, garlic, or goat's rue.

See Part Three if you take prescription medication.

UNDERSTANDING THE HEALING PROCESS

Breastfed babies have fewer illnesses, fewer doctor visits, and fewer hospitalizations.[3] They have less frequent ear, gastrointestinal, and respiratory infections due to antibodies transferred from mother to child through breast milk.[4] Breastfeeding also decreases the risk of juvenile

diabetes,[5] Crohn's disease,[6] and lymphoma.[7] It enhances the emotional bond that develops between mother and child. However, only 60 percent of mothers in the United States breastfeed their children at all, and only 20 percent breastfeed for 6 months or more.[8] One of the most important reasons many women do not nurse their babies is fear of not producing enough milk.

For most women, this concern is unfounded. The more milk is removed from the breasts through breastfeeding or milk expression, the more milk the breasts make. The problem is not that the mother does not have enough milk, but that the baby does not get the milk that the mother has. Women who give 8–12 breastfeedings in a 24-hour period usually produce enough milk,[9] but women who skip feedings or who do not feed long enough may not make enough milk.

Ten to 20 minutes is usually enough time for a baby to feed. Eight to 12 feedings a day is normal. When a baby is breastfed often enough and long enough but still fails to gain weight, the problem may be improper positioning. A baby who is well positioned at the breast will:

• Open mouth wide like a yawn,

• Touch the breast with cheeks, chin, and nose,

• Touch the breast with chest and head,

• Turn lips out like a fish.

A baby who is well fed will:

• Gain 4–8 ounces (250–500 grams) a week after the first week,

• Get back to birth weight within 14 days,

• Have at least 3 stools and 3 wet diapers during the first 3 days, and at least 4 stools and 6 wet diapers a day during the next 4 weeks,

• Lose less than 7 percent of birth weight the first 5–7 days,

• Show contentment after breastfeedings,

• Stay active and alert between breastfeedings,

• Swallow while breastfeeding.

Relatively few foods have a direct influence on the production of breast milk. Fava beans increase the brain's production of dopamine and in turn inhibit the production of prolactin, the hormone that stimulates milk production. Consumption of very large quantities of miso or yogurt could supply enough of the amino acids L-phenylalanine and L-tyrosine to have a similar effect. Avoid these foods if you fail to produce enough milk for breastfeeding.

There is disagreement in the scientific community over whether cabbage leaves can relieve breast irritation, but many mothers report that they work. *People's Pharmacy* talk show hosts Joe and Terry Graedon speculate that compounds called isothiocyanates in cabbage leaves are responsible for this effect.

Fennel is used in European herbal medicine as a galactagogue, a stimulant to milk production. Its effects on lactation have not been scientifically documented, but the calming influence of some of its chemical constituents on the digestive tract has been documented in several studies.

Fennel oil and fennel seed teas are of similar therapeutic value, but undiluted fennel seed oil can cause intestinal inflammation. Never give fennel seed oil to an infant.

Fenugreek has been used since 1500 B.C. as a galactagogue. Despite centuries of use, evidence that it actually increases lactation is only anecdotal, but abundant. Fenugreek capsules are preferred to fenugreek teas, which can have a bitter aftertaste.

When you are taking the right dosage of fenugreek, your sweat and urine will smell like maple syrup. Too much fenugreek can cause diarrhea, which goes away when the herb is discontinued. The dosages of the herb recommended to encourage lactation are much lower than the dosages recommended for other applications.

Fenugreek can cause uterine contractions, and so should not be used by women who are pregnant. Diabetic mothers should use fenugreek with caution since it can lower blood sugar levels. Fenugreek poultices are sometimes used externally to ease inflammation, but should not be used on the breasts by nursing mothers, since they will leave a bitter taste for the baby.

As its name suggests, milk thistle is another traditional remedy for insufficient milk production. No scientific studies back up centuries of practical experience with this application of the herb. It is extraordinarily nontoxic, however, and has many beneficial effects on the liver. (For additional information, see HEPATITIS C.)

Chaste tree fruit is a traditional remedy for missed periods. It has been used to relieve the pain of mastodynia (pain in the breasts) associated with nursing. The problem with using chaste tree fruit to treat breast pain is that it stops the production of breast milk. Women

who have problems producing enough breast milk should not use it at all.

Unlike other herbs, garlic has been scientifically studied for its use as a galactagogue. The study found that colicky babies nursed longer when mothers took garlic, although they did not take in more milk. After several exposures to garlic-flavored breast milk, nursing times were diminished.[10] This would result in the baby taking less milk.

Goat's rue tinctures have found favor among some lactation consultants as a stimulant to milk production. There is no organized scientific research supporting their use as a galactagogue, however, and, like fenugreek, they can lower blood sugars in diabetic mothers.

CONCEPTS FOR COPING WITH INSUFFICIENT LACTATION

○ The Chinese herbal remedies Three Treasures (a variation of Xiao Yao San powder) and Women's Treasure (a variation of Yue Ju Wan pill), their names not to be confused with similar-sounding brand names, are ancient formulas modified to stimulate milk production in nursing mothers who may have had difficulties nursing in the first few days after birth. These and other herbal formulas are available from practitioners of Traditional Chinese Medicine.

○ The acupressure points for stimulating lactation are about a finger's width directly below the eyes on a line with the pupils when the eyes are fixed looking straight ahead. Gently stimulating this area for 5–10 minutes several times a day is thought to disperse toxins associated with infection and emotional stress and to increase the flow of milk. Massaging the clavicle directly above the midline of the breasts is also helpful.

○ It is not normal for breastfeeding to hurt. Some tenderness during the first few days is relatively common, but pain that is more than mild is usually due to the baby latching on improperly. A new onset of pain that occurs after nursing for several weeks is usually a sign of mastitis (see MASTITIS).

○ Washing the nipples before breastfeeding is unnecessary and depletes breast skin of protective oils. Breast milk protects the baby against infection.

○ Avoid giving a baby water and supplements during the first 4 weeks of life. Supplements can confuse the baby and limit breast milk production.

○ Breastfeed as long as the baby wants on the first breast before offering the second breast. When the baby stops suckling and swallowing or falls asleep at the first breast, break the suction, burp and wake the baby, and offer the second breast. If necessary, express by hand or pump the second breast to relieve fullness.

○ If the baby does not wake at least 8–12 times every 24 hours during the first 4 weeks of life, watch for early signs of hunger, such as wiggling, finger sucking, lip smacking, coughing, or yawning. Offer a breast at those times.

○ If other measures fail, your doctor may recommend a nasal spray of oxytocin to stimulate milk production.

○ The best way to offer expressed breast milk, formula, water, or glucose water with added colostrum (the latter usually offered when a baby is 1–2 days old) is with a lactation aid, a container with a long, thin tube to be slipped into the baby's mouth after he or she has begun nursing at the breast. Lactation aids avoid the use of artificial nipples, and prevent the baby's becoming "bottle spoiled" or "nipple confused," not wanting to nurse naturally. Lactation aids are not inexpensive, costing about as much as 2 weeks-worth of formula, but may reduce cost in the long run by keeping the baby interested in breastfeeding and keeping the breasts productive.

Lactose Intolerance
See **Bloating; Flatulence.**

Laryngitis

SYMPTOM SUMMARY

○ Hoarseness

○ Inability to speak

○ Usually follows other symptoms of upper respiratory infection, such as runny nose, sore throat, shortness of breath, fever

UNDERSTANDING THE DISEASE PROCESS

Laryngitis is an inflammation of the larynx, the "voice box" of the throat that produces speech. Although the medical literature identifies at least 2,286 conditions that cause laryngitis,[1] acute or short-term laryngitis is usually the result of a viral infection (although laryngitis following bacterial sinusitis is sometimes especially severe). White blood cells attempt to isolate infectious microorganisms in the throat by secreting chemicals that cause tissues to swell around them. The membrane covering the folds of the larynx become red and swollen. Irregularities in this membrane lower the pitch of the voice.

Vibration of the larynx is also reduced. The threshold pressure for sound is increased so that generating a steady flow of pressure over the larynx becomes difficult, resulting in hoarseness. The pressure required to set the folds of the larynx in motion can become so great that the person becomes voiceless. Typically the effects of laryngitis are most noticeable for vocal sounds of higher pitch (requiring more vibrations) or the vowels a, e, o, i, and u, requiring prolonged vibration.

Chronic laryngitis, as its name suggests, develops over a longer time, a period of at least several weeks. This form of laryngitis may be caused by environmental factors such as inhalation of cigarette smoke or polluted air, irritation from asthma inhalers (especially the steroid fluticasone),[2] reflux of stomach acids through the esophagus, or vocal abuse, that is, prolonged use of the voice at an abnormal volume or pitch. Vocal abuse results in an increased adhesive force and friction between the folds of the larynx. The area of contact between the folds becomes swollen.

Although acute laryngitis usually is not a result of vocal abuse, the contrary is often true. The underlying infection or inflammation results in a hoarse voice. Typically, people with laryngitis aggravate the condition by attempting to speak or sing as if their throats were well.

TREATMENT SUMMARY

In addition to treatment for colds or sinusitis, use any herbs for symptoms of concern to you.

HERBS

To relieve cough (antitussives):

○ Lobelia

  • Ointments: apply to the chest 2–3 times a day, *or*

  • Vinegar extract (acetract): no more than ¹/₂ teaspoon 3 times a day. Take less if you experience nausea. *Do not give to children.*

○ Marshmallow

  • Tea: a rounded teaspoon of the herb in a cup of water as often as desired, *or*

  • Tincture: 1–3 teaspoons up to 4 times a day.

To treat sore throat (demulcents):

○ Colt's foot, couch grass, or elecampane

  • Tea: no more than $1/4$ teaspoon in a cup of water allowed to brew for 15 minutes, up to 3 times a day. *Strain before drinking.*

○ Ivy leaf (Hedera)

  • Extract: a dropperful by itself or in a small amount of water, 2–3 times a day.

○ Marshmallow

  • Tea: a rounded teaspoon of the herb in a cup of water as often as desired, *or*

  • Tincture: 1–3 teaspoons up to 4 times a day.

○ Plantain

  • Cough syrup: $1/2$ teaspoon 3 times a day, *or*

  • Tea: $1/4$–$1/2$ teaspoon of the herb brewed in hot water for 15 minutes.

○ Scutellaria (Chinese skullcap)

  • Fluid extract: $1/2$–2 teaspoons 1–3 times per day.

○ Slippery elm

  • Tea: 1 teaspoon in 1 cup of water as often as desired.

To break up phlegm (expectorants):

○ Anise

  • Aromatherapy: 10–20 drops of essential oil in a basin of hot water, vapors inhaled for several minutes once or twice a day. *Never drink essential oils of anise.*

  • Tea: bagged anise tea brewed in 1 cup of hot, but not boiling, water.

○ Mullein

  • Tincture: $1/4$–$3/4$ teaspoon up to 4 times a day.

○ Mustard

  • Apply as poultice or plaster once or twice a day.

To stop coughing fits (spasmolytics):

○ Lobelia

  • Ointments: apply to the chest 2–3 times a day.

  • Vinegar extract (acetract): no more than $1/2$ teaspoon 3 times a day. Take less if you experience nausea. *Do not give to children.*

○ Thyme

  • Tea: $1/4$–$1/2$ teaspoon of the kitchen herb in 1 cup of hot water, 2–3 times daily.

  • Tincture: $1/3$–1 teaspoon, 2–3 times daily.

AROMATHERAPY

○ Add 5–10 drops of eucalyptus oil to the water in a vaporizer operated in your bedroom as your sleep.

UNDERSTANDING THE HEALING PROCESS

If your voice is especially important to your personal or professional life, the first rule for treating laryngitis is "Do no harm. Tomorrow is important, too." Avoid any situation requiring you to strain your voice. If you use over-the-counter cough syrups, choose a brand that includes guaifenesin. This mucolytic breaks up the phlegm constraining the vocal cords.

There are a number of herbs that help relieve laryngitis. The best way to use them is to treat the symptoms that are the most bothersome to you. Anise and the related herb star anise contain an antimicrobial chemical, anethole.[3] The essential oil is especially deadly to molds and yeast infections,[4] which are a special problem for people who use steroid asthma inhalers. Since anise stimulates production of secretions, it should be used to treat dry coughs rather than productive coughs.

Colt's foot and couch grass, used as teas, are traditional remedies for laryngitis. Elecampane mostly consists of the sugar inulin (not to be confused with insulin), the same carbohydrate found in Jerusalem artichokes. The inulin in elecampane coats and soothes the throat. The herb also contains small amounts of volatile oils that act as counterirritants, desensitizing the throat to pain. (Do not to try speaking in a loud voice just because pain has stopped. Avoid speaking or singing in a loud voice until you feel normal pressure at the base of your throat.)

It is important not to use too much elecampane. The volatile oils in the herb can irritate the mouth and the bowel. There has been a single report in the medical literature of a potentially life-threatening allergic reaction to foods containing the same carbohydrates as elecampane. This experience has been cited as a reason not to use elecampane, but this allergy was to inulin, possibly to Jerusalem artichokes, rather than to any herb. There is no evidence whatsoever that the man who experienced a severe allergic reaction after eating foods containing inulin took any herb, including elecampane.[5] Nonetheless, if you are allergic to Jerusalem artichokes, do not take elecampane. There is also a report in the medical literature of a severe allergic reaction to Inutest, a highly refined form of inulin used to measure kidney function. Although this report also has been cited as a reason not to use elecampane, Inutest is not made from this herb, and the allergic reaction to Inutest occurred after it was *injected* into a sensitive patient.[6]

Ivy leaf, also known as Hedera, is a common remedy for laryngitis in the Azores. Researchers have identified at least six chemicals in ivy leaf that stop bronchial spasms.[7] These compounds are not water soluble so the herb must be taken as an extract, although it can be mixed with water to make the extract easier to swallow. Ivy leaf is used to stop "coughing fits" caused by phlegmy coughs rather than dry coughs. Some samples of the herb can contain very small amounts of a nausea-inducing chemical known as emetine, so the herb should not be used by pregnant women or small children.

Lobelia contains the phlegm-dissolving plant chemical lobeline. This chemical acts on the same centers in the brain as nicotine, giving somewhat the same sense of satisfaction as smoking.[8] Unlike nicotine, this plant chemical makes breathing deeper and stronger. It also stimulates the flow of blood to the heart by activating nerves in the carotid sinus.[9] In overdose, however, it can also activate the vagus nerve, which has roughly the same effect as a punch in the stomach. Too much lobeline, and too much lobelia, can cause nausea and vomiting.

Lobelia makes the brain less sensitive to amphetamines,[10] so it should not be taken by anyone who takes amphetamine or dextroamphetamine (Adderall), methamphetamine (Desoxyn), methylphenidate (Ritalin), or pemoline (Cylert). There is a widely held misconception that lobelia is toxic, but a systematic search of the medical literature failed to find any reports of lobelia poisoning.[11] Ear infections make it more likely that lobelia will cause stomach upset.

According to the herbal reference work *The Complete German Commission E Monographs,* marshmallow contains healing sugars that line and soothe the throat and stop dry cough.[12] Marshmallow teas are more effective in stopping coughs than marshmallow cough drops or tinctures.[13] Marshmallow does not interact with medications, but as it is nearly pure sugar it should be used with caution by people who have diabetes.

Mullein contains chemicals that kill bacteria and stop pain.[14] Taken at the same time as a flu treatment such as amatadine (Symmetrel), it greatly increases the probability that the flu treatment will work.[15] The combination of mullein and zanamivir (Relenza) has not yet been tested. Mullein does not generally cause any side effects, although some people may be allergic to it.

Plantain is both soothing and astringent. It contains both mucilages, slimy complex carbohydrates that coat the throat, and tannins, the same chemicals that are found in tea and that tighten the lining of the throat. One of its chemical components is aucubin, a chemical that locks itself to the proteins in the lining of the throat[16] and possibly forms a protective barrier against infection. Another of its components is a pectin, a sugar closely related to the pectin used in making jams and jellies, that in its purified form is as potent a stimulator of the immune system as gamma globulin.[17] Plantain is more useful in helping phlegm come up rather than in relieving dry cough. There are no interactions between plantain and prescription drugs, although it should not be taken at the same time as prescription drugs because it can interfere with their absorption.

Scutellaria is one of Traditional Chinese Medicine's most important herbs for treating respiratory infections. It contains a variety of anti-inflammatory chemicals that are antioxidant in some situations, protecting red blood cells, and prooxidant in others, activating the immune process.[18] It contains several chemicals that are effective in treating laryngitis that is secondary to infection with respiratory syncitial virus (RSV),[19] the most common cause of croup. That is, unlike most other herbs and most other medications, scutellaria is antiviral rather than only antibacterial.

Slippery elm makes the lining of the throat "slippery" and reduces inflammation caused by eating and drinking. The complex carbohydrates in slippery elm are completely digestible and the product is wholly nontoxic. Teas can be made with 1/2–2 teaspoons of the bark depending on personal preferences. Slippery elm is also found in many herbal cough lozenges.

Thyme releases an essential oil known as thymol, which travels through the bloodstream to be exhaled through the lungs. Of all the herbs studied in the treatment of bronchitis, thyme has the longest half-life, lasting in the body for up to 20 hours.[20] There are reports that the essential oil of thyme, combined with essential oils of cinnamon, cloves, lavender, and mint, may reduce repeated infections in people who have bronchitis. The most common use of thyme, however, is in treating coughing spasms in children.

Never take the essential oil of thyme by mouth. The essential oil should only be used in aromatherapy. The chopped herb can be used in teas. There are also commercially available fluid extracts and tinctures of thyme that are safe for use with either children or adults. In Europe, thyme is frequently combined with an extract made from a carnivorous plant, the sundew, to make cough drops such as Ricola.

Not to be neglected in taking care of laryngitis is aromatherapy. Although the concept of aromatherapy sounds exotic to many people, it is actually very basic: if you use a vaporizer, you use aromatherapy. Eucalyptus oil is a standard ingredient in cough drops and in oils added to humidifiers and vaporizers. While it does not increase breathing capacity, a study of 246 people with chronic bronchitis found that eucalyptus oils stop the worsening of cough that commonly occurs in the winter (in wet climates where heaters are used) or summer (in desert climates).[21] Eucalyptus is especially helpful for laryngitis following croup in small children.

CONCEPTS FOR COPING WITH LARYNGITIS

❍ Rest your voice, completely if possible. If you must speak, use a soft "sighing" intonation. Avoid whispering, which strains the larynx. Also avoid clearing the throat, which is traumatic to the larynx.

❍ Drink 8 glasses of water daily to maintain hydration for the throat. Laryngitis is also helped by a cool vaporizer—but not by hot baths.

❍ Hearing loss is an often overlooked contributing factor in laryngitis. Sometimes distorted perception of pitch causes the person to attempt to lower the voice to how it "should" sound, resulting in laryngitis.

❍ Painless gastroesophageal reflux disease (GERD), or "heartburn without the burn," is a frequent cause of laryngitis. Indications that laryngitis is caused by reflux of stomach acid are hoarseness, halitosis, or a bitter taste in the mouth in the morning, lump in the throat, or a chronic need to clear the throat without other signs of

infection. Treatment for GERD-induced laryngitis is the same as for heartburn. (See HEARTBURN.)

❍ Loss of vocal range is sometimes symptomatic of hypothyroidism. (See HYPOTHYROIDISM.)

❍ Both PMS and pregnancy affect abdominal support and alter the quality of women's singing voices. Rescheduling performances is usually the simplest way to deal with the problem.

❍ Antihistamines usually do not help laryngitis. People who use antihistamines may gain the false impression that the laryngitis is resolving and continue to use the voice, causing injury to the vocal cords. The drying effect of antihistamines is also harmful.

❍ You cannot hear your own voice the way others hear it when you have inflammation of the ears, nose, or throat. If you are a professional speaker or singer, find people you can trust to make an assessment of the quality of your voice when your have an allergy or upper respiratory infection.

❍ Prescription beta-blockers have become popular among professional speakers and singers for controlling nervous tension before a performance. There are two important drawbacks to their use: they lower the threshold for an asthmatic attack, and they have unpredictable effects on the quality of the voice the first time they are used. Taking a beta-blocker to control anxiety for the first time just before a performance can have professionally disastrous results.

❍ Avoiding tobacco smoke accelerates recovery.

❍ If you have frequent heartburn or GERD, be sure to avoid caffeine. Try sleeping with the head of your bed elevated 2–4 inches (5–10 centimeters) by placing a brick under the castors supporting the head of your bed. Reducing stomach acid will accelerate your recovery from laryngitis.

❍ Horehound, also known as marrubio, is a traditional remedy for laryngitis in the southwestern United States and Mexico but should be strictly avoided by people who have GERD.

❍ There are a number of homeopathic remedies for colds and other upper respiratory conditions that cause laryngitis. Usually it is best to start with a single dose of the lowest strength (6C, 6X, or 12C) of the remedy matching the symptoms to be treated, and then wait for a response. If there is an improvement in symptoms, let the remedy continue to work until there is no more improvement, then take another dose. If there is no improvement, try a different potency (30X or 30C). Sometimes homeopathic medicines work for a few minutes, and sometimes they work for an entire day before another dose is needed.

- Aconitum napellus is recommended when symptoms come on suddenly, especially after a stressful or traumatic experience. Symptoms relieved by this homeopathic formula include scratchy throat, choking cough, tightness across the chest, and dry, stuffy nose.

- Alium cepa is recommended for runny nose with a clear discharge, watery eyes, burning eyes, and sneezing.

- Arsenicum album is recommended for people who have frequent colds and sore throat. It is most effective when symptoms are worse at night and when there is thick, burning mucus.

- Baryta carbonica is recommended for people who catch colds easily after getting chilled. It treats runny nose, swollen lips, swollen tonsils, and adenoids.

- Belladonna is recommended when cold comes on suddenly with flushed face and restlessness. It relieves "dried out" sinuses and earache.

- Dulcamara is recommended for colds occurring in chilly, wet weather. It is also helpful for allergies.

- Euphrasia relieves red eyes and frequent sneezing with a clear discharge. It is helpful when symptoms interrupt sleep and when the person feels better after eating.

- Ferrum phosphoricum is said to stop a cold from developing if taken immediately after symptoms are first noticed. It is used to relieve hacking cough after a cold has set in.

- Gelsemium treats fatigue, headache, fever, and chills. It is especially recommended when the person with the cold feels shaky. Gelsemium treats colds occurring in hot weather.

- Kali bichromicum helps break up thick, stringy mucus in the nose and throat.

- Mercurius solubilis treats colds in people who wake up sweaty. It also treats bad breath, swollen lymph nodes, and earache.

- Natrum muriaticum treats colds with a white (not clear) discharge, sneezing that is worse early in the morning, and chapped lips.

- Nux vomica treats stuffy head and runny nose.

- Phosphorus keeps colds from going to the chest, and is useful when one nostril is blocked and the other is clear. Phosphorus is recommended for people who tend to get nosebleeds.

- Pulsatilla helps when the nose is stopped up indoors and runs outdoors. It treats colds causing thick green or yellow mucus that are worse in the evening.

- Rhus toxicodendron treats colds that begin with stiffness and body aches before sneezing, tearing, cough, and sore throat occur.

Lead Exposure

SYMPTOM SUMMARY

○ Vague symptoms, principally abdominal pain, constipation, loss of appetite, and vomiting with slow mental and physical development

Lead poisoning is diagnosed by blood test.

UNDERSTANDING THE DISEASE PROCESS

Lead poisoning is a worldwide problem, principally among children. In the United States, about 1 in 25 of all children under the age of 5 has been exposed to toxic levels of lead. Approximately 1 in 5 children living in houses built before 1946 has been exposed to toxic levels of this heavy metal.[1]

In the United States, the most common source of toxic lead is paint. Although lead has been banned in household paints since 1978, older layers of paint may contain lead, entering the environment as the paint chips and flakes. Toddlers find the chips and put them in their mouths. Fine dust released in stripping old paint enters the air and is inhaled; the lungs of small children are less able to "cough up" the lead paint. The finer the particle, the more lead is absorbed. Nutritional deficiencies of calcium, copper, zinc, and protein accelerate the absorption of lead, as does excessive consumption of dietary fats and oils. The phytates in beans, whole grains, and leafy vegetables bind to lead and increase its elimination.

Lead destroys sulfur-dependent enzymes. Muscles, nerves, and bones of infants and toddlers are in a state of rapid development, making them especially susceptible to the toxic effects of heavy metals. Lead poisoning usually causes a large number of vague symptoms, principally abdominal pain, constipation, anorexia, nausea, and vomiting. It also causes retardation of mental and physical development.

TREATMENT SUMMARY

DIET

❍ Include green, leafy vegetables and whole grains or beans in meals every day.

NUTRITIONAL SUPPLEMENTS

❍ Any multivitamin and mineral supplement daily.

❍ Selenium: 100 micrograms *weekly*.

UNDERSTANDING THE HEALING PROCESS

Including whole foods and vegetables in the child's diet and preventing mineral deficiencies reduces the absorption of lead. Additionally, selenium protects sulfur-containing enzymes from the chemical effects of lead.[2] Laboratory research suggests that selenium ensures that the DNA in cells in rapidly growing tissues keeps up with the demands of growth and multiplication.[3]

CONCEPTS FOR COPING WITH LEAD EXPOSURE

❍ Tetraethyl lead in gasoline, no longer used in the United States, rapidly enters the skin. Take more than usual care to avoid gasoline spills when traveling in countries where leaded gasoline is still sold.

❍ Blood samples are more accurate than hair samples for detecting lower levels of lead exposure.

❍ Lead leaches into acidic liquids, such as juices and vinegars. Store these and other acid foods in glass rather than in glazed pottery. Mexican pottery and sour (notably tamarind) candies stored in Mexican pottery are among the most common sources of serious lead poisoning in children in the United States.[4]

❍ EDTA chelation was approved in 1955 as a treatment for lead poisoning. EDTA chelation is still the primary medical treatment for toxic exposure to lead, although other chelating agents are now preferred.

Leg Cramps
See **Peripheral Vascular Disease; Phlebitis.**

Lennox-Gastaut Syndrome

SYMPTOM SUMMARY

❍ Tonic (stiffening of the body, dilation of the pupils), clonic (sudden muscle jerks), or atonic (loss of muscle tone and/or consciousness) seizures

UNDERSTANDING THE DISEASE PROCESS

Lennox-Gastaut syndrome is a severe form of epilepsy, usually occurring in children between 1 and 8 years old. It can cause tonic, clonic, or atonic seizures, and is usually accompanied by severe developmental delays and attention deficit disorder. The cause of the condition is not known, but it may be related to brain injury or severe infections in infancy or early childhood.

TREATMENT SUMMARY

NUTRITIONAL SUPPLEMENTS

❍ Vitamin B_6: dosage selected in consultation with a physician.

UNDERSTANDING THE HEALING PROCESS

Lennox-Gastaut syndrome is difficult to control with conventional medications, but up to approximately 35 percent of children with Lennox-Gastaut syndrome respond to high doses of vitamin B_6. Perhaps 15 percent of children on vitamin therapy will eventually have normal EEGs.[1] Since high-dose vitamin B_6 therapy can cause diarrhea, vomiting, and liver dysfunction, monitoring by a doctor is essential.

CONCEPTS FOR COPING WITH LENNOX-GASTAUT SYNDROME

❍ Vitamin B_6 therapy can be extremely helpful in Lennox-Gastaut syndrome but can actually cause seizures in other forms of epilepsy. Do not use vitamin B_6 unless the diagnosis has been confirmed with a physician.

Leukoplakia

SYMPTOM SUMMARY

Smoker's keratosis:

❍ Sore or lesion on a mucous membrane

- Usually on the tongue
- May be on inside of cheeks or genitals
- Gray or white coloration
- Hard surface
- Usually soft and flat
- Thick, slightly raised

"Hairy" leukoplakia:

❍ Fuzzy white patches on tongue

❍ Painless

UNDERSTANDING THE DISEASE PROCESS

Leukoplakia is a gray or white growth anywhere in the mouth. It is usually a reaction of the mucous membrane or skin of the tongue to irritation caused by smoking, although it can also be caused by constant irritation from irregular surfaces on dentures or fillings, and it can be a complication of a kind of sunlight-induced skin damage known as actinic cheilitis or "farmer's lip." Leukoplakia can also occur on the genitals in women.

Leukoplakia is frequently referred to as a precancerous condition, but it usually isn't. About 97 percent of leukoplakias are the result of hyperkeratosis or hyperplasia, a benign buildup of cells in the outermost layer of the mucous membrane. Only about 3 percent of leukoplakias damage one or more of eleven genes to cause dysplasia of the connective tissues beneath the mucous membrane, and develop into oral cancers.[1]

Even though most leukoplakias are noncancerous, most smokers develop leukoplakias more than once. The disease is so common among smokers that there are more cases of cancerous leukoplakia than there are of skin cancer. Over 80 percent of cases are in men, virtually all of them smokers of cigarettes or cigars. Six million people in the United States will develop leukoplakia at some point in their lives.

Two other forms of leukoplakia are much less common. Every year in the United States, about 1,500 male and 50 female users of chewing tobacco develop the form of leukoplakia known as smokeless tobacco keratosis.[2] Another form, "hairy" leukoplakia, is a fuzzy growth on the tip of the tongue. This form of leukoplakia is caused by infection with the Epstein-Barr virus (EBV) in people with HIV whose T-cell counts have dropped below 200. Its treatment differs substantially from other forms of leukoplakia. For more information about "hairy" leukoplakia, see HIV AND AIDS.

TREATMENT SUMMARY

DIET

❍ Eat curries made with turmeric, fruits (especially papaya, pink grapefruit, and pink guava), vegetables (especially cooked tomatoes and tomato paste), and whole grains. Tomatoes cooked in olive oil are an especially good source of lycopene, in which most men with leukoplakia are deficient. Adding black pepper to tomatoes or eating black pepper at the same meal as a curry diminishes absorption of the antioxidants they contain.

NUTRITIONAL SUPPLEMENTS

❍ Beta-carotene: 30 milligrams daily.

❍ Curcumin: 500 milligrams 3 times a day with meals.

❍ Lycopene: 5 milligrams per day.

❍ Vitamin A: see comments in Understanding the Healing Process.

❍ Vitamin C (especially important for women who smoke): 2,000–3,000 milligrams daily.

❍ Vitamin E: 400 IU daily.

❍ Zinc picolinate (especially important for men who smoke): 30 milligrams per day.

UNDERSTANDING THE HEALING PROCESS

The most important thing you can do to take charge of the healing process in leukoplakia is to quit smoking. Various studies find that there is between a 70 and 90 percent chance precancerous leukoplakias will disappear within 12 months of smoking cessation. Studies of leukoplakia related to chewing betel nuts, rather than smoking, report that eating fruits, vegetables, and fiber lowers risk for the disease, and that adequate intake of zinc is especially important for men and adequate intake of vitamin C is especially important for women.[4] While eating fruits and vegetables and getting adequate zinc and vitamin C is likely to be helpful in preventing and treating leukoplakia in smokers, this fact is not scientifically established.

Beyond smoking cessation, nutritional treatment is very helpful. There is some confusion in interpretations of the medical literature due to the fact that the levels of antioxidants needed to *treat* leukoplakia are very high, while the doses needed to *prevent* leukoplakia are relatively low. Researchers at the M.D. Anderson Cancer Center in Houston report in *The New England Journal of Medicine* that a "knock-out" treatment with high-dose vitamin A derivatives under medical supervision preceding nutritional treatment makes nutritional therapy to prevent cancer much more effective.[5]

Vitamin A has been used to treat leukoplakia since the 1950s. The early studies of nutritional treatment of leukoplakia involved giving massive amounts of vitamin A, up to 900,000 IU a day (180 times the dosage usually given today). The doctors got good results, but the treatment produced side effects, such as dry skin, chapped lips, headaches, and joint pain. Women of reproductive age cannot be given this level of vitamin A, since it can cause birth defects if taken during the first 3 months of pregnancy. Doctors today still use high-dose vitamin A therapy in the form of synthetic vitamin A, also known as tretinoin or Accutane. In one study, a physician-prescribed vitamin A (tretinoin) gel applied directly to the mouth resulted in complete remission in 27 percent of patients, and an average 50 percent reduction in the number of patches overall.[6]

Studies in the 1980s tested giving much smaller doses of vitamin A to both men and women. Scientists working in the Philippines found that taking 15,000 IU of vitamin A and 45,000 IU of beta-carotene daily for 3 months was enough to reverse precancerous changes to DNA in 37 out of 40 tobacco chewers tested.[7] Another study in India confirmed that the combination of vitamin A and beta-carotene was more effective than vitamin A alone in reversing leukoplakia in betel nut chewers.[8]

Success in treating tobacco chewers overseas led to clinical trials treating tobacco smokers in the United States. Of 10 combinations of nutritional supplements tested, the best combination was 30 milligrams of beta-carotene, 1,000 milligrams of vitamin C, and 800 IU of vitamin E. Clinical trials at the Medical College of Virginia found that taking this combination for 9 months resulted in clinical improvement in 55.7 percent of patients who took it. The best results were found among patients who quit smoking and drinking, but even among patients who continued to smoke and drink,

about half improved noticeably.[9] Another study at the M.D. Anderson Cancer Center found vitamin E used alone is nearly as effective as the combination of C, E, and beta-carotene. The M.D. Anderson Cancer Center researchers found that 800 IU of vitamin E daily for 6 months significantly reduced numbers of micronuclei, tangled knots of DNA within chromosomes that are found in leukoplakia.[10] Two out of three patients in the study showed improvement on a microscopic level, and 46 percent showed visible reduction in the size of plaques.[11]

The most recent studies have found that men who have leukoplakia tend to have *significantly* low bloodstream levels of beta-carotene and lycopene, while women tend to have low levels of these nutrients that cannot be linked to leukoplakia with statistical certainty.[12] Taking beta-carotene, however, definitely helps. Studies at the Arizona Cancer Center in Tucson have found that leukoplakia plaques in 4 out of 5 people who take 60 milligrams of beta-carotene a day for 6 months improve or at least do not get worse. Bringing the body's supply of beta-carotene up to normal levels takes about 9 months, but the benefits of taking beta-carotene last for up to a year even if it is discontinued.[13]

Curcumin and green tea polyphenols are generally helpful in leukoplakia, but they are essential when leukoplakia is treated with tretinoin (Accutane). In proliferative verrucous leukoplakia (described in Concepts for Coping with Leukoplakia), the body attempts to control the spread of the plaque by activating a gene called p53.[14] Gene p53 ordinarily makes sure dividing cells "rest for repairs" if there are other defects in their genetic material. Even in less virulent forms of leukoplakia, stress on gene p53 is directly related to the size and number of the plaques.[15] If p53 is not active, vitamin A, beta-carotene, and tretinoin (Accutane) are effective about 14 percent of the time. If p53 is active, vitamin A, beta-carotene, and tretinoin are effective about 70 percent of the time.[16]

Curcumin is a well-known activator of p53. It helps p53 deactivate defective cells at G2, a second gap or resting phase in the process of cell division just before the cell divides. Scientists at New York's Memorial Sloan-Kettering Cancer Center have found that, at least in the test tube, green tea is a perfect complement for curcumin, since it activates p53 at G1, the first gap in the process of cell division.[17] Scientists in China have partially confirmed with clinical studies what scientists at

Sloan-Kettering found in the laboratory. A clinical study at the Chinese Academy of Preventive Medicine in Beijing found that giving smokers 3 grams (approximately 1½ teaspoons) of green tea every day, plus painting plaques with a green tea tincture every day, significantly reduced DNA damage over a period of 6 months.[18]

CONCEPTS FOR COPING WITH LEUKOPLAKIA

O In rare instances, food allergies (a reaction to cinnamon is reported in the medical literature) can cause leukoplakia in nonsmokers.[3] If you know you have food allergies and develop white patches on your tongue or in your mouth, try eliminating known allergy-provoking foods for 3–4 weeks.

O Reverse smoking, the practice of smoking with the lit end of a cigarette or cigar in the mouth, increases the risk of leukoplakia becoming cancerous.

O Human papillomavirus (HPV) can cause an especially rapid form of leukoplakia known as proliferative verrucous leukoplakia (PVL). This form of leukoplakia quickly spreads over a large part of the mouth (in women) or tongue (in men) and frequently becomes cancerous. Most people who develop PVL do not use tobacco. Any rapidly spreading white plaque in the mouth should be examined by a physician as a potential cancer. To prevent PVL, persons who engage in oral contact with partners who have diseases caused by HPV should follow the nutritional recommendations for those conditions, in addition to the recommendations for leukoplakia. See ABNORMAL PAP SMEAR and GENITAL WARTS for further information.

Liposuction, Healing after

SYMPTOM SUMMARY

O Bleeding

O Bruising

O Discoloration of skin

O Pain

O Swelling, area may appear larger than before surgery

O Tingling or numbness

UNDERSTANDING THE DISEASE PROCESS

Liposuction is a common surgical procedure for the removal of fatty tissue. First-time users of the procedure are often surprised to learn that the immediate result of the surgery is not a svelte contour. Immediately after surgery, the area operated on swells. For several days, it may be larger than it was before surgery. There may also be bleeding, bruising, and discoloration.

TREATMENT SUMMARY

O Follow recommendations for diet, herbs, and nutritional supplements listed under BRUISES.

O Magnet therapy, as described in Understanding the Healing Process.

UNDERSTANDING THE HEALING PROCESS

One of the more exciting points of contact between conventional medicine and complementary healing is the use of magnets. Grave concerns have been raised about the potentially harmful health effects of magnetic fields in the environment. On the other hand, local applications of magnetic fields are becoming generally accepted in the treatment of a variety of painful conditions, including recovery from liposuction.

Experimental studies with animals have found that magnetic fields accelerate healing and increase the strength of the fibrin net covering wounds. Magnetic fields increase the deposition of collagen. They encourage fibroblasts to migrate to the wounds to spin the protein net on which collagen is collected. They attract leukocytes and macrophages that control infectious bacteria. They decrease vasoconstriction, increasing blood supply, and they stimulate the growth of skin over wounds.[1,2]

Plastic surgeons Boris Man, Daniel Man, and Harvey Plosker have studied the treatment of liposuction wounds with magnet patches. The magnets they used are commercially available in square and rectangular patches of 5 x 15 to 20 x 30 centimeters (2 x 6 to 8 x 12 inches) with strengths of 150–400 gauss. In a pilot study conducted at their Florida clinic in 1999, they found that magnets greatly reduced discoloration, swelling, and pain, especially during the first 1–7 days after surgery. While magnets did not completely eliminate post-operative trauma—patients treated with magnets still had some bruising, swelling, and pain—the effects are visually obvious. Bruises that typically take 2–3 weeks to heal disappeared in 48–72 hours.

Drs. Man and Dr. Plosker believe that the magnetic fields enhance blood flow to the site of liposuction. This increases oxygen and accelerates the overall healing process, and also allows the circulation of the body's natural anti-inflammatory hormones. Best of all, magnet therapy has no side effects.[3]

CONCEPTS FOR RECOVERY FROM LIPOSUCTION

❍ Be sure to wear any elastic dressing, stocking, or girdle the doctor prescribes. This reduces bleeding and swelling and helps skin shrink to fit the new contour.

❍ Walk as soon as the surgeon gives you the OK. Walking helps prevent blood clots.

Liver Cancer

SYMPTOM SUMMARY

❍ Bloating, abdominal swelling may be severe

❍ Fever

❍ Loss of appetite

❍ Nausea and vomiting

❍ Pain in the upper abdomen on the right side; the pain may extend to the back and shoulder

❍ Weakness or severe fatigue

❍ Weight loss

❍ Yellow skin and eyes, and dark urine (jaundice)

❍ Liver cancer may present no symptoms in its early stages. The symptoms of liver cancer are also symptoms of other, less serious liver diseases.

UNDERSTANDING THE DISEASE PROCESS

The liver is the largest internal organ of the body, and weighs less than the skin. It lies under the right rib cage just beneath the right lung and diaphragm. If you were to poke your fingers up under your right ribs, you would almost be touching it. The liver is shaped like a pyramid and is divided into right and left lobes. Unlike most other organs, the liver receives blood from 2 sources. The hepatic artery supplies the liver with blood that is rich in oxygen. The portal vein carries nutrient-rich blood from the intestines.

Because the liver has an extensive blood supply, it is especially subject to acquiring cancer cells from other organs. Cancers of the breast, colon, and lung frequently migrate to the liver. The liver can also be a site of primary cancer, especially in people who have cirrhosis of the liver following alcoholism or infection with hepatitis C.

The controllable factors in liver cancer are cumulative. People who both drink and smoke are at considerably greater risk for liver cancer than people who only drink or smoke.[1] Various dietary factors also interact with personal habits. In one study, heavy drinking was found to be a risk factor for liver cancer only among people who had low bloodstream levels of the antioxidants alpha-carotene, beta-carotene, glutathione, and lycopene.[2] In another study, smoking was found to be an especially high risk factor among people who had low levels of selenium as well as beta-carotene, but not if levels were adequate. (Interestingly, this study found that extremely high levels of antioxidants were also a risk factor for liver cancer.)[3]

Consuming large amounts of iron, which neutralizes antioxidants, can be an extraordinary risk factor for liver cancer. In South Africa, where food is cooked in iron pots and the most popular brands of beer are extremely high in iron, the combination of a high-iron diet (emphasizing meat) and exposure to aflatoxins in moldy food increases the risk of getting liver cancer up to 154 times.[4]

TREATMENT SUMMARY

NUTRITIONAL SUPPLEMENTS

❍ Coenzyme Q_{10}: 100 milligrams.

❍ Vitamin E: not more than 400 IU per day.

❍ Vitamin C: not more than 1,000 milligrams per day.

HERBS

❍ Maitake-D: 4–10 grams (4,000–10,000 milligrams daily).

❍ *Sho-saiko-to:* as directed on label.

❍ Silymarin: 360 milligrams daily.

UNDERSTANDING THE HEALING PROCESS

It is important to understand that while adequate levels of alpha-carotene, beta-carotene, lycopene, and lutein in the diet reduce the risk of developing liver cancer and partially compensate for bad health habits, different antioxidants are required once liver cancer has occurred. Cirrhosis, hepatitis, and liver cancer all put heavy stress on the nutrient ubiquinone (coenzyme Q_{10}), forcing it to remove oxidants throughout the body.[5] The combination of vitamin C and vitamin E is known to stop multiplication of liver cancer cells in the test tube,[6] but has not been tested in living patients. Similarly, conjugated linolenic acid (CLA) stops growth of liver cancer cells even when vitamins C and E are deficient in laboratory studies,[7] but has not been clinically tested.

There is considerable likelihood that *moderate* amounts of these supplements will be helpful and there is no evidence they will be harmful. Massive doses of antioxidants, however, can have unexpected side effects. The liver is an important site for activity of the immune system. "Clean-up" cells known as Kupffer cells migrate to the liver to remove bacteria from its large blood supply. These clean-up cells are activated by free radicals, which are suppressed by antioxidants. Taking very large doses of CoQ_{10}, CLA, or vitamins C or E could have unexpected side effects.

There is more evidence for maitake-D, *sho-saiko-to*, and silymarin. A series of case studies in Japan found that maitake-D helped 7 out of a total of 12 liver cancer patients treated with it. The most notable effect of treatment with maitake-D is improvement of prothrombin activation, making additional clotting factors for the blood. Maitake-D is also immunostimulant; for 9 patients for whom measurements were recorded, maitake-D treatment increased interleukin-2 production by 29 percent and increased CD4+ (T-cell) counts by 42 percent. There was one complete remission, and some patients classified as stage III (a tumor more than 4 centimeters in diameter, not metastasized to another organ) were classified as stage I (a tumor no more than 2 centimeters in diameter).[8] No side effects have been noted.

In 2001 the prestigious Sloan-Kettering Institute in New York started a clinical trial of the Japanese herbal formula *sho-saiko-to* for the treatment of advanced liver cancer. Japanese research in the 1990s found that this formula has hepatoprotective, antiproliferative and immunostimulant effects in the laboratory. A Japanese clinical trial found that hepatitis C and cirrhosis patients receiving the formula had a lower incidence of developing liver cancer (and improved liver health even without interferon treatment). The Sloan-Kettering Study will show whether *sho-saiko-to* will help patients who have already developed liver cancer and cannot be treated by conventional means.

Other clinical studies of people with hepatitis B have found that *sho-saiko-to* increases the immune system's production of interferon, a chemical that interferes with the reproduction of the virus.[9] The key drawback to the use of *sho-saiko-to* is that it can overstimulate the body's production of interferon when used in combination with interferon therapy. An autoimmune form of pneumonia can result. Do not use *sho-saiko-to* at any time during the months you take interferon therapy. *Sho-saiko-to* is available in the United States and Canada as:

- Liver Kampo (Honso)
- Minor Bupleurum Combination (Lotus Classics, Qualiherb, Sun Ten)
- Minor Bupleurum Formula (Chinese Classics, Golden Flower Chinese Herbs)
- Minor Bupleurum Formulation (Kan Traditionals)
- Sho-saiko-to (Honso, Tsumura)

Silymarin from milk thistle has been associated with a single case of complete remission from liver cancer.[10] At the time of this report, there had been only 9 cases of liver cancer ever known to go into remission, so the finding about silymarin electrified the herbal community. Later laboratory research failed to yield an easy explanation of how silymarin works—in fact, milk thistle was found to be a prooxidant, accelerating destruction of DNA in liver cells and, presumably, in liver cancer cells.[11] In some cases, silymarin can cause mild diarrhea. Reduce the dosage if diarrhea occurs.

CONCEPTS FOR COPING WITH LIVER CANCER

❍ If members of your family have had liver cancer, you are at a greater risk. A 24-year study in France found that the people least likely to develop liver cancer had the lowest levels of insulin, that is, they avoided severe overweight, did not binge on sugars, and exercised regularly. Drastic changes in lifestyle are not necessary or proven to reduce the risk of liver cancer, but simply avoiding sugar binges is likely to help.[12]

Loss of Sexual Desire in Men

SYMPTOM SUMMARY

○ Decreased desire for or frequency of sexual relations, as perceived by the man

UNDERSTANDING THE DISEASE PROCESS

Diminished interest in sex in both men and women has been a problem in relationships through the centuries. Some people experience this condition in midlife, but loss of libido is increasingly reported among people in their 20s. A loss of interest in lovemaking frequently results in problems in relationships, especially if sexual activity at one time was frequent.

Sexual desire in both men and women is powered by testosterone, the hormone usually associated with male sexuality. Men with intact testes produce testosterone throughout life, but in gradually declining quantities as they age. After 40, most men go through a stage sometimes termed "andropause." After 40, men's bodies produce about 1 percent less testosterone each year.[1] Memory skills, muscle growth, and sperm production, are all reduced, but a majority of normal-weight men pass through andropause with their sex drives largely intact.

Overweight men, however, lose testosterone production and sex drive at a much faster rate. Oxygen deprivation during sleep, however, interferes with the release of luteinizing hormone which in turn greatly reduces the production of testosterone at night. In many cases, sleep apnea caused by overweight leads to levels of testosterone as low as those of men who have had their testicles removed. About 40 percent of overweight men who snore have chronically low levels of testosterone and experience loss of desire for sex,[2] without regard to the diminished interest of their sleep-deprived spouses.

Overweight is the most common cause of loss of libido in men, but it is one among many. Alzheimer's disease, cancer and cancer treatment, cirrhosis of the liver, diabetes, Guillain-Barré syndrome, hemochromatosis, hyperthyroidism, hypothyroidism, scleroderma, many medications (especially medications for depression and prostate conditions), and major surgery can all rob men of sexual desire. When correcting these problems does not restore sexual desire, however, the most common and correctable cause is obesity.

TREATMENT SUMMARY

NATURAL SUPPLEMENTS

○ Chrysin: 500–1,000 milligrams per day.

UNDERSTANDING THE HEALING PROCESS

Weight loss often works wonders in restoring the male sex drive, and sexual possibilities can be a powerful motivator for staying on diets. Because weight loss has only beneficial side effects, any man suffering loss of sex drive should try diet and exercise before trying testosterone replacement.

One natural product also helps. The passionflower extract chrysin preserves the testosterone a man's body already makes. Since it preserves existing testosterone rather than stimulating additional testosterone, there is no danger of causing prostate disease. As a precaution, however, men with existing prostate enlargement or prostate cancer should avoid it.

CONCEPTS FOR COPING WITH LOSS OF SEXUAL DESIRE IN MEN

○ Testosterone replacement therapy must be medically monitored. Excessive testosterone levels contribute to diseases of the prostate. Testosterone replacement is almost never indicated for men under 40 who have intact testes.

○ Androstenedione is clinically proven to raise testosterone levels—in women. A recent study found that 300 milligrams of androstenedione a day significantly raises estrogen levels in young men.[3] Some scientists believe that androstenedione might raise testosterone levels in older men, but only if taken in doses under 300 milligrams per day. It is not known whether increases in estrogen levels in these men would offset the benefits of increased testosterone.

○ Androstenediol is converted into testosterone in both men and women. The problem with the use of androstenediol is timing: increases to serum testosterone levels are short-lived, and may not increase sex drive or muscle mass. Safe dosages of androstenediol for men at risk of prostate cancer are not known, and men with existing prostate problems should not use this supplement.

○ DHEA effects on testosterone are minimal in men, but potentially harmful in women. This supplement may alter mood and indirectly increase sex drive in men, but it does not have demonstrable direct benefits in maintaining or increasing testosterone levels.

○ The herb *Tribulus terrestris* contains a plant chemical, protodioscine, which is converted into DHEA, which in turn can be converted into testosterone. The beneficial effects and side effects of *Tribulus* are probably minimal in most men.

○ Don't drink beer. Hops contain compounds very similar to estrogen. In the Middle Ages, hops were used in Central Europe to discourage sexual activity in young men and unmarried women. They were also very popular among monks struggling to keep vows of celibacy. Heavy marijuana smoking has a similar effect.

Loss of Sexual Desire in Women

SYMPTOM SUMMARY

○ Decreased desire for or frequency of sexual relations, as perceived by the woman

UNDERSTANDING THE DISEASE PROCESS

Diminished interest in sex in both men and women has been a problem in relationships through the centuries. Some people experience this condition in midlife, but loss of libido is increasingly reported among people in their 20s. A loss of interest in lovemaking frequently results in problems in relationships, especially if sexual activity at one time was frequent.

Sexual desire in both men and women is powered by testosterone, the hormone usually associated with male sexuality. Women's bodies contain testosterone throughout their lives, but only in vanishingly small quantities until puberty. About the time of a woman's first period, the adrenal glands begin to make massive quantities of dehydroepiandrosterone (DHEA) from cholesterol. Most of the young woman's DHEA is processed by the adrenal glands into the stress hormones so well known in adolescence. Some of the DHEA goes to the ovaries and uterus to form the female hormones estrogen and progesterone. Trace amounts of DHEA accumulate as a byproduct, DHEA sulfate. When a woman's adrenal glands and ovaries turn this byproduct into testosterone, she begins to experience sexual desire.[1] Sexual desire is highest in the middle of a woman's menstrual cycle, when her body is producing the greatest amount of progesterone and DHEA sulfate, and when she is most likely to ovulate.

A healthy woman's production of testosterone is always small. Even very young women can suffer testosterone deficiency. High-progesterone birth control pills replace the body's production of progesterone, and eliminate the production of the DHEA sulfate byproduct that becomes testosterone. Women on the Pill continue to menstruate, but lose their cycles of intense sexual interest. The effect of the Pill on a woman's libido is greater when she reaches her early 30s. Testosterone production in a woman's adrenal glands peaks at about age 30, although it continues in her ovaries until well after menopause.

As testosterone production finally tapers off, there is usually a lessening of sexual desire, decreased sexual responsiveness, and decreased sexual activity. At the same point in a woman's life, her body makes much less estrogen, so that the vagina becomes dry and intercourse may become painful. Aging male partners may be completely absent from her life or unable to perform intercourse. Hormone production may be diminished even more by hysterectomy or oophorectomy (removal of the ovaries), and sexual response may be muted by use of medications for allergy, anxiety, cancer, depression, or fluid retention. Estrogen replacement therapy can lubricate the vulva and vagina and make intercourse more comfortable, but does nothing to stimulate sexual desire. In fact, estrogen replacement therapy, like high-progesterone contraceptives, can reduce the amount of testosterone in circulation and lessen sexual desire.

TREATMENT SUMMARY

NUTRITIONAL SUPPLEMENTS

○ DHEA: 50 milligrams daily.

HERBS

○ Ginkgo: 70 milligrams 3 times a day.

Combination products:

○ Arginine, damiana, ginkgo, ginseng, and multiple vitamins and minerals.

UNDERSTANDING THE HEALING PROCESS

The obvious answer for a testosterone deficiency would seem to be testosterone replacement. There are clinical studies that suggest that adding testosterone to estrogen replacement therapy offers better protection against osteoporosis[2] and lowers total cholesterol, LDL or "bad" cholesterol, and triglycerides.[3] Only one clinical study, however, has found that testosterone replacement therapy can restore women's sexual desire. This study used very high doses of testosterone, 4 to 5 times the normal level of the hormone in healthy men, and only involved women who had had their ovaries removed.[4] In men, normal levels of testosterone are involved in hair loss on the scalp and hair growth elsewhere on the body, weight gain, deepening voice, hostility, abnormal levels of liver enzymes, and lower levels of HDL or "good" cholesterol. All of these detrimental side effects can occur in women who are given testosterone therapy.[5,6]

A better approach is to give the body the materials it needs to make its own testosterone. Scientists at the School of Medicine of the University of California at La Jolla found that giving 50 milligrams of DHEA nightly to 30 men and women aged 50–60 for 6 months doubled the concentration of testosterone and hormones that the body can convert into testosterone (androstenedione and dihydrotesterone) in women, bringing them to levels approximately normal for 30-year-old women. The women's weight, fat, and estrogen levels were unaffected, but 14 of the 17 women reported significant improvement in their psychological well-being.[7] It is important not exceed 50 milligrams per dose, since very high (1,500 to 3,000-milligram) doses may cause masculinizing side effects.

Scientists at the University of California at San Francisco conducted a preliminary study of the use of ginkgo in treating loss of libido connected with the use of antidepressants. Women included in the study were treated with the newer selective serotonin uptake inhibitors, Luvox, Paxil, Prozac, and Zoloft, or with the older MAOIs or tricyclic antidepressants. While some of the women in the study experienced headache or acid stomach, 28 out of 31 women reported a positive effect on all 4 phases of the sexual response cycle: desire, lubrication, orgasm, and afterglow.[8]

Scientists at the University of Hawaii supervised a study of ArginMax for Women, a product containing arginine, damiana, ginkgo, ginseng, and multiple vitamins and minerals. Nearly 3 out 4 women given ArginMax for 4 weeks reported increased sexual desire, reduced vaginal dryness, greater frequency of sexual intercourse and orgasm, and enhanced clitoral sensation. None of the women reported side effects.[9]

Yohimbine, a chemical extracted from the herb yohimbe, is probably highly effective in treating women's sexual dysfunction resulting from treatment for depression, but cannot be recommended here. Anxiety, surges in blood pressure, and heart palpitations can occur after taking even a single dose of yohimbine. These effects are worse when yohimbine is taken after consuming foods that contain the amino acid tyramine (chocolate, most French cheeses, liver, organ meats, or red wine), nasal decongestants, or weight-loss aids containing phenylpropanolamine. Even when the herb yohimbe is safe, it often is not effective. An unpublished study in the mid-1990s found that 13 out 14 "yohimbe" products tested did not contain the herb advertised.

If you still feel yohimbe could be effective for you, your best bet is to take the South American herb quebracho. This plant contains yohimbine, and is available from reliable manufacturers. There are numerous reports from satisfied buyers of Jaguara, available from Rainforest Herbs. More information is available from their web site at www.rain-tree.com. Other potentially useful herbs include pine pollen (taken in a dosage of 3,000–4,000 milligrams daily), which is anecdotally reported to increase testosterone levels in women, and stinging nettle root (taken in a dosage of 500–1,000 milligrams 3 times a day), which blocks a biochemical process that converts testosterone to 5-dihydrotesterone, a less potent form for sexual stimulation. Younger women who take the Pill may benefit from Tribestan (*Tribula terrestris*), taken as directed on the label.

CONCEPTS FOR COPING WITH LOSS OF SEXUAL DESIRE IN WOMEN

❍ Don't drink beer. Hops contain compounds very similar to estrogen. In the Middle Ages, hops were used in Central Europe to discourage sexual activity in young men and unmarried women.

❍ Chocolate is in fact an aphrodisiac. It contains large quantities of the amino acid L-arginine, included in ArginMax for Women.

❍ Androstenediol is converted to testosterone by both men and women. The problem with the use of androstenediol is timing: increases to serum testosterone levels are short-lived, and may not increase sex drive while it could cause other side effects.

❍ Women who have a diminished sex drive should avoid herbs that increase estrogen production, including dong quai (tang-kuei), fennel, hops, licorice, peony, soy isoflavones, and white willow.

Lung Cancer

SYMPTOM SUMMARY

❍ New onset of persistent cough, especially if you smoke

❍ Shortness of breath

❍ Dull chest pain (does not always occur)

❍ Coughing up blood (does not always occur)

UNDERSTANDING THE DISEASE PROCESS

Lung cancer is the number one cause of cancer deaths in the United States, Canada, and China. In Australia, New Zealand, the United Kingdom, and Europe lung cancer is the leading cause of cancer deaths among men. Only about 1 in 7 people who develops lung cancer survives 5 years.

Scientists have known for over 50 years that smoking cigarettes causes lung cancer. Over 85 percent of all cases of lung cancer occur in smokers. Smoking 1 pack of cigarettes a day increases the risk of lung cancer 25-fold, and just living in the same household with a smoker doubles the risk of lung cancer. Former smokers have an increased risk of cancer of the lungs for up to 15 years after they quit.[1] Nonetheless, quitting smoking is the best way to prevent lung cancer.

Although nearly all people who get lung cancer are smokers, not all smokers get lung cancer. The critical difference may be nutrition. Scientific studies generally indicate that as consumption of fruits and vegetables increases, risk of lung cancer decreases. Complex sugars from fruit are being investigated as a potential treatment for lung cancer.[2] On the other hand, regular consumption of cured meats (especially ham), eggs, French fries, and foods made with shortening increases the risk of lung cancer, even in people who never smoked.[3]

There has been considerable controversy has con-

tinued for years over the use of supplements in the prevention of lung cancer. Beta-carotene supplementation, in particular, has been found to increase the incidence of lung cancer in smokers, although fruits and vegetables rich in beta-carotene unequivocally lower the risk of lung cancer in smokers. The reason for these confounding findings seems to be that lung health requires a balanced supply of antioxidants, enough to undo the toxic effects of inhaled chemicals, but not so much as to limit the free-radical activation processes of the immune system. Without further evidence, use of nutritional supplements to prevent lung cancer is not advised.

TREATMENT SUMMARY

NUTRITIONAL SUPPLEMENTS

❍ Melatonin: 20 milligrams per day, taken 60 minutes before going to bed.

❍ Vitamin A: 300,000 IU per day. Women who are or who may become pregnant should strictly limit their intake of vitamin A to 5,000 IU per day or less.

UNDERSTANDING THE HEALING PROCESS

Once lung cancer has developed, at least two supplements may be helpful in some cases. A clinical study in Italy found that a very high dose of melatonin, 20 milligrams per day for 2 months, reduced the production of vascular endothelial growth factor, a chemical tumors need to grow the vessels for their own blood supply. Melatonin supplementation extended life in stable patients, but did not help "progressing" patients.[4] This dosage of melatonin often causes a daytime "hangover" and can aggravate depression. Melatonin is not recommended for any patient receiving interferon or any other form of immunotherapy.

Research is underway for the use of chemical compounds closely related to vitamin A as a form of chemotherapy for lung cancer. These compounds tend to be of significant but short-term benefit.[5] Clinical studies with vitamin A have found that high doses of the vitamin neither cure nor prevent recurrence of lung cancer, but they may slow the return of surgically treated lung cancer by a few months. The 300,000 IU per day of the vitamin needed for this effect can cause side effects of its own, notably dry skin and chapped lips. If skin changes occur, the vitamin should be stopped. Toxic levels of the vitamin cause joint pain, headaches, and liver damage.

Avoid vitamin A if you are receiving chemotherapy with doxorubicin (Adriamycin).

CONCEPTS FOR COPING WITH LUNG CANCER

While complementary treatment is of limited value as a sole therapy for lung cancer, it is of great benefit for enhancing the effectiveness and limiting the side effects of chemotherapy with doxorubicin (Adriamycin). Why would a book entitled *Healing without Medication* discuss chemotherapy? This book includes this topic because hundreds of thousands of cancer sufferers choose to take Adriamycin, and the usual attitude of doctors during all kinds of chemotherapy is wait and see. Doctors expect you either to tolerate complications or to come back to the hospital for emergency care. If you choose to be treated with this drug, an antioxidant supplement program during chemotherapy can both reduce your risk of complications and increase your chances of recovery from cancer.

O A number of studies with animals have confirmed that coenzyme Q_{10} reduces the risk of heart damage during chemotherapy with Adriamycin. One study with humans found that taking 50–100 milligrams of CoQ_{10} a day reduced the risk of heart damage by 20 percent and also prevented diarrhea and mouth sores.[6]

If you take CoQ_{10} during chemotherapy, you should avoid black pepper. The combination of CoQ_{10} and the spice makes CoQ_{10} less available in your body. If you are taking heparin, clopidogrel (Plavix), or warfarin (Coumadin), you need to let your doctor know you are taking CoQ_{10}, since the combination can make these anticlotting drugs less effective.

O N-acetyl cysteine (NAC) is often recommended during chemotherapy. Unfortunately, for Adriamycin therapy, this can be bad advice. NAC reduces heart damage during Adriamycin treatment in mice,[7] but even massive doses of NAC do not prevent heart damage during Adriamycin treatment in people.[8] One animal study found that NAC can actually interfere with the anticancer effect of Adriamycin.[9] Since NAC doesn't help and may hurt, it should be avoided during chemotherapy with Adriamycin.

O Quercetin is also often recommended during cancer treatment. People who take Adriamycin, however, should not take quercetin. Laboratory studies have shown that quercetin makes Adriamycin more effective in treating multidrug-resistant breast cancer,[10] but less effective in treating breast cancer that isn't multidrug resistant.[11] If you don't know whether you have a drug-resistant cancer, you definitely should not take quercetin. Green tea polyphenols, which are chemically similar to quercetin, pose the same problem. Since these supplements can also be harmful, don't take them while you are taking Adriamycin. An occasional cup of green tea as a beverage does not interfere with the drug.

O The bottom line on vitamin A and Adriamycin is that you should take this vitamin if you are being treated with Adriamycin for any form of cancer *except* lung cancer. Test tube studies have found that vitamin A actually makes lung cancer more resistant to Adriamycin.[12]

O Generally speaking, vitamin C will make Adriamycin more effective when cancer cells are susceptible to it. It will also make Adriamycin less effective when cancer cells are resistant to it. Animal experiments have found that taking large doses of vitamin C with Adriamycin reduces the risk of heart damage,[13] but consult with your physician before taking vitamin C. If your doctor believes you have a multidrug-resistant cancer, you should not take both Adriamycin and vitamin C.

Vitamin C taken in the form of vitamin C with bioflavonoids can interfere with the liver's ability to process statin drugs for controlling cholesterol, calcium channel blockers such as nifedipine (Procardia) for hypertension, or cyclosporine for preventing transplant rejection.

O Vitamin E appears to be extremely useful in preventing side effects from Adriamycin. Several experiments have confirmed that vitamin E keeps Adriamycin from destroying all kinds of cells with free radicals forming hydrogen peroxide, but allows Adriamycin to damage DNA in ways that restore cells to a normal life cycle.[14,15]

Vitamin E can reduce the risk of bleeding, so you need to consult with your physician before taking it, especially if you have had cancer surgery.

Lupus

SYMPTOM SUMMARY

O Butterfly-shaped rash across the nose and cheeks

O Diarrhea

○ Fatigue

○ Fever

○ Joint pain

○ Loss of appetite

○ Weight loss

○ Hair loss

○ Blood-vessel damage to kidney, lung.

○ Mouth sores

○ Rashes activated by exposure to sunlight

○ Seizures

○ Swelling

UNDERSTANDING THE DISEASE PROCESS

Systemic lupus erythematosus (SLE), more commonly called "lupus," is a chronic illness induced by an overactive immune system. It causes a characteristic butterfly-shaped rash across the nose and cheeks, accompanied by inflammation of joints and ligaments throughout the body. Lupus almost always occurs in women of child-bearing age. The causes of lupus are not known, although attacks can be triggered by eating alfalfa sprouts or using zinc supplements.

TREATMENT SUMMARY

NUTRITIONAL SUPPLEMENTS

○ DHEA: 200 milligrams per day, used under medical supervision.

UNDERSTANDING THE HEALING PROCESS

Dehydroepiandrosterone, commonly abbreviated as DHEA and also known as prasterone, is a steroid hormone made by the adrenal glands. For reasons that are not completely understood, low levels of DHEA are associated with especially severe symptoms of lupus. The latest clinical research finds that about half of women with lupus who take 100 or 200 milligrams of DHEA per day for 9 months can reduce their dosage of steroid medications for relief of joint pain—but nearly as many women got better on placebo.[1] Side effects of this dosage of DHEA are usually limited to acne, but because DHEA can cause liver damage and increase the risk of breast cancer when taken for a long time, its use should be medically monitored.

CONCEPTS FOR COPING WITH LUPUS

○ In one clinical study, 14 out of 17 patients taking a very high dose of fish oil (MaxEPA)—20 grams a day—experienced remission of symptoms of lupus over the course of 34 weeks.[2] Other studies using lower doses (even 15 grams per day) have failed to find benefit, and eating cold-water fish, while frequently recommended, is not scientifically proven to be helpful. If you choose to try high doses of fish oil as a treatment for lupus, be sure to check with your doctor to make sure none of your medications increase risk of bleeding. Be aware that taking a dosage of fish oil high enough to help lupus is likely to aggravate diarrhea and cause fishy burps.

○ There are a number of reports that the Chinese herb *Tripterygium wilfordii,* or thundervine, reduces the symptoms of lupus by suppressing immune function. Severe side effects and even death from using the herb are not unknown, and treatment with the herb should only be undertaken with the guidance of a knowledgeable professional.

Lyme Disease

SYMPTOM SUMMARY

○ Rash at the site of a tick bite, usually a flat or slightly raised red lesion at least 1–2 inches (3–5 centimeters) in diameter with a clear area in the center.

○ Unexplained fever, sweats, and chills

○ Headache

○ Fatigue

○ Buzzing or ringing in the ears

○ Disturbed sleep

○ Dizziness, wooziness, difficulty walking or standing up

○ Dry cough

○ Hair loss

○ Irritable bladder

○ Loss of vision, double vision, blurred vision

○ Mental confusion, memory loss, or difficulty concentrating or reading

- ○ Mood swings
- ○ Motion sickness
- ○ Muscle pain or cramps
- ○ Neck stiffness or crepitation (creaking)
- ○ Pelvic or testicular pain
- ○ Racing heart
- ○ Shortness of breath
- ○ Sore throat
- ○ Stiff joints
- ○ Swollen glands
- ○ Tingling, numbness, burning, stabbing sensations
- ○ Tremors
- ○ Unexplained lactation
- ○ Unexplained menstrual irregularity
- ○ Unusually severe hangover after drinking alcohol

UNDERSTANDING THE DISEASE PROCESS

Lyme disease is a bacterial infection causing an astonishing number of seemingly unrelated symptoms. Transmitted by bites from ticks that normally live on deer, Lyme disease is most commonly acquired during tick season, roughly from May through October. Infection with the bacteria that cause Lyme disease is most common in people who spend a lot of time out of doors. The infection is more likely to cause symptoms in children aged 15 and younger and adults aged 30 and older. Although cases have been reported in every state in the United States except Hawaii, more than 80 percent of cases are found in eight states—Connecticut, Maryland, Massachusetts, New Jersey, New York, Pennsylvania, Rhode Island, and Wisconsin. The number of cases reported increased from 7,943 in 1993 to 16,273 in 1999, and over 120,000 people in the United States have ongoing symptoms of the disease.[1]

Not every tick carries *Borrellia burgdorferi,* the bacterium that causes Lyme disease, and not every bite from an infected tick transmits the disease to a human host. *B. burgdorferi* tends to localize in the stomach of the tick. It only migrates to the tick's salivary glands after the tick has made a bite. If the tick is removed quickly, there is less time to transmit the bacterium. Researchers believe that few infections occur if the tick is removed in the first 24 hours, but the chance of infection is high if the tick is allowed to remain on the skin for 72 hours or more.

After *B. burgdorferi* enters the human body, the immune system attempts to trap it at the site of the bite. A ring of inflammation surrounds the invading bacteria. This makes the characteristic *erythema migrans,* or target lesion, a ring-shaped rash. Sometimes the lymphatic system is able to contain the infection, but frequently it escapes to infect the central nervous system and the joints. Whether the bacterium is trapped or escapes depends in part on whether the skin has an adequate supply of vitamin D. Skin cells that have an adequate supply of vitamin D are better able to secrete an immune hormone known as interleukin-8 (IL-8), which signals white blood cells that a bacterium has invaded the skin.[2] Vitamin D continues to be important in fighting Lyme disease as the infection spreads beyond the skin, enabling cells in other tissues to send out an alarm to the immune system.

Once inside the body, *B. burgdorferi* becomes a stealth invader. In the ticks and mice that host the bacterium through much of its life cycle, the bacterium has a thick cell wall and a spiral shape. If it maintained its thick cell wall and its spiral shape, an antibiotic could be found to control it. However, in the human body *B. burgdorferi* can shed its cell wall and take on a different shape. When under attack from antibiotics or the immune system, it simply changes shape so it is not recognized.

Unfortunately, the stealth bacterium produces a "shock protein" the immune system does recognize. The immune system senses this protein on the surface of nerves. It sends antibodies to latch onto the protein and neutralize it. However, in the process of attempting to neutralize the protein it interferes with the function of the nerves in ways that produce a bewildering array of symptoms. Certain nerves are immune to this process: those that have an adequate supply of the messenger chemical cAMP and those that have adequate supplies of vitamin A.[3]

TREATMENT SUMMARY

NUTRITIONAL SUPPLEMENTS

○ Vitamin A: 50,000 IU per day. Women who are or who may become pregnant should strictly limit their intake of vitamin A to 5,000 IU per day or less.

○ Vitamin D: 200–600 IU daily.

○ Zinc picolinate: 30 milligrams daily.

HERBS

○ Forskolin: 5–10 milligrams 3 times a day (or 50 milligrams of 18% forskolin extract 3 times a day).

○ Ginseng: 100 milligrams of ginsenoside extract, or 4 grams of ginseng root, daily.

○ Milk thistle: 70 milligrams of silymarin phytosomes 3 times a day.

UNDERSTANDING THE HEALING PROCESS

Since Lyme disease has only been recognized since the 1990s, both conventional medicine and complementary medicine are just beginning to understand it. No clinical studies have been conducted to confirm the value of the treatments recommended here. Nonetheless, there are anecdotal reports and a rationale for their use in the supportive care of the condition.

As noted above, laboratory tests suggest that nerve cells provided with adequate supplies of vitamin A are less likely to suffer damage from autoimmune attack when bacterial proteins lodge on their surfaces. Additionally, relatively low doses of vitamin A are sufficient to prevent "burnout" due to stress on the immune output of the thymus.[4] Vitamin A also enhances antibody response, increases the rate at which macrophages destroy bacteria, and stimulates natural killer cells.[5]

This dosage of vitamin A can cause side effects, such as dry skin, chapped lips, headaches, and joint pain. Discontinue vitamin A immediately if any of these symptoms appear. Women who are or who may become pregnant should strictly limit their intake of vitamin A to 5,000 IU per day or less, since it can cause birth defects if taken during the first 3 months of pregnancy.

Cells throughout the body that have adequate supplies of vitamin D can signal the immune system for help. Although the B. burgdorferi bacterium can change forms so that it is not recognized by the immune system, at any given time at least some of the bacteria circulating through the body can be neutralized by white blood cells. A dosage of 200 IU per day for children to 600 IU per day for adults is enough to prevent deficiency, even in the cloudy states of the northeastern United States where vitamin D deficiency is most likely to occur.

Zinc is an important cofactor for vitamin A. When zinc is deficient, the immune system's ability to produce white blood cells in response to infection is reduced, thymic hormone levels are lower, and phagocytosis, the process in which bacteria are engulfed and digested, is slowed. When zinc is deficient, all of these processes can be corrected by taking zinc supplements.[6]

A quick method for detecting zinc deficiency is a taste test. Powder a tablet of any zinc-based supplement or cold medication and mix with $\frac{1}{4}$ cup (50 milliliters) of water. Slosh the mixture in the mouth. People who notice no taste at all or who notice a "dry," "mineral," or "sweet" taste are likely to be zinc deficient. Anyone who notices a definite strong and unpleasant taste that intensifies over time is not likely to be zinc deficient.

Zinc picolinate is the most readily absorbed form of zinc. Do not take more than 50 milligrams of any zinc supplement daily. In rare cases, excessive intake of zinc depletes copper to cause anemia, that is, a deficiency of red blood cells, and neutropenia, a serious deficiency of white blood cells.

Forskolin activates the enzyme adenylate cyclase, which increases the amount of the regulator cyclic adenosine monophosphate (cAMP) in cells.[7] This enzyme is found in all cell membranes and is crucial to preventing autoimmune damage to the membrane. It is likely that taking forskolin can offset some of the symptoms of Lyme disease associated with nerve cell irritation, such as headache, tingling, burning, numbness, stabbing sensations, tremor, unexplained lactation, or severe hangover. People who have unusually low blood pressure or who have peptic ulcers should not take forskolin. Forskolin also should be used with caution by people who take the asthma medication theophylline (Theo-Dur), since it increases the medication's effects on the lungs.

Ginseng balances the body's production of stress hormones by increasing the production of cAMP. This action also enables nerve cells under attack by the immune system to attract and bind anti-inflammatory hormones to protect themselves from damage. It also stimulates the production and activity of white blood cells to fight infection.[8]

Side effects from the use of ginseng are possible. These include morning diarrhea, elevated blood pressure, nervousness, sleep disturbance, skin outbreaks, and euphoria. Side effects are most common in warm weather and in physically active people. Although it defies intuition, side effects are eliminated by taking a higher dose of the herb.

Milk thistle is an especially potent deactivator of cyclic AMP phosphodiesterase, the enzyme that breaks down the cAMP protecting the lining of nerve cells.[9] In addition to its benefit to nerve tissue, it prevents inflammatory reactions in the liver. Some people experience mild diarrhea when first taking the herb, but it is nontoxic and does not interfere with the action of prescription medications.

CONCEPTS FOR COPING WITH LYME DISEASE

○ If you choose to take antibiotics, bromelain increases the absorption. Take 500–750 milligrams of bromelain between meals. It is also helpful to take 1–2 capsules of *Lactobacillus* every day to restore friendly bacteria that are lost during antibiotic treatment.

CONCEPTS FOR REDUCING THE RISK OF CONTRACTING LYME DISEASE

○ The ticks that carry Lyme disease are small, brown, and pear-shaped, and have black legs. Remove an attached tick as soon as it is detected. Ticks usually bite in folds of skin or where creases in clothing stop their movement. To remove the tick, place *one end* of a pair of tweezers under the tick as close to the skin as possible and pull upward with steady pressure. Do not squeeze the tick, since this can force the contents of the tick's stomach into the bite and infect the wound. Do not use alcohol, turpentine, or a hot match to remove ticks, since these methods can cause the tick to vomit into the wound, transmitting the bacteria that cause Lyme disease.

○ Perform daily checks of your skin for ticks. Pay special attention to hairy areas.

○ Keep pets tick-free.

○ Keep deer out of residential properties.

○ Tuck long pant legs into socks.

○ Wear long-sleeved shirts that are tight at the wrists.

○ Wear a hat when walking through woods.

○ Wear white or light clothes. This makes it easier to see ticks.

○ Walk in the center of trails.

○ Avoid sitting on the ground in tick-infested areas.

○ Clear away brush and trees near your home. Do not stack piles of leaves in the yard.

Lymphedema

SYMPTOM SUMMARY

○ Chronic swelling of the arm or leg, or of the scrotal sac in men.

UNDERSTANDING THE DISEASE PROCESS

Approximately 2 out of 5 women who have surgical treatment for breast cancer subsequently develop lymphedema, swelling in the arm nearest the mastectomy.[1] The circulation of the lymph is regulated by a series of valves that allow for unidirectional flow. When lymph nodes are removed to test for or treat cancer, the circulation of lymph is stopped, causing fluid to accumulate in the affected arm or arms. Lymph is forced to leak slowly into the surrounding tissues and then into the bloodstream. The resulting swelling can cause the arm to swell to several times its original size. It may occur immediately after surgery or as much as 20 years later. Women of the greatest weight before surgery are at the highest risk for developing the condition.[2]

Although breast cancer surgery is the most common cause of lymphedema in the United States, any cancer surgery involving dissection of the lymph nodes can cause lymphedema. Surgical treatment of cervical or uterine cancer or melanoma sometimes results in lymphedema of the legs. Removal of the prostate can cause lymphedema in the legs or penis or a swelling of the scrotum known as hydrocele.

Lymphedema can be complicated by lymphangitis, a cellulitis infection that interrupts the normal flow of lymph. A severe traumatic injury to an arm or leg may also trigger lymphedema. As many as 200 million people in southeast Asia, India, and Africa suffer lymphedema from a chronic infection called filariasis. When the filarial larvae of a mosquite bite enter the lymph canal, the larvae mature into worms causing severe lymphedema of the arms, legs, and genitals.

TREATMENT SUMMARY

For lymphedema of all causes:

NUTRITIONAL SUPPLEMENTS

○ Wobenzym (Nutri World): as directed on label.

HERBS

○ Sweet clover (Le Thalasso Bain Leg Health Gel by Goemar): apply as an ointment daily.

DIET

○ Avoid long-chain triglycerides, any fat that stays solid at room temperature (shortening, butter, and so on).

For filiariasis:

NUTRITIONAL SUPPLEMENTS

○ Vitamin E: 400 IU per day.

○ Avoid iron supplements.

UNDERSTANDING THE HEALING PROCESS

Two supplements are generally helpful in treating lymphedema after cancer surgery. Clinical studies of recovering breast cancer patients in Austria have found that Wobenzym typically begins to reduce swelling after about 2 months of regular use.[3] Adverse reactions to Wobenzym have never been reported. If this product is unavailable, bromelain or papain (taken as directed on the label) may also help. Sweet clover contains "thinners" known as coumarins that accelerate the circulation of lymph through the wall of the remaining lymphatic system and into the bloodstream.[4] Consult your physician before using sweet clover ointments if you are taking a prescription coumarin such as Lympedim.

Anyone suffering from lymphedema can benefit from avoiding long-chain triglycerides, fats that remain solid at room temperature, such as butter, lard, or shortening.[5] Since lymphedema is an accumulation of a protein-rich fluid, extreme low-protein diets are sometimes recommended for reducing swelling, but resulting muscle tissue breakdown can actually increase, rather than decrease, overall edema.

Studies of lymphedema caused by filariasis show that the intensity of the infection is less when vitamin E is adequate and greater in the presence of excessive iron.[6] No one with lymphedema of infectious origins should take iron supplements.

CONCEPTS FOR COPING WITH LYMPHEDEMA

○ Of all the therapies for leg lymphedema, the most effective is a combination of magnet therapy, compression, and moist warmth. In a clinical test in Japan, 6 out of 10 legs treated with the therapy returned to normal size.[7] Physical therapists may begin offering this treatment in the United States in 2003.

○ Lymphatic drainage by applying rollers to the affected limb, rather than manual massage, has yielded impressive results in clinical trials in Brazil.[8] This method may also be introduced into the United States in the near future.

○ If you notice a rash, blistering, redness, increase of temperature or fever, see your physician immediately. An inflammation or infection in the affected limb could be the worsening of lymphedema or the beginning of lymphangitis, a particularly serious form of cellulitis.

○ If itching under a compression sleeve, stocking, or bandage is a problem, try moisturizing the skin before replacing the bandage. Be sure to change sleeves, stockings, and bandages every 12 hours, and only use sleeves and stockings that are freshly laundered.

○ Regular exercise is helpful for many health reasons, but it will not improve circulation of lymph. Excessive exercise can transport additional lymph to the limbs and cause swelling. If you are beginning an exercise program, increase your amounts of daily exercise slowly to avoid overloading your lymphatic channels.

○ Swimming is the best exercise for lymphedema, but it is important to dry thoroughly and to apply moisturizing lotion to the skin. Talcum powder, especially behind the knee, makes is easier to put on compression stockings.

○ Many people do not realize it is possible to get a sunburn through a compression garment. Skin over a lympedema-affected limb is at greater risk for skin cancer.[9] Burned skin on a swollen limb takes longer to heal. Before going outdoors, apply a sunscreen with an SPF of 30 to the skin beneath the garment.

○ Avoid acupuncture in affected limbs.

○ If you develop poison ivy or poison oak, put on gloves before washing affecting areas. Do not bandage.

○ Liposuction is not a cure for lymphedema.

○ Chronic lymphedema in the legs can cause warty growths on the toes. Compression bandages applied to the toes can reduce draining and swelling.

○ Travel by air can trigger lymphedema in surgically treated cancer patients who previously did not have symptoms. When traveling by air, be sure to wear a compression sleeve. Affected limbs may swell when exposed to reduce air pressure.

❍ Take warm, not hot, baths and showers. Hot water can cause dry skin, leading to infection. After taking a bath or shower, apply Eucerin or Nivea cream to the skin on the affected limb. This protects the skin from chapping and infection. Dove unscented soap or a glycerin soap keeps the skin from becoming too alkaline. Avoid body washes, which can dry the skin.

❍ Avoid any type of trauma to a limb affected by lymphedema: bruises, cat scratches, cuts, insect bites, sports injuries, or sunburn.

❍ Do not wear tight anklets, bracelets, rings, or watch bands over affected tissue.

❍ Never carry heavy handbags or bags with over-the-shoulder straps with an affected arm.

❍ Wear gloves while doing gardening, housework, or any other kind of work that could result in even a minor injury.

❍ A heavy breast prosthesis can place too much pressure on the collar bone. Use the lightest prosthesis available.

❍ Never remove hair from an affected limb with a straight-edged razor. Always use an electric razor.

Macular Degeneration

SYMPTOM SUMMARY

❍ Blurred or absent central vision (peripheral vision is unaffected)

UNDERSTANDING THE DISEASE PROCESS

The macula is the circular disk in the center of the retina that recognizes fine details in the center of the field of vision. In the less common form of macular degeneration, "wet" macular degeneration, misplaced blood vessels grow behind the retina. These weakened blood vessels tend to leak. In the worst cases, the accumulation of fluids can physically lift the macula from its moorings to create a distorted field of vision. Wet macular degeneration accounts for 10 percent of cases of the disease but 90 percent of the cases of blindness caused by the condition. In the more common "dry" form of the dis-

ease, damage occurs without hemorrhage and without scarring. Both types of macular degeneration cause the destruction of rods and cones in the retina, resulting in loss of vision.

Risk factors for macular degeneration include smoking cigarettes, working with chemicals, and exposure to bright sunlight. People who are farsighted are more likely to get the disease than people who are nearsighted or who have normal vision, and people of European descent are more likely to get the disease than people of African descent. A family history of the disease increases the risk. Many people who have macular degeneration have a history of heart disease and a weak hand grip.

TREATMENT SUMMARY

DIET

❍ Eat your greens, especially collard greens and spinach, as well as orange and yellow fruits and vegetables, including corn.

❍ Drink wine in moderation. Avoid beer.

NUTRITIONAL SUPPLEMENTS

❍ Lutein: 5 milligrams per day.

❍ Mixed carotenoids: 50,000 IU per day.

❍ Selenium: 400 micrograms per day.

❍ Vitamin C: 1,000 milligrams 3 times a day.

❍ Vitamin E: 600–800 IU per day.

❍ Zinc picolinate: 80 milligrams (a 30-milligram capsule plus a 50-milligram capsule) per day.

HERBS

❍ Bilberry: 40–80 milligrams of 25% anthocyanidin extract, 3 times a day.

❍ Ginkgo: 40–80 milligrams 3 times a day.

❍ Grape seed extract (with 95% procyanidols): 150–300 milligrams per day.

UNDERSTANDING THE HEALING PROCESS

Conventional medicine offers no effective prevention for macular degeneration. Over 40 scientific studies, however, confirm the value of nutritional supplements and herbs in preventing the condition.

The National Health and Nutrition Examination Survey found that the more survey respondents ate fruits and vegetables high in beta-carotene, the less likely they were to develop macular degeneration.[1] Eating collard greens and spinach, in particular, is associated with a lower rate of the disease.[2] The Beaver Dam Eye Study examined the diets of 2,003 individuals aged 43–84 and found that consumption of foods containing either beta-carotene (the collard greens and spinach previously mentioned, as well as apricots, carrots, mangoes, and squash) or vitamin E (such as nuts) prevented the formation of drusen, spots of pigmentation that precede the development of macular degeneration.[3]

Drinking as little as one glass of wine a month seems to confer some protection against macular degeneration. In its nutritional assessment of 3,072 adults aged 45–74, the National Health and Nutrition Examination Survey found that only 4 percent of adults who drank wine developed macular degeneration, compared to 9 percent who drank no alcohol at all. The Beaver Dam Eye Study, on the other hand, found that men who consumed at least one beer a week had a higher (11 percent) rate of early development of age-related macular degeneration than men who did not drink beer (7 percent). Beer drinking was also associated with the development of predegenerative drusen.

Lutein is a chemical relative of beta-carotene that is found in carrots, corn, greens, potatoes, tomatoes, and most fruits. Zeaxanthin is another relative of beta-carotene found in corn, fruit, paprika, and spinach. Both compounds are strong antioxidants. Along with three other antioxidants, vitamins A, C, and E, they are found in relatively high concentrations in the retina. Lutein and zeaxanthin give the macula its characteristic yellow color, lutein tending to accumulate around the edges of the eye, and zeaxanthin accumulating in the center of the eye.

Individually, none of these five antioxidants—lutein, zeaxanthin, or vitamins A, C, or E—confers protection against macular degeneration. Taken together, these five antioxidants offer significant protection against macular degeneration,[4] but even when taken separately, antioxidants have important benefits. Experiments with laboratory animals have found that vitamin C protects the visual pigment rhodopsin from degradation by intense light—provided vitamin C is available in adequate amounts *before* exposure to the bright light.[5] A study enlisting 976 participants found that just having high bloodstream concentrations of vitamin E (as alpha-tocopherol) was protective against macular degenera-

tion.[6] The Physician's Health Study evaluated 21,120 individuals over a period of $12\frac{1}{2}$ years. None of the 21,120 participants had a diagnosis of macular degeneration at the beginning of the study. Taking vitamin E regularly resulted in a 13 percent reduced risk of developing macular degeneration (which was statistically insignificant).[7] Vitamin E in the form of dihydrolipoic acid also regenerates vitamin C by releasing it from its end-product, dehydroascorbate.[8]

Zinc and selenium together help renew antioxidants in the eye, although they are probably more important in the "dry" form of macular degeneration. One hundred fifty-one subjects aged 42–89, all of whom had dry macular degeneration with vision of less than 20/80 in at least one eye, were enlisted in a study in which they received either 40 milligrams of elemental zinc or a placebo every day for 2 years. At the 1-year and 2-year evaluations, the participants receiving zinc had lost less vision than those receiving a placebo.[9] A follow-up study involving patients with "wet" macular degeneration failed to find a similar benefit.[10] *Injections* of zinc and selenium together, however, sometimes produce dramatic results. Injections must be administered by a physician.

Bilberry, ginkgo, and grape seed extracts complement antioxidant supplements by strengthening blood vessels and by improving the circulation of blood through the retina. Bilberry anthocyanosides are especially valuable in the treatment of the "dry" form of the disease, possibly even reversing macular degeneration.[11] Ginkgo is probably most useful when there are also signs of cerebrovascular insufficiency, such as memory loss, hearing loss, or dizziness. Grape seed extract may be the most useful when there is impairment of night vision.[12]

CONCEPTS FOR COPING WITH MACULAR DEGENERATION

○ Smoking is extremely detrimental in macular degeneration. A study comparing 34 smokers and 34 non-smokers found that nonsmokers had more than twice the amount of healthy pigment in their retinas as non-smokers. The more cigarettes smoked, the thinner the pigment.[13] The effects of smoking are more severe in women than in men. A clinical study found that women smokers had 38 percent less pigment in their eyes than male smokers, despite similar antioxidant levels.[14]

Maculopathy

See **Macular Degeneration.**

Malabsorption

See **Celiac Disease; Cirrhosis of the Liver; Cystic Fibrosis; Inflammatory Bowel Disease; Pancreatitis.**

Male Infertility

SYMPTOM SUMMARY

○ Failure to achieve pregnancy after 1 year of unprotected sexual intercourse and medically demonstrated deficiencies in the number, motility (movement), or quality of sperm

UNDERSTANDING THE DISEASE PROCESS

Varying degrees of infertility affect about 1 in 16 men in the United States and other developed countries. The condition can be caused by vasectomy, inflammation or blockage of the ducts carrying sperm out of the testes, or ejaculatory disorders, but in about 90 percent of cases, infertility is due to deficient sperm production of unknown causes.[1] Chemotherapy, drugs for epilepsy and tuberculosis, the antibiotic nitrofurantoin (Macrobid), steroids, and recreational use of cocaine and marijuana reduce fertility. Hemochromatosis, hypothyroidism, and cirrhosis of the liver also reduce fertility. Infection with chlamydia, which produces antisperm antibodies, affects up to 70 percent of infertile men.[2]

TREATMENT SUMMARY

NUTRITIONAL SUPPLEMENTS

○ Folic acid: 5 milligrams per day.

○ Zinc: 75 milligrams per day.

Other treatments are effective for specific indications of male infertility.

UNDERSTANDING THE HEALING PROCESS

All men attempting to improve their fertility should wear boxer shorts and trunks instead of briefs or bikinis, avoid tight-fitting pants, and steer clear of strenuous workouts, hot tubs, and hot baths. Keeping scrotal temperature low by keeping clothing loose increases production of live sperm.

The combination of zinc and folic acid offers the greatest general usefulness in treating male infertility. A study at the University Medical Centre at Nijmegen in the Netherlands reported in 2002 that sperm counts increased an average of 74 percent in 108 fertile and 103 subfertile men given 5 milligrams of folic acid and 66 milligrams of zinc daily for 6 months. The treatment was effective even though blood tests before the trial found that men were not deficient in these nutrients.[3]

L-carnitine is helpful when infertility is due to athenospermia, a condition of poor motility or "swimming" ability rather than a low sperm count. This naturally occurring compound provides energy for the sperm to travel from the cervix to the egg in the uterus. In one clinical trial, 100 men with sperm motility problems were given 3,000 milligrams of L-carnitine per day for 4 months. At the end of the study, the average number of motile sperm per sample increased from 26–37 percent, enough to ensure normal fertility.[4] L-carnitine treatment helps about three-quarters of men with athenospermia.[5]

Clinical studies have found benefits from calcium, coenzyme Q_{10}, L-arginine, vitamin B_{12}, vitamin C, and vitamin E. The majority of scientific research supports the use of folic acid, zinc, and L-carnitine.

CONCEPTS FOR COPING WITH MALE INFERTILITY

○ A normal sperm count is 20 million sperm per cubic centimeter (cc) of seminal fluid. A low sperm count, however, does not always mean infertility. One study found that 52 percent of men with a sperm count below 20 million per cc were able to impregnate their partners and 40 percent of men with a sperm count below 10 million per cc were also able to conceive.[6]

○ If you smoke, quit. If you can't quit smoking, take vitamin C. A study at the University of Texas found that taking 1,000 milligrams of vitamin C daily improved motility and quantity of sperm.[7]

○ Cottonseed oil, now seldom used for cooking in the United States, can have a devastating effect on male fertility. Cottonseed contains gossypol, used experimentally in China as a male contraceptive. Male workers on cotton farms and in cotton gins may also have reduced fertility.

O Men who become infertile after chemotherapy with doxorubicin (Adriamycin) sometimes recover fertility after use of the Japanese herbal formula *hochu-ekki-to*. In a clinical study in Japan, 20 percent of participating couples achieved conception within 12 weeks, and 51 percent of the men taking the formula had increased sperm counts.[8] Laboratory studies with animals indicate that the formula works by stimulating the production of proteins that enable sperm to reach functional maturity. In the United States and Canada, this herbal formula is available under the following trade names:

- Added Flavors Supplement the Center & Boost Qi (Blue Poppy Herbs)
- Arouse Vigor (Kan Herbals)
- Breaking Clouds (Three Treasures)
- Bu Zhong Yi Qi Tang (Asian Patents, Blue Poppy Herbs, Chinese Classics, Golden Flower Chinese Herbs, Health Concerns, Kan Herbals, Lotus Classics, ProBotanixx, Qualiherb, Sun Ten, Three Treasures)
- Central Chi Tea (Asian Patents)
- Ginseng & Astragalus (Qualiherb)
- Ginseng & Astragalus Combination (Sun Ten)
- Ginseng & Astragalus Formula (Golden Flower Chinese Herbs)
- Hochuekkito Formula 017 (Kampo Institute)
- Raise Qi (Health Concerns)
- Tonify Qi & Ease the Muscles (Three Treasures)
- Yi Qi (Probotanixx)

Manic Depression

See **Bipolar Disorder (Manic Depression)**.

Mastitis

SYMPTOM SUMMARY

O Breast enlargement in one breast only

O Breast lump

O Breast pain

O Fever

O Heat, redness, swelling, and tenderness in breast tissue

O Itching

O Nipple discharge

O Shiny or red-streaked skin on the breast

O Tender or swollen lymph nodes on the same side as the affected breast

Shooting pains in the breast without an area of hardness do not indicate mastitis. These are more likely due to a yeast infection.

UNDERSTANDING THE DISEASE PROCESS

Mastitis is a bacterial infection of the breast. Mastitis most commonly occurs in women who are breastfeeding, but it can occur in women who are not breastfeeding and even in small babies.[1] No one knows why some women get mastitis and others do not, but the condition is usually caused by *Staphylococcus aureus* entering through a break or crack in the nipple.[2] The bacterium may be transmitted from the baby's mouth to the nipple, especially from a teething infant, although it typically grows on the skin. Since the baby frequently is the source of the infection, nursing during mastitis does not harm the infant. About 1 in 20 nursing mothers gets mastitis.[3]

It is important to distinguish mastitis from a plugged or blocked milk duct. A plugged duct presents itself as a firm, painful, swollen mass in the breast. The reddening of the skin due to a clogged duct is less intense than the reddening caused by mastitis. Mastitis causes a more intense pain and is usually accompanied by fever. It is not always easy to distinguish a blocked duct from mastitis, and a blocked duct may lead to mastitis. Blocked ducts, however, will almost always resolve spontaneously within 24–48 hours after onset.

TREATMENT SUMMARY

DIET

O Avoid foods to which you may be allergic. Limit consumption of simple sugars to 50 grams (2 ounces) per day. Be sure to include whole, natural foods, such as fruits, vegetables, legumes, and whole grains in your diet. Drink at least six 8-ounce glasses of water daily.

NUTRITIONAL SUPPLEMENTS

○ Coenzyme Q_{10}: 30 milligrams per day.

○ Thymus extract: 500 milligrams of crude polypeptides daily.

○ Vitamin A: 5,000 IU per day.

○ Vitamin C: 1,000 milligrams 3 times per day.

○ Zinc picolinate: 30 milligrams per day.

HERBS

○ Aloe gel: apply to skin 2–3 times a day after abscesses have burst. *Note:* breast abscesses require medical attention. Treatment with aloe is not a substitute for a physician's care.

○ Astragalus: solid extract (0.5% 4-hydroxy-3-methoxy isoflavone), 100–150 milligrams 3 times a day, or dried root or tincture, as recommended on the label.

○ Echinacea: 150–300 milligrams of solid extract (3.5% echinacosides) 3 times a day, or dried root, freeze-dried plant, juice, fluid extract, or tincture, as recommended on the label.

For infections affecting the end of the nipple:

Tea tree oil: creams containing 8–20% tea tree oil or 40% solution, applied to the skin with a cotton swab 2–3 times daily. Be sure to discard the applicator in a plastic bag so that the infection is not spread.

UNDERSTANDING THE HEALING PROCESS

Healing mastitis takes place from the inside out. Enhancing and maintaining the strength of the immune system is key to controlling recurring infections. Amoxicillin, plain penicillin, and other antibiotics are often ineffective because they have been prescribed too frequently and bacteria have become resistant to them.[4]

Moreover, because staph infections tend to be most active below the surface of the skin, topical treatment is of limited value, except for treating blisters at the end of the nipple. Of the natural products that may be applied to the skin, only aloe and tea tree oil have been scientifically demonstrated to heal staph infections, although poultices of barberry, coptis, goldenseal, or Oregon grape root are likely to be helpful when a different kind of bacteria is causing the infection.

Simply maintaining the hydration of the breast by drinking adequate amounts of water can be of great val-ue in treating boils. Well-hydrated breast tissue is supple, more resistant to reinfection, and releases accumulated white blood cells and pus more easily. Whole grains, fruits, and vegetables are natural sources of flavonoids, which help vitamin C in fighting infection.[5]

In laboratory experiments with mice, coenzyme Q_{10} (CoQ_{10}) increased the immune response to infection with *Staphylococcus aureus*.[6] CoQ_{10} supplementation is especially useful for persons who take statin drugs to control cholesterol levels, since the statins interfere with the body's ability to produce both CoQ_{10} and cholesterol.

There are very few precautions to take in the use of CoQ_{10}. The medical literature contains one report of CoQ_{10} decreasing the effectiveness of warfarin (Coumadin). It may improve sugar control in some cases of diabetes. If you are diabetic, check your blood sugars regularly when you take CoQ_{10}. Black pepper increases bloodstream levels of CoQ_{10} and seasoning your food with pepper would be helpful when you take CoQ_{10}, provided your baby does not object.

Although there are no studies that directly confirm the usefulness of thymus extracts in treating staph infections, there is considerable evidence that thymus extracts correct low immune function. In particular, research has shown that thymus extract normalizes the ratio of T-helper cells to T suppressor cells, maintaining a healthy immune response that neither destroys healthy tissue nor allows infectious microorganisms to flourish.[7]

Relatively low doses of vitamin A are sufficient to prevent "burnout" due to stress on the immune output of the thymus.[8] Vitamin A also enhances antibody response, increases the rate at which macrophages destroy bacteria, and stimulates natural killer cells.[9]

Birth defects due to taking vitamin A supplements are extremely rare, having occurred fewer than 20 times in the United States. Nonetheless, women who could become pregnant—unlikely while breastfeeding—should not take more than 5,000 IU of supplemental vitamin A daily. Overdoses of vitamin A can cause dry skin and chapped lips, especially in dry weather. Later signs of toxicity are headache, mood swings, and pain in muscles and joints. In massive doses, vitamin A can cause liver damage. Discontinue vitamin A at the first sign of toxicity, and never use it for more than 3 months at a time.

Vitamin C levels are quickly depleted during the stress of infection.[10] In combination with the anthocyanidins and proanthocyanidins found in blue and dark red fruits, vitamin C helps increase the stability of the ground substance, the "glue" between the skin and the tissues below it.[11]

Women with mastitis are seldom prescribed any drugs that interact with vitamin C, but some cautionary notes are in order. Vitamin C taken in the form of vitamin C with bioflavonoids can interfere with the liver's ability to process statin drugs for controlling cholesterol, calcium channel blockers such as nifedipine (Procardia) for hypertension, or cyclosporine for preventing transplant rejection.

Zinc is an important cofactor for vitamin A. When zinc is deficient, the immune system's ability to produce white blood cells in response to infection is reduced, thymic hormone levels are lower, the immune response in the skin is especially reduced, and phagocytosis, the process in which bacteria are engulfed and digested, is slowed. When zinc is deficient, all of these processes can be corrected by taking zinc supplements.[12]

Zinc is also essential to dozens of enzymatic processes, including those that send a signal to polymorphonuclear leukocytes to fight bacterial infection. Zinc helps breast tissue make enzymes that slow down the process of tissue destruction initiated by endotoxins released by bacteria.[13]

While it is important to take zinc in treating mastitis, it is equally important not to take too much. Except where otherwise directed, do not take more than 50 milligrams of any zinc supplement daily. In rare cases, excessive intake of zinc depletes copper to cause anemia, that is, a deficiency of red blood cells, and neutropenia, a serious deficiency of white blood cells. Zinc should not be taken with antibiotic drugs. It can interfere with their absorption or possibly cause rheumatoid inflammation of joints.

Aloe is especially useful treating abscesses that have burst. It contains a number of compounds necessary for healing wounds, including vitamin C, vitamin E, and zinc. Gels that are at least 70 percent aloe are bactericidal against both *Pseudomonas aeruginosa* and *Staphylococcus aureus,* the two most common infections causing boils and carbuncles.[14]

Allergies to aloe are extremely rare. There are no known drugs that cause adverse reactions when used with aloe.

Astragalus is a traditional Chinese treatment for boils. It is especially useful in reversing damage to the immune system caused by chemicals or radiation.[15] In laboratory studies with test animals, it increases the number and activity of monocytes and macrophages, responsible for controlling bacterial infection.[16]

Astragalus is an extremely useful immune stimulant, but not everyone should take it. Anyone who is on an immune suppressant (for example, people who have had organ transplants) or who takes immune suppressant drugs for multiple sclerosis, myasthenia gravis, rheumatoid arthritis, scleroderma, Sjögren's syndrome, or similar diseases, should not take astragalus. (If you develop an abscess while taking drugs for any of these conditions, you should seek medical care.) It is theoretically possible that astragalus could cause excessive bleeding when taken with drugs such as Coumadin (warfarin), heparin, Plavix (clopidogrel), Ticlid (ticlopidine), Trental (pentoxifylline), or aspirin. Be especially careful not to overdose astragalus if you take any of these prescription drugs. Stop taking astragalus if you notice a bruise or a bleeding cut.

Echinacea is a well-known immune stimulant. It is especially useful in stimulating phagocytosis, the process by which white blood cells surround and digest infectious microorganisms. A study of oral administration of an *Echinacea purpurea* root extract (30 drops 3 times per day) to healthy men for 5 days resulted in a 120 percent increase in phagocytosis.[17] In laboratory tests, caffeic acid and echinacoside, two important chemical constituents of the herb, have been found to have specific antibacterial action against *Staphylococcus aureus.*[18]

While this precaution is not likely to apply to breastfeeding mothers, women who are trying to get pregnant should avoid *Echinacea purpurea.* It contains caffeoyl esters that can interfere the action of hyaluronidase, an enzyme essential to the release of unfertilized eggs into the fallopian tube.

There is laboratory evidence that *Echinacea angustifolia* deactivates the liver enzyme CYP3A4. This compound enables the liver to detoxify a wide range of medications, including anabolic steroids, the chemotherapy drug methotrexate (Methotrex), which is used in treating cancer, lupus, and rheumatoid arthritis, astemizole (Hismanal) for allergies, nifedipine (Adalat) and captopril (Capoten) for high blood pressure, and sildenafil (Viagra) for erectile dysfunction in men and failure to achieve orgasm in women, as well as many other drugs. *Echinacea angustifolia* might help maintain levels of these drugs in the bloodstream and make them more effective, or it might also cause them to accumulate to levels at which they cause side effects. If you take any of these drugs, you should not take *Echinacea angustifolia,* but neither should you be breastfeeding. Similarly you should avoid echinacea products if you are being treated for HIV, but you should not breastfeed your baby if you have this disease.

Naturopathic physicians Michael Murray and Joseph Pizzorno write that an Australian study conducted in the 1960s found that tea tree oil accelerated the healing process and prevented scarring in other kinds of staph infections. The method of application included cleaning the site, then painting the infected skin with tea tree oil 2 or 3 times a day.[19]

While tea tree can help cure mastitis, you must stop breastfeeding while you use it. Never expose an infant to tea tree oil. There have only been two recorded cases in which quantities of tea tree oil were found to poison children, both involving a child swallowing 10–70 times the amount that would be used to treat mastitis. Nonetheless, tea tree oil can cause loss of coordination in a young child, so you should never breastfeed your baby unless every trace of tea tree oil has been washed from the breast.

CONCEPTS FOR COPING WITH MASTITIS

Care for mastitis:

❍ Continue breastfeeding from the affected breast unless it is too painful to do so. Continuing breastfeeding helps mastitis resolve more rapidly. This species of bacteria will not grow in the baby's digestive tract.

❍ Do not rush feeding, so the breast will be more fully drained.

❍ Do not treat fever unless you are uncomfortable because of it. Fever slows the rate at which the infectious bacteria reproduce and accelerates recovery.

❍ Apply hot, wet compresses to relieve pain. Repeated application of compresses will make it easier for your healthcare professional to lance an abscess.

❍ Avoid external friction, such as that caused by a tight-fitting brassiere.

❍ Avoid sleeping face down.

❍ Never squeeze bumps (other than a blister at the end of the nipple, associated with a blocked duct) or cut open an abscess.

❍ Do not share clothes.

❍ Use clean washcloths. Change sheets and towels daily.

❍ Wash your hands frequently, especially after changing a dressing or applying ointment.

❍ Women who take antibiotic treatment should also take 10–40 million units of *acidophilus* or *Lactobacillus* (or combinations thereof) daily to maintain friendly bacteria.

❍ Some doctors who prescribe antibiotics for mastitis recommend giving nonantibiotic methods 8–12 hours to see if symptoms improve. If the condition begins to resolve on its own, antibiotics should not be taken. If symptoms do not improve in 8–12 hours, they recommend taking antibiotics.

❍ Rest as much as possible.

❍ The acupressure points for relieving breast pain lie about half a hand's width to the left and to the right of the midline of the front of the body, between the third and fourth ribs. Gently stimulating this area for 5–10 minutes several times a day is thought to disperse toxins associated with infection and emotional stress and move them out of the breasts.

Care for a blocked duct:

❍ Continue breastfeeding from the breast with the blocked duct. An oversupply of milk will worsen pain. Keep breasts draining by expression or by waking the baby for a feeding if he or she sleeps for long periods of time.

❍ Gently but firmly massage the lump in the direction of the nipple during and after feedings.

❍ Apply a hot water bottle to the affected nipple.

❍ Do not rush feeding, so the breast will be more fully drained.

❍ Drain the breast by positioning the baby's head so that the chin points to the area of hardness. The baby may be fussy about feeding when nursing on the affected side, since milk will flow more slowly.

❍ If a blocked duct has not corrected itself within 48 hours, therapeutic ultrasound is often helpful. This treatment is available from a physiotherapist or a sports medicine clinic. Since many ultrasound therapists are not aware of this application of ultrasound, it may be helpful to mention that the dose of ultrasound is 2 watts per square centimeter for 5 minutes continuously to the affected area of the breast, with one repeat treatment in any given day.

❍ If a blocked duct is associated with a small blister on the end of the nipple, gently squeeze the blister to allow flow of milk. This usually relieves nipple pain and may result in immediate opening of the duct.

❍ Use breast compression while the baby is feeding from the affected breast.

❍ Rest as much as possible.

❍ To prevent recurrences of blocked ducts, take 1 capsule (1,200 milligrams) of lecithin 3 or 4 times a day.

Specialized concerns:

❍ Women with HIV should not breastfeed. Mastitis increases the risk of transmitting the virus to the child, especially if the child is fed a mixture of breast milk and other foods.[20]

Measles

SYMPTOM SUMMARY

❍ Fever

❍ Cough

❍ Red eyes

❍ Fatigue

Followed by:

❍ Appearance of a red rash on the head spreading to the rest of the body

❍ Rash is usually not itchy

UNDERSTANDING THE DISEASE PROCESS

Measles, also known as rubeola, is a viral infection of the respiratory system that is usually accompanied by a red rash. Rubella, or German measles, is caused by a different virus. Since the advent of vaccination, measles has become a very rare condition in the United States, but outbreaks occur almost every year among unvaccinated children.

The measles virus is spread by coughs and sneezes. Symptoms begin 8–12 days after exposure, and the rash appears about 14 days after exposure. Infectees are con-

tagious 1–3 days before any symptoms appear, 3–5 days before the rash starts, and then continue to be infectious for up to a week.

TREATMENT SUMMARY

NUTRITIONAL SUPPLEMENTS

❍ Vitamin A: at least 100,000 IU and up to 200,000 IU exactly 2 times. Do not give this dosage of vitamin A to any child who may be pregnant. Women who are or who may become pregnant should strictly limit their intake of vitamin A to 5,000 IU per day or less.

UNDERSTANDING THE HEALING PROCESS

The primary complication of measles is pneumonia. A review of clinical studies found that deaths from pneumonia as a complication of measles in children under 2 years old were reduced by 82 percent by giving just 2 doses of vitamin A. At least 2 separate doses seem to be required for the effect.[1] Do not give more than 2 doses of vitamin A to any child who has measles, and never give vitamin A to a child who has liver disease or who may be pregnant.

CONCEPTS FOR COPING WITH MEASLES

❍ Some studies report that Vitamin A also increases the effectiveness of measles vaccinations, especially in boys, but the findings are inconsistent. Only a single dose of the vitamin would be required to stimulate the immune response to the vaccination.

❍ Provide plenty of fluids to prevent dehydration.

❍ Use of a vaporizer may reduce cough.

❍ Bed rest is usually required for measles. Children who have not been vaccinated for measles should be kept at home when it is known they have been exposed, until the rash disappears.

Memory Loss

SYMPTOM SUMMARY

❍ Inability to remember names and dates.

❍ Not a major problem in daily living.

❍ Not rapidly progressive.

UNDERSTANDING THE DISEASE PROCESS

Memory loss is a normal, if not natural, consequence of aging. Age-related memory loss occurs gradually. Illnesses such as Alzheimer's disease destroy memory quickly. In contrast, many people suffering age-related memory loss retain most of their intellectual faculties throughout life.

Doctors debate whether age-related memory loss—also known as age-associated memory impairment, age-consistent memory decline, and benign senescent forgetfulness—is a distinct clinical entity or a milder form of Alzheimer's disease. Older people who have not retired sometimes believe they suffer impaired memory when they do not, simply because of the increasing complexities of daily life. Psychologists and psychiatrists employ sophisticated measurement techniques to determine whether loss of memory capacity has actually occurred. A professional diagnosis is best when memory loss is suspected.

TREATMENT SUMMARY

NUTRITIONAL SUPPLEMENTS

❍ Acetyl-L-carnitine: 1,000 milligrams 3 times a day.

❍ Phosphatidylserine: 300–600 milligrams per day.

HERBS

❍ Ginkgo: 70–80 milligrams 3 times a day.

UNDERSTANDING THE HEALING PROCESS

Three nutritional supplements are particularly helpful in treating benign memory loss. Acetyl-L-carnitine (ACL) is a modification of the amino acid derivative L-carnitine, chemically modified so that it is more easily absorbed by the brain. ACL seems to slow the life cycle of brain cells so that fewer die. The usefulness of ACL in treating memory loss has been established by its use in treating Alzheimer's disease. People with Alzheimer's under the age of 65 who take ACL sometimes improve. Alzheimer's patients over the age of 65 who take ACL generally get worse more slowly.[1] People with benign memory loss almost always benefit from the supplement.

Any dosage of ACL high enough to slow the progression of memory loss can cause mild stomach upset, abdominal cramps, and diarrhea. In rare instances it causes intense dreams, and a small number of people taking it in the early stages of Alzheimer's will become agitated. ACL can make seizures more frequent in epileptics, and can induce a manic state in people who have bipolar disorder.

Phosphatidylserine (PS) is a major component of the membranes lining nerve cells, particularly at their junctures with other nerve cells. Experiments with animals indicate that PS somehow encourages the regrowth of nerve networks within the brain. At its peak performance state, usually around the age of 30, the human brain may have up to 10,000 connections for every one of its approximately 100 billion nerve cells, yielding as many as 1,000 trillion cell-to-cell connections, that is, a quadrillion nerve pathways. In severe conditions of memory loss such as Alzheimer's disease, up to 90 percent of these connections are lost.[2] By the end of life, an Alzheimer's patient may have virtually nothing remaining of the CA_1 region of the hippocampus, the region of the brain in which memories are formed.[3]

PS seems to stimulate nerve growth factor in the cerebral cortex and the hippocampus, the two regions of the brain most affected by AD.[4] Loosely controlled clinical testing in the United States has found that it helps sufferers of age-related memory loss (not just Alzheimer's disease) recover their abilities of verbal association and recall.[5] It helps restore hormone rhythms that help the individual deal with emotional stress.[6]

A dosage of 300 milligrams per day helps memory and a dosage of 600 milligrams per day lowers anxiety. PS is completely nontoxic and does not interfere with medications. Since European brands of PS are extracted from cow brain, there has been concern about mad cow disease, but functionally equivalent formulations made from soy are also available.

A controversy concerning the use of ginkgo as a memory aid arose in August 2002 through a highly-publicized article published in the *Journal of the American Medical Association*. Researchers at Williams College in Williamstown, Massachusetts tested healthy older adults for changes in learning, memory, attention, concentration, and verbal fluency after taking a dose of 120 milligrams of ginkgo extract per day for 6 weeks. The authors concluded that ginkgo did not help.[7]

In all likelihood, the conclusions of this study were correct. However, the researchers used a dosage of ginkgo much smaller than the 360 milligrams a day used as a memory aid in young adults. In a study published the same year in *Human Psychopharmacology* using a similar design with a higher dosage (180 milligrams per day), researchers observed clinically significant cognitive benefits in healthy individuals.[8] An optimal dosage of ginkgo for benign memory loss is probably 180–240 milligrams per day in most adults.

Never take a whole-leaf preparation of ginkgo. The whole leaf of the herb can contain toxins that can be especially detrimental to AD patients. Always take ginkgo extract. Do not take ginkgo with high dosages of vitamin E, since the combination can increase the risk of bleeding.

CONCEPTS FOR COPING WITH MEMORY LOSS

○ The old adage "Use it or lose it " applies to the brain. The more dense the brain circuitry is earlier in life, the more that can be lost later in life before function becomes seriously compromised. The *Journal of the American Medical Association* reported a study of nuns that found those who wrote in journals in the most complex language early in life were the least likely to develop AD later in life.[9] In the very early stages of AD, working crossword puzzles, maintaining social ties, and attempting intellectual tasks can slow intellectual decline.

○ Avoiding head trauma helps lower the risk of developing AD. One study has found that injury to the head increases the risk of AD predicted by genetics 10-fold.[10]

Ménière's Disease

SYMPTOM SUMMARY

○ Waxing and waning hearing loss (As disease progresses, hearing loss may become permanent, with sensitivity to loud noises.)

○ Difficulty understanding speech

○ Acute attacks signaled by a feeling of fullness in one or both ears, followed by:

• Vertigo (sensation of room spinning around)

• Cold sweats

• Headache

• Nausea

• Vomiting

• General weakness

○ Attacks that tend to last several hours, but hearing loss that continues for up to a day and headache that may last for several days

UNDERSTANDING THE DISEASE PROCESS

A condition of dizziness accompanied by auditory and visual distortion first described by the French physician Prosper Ménière in 1861, Ménière's disease is still poorly understood by medical science. The condition causes an accumulation of lymph causing increased pressure in the inner ear. When lymphatic fluid builds up to a critical level, expansion of the labyrinth of the inner ear can cause a loss of balance, leading to accidents and falls, and vertigo, a sense of being trapped in a spinning container. Repeated episodes of inner ear inflammation gradually cause loss of hearing.

TREATMENT SUMMARY

NUTRITIONAL SUPPLEMENTS

○ Hydroxyethylrutosides: 2 grams per day.

UNDERSTANDING THE HEALING PROCESS

Rutin is the primary nutritional supplement for treating Ménière's disease. This supplement is more commonly identified as hydroxyethylrutosides. A clinical study found that using hydroxyethylrutosides for 3 months reduced hearing loss at all frequencies and also reduced attacks of vertigo.[1]

Hydroxyethylrutosides cause no side effects in and of themselves, although most authorities advise that they should not be used in pregnancy. The drawback to using hydroxyethylrutosides is that they are incompatible with many antibiotics, including:

• ciprofloxacin (Cipro, Baycip, Cetraxal, Ciflox, Cifran, Ciplox, Cyprobay, Quintor)

• enoxacin (Penetrex)

• gatifloxacin (Tequin)

• gemifloxacin (a relatively new drug)

• grepafloxacin (Raxar)

• levofloxacin (Levaquin)

• lomefloxacin (Maxaquin)

• moxifloxacin (Avelox)

• norfloxacin (Amicrobin, Anquin, Baccidal, Barazan, Biofloxin, Floxenor, Fulgram, Janacin, Lexinor, Norofin, Noroxin, Norxacin, Orixacin, Oroflox, Urinox, Zoroxin)

• ofloxacin (Floxin)

- sparfloxacin (Zagam)
- temafloxacin (Omniflox)
- trovafloxacin (Trovan)

CONCEPTS FOR COPING WITH MÉNIÈRE'S DISEASE

❍ Ménière's disease shares some symptoms with stroke. If double vision, slurred speech, or tingling, numbness, or paralysis on one side of the body occur, seek immediate medical attention.

❍ If your doctor recommends a low-salt diet with or without furosemide (Lasix), be sure to take a complete B vitamin and a complete multivitamin and mineral supplement daily. You should also eat at least 5 servings of fruits and vegetables a day when taking diuretics. Lasix depletes B vitamins and potassium, and the resulting deficiencies can cause burning feet and memory loss.

❍ Some people with Ménière's disease benefit from a low-sugar diet. Ancient Egyptian and ancient Chinese medicine both identified eating sweets as a cause of hearing loss, and a series of studies over the past 30 years has correlated insulin resistance, an abnormal processing of sugar, with Ménière's disease and tinnitus.[2] If your symptoms are particularly bad when you eat a lot of sugar (around holidays, for example), try gradually increasing exercise and lowering total calorie consumption, especially of sweets. Taking 1,000 micrograms of chromium from brewer's yeast may also help. Together, increased exercise, decreased consumption of total calories and sugar, and chromium supplementation may increase the body's ability to respond to insulin, and, according to that theory, moderate the biochemical processes that lead to accumulation of lymphatic fluid in the inner ear.

❍ There are numerous reports of improvement in symptoms of Ménière's disease after consistent use of transcutaneous electroneural stimulation, or TENS. The "electricity" used to treat Ménière's disease is typically applied to the hand, not the ear. TENS may be most useful when used in combination with relaxation exercises, taught in 1 or 2 sessions by a therapist.

❍ Tinnitus is a common complication of Ménière's disease. In one of the few scientific studies of the use of homeopathy in the treatment of tinnitus, researchers at the Medical School of the University of Birmingham in England noted that test participants preferred the homeopathic remedy over placebo, but audiologists could not find a measurable difference between homeopathic treatment group and the placebo group.[3] This is probably because both the discomfort of tinnitus and the practice of homeopathy are highly subjective. Substantial relief from tinnitus may occur by changes in the sensory apparatus in the ear, or by emotional changes leading to lesser irritation by sound, thought to be produced by classical homeopathy. Homeopathic remedies frequently used in the treatment of tinnitus include the following:

- Calcarea carbonica treats tinnitus compounded by dizziness. The individual who benefits from calcarea carbonica may have cracking and throbbing sensations in the ears or may be hard of hearing. People who benefit from this remedy usually have a "sweet tooth" and are sensitive to cold drafts.

- Carbo vegetabilis is recommended for nausea occurring at the same time as ringing in the ears. It is also useful for tinnitus occurring during recovery from the flu, especially if recovery is slow.

- Cinchona officinalis was originally used to treat malaria. As a homeopathic remedy, it is used to treat tinnitus occurring with some of the same symptoms as malaria, such as chills and dizziness causing buzzing and ringing sounds to seem louder.

- Chininum sulphuricum relieves ringing and roaring sounds that are loud enough to interfere with normal hearing. Like cinchona officinalis, it treats chills and dizziness that make sounds seem louder.

- Cimicifuga (black cohosh) was used in Traditional Chinese Medicine to treat neck pain and is used in modern herbal medicine to treat menstrual irregularities. It is also used in homeopathy to treat tinnitus occurring with pain or tightness in the neck and/or shoulder muscles or during the menstrual period. Women who benefit from this remedy tend to be naturally outgoing but moody when they do not feel well.

- Coffea cruda treats tinnitus occurring with symptoms that could be caused by overconsumption of coffee, such as a "buzz" in the back of the head and insomnia. People who respond well to this remedy tend to be excitable and nervous.

- Graphites treat symptoms that need "lubrication,"

such as crackling or creaking sounds, gunshot sounds, or hissing with accompanying deafness. People who respond well to this remedy tend to be constipated and have poor concentration.

• Kali carbonicum is a chemical fertilizer applied to "sour" soils. In homeopathy, it treats tinnitus accompanied by "sour" symptoms, such as rigid conservatism, tension in the stomach, and dizziness when turning.

• Lycopodium relieves echoes and hums. People who respond well to this remedy tend to have urinary tract ailments.

• Natrum salicylicum and salicylicum acidum treat tinnitus occurring with Ménière's disease. As a form of aspirin, salicylicum acidum is used under the principle of "like treats like" to relieve tinnitus occurring after overconsumption of acetylsalicylic acid (aspirin).

Menke's Disease

SYMPTOM SUMMARY

O Kinky, white hair

O Soft bones

O Growth retardation

O Mental deterioration

UNDERSTANDING THE DISEASE PROCESS

Menke's disease, also known as steely-hair syndrome, is a rare hereditary disorder caused by a deficiency of copper only affecting boys. Copper is often described as a Jekyll-and-Hyde element in the human body. In small quantities it has an essential and benign role in normal development and metabolism, but in excess or deficiency, it can be a killer. In Menke's disease, varying segments of the MNK gene coding a protein for carrying copper are deleted. If only a small portion of the MNK gene is damaged, the child may produce some proteins for carrying copper. In these cases, with therapy, the child may suffer only a group of symptoms called occipital horn syndrome: arterial weakness, soft bones, and mild mental retardation. If a large portion of the MNK gene is damaged, treatment is extremely difficult and death is common.

Until about 20 years ago, Menke's disease was invariably fatal. Now the disease can be identified by prenatal testing and treated even before birth, although treatment begun after infancy is unlikely to be successful.

TREATMENT SUMMARY

NUTRITIONAL SUPPLEMENTS

O *Injectable* copper, administered by a physician.

UNDERSTANDING THE HEALING PROCESS

Since Menke's disease is caused by a shortage of copper, it would be logical to treat it with copper supplements. However, in Menke's disease, copper supplements taken by mouth do not bind with the carrier protein ceruloplasmin and do not build up in the bloodstream.[1] Menke's disease must be treated with injectable copper administered by a physician.

CONCEPTS FOR COPING WITH MENKE'S DISEASE

O Do not attempt to treat Menke's disease on your own with nutritional supplements. Copper levels can build up to toxic levels and cause the array of symptoms associated with Wilson's disease. (See WILSON'S DISEASE.)

O Boys who are successfully treated for Menke's disease are still at risk for arterial problems including increased risk of aneurysm. For additional information, see ANEURYSM.

Menopausal Complaints

See **Hot Flashes; Loss of Sexual Desire in Women; Osteoporosis; Vaginal Dryness.**

Menorrhagia

See **Heavy Periods (Menorrhagia).**

Menstrual Conditions

See **Amenorrhea; Dysmenorrhea; Premenstrual Syndrome (PMS).**

Migraine

SYMPTOM SUMMARY

○ In many cases, an "aura" of personality changes or altered vision (shooting stars, curtain falling, kaleidoscope) several hours before headache begins

○ In most but not all cases, throbbing or pulsating headache usually on one side of the head, beginning at the front and extending backward as pain intensifies

○ Nausea, often with clamminess

○ Vomiting

○ Sensitivity to light and sound

○ Pain may last several hours to several days, ending after a period of sleep

UNDERSTANDING THE DISEASE PROCESS

Migraine headaches are an inherited disorder causing varying degrees of throbbing headache pain, distorted vision or hearing, depression, mood swings, and sleepiness on a periodic basis. Not everyone who has migraines has all the symptoms of migraine. For instance, some people have migraines with severe visual disturbance but without headache, others only experience severe mood swings, and some experience temporary loss of sight or speech similar to stroke.

The most recent thinking on the cause of migraine is that it involves an overload of the locus coeruleus, the "switchboard" of the brain. The locus coeruleus anchors nerve fibers that generate the chemical serotonin. When the production of serotonin along these fibers gets out of sync with the brain's needs, various processes that "gate" the sensation of pain cease to function. As the imbalance spreads through the cerebral cortex, the permeability of the outer layers of the brain to blood is also altered, and a throbbing headache typically ensues.[1]

The Centers for Disease Control report that 6 percent of men and 17 percent of women in the United States suffer at least an occasional migraine headache.[2] Migraines typically begin in the late teens or 20s and remits by age 50. Almost all people who suffer migraines have a normal neurological examination.

TREATMENT SUMMARY

NUTRITIONAL SUPPLEMENTS

○ Magnesium: 600 milligrams per day.

○ Women of child-bearing age should not take any calcium supplement that does not also contain magnesium.

○ Melatonin: 5 milligrams per day, taken 30 minutes before bedtime.

○ Riboflavin: 400 milligrams per day.

HERBS

○ Feverfew: 250 micrograms of parthenolide per day.

UNDERSTANDING THE HEALING PROCESS

There are at least 20 prescription medications used to abort migraine headaches, many of them with considerable success. The problem with using drugs more than once a week on a regular basis to prevent migraines is the potential for "rebound headaches," intense, untreatable pain caused by overuse of medication. Nutritional supplements and herbs are useful for reducing the need for medication and reducing the risk of rebound pain.

Both men and women who suffer migraine are typically deficient in magnesium.[3] An imbalance between magnesium and calcium is an important factor in premenstrual migraine.[4] Intravenous magnesium often produces complete symptom relief during acute migraines, usually within 15 minutes or less, although it is more useful for migraine sufferers who experience an "aura" before the onset of headache.[5]

The regular use of magnesium supplements is of clear benefit to women who suffer premenstrual or perimenstrual migraine headaches. At least one study has found that taking 600 milligrams of magnesium a day reduces the frequency of migraine headaches,[6] and since magnesium is safe and inexpensive, any migraine sufferer should give it a try. The only drawbacks to using magnesium are that high doses can aggravate diarrhea, and the supplement should be discontinued when taking antibiotics.

Unlike magnesium, melatonin is usually not deficient in people who suffer migraine. However, the administration of melatonin may resynchronize the production of serotonin and prevent migraines, especially for people who awaken with migraine in the middle of the night.[7] Be sure not to take melatonin during the day, since sleep disturbance may result.

One clinical trial found that taking large doses of the B vitamin riboflavin for 2 months led to at least a 50 percent reduction in the number of attacks in 59 percent of people taking it.[8] Riboflavin may be especially helpful for women who take birth control pills and for both men and women on cholesterol-lowering medications.

Feverfew is the most commonly used herb for migraine. Three clinical studies have found that regular use of the herb reduces the frequency and severity of migraine attacks. Results may not be noticeable until the herb has been taken for 4–6 weeks. It is important only to take encapsulated formulations of the freeze-dried herb. Other forms of feverfew may cause stomach upset.

Several other supplements reduce the frequency of migraines, notably 5-HTP and SAM-e, but they are incompatible with migraine medications. Vitamin D has been used to treat migraine in women, but the doses required are so high that they should only be taken under medical supervision.

CONCEPTS FOR COPING WITH MIGRAINE

❍ Excesses of the amino acid tyramine can aggravate migraine attacks. Try avoiding foods containing tyramine, including anchovies, beer, hard cheeses, chocolate, corned beef, dried meats, fava beans, fermented beans such as miso and soy sauce, lima beans, pickled herring, red wine, sardines, sauerkraut, and yeast.

❍ Many migraine sufferers benefit from the use of ice packs. Ice "pillows" that can be kept in the freezer are available from drugstores.

❍ Homeopathic medicine offers a number of remedies for migraine, tailored to individual symptoms.

• Belladonna treats migraines causing dilation of the pupils. Some authorities teach that this remedy is best for migraines that peak in the middle of the afternoon.

• Bryonia treats headache that begins over the left eye and spreads over the entire head. The person benefiting most from this remedy usually suffers dry mouth during the migraine attack.

• Cimicifuga is indicated when neck muscles are also involved. Eating relieves symptoms.

• Gelsemium treats migraines precipitated by emotional stress and relieved by going to the bathroom.

• Ignatia treats "pounding" headaches focused on one side of the face. It is frequently recommended for people experiencing illness while dealing with grief.

• Iris versicolor relieves headaches heralded by visual distortion. It is especially useful for headaches set off by motion sickness.

• Kali bichromicum treats pain that is focused rather than spread across the head and face. It is recommended for people who tend to get chills easily.

• Lachesis treats migraines on the left side of the face, especially if there is blushing or flushing just before pain begins.

• Sanguinaria relieves vomiting. Pain relieved by sanguinaria is made worse by lying on the affected side.

• Silicea (silica) is recommended for headaches occurring before, during, or just after menstruation. It is also used to treat right-sided headaches in men.

• Spigelia treats pain in the eye. It is best for pain that is relieved by supporting and immobilizing the right side of the head.

Mitral Valve Prolapse

SYMPTOM SUMMARY

❍ Irregular heartbeat or palpitations, especially when lying on your left side

❍ Chest pain (sharp or dull), lasting a few seconds to a few hours

❍ Dizziness after rising from a chair or bed

❍ Fatigue after slight exertion (often misdiagnosed as chronic fatigue syndrome)

❍ Shortness of breath

❍ Most people with mitral valve prolapse do not experience heart symptoms.

❍ Forty percent of people with mitral valve prolapse also experience general anxiety, panic attacks, migraines, or irritable bowel syndrome.

❍ Seventy percent of people with mitral valve prolapse have depression.

UNDERSTANDING THE DISEASE PROCESS

The mitral valve regulates the flow of blood between the left atrium and the left ventricle of the heart, keeping blood from flowing backward or "regurgitating." This valve consists of two leaflets that touch to stop the flow of blood and separate to allow the flow of blood. When the valve is prolapsed, excessive mucus has stretched the leaflets of the valve so that they do not fit properly. Because of the uneven size, the valve expands and "prolapses" into the atrium in the shape of a balloon. The prolapse causes a backward flow of blood and an identifiable "click" or murmur.

About 4 percent of the population of the United States and worldwide have mitral valve prolapse (MVP). The condition begins between ages 10 and 16 and is most commonly diagnosed between the ages of 20 and 40. It is 3 times more common in women than in men. Women with MVP tend to have narrow hips.

The cause of MVP is unknown. Some people seem to inherit the condition. Sometimes it is a complication of coronary artery disease, cardiomyopathy, Marfan's syndrome, Duchenne muscular dystrophy, hyperthyroidism, sickle-cell disease, rheumatoid arthritis, or hypomastia (unusually small breasts). More than half the time, MVP causes no symptoms and does not interfere with good health. Nonetheless, MVP is a leading cause of transient ischemic attacks, strokes in the young, and sudden death.

TREATMENT SUMMARY

NUTRITIONAL SUPPLEMENTS

○ Coenzyme Q_{10}: 150–300 milligrams daily.

○ L-carnitine: 500–1,000 milligrams 3 times per day.

○ Magnesium: 400–500 milligrams per day.

UNDERSTANDING THE HEALING PROCESS

There has been very little research into the nutritional treatment of MVP, but the few studies there are present encouraging results. *The American Journal of Cardiology* reported a study of 85 people with severe MVP who were found to be deficient in magnesium. Each person received magnesium supplements for 5 weeks and a placebo for 5 weeks. When participants received magnesium, but not when they received a placebo, they experienced reduction in anxiety, chest pains, shortness of breath, and palpitations.[1] The key to successful use of magnesium seems to be that sooner is better than later. The greatest enhancement to health occurs by preventing irregular heartbeat rather than treating it.

Don't overdose magnesium. It is the primary ele-

ment in milk of magnesia, and magnesium supplements can cause diarrhea. Usually the effect is short term and takes places the first 2 or 3 days the supplement is taken. In heart patients, supplemental magnesium can interfere with the body's ability to absorb quinolone (Cipro). Magnesium supplements can also interfere with the absorption of tetracycline. You should not use magnesium supplements if you have myasthenia gravis. They may exacerbate muscle weakness and precipitate a myasthenic crisis.

A Japanese study in the mid-1980s found that children with MVP (a relatively rare condition) improved when given 1.5 milligrams of coenzyme Q_{10} for every pound of body weight.[2] Coenzyme Q_{10} is most likely to be helpful to adults taking statin drugs to lower cholesterol. Diabetics taking this supplement should monitor blood sugars carefully.

There are isolated reports of improvement in MVP in adults after administration of L-carnitine. People with seizure disorders should consult with their physicians before taking L-carnitine.

CONCEPTS FOR COPING WITH MITRAL VALVE PROLAPSE

○ Avoid coffee and other stimulants that may induce irregularity in the heartbeat. Cocaine is especially detrimental in MVP.

○ Be sure to inform your dentist you have MVP before dental surgery, so that appropriate measures may be taken to prevent infections of the mitral valve.

○ Consult a physician immediately if you experience signs of congestive heart failure, such as swollen ankles and legs.

Morning Sickness

SYMPTOM SUMMARY

○ Nausea

○ Vomiting

○ Excessive salivation

○ General weakness

UNDERSTANDING THE DISEASE PROCESS

Morning sickness is a condition of nausea and vomiting in pregnancy. The symptoms of morning sickness are not necessarily confined to the morning. Surveys have found that up to 89 percent of pregnant women experience nausea and up to 57 percent of pregnant women experience vomiting, usually during the ninth through fourteenth weeks of pregnancy.[1] Especially severe nausea and vomiting is known as hyperemesis gravidarum, hyperemesis referring to "hyper-vomiting" and gravidarum referring to pregnancy.

Nausea and vomiting during pregnancy is not a psychosomatic illness. Increased production of estrogen during the first trimester of pregnancy makes the esophagus, stomach, and small bowel more sensitive to chemical cues that could be associated with contaminated food. Supersensitivity to food protects the embryo from potential exposure to mutagenic chemicals. As the embryo matures, the mother's sensitivity to food gradually returns to normal, almost always by the twentieth week of pregnancy.

TREATMENT SUMMARY

NUTRITIONAL SUPPLEMENTS

O Any multivitamin and mineral supplement daily.

O Vitamin B_6: 30 milligrams daily.

HERBS

O Ginger: 250 milligrams 3 times a day.

UNDERSTANDING THE HEALING PROCESS

The medical community is beginning to agree that multivitamin supplements, vitamin B_6, and ginger are safe and effective for controlling nausea and vomiting during pregnancy.[2] Vitamin B_6[3] prevents nausea but not vomiting, while ginger is more effective for vomiting than nausea.[4] Multivitamin and mineral supplements replace nutrients lost through vomiting.

CONCEPTS FOR COPING WITH MORNING SICKNESS

O Vitamin K in very large doses (5 milligrams per day) and vitamin C in very small doses (25 milligrams per day) are sometimes recommended for morning sickness, but there is no evidence they help. Red clover is not effective; estrogenlike compounds in red clover may actually make morning sickness worse.

O Acupressure to the "Inner Gate Point" (known in Traditional Chinese Medicine as the Neiguan point) often relieves nausea and vomiting caused by any kind of pressure on the pelvis. Acupressure is best done by a trained massage or shiatsu therapist, but you can also massage this point yourself. You can find your "Inner Gate" by laying your hand flat and then moving up your arm the width of three fingers from the crease of your wrist. You will know you found the right point when you feel slight but distinct soreness when you apply pressure. Massage the point at least 20 minutes 3 times a day. Acupressure wristbands sometimes give relief but are not as effective as acupressure massage.

O Other suggestions for reducing nausea include:

- Eat small meals several times a day.

- Eat when hungry, regardless of mealtimes.

- Increase consumption of carbonated beverages, especially mineral water.

- Ginger ale, broth, unbuttered toast, gelatin, and frozen desserts are usually tolerated. Dry carbohydrates such as crackers usually stay down.

- Avoid strong food tastes and smells.

- In severe morning sickness (hyperemesis gravidarum), discontinue multivitamin and mineral supplements. Take special care to avoid supplements containing iron.

Motion Sickness

SYMPTOM SUMMARY

O Abdominal awareness and/or abdominal pain

O Breaking out into a cold sweat

O Fatigue

O Flushing

O Headache

O Nausea

O Racing pulse

O Vomiting

UNDERSTANDING THE CONDITION

Motion sickness is a motion-induced condition that manifests itself in some or all of a number of unpleasant symptoms associated with the activation of nerve cell receptors for histamine. Motion sickness occurs in cars, planes, trains, submarines, spacecrafts, amusement park rides, and virtual reality simulators. Its symptoms may be mildly uncomfortable, or it may cause complete incapacitation and dehydration from unrelenting vomiting.

Most of the theories on the cause of motion sickness claim that the condition arises when the brain is unable to resolve conflicts among various sensory inputs regarding position and movement of the body. The modes of information that are in conflict include the sensation of forward acceleration from the otolith organs of the middle ear, the sensation of angular movement from the semicircular canals, visual information, and the sense of touch. A common example is reading a book while riding in a car. The eyes are fixed on the book, which does not move relative to the rider. The car, on the other hand, accelerates, decelerates, and turns, providing conflicting information through the sense organs of the ear and the sense of touch. A sailor below deck on a ship, an airline passenger in a rapidly turning aircraft, or the user of a virtual reality game has a similar set of conflicting sensory signals.

The part of the brain known as the area postrema somehow interprets the incompatible sensory inputs as "poisonous." It activates the same neurotransmitters used to empty the digestive tract when a poisonous plant or food is accidentally ingested, and it accelerates the nervous system as if to compensate for intoxication.[1] For this reason, actual intoxication with alcohol or other drugs makes motion sickness much worse.

TREATMENT SUMMARY

DIET

○ Avoid high-sodium foods, such as frankfurters, luncheon meats, and potato chips, and high-thiamine foods, such as beef, eggs, fish, and pork. Do not snack between meals. Avoid alcohol for 24 hours before traveling and during the trip itself.

NUTRITIONAL SUPPLEMENTS

○ Vitamin B_6 (pyridoxine): 50 milligrams per day, starting 2–3 days before travel. Do not take a complete vitamin B supplement in lieu of a vitamin B_6 supplement.

HERBS

○ Ginger: 1 or 2 days before travel, take 1,000 milligrams (1 gram) of powdered ginger 3–4 times daily.

UNDERSTANDING THE HEALING PROCESS

The armed forces take no chances with motion sickness interfering with military operations. Flight medics typically prevent symptoms with intramuscular injections of diphenhydramine, promethazine, or the herb-derived scopolamine. These drugs are highly effective. However, they are also central nervous system depressants and cannot be used by drivers or passengers who need to stay alert.

A study of airline pilots found that eating high-sodium foods, such as preserved meats, corn chips, and potato chips, or high-thiamine foods, such as beef, eggs, fish, or pork, or high-calorie foods in general, increased the risk of airsickness. In men, high-protein foods such as cheeses, milk products, and preserved meats also positively correlated to airsickness. Eating fewer meals and eliminating snacks also reduced the risk of motion sickness in the air.[2]

Experiments by the British Royal Air Force have found that the use of alcohol in the 24 hours before a flight increases the risk of motion sickness.[3] Passengers under the influence of alcohol are less able to control head movements that minimize motion sickness.

Laboratory experiments with animals have found that vitamin B_6 increases oxygenation to the brain in motion sickness.[4] This could account for anecdotal reports that it reduces motion sickness.

Herbalists have prescribed ginger for motion sickness for generations. The first scientific tests, commissioned by NASA, failed to find a significant benefit for the herb, but these tests involved placing subjects in a high-speed rotating chair for 2 hours until vomiting occurred.[5,6] Travelers other than astronauts (and even some astronauts) do not encounter these conditions.

Later tests in more realistic conditions confirm the value of ginger in treating motion sickness. One study found the effects of ginger and the over-the-counter remedy dimenhydrinate to be roughly equivalent in a group of 60 passengers on a cruise through rough seas.[7] A study of 79 Swedish naval cadets found that ginger decreases the incidence of vomiting and cold sweating, although it does not decrease nausea and vertigo.[8] In addition, a small double-blind study to evaluate whether ginger could help with experimentally induced vertigo found that ginger root powder significantly reduced vertigo compared to the placebo.[9]

Chinese scientists believe that ginger acts on both the brain and the peripheral nervous system. The pungent compounds in ginger act on nerve fibers so that they are less sensitive to the neurotransmitters acetylcholine and histamine, both of which are involved in the reflexes that cause nausea and vomiting.[10]

It is theoretically possible that ginger could cause excessive bleeding when taken with drugs such as Coumadin (warfarin), heparin, Plavix (clopidogrel), Ticlid (ticlopidine), Trental (pentoxifylline), or aspirin. Be especially careful not to overdose ginger if you take any of these prescription drugs.

CONCEPTS FOR COPING WITH MOTION SICKNESS

❍ If you are a passenger in a boat, train, or car, maintain a visual reference to the horizon (which does not move).

❍ Take a seat on a plane near the wing or in the center of the plane.

Mouth Ulcers
See Canker Sores.

MS
See Multiple Sclerosis.

MSG Sensitivity

SYMPTOM SUMMARY

❍ Diarrhea

❍ Migraine

❍ Nausea

❍ Sensitivity to light

❍ Tightness in the chest

❍ Tingling

❍ Visual disturbances

❍ Vomiting

❍ Symptoms occur 2–3 hours after eating food prepared with MSG

UNDERSTANDING THE DISEASE PROCESS

MSG (monosodium glutamate) is the term for a group of chemicals containing glutamic acid that are used to add flavor to food. For thousands of years the Chinese used certain seaweeds in cooking. In 1908, the Japanese company Ajinomoto Sanyo developed a process for extracting the glutamic acid from the seaweeds, and the resulting product became popularly known as MSG.

In 1968 Dr. Robert Ho Man Kwok, an American physician who was born in China, experienced a severe reaction after eating food in a Chinese restaurant. Noting that similar symptoms were unknown in China, he coined the term "Chinese restaurant syndrome" to describe toxicity of MSG. A controversy over the validity of the syndrome ensued, but in 1995 a panel of experts convened by the FDA agreed that MSG could cause short-term effects when consumed in a dose of at least 3 grams, roughly equivalent to the amount of MSG in 6 servings of commercially prepared Chinese food. The long-term effects of MSG continue to be debated. (See HUNTINGTON'S DISEASE and AMYOTROPHIC LATERAL SCLEROSIS.)

TREATMENT SUMMARY

NUTRITIONAL SUPPLEMENTS

❍ Vitamin B_6: 50 milligrams per day for at least 3 months.

UNDERSTANDING THE HEALING PROCESS

The most important step in stopping the symptoms of MSG sensitivity is avoiding MSG. In the United States, MSG appears in canned and packaged broth, calcium caseinate, casein, gelatin, hydrolyzed and textured vegetable protein, liquid smoke, meat tenderizers, soy sauce, malt extracts, autolyzed yeast, yeast extracts, "natural flavoring," and whey. Additionally, it is important to know whether or not restaurant foods are prepared with MSG.

In addition to avoidance, taking vitamin B_6 may be helpful. In a clinical study conducted in the early 1980s, 8 out of 9 people stopped reacting to MSG after taking 50 milligrams of vitamin B_6 per day for at least 12 weeks.[1] A later study confirmed that a deficiency of the vitamin explained the reactions to MSG.[2]

CONCEPTS FOR COPING WITH MSG SYNDROME

❍ Some foods, including fresh tomatoes, tomato paste, and Parmesan cheese, naturally contain free glutamates, and may also trigger MSG sensitivity.

Multiple Sclerosis (MS)

SYMPTOM SUMMARY

Relatively common symptoms:

○ Clumsiness

○ Dragging legs when walking

○ Fatigue

○ Tendency to drop things

○ Weakness

Less common symptoms:

○ Blurred vision

○ Double vision

○ Eyeball pain

○ Loss of balance, sensation of spinning

○ Nausea and vomiting

○ Numbness

○ Tingling, "pins and needles" sensation or feeling of "electricity" on the skin

Relatively rare symptoms:

○ Loss of bladder control

○ Loss of sexual function

UNDERSTANDING THE DISEASE PROCESS

Multiple sclerosis (MS) is a condition of perioic inflammation at various places along the fatty white sheath covering the nerves of the brain and spinal cord. Made of a material called myelin, this sheath normally insulates the nerve fibers, allowing electrical impulses to move without "static" between the brain, spinal cord, and the muscles and sense organs. In MS, immune cells made in the thymus (T cells) enter the brain and strip away their myelin insulation, sometimes causing myelin to be replaced by scar tissue and sometimes destroying the nerve completely. This slows, distorts, or blocks nerve signals.

Worldwide, MS affects over 1 million people, and about 250,000 in the United States.[1] Every year about 3,000 people die of complications of the disease.[2] MS usually begins between the ages of 20 and 40, although it can begin as late as age 60 and as early as age 2, and it is more common in women than in men. The disease is 10 times more frequent in countries above 45°N lati-

tude (there being no countries with appreciable land mass above 45°S latitude) than it is in the tropics, and it is more frequent in inland communities than along coasts. Persons who move from a low-risk area to a high-risk area before age 15 acquire a high risk for developing MS, but those who make the same move after age 15 retain their low risk.[3]

The prevalence of cases at northerly latitudes suggests that at least one factor in developing MS is a deficiency of vitamin D, but no single genetic or environmental factor adequately explains the disease. MS has been linked to infection with chlamydia, mycoplasmas, human herpesvirus type 6 (HHV-6), and at least 3 other classes of viruses. Suspected environmental causes include exposure to x-rays, solvents, or pesticides, and ownership of cats, dogs, or caged birds.[4]

MS is an insidious disease. In its early stages, it causes leg dragging, weakness, feelings of heaviness, weakness, stiffness, and a tendency to drop things. There may be a feeling of "pins and needles" or other electrical sensations. Symptoms may occur alone or in combination, but as soon as they appear, they recede. The sense organs may be involved. There may be double vision or blurred vision, and problems with the inner ear may cause dizziness, nausea, or vomiting. Typically, symptoms develop over a few days, remain stable for a few weeks, and then go away.

The appearance and disappearance of symptoms makes MS difficult to diagnose during its earliest and most treatable stages. As the disease progresses, damage to genitourinary nerves often leads to loss of bladder, sexual, and bowel function. As more and more lesions are formed, the person with MS usually becomes progressively disabled.

Patterns of MS progression vary. About 80 percent of people with MS are relapsing-remitting, that is, they experience flare-ups and relief, and a small minority of people with MS have symptoms that are primary-progressive, that is, progressively worse. After 7–15 years, the overwhelming majority of people with relapsing-remitting MS develop some symptoms that are secondary-progressive, that is, bad all the time. Periods of remission become shorter and less frequent and eventually do not occur at all.

TREATMENT SUMMARY

DIET

○ Swank diet (see the inset on page 412).

NUTRITIONAL SUPPLEMENTS

Several supplements are appropriate for specific symptoms (see Understanding the Healing Process).

See Part Three if you take prescription medication.

UNDERSTANDING THE HEALING PROCESS

The cyclical nature of MS complicates the evaluation of both conventional and complementary treatments. In the early stages of relapsing-remitting MS, almost any intervention works—for a time. Knowing which treatments are truly effective requires patient use for a period of months or years.

No natural intervention for MS has been studied longer than the Swank diet. Developed by physician R. L. Swank in his private medical practice from the 1940s through the 1970s, this low-fat diet replaces the saturated fat in animal fats and hydrogenated vegetable oils with unsaturated fat from canola (rapeseed), corn, grape seed, linseed, olive, peanut, safflower, sesame, soy, sunflower and walnut oils, and seeds, nuts, and cold-water fish (such as salmon and trout). Hydrogenated oils, oils that are stable at room temperature due to chemical processing, are not strictly prohibited but limited to the equivalent of 1 tablespoon (or 100 calories) per day. Unsaturated oils are *required,* at least 1 tablespoon to as much as 3 tablespoons (100–300 calories) per day. Other Swank diet rules are summarized in the inset.

While the Swank diet has not and cannot be subjected to strict scientific testing (since it is not possible to confine MS patients for a decades-long trial), Dr. Swank and his colleagues followed 144 patients for 34 years. Patients who consumed less than 20 grams of saturated fat had much lower rates of death and disability than patients who consumed more than 20 grams of saturated fat per day. Among patients following the low-fat protocol, fewer than 5 percent became disabled during the 34 years of the study.[5] Dr. Swank himself followed the diet and was still publishing in the medical journals at the age of 87, and at the time this book was being written, was still active at the age of 92.

Dr. Swank's findings are not unique. In the late 1990s, doctors at the Haukeland Hospital in Bergen, Norway, gave 16 patients newly diagnosed with MS instructions to take 3.5 rams of fish oil every day and to eat 3 or 4 fish meals per week, as well increasing their consumption of fruit and vegetables. At the end of 1 year, the frequency of MS attacks had decreased 95 percent. At the end of 2 years, the patient's disability index decreased 25 percent, meaning the patients regained a significant measure of mobility.[6] Since MS patients usually do not get better over time, scientists found these results to be startling.

Probably the simplest effective diet for MS is a vegan diet, whole-food diets supplemented by 3–10 grams of pharmaceutical-grade fish oil, or, for those who eschew animal products, 3–10 grams of DHA from microalgae. Scientists believe this diet encourages T cells to progress through their normal life cycle, dying and being replaced before they can damage myelin.[7] Key to any effective diet is avoiding saturated animal fats and including essential fatty acids, as well as avoiding excessive consumption of sugary foods.

Several supplements are helpful in managing specific symptoms. A Tibetan herbal formula, Padma-28, given over the course of a year, has been shown to help correct visual problems related to MS, specifically the ability to follow a moving object (or read) without moving the head to one side and then the other. In the test, Padma-28 caused no side effects.[8]

The essential amino acid phenylalanine makes transcutaneous electrical nerve stimulation (TENS) more effective in treating pain related to MS. Patients treated with phenylalanine and TENS experienced less muscle spasticity, fewer bladder symptoms, and less depression after 4 weeks of treatment than those treated with TENS and placebo, with improvements in 49 out of 50 MS patients participating in one clinical trial.[9] Threonine, a naturally occurring amino acid, may decrease the muscle spasticity. Two clinical studies found benefits from taking threonine over a period of 2–8 weeks.[10,11] Interestingly, a lower dosage of the supplement, 6 grams rather than 7.5 grams per day was more effective. Calcium, magnesium, niacin, thiamine, and vitamin D have been tested in treating MS. All of these supplements are harmless, but none is known with certainty to have long-term benefits.

CONCEPTS FOR COPING WITH MS

○ Dental amalgams containing mercury have been suggested as a contributing factor in MS. Amalgam fillings generally contain approximately 50 percent mercury mixed with copper, silver, tin, and zinc. This alloy continually emits mercury vapor, especially after chewing, eating, brushing, and drinking hot liquids. Spinal taps

---

The Swank Diet for MS

All grains and cereals are permitted, but whole-grain products are preferable. All hot cereals are permissible, including Cream of Wheat, Cream of Rice, and oatmeal. Choose breakfast cereals that are low in fat, such as Cheerios, Grapenuts, puffed rice, or shredded wheat. Avoid high-fat granola.

Angel food cake is an acceptable desert. Other desserts include butter, margarine, and eggs, and are too high in fat.

Up to 3 eggs per week are permitted, but no more than 1 egg per day.

Catsup, mustard, and salsa can be consumed without limitation, but mayonnaise must be counted against your daily allowance of saturated fat. Two tablespoons of mayonnaise, containing 1 tablespoon of saturated fat is your entire allowance of saturated fat for 1 day. Two tablespoons of a mayonnaise-based salad dressing is likewise your entire allowance of saturated fat for 1 day.

Avocados, olives, nuts, and seeds are good sources of unsaturated fat, required in the diet. One third of your daily allowance of unsaturated fat may be obtained from:

- Avocados. $\frac{1}{8}$ of an avocado = 1 teaspoon of unsaturated fat (oil)

- Olives. 3 medium black olives = 1 teaspoon of unsaturated fat (oil)

- Olives. 6 medium green olives = 1 teaspoon of unsaturated fat (oil)

- 3 teaspoons sunflower seeds

- 3 teaspoons pumpkin kernels

- 2 teaspoons peanut butter or other nut butters (self-ground, not processed) = 1 teaspoon oil

- $\frac{1}{3}$ ounce energy snack mix (mix together almonds, walnuts, hazelnuts, pumpkin seeds, sunflower seeds, and sesame seeds) = 1 teaspoon oil

- $\frac{1}{3}$ ounce (about 10) of any other kind of nuts (walnut and pecan halves, filberts, hazelnuts)

- $\frac{1}{2}$ ounce (about 10) peanuts, almonds, or cashews

Choose 3 servings from the list above every day.

All *nonfat* dairy products are permitted. Two servings per day are recommended.

All fruits are permitted. Two servings per day are recommended.

All white fish and shellfish (abalone, cod, flounder, haddock, mahi mahi, perch, smelt, snapper, sole, sturgeon, tuna canned in water) are permitted in unlimited quantities. Fatty fish such as salmon and tuna packed in oil are limited to 3 tablespoons per day.

Red meat (beef, pork, and game) is not permitted the first year of the diet. One 3-ounce serving per week is permitted after the first year.

Dr. Swank also recommends taking 5 grams of fish oil, 1,000 IU of vitamin C, and 400 IU of vitamin E per day.

---

done before and after removal of fillings from MS patients demonstrate that removing amalgam removes mercury from circulation in the spinal fluid,[12] and it is known that mercury is especially destructive to the nerves that control motor function.

However, removal of fillings produces more failures than favorable results. This is probably due to failure to take precautions to keep the patient from swallowing any part of the filling after it is drilled out. It could also be due to failure to use a negative ion generator in the dentist's office to keep mercury from forming mercuric oxide, the more toxic form of the metal. MS patients who have been successfully treated with amalgam removal usually have been given vitamin C after the procedure, and are not scheduled for follow-up visits on the seventh, fourteenth, or twenty-first days after the first procedure, days when their body's concentrations of previously released mercury are highest.

○ Several studies have found that a skin cream made with the amino acid histamine, the chemical responsible for allergies, can relieve MS symptoms. A skin cream (Procarin), developed by Elaine Delack, RN, herself afflicted with MS, was administered through Tahoma

Clinic in Kent, Washington, to 55 MS patients. Delack and her colleagues report that in two out of three cases it improved some symptoms. They included recovery of the ability to move an affected limb, increase in the strength of an affected limb, disappearance of numbness, recovery of the ability to stand without assistance, increased ability to transfer or reposition oneself in bed, recovery of the ability to walk, recovery of the ability to drive an automobile, increased walking distance, decrease in the number of falls, and recovery of bladder control or significant decrease in urgency and frequency of voiding. Roughly 10 percent of patients commented they had seen an improvement in every symptom of their MS. Several patients were able to return to work full- or part-time.[13] Researchers theorize that histamine provides a "booster" to the electrical circuits that transmit nerve messages,[14] and slows the activities of the kind of T cells that cause nerve damage in MS.[15] The problem with the study is that it was conducted over a period of only 6 weeks, during which time symptoms in relapsing-remitting MS might be expected to improve with no special treatment. Some patients taking the cream noted a return of symptoms 36 hours after stopping it. However, in some cases, continued use of Procarin may be helpful. Current cost of the therapy in the United States is $249 per month. The skin cream has been renamed Prokarin and is available from compounding pharmacies across the United States, Canada, and Australia. For more information, see http://welcome.to.prokarin.com or call the International Academy of Compounding Pharmacists (IACP) at 1-800-927-4227.

Multisystem Vasculitis
(Behcet's Disease)

SYMPTOM SUMMARY

○ Canker sores

○ Genital ulcers

○ Eye inflammation

○ Hypersensitivity to skin injury, redness and pus occurring within 24 hours of a cut, scrape, scratch, or pin prick

UNDERSTANDING THE DISEASE PROCESS

Multisystem vasculitis (MV), also known as Behcet's disease, BD, and Silk Road disease, is a rare, chronic, lifelong disorder that involves inflammation of blood vessels throughout the body. This hard-to-treat condition causes oral inflammation resembling canker sores, genital ulcers, and changes in the circulation of the eyes, frequently leading to blindness. It can also cause inflammatory bowel disease, arthritis, and meningitis. The symptoms of MV tend to relapse and remit, gradually getting worse after age 30. At least 50,000 people in the United States have MV.

TREATMENT SUMMARY

HERBS

○ Kampo formulas, chosen with the help of a specialist.

UNDERSTANDING THE HEALING PROCESS

Japanese physicians report remissions of MV after treatment with Kampo, the various formulas of Japanese herbal medicine, especially *shi-kunshi-to*.[1] Choice of the specific formula must be made with the initial assistance of an herbalist or physician knowledgeable about Kampo or Traditional Chinese Medicine.

CONCEPTS FOR COPING WITH MULTISYSTEM VASCULITIS

○ Rutin, quercetin, and hydroxyethylrutosides are incompatible with the medications most commonly used to control MV.

Mumps, Complications of

See **Epididymitis; Lymphedema.**

Muscle Contraction Headache

See **Tension Headaches.**

Myasthenia Gravis

SYMPTOM SUMMARY

○ Weakness of the facial muscles

○ Horizontal smile

○ Drooping eyelids

○ Furrowed eyebrows (from compensation for weakness in facial muscles)

○ Nasal twang to the voice

○ Nasal regurgitation of food and liquids

○ Double vision

○ General weakness of arms and legs

○ Difficulty breathing

UNDERSTANDING THE DISEASE PROCESS

Myasthenia gravis (MG) is a rare neuromuscular disorder caused by a misdirected attack by T cells, white blood cells manufactured in the thymus, against the nerves controlling movement of the facial muscles, throat, and lungs. It may occur with hyperthyroidism, lupus, or scleroderma, which must also be treated for improvement in symptoms. MG was once frequently fatal but is now almost always successfully treated with immunosuppressive medication.

TREATMENT SUMMARY

NUTRITIONAL SUPPLEMENTS

○ Calcium citrate: at least 1,000 milligrams per day.

○ Vitamin D: 400–800 IU per day.

UNDERSTANDING THE HEALING PROCESS

There are no nutritional interventions that affect the course of MG. Supplementation with calcium and vitamin D, however, is essential for preventing osteoporosis caused by the drugs used to treat the condition.[1]

CONCEPTS FOR COPING WITH MYASTHENIA GRAVIS

○ Since myasthenia gravis is a condition caused by T cells, herbs that stimulate the production of T cells, such as echinacea and wild indigo, absolutely must be avoided.

○ Grapefruit juice, onions, and supplemental quercetin interfere with the metabolism of many of the drugs used to treat MG and absolutely must be avoided.

Myocardial Infarction

See **Angina; Atherosclerosis; Cardiomyopathy; Congestive Heart Failure; Irregular Heartbeat; Mitral Valve Prolapse.**

Nail Infections

SYMPTOM SUMMARY

○ Nails marked by:

- Thickening

- Chalkiness

- Crumbling

- White discoloration

UNDERSTANDING THE DISEASE PROCESS

Fungal and bacterial infections of fingernails or toenails are persistent and hard to treat. Infections can cause nails to become thickened, discolored, disfigured, and split. When the problem is caused by a fungus, the term onychomycosis is used. When caused by a bacterium, the condition is properly called paronychia.

Infected nails are a concern initially for cosmetic reasons. Without treatment, however, they can become so thick that they press against the inside of the shoes, causing pressure, irritation, and pain.

The two primary fungi that cause onychomycosis are *Trichophyton rubrum* and *Trichophyton mentagrophytes.* They feed on the keratin in nail tissue. The infections they cause normally are confined to the nails, but occasionally spread to the surrounding skin. Another type of onychomycosis is caused by a yeast, either *Candida albicans* or *Candida parapsilosis*. These infections are less common, but produce similar symptoms.

Paronychia infections normally are caused by *Pseudomonas, Staphylococcus,* or *Streptococcus* bacteria. Unlike fungal infections, bacterial infections typically inflame the skin adjacent to the nail.

Deformities in the nails are sometimes symptoms of

more serious health conditions. A listing of nail symptoms and corresponding systemic illnesses is found in the following table.

TREATMENT SUMMARY

HERBS

○ Tea tree oil (in 40 percent solution): apply to the nails 2–3 times daily, with debridement by a nail care specialist every 1–2 months.

○ Calendula: wash affected hands or feet with calendula soap 2–3 times daily.

NAIL DEFORMITIES INDICATING SYSTEMIC ILLNESS

"Clubbing": nail bulges outward like the back of a spoon	Heart valve problems, chronic pulmonary obstruction
Brittle nails	Thyroid problems (both hypothyroidism and hyperthyroidism)
Horizontal depressions (Beau's lines)	Recovery from surgery or internal trauma
Loss of luster	Chronic hepatitis
Ridging and pitting	Rheumatoid arthritis, lupus, or other autoimmune disease

UNDERSTANDING THE HEALING PROCESS

Physicians frequently treat nail infections with Lamisil or Sporanox, which are taken orally. Because the nail grows slowly, these medications work slowly. They usually require several months to completely eliminate the infection.

Prescription medications are a far better alternative to a lifetime of nail problems or nail removal. However, both of these medications can produce adverse side effects on the liver. It is necessary to have a blood test before starting treatment to establish a liver enzyme baseline. After a few weeks, the test is repeated to check liver function. If liver enzymes are elevated during treatment, the medication must be discontinued.

Natural treatments for nail infections also work slowly, and none is effective without debridement, the surgical removal of diseased tissue under the nail every 1–2 months. They do not, however, pose the risk of severe side effects sometimes encountered wth Lamisil and Sporanox.

Tea tree oil used by itself has little effect on nail infections. Tea tree oil combined with debridement, however, provides excellent improvement in nail appearance.

Physicians at Highland Hospital in Rochester, New York treated 117 onychomycosis patients with infected toenails with either clotrimazole or 100 percent tea tree oil for 9 months. The patients received debridement and a clinical evaluation at 1, 3, and 6 months. At 6 months, 11 percent of clotrimazole patients and 18 percent of tea tree oil patients showed abatement of infection. At the end of the study, 55 percent of patients treated with clotrimazole and 56 percent of patients treated with tea tree oil had either continued improvement or complete restoration of the appearance of nails.[1]

Calendula soaps are a useful complement to tea tree oil. They kill *Staphylococcus aureus,*[2] which is not affected by tea tree oil.

CONCEPTS FOR COPING WITH NAIL INFECTIONS

○ Avoid tight-fitting shoes or gloves. Good circulation to the fingers and toes is needed to fight nail infections.

○ Do not bite, pick, or tear the nails.

○ Do not use Clorox or similar (sodium hypochlorite) solutions to treat infected nails. Hypochlorite solutions can be extremely irritating to the skin, even when diluted.

○ Take *acidophilus* or *Lactobacillus* daily, especially if you have been taking antibiotics. These probiotics restore beneficial bacteria that control bacterial and yeast infections.

Nausea
See **Morning Sickness; Motion Sickness.**

Nephrolithiasis
See **Kidney Stones.**

Nervousness
See **Anxiety (Generalized Anxiety Disorder).**

Neuropathy
(Diabetic Complication)

SYMPTOM SUMMARY

Peripheral neuropathy:

○ Numbness or insensitivity to pain or temperature

○ Tingling, burning, or prickling

○ Extreme sensitivity to touch, even light touch

○ Loss of balance and coordination

○ Sharp pains or cramps

○ Carpal tunnel syndrome

Autonomic neuropathy (usually only one symptom predominates):

○ Bloating, alternating constipation and diarrhea (diarrhea is worse at night), nausea and vomiting, loss of appetite

○ Copious sweating while eating

○ Dizziness when moving from seated to standing position

○ Overheating

○ Problems with bladder control

Focal neuropathy:

○ Aching behind an eye

○ Chest or abdominal pain sometimes mistaken for angina, heart attack, or appendicitis

○ Double vision

○ Inability to focus the eye

○ Pain in the chest, stomach, or flank

○ Pain in the front of a thigh

○ Paralysis on one side of the face (Bell's palsy)

○ Severe pain in the lower back or pelvis

○ Problems with hearing

UNDERSTANDING THE DISEASE PROCESS

Diabetic neuropathy is a progressive degeneration of the nerves that is caused by diabetes. Symptoms of neuropathy include numbness or, less frequently, pain in the hands, feet, or legs. Nerve damage caused by diabetes can also lead to problems with internal organs such as the digestive tract, heart, and sexual organs. It can cause bladder infections, constipation or diarrhea, dizziness, and erectile dysfunction.

The most common type of neuropathy is peripheral neuropathy. This form damages the nerves of the limbs, especially the feet. The foot often becomes wider and shorter. The stride becomes longer or shorter. Foot ulcers appear as pressure is put on parts of the foot that are less protected. Because of the loss of sensation, injuries may go unnoticed and often become infected. If ulcers or foot injuries go untreated, the infection may involve the bone and require amputation. However, problems caused by minor injuries can usually be controlled if they are caught in time.

Diabetes can also damage the autonomic nervous system. Autonomic neuropathy affects the nerves that serve the heart and internal organs and produces changes in many processes and systems. Diabetic nerve damage may stop the bladder from emptying completely, so bacteria have a chance to grow in the bladder and kidneys. Circulatory problems caused by diabetes frequently lead to a loss of sexual response in both men and women, although sex drive is unchanged. Men may become impotent or may reach sexual climax without ejaculating normally.

A particularly serious consequence of autonomic neuropathy is damage to the vagus nerve. This keeps the heart from receiving signals from other parts of the body that there is a need for increased blood pressure. The result may be orthostatic hypotension, a sharp decrease in blood pressure after sitting or standing, causing dizziness or fainting. Diabetics may not feel the pain of angina and have painless heart attacks. Nerve damage can also impede the body's control of the sweat glands, so there is overheating in hot weather or sweating while eating. And autonomic neuropathy can stop the signals of low blood sugar, so diabetics can have severe insulin reactions without early symptoms.

Focal neuropathy expresses itself in limited areas of the body. It most often occurs in older people who have mild diabetes. Although its symptoms are painful, they usually go away on their own in a few weeks.

All of the various kinds of nerve damage in diabetes result from a combination of antioxidant deficiency, high blood sugars, and high concentrations of blood fats and salt.[1] High blood sugars cause an accumulation of superoxides, peroxinitrites, and highly reactive hydroxyl radicals, the injurious compounds that are controlled by antioxidants. If there are adequate supplies of vitamin E and other antioxidants in nerve tissue, free radicals do not usually damage nerve tissue. When there is a deficiency of antioxidants, free radicals disrupt the structure of the nerve, causing them to become riddled with vacant areas, or vacuoles. These free radicals can cause a disruption of the nerve's DNA so that it initiates apoptosis, a "death sequence."

Apoptosis accounts for some but not all of the destruction of nerve cells. If there is also a high bloodstream concentration of sodium (from table salt and salty foods), the nerve cells acquire an intense electrical charge, drawing still more free radicals inside. When enough free radicals accumulate, the cell membrane loses its charge and can no longer attract and transport the nutrients it needs to survive.[2] Over time, the nerve cell weakens or dies.

TREATMENT SUMMARY

NUTRITIONAL SUPPLEMENTS

O Alpha-lipoic acid: 400 milligrams twice a day for 4 months, then 100 milligrams 3 times a day thereafter.

HERBS

O Chinese herbal teas: prescribed by a Traditional Chinese Medicine specialist.

See Part Three if you take prescription medication.

UNDERSTANDING THE HEALING PROCESS

The most important thing any diabetic can do to prevent neuropathy is to keep tight control over blood sugars. While several years of blood sugars running 250 mg/dl (13.8 mM) and higher practically guarantees the development of this complication, just a few weeks of keeping blood sugars below 100 mg/dl (5.5 mM) begins to reverse the damage. Equally as important as maintaining low blood sugars is maintaining low blood lipids, that is, low cholesterol and low triglycerides. High levels of blood fats are just as injurious as high blood sugars.[3] It is also important to stop smoking and limit drinking. While high blood sugars and high blood lipids are more important risk factors for neuropathy, either smoking or drinking more than doubles a diabetic's risk of developing neuropathy, from 1 in 6 to about 1 in 2.

Doctors in Germany have used alpha-lipoic acid to treat diabetic neuropathy since the 1960s. Although all clinical studies have shown the benefits of taking the *injected* form of the supplement in relatively high doses (600–1,800 milligrams per day), at least one study found that alpha-lipoic acid was more likely to restore sensation than to relieve pain.[4] There is general agreement that high doses of the supplement relieve pain, burning, and numbness in 3–4 weeks.

Sodium Restrictions

Many doctors recommend sodium restriction to prevent the progress of diabetic neuropathy. You can lower the amount of sodium in your bloodstream by reducing or eliminating your consumption of the following items:

- All drugs containing sodium, such as Alka-Seltzer and aspirin.

- Anchovies, canned salmon, sardines, and shellfish in general.

- Any "fizzy" drink not specifically labeled as low-sodium.

- Any kind of salted grilled meat, soup, or consommé.

- Bacon, ham, sausages, and all cured meats, pork or otherwise.

- Beets, celery, and spinach.

- Beer, carbonated beverages whether sweetened with sugar or aspartame, and mineral water.

- Breakfast cereals, bread, biscuits, pancakes, and waffles.

- Cheeses and other processed dairy products.

- Chocolate.

- Dried fruit and nuts.

- Peanuts, whether salted or not.

- Popcorn.

- Prepared foods of all types, especially salad dressings.

The scientific evidence shows that the most effective form of alpha-lipoic acid for treating diabetic neuropathy is an injection, but over-the-counter preparations of alpha-lipoic acid can never be used for this purpose. To compensate for the limited absorption of alpha-lipoic acid through the digestive tract, German physicians recommend taking 800 milligrams of encapsulated alpha-lipoic acid for 4 months, and 100 milligrams 3 times a day thereafter.[5] Up to 1,800 milligrams of alpha-lipoic acid a day may be helpful during the first 3 weeks, but since very high doses of the supplement can lower blood sugars unpredictably, you should not take this large a dose without consulting your physician.

CONCEPTS FOR COPING WITH DIABETIC NEUROPATHY

○ Acupuncture is gaining favor as a treatment for diabetic neuropathy. There is some evidence that whether acupuncture succeeds or fails depends on the nervous system's having adequate supply of the neurochemical serotonin.[6] If you are not already on a prescription antidepressant, you should start taking 5-HTP several weeks before beginning acupuncture. Begin with a dose of 50 milligrams per day and build up to 200 milligrams per day over a period of 2 weeks. Do not take 5-HTP if you take the migraine medications naratriptan (Amerge), rizatriptan (Maxalt), sumatriptan (Imitrex), or zolmitriptan (Zomig).

○ Painful neuropathy in the feet and hands is often treatable with transcutaneous electronic nerve stimulation (TENS). In this treatment, small amounts of electricity block pain signals as they pass through a patient's skin. TENS is available from physicians and sometimes from massage therapists.

○ If dizziness is a problem, try wearing elastic stockings. The stockings help keep blood in the upper half of the body and, therefore, available to the brain. Doctors frequently recommend adding salt to the diet to treat dizziness, or prescribe hormones that increase the body's retention of salt such as fludrocortisone. This approach reduces dizziness but can accelerate the process of neuropathy.

○ For general information about coping with digestive problems associated with diabetes, see GASTROPARESIS (DIABETIC COMPLICATION). For general information about men's sexual problems in diabetes, see ERECTILE DYSFUNCTION.

Night Blindness
See **Night Vision, Impaired.**

Night Terrors in Children

SYMPTOM SUMMARY

○ Hyperventilation

○ Racing pulse

○ Sudden screaming

○ Sweating

○ Occur during the first 3–4 hours of sleep

UNDERSTANDING THE DISEASE PROCESS

Night terrors, also known as *pavor nocturnus,* primarily affect small children during the first several hours after they fall asleep. The child suddenly screams and seems to be in a panic. Night terrors do not cause the child to wake up, and they are not remembered the next morning.

TREATMENT SUMMARY

HERBS

○ Licorice, Wheat, and Jujube Formula. This herbal formula is sold as:

- Gan Mai Da Zao Tang (Herbal Times, Kan Traditionals, Lotus Classics, Qualiherb, Sun Ten)
- Kanbaku-taiso-to (Honso, Tsumura)
- Licorice & Jujube Combination (Lotus Classics, Qualiherb, Sun Ten)
- Rescue Formula (Kan Traditionals)

UNDERSTANDING THE HEALING PROCESS

Textbooks of medicine usually recommend treatment of night terrors by way of reassurance by parents. However, Traditional Chinese Medicine offers an herbal treatment.

In the conception of traditional East Asian medicine, the causes of night terrors are emotional, and the results of the condition are also emotional. In children, the only observable symptoms may be night terrors, but in adults the same imbalance may cause anxiety, disorientation, impulsiveness, and insomnia. During acute attacks of this syndrome, the person is upset to the point of uncontrollable crying, disorientation, or manic behavior. Chinese medicine explains that this condition is a futile attempt of the Yang of the body to reunite with the Yin.

Pharmacology, however, offers a scientific explanation. Both milk and wheat (as well as beef) have pharmacological actions surprisingly similar to those of opium. Opiumlike alkaloids in wheat bind to the same receptor sites in the brain as heroin, morphine, and opium. This pharmacological property of wheat accounts for the calming effect of the formula.[1] A cheeseburger actually would have a greater effect than either a warm glass of milk or the herbal formula, but cannot be recommended as a bedtime snack because of excessive fat content.

Recurrent night terrors are rare. If your child experiences frightening experiences during the first half hour of sleep, or if he or she can tell you about the bad dream the next day, the problem is nightmares or anxiety. These conditions require greater care.

CONCEPTS FOR COPING WITH NIGHT TERRORS IN CHILDREN

○ Children benefit from a warm glass of milk—not cocoa—before going to bed.

Night Vision, Impaired

SYMPTOM SUMMARY

○ Difficulty seeing clearly at night
○ Slow visual adjustment to dark surroundings

UNDERSTANDING THE DISEASE PROCESS

A substance called visual purple or rhodopsin enables sight in poor light. This compound is broken down by bright light but rapidly regenerates in the dark. For some people, however, restoration of normal levels of rhodopsin takes an unusually long time. There are no medical treatments for this condition.

TREATMENT SUMMARY

NUTRITIONAL SUPPLEMENTS

○ Vitamin A: 15,000 IU per day. Women who are or

who may become pregnant should strictly limit their intake of vitamin A to 5,000 IU per day or less.

○ Zinc picolinate: 30 milligrams per day.

HERBS

○ Bilberry: 160 milligrams of bilberry anthocyanosides, daily.

UNDERSTANDING THE HEALING PROCESS

Some authors have criticized the use of natural approaches to treating impaired night vision on the grounds that the most recent research failed to find any benefits of taking them—for Navy SEALS[1] and Israeli fighter jet pilots[2] who already have excellent vision. For many people who have uncomplicated cases of poor night vision, however, nutritional supplementation yields results in about 1 week.

The author of this book, growing up in the 1950s and 1960s, was admonished with Bugs Bunny stories to get him to eat his carrots so he could see better at night. The advice to eat carrots for good night vision has scientific validity. Carrots are an excellent source of vitamin A. Night blindness is a serious health problem in societies in which women, in particular, are chronically deficient in vitamin A.[3] Vitamin A supplementation greatly reduces but does not eliminate the problem. Zinc supplements added to vitamin A, however, nearly completely eliminate night blindness when the underlying cause is nutritional deficiency.

Supplemental vitamin A treats night blindness in doses that are essentially nontoxic. In women who have night blindness that is not explained by any other condition, vitamin A supplementation of up to 15,000 IU per day is even appropriate during the last 3 months of pregnancy (when night blindness is most likely to be a problem). Side effects from accidental overdosing of vitamin A are rare, but they are significant. The first signs of vitamin A overdose are dry skin and chapped lips, especially in dry weather. Later signs of toxicity are headache, mood swings, and pain in muscles and joints. In massive doses, vitamin A can cause liver damage. In the first 3 months of pregnancy, it can cause birth defects. Women who are or may become pregnant should strictly limit their intake of vitamin A to 5,000 IU per day or less. Discontinue vitamin A at the first sign of toxicity.

Zinc supplementation is most likely to help those

who are zinc deficient. A quick method for detecting zinc deficiency is a taste test. Powder a tablet of any zinc-based supplement or cold medication and mix with ¼ cup (50 milliliters) of water. Slosh the mixture in the mouth. People who notice no taste at all or who notice a "dry," "mineral," or "sweet" taste are likely to be zinc deficient. Anyone who notices a definite strong and unpleasant taste that intensifies over time is not likely to be zinc deficient.

Bilberry has been used as a remedy for poor night vision at least since World War II, when pilots in the Royal Air Force reported that an extra serving of bilberry jam with breakfast dramatically improved their night vision.[4] French physicians examined the RAF pilots and found that administration of bilberry extract resulted in improved nighttime visual acuity, faster adjustment to darkness, and faster restoration of visual acuity after exposure to glare.[5] In the 1960s and 1970s French scientists attempted to demonstrate the benefits of bilberry in noncombat conditions. A study involving 14 air traffic controllers found that the 5 who had poor night vision had better night vision after taking bilberry for 8 days.[6]

Many bilberry products combine the herb extract with lutein, which also improves night vision. Bilberry extracts are extremely nontoxic and difficult to overdose, although no added benefit can be expected from taking more than 540 milligrams per day.

Nocturnal Enuresis
See **Bedwetting**.

Nosebleeds

SYMPTOM SUMMARY

○ Bleeding from one or both nostrils

○ Frequent swallowing

○ Sensation of fluid in the back of the nose or throat

Related term: Epistaxis

UNDERSTANDING THE DISEASE PROCESS

At some time or another nearly everyone has had a nosebleed, whether a terrifying torrent or a speck of

blood on a tissue. Nosebleed can be caused by allergies, colds, sinusitis, very dry or very cold air, trauma (such as a punch in the nose), forceful nose blowing, or picking one's nose. A deviated septum or foreign objects in the nose may also cause bleeding. Blood disorders such as sickle-cell anemia and leukemia, arteriosclerosis, high blood pressure, a condition called hereditary hemorrhagic telangiectasia (a disorder involving a growth of blood vessels similar to a birthmark in the back of the nose), and strenuous exercise can also cause nosebleeds, as can taking large quantities of aspirin or blood thinning medications, nasal sprays, garlic, ginkgo, or vitamin E. Nasal sprays containing corticosteroids thin the collage in the mucous membranes lining the nose and cause nosebleeds. Most of the time, however, no single cause can be determined with confidence.

Nosebleeds are most common during childhood, and they most commonly occur at Kiesselbach's plexus. This is the spot on the tip of the nasal septum, the midline, vertical cartilage that separates the nasal chambers. The septum is home of numerous small, fragile blood vessels. Despite the large number of blood vessels serving Kiesselbach's plexus, this tissue is poorly oxygenated, especially in younger noses, so it gets dry and scabby easily in cold weather. Picking at the scabs causes bleeding.

Rarely, nosebleeds may occur higher on the nasal septum or deeper in the nose. These nosebleeds are usually much more difficult to control. A nosebleed that persists after 15–20 minutes of first aid care, recurrent nosebleeds, or blood draining persistently down the throat require emergency medical assistance.

TREATMENT SUMMARY

NUTRITIONAL SUPPLEMENTS

○ Citrus bioflavonoids containing diosmin and hesperidin: 500 milligrams twice a day.

○ Vitamin C: at least 500 milligrams a day.

UNDERSTANDING THE HEALING PROCESS

Healing broken blood vessels in the nose requires giving them time to recover without injuring them again. It is especially important to avoid blowing the nose or trying to clear clots during the first 4 hours after a nosebleed.

One double-blind study found that the citrus bioflavonoids diosmin and hesperidin decreased symptoms of capillary fragility, such as nosebleeds and easy bruising. The study did not specifically measure how much nosebleeds improved.[1] It may be necessary to take citrus bioflavonoids for 6 weeks to begin to stop recurrent nosebleeds.

Scientists are unsure of the interaction between citrus bioflavonoids and vitamin C. Citrus bioflavonoids and vitamin C were once thought to be synergistic, but some recent studies suggest that diosmin and hesperidin may actually interfere with the body's ability to absorb vitamin C. To be sure vitamin C requirements are met, take at least a small dose (500 milligrams) of vitamin C when taking citrus bioflavonoids.

If you are taking tamoxifen (Nolvadex) for breast cancer, you should avoid both citrus bioflavonoids and citrus juices. Although citrus bioflavonoids have been used to treat hemorrhoids during pregnancy, most authorities recommend that pregnant women and nursing mothers take no more than 20 milligrams of diosmin and hesperidin daily.

First Aid for Nosebleed

1. Reassure the victim. Encourage him or her to breathe through the mouth.

2. Have the person with the nosebleed sit and lean forward slightly. This keeps blood from going down the back of the throat.

3. Gently pinch the soft part of the nose for 5 to 10 minutes without releasing.

4. Place a cold compress on the bridge of the nose.

5. Release the nostrils slowly. Encourage the person with the nosebleed to avoid blowing the nose or clearing clots for at least 4 hours.

6. If bleeding has not stopped after 15 minutes, repeat this procedure one more time. If the nose is still bleeding after a second attempt, seek medical attention.

While citrus bioflavonoids are the only supplement that has been scientifically tested as a treatment for nosebleeds, many other nutritional supplements have similar activity. OPCs (oligomeric proanthocyanidins) such as those found in grape seed extract protect collagen by stopping an enzyme that breaks it down.[2]

Anthocyanosides, such as those found in high concentrations in bilberry, also strengthen fragile capillaries by protecting collagen. Additionally, anthocyanosides reduce capillary flow.[3] These supplements are likely to help reduce recurrent nosebleeds. The herb shepherd's purse (*Capsella bursae pastoris*) is a traditional topical treatment for nosebleeds. It should not be used during pregnancy since it may induce premature labor.

CONCEPTS FOR COPING WITH NOSEBLEEDS

○ Use a humidifier to prevent dryness.

○ Avoid putting fingers in the nose.

○ For minor recurrent nosebleeds, dab a small amount of petroleum jelly in the nostrils at night for 1–2 weeks.

○ Ice applied to the back of the neck may not stop nosebleed but does not cause harm.

○ Nosebleeds are usually benign, but nosebleeds that happen over and over again can be a sign of a serious blood disorder. See a doctor if nosebleeds become a weekly or daily occurrence, especially during damp weather.

○ Yarrow powder can stop minor nosebleeds. Open a yarrow capsule if the powder form is not available.

Obesity
See **Weight Control.**

Obsessive-Compulsive Disorder (OCD)

SYMPTOM SUMMARY

○ Persistent or recurrent ideas or impulses that cause distress

○ Intentional, purposeful, and repetitive behaviors performed in response to an obsession

---

UNDERSTANDING THE DISEASE PROCESS

Obsessive-compulsive disorder (OCD) is a form of anxiety characterized by an inability to stop intrusive thoughts combined with repetitive, ritualistic, and involuntary defensive behaviors. Obsession involves recurrent and persistent ideas, images, or thoughts that are unwelcome entrants to conscious awareness. These thoughts may concern contamination (commonly "germs"), violence, or anticipation of a tragic event. Compulsion is the action the individual feels compelled to take in response to the obsession, even though it may be senseless or harmful. If this act cannot be performed, the result is extreme anxiety.

While most authorities consider OCD to be a relatively rare disorder, some experts estimate that it may affect as many as 5 million people in the United States.[1] The onset of the condition usually occurs in late adolescence or early adulthood. Men and women are affected with equal frequency.

TREATMENT SUMMARY

SUPPLEMENTS

❍ 5-HTP: 100–200 milligrams 3 times a day.

UNDERSTANDING THE HEALING PROCESS

The most commonly prescribed medication for OCD in the United States is fluvoxamine (Luvox), a medication in the same class as Paxil, Prozac, and Zoloft. In 1991 a double-blind clinical study conducted in Switzerland found that 5-HTP offered comparable to slightly better results in the treatment of OCD than the prescription drug.

In the study, subjects received either 100 milligrams of 5-HTP or 50 milligrams of fluvoxamine 3 times a day for 6 weeks. Psychiatrists supervising the study measured effectiveness of treatment with the Hamilton Depression Rating Scale as well as subjective ratings by both patients and doctors. At 2, 4 and 6 weeks, patients taking 5-HTP had better ratings on the Hamilton Depression Rating Scale than patients taking fluvoxamine. For physical symptoms, 5-HTP produced a 47.6 percent decrease in severity compared with 37.8 percent for fluvoxamine. For depressed mood, 5-HTP produced a 65.7 percent reduction in severity compared with 61.8 percent for fluvoxamine. The most impressive effect of treatment with 5-HTP, however, was improvement in the quality of sleep. 5-HTP produced a 61.7 percent reduction in the severity of insomnia compared to a 55.9 percent decrease for fluvoxamine.

5-HPT is not entirely free of side effects, but its side effects are much less severe than those of fluvoxamine and other drugs similar to Paxil, Prozac, and Zoloft. In the Swiss study, the doctors commented, "Whereas the two treatment groups did not differ significantly in the number of patients sustaining adverse events, the interaction between the degree of severity and the type of medication was highly significant: fluvoxamine predominantly produced moderate to severe, [5-HTP] primarily mild forms of adverse effects."[2]

The most common side effects from 5-HTP are heartburn, nausea, and various kinds of stomach upset including, bloating, flatulence, and stomach rumbles. This complication is due to the fact that the digestive tract makes its own serotonin, which may be overabundant until it adjusts to the supplemental supply. About 2 in 5 people who use the supplement experience these effects during the first 2 weeks of using it. To avoid this complication, begin by taking a 50-milligram dose once or twice a day, gradually building up to a 100-milligram dose after 3 or 4 weeks.

There are no reports of adverse effects on the central nervous system from taking even high doses of 5-HTP. Theoretically, however, large doses of 5-HTP taken with the migraine medications naratriptan, sumatriptan, or zolmitriptan or any prescription medications for depression could cause "serotonin syndrome." In this rare condition of excess serotonin there may be agitation, confusion, heightened physical reflexes, racing pulse, and excessive sweating leading to hypertension, coma, and death. This condition has never been observed from supplementation with 5-HTP, but as a precaution, avoid using 5-HTP if you take any prescription drugs for depression or migraine. Persons who have angina, heart attack, uncontrolled high blood pressure, or a rare form of migraine known as Prinzmetal's angina should also avoid 5-HTP.

CONCEPTS FOR COPING WITH OBSESSIVE-COMPULSIVE DISORDER

Psychotherapy for OCD is usually a long-term process. Therapeutic techniques include:

❍ Aversion therapy—application of a painful stimulus when the obsession occurs to stop the associated compulsion.

❍ Flooding—frequent exposure to an object that triggers symptoms.

○ Thought stopping—teaching the individual to stop unwanted thoughts and focus attention on relieving anxiety.

Osgood-Schlatter's Disease

SYMPTOM SUMMARY

○ Persistent pain just below the knee in teens and preteens undergoing growth spurts

UNDERSTANDING THE DISEASE PROCESS

Osgood-Schlatter's disease is the most common cause of knee pain among preteen and teenage athletes. It causes swelling, pain, and tenderness just below the knee, over the shin bone (also called the tibia). Since the disease occurs mostly in girls aged 10–11 or boys aged 13–14 at the time of their growth spurt, the condition is sometimes referred to as "growing pains." Osgood-Schlatter's disease affects only one knee about 75 percent of the time, but both knees can be affected.[1]

Researchers believe that Osgood-Schlatter's disease results from the femur, or thigh bone, growing faster than the quadriceps, the muscles of the thigh. The quadriceps join with patellar tendons, passing through the knee and into the tibia, to connect the muscles to the knee. When the quadriceps contract, the patellar tendons can start to pull away from the shin bone to form a "shell" around the muscle; Osgood-Schlatter's disease does not affect the knee joint itself.[2] This muscular tension causes pain. Osgood-Schlatter's disease is most noticeable during activities that require jumping, running, or going up or down stairs. The problem is common in teens who play basketball, football, or soccer, or who are involved in ballet or gymnastics.

TREATMENT SUMMARY

NUTRITIONAL SUPPLEMENTS

○ Any multivitamin product including B vitamins, vitamin E, manganese, selenium, and zinc. Additional supplementation with 400 IU of vitamin E may be helpful.

UNDERSTANDING THE HEALING PROCESS

Within limits, strength training for the thighs and knees

prevents Osgood-Schlatter's disease.[3] Once the condition develops, the teen may need to avoid any activity that requires deep knee bending for 2–4 months. It may be necessary to walk with crutches while the knee heals. It is important to see a physician to make sure knee pain is not caused by a fracture or tumor before treating for this condition.

There has been very little research into nutritional interventions for Osgood-Schlatter's disease. There are numerous anecdotal reports of good responses to supplementation with B vitamins, vitamin E, manganese, selenium, and zinc. Of these supplements, vitamin E seems to have the greatest anti-inflammatory effect.

The prognosis for Osgood-Schlatter's disease is good. Even without treatment, the condition usually resolves by itself in a few months to a year. Some teens will experience pain for 2–3 years until the tibial growth plate closes. Without treatment, however, physical activity will constantly cause pain.

CONCEPTS FOR COPING WITH OSGOOD-SCHLATTER'S DISEASE

○ The standard treatment for knee pain in Osgood-Schlatter's disease is RICE: rest, ice, compression, and elevation.

- **R** = Rest the knee from the painful activity.
- **I** = Ice the affected area for 20 minutes, 3 times a day.
- **C** = Compress the painful area with an elastic bandage.
- **E** = Elevate the leg.

○ Don't offer teens aspirin or willow bark for pain relief. In rare instances, children and teens with viral infections who are given aspirin or herbs containing salicylates can develop Reye's syndrome, a devastating neurological condition. Acceptable aspirin substitutes are Advil and Tylenol. They can be supplemented with the following herbs.

- Boswellic acids: 400 milligrams per day.
- Capsaicin cream: apply to the knee daily. Be careful not to get capsaicin under fingernails, on the face, or in the eyes. If you are sensitive to capsaicin, substitute diluted essential oils of peppermint, eucalyptus, rosemary, or wintergreen.
- Devil's claw (as an alternative to NSAIDs or aspirin): 405–520 milligrams up to 4 times a day
- Yucca (leaf): 2–4 grams (1–2 teaspoons) per day.

○ If the child uses aspirin or NSAIDs on a regular basis, offer:

- DGL (deglycyrrhizinated licorice): chew and swallow 1–2 380-milligram tablets of DGL 20 minutes before meals, 3 times a day.

See Part Three if you take prescription medication.

Osteoarthritis

SYMPTOM SUMMARY

○ Joint pain
  - Gradual onset over a period of months or years
  - More noticeable in the morning
  - Relieved by rest
  - Usually in the elbow, foot, knee, or wrist
  - Worse after exercise or picking up heavy objects

○ Limited movement

○ Crepitation, a grating or crackling sound or sensation (as that produced by the fractured ends of a bone moving against each other)

○ Painful bony growths in fingers or toes

○ X-rays of the joint will show narrowed space within the joint

UNDERSTANDING THE DISEASE PROCESS

No illness is more likely to cause disability than osteoarthritis (OA). This well-known degenerative disease of the joints causes pain and incapacity to 40 million people in the United States alone, including 80 percent of people over the age of 50. Arthritis of the knee, referred to in the literature of sports medicine as *chondromalacia patellae,* strikes men and women at early in life, often before the age of 30.[1] The greatest risk factors for OA are intense physical activity at work, and overweight.[2]

Primary osteoarthritis is a condition due simply to the cumulative wear and tear of joints. The joints most likely to be affected by primary OA are those that bear weight and those that are in constant motion, such as the joints of the fingers and toes. Years of use stress the collagen matrix of the cartilage. The joint's natural repair system sends out enzymes to dissolve defective components of cartilage, but eventually the joint's ability to generate new collagen cannot keep up with the damage.[3]

Secondary osteoarthritis is associated with some predisposing factor, such as obesity, fractures along the linings of a joint, congenital abnormalities in the structure of a joint (such as "double joints" or abnormally shaped joint surfaces), trauma, or prior inflammation of the join by gout, rheumatoid arthritis, or septicemia. Estrogen replacement therapy, diabetes, and thyroid disease also increase the risk of OA.

TREATMENT SUMMARY

NUTRITIONAL SUPPLEMENTS

○ Boron: 6 milligrams a day.

○ Copper: 1 milligram a day.

○ Glucosamine sulphate: 1,500 milligrams per day.

○ Chondroitin: 1,200 milligrams per day.

○ SAM-e: 400 milligrams 3 times a day.

○ Vitamin A: 5,000 IU per day.

○ Vitamin B_6: 50 milligrams per day.

○ Vitamin C: at least 1,000 milligrams per day.

○ Vitamin E: 600 IU per day.

○ Zinc: 30–60 milligrams a day.

HERBS

○ Boswellic acids: 400 milligrams per day.

○ Capsaicin cream: apply to the back daily. If you are sensitive to capsaicin, substitute diluted essential oils of peppermint, eucalyptus, rosemary, or wintergreen.

○ Devil's claw (as an alternative to aspirin or NSAIDs): 405–520 milligrams up to 8 times a day.

○ Willow bark (as an alternative to aspirin or NSAIDs): 1 teaspoon in a cup of hot water or tea, as desired.

○ Yucca (leaf): 2–4 grams (1–2 teaspoons) per day.

If you use aspirin or NSAIDs on a regular basis, take:

○ DGL (deglycyrrhizinated licorice): chew and swallow 1–2 380-milligram tablets of DGL 20 minutes before meals 3 times a day.

See Part Three if you take prescription medication.

UNDERSTANDING THE HEALING PROCESS

The good news about OA is that, if it is treated early enough, it is frequently reversible. In fact, even advanced OA sometimes reverses itself with no treatment at all, natural or otherwise. In the 1960s, research physicians followed a group of patients whose x-rays identified narrow joint spaces indicating advanced OA in the hip. The doctors intentionally gave the patients no treatment at all for a period of 10 years. At the end of the 10-year study, 14 of 31 examinations showed that the hip had recovered its normal joint space with no treatment at all. The researchers commented that most patients showed marked clinical improvement.[4]

For those who cannot take 10 years off to rest, natural therapies probably represent their best bet. Conventional medical treatment of OA consists primarily of nonsteroidal anti-inflammatory drugs (NSAIDs) and other pain relievers, such as piroxicam (Feldene). These medications often relieve symptoms, but they can cause serious side effects. NSAIDs can cause peptic ulcer and, less commonly, kidney or liver failure. And there is even evidence from both laboratory experiments with animals with experimental OA and clinical observation of humans that some (but not all) NSAIDs may actually accelerate joint destruction (see the table below).[5]

PAIN RELIEVERS THAT HELP AND PAIN RELIEVERS THAT HURT RECOVERY OF CARTILAGE IN OSTEOARTHRITIS		
Stimulate the Recovery	No Effect on Recovery	Interfere with Recovery
Aceclofenac	aspirin	ibuprofen (Motrin)
Tenidap	piroxicam (Feldene)	indomethacin (Indocin)
Tometin	Tiaprofenic acid	naproxen (Naprosyn) Nimezulide

The newer pain relievers celecoxib (Celebrex) and rofecoxib (Vioxx) do not cause stomach upset, but whether they cause joint damage over the long run is not known. For that reason, acetaminophen (Tylenol) is the safest available pain reliever for OA.[6] Even Tylenol, however, can cause constipation, dizziness, drowsiness, nausea, vomiting, dependency, and fatigue.

Boron, copper, vitamins A, B$_6$, C, and E, and zinc are required for the synthesis of collagen in the joints, and deficiency in any of these nutrients causes accelerated joint destruction. Of these nutrients, boron is the most frequently neglected. One clinical trial found that approximately 70 percent of people who take boron will notice pain relief. Vitamin C may duplicate one of the newest treatments for OA, the injection of hyaluronic acid directly into the joint. This relatively expensive medication offers long-term pain relief with few side effects. However, studies in ophthalmology suggest vitamin C supplementation encourages the body to make its own hyaluronic acid.[8] The provision of hyaluronic acid to the joint encourages chondrocytes to release collagen needed to restore the lining of the afflicted joint.

None of these supplements is likely to cause problems. Boron is almost completely nontoxic in dosages of up to 20 milligrams per day and does not interact with prescription drugs. Taking too much copper can cause stomachache, nausea, diarrhea, and vomiting. Eating too much molasses or leafy green vegetables on a regular basis can cause copper deficiency, as can taking a daily dose of more than 50 milligrams of supplemental zinc. Women who use oral contraceptives and people who take prescription medications for bipolar disorder, unipolar depression, tuberculosis, or seizures are at risk for vitamin B$_6$ deficiency. If you take theophylline (Theo-Dur) for asthma and have any history of seizure disorder or unexplained loss of consciousness, you should not take vitamin B$_6$.

If you take certain prescription drugs, you should ask a doctor or nutritionist before taking vitamin C. Vitamin C taken in the form of vitamin C with bioflavonoids can interfere with the liver's ability to process statin drugs for controlling cholesterol, calcium channel blockers such as nifedipine (Procardia) for hypertension, or cyclosporine for preventing transplant rejection. Reduce your daily dosage of vitamin E to 200 IU per day if you take aspirin, clopidogrel (Plavix), or warfarin (Coumadin) on a daily basis. Don't take zinc supplements with foods rich in oxalic acid (beans, rhubarb, spinach, or sweet potatoes), phytic acid (matzo, nuts, or seeds), coffee, tea, or caffeinated soft drinks. These foods interfere with the absorption of zinc. People who have arthritis should also be careful not to take zinc with quinolone antibiotics, such as:

- ciprofloxacin (Cipro, Baycip, Cetraxal, Ciflox, Cifran, Ciplox, Cyprobay, Quintor)

- enoxacin (Penetrex)

- gatifloxacin (Tequin)

- gemifloxacin (a relatively new drug)

- grepafloxacin (Raxar)

- levofloxacin (Levaquin)

- lomefloxacin (Maxaquin)

- moxifloxacin (Avelox)

- norfloxacin (Amicrobin, Anquin, Baccidal, Barazan, Biofloxin, Floxenor, Fulgram, Janacin, Lexinor, Norofin, Noroxin, Norxacin, Orixacin, Oroflox, Urinox, Zoroxin)

- ofloxacin (Floxin)

- sparfloxacin (Zagam)

- temafloxacin (Omniflox)

- trovafloxacin (Trovan)

Taking zinc and the antibiotic together can reduce absorption of the antibiotic and set off an immune reaction that is destructive to cartilage or initiates another form of arthritis, rheumatoid arthritis.

Glucosamine stimulates the production of glycosaminoglycans, the building blocks of the collagen that lines the joints. There are indications that the joints lose their ability to make glucosamine as they age. There is wide agreement that a lack of glucosamine may be one of the most important contributing factors to the development of OA.

Three studies confirm that glucosamine gives better results than aspirin or other NSAIDs in the long-term relief of pain.[9,10,11] Glucosamine has no anti-inflammatory effect and does not affect the central nervous system. Instead, it corrects the underlying problem to relieve pain. One of the studies found that glucosamine is more effective than piroxicam (Feldene) or even a combination of glucosamine and piroxicam.[12] Glucosamine relieves symptoms of pain at rest, during exercise, on standing, and during stretching and passive movement.[13]

Probably the only drawback to using glucosamine is that people who are overweight may not respond as well to it. There are some indications that overweight people need a higher dose. Overweight people who have diabetes, however, should not take a higher than recommended dose, since glucosamine increases the need for insulin. Anyone who has diabetes and takes glucosamine should monitor blood sugars carefully to make sure they do not need additional insulin or diabetes medication.

Chondroitin is one of the glycosaminoglycans glucosamine stimulates the body to make. Found in fish, shark, and human cartilage, chondroitin was long thought to be too large a molecule to be absorbed if taken orally. Recent research, however, has found that a large percentage of the chondroitin taken in supplements is actually absorbed into the body.

Like glucosamine, chondroitin relieves pain by helping heal joints. One study found that people with arthritis of the knee who took chondroitin were able to increase their maximum walking speed, and that pain relief was noticed in as little as 1 month. More important, at the end of 12 months, study participants who had been taking chondroitin were found to have no worsening of the joints.[14] Chondroitin seems to protect joints from damage, perhaps halting the course of the disease.

SAM-e also relives pain. Various studies have found SAM-e to be as good or better for pain relief as Advil, Motrin, Naprosyn, and Nuprin. A study involving 20,641 people with osteoarthritis of the finger, hip, knee, and spine found that SAM-e alone was as effective as their ordinary pain relievers.[15] Another study involving 734 subjects found that SAM-e was more effective than Naprosyn (naproxen sodium).

The advantage of SAM-e is that it very seldom causes side effects. In the longest-running study involving the supplement, various minor side effects occurred in 20 out of 97 patients from time to time during the first 18 months of the intervention. In the final 6 months of the study, however, no patients experienced any side effects from SAM-e. Patients received relief of morning stiffness, pain at rest, and pain on movement, as well as depression.[16]

Although herbal treatments for OA are not especially well documented, several herbs are likely to be helpful if used on an occasional basis. Animal studies show that boswellic acid extracts (produced from the Ayurvedic herb guggul) stop inflammation, increase glycosaminoglycan synthesis, and improve blood flow to joints.[17] When used at a dosage of 400 milligrams per day, there are no reported side effects from this product. The Ayurvedic formula Yogaraj Guggulu has the same effect.

Both boswellic acids and Yogaraj Guggulu alter the body's production of thyroid hormone, and should be avoided by people who have Graves' disease or hyperthyroidism. They also should be avoided by persons taking beta-blockers, especially propanolol (Inderal, Inderide), or calcium channel blockers, especially diltiazem (Cardizem), for high blood pressure, since either product can make these drugs less available to the body.[18]

Capsaicin, devil's claw, and willow bark offer pain relief. Capsaicin is the chemical that gives hot peppers their heat. As anyone who has cooked with chiles knows, capsaicin can cause burning, redness, and inflammation, especially to the eyes and mouth. The first time capsaicin cream is applied to the skin over a painful area, it causes these symptoms, but the nerve fibers serving the area become insensitive to it—and to back pain.[19]

Capsaicin works best when there is good circulation to the skin to which it is applied.[20] Do not apply capsaicin to your feet if you have diabetes, and never apply capsaicin to ulcerated skin. It is also important to keep capsaicin out of your nose and eyes. Allergic reactions to the herb are rare but are not unknown, and there have been cases of hypothermia in people who used capsaicin in an especially cold room. It is theoretically possible that capsaicin absorbed into the bloodstream could reduce the bioavailability of aspirin; if you use capsaicin, use pain relievers other than aspirin.

Devil's claw relieves joint pain, but only if it is taken in an enteric-coated form that protects its analgesic compounds from being digested in the stomach. Do not use devil's claw with NSAIDs such as aspirin and Tylenol, and avoid it entirely if you have duodenal or gastric ulcers.

Willow bark is a natural substitute for aspirin. It contains silicon, a less potent pain reliever than the salicylates found in aspirin that does not generally cause bleeding or stomach irritation. Do not use willow bark during pregnancy, if you have tinnitus (ringing in the ears), or if you are allergic to aspirin. Do not give willow bark or aspirin to children who have colds or flu.

Natural health experts Dr. Michael Murray and Dr. Joseph Pizzorno suggest that yucca reduces inflammation in OA through a unique pathway, stopping the production of bacterial toxins in the intestines. They base their suggestion on the scientific observation that bacterial endotoxins stop proteoglycan synthesis, and that yucca contains natural soaps that break up the fat components of the bacterial endotoxins.[21] Although research has not yet confirmed their theory, many sufferers of OA report that yucca seems to help if it is used over a period of several months.

CONCEPTS FOR COPING WITH OSTEOARTHRITIS

○ Preliminary clinical research in France has found that a combination of phytonutrients found in avocado and soybean that are not dissolved in their oils reduces damage to joints in *advanced* arthritis.[22] The research did not offer an answer as to whether different daily doses of the two oils might be helpful for OA in its earlier stages. For people with OA, results from including more soybean and avocado in the diet are real but likely to take 1–2 years and will be hard to distinguish from results of other self-help measures.

○ Especially during the early stages of OA, resting affected joints gives them time to heal. If at all possible, do not stress painful joints.

○ Recent clinical studies suggest that acupuncture for advanced OA is reliably better than receiving no treatment at all. One study found that giving acupuncture to OA patients waiting for knee replacement surgery improved flexibility and walking distance, and relieved pain.[23] Older and better educated people with OA are more likely to respond to acupuncture, while anxious and fatigued people with OA are less likely to respond to acupuncture.[24]

○ Bee venom therapy (BVT) is another method of pain relief for OA. A Korean clinical study found that BVT lowered pain and improved circulation in affected joints, and was more effective than the more commonly used (in Korea) method of acupuncture.[25] One of the components of bee venom, alodapin, is a COX-2 inhibitor, that is, a pain reliever in the same class as celecoxib (Celebrex) and rofecoxib (Vioxx). Purifying the venom before injection makes it possible to treat OA without causing many of the complications of bee stings, although BVT cannot be used by people who are allergic to bee stings. More information is available from The American Apitherapy Society at their website, www.apitherapy.org. Apitherapy should be attempted only under the supervision of a knowledgeable health practitioner with provisions for emergency treatment in case of allergic reactions.

○ Long-distance runners frequently develop OA. Recent research suggests that runners who develop arthritis have preexisting lesions in the meniscus, the shock absorber, of the knee.[26] For this reason, careful attention to the nutrients that nourish cartilage is important *before* long-distance training and especially before competition. Start taking glucosamine, chondroitin, boron, copper, vitamins A, B$_6$, C, and E, and zinc at least 6 weeks before beginning training for a long-distance event.

○ Pain is not necessarily related to deformity. That is, joints that still move freely can be extremely painful. If you have intense joint pain without limitation of mobility, do not allow a health practitioner to tell you "it's all in your head."

○ There are numerous anecdotal reports that eliminating vegetables in the Nightshade family—peppers, potatoes, and tomatoes—slows the progress of OA.

○ Diabetics have more frequent and more severe OA than non-diabetics. Insulin therapy can have the side effect of relieving the disease. Insulin stimulates the chondrocytes to use glucosamine to make cartilage.

○ People with hypothyroidism also have a higher incidence of OA, and treating thyroid problems often improves OA.

○ Certain kinds of medications, such as those used to treat seizure disorders, excessive consumption of alcohol, and chemical exposure, inhibit the liver's ability to secrete somatomedins, hormonal messengers that stimulate the repair of joints. If you drink, smoke, or work around chemicals and have OA, you will benefit from taking 210–500 milligrams of silymarin (milk thistle) phytosomes daily to stimulate liver function.

○ Women who have passed menopause benefit from the inclusion of apples, celery, fennel, parsley, soy, and whole grains in the diet. These foods help maintain estrogen levels and reduce the number of erosive lesions caused by OA.

○ DMSO (dimethyl sulfoxide) applied to the skin can relieve arthritis pain, although weaker solutions (70%) offer greater pain relief than stronger solutions (the more usual 90%). With respect to the joints (and only with respect to the joints), DMSO works like a fast-acting vitamin C. In as little as 30 seconds after application, the bloodstream carries DMSO to the joints, where it protects hyaluronic acid from damage by free radicals.[27] Unfortunately, DMSO also can dissolve any toxin on the skin and send it into circulation throughout the body in under 30 seconds. Industrial-grade DMSO, the form most commonly sold in flea markets, can contain toxic byproducts of the manufacturing process and should not be applied to the skin. MSM (methylsulfonylmethane) is a byproduct of DMSO, as it is metabolized by the body, that is also found in alfalfa sprouts, corn, most fruits, tomatoes, coffee, tea, and milk. MSM is also used to treat arthritic pain, and unlike DMSO, is almost completely nontoxic. Most naturopaths recommend 1,000–2,000 milligrams of MSM daily to prevent OA pain and 3,000–5,000 milligrams of MSM daily to treat OA pain.

○ Homeopathic physicians typically recommend ledum for foot and ankle pain (200C for relief of acute pain, 6C to 30C for prevention), lycopodium for arthritis that is relieved by application of warmth and for joint pain on the right side of the body, and cell salts, especially calcarea sulphurica (Calc Sulf) for general relief of OA.

○ Ice massage, moist heat, and transcutaneous electrical nerve stimulation (TENS) all help relieve the pain of OA.

Osteomalacia

SYMPTOM SUMMARY

○ "Bow legs" or bowing of the bones in the arms

○ Pain in the bones of the arms, legs, pelvis, and spine

○ Weakening of the bones

○ Fractures (more common in adults than in children)

○ Progressive weakness

UNDERSTANDING THE DISEASE PROCESS

Osteomalacia is a progressive softening of the bones resulting from the loss of calcium from the skeleton. The bones become flexible and are slowly molded by the weight-bearing forces placed on them. Bone deformities result.

Osteomalacia became widely known to the American public during the coverage of the Afghanistan war, in which reports of women suffering from the disease due to deprivation of sunlight reached the news media. Osteomalacia is actually a relatively common condition even in North America and Europe, although it seldom results from sunlight deprivation. The most common cause of osteomalacia is a failure to absorb fat, called steatorrhea. In this condition, fats are passed directly out the body in the stool instead of being absorbed. As a result, vitamin D, which is usually absorbed with fat, and calcium are poorly absorbed. This poor absorption can be a result of digestive disorders, especially celiac disease, or cystic fibrosis.

Osteomalacia may also occur as a result of a condition known as tubular acidosis. This condition causes an increased concentration of acids in body fluids as the tubules of the kidneys are unable to clear them. The excess acid literally dissolves the skeleton. Tubular acidosis can occur as a result of chemotherapy or may be due to a genetic condition.

TREATMENT SUMMARY

NUTRITIONAL SUPPLEMENTS

O Calcium citrate: variable dosage, see Understanding the Healing Process.

O Taurine: in children, 30 milligrams for each kilogram of body weight per day (150 milligrams for every 10 pounds of body weight per day). In adults, 500 milligrams 3 times a day.

O Vitamin D: variable dosage, see Understanding the Healing Process.

O Vitamin K: 5 milligrams every other week, especially if taking antibiotics.

UNDERSTANDING THE HEALING PROCESS

The first step in treating osteomalacia is making sure of the diagnosis. Cushing's disease, hyperthyroidism, hyperparathyroidism, neurofibromatosis, and osteoporosis cause similar symptoms but require different treatments. Chronic use of seizure medication and verylow-fat diets can also cause symptoms similar to osteomalacia.

The two most important nutrients in treating osteomalacia are calcium and vitamin D. Appropriate dosages vary by the contributing causes of the condition. When osteomalacia occurs after deprivation of sunlight, such as after a long period of confinement indoors, it is usually necessary to take 800–4,000 IU of the vitamin daily for 6 weeks, tapering off to a dosage of 200–600 IU a day thereafter to prevent deficiency. Healing of fractures, leading to reductions in pain, usually begins in 3–4 weeks. Complete healing can occur in 6 months.

When osteomalacia is due to sunlight deprivation, calcium supplements usually are not necessary except when there is muscle pain. In this case, 1,000 milligrams of any calcium supplement is sufficient.

When osteomalacia is due to an intestinal absorption disease or kidney failure, calcium and vitamin D are usually needed in very large doses. If there is celiac disease, it may be necessary to take as much 15,000 milligrams of calcium lactate or 4,000 milligrams of calcium carbonate daily. Vitamin D in doses of up 50,000 IU per day may be required. Renal dialysis patients who develop osteomalacia may also need phosphorus. Since the dosages of calcium and vitamin D required to do any good can also cause serious side effects in people who don't need them, consult a nutritionally oriented physician before attempting to treat osteomalacia due to any cause other than sunlight deprivation.

Taurine and vitamin K are safe to use in osteomalacia. Taurine is especially useful when there are absorption problems. It is an amino acid that latches onto bile salts to carry them away from the liver. Once the bile salts reach the intestine, taurine helps them attach onto essential fatty acids to be reabsorbed into the body. This keeps nutritional fats from being excreted with stool. In one study, 92 percent of children given 30 milligrams of taurine for every kilogram of their body weight each day had fewer symptoms of steatorrhea (floating, foul smelling, and pale or clay-colored stools) and better reabsorption of bile salts.[1] Another study suggests that taurine supplementation increases absorption in the segment of the intestines known as the ileum, where 80 percent of bile acids reenter the bloodstream.[2] When fats are not lost in the stool, calcium and vitamin D are better absorbed.

Vitamin K is necessary for the bones to make osteocalcin, a protein that controls the uptake of calcium. Deficiencies of osteocalcin result in increased risk of fractures, especially in the hips.[3] Vitamin K is synthesized by bacteria in the intestine, so vitamin K levels go down during antibiotic treatment. However, taking vitamin K supplements as infrequently as every other week is usually sufficient.[4]

CONCEPTS FOR COPING WITH OSTEOMALACIA

O Homeopathic remedies treat osteomalacia with minute amounts of substances beneficial to bone health. Common homeopathic remedies for the condition include:

- Calcarea carbonica for back pain and swollen joints, particularly in people who tend to sweat easily.

- Calcarea phosphorica for fractures and bone spurs in the neck, upper back, and hips.

- Phosphorus for pain between the shoulder blades, particularly in people who enjoy cold drinks.

- Symphytum, a homeopathic dosage of the herb comfrey (also known as knitbone), for fractures in weakened bones.

Osteoporosis

SYMPTOM SUMMARY

○ Dull pain in back or muscles (in early stages)

○ Sharp pain upon putting weight on a joint or bone, subsiding in 1–3 weeks (in advanced stages)

○ Stooped posture due to compression fractures of the spine

○ Fractures

UNDERSTANDING THE DISEASE PROCESS

Osteoporosis is a loss of bone due to a failure to make bone or excessive destruction of bone through natural processes. Bone is constantly remodeled throughout life to compensate for microscopic trauma, the process of bone destruction, known as resorption, always followed by a process of bone formation. When resorption and formation get out of balance, osteoporosis results.

Risk factors for osteoporosis in women include use of tobacco or alcohol, history of anorexia, history of irregular menstrual periods, advanced age, white or Asian ethnicity, small frame, early menopause, not having borne children, estrogen deficiency, and calcium deficiency. Over 50 diseases cause secondary osteoporosis in men, but it is most common in men who are on hormone therapies for prostate cancer. Estrogen replacement therapy in women is associated with a 2 to 4 percent increase in bone mass each year during the first 1–3 years it is used, and a 75–80 percent reduction in fractures over the course of 10 years.[1] Estrogen replacement, however, elevates risk of several kinds of cancer.

TREATMENT SUMMARY

NUTRITIONAL SUPPLEMENTS

○ Calcium citrate: 1,200–1,500 milligrams a day, but no more than 600 milligrams in any single dose.

○ Copper: 3 milligrams per day.

○ Ipriflavone: 600 milligrams per day.

○ Vitamin D: 800 IU per day.

○ Vitamin K: 1 milligram per day to prevent osteoporosis; 45 milligrams per day to treat osteoporosis.

○ Zinc picolinate: 30 milligrams per day.

○ Any multivitamin and mineral formula containing trace minerals, daily.

UNDERSTANDING THE HEALING PROCESS

One of the simplest and least expensive ways to treat osteoporosis is to reduce consumption of meat and increase consumption of fruits and vegetables. A diet high in animal protein and low in plant foods tends to make the blood acidic, leaching calcium out of the bones.[2] It is important to replace meat with other sources of protein, such as soy, since normal bone formation requires adequate dietary protein, and low dietary protein intake has been associated with low bone mineral density.[3] It is probably helpful to avoid or even eliminate salty foods from the diet. Short-term increases of sodium increase the amount of calcium excreted into the urine, and long-term consumption of salt can be presumed to have the same effect. Overweight is sometimes linked to osteoporosis, but the detrimental factor is probably not total weight but the amount of fat under the skin. Subcutaneous fat absorbs the vitamin D made by the skin and keeps it from entering circulation.[4]

No single supplement is enough to prevent or treat osteoporosis. Calcium, of course, is essential to the formation of bone. There is disagreement among researchers regarding which source of calcium is best. Soy products and leafy green vegetables such as bok choy, broccoli, collard greens, Chinese cabbage, and mustard greens are unquestionably safe as sources of calcium for people at risk for osteoporosis. Nonfat milk and yogurt are more questionable as sources of calcium, since their high protein content might increase urinary acidity and encourage calcium excretion, although no experts recommend excluding them from the diet to prevent osteoporosis. Cottage cheese, hard cheeses, and yogurt are probably undesirable because of their high content of both protein and salt. Calcium-fortified milk by itself slows the course of osteoporosis, but, for reasons not explained, only in the spine and not in the arms and legs.[5]

Calcium supplements by themselves have very little effect on bone mass. Taking supplemental calcium during estrogen replacement therapy, however, has considerably greater benefit to bones than estrogen replacement by itself.[6] In at least 10 clinical trials, taking both calcium and the soy extract ipriflavone stops bone loss, reduces bone pain, and reduces the risk of fracture.

Vitamin D increases the absorption of calcium and strengthens bone.[7] Mild vitamin D deficiencies are common in active elderly persons who avoid the sun because of concerns about wrinkles or skin cancer. Severe vitamin D deficiencies are common among persons confined to nursing homes.

Vitamin K makes estrogen replacement therapy much more effective in treating osteoporosis.[8] It is also useful for preventing bone loss in women who have hepatitis C.[9] In combination with estrogen, a typical dosage of vitamin K for treating osteoporosis is 45 milligrams per day. A dosage for preventing deficiency is 1 milligram per day.

Zinc is particularly important for preventing fractures in men.[10] It is only effective when used in combination with calcium and copper supplementation. Bones need copper to absorb calcium, and supplemental zinc can deplete the body's copper stores. Do not take supplemental zinc for prevention or treatment of osteoporosis unless you also take copper.

Various studies and anecdotal reports support the use of trace amounts of boron, magnesium, silicon, strontium, and B vitamins in the prevention and treatment of fractures. To avoid imbalances, take a multivitamin and mineral supplement containing trace elements rather than individual doses of these health aids.

CONCEPTS FOR COPING WITH OSTEOPOROSIS

○ A beneficial side effect of taking red yeast rice (Cholestin) for lowering cholesterol may be slowing osteoporosis by increasing bone formation. Cholestin is chemically identical to statin medications found to have this effect.[11]

○ The soy extract ipriflavone could be extremely useful for women who have breast cancer. Experiments with animal models of breast cancer have found that treatment with ipriflavone prevents the infiltration of the cancer into the bones, preventing bone pain and debilitating fractures.[12]

○ Homeopathy treats osteoporosis with minute amounts of substances beneficial to bone health. Common homeopathic remedies for the condition include:

• Calcarea carbonica for back pain and swollen joints, particularly in people who tend to sweat easily.

• Calcarea phosphorica for fractures and bone spurs in the neck, upper back, and hips.

• Phosphorus for pain between the shoulder blades, particularly in people who enjoy cold drinks.

• Symphytum, a homeopathic dosage of the herb comfrey (also known as knitbone), for fractures in weakened bones.

Ovarian Cancer

SYMPTOM SUMMARY

○ Abdominal swelling

○ Lumps or masses in the abdomen

○ Vaginal bleeding

○ Difficult urination

○ Lower back pain

These symptoms are caused by many conditions in addition to ovarian cancer.

UNDERSTANDING THE DISEASE PROCESS

Ovarian cancer is among the most deadly of all cancers for women. According to the American Cancer Society, 1 out of every 70 women will be diagnosed with the disease, and 70 percent of women with the most common form of ovarian cancer are not diagnosed until the disease is advanced and very difficult to treat. The American Cancer Society estimates that there were 23,400 new cases and 13,900 deaths in 2001. The death rate for this disease has not changed much in the last 50 years.

The symptoms of ovarian cancer, abdominal swelling, masses in the abdomen, bleeding, lower back pain, and urinary difficulties, overlap with those of many other conditions. The risk factors for ovarian cancer likewise overlap with those of many other conditions. Most (but not all) epidemiological studies have found that the women at greatest risk of ovarian cancer have the highest dietary consumption of fat and milk products. Women who consume more than 4 eggs per week are nearly twice as likely to develop ovarian cancer as women who consume one or fewer eggs per week.[1] Women who develop this form of cancer typically have very high levels of iron in their blood.[2] Surveys have also found that the risk of ovarian cancer is lowest in women who consume the most dietary fiber, vitamin A, vitamin E, beta-carotene, and lycopene. Food items strongly related to decreased risk for ovarian cancer are raw carrots and tomato sauce.[3]

Even very low doses of vitamin C and E taken as supplements may reduce the risk of ovarian cancer. One study found that taking just 90 milligrams of vitamin C a day (less than the smallest commercially available tablet) was associated with a 68 percent reduction of ovarian cancer risk in women who smoked, and a 19 percent reduction in risk in women who do not smoke. The same study found that taking 45 IU of natural vitamin E a day (also less than the smallest commercially available capsule) reduced women's risk of ovarian cancer by 67 percent.[4]

TREATMENT SUMMARY

NUTRITIONAL SUPPLEMENTS

❍ Quercetin: 125 milligrams 3 times a day with meals.

❍ Selenium: 200 micrograms daily.

❍ Soy isoflavones: 3,000 milligrams daily.

Nutritional supplementation does not replace medically directed therapy for ovarian cancer.

See Part Three if you take prescription medication.

UNDERSTANDING THE HEALING PROCESS

There are no magic bullets in either conventional or complementary medicine for ovarian cancer. Once ovarian cancer has developed, the most important dietary principle is to ensure adequate calories. Women with ovarian cancer develop a very fast metabolism, and their bodies will convert the protein in muscle tissue into energy if adequate nutrition is not maintained.[5]

Three nutritional supplements may be of modest benefit in treating ovarian cancer. Laboratory experiments have found that quercetin and genistein, a soy isoflavone, stop growth of ovarian cancer cells at different stages in their process of multiplication.[6] It is not known whether they have the same effect in a woman's body, but it is at least theoretically possible they will help. Do not take quercetin if you are also receiving antibiotic treatment.

Russian laboratory research has found that selenium disables an "unzipping" step critical to the ovarian cancer cell's replication of the double helix of DNA. Once again, it is not known whether selenium has a similar effect in a woman's body but net benefit is possible. Do not take selenium while taking chemotherapy or radiation.

CONCEPTS FOR COPING WITH OVARIAN CANCER

❍ A recent study that followed 44,241 postmenopausal women for approximately 20 years concluded that estrogen use is associated with an increased risk of ovarian cancer. In this study, women who used estrogen alone for 10–19 years were twice as likely to develop ovarian cancer than women who did not use hormones during and after menopause. For women who used estrogen for 20 or more years, the risk of ovarian cancer increased to 3 times that of women who did not use postmenopausal hormones. The risk of ovarian cancer may be elevated as long as 29 years after a woman quits using estrogen replacement therapy.[7]

❍ An outbreak of acne or growth of hair on the chest or chin with galactorrhea is a symptom requiring urgent medical attention. This combination of symptoms can result from ovarian cysts or ovarian cancer in a relatively early, treatable stage.

❍ The antioxidant glutathione can greatly reduce the risk of kidney damage during chemotherapy with Platinol (cisplatin), a commonly prescribed treatment for ovarian cancer.[8] Since glutathione must be administered intravenously in relatively high doses (3,000 mg/m_2) immediately before chemotherapy, the oncologist's approval is required. Smaller doses do not protect against kidney damage but significantly increase the likelihood of tumor reduction.[9] Similar benefits have been found when glutathione was given to women treated with a combination of cisplatin and cyclophosphamide (Cytoxan).[10]

Paget's Disease

SYMPTOM SUMMARY

- Bone pain (may be severe and persistent)
- Barrel-shaped chest
- Blindness
- Bowed legs
- Headache
- Hearing loss
- Joint pain and stiffness
- Legs or arms of different lengths
- Neck pain
- Reduced height
- Spinal curvature
- Sometimes causes no symptoms

UNDERSTANDING THE DISEASE PROCESS

Paget's disease is a condition in which too much bone tissue is broken down. When the bones send out hormonal signals that too much bone is being broken down, the body increases the rate at which new bone is formed. In Paget's disease, the new bone is replaced so fast that its collagen fibers are laid down in a disordered pattern. It is softer than normal bone. As in osteoporosis, the bones grow weak and deformed and may fracture. Excessive growth of the bones may also tear the cartilage lining the joints.

TREATMENT SUMMARY

NUTRITIONAL SUPPLEMENTS

- Ipriflavone: 600–1,200 milligrams daily.

UNDERSTANDING THE HEALING PROCESS

Modern medical treatment of Paget's disease seeks to stop the dissolution of bone by inhibiting and shortening the life span of the osteoclasts, specialized cells that remove old bone tissue to make room for new bone. The biphosphonate drugs used to control osteoclasts have to be taken on an empty stomach and can cause constipation, diarrhea, heartburn, acid reflux, and difficulty swallowing. Despite the side effects of these drugs, natural medicine has no comparable healing agents.

It may be possible to reduce the dosage of biphosphonates, however, by taking the nutritional supplement ipriflavone. A chemically altered form of the soy isoflavone genistein, this isoflavone hormone prevents the loss of bone not by shortening the life span or osteoclasts or inhibiting their normal activity, but by blocking the chemical signals that attract them to susceptible bones.[1] In one study in Italy, *all* the Paget's disease patients taking 1,200 milligrams of ipriflavone daily experienced a reduction in bone pain within 3 months.[2]

Ipriflavone enhances and improves the effects of biophosphonates and calcitonin used in the treatment of Paget's disease. It also adds to the effects of estrogen replacement therapy. However, it should not be taken by anyone who uses the drug tolbutamide (Orinase) for diabetes, since ipriflavone interferes with the biochemical process by which tolbutamide is broken down in the liver. Taking ipriflavone and tolbutamide together can result in unexpected drops in blood sugars. Ipriflavone also must not be taken with the asthma drug theophylline (Theo-Dur), since ipriflavone can cause theophylline to build up to toxic levels in the bloodstream.

CONCEPTS FOR COPING WITH PAGET'S DISEASE

- Many people with Paget's disease have no symptoms. Sometimes the condition is discovered by accident from an x-ray or a routine blood test. Many times Paget's disease only affects bone in one part of the body, most frequently the lower legs, pelvis, spine, skull, or thighs. Paget's disease can also affect multiple bones. People with Paget's disease live out normal life spans but suffer severely diminished quality of life. A historical example of Paget's disease is thought to be the life of the composer Ludwig van Beethoven—he was short, 5'4" (138 centimeters), began losing his hearing at the age of 25, and had to wear his hat on the back of his head because continuing growth of the bones in his skull made his hat too small.[3]

Pancreatic Cancer

SYMPTOM SUMMARY

The outward symptoms of pancreatic cancer are especially vague and are associated with many other diseases. Most patients with treatable pancreatic cancer have very few symptoms. Having any or all of these symptoms should not be interpreted as evidence of pancreatic cancer.

❍ Blood in stool

❍ Dark urine and light stools

❍ Loss of appetite

❍ Pain over the stomach that is worse after eating

❍ Weight loss

❍ Yellowing of the skin

UNDERSTANDING THE DISEASE PROCESS

The pancreas is an enzyme-excreting and hormone-secreting gland located in the upper abdomen. Anatomically, it consists of a head, neck, body, and tail, along with a duct through which it excretes digestive enzymes into the intestines. The pancreas also contains islets of Langerhans that secrete insulin into the bloodstream.

Most pancreatic cancers are carcinomas located in the duct. Blocking the flow of pancreatic enzymes into the duodenum, these tumors deprive the digestive tract of chymotrypsin, pancreatin, and trypsin as well as other digestive enzymes. The digestion of carbohydrates, fats, and proteins is impeded and the body has less energy. The early stages of pancreatic cancer typically only cause loss of appetite and weight loss, so there is usually a 2- to 6-month delay in diagnosing the disease. As the cancer grows, there are problems with tissue repair, breaking down blood clots, and immune response, eventually causing enough outward symptoms that medical attention is sought.

On a molecular level, pancreatic cancer, like all other cancers, results from genetic defects or faulty genes that are not adequately compensated by the body's genetic repair systems. More than 90 percent of pancreatic cancers involve a mutation in the p16 gene and more than 75 percent of pancreatic cancers involve a mutation in the p53 gene. Normally, these two genes regulate the G_1/S checkpoint, a point in the life of the cancer cell at which it "decides" whether it will make new DNA with which it could multiply itself. These genes also have a great deal to do with apoptosis, the normal process of retiring a cell that has completed its life cycle. In cancer, healthy p16 and p53 genes can

instruct a cancer cell that it has completed its task and should die. In those cases of pancreatic cancer in which one or the other of these genes is intact, stimulating it by natural means can greatly influence the course of the disease.

TREATMENT SUMMARY

DIET

❍ Sodi-Pallares diet, described in Understanding the Healing Process.

UNDERSTANDING THE HEALING PROCESS

Most pancreatic cancer patients are given a bleak prognosis. However, at least a few people with pancreatic cancer, interviewed by the author of this book, have lived healthy and productive lives for as long as 12 years after diagnosis. There is medical confirmation of the original diagnosis and subsequent remission of the primary tumor, but none of the cases involved metastases to the liver and peritoneum. Since the treatment method does not interfere with any standard medical procedures or treatment, costs very little, and has no side effects, it is reported here.

Demetrio Sodi-Pallares is a physician who has been practicing medicine 12 hours a day 6 days a week in a private clinic since 1936. A professor of medicine and president of the Mexican National Academy of Medicine, Dr. Sodi-Pallares is the author of hundreds of medical papers, several books, and an internationally recognized authority on diagnosis of diseases of the heart by EEG.

He developed a diet with remarkable effects in the treatment of congestive heart failure (see CONGESTIVE HEART FAILURE). He pioneered emergency treatments for heart attack which, 45 years after he developed them, received a recommendation from the American Heart Association.

In the 1960s Dr. Sodi-Pallares observed that the low-sodium diets he prescribed for heart patients sometimes had remarkable effects in cancer patients. As an expert in the measurement of the electrical activity of the heart, he began to try to understand his observations of cancer in terms of what was then known about the electrodynamics of various kinds of cells. The most important finding of the cell physiology of that time seemed to be that cells have to maintain a negative charge in order to transport nutrient molecules across the cell membrane. Also, every time the cell produces a molecule of the energy storage chemical ATP, two positively charged ions of potassium have to come into the cell and three positively charged ions of sodium have to go out. This allows the cell to keep an overall negative charge that attracts the glucose and amino acids it requires to function.

Cancer cells have weak electrical charges. Dr. Sodi-Pallares's colleagues noted that a healthy muscle cell typically carries a charge of –90 millivolts, for instance, while a myosarcoma (muscle cancer) cell has a charge of only –10 millivolts. While a buildup of sodium cannot be said to be the "cause" of cancer, cancer cells typically contain many times the normal level of sodium, every sodium ion carrying a positive charge. They cannot attract the nutrients they need to function normally. Additionally, the high degree of positive charge within the cell encourages the separation of strands of DNA, uncouples the DNA from the "watchdog" genes p26 and p53, and encourages multiplication of sick cells.

Through years of trying to treat cancer patients who did not have income or insurance, Dr. Sodi-Pallares learned that low-sodium diets deprive cancer cells of sodium and sometimes arrest the disease. All kinds of cancer cells are not equally response to low-sodium diets. Skeletal muscle needs a great deal of glucose and normally carries a highly negative –90-millivolt charge. It is relatively difficult to recharge a cell from –10 millivolts back to –90 millivolts, so muscle cancer is not especially responsive to a low-sodium diet. Bone cells and pancreatic cells, on the other hand, have relatively low energy requirements. In a healthy state, a pancreatic cell carries an electrical charge of only –20 millivolts. It is relatively easy, in Dr. Sodi-Pallares's experience, to restore normal electrical charge to pancreatic tissue through a sodium-restricted diet.

In a case the author of this book observed personally, simply following a *severe* sodium-restricted diet has allowed a woman diagnosed with pancreatic cancer to live normally for 12 years. In other cases supervised by Dr. Sodi-Pallares, patients achieved remission from pancreatic cancer on a combination of sodium restriction, potassium supplementation, and magnetic therapy (whole-body exposure to a field of 130–140 Gauss for 4 hours daily). In every case in which the patient resumed eating salty foods, usually at the permission of another physician, the pancreatic cancer came back and death occurred in a matter of weeks. In one case, a woman

decided to celebrate a new marriage with a stay at a beach resort, eating large quantities of seafood. She died 2 weeks later. In another case, a man who had been very near death decided that he had to work to support his family, and he had to eat the lunch offered by his company cafeteria. He died a month later. The cancer is held in check only as long as the cancer cells are deprived of sodium. There must be no exceptions to the diet, ever.

The Sodi-Pallares diet absolutely forbids:

• All drugs containing sodium, such as Alka-Seltzer and aspirin.

• Anchovies, canned salmon, sardines, and shellfish in general.

• Any "fizzy" drink not specifically labeled as low-sodium.

• Any kind of salted grilled meat, soup, or consommé.

• Bacon, ham, sausages, and all cured meats, pork or otherwise.

• Beer, carbonated beverages whether sweetened with sugar or aspartame, and mineral water.

• Beets, celery, and spinach.

• Breakfast cereals, bread, biscuits, pancakes, and waffles.

• Cheeses and other processed dairy products.

• Chocolate.

• Dried fruit and nuts.

• Egg *whites*. Egg yolks are permissible.

• Peanuts, whether salted or not.

• Popcorn.

• Prepared foods of all types, especially salad dressings.

Dr. Sodi-Pallares notes that, unlike most cardiologists, he encourages his patients to eat egg yolks but not egg whites. Egg whites are not allowed because their sodium content is about 2 milligrams per gram, whereas egg yolks have a sodium content of about 0.3 milligrams per gram. Nuts, peanuts, and dried fruits are forbidden because they tend to have a high sodium content even when they are packed without salt. Prepared foods typically contain sodium benzoate as a preservative.

Dr. Sodi-Pallares recommends that his patients consume fresh fruit and fresh fruit juices as desired, and rice, raw vegetables (except beets, celery, and spinach) served in salads with oil, vinegar, and pepper, artichokes, avocados, carrots, cauliflower, green beans, lentils, lettuce and field greens, potatoes, radishes and turnips in any amounts that do not cause indigestion. He recommends eating 1 egg yolk and 5 ounces of fresh beef, chicken, lamb, veal, red snapper, sea bass, or white fish daily. He recommends boiled prunes as a rich source of potassium, but forbids packaged prunes that have not been washed to remove sodium benzoate. Wine is encouraged because it is low in sodium and high in potassium. Dr. Sodi-Pallares also recommends drinking at least 8 glasses of water every day.

Success on the diet can be measured by blood tests for sodium and potassium. Sodium levels of 136–137 mEq and potassium levels of 4.8–5.0 mEq indicate adherence to the diet. Any sodium level above 140 mEq is a sign that further sodium restriction is necessary.

Pancreatitis

SYMPTOM SUMMARY

○ Bulky, foul-smelling stools that stick to the side of the bowl or are hard to flush

○ Oil droplets floating in the bowl after bowel movements

UNDERSTANDING THE DISEASE PROCESS

Pancreatitis is a process of inflammation, fiber formation, and obstruction of the pancreas, the organ that produces both insulin and digestive enzymes. As the channels used by the pancreas to release digestive enzymes into the intestine become blocked, normal digestion ceases to occur. Fat that is not absorbed from food remains in the stool, causing intensely odorous diarrhea.

Acute pancreatitis is a short-term condition usually caused by gallstones, abdominal injury, high triglycerides, or a single event of excessive consumption of alcohol. Chronic pancreatitis is sometimes a complication of cystic fibrosis or extremely high triglycerides, but about 90 percent of cases of chronic pancreatitis are tied to alcoholism. Only about 10 percent of alcoholics, however, develop pancreatitis.

Alcoholics who are prone to pancreatitis generate large quantities of acetate, the chemical responsible for hangover. Acetate builds up in the pancreas and reacts with oxygen to release inflammatory chemicals that eventually cause calcification and fibrosis of the microscopic ducts through which the pancreas delivers digestive enzymes to the intestines. Exposure to other chemicals that deplete the enzymes that detoxify acetate, including industrial solvents (especially carbon tetrachloride), anesthetics, nitrosamines from cured meats such as bacon and ham, and chemicals in tobacco smoke, accelerates the process.[1]

TREATMENT SUMMARY

NUTRITIONAL SUPPLEMENTS

○ Lipase: 30,000 units or more, as prescribed, before each meal.

○ Grape seed or pine bark OPCs (Pycnogenol): 100 milligrams 3 times per day.

HERBS

○ Deglycyrrhizinated licorice (DGL): 2 tablets (500 milligrams) *chewed* and swallowed 15 minutes before meals and 1 hour before bedtime.

UNDERSTANDING THE HEALING PROCESS

Key to coping with pancreatitis is replacing the digestive enzymes that the pancreas cannot provide. Most people will need at least 30,000 units of lipase at every meal to prevent "leakage" of food fats into the stool. Sometimes much higher doses of lipase (100,000 units) will relieve pain, but it is important to avoid high doses of lipase in acute pancreatitis caused by gallstones.[2]

For digestive enzymes to work, however, they must be enteric-coated to make them resistant to high acidity in the stomach, or the stomach acid must be kept to a minimal level. DGL, an extract made from licorice, helps lower stomach acid. DGL must be chewed and mixed with saliva before it is swallowed to be effective. Lipase supplements, in most cases, must be discontinued if there is diarrhea. Some authorities recommend taking bromelain with lipase before meals to prevent diarrhea, although the evidence for doing so is purely from personal experiences.

There is growing evidence that oligomeric proanthocyanidins (OPCs), such as those found in grape seed or pine bark extracts (Pycnogenol), have the potential to reverse the biochemical imbalances that cause chronic pancreatitis. Researchers at Creighton University have found that grape seed extracts help preserve the enzyme p450 2E1 that the body needs to deal with the toxic effects of alcohol, industrial solvents, and nitrosamines.[3] There are no potential side effects from the use of OPCs in the treatment of pancreatitis, although most authorities warn that they should not be used by pregnant women.

A very small clinical trial at the Manchester Royal Infirmary in England in the late 1980s found that a mixture of antioxidants completely prevented pain in chronic pancreatitis. Volunteers were given a mixture containing 9,000 IU of beta-carotene, 2,000 milligrams of SAM-e, 600 micrograms of selenium from yeast, 5,400 milligrams of vitamin C, and 270 IU of vitamin E, or a placebo daily for 10 weeks. No patient experienced pain while taking the antioxidant formula, and no benefit was observed from the placebo. The likelihood of side effects from this formula is minimal, although it is expensive. Check the cost of having the formula made for you by a compounding pharmacist if you wish to try antioxidant therapy for pancreatitis.

CONCEPTS FOR COPING WITH PANCREATITIS

O Giving up drinking and smoking are essential to recovery from pancreatitis. In the early stages of chronic pancreatitis caused by alcoholism, giving up alcohol results in lasting pain relief. People with pancreatitis who continue to drink have a 300 percent higher mortality rate than those who quit.

O There is a long list of herbs used to treat indigestion that should not be used to treat pancreatitis. Bitters that stimulate the production of stomach acid should be avoided. These include absinthe, andrographis (used as a tea), Angostura bitters, barberry, bitter orange, blessed thistle, boldo, centaury, devil's claw (enteric-coated capsules for arthritis pain relief are OK), gentian, goldenseal, greater celandine, horehound, Oregon grape root, prickly ash, vervain, wormwood, yellow dock. People with pancreatitis should also avoid betaine HCl.

O Neither acupuncture nor TENS (transcutaneous electroneural stimulation) relieves pain in pancreatitis.

Panic Attack
See **Anxiety (Generalized Anxiety Disorder).**

Parasites, Intestinal

SYMPTOM SUMMARY

O Passing worms in stool

O Worms exiting nose or mouth

O Vomiting up worms

O Bloody sputum

O Cough

O Low-grade fever

O Shortness of breath

O Stomach pain

O Vomiting

O Wheezing

UNDERSTANDING THE DISEASE PROCESS

Intestinal parasites are a surprisingly common affliction. In the United States, the most common intestinal parasite is the pinworm, *Enterobius vermicularis*. The pinworm is a long, white, slender nematode that lives in the descending colon or the appendix. Pinworms primarily affect children and are transmitted through fecal contact, shared clothes, and doorknobs. In adults, pinworms can be sexually transmitted. Pinworms cause anal irritation as they pass out the anal canal, but they are a serious threat to health only when there is inflammatory bowel disease. About 1 percent of Americans carry pinworms, but in some areas the infection rate approaches 12 percent.[1]

Worldwide, the most common intestinal parasite is *Ascaris,* the roundworm. According to the Centers for Disease Control, as many as 1 billion people are affected by *Ascaris* worldwide, children more severely than adults. Infection with roundworms, is only found in humans and pigs, which can pass the infection to humans through their manure.

Roundworms most often enter the digestive tract as a result of the contamination of food or fingers by human fecal matter containing mature roundworm eggs. Roundworm contamination of food is a special problem in parts of the world where night soil, or human feces, is used as a fertilizer. When the eggs are swallowed, they hatch larvae that are capable of penetrating the wall of the small intestine. From the small intestine they begin to migrate through the mesenteric venules and the lymphatic system to the heart and lungs. From the lungs, the larvae burrow through the alveoli and migrate into the trachea and throat, where they are swallowed to return back to the intestine to become mature worms. Two to three months later, the mature female roundworm releases hundreds of thousands of eggs which are released into the feces, perpetuating the cycle. Adult female worms can grow to 12 inches (30 centimeters) in length; male worms are smaller.

Ascariasis causes a variety of symptoms. As the worms pass through the lungs, they cause damage to the alveoli. This may result in eosinophilic pneumonia (recognized medically by increases in the numbers of eosinophils in the complete blood count), with coughing, wheezing, fever, and shortness of breath. Even when ascariasis does not cause pneumonia, it can aggravate allergies and asthma. The slimy polysaccharides secreted from the coats of the roundworms are highly allergenic. They can provoke allergic reactions to themselves, or to other common allergens. Several studies suggest that seasonal allergies in children can be made worse by exposure to the allergenic substances released by roundworms.[2] Roundworms may also aggravate asthma, especially in children.[3]

Both before and after passing through the lungs, roundworms can interfere with the absorption of nutrients from food. Covering the surface of the intestines, the worms may physically block the absorption of food. Irritation at the sites where the worms enter the mesentery and lymphatic system also interferes with the absorption of proteins and fats. Nausea and vomiting induced by ascariasis cause anorexia. Roundworms also secrete an enzyme to keep themselves from being digested, with the result that the host cannot absorb proteins.[4] Children with roundworms tend to be lactose intolerant and have impaired absorption of vitamin A.[5]

TREATMENT SUMMARY

DIET

○ During days 1–3 of treatment, eat as little as possible and only eat highly fibrous whole grains, fruits, nuts, and vegetables, with no meat, dairy, or sweets.

○ On day 4 of treatment, eat a candy bar or raisins about an hour before taking the laxative.

NUTRITIONAL SUPPLEMENTS

On days 1–3, take the following supplements on an empty stomach:

○ Bromelain: 500 milligrams.

○ *Lactobacillus*: 10 million units per day for children; 40 million units per day for adults.

○ Papain: 500–1,000 milligrams.

HERBS

All herbs taken on days 1–3:

Children:

○ Elecampane (*Inula helenium*): $1/2$–1 teaspoon of fluid extract or 1,000–2,000 milligrams of powdered root, 3 times a day.

Adults:

○ Wormwood (*Artemisia absinthium*): 1–5 drops of oil in $1/4$ cup (75 milliliters) of water, 3 times a day, *or*

○ Quassia (*Picraena excelsior*): 1,000–2,000 milligrams of powdered wood, 3 times a day.

UNDERSTANDING THE HEALING PROCESS

Both pinworm and roundworm infections are relatively common in childhood, and often cause very mild symptoms. For this reason, a gentle, natural treatment may be preferable to toxic vermifugal drugs for children. The drugs commonly prescribed for treating roundworms in adults are not only toxic but can induce adult roundworms to leave the intestines for other tissues, causing considerably more tissue damage as adults than they did as larvae.

The objective of the first 3 days of treatment for any kind of parasitic worm is to create an inhospitable environment for the worms. Worms prefer an acidic, sweet environment such as is created by consuming meat, dairy products, highly refined carbohydrates, and sugar. Eating vegetables, fruits, and whole grains creates an alkaline environment the worms find inhospitable. Of course, fasting, offering the worms no food at all, is preferable even to a high-fiber diet.

The supplements taken during the first 3 days of treatment literally dissolve parasitic worms. Bromelain and papain, as well as other proteolytic enzyme complexes, interfere with the enzyme system that protects the worms from digestive acids.[6] *Lactobacillus* competes with the worms for sugars, and encourages regularity, increasing the likelihood that "loose" worms will be flushed out with stool.

Elecampane and wormwood literally cause a worm to "lose its grip" on the lining of the intestine, paralyzing the worm's central nervous system.[7] They also contain bitters which induce a nerve reflex in the gastric tract to propel food, and worms, downward. Many other herbs, including wormseed (*Chenopodium abrosoides*, not to be confused with wormwood), pinkroot, and tansy, contain similar chemicals, but are potentially toxic—especially tansy.

After roundworms have been "softened up," laxatives are given on day 4 to expel them from the intestine. Eating a candy bar or dried fruit such as raisins about an hour before taking the laxative encourages the worms to gather in the lumen, or central cavity, of the intestine, so they can be easily flushed. Herbal stimulant laxatives such as buckthorn, cascara sagrada, and senna are readily available and highly effective, but milk of magnesia is also useful.

One treatment usually does not get rid of all of the worms. Repeat the entire 4-day program 2 more times at 2-week intervals. Avoid meat, dairy, and sugars between treatments to avoid nourishing the worms.

CONCEPTS FOR COPING WITH INTESTINAL PARASITES

○ Never use santonin crystals (*Artemesia maritima*) to treat roundworms in children. While it is an effective treatment, it is easy to overdose. A dosage of santonin crystals that is just adequate to treat roundworms in an adult may be highly toxic or even fatal to a child.

○ Never use tansy oil internally under any circumstances. A dosage of up to 10 drops of tansy oil is required to have an effect on roundworms, but 2 teaspoons is fatal.

○ Once the worms have been expelled, it is important to avoid reinfection.

○ Do not touch soil that may be contaminated with human feces or pig waste.

• Do not defecate outdoors.

• Wrap disposable diapers before throwing them away; launder cloth diapers in hot, soapy water.

• Wash hands with soap and water before handling food.

• When traveling to countries where night soil is used as a fertilizer, wash, peel, or cook all raw vegetables and fruits before eating.

○ Isolating a child who has roundworms is not necessary, as long as good hygiene is observed at all times.

○ If roundworms recur, the most likely cause is poor hygiene. However, constipation sometimes interferes with treatment. If roundworms reappear after following the treatment plan above, repeat the 4-day treatment after treating constipation (see CONSTIPATION).

Parkinson's Disease

SYMPTOM SUMMARY

○ Tremors at rest

○ Rigidity

○ Slow initiation of movement (bradykinesia)

○ Two out of 3 symptoms is required to make a diagnosis of the disease.

○ Postural instability, difficulty remaining upright, occurs 8 or more years after the disease begins.

○ Other possible symptoms include:

• Freezing when starting to walk, turning, or entering a doorway

• Altered vision

• Altered mental status

• Flexed posture of arms and neck

UNDERSTANDING THE DISEASE PROCESS

Parkinson's disease (PD) is the most common disorder of motion in adults. The onset of PD is typically lopsided, with the most common initial finding being a tremor in one arm. At first tremors only occur in resting muscles. There may be a subtle loss of dexterity or difficulty participating in sports or performing hand work. The first-affected arm may not swing when the person with PD walks, and the foot on the same side may scrape the floor.

As the condition progresses, posture becomes increasingly hunched and tremors may affect both sides of the body. A person with PD may need a "jump start" (usually slapping the leg) to get out of a chair or to resume a walk after stopping for any reason. Reduced swallowing may cause drooling, and speech, vision, memory, and mental status are eventually affected.

The current scientific explanation for PD is the "oxidation hypothesis," a combination of genetic susceptibility and exposure of brain tissue to the effects of free radicals. The brain chemical dopamine breaks down in the presence of oxygen to form hydrogen peroxide. If there is a shortage of the free-radical quencher glutathione, the hydrogen peroxide "fizzes" and destroys the lining of brain cells. This effect is greatest in the portion of the brain that produces the most dopamine, the substantia nigra. When 85 percent of the substantia nigra has been destroyed by hydrogen peroxide, shortages of dopamine produce the initial symptoms of PD.

PD can also be induced by drugs that reduce the brain's supply of dopamine. Almost all medications used to treat schizophrenia, as well as valproic acid (Depakote) used to treat seizures, can cause reversible symptoms of Parkinson's disease. For reasons that are not fully understood, the risk of PD is increased by being exposed to pesticides, herbicides, or wood pulp mills, living in a rural area, or drinking well water.

TREATMENT SUMMARY

NUTRITIONAL SUPPLEMENTS

○ CDP-choline: 1,000 milligrams twice a day.

○ NADH: 5 milligrams twice a day (coated capsules are preferable).

UNDERSTANDING THE HEALING PROCESS

Two nutritional supplements are frequently helpful in managing PD. CDP-choline taken in a dose of 1,000–2,000 milligrams may help correct impaired memory and double vision.[1] CDP-choline does not have a long shelf life so it is better to use a product with a use-by date.

Scientists speculate that NADH stimulates the mitochondrial energy centers of brain cells in PD patients to make more dopamine. An open-label trial (a clinical study in which patients knew they were receiving a potentially helpful compound) found that 77 percent of PD patients experienced various improvements in symptoms. NADH is most effective for people who developed PD before the age of 60 and for those who have had the disease for fewer than 5 years.[2] In a few cases, NADH can cause nausea or loss of appetite, but this side effect is rare.

CONCEPTS FOR COPING WITH PARKINSON'S DISEASE

○ Young people with PD usually have worse tremor, but keep their ability to walk longer. Older people with PD develop difficulty walking at an earlier stage of the disease and suffer more falls.

○ Many people with PD develop constipation, sexual dysfunctions, sleep disturbances, and osteoporosis of the hip. Attention to these conditions greatly increases quality of life.

○ Fava beans contain measurable quantities of dopamine. Consumption of legumes is associated with a lower risk of developing PD.

○ There is a much longer list of supplements to avoid than supplements to use for PD.

○ 5-HTP increases the production of serotonin in the brain. Without a corresponding increase in the production of dopamine, PD symptoms get worse. Do not take 5-HTP for depression unless you are being treated with carbidopa (Sinemet).

○ Copper, iron, and zinc taken in excess increase the production of hydrogen peroxide in the brain and worsen symptoms of PD.

○ D-phenylalanine reduces tremors in PD patients who are not on medication, but interferes with the transfer of L-dopa into the brain and counteracts carbidopa (Sinemet).

○ L-tyrosine is a precursor for L-dopa, and if injected directly into the brain could increase the production of dopamine. Taken as an oral supplement, however, L-tyrosine interferes with the transport of L-dopa into the brain and counteracts treatment with carbidopa (Sinemet).

○ Octacosanol may increase endurance, but sometimes aggravates motion problems in PD.

○ Phosphatidylserine extracted from cow brain has been shown to improve mood (although not motor control) in PD, but has also been linked to Creutzfeldt-Jakob disease (mad cow disease).

○ Vitamin B_6 must not be used by people who are not taking carbidopa (Sinemet) or selegiline (Eldepryl, Atapryl). Without these medications, it increases the production of dopamine *outside* the brain, making symptoms worse.

Pelvic Adhesions

SYMPTOM SUMMARY

○ Infertility

○ Intestinal obstruction, constipation that does not respond to fiber or laxatives

○ Menstrual pain

○ Pelvic pain

UNDERSTANDING THE DISEASE PROCESS

An adhesion is a fibrous growth binding two tissues after trauma or inflammation. Adhesions are similar to scars except they occur *inside* the body. While adhesions can result from almost any kind of major surgery, they are a special problem of women who have had dilatation and cuterrage (D & C), hysterectomy, or other surgeries of the pelvic region.

Despite meticulous care during surgery, adhesions occur in 55–95 percent of women who have pelvic operations.[1] Adhesions occurring after D & C are so common they even have their own name, Asherman's syndrome. Menstruation, urination, and defecation can become painful and difficult once adhesions have formed. Even though adhesions are among the most common complications of surgery, few women know about them, and fewer seek medical help.

Adhesions result from abnormal healing. About 3 hours after surgery, injured tissues begin to release histamine to make capillaries "leak" fluid to cushion the site of the incision. This protein-filled fluid slowly coagulates, forming fibrous bands. About 3 days after surgery, the same chemical processes that clear blood clots should dissolve these bands.[2] Unfortunately, this usually does not happen. "Primitive cells" that create the cartilage supporting the uterus migrate to the bands formed after surgery. The bands turn into misplaced cartilage that can hold the uterus and smooth muscles in a contorted position. Once adhesions have fully formed, only surgery can remove them.[3]

TREATMENT SUMMARY

NUTRITIONAL SUPPLEMENTS

○ Beta-carotene: 25,000 IU per day.

○ Bromelain: 500 milligrams 3 times a day.

○ Quercetin: 250–600 milligrams 3 times a day, taken at the same time as bromelain.

○ Vitamin C: 2,000 milligrams daily.

Begin taking supplements 3 weeks before surgery.

UNDERSTANDING THE HEALING PROCESS

There is nothing you can do nutritionally to reverse adhesions once they have formed, although magnet therapy and sitz baths can reduce pain. (See Concepts for Coping with Adhesions) But if you can plan before surgery, there is a great deal you can do nutritionally to prevent adhesions from ever occurring.

Adhesions are much less likely to form if the ovary is producing the hormone progesterone at the time of surgery.[4] Progesterone stops the movement of white blood cells into the bands that form after surgery.[5] It also keeps capillaries from releasing fluids around the wound to cause swelling.[6]

Women of reproductive age who are not pregnant produce the greatest amount of progesterone at the midpoint of the menstrual cycle. This is typically the best time for pelvic surgery. In addition to timing surgery to match the rhythms of the body, it is also important to provide the nutritional support the body needs to produce progesterone. No function of the human body requires more beta-carotene than the production of progesterone by the corpus luteum of the ovary. Supplementation with beta-carotene ensures that the greatest amount of progesterone is in circulation at the midpoint of the menstrual cycle, and offers the greatest degree of hormonal protection possible short of progesterone injections.

Since the late 1980s, researchers have been trying to find a drug that will break down fibrin, the protein net on which adhesions form. Over 15 years of laboratory testing has failed to yield a pharmaceutical treatment without significant side effects.[7] However, the current generation of medical research seems to have forgotten research in the 1960s on the natural anti-inflammatory bromelain.

Bromelain is a protein-dissolving enzyme refined from the stem of the pineapple plant. It helps reverse tissue damage inflicted by the immune system in response to incision by enhancing the production of plasmin, a chemical that causes the protein chains that make up fibrin to unlink. This stops the formation of an adhesion in its early stages. It allows blood to flow to the wound.

Blood carries away the monocytes, plasma cells, polymorphonuclear cells, and histiocytes that can get caught on the fibrin net and cause inflammation. Bromelain also counteracts the bradykinin system that makes the healthy capillaries near the site of inflammation "leak" fluid, keeping it from causing swelling and pain.[8]

A double-blind, placebo-controlled study of 160 women receiving episiotomies after childbirth found that bromelain reduces inflammation.[9] A similar study failed to provide statistics to confirm these results,[10] but bromelain has become widely accepted among midwives and naturopaths as a means of treating pelvic inflammation.

Allergies to bromelain are very rare but not unheard of, so don't take bromelain immediately after surgery if you have never taken it before. Allergic reactions to this supplement are most likely in people who are already allergic to pineapple, papaya, wheat flour, rye flour, or birch pollen. It's also important that you let your surgeon know you intend to take bromelain and that you do not take it if your surgeon advises you not to do so. As a precaution, women who have severe bleeding as a complication of surgery should not take bromelain.

There has never been a report of an anaphylactic reaction to bromelain. Neither has there ever been a report of postsurgical bleeding directly linked to the use of this supplement. There have been isolated reports of heavy periods, nausea, vomiting, and hives when bromelain is taken in very large overdoses (2,000 milligrams and higher).

Surgeons are also studying the prevention of adhesions with hyaluronic acid. This chemical is similar to glucosamine in that it forms a protective coat around sites of injury. Laboratory experiments with white mice have failed to find that spraying hyaluronic acid on the site of an incision prevents adhesions.[11] Providing hyaluronic acid before surgery, on the other hand, does prevent adhesions.[12]

You can enhance your body's supply of hyaluronic acid by taking quercetin, a flavonoid compound found in a wide variety of vegetables and herbs. Quercetin blocks the action of hyaluronidase, an enzyme that breaks down hyaluronic acid. Hyaluronidase also breaks down collagen in the linings of the walls of capillaries so that they can leak fluid and cause swelling around a point of irritation.

For best results, take bromelain and quercetin together 5–10 minutes before meals. Bromelain increases the absorption of quercetin.[13]

Another way of preventing inflammation after pelvic or abdominal surgery is by taking antihistamines. Vitamin C is an overlooked antihistamine. It prevents the secretion of histamine by mast cells at the site of a wound.[14] Laboratory experiments have found exponential increases in the release of histamine when vitamin C is deficient.[15] Vitamin C also accelerates healing of wounds.

Therapeutic dosages of vitamin C for postsurgical care have not been scientifically established, but experts agree that 2,000 milligrams a day is adequate. You should begin taking vitamin C at least 3 weeks before surgery, if at all possible. Very few people experience any side effects with this dosage, and those who do are only likely to have diarrhea or abdominal swelling for a few days after beginning the vitamin. Take vitamin C with caution if you also take certain prescription drugs. Vitamin C taken in the form of vitamin C with bioflavonoids can interfere with the liver's ability to process statin drugs for controlling cholesterol, calcium channel blockers such as nifedipine (Procardia) for hypertension, or cyclosporine for preventing transplant rejection.

CONCEPTS FOR COPING WITH ADHESIONS

❍ Always tell your surgeon about any vitamins, minerals, herbs, and supplements you take before you have surgery. Interactions between supplements and anesthesia are rare, but are not unknown.

❍ Acupressure can relieve nausea and vomiting during recovery from pelvic surgery, without the expense and potential side effects of frequently prescribed antiemetic drugs. A study of 102 women who had laparoscopy at the Rotunda Hospital in Dublin found that acupressure reduced the rate of nausea and vomiting from 42 percent to 19 percent,[16] and a study of 94 women who had cesarean sections found that acupuncture reduced the rate of postoperative nausea and vomiting from 53 percent to 23 percent.[17] A study at a hospital in Taiwan found even better results. No woman given acupressure to the "Inner Gate Point" (known in Traditional Chinese Medicine as the Neiguan point) after cesarean section had digestive problems after surgery in the Chinese study.[18] Acupressure is best done by a trained massage or shiatsu therapist, but you can also massage this point yourself. You can find your "Inner Gate" by laying your hand flat and then moving up your arm the width of three fingers from the crease of your wrist. You will know you have found the right point when you feel slight but distinct soreness when you apply pressure. Massage the point at least 20 minutes 3 times a day during recovery from surgery. Do not apply acupressure to the arm through which you have received an IV. Acupressure wrist bands sometimes give relief but are not as effective as acupressure massage.

○ If you have chronic pain from existing pelvic adhesions, try magnet therapy. A clinical trial conducted by Dr. Candace Brown of the University of Tennessee in Memphis found preliminary scientific evidence that magnets can relieve chronic pelvic pain. In this study, the longer women used magnets, the more likely the magnets were to give relief.[19] If you have noticed particular points on your abdomen that cause pain when touched, apply the magnets there. It may be necessary to use magnets for several weeks before you notice results.

○ Sitz baths relieve pain caused by adhesions. Ideally, two tubs are used to produce three alternations of hot to cold. The hot tub is warmed to 105–115°F (40–45°C). The cold tub is chilled to 55–85°F (12–30°C). The water level in the hot tub is 1 inch (2.5 centimeters) higher than in the cold tub. Sit in the cold tub for 30 seconds and in the hot tub for 3 minutes, finishing with the cold.

Pelvic Inflammatory Disease

SYMPTOM SUMMARY

○ Abdominal pain

○ Bleeding after sexual intercourse

○ Chills

○ Fatigue

○ Fever (may be slight or intense, periodic or continuous)

○ Frequent urination

○ Increased menstrual cramping

○ Joint pain and tenderness

○ Loss of appetite

○ Lower back pain

○ Missed periods

○ Nausea

○ Pain during sexual intercourse

○ Painful urination

○ Spotting during menstrual period

○ Vaginal discharge with abnormal consistency, color, or odor

UNDERSTANDING THE DISEASE PROCESS

Pelvic inflammatory disease is a complication of infection with *Neisseria gonorrhea* or *Chlamydia trachomatis,* the microorganisms that cause gonorrhea and chlamydia, respectively. These are the two most common sexually transmitted diseases in the United States. It causes women to make an estimated 2.5 million visits to physicians each year. One-fourth of women treated for PID develop serious complications.[1] Gonorrheal infection of the Fallopian tubes can have an especially devastating effect on women's fertility. A single episode of PID increases the risk of ectopic pregnancy by 600 percent. One episode of PID causes an average 13 percent loss of fertility. Three occurrences of PID reduce fertility by 70 percent.[2]

Gonorrhea is especially contagious. There are almost 400,000 cases of gonorrhea reported each year to the Centers for Disease Control in the United States, and there are probably many more cases that go undiagnosed. As many as 80 percent of women exposed to gonorrhea develop the disease.[3] The gonococcus can establish itself in the lining of the urethral mucous membrane less than an hour after intercourse, making itself resistant to douching or being washed away by the flow of urine.[4] Cervical mucus is an effective barrier to bacterial infection. Gonorrhea bacteria attached to sperm, however, flow into the uterus during menstruation, although not during other phases of the menstrual period. Sperm can carry cytomegalovirus, the organism causing toxoplasmosis,[5] and chlamydia.[6] A common urinary tract infection, trichomoniasis, can carry gonorrhea "piggy back" into the Fallopian tubes.[7]

About 20 percent of cases of PID are caused by chlamydia.[8] Another 45–50 percent of cases involve a mild infection with chlamydia in addition to infection with gonorrhea.[9] A few cases are caused by the microorganisms *Haemophilus influenzae* or streptococci.[10]

As noted previously, PID can have devastating consequences on women's fertility. Additionally, a cycle of inflammation and scar tissue caused by chlamydia infection can encase the liver, and, in rare instances, the Fallopian tubes can burst, endangering life itself.

TREATMENT SUMMARY

NUTRITIONAL SUPPLEMENTS

❍ Beta-carotene: 100,000 IU per day for the first 2 months.

❍ Bioflavonoids: 1,000 milligrams per day.

❍ Chlorophyll: 10 milligrams of a fat-soluble form 4 times a day for 1 month. Chlorophyll should not be taken orally before infection has been confirmed.

❍ Thymus extract: 500 milligrams of crude polypeptides daily.

❍ Vitamin A: 5,000 IU per day.

❍ Vitamin C: 500 milligrams 3–4 times a day.

❍ Vitamin E: 400 IU per day for the first 2 months.

❍ Zinc picolinate: 30 milligrams per day.

HERBS

❍ Bromelain: 250 milligrams 4 times a day between meals and at night before bedtime.

❍ Comfrey: 500 milligrams of freeze-dried herb 3 times a day, or 30 drops of 1:1 fluid extract twice a day.

❍ Echinacea: 150–300 milligrams of solid extract (3.5% echinacosides) 3 times a day, or dried root, freeze-dried plant, juice, fluid extract, or tincture, as recommended on the label.

❍ Epimedium: as recommended on the label.

❍ Goldenseal: as recommended on the label.

For difficulty in urination:

❍ Polyporus Formula: as directed on the label. This product has several common brand names in the United States, including:

- Chorei-to (Tsumura)
- Polyporus Combination (Lotus Classics, Sun Ten)
- Zhu Ling Tang (Lotus Classics, Sun Ten)

In Traditional Chinese Medicine, it is referred to as *zhu ling tang.*

UNDERSTANDING THE HEALING PROCESS

The goals of treatment in PID are to stop the infection and to heal damaged tissues. Women should avoid sexual intercourse until acute symptoms have passed and their male partners have been examined and treated. All sexual partners from up to 3 months prior to the onset of the illness should receive medical attention. Women who have PID need increased bed rest while symptoms are active.

Although there are no studies that directly confirm the usefulness of thymus extracts in treating PID, there is considerable evidence that thymus extracts correct low immune function. In particular, research has shown that thymus extract normalizes the ratio of T-helper cells to T suppressor cells, maintaining a healthy immune response that neither destroys healthy tissue nor allows infectious microorganisms to flourish.[24]

Relatively low doses of vitamin A are sufficient to prevent "burnout" due to stress on the immune output of the thymus.[25] Vitamin A also enhances antibody response, increases the rate at which macrophages destroy bacteria, and stimulates natural killer cells.[26]

The related compound beta-carotene is especially important to the health of the ovary. When gonorrhea infects the ovary, beta-carotene helps limit cell damage caused by inflammation. Beta-carotene is also useful in limiting tissue damage in other organs, and enhancing various immune functions such as antibody levels, the beneficial effects of interferon, and the activity of white blood cells.

To a limited extent, chlorophyll taken orally increases the iron supply available to the gonococcus before it "takes root" in the reproductive tract, by stimulating the production of hemoglobin. For this reason, women who merely suspect they have been exposed to gonorrhea should avoid oral chlorophyll supplements and chlorophyll chewing gums. A chlorophyll douche taken after suspected contact lowers the risk of infection. Chlorophyll breaks down carbon dioxide into oxygen and creates an environment unfavorable to the anaerobic gonorrhea bacteria.

After infection, orally administered chlorophyll is helpful. It is theorized to create an oxygenated environment on the soft tissues lining the reproductive tract that is unfavorable for strong development of bacterial colonies.[27]

Vitamin C levels are quickly depleted during the stress of an infection.[28] In combination with bioflavonoids, it helps increase the stability of the collagen matrix of the connective tissues, the "glue" between the reproductive tract and the tissues around it.[29] Its anti-inflammatory activity helps prevent urethral stenosis and pelvic scarring.

Zinc is an important cofactor for vitamin A. When zinc is deficient, the immune system's ability to produce white blood cells in response to infection is reduced, thymic hormone levels are lower, the immune response in the skin is especially reduced, and phagocytosis, the process in which bacteria are engulfed and digested, is slowed. When zinc is deficient, all of these processes can be corrected by taking zinc supplements.[30]

A quick method for detecting zinc deficiency is a taste test. Powder a tablet of any zinc-based supplement or cold medication and mix with $\frac{1}{4}$ cup (50 milliliters) of water. Slosh the mixture in the mouth. People who notice no taste at all or who notice a "dry," "mineral," or "sweet" taste are likely to be zinc deficient. Anyone who notices a definite strong and unpleasant taste that intensifies over time is not likely to be zinc deficient.

Zinc picolinate is the most readily absorbed form of zinc. Do not take more than 50 milligrams of any zinc supplement daily. In rare cases, excessive intake of zinc depletes copper to cause anemia, that is, a deficiency of red blood cells, and neutropenia, a serious deficiency of white blood cells.

Bromelain serves as an all-purpose inflammation treatment. Bromelain stops the production of kinins and prostaglandins that cause inflammation, and accelerates recovery time. It increases the effectiveness of antibacterial herbs by increasing the permeability of the barrier between the bloodstream and the reproductive organs.[31] Bromelain is especially useful in preventing adhesive scar tissue from forming in the ovaries and urethra.

Comfrey contains allantoin, a stimulant to cell regeneration. Allantoin also stops the infiltration of white blood cells into the linings of the reproductive organs, limiting inflammation.[32] It should not be used by women who are or who may become pregnant, or by nursing mothers. Never gather comfrey in the wild for personal use; the aerial parts of the plant are reliably nontoxic, but the other parts of the plant are highly toxic.

Echinacea relieves inflammation. One study found that a teaspoon of *Echinacea purpurea* juice is as effective in relieving pain and swelling as 100 milligrams of cortisone.[33] Echinacea also enhances the immune system's response to bacterial infections. It is especially useful in stimulating phagocytosis. A study of oral administration of an *Echinacea purpurea* root extract (30 drops 3 times per day) to healthy men for 5 days resulted in a 120 percent increase in phagocytosis.[34] Similar effects are likely in women.

Women who are trying to get pregnant should avoid *Echinacea purpurea*. It contains caffeoyl esters that can interfere with the action of hyaluronidase, an enzyme essential to the release of unfertilized eggs into the fallopian tube.[35]

There is laboratory evidence that *Echinacea angustifolia* contains chemicals that deactivate CYP3A4. This is a liver enzyme that breaks down a wide range of medications, including anabolic steroids, the chemotherapy drug methotrexate used in treating cancer and lupus, astemizole (Hismanal) for allergies, nifedipine (Adalat) and captopril (Capoten) for high blood pressure, and sildenafil (Viagra) for impotence, as well as many others. *Echinacea angustifolia* might help maintain levels of these drugs in the bloodstream and make them more effective, or it might also cause them to accumulate to levels at which they cause side effects. Switch to a brand of echinacea that does not contain *Echinacea angustifolia* if you experience unexpected side effects while taking any of these drugs.[36]

Avoid all forms of echinacea if you have HIV. Echinacea stimulates immune function, but it also slightly increases production of T cells.[37] These are the immune cells attacked by HIV. When there are more T cells, the virus has more cells to infect. This gives it more opportunities to mutate into a drug-resistant form. This effect also makes echinacea inadvisable in autoimmune conditions, such as lupus, rheumatoid arthritis, and Sjögren's syndrome.

The combination of echinacea and goldenseal is especially useful in treating conditions that involve drainage. A 1999 study reported that the combination of the two herbs stimulates the production of the immunoglobulins IgG and IgM, infection fighters that "remember" specific infections.[38] Goldenseal contains the general antibacterial compound berberine. This alkaloid kills a wide range of bacteria, including those in the same family as *Chlamydia*.

People's Pharmacy authors Joe and Teresa Graedon warn that goldenseal reportedly limits the effectiveness of the anticoagulants heparin and warfarin (Coumadin). Do not take goldenseal with these medications. Avoid supplements containing vitamin B_6 or L-histidine if you take goldenseal, since they can interfere with goldenseal's antibacterial action.

Epimedium is a traditional East Asian treatment for venereal infections. It stimulates the production of urine so that *Chlamydia* or *E. coli* bacteria cannot lodge in the lining of the urethra. Japanese physicians report that epimedium stimulates muscle growth in the sphincter muscles. It is also directly antibacterial against *Chlamydia* and *N. gonorrhea,* stimulating macrophages from the immune system to engulf and digest the bacteria.[39]

Japanese medicine has considerable experience in using Polyporus Formula to treat urinary tract infections. Tsumura & Company confirms that approximately two-thirds of female patients who have a combination of symptoms modern Japanese doctors call "urethral syndrome," painful urination and/or a sense of retained urine, find relief when taking this formula. About 6 percent of patients experience some degree of stomach upset when first taking the formula, but this side effect is not so great that they choose to discontinue the herbal formula.

CONCEPT FOR COPING WITH PELVIC INFLAMMATORY DISEASE

❍ One survey found that women who have multiple sex partners are 4.6 times more likely to develop PID than women in monogamous relationships.[11]

❍ The greatest risk of recurrence of PID caused by chlamydia infections occurs at or shortly after menstruation.[12] Being sure to take supplements several days before the period, lessens the probability of a relapse.

❍ Abortion, cervical dilation, curettage, hysterosalpingography, insertion of an IUD, or tubal insufflation can disturb the microbial balance of the Fallopian tubes and induce a recurrence of PID.

❍ Sitz baths relieve pain during the acute phase of PID. Ideally, two tubs are used to produce three alternations of hot to cold. The hot tub is warmed to 105–115°F (40–45°C). The cold tub is chilled to 55–85°F (12–30°C). The water level in the hot tub is 1 inch (2.5 centimeters) higher than in the cold tub. Sit in the cold tub for 30 seconds and in the hot tub for 3 minutes, finishing with the cold.

❍ Avoid iron supplements. Gonorrhea bacteria "seek out" iron-bearing proteins such as transferrin in attaching themselves to the lining of the urethra.[13] They compete with their host for iron supplies. Deprived of iron, gonorrhea cannot cause inflammation.[14]

❍ Survey data show that many adolescent males and young men who have gonorrhea are unwilling to use condoms and unwilling to have sex with a single partner.[15] These are the major risk factors for the disease. As many as 75 percent of men who carry gonorrhea show no symptoms.[16]

❍ In the United States, uncircumcised men contract gonorrhea at a rate approximately 60 percent higher than circumcised men,[17] and are proportionately more likely to spread it.

❍ Women who have gonorrhea should avoid or cut down on smoking. A study of 197 women hospitalized for their first PID infection found that women who smoke were 1.7 times more likely to have PID than women who did not, regardless of the number of cigarettes smoked per day.[18] Another study found that women who smoke more than 10 cigarettes per day were more likely to develop PID than women who smoke fewer than 10 cigarettes per day.[19]

❍ Unprotected intercourse during the menstrual period increases the risk of infection for both partners. The endometrium both offers the woman protection against disease and hosts any gonorrheal bacteria previously infecting her. It is this layer that is sloughed off during menstruation, increasing the risk of infection.

❍ Overfrequent use of douches is not recommended for women, since they disturb the protective bacteria that naturally reside in the vagina and cervix. A woman who believes she has been exposed to gonorrhea may benefit from a single douche with water-soluble chlorophyll solution. One study found that use of douches 3 or more times per month was associated with a 360 percent increase in risk for PID, although that number may reflect exposure to the infection.[20]

❍ The use of IUDs for contraception greatly increases a woman's risk of contracting gonorrhea. The surface of the IUD hosts colonies of infectious bacteria while the presence of the device reduces immune capacity.[21]

○ The use of oral contraceptives (the Pill) reduces a woman's risk of infection with gonorrhea. Estrogens cause the cervix to secrete a thicker protective mucus, and diminish blood flow during the period.[22] On the other hand, use of the Pill increases a woman's risk of becoming infected with *Chlamydia,* especially during the second half of her period. The progesterone in the Pill causes the cervix to grow tissues in such a way that a tissue layer favored by *Chlamydia* is more exposed.[23]

Peptic Ulcer Disease

SYMPTOM SUMMARY

○ Dull, gnawing abdominal pain

- Usually comes and goes for several weeks
- May cause nighttime wake-ups (when the stomach is empty)
- Is usually relieved by eating a meal or by taking antacids or milk
- May occur 2–3 hours after a meal
- Is worse when meals are skipped

○ Dark, tarry stools

○ Fatigue

○ Nausea

○ Vomiting

○ Weight loss

In some cases there may also be:

○ Belching

○ Bloody stools

○ Chest pain

○ Heartburn

See a doctor immediately if you experience "coffee ground" vomit or tarry black stools.

UNDERSTANDING THE DISEASE PROCESS

Burning stomach pain associated with fasting and relieved by eating is the cardinal symptom of peptic ulcer disease (PUD). A peptic ulcer is a sore on the lining of the stomach, usually where the stomach curves, or the duodenum, the uppermost part of the small intestine, sometimes in a "pocket." Ulcers replace healthy tissue with fibers and debris. PUD is very common, affecting 12 percent of men and 10 percent of women at some time in the course of their lives.[1]

Stomach acid is essential to health. It serves as a barrier against infection by bacteria, fungi, viruses, and parasites. It makes it possible for the body to absorb proteins, calcium, copper, folic acid, iron, and vitamin B_{12}. PUD is usually but not always associated with excessive production of stomach acid. In some cases ulcers related to vitamin deficiencies are caused by infection with a bacterium called *Helicobacter pylori* (sometimes called *Campylobacter pylori* in older natural medicine books), and stomach acid is actually deficient.

After the discovery that the classic rule "No acid, no ulcer" was not necessarily true, scientists began to look for a cause of ulcers other than spicy food or stress (both of which increase the production of stomach acid). It is now believed that most ulcers are caused by infection with *H. pylori.* Some ulcers are caused by long-term use of nonsteroidal anti-inflammatory drugs (NSAIDs) such as aspirin and ibuprofen. In a relatively rare condition known as Zollinger-Ellison syndrome, peptic ulcers result from tumors of the pancreas or stomach. Ulcers can also result from extreme trauma, such as extensive burns, major surgery, or pressure within the brain.

Researchers do not know how *H. pylori* is transmitted, but it is believed to be spread through food or water. The bacterium has been observed in saliva, so it may be spread by kissing.

TREATMENT SUMMARY

DIET

○ Vegetables in the cabbage family, especially raw cabbage juice, greatly relieve ulcer pain and accelerate healing by stimulating production of mucus. They are not recommended, however, for ulcer sufferers who also have inflammatory bowel syndrome, who benefit from glutamine supplements instead.

○ For gastric ulcers, eat bananas (sometimes referred to as plantain bananas) that have not ripened so much that they are soft.

NUTRITIONAL SUPPLEMENTS

○ Bioflavonoids: 500 milligrams 3 times daily.

○ Glutamine: 500 milligrams 3 times daily.

○ *Lactobacillus* (especially during the first week of any antibiotic treatment): 1–2 billion live organisms daily.

❍ Vitamin A: 20,000 IU 3 times daily. Women who are or who may become pregnant should strictly limit their intake of vitamin A to 5,000 IU per day or less.

❍ Vitamin B_{12} (until *H. pylori* infection is eliminated): 1 milligram per day.

❍ Vitamin C: 5,000 milligrams taken in 4 doses (1 dose of 2,000 milligrams, then 3 doses of 1,000 milligrams each) every day for 1 month. Take 500 milligrams 3 times daily thereafter.

❍ Vitamin E: 400 IU daily.

❍ Zinc: 100 milligrams per day for 2 weeks, then 30 milligrams per day thereafter.

HERBS

❍ Licorice: chew and swallow 1–2 380-milligram tablets of DGL 20 minutes before meals, 3 times a day.

❍ Mastic: 500 milligrams, twice a day. Mastic gums would also be effective, but capsules disguise the taste.

UNDERSTANDING THE HEALING PROCESS

Medical studies including 4,329 peptic ulcer patients have concluded that eradicating *H. pylori* accelerates healing of ulcers.[2] Wiping out the infection greatly reduces the risk of relapse. Approximately 60–70 percent of PUD patients with *H. pylori* infections develop a recurrence after initial healing, while only 5–10 percent of PUD patients in whom *H. pylori* infection has been controlled get ulcers again after the original ulcers have healed.[3]

The treatment guidelines formulated for physicians by the American College of Gastroenterology state that "antibiotic therapy is indicated for all *H. pylori*-infected ulcer patients."[4] Ulcer sufferers who have to take nonsteroidal anti-inflammatory agents for pain relief, however, heal more slowly if they are given antibiotics than if they are not.[5]

Garlic may have some effect on *H. pylori*. In the mid-1990s a series of reports emerged that garlic oil could stop the growth of the bacterium under test-tube conditions. Then investigators tried to confirm the usefulness of garlic oil in treating peptic ulcers in humans.

A study at the Baylor College of Medicine in Texas found that feeding garlic-laced fajitas to volunteers who did not have ulcers did not have any immediate effect on the bacterium. (The Baylor College researchers measured effects of garlic oil after a single meal containing garlic.)[6] A researcher in England found that giving ulcer sufferers garlic as the only treatment for *H. pylori* cured only 1 out of 8 volunteers by the end of an 8-week study.[7] A holistically oriented practice in Stroud (Gloucestershire), England, gave dyspeptic patients with positive tests for *H. pylori* one 4-milligram garlic capsule with a meal 4 times a day for 14 days. The amount of the bacterium in their stomach was measured by a breath test measuring changes in the carbon-13 concentration of the air they exhaled. At the end of the 14-day test period, not even one of the patients showed as much as 50 percent reduction in the amount of the bacterium in their systems.[8]

The disappointing results of the garlic tests do not mean that garlic has no value in treating ulcers. There is only one antibiotic, clarithromycin, that is effective against *H. pylori* when used by itself, so it is possible that garlic is useful against the infection when it is used with other treatments.

It is not necessary to avoid chili peppers if you have peptic ulcers. In fact, studies with lab rats[9] and with human volunteers[10] have even found that capsaicin in chili peppers protects the lining of the stomach from damage from aspirin and other NSAIDs. The capsaicin in chili peppers activates nerve fibers that release chemicals that greatly reduce the damage caused by these common pain relievers.

In at least two animal studies, the dried extract of green banana stopped the formation of ulcers by stimulating the growth of protective mucosal cells in the lining of the stomach.[11,12]

At least under test-tube conditions, the bioflavonoids flavanone, flavone, and quercetin have a variety of beneficial effects on peptic ulcers. All three substances reduce the stomach's natural tendency to produce more acid under conditions of injury or stress. All three substances also reduce the production of stomach acid through a mechanism similar to drugs like Zantac.[13]

Lactobacillus is extremely helpful during the first week of any antibiotic treatment for *H. pylori*. At the Catholic University in Rome, 120 people were enrolled in a study on preventing side effects of eradicating *H. pylori* with a standard therapy consisting of three antibiotics—clarithromycin, pantoprazole, and tinidazole—for 1 week. Sixty participants were given *Lactobacillus* supplements for 2 weeks, and 60 were given a placebo. The antibiotics caused bloating, diarrhea, and taste disturbances in both groups, but these unpleasant effects were greatly reduced in the group given *Lactobacillus*.[14]

However, *Lactobacillus* not only counteracts the side effects of antibiotics, it is itself a natural antibiotic, as well as an anti-inflammatory. Thirty patients followed in an 8-week study at Tokai University School of Medicine in Japan were found to have lowered levels of *H. pylori* and reduced inflammation after treatment with *Lactobacillus* alone.[15] The Japanese study used yogurt, eaten in quantities as desired but eaten every day, as the source of the friendly bacteria.

Vitamins A[16] and E[17] stop the development of stress ulcers in lab rats, probably by helping the stomach maintain the mucosal barrier as a seamless shield. While there is no direct evidence these vitamins are of benefit to humans who have ulcers, they are unlikely to be harmful when used as directed. Side effects from using up to 300,000 IU of vitamin A per day are rare, but they are significant. The first signs of vitamin A overdose are dry skin and chapped lips, especially in dry weather. Later signs of toxicity are headache, mood swings, and pain in muscles and joints. In massive doses, vitamin A can cause liver damage. In the first 3 months of pregnancy, it can cause birth defects. Women who are or who may become pregnant should strictly limit their intake of vitamin A to 5,000 IU per day or less. Discontinue vitamin A at the first sign of toxicity, and never use it for more than 3 months at a time.

Vitamin B_{12} is absorbed poorly in PUD. A study of 159 patients with low B_{12} levels and 43 healthy controls found that *H. pylori* infection was associated with low vitamin levels.[18] Simply eradicating the bacterium will correct the deficiency, but until the infection is eliminated, supplementation is needed.[19]

There is at least some evidence that vitamin C controls *H. pylori.* In one clinical study in which 51 PUD patients were given 5,000 milligrams of vitamin C a day (divided into 4 doses), 30 percent were free of infection by the end of 1 month.[20] It has not been scientifically determined that taking this relatively high dose of vitamin C for more than a month will do additional good. It is important to drink 8 glasses of water a day when taking this much vitamin C. A few people will experience diarrhea when taking 5,000 milligrams of vitamin C a day; do not take this much C if you have a history of kidney stones.

In the long run, vitamin C it is probably extremely important in the prevention of stomach cancer. The concentration of vitamin C in gastric juice is lower in people who have *H. pylori* infections that in those who do not.[21] This is probably due to the bacterium's destruction of tissues in the lining of the stomach that secrete vitamin C.[22] When *H. pylori* bacteria are eliminated, vitamin C levels go up. Since vitamin C prevents the conversion of dietary nitrites into carcinogenic nitrosamines, vitamin C is probably important in protecting against carcinomas of the stomach.[23]

Zinc is a well-known lysosomal stabilizer, that is, it deactivates destructive enzymes in the membranes lining cells. In studies in Brazil[24] and Russia[25], zinc treatments have a strong stabilizing effect on the gastric membranes of patients given 100 milligrams of zinc a day for up to 2 weeks.

Two studies have found that deglycyrrhizinated licorice (DGL) is as effective as drugs in the same family as Zantac in controlling ulcers.[26,27] It is believed to accelerate the growth of healthy cells and to increase the production of protective mucus. It also slows the growth of *H. pylori.* To be effective, DGL must be mixed with saliva by chewing before it is swallowed.

Mastic is a resin taken from the leaves and stems of the mastic tree, an evergreen shrub found around the northern and eastern shores of the Mediterranean Sea. It is used to make chewing gum in Syria and Lebanon, although most Americans would find the taste unpleasant. Encapsulated extracts disguise the taste. A pilot study of 6 patients with gastric ulcers found that taking a gram of mastic extract every day for 4 weeks promoted ulcer healing.[28] A double-blind trial involved 38 patients with duodenal ulcers showed healing in 78 percent of patients taking mastic gum for 2 weeks.[29]

CONCEPTS FOR COPING WITH PEPTIC ULCER DISEASE

○ Don't smoke. Smoking causes the bile in the intestine to erupt upward into the stomach. Bile dissolves fats, such as those making up the linings of the cells protecting the stomach.

○ Bismuth preparations such as Pepto-Bismol coat the lining of the stomach and "smother" *H. pylori.* Children should take bismuth subcitrate rather than bismuth subsalicylate (Pepto-Bismol), since bismuth subsalicylate can mask Reye's syndrome, a potentially dangerous complication of colds and flu. Bismuth subcitrate is available from compounding pharmacists, who can be located through the International Academy of Compounding Pharmacists, 1-800-927-4227.

Periodontal Disease

See **Gingivitis**.

Peripheral Vascular Disease

SYMPTOM SUMMARY

○ Claudication (intense muscle pain triggered by activity and relieved by rest)

UNDERSTANDING THE DISEASE PROCESS

Peripheral vascular disease (PVD) is the common complication of atherosclerosis (see ATHEROSCLEROSIS). During rest, the blood vessels carry 300–400 milliliters (about 2 cups) of blood every minute to the lower legs and feet. During even mild exercise, the muscles' demand for oxygen requires a 10-fold increase of circulation, to about 3 or 4 liters (3 or 4 quarts) of freshly oxygenated blood every minute. Atherosclerotic arteries are capable of delivering the blood the leg muscles need during rest. They are not capable of delivering enough oxygenated blood to support exercise, and the result is intense muscle pain relieved by rest. As a general rule, doctors diagnose peripheral vascular disease when the patient cannot walk more than 2 blocks (100 meters) without resting to relieve muscle pain, provided there has been no muscle injury.

TREATMENT SUMMARY

HERBS

○ Padma: as directed on the label.

UNDERSTANDING THE HEALING PROCESS

Most people with peripheral vascular disease mistakenly believe it is a normal part of aging. It is more often a complication of unhealthy lifestyle. More than any other single cause, smoking is a correctable source of vascular pain. When people with PVD stop smoking, the arteries often are able to compensate for oxygen stress during exercise without causing pain.

The Tibetan herbal formula padma was banned by the FDA because of fraudulent labeling on a single lot of a single brand by a single foreign manufacturer in the late 1980s. Having reappeared on the United States market in 2000, padma is the best natural treatment for PVD for people who have had it for 5 years of more. Clinical studies in Denmark found that using the herb for 4 months increased pain-free walking distance by an average of approximately 50 percent and maximum walking distance by approximately 100 percent.[1] Padma does not alter blood pressure (measured in the arm or the ankle), and has a beneficial side effect of counteracting stomach irritation from use of aspirin.

CONCEPTS FOR COPING WITH PERIPHERAL VASCULAR DISEASE

○ Walking 45–60 minutes every day eventually reduces PVD pain. Studies have found 80 to 234 percent increases in walking range after regular exercise.

○ Inositol nicotinate is often used to treat PVD. The drawback to using inositol is that it increases blood flow more to the chest and face than to the legs. Medical examination to rule out obstruction to the carotid arteries is essential before using inositol nicotinate to treat PVD. Niacin, a faster-acting form of the same B vitamin, should not be used in PVD.

○ If aspirin causes stomach upset, the solution is not to stop taking aspirin, but to chew and swallow 1–2 380-milligram tablets of deglycyrrhizinated licorice (DGL) 20 minutes before meals, 3 times a day.

○ The location of leg pain indicates the location of the hardened cholesterol plaque. Atherosclerosis in the femoral artery, just above the knee, causes pain in the calf. Atherosclerosis in the sacroilial arteries causes pain in the thigh and buttocks.

Peyronie's Disease

SYMPTOM SUMMARY

○ Curvature of the penis during erection (only during erection)

○ May have hourglass deformity with flaccidity in the tip

○ Fibrous mass in the midline of the shaft of the penis

UNDERSTANDING THE DISEASE PROCESS

Peyronie's disease is a surprisingly common but seldom discussed condition causing curvature of the penis during erection. Described in a historical medical text as "a rare affection of the genitals in people with excessive sexual intercourse"[1] and made a matter of public record during a recent American political scandal, Peyronie's disease begins when microscopic blood vessels in the penis are damaged during excessively vigorous sexual intercourse. Immune-mediated inflammation leads to the deposit of fibers that eventually accumulate in a plaque about an inch (2.5 centimeters) wide, causing a curvature of the penis during erection.

The lump in the penis associated with Peyronie's disease can appear "overnight," but men with the condition more commonly notice an increasing curvature of the penis during erection. Eventually Peyronie's disease causes intense pain during erection, and it may lead to impotence.

Approximately 1 in 250 men in the United States has Peyronie's disease. About 10 percent of men with Peyronie's disease have Dupuytren's contracture, and about 3 percent of men with Dupuytren's contracture have Peyronie's disease. Men who get Peyronie's disease tend to have thick knuckles. The condition is more common among Caucasians than in other racial groups. Peyronie's disease seldom appears before the age of 30, and most commonly begins between the ages of 40 and 60.

TREATMENT SUMMARY

DIET

○ Include soy foods in your daily diet.

NUTRITIONAL SUPPLEMENTS

○ Para-aminobenzoic acid (PABA): 12 grams daily.

○ Vitamin E: at least 200 IU per day.

UNDERSTANDING THE DISEASE PROCESS

Peyronie's disease sometimes resolves on its own if there is complete abstinence from all forms of sexual activity for 2–3 years. Many men opt for surgical correction of the condition. Otherwise, certain nutritional interventions are helpful.

The process of fibrosis in the penis leading to curvature is accelerated by estrogen, the female hormone present in men's bodies in trace amounts. Men with Peyronie's disease should avoid supplements that increase estrogen levels, such as androstenedione (which also increases testosterone levels), and should include soy foods in their daily diet. Some physicians note improvement when men eat soy food, and it is theoretically possible that soy phytochemicals "lock" receptor sites in the penis that would be occupied by estrogen. The evidence for vitamin E is also anecdotal, but there are no side effects from a small dose. Be sure to inform your doctor that you take vitamin E if you are planning to have surgery, since vitamin E could increase bleeding.

A clinical study confirmed that treatment with a compound similar to the B vitamins, para-aminobenzoic acid, helps about 50 percent of men who take it. Clinicians gave 32 men with Peyronie's disease 12 grams of a potassium salt of PABA daily for 8–24 months. Penile angulation improved in 18 of 31 patients, plaque size decreased in 18 of 32 patients, and pain during erection was diminished in 8 of 32 patients.[2] Loss of appetite, nausea, vomiting, fever, and rashes occasionally occur when PABA is taken at this dosage. The side effects stop when the supplement is discontinued.

CONCEPTS FOR COPING WITH PEYRONIE'S DISEASE

○ The greatest damage to the penis occurs when vigorous intercourse is attempted with a weak erection.

○ Peyronie's disease never leads to penile cancer. It is a long-term condition, but it sometimes completely resolves without surgery.

Phenylketonuria (PKU)

SYMPTOM SUMMARY

In infants:

○ Excessive sleep

○ Lethargy

○ Skin outbreaks

○ Unusual odor of urine

In children not receiving adequate treatment:

○ Diminished mental capacity

○ Attention deficit

○ Seizures

UNDERSTANDING THE DISEASE PROCESS

PKU, or phenylketonuria, is a rare genetic condition causing the amino acid phenylalanine to build up and the amino acid tyrosine to become depleted in the bloodstream. If it is untreated, high levels of phenylalanine deplete antioxidants in the brain and central nervous system, which can cause severe mental retardation and psychological disturbances.[1] Blood-screening programs in the United States and other countries usually identify the condition at birth.

TREATMENT SUMMARY

DIET

○ Low phenylalanine diet with amino acid supplements, prescribed and monitored by a medical nutritionist.

NUTRITIONAL SUPPLEMENTS

○ Branched-chain amino acids: See Understanding the Healing Process.

○ Fish oil: See Understanding the Healing Process.

○ L-tyrosine: See Understanding the Healing Process.

○ Selenium: See Understanding the Healing Process.

○ Vitamin B_{12}: See Understanding the Healing Process.

○ Vitamin K: See Understanding the Healing Process.

UNDERSTANDING THE HEALING PROCESS

Strict adherence to a low-phenylalanine diet is essential in treating PKU. High-protein foods such as eggs, fish, legumes, meat, nuts, and soy are eliminated. Low-protein foods are allowed in measured amounts, and amino acid supplements not containing phenylalanine ensure the child receives adequate protein. Following the PKU diet improves muscle control and supports intellectual development.

Phenylalanine restriction is of greatest benefit when it is started during the first few days of life, but older children whose PKU is diagnosed late still benefit from a low-protein diet.[2] A few experts believe that older children and adults do not need to follow a strict diet, but the overwhelming majority of doctors who treat PKU maintain that the diet must be followed for life. Teenagers with PKU are at special risk for dangerously elevated phenylalanine levels, 80 percent of teenagers failing to follow their diet.[3]

Supplementation with branched-chain amino acids (isoleucine, leucine, and valine) may limit damage to the brain caused by failures in strictly observing the PKU diet. These amino acids may inhibit entry of phenylalanine into the brain and reduce its toxic effects on the central nervous system. In a study at Children's Hospital in Cincinnati, Ohio, 16 adolescents and young adults with phenylketonuria participated in double-blind trials in which a valine, isoleucine, and leucine mixture or a control mixture was given for four 3-month periods. They performed better on an intelligence test (the Attention Diagnostic Method) when they were receiving branched-chain amino acids than when they were receiving a control mixture.[4]

The amounts of amino acids used in the study were 150 milligrams per kilogram (2.2 pounds) of body weight each of valine and isoleucine, and 200 milligrams per kilogram of body weight of leucine, taken with meals and at bedtime. This is 3–5 times the usually recommended dosage of branched-chain amino acid supplements. Do not use amino acid combination products that contain phenylalanine.

The low-protein diet required in PKU is sometimes deficient in essential fatty acids essential for normal brain development. In one clinical study of children with PKU who were deficient in fatty acids, supplementation with fish oil, but not with black currant seed oil, for 6 months corrected the deficiency. The children received 500 milligrams of oil for every 4 kilograms (8.8 pounds) of body weight each day for 6 months. This amount of fish oil can cause diarrhea or burping, so it is important to use pharmaceutical-grade fish oils if available.[5]

The severely restricted diet for PKU can also cause deficiencies of selenium, vitamin B_{12}, and vitamin K throughout life. Unlike some conditions, PKU responds better to "unnatural" selenium rather the natural selenium found in sprouts. One study found that sodium selenite corrected selenium deficiency in phenylketonurics but selenomethionine did not.[6] Children over age 3 should receive 100 micrograms of selenium once a week, children up to age 12, twice a week, teens and adults, once a day.

The PKU diet is largely vegan and usually deficient in vitamin B_{12}. Anemia can result from vitamin B_{12} deficiency. The best approach to remedying B_{12} deficiency in PKU is to treat initial deficiency with a vitamin B_{12} injection administered by a physician, and then to take 1,000–2,000 micrograms (1–2 milligrams) of vitamin B_{12} a day to prevent recurrences of deficiency.

Fat-soluble vitamin K is also frequently deficient in the PKU diet. Taking 5 milligrams every other week is sufficient.

CONCEPTS FOR COPING WITH PKU

○ Experts disagree whether people with PKU can safely use aspartame (NutraSweet), a no-calorie substitute that is about half phenylalanine. Clinical studies show that phenylketonurics following a prescribed diet are unaffected by the amount of aspartame contained in a 12-ounce can of Diet Coke.[7] All the studies of the use of NutraSweet by people with PKU, however, have focused on the effects of "loading" aspartame with a single serving of a sugar-free beverage. The long-term effects of using NutraSweet on a daily basis in PKU are not known.

○ Breastfeeding is preferable to formula for infants with PKU. Most infant formulas contain a much higher concentration of the trace element molybdenum than is found in mother's milk. Babies with PKU cannot eliminate molybdenum, and, if given formula, can accumulate the element to toxic levels.[8]

Phlebitis

SYMPTOM SUMMARY

○ Pain and/or tenderness over a vein

○ Reddened skin (may or may not be present)

Alternative names: Thrombophlebitis

UNDERSTANDING THE DISEASE PROCESS

Phlebitis is an inflammation of a vein. Thrombophlebitis is an inflammation of a vein related to a blood clot. Common causes of vein inflammation include local irritation from an IV line, infection, or blood clots.

TREATMENT SUMMARY

NUTRITIONAL SUPPLEMENTS

○ Bromelain: 500–900 milligrams daily, taken between meals in divided doses.

UNDERSTANDING THE HEALING PROCESS

In Europe, bromelain is widely accepted as a safe, effective, side effect–free treatment for phlebitis. It helps the body absorb antibiotics and other medications,[1] but it is itself as effective as many first-generation antibiotics in treating abscesses, bronchitis, pneumonia, and staph infections.[2] It prevents the synthesis of proinflammatory prostaglandins, which otherwise stop white blood cells from "cleaning up" cellular debris in blood vessels.[3] Most important, bromelain blocks the biochemical reactions that cause blood clots to form under conditions of stress, by enhancing the activity of plasmin.[4]

Research in the 1960s found that bromelain used with over-the-counter pain relievers reduced pain, swelling, redness, tenderness, and elevated skin temperature in acute thrombophlebitis. In this study involving 73 patients, relief was achieved with a relatively small dose, only 60–160 milligrams per day.[5] Due to the wide variations in the strength of bromelain products, however, a dose of 500–900 milligrams a day would ensure results.

Bromelain has no known side effects, and can be used on an ongoing basis. People who are allergic to pineapple or papaya should avoid bromelain, since they could experience allergic reactions. While there has never been a report of anaphylactic reaction to bromelain, skin rashes and hives have occurred.

CONCEPTS FOR COPING WITH PHLEBITIS

○ Elevate the affected area to reduce swelling. Keep pressure off it to reduce pain and to avoid further damage.

○ Moist heat, such as a hot water bottle wrapped in a cloth, relieves inflammation and pain.

○ Changing IV lines frequently reduces the risk of phlebitis.

○ Phlebitis in the feet and legs usually benefits from support stockings.

○ Phlebitis can be a medical emergency. Make an appointment with your healthcare provider if symptoms do not improve with treatment. Seek emergency care if an entire arm or leg becomes cold, pale, or swollen, or if you develop fever and chills.

Pinkeye

See **Conjunctivitis**.

Pinworms

See **Parasites, Intestinal.**

PKU

See **Phenylketonuria (PKU).**

Plummer-Vinson Syndrome

SYMPTOM SUMMARY

○ Choking spells after eating

○ Iron-deficiency anemia

- Nail deformities ("spoon nails")
- Pale skin
- Weight loss

UNDERSTANDING THE DISEASE PROCESS

Plummer-Vinson syndrome (PVS) was once a relatively common disease among middle-aged women of Scandinavian descent. Causing the formation of webs of fibrous tissue in the esophagus, PVS results in regular choking spells after eating solid foods. The precise cause of PVS has never been determined, but it seems to be a combination of genetic factors causing overactivity in the immune system, and iron deficiency, possibly due to a mild form of celiac disease.

TREATMENT SUMMARY

DIET

○ If you are not a vegetarian, eat 3–4 servings of pureed lean meat, poultry, or fish daily. If you are a vegetarian, eat purees of dried fruit, leafy green vegetables, and molasses as often as possible.

○ Cook in iron pots and pans. Use vinegar and juices in cooking as much as possible.

NUTRITIONAL SUPPLEMENTS

Medically prescribed iron supplements, plus:

○ Vitamin A: 5,000 IU per day for women of reproductive age; 10,000 IU per day for all others.

○ Vitamin C: 500 milligrams, every time you take an iron supplement.

UNDERSTANDING THE HEALING PROCESS

Treating PVS is largely a matter of correcting the related problems, celiac disease, if it exists, and iron-deficiency. Iron supplements for PVS should be medically prescribed. At least 11 clinical studies have found that taking vitamin A enhances your body's ability to absorb iron supplements.[1] Vitamin C does not increase iron absorption, but taking vitamin C and iron together results in an increase in levels of ferritin, the iron-binding protein, in the blood. The dosages recommended here are not likely to cause side effects or to interfere with medications.[2]

CONCEPTS FOR COPING WITH PLUMMER-VINSON SYNDROME

○ The esophageal webs causing choking are easily removed by a medical instrument known as a bougie. The procedure is done without general anesthesia and usually causes only transient discomfort.

PMS

See **Premenstrual Syndrome (PMS).**

Pneumonia

SYMPTOM SUMMARY

Common symptoms:

○ Cough, frequently with thick greenish yellow phlegm

○ Chest pain described as sharp or stabbing, made worse by coughing

○ Fever and chills, shaking with chills

○ Severe fatigue

Occasional symptoms:

○ Clammy skin, excessive sweating

○ Coughing up blood

○ Nausea and vomiting

○ Rapid breathing

UNDERSTANDING THE DISEASE PROCESS

Pneumonia is a lung disease that can be caused by a variety of bacteria, fungi, and viruses. The Centers for Disease Control and Prevention estimate that nearly 900,000 people in the United States contracted pneumonia and 87,000 people died of pneumonia in the most recent year for which there are data, making it the nation's fifth leading cause of death. Rates of infection are 3 times higher among African-Americans than the nation as a whole and 10 times higher among Native American children. Pneumonia is not an uncommon complication of HIV or chemotherapy for cancer, but it is most common in persons over the age of 65.[1]

The most common form of pneumonia is an infection of the lungs caused by bacteria called *Streptococcus pneumoniae,* the same microorganism that causes inner ear infections and bacterial meningitis. Almost every adult is infected with the bacteria that cause pneumococcal pneumonia. The bacteria are spread by coughing, sneezing, kissing, and shared drinking and eating utensils. The overwhelming majority of people carrying *S. pneumonia* don't get sick, but in some people the bacterium invades the upper respiratory tract, lungs, and bloodstream to cause disease.

Pneumococcal pneumonia begins as a severe shaking chill followed by a deep cough and a high fever. In adults, the bacterium usually settles into one or more sections of the lungs known as lobes, causing lobar pneumonia. Infants, young children, the elderly, and people with compromised immune systems may develop milder forms of the disease involving the bronchi, or bronchial pneumonia.

Pneumonias caused by chlamydia, fungi, or viruses present similar symptoms. Susceptibility to pneumonia is enhanced by viral infections such as colds and flu, cigarette smoke, air pollution, and choking. Especially when pneumonia strikes an infant, young child, elderly person, or person with an immune system impaired by chemotherapy or HIV, medical attention is highly desirable.

TREATMENT SUMMARY

NUTRITIONAL SUPPLEMENTS

○ Bromelain: 500–750 milligrams 3 times per day between meals.

○ Vitamin C: 500 milligrams daily.

○ Vitamin E: 200 IU per day.

HERBS

○ *Echinacea purpurea*: 150–300 milligrams daily.

UNDERSTANDING THE HEALING PROCESS

Pneumonia is a condition that is especially responsive to the support care of nurses and family members. There is a great deal you can do to care for a friend or family member whose symptoms are mild enough not to be hospitalized.

Heat loosens phlegm. The simplest way to apply heat to the chest is with a hot water bottle placed in a towel and laid on the chest. Never place a hot water bottle directly on the skin. Moist heat should be applied several times a day while the patient is awake. If the patient is able to sit up, a hot bath offers the same benefits.

A more effective means of providing heat is diathermy, a technique using high frequency sound to heat deep-seated tissues. Naturopathic physicians maintain that diathermy increases blood flow by dilating blood vessels. This increases oxygen supply and allows the free transit of white blood cells to deal with the infection. It also relaxes the diaphragm so that phlegm is expectorated with less effort. Diathermy is typically used for 30 minutes in the morning after the patient awakes. This technique should not be used in people who have bleeding disorders, who take or have recently taken blood thinners, or by people who have cancer. Home diathermy treatments are usually arranged by contacting chiropractors, naturopaths, or holistically oriented physicians.

Inhaling warm vapors also loosens phlegm. A vaporizer should be run 24 hours a day in the patient's bedroom. Mustard plasters are an especially potent source of healing vapors and should be applied once a day. A plaster is a thick, moist, warm herbal paste placed between two layers of cloth or in a cloth pouch. To make a plaster, grind 1/4 cup of black or white mustard seed, taking care not to get the powder under your fingernails or in your eyes. It is important to grind the herb just before making the plaster, because the action of grinding releases healing volatile oils that quickly escape. When you have ground the herb, add just enough (1/4 cup or about 25 milliliters) of *lukewarm* water to make a slurry. It is important not to use hot water, since temperatures over 140°F (60°C) deactivate an enzyme that unlocks the volatile oils from the waxes that hold them in the mustard seed.[2] Place the mixture between two layers of light cloth and apply to the chest.

Applied to the chest, the ground mustard will induce an intense burning sensation as part of the healing process. A strong but bearable sensation of burning is a signal that the allyl mustard oils in the mustard seed released by grinding have entered the deeper layers of the skin. The plaster should only remain on the skin until the burning sensation *begins,* and then should be removed immediately to avoid skin irritation. Mustard plasters help in all types of pneumonia, but they are most effective in bronchial pneumonia.

After the application of heat and vapor therapy, the next step in the daily care of someone with pneumonia is postural drainage. This technique uses gravity to move phlegm in various reaches of the lungs in sequence so that it is more easily coughed up. The first step in postural drainage is to move phlegm in the right upper lobe. To do this, the patient needs only to sit up in bed, bend the knees, and place the right arm across the stomach. This position is held as long as comfortable, preferably for 3–5 minutes. To move the phlegm in the upper left lobe, the right arm is return to the side and the left arm is placed across the stomach, keeping the knees bent. This position is also held for 3–5 minutes.

The next step in postural drainage is to move phlegm in the middle lobes. The bed is elevated so that the foot of the bed is 1 foot (30 centimeters) higher than the head of the bed. The patient lies down so that his or her feet are higher than the head. The patient rolls onto his or her left side, bends the left arm at the elbow, letting it lie in front of the chest, and holds this position for 3–5 minutes. The procedure is repeated for the right side.

The final step in postural drainage is to move phlegm in the lower lobes. Keeping the foot of the bed elevated, the patient rolls onto his or her stomach, elevating one side and then the other to allow breathing. Holding these final two positions for 3–5 minutes each completes the sequence.

Never attempt to drain the lungs immediately after the patient has eaten, or if the patient has nausea or vomiting. Postural drainage should never be performed on someone who has an actively bleeding wound or a head or neck injury. Do not elevate the head of the bed for a patient who has uncontrolled high blood pressure or has had recent eye surgery. Stop postural drainage if difficulty breathing or pain increases. Never leave a pneumonia patient unattended during postural drainage.

Nutritional therapy complements physical therapy. All of the nutritional supplements recommended for pneumonia are most effective if they are begun *immediately* when symptoms are first noticed.

Bromelain is a chemical found in pineapple that can break up mucus. Bromelain treatment makes the mucus more fluid. In one study of the use of bromelain in the treatment of chronic phlegm, patients who took the supplement demonstrated less frequent cough and greater lung capacity.[3] Bromelain also increases the absorption of antibiotics through the intestinal tract.

Allergies to bromelain are very rare but not unheard of. Allergic reactions to this supplement are most likely in people who are already allergic to pineapple, papaya, wheat flour, rye flour, or birch pollen. There has never been a report of an anaphylactic reaction to bromelain. There have been isolated reports of heavy periods, nausea, vomiting, and hives when bromelain is taken in very large overdoses (2,000 milligrams and higher).

Clinical studies have found that giving very low doses of vitamin C improves the immune response to pneumonia, especially in the elderly.[4] The acute phase of pneumonia also drains the body's supply of vitamin E.[5] There is no question that supplementing these two antioxidants is helpful in pneumonia, but more is not necessarily better. Many people are unaware that the free radicals quenched by vitamins C and E are not always harmful, but they are involved in many defense reactions of the cells, especially the action of the white blood cells known as macrophages to surround and digest bacteria. High levels of antioxidants may disturb these reactions with unpredictable and unexpected consequences. Therefore, only low doses of vitamins C and E are recommended for pneumonia.

There is no specific clinical evidence that echinacea can effect the course of pneumonia, but there is considerable evidence that echinacea can relieve the symptoms of pneumonia. German studies have found that *Echinacea purpurea* stimulates the immune system to produce macrophages, the white blood cells specifically responsible for removing infectious bacteria (and that depend on the generation of free radicals for their work), without increasing the numbers of other kinds of white blood cells that generate inflammatory hormones.[6] This targeted immune stimulation fights infection but avoids inflammation. In fact, echinacea relieves inflammation. One study found that a teaspoon of *Echinacea purpurea* juice is as effective in relieving pain and swelling as 100 milligrams of cortisone.[7]

Some drugs should not be combined with echinacea. There is laboratory evidence that *Echinacea angustifolia* contains chemicals that deactivate CYP3A4. This is a liver enzyme that breaks down a wide range of medications, including anabolic steroids, the chemotherapy drug methotrexate used in treating cancer and lupus, astemizole (Hismanal) for allergies, nifedipine (Adalat) and captopril (Capoten) for high blood pressure, and sildenafil (Viagra) for impotence, as well as many others. *Echinacea angustifolia* might help maintain levels of these drugs in the bloodstream and make them more effective, or it might also cause them to accumulate to levels at which they cause side effects. Switch to a brand of echinacea that does not contain *Echinacea angustifolia* if you experience unexpected side effects while taking any of these drugs.[8]

CONCEPTS FOR COPING WITH PNEUMONIA

○ Avoid all forms of echinacea if you have pneumonia while you have HIV. As unlikely as it may seem, immune stimulation is a frequent cause of severe, untreatable pneumonia during HIV and AIDS.

Poison Ivy, Poison Oak, and Poison Sumac

SYMPTOM SUMMARY

○ Red pimples, weeping blisters, and extreme itching on areas of skin exposed to plant

○ Inflammation appears in streaks or patches

○ Symptoms first appear 1 day to 3 weeks after exposure and last 1–2 weeks

○ Reactions vary greatly among individuals, ranging from none at all to symptoms requiring hospitalization

UNDERSTANDING THE DISEASE PROCESS

Skin reactions to poison ivy, poison oak, and poison sumac constitute a form of contact dermatitis, an allergic sensitivity to volatile oils found in their leaves. The actual injury of the skin is carried out by the release of inflammatory hormones from memory T cells, white blood cells that carry a chemical coding from prior exposure to the plant. When the skin is exposed to volatile oils from the plant for a second time, the memory T cell for that plant is reactivated. But since the immune system normally only has a very small number of memory T cells for each noxious agent, itching, swelling, and blistering are not noticed for several days to several weeks while the memory T cells multiply.

Poison ivy, poison oak, and poison sumac are especially persistent on dry skin. While the blisters they cause are not infectious, the inflammation causing volatile oils can be spread from person to person by touching the skin or affected clothing. Burning poison ivy, poison oak, and poison sumac plants is especially hazardous, since the irritant resins they contain can be spread by smoke and even inhaled.

Recognizing Poisonous Plants

Poison ivy is found on the banks of streams and rivers throughout the United States except in the Desert Southwest, Hawaii, and Alaska. Many Americans are familiar with the childhood warning, "Leaves of three, leave it be." Poison ivy can be recognized by its leaves in groups of three on a red stem.

Poison oak is found primarily in California, Oregon, and Washington, although it also appears in Oklahoma and Texas. It grows as a shrub and, like poison ivy, has leaves in groups of three.

Poison sumac is most abundant in the Mississippi Delta, although it is occasionally found throughout the eastern two-thirds of the United States. Like poison oak, it grows as a shrub, but has groups of 7–13 leaves arranged in pairs.

TREATMENT SUMMARY

HERBAL FIRST AID

○ Simicort or other cream containing glycyrrhetinic acid, or cream containing chamomile or witch hazel, or zinc oxide cream, daily. Do not apply zinc oxide creams to "oozing" skin.

NUTRITIONAL SUPPLEMENTS

○ Evening primrose oil: 3,000 milligrams per day.

○ Quercetin: 400 milligrams 3 times per day, before meals.

○ Vitamin A: 50,000 IU per day. Women who are or who may become pregnant should strictly limit their intake of vitamin A to 5,000 IU per day or less.

○ Vitamin E: 400 IU per day.

○ Zinc picolinate: 50 mg per day until symptoms subside.

HERBS

○ Burdock (*Arctium lappa*) or dandelion (*Taraxacum officinale*): 500 milligrams solid extract capsules 3 times per day.

○ Coleus forskolii: 50 milligrams of 18% forskolin extract 3 times per day.

○ Licorice: 250–500 milligrams of solid extract (4:1) capsules 3 times per day.

UNDERSTANDING THE HEALING PROCESS

The most important consideration in getting over a case of poison ivy, poison oak, or poison sumac is avoiding new inflammation. Launder any clothing that could carry volatile resins in hot, soapy water before using again. Avoid exposure to chemical agents that activate the immune system in the skin (causing memory T cells to multiply): colognes and perfumes, thimerosal in contact lens solution, formaldehyde, and, surprisingly, the skin cream neomycin.

Licorice creams such as Simicort perform many of the same functions as steroid creams without their side effects. One of the components of licorice, glycyrrhetinic acid, potentiates the effects of the natural anti-inflammatory hormone cortisol by inhibiting the enzyme 11-beta-hydroxysteroid dehydrogenase, which converts cortisol to an inactive form.[1]

In the early 1980s nutritionally oriented physicians recognized that if the underlying metabolic problem in dermatitis is a failure to convert linoleic acid (the n-6 fatty acid found in animal fats and corn oil, among many other sources) to gamma-linolenic acid (GLA), supplementing with GLA should help. British studies found that giving 2, 4, or 6 grams of evening primrose oil (EPO) daily to adults with dermatitis corrected their fatty acid profiles measured by blood tests.[2] Other studies found that taking EPO for a month lowered the levels of the stress hormones epinephrine and norepinephrine in the skin,[3] and reduced roughness of inflamed skin.[4]

Quercetin was once known as "vitamin P," an essential cofactor for vitamin C. Quercetin stops the biological signals that tell mast cells to release histamine, the inflammatory agent in delayed hypersensitivity reactions, such as those in poison ivy, poison oak, and poison sumac.[5] It also short-circuits a series of biochemical steps necessary for the formation of leukotrienes, other slow-acting agents of allergic inflammation.[6]

Quercetin interacts with a number of medications. It increases the toxicity of the cancer chemotherapy drug Platinol (cisplatin), the antirejection drug cyclosporine (Neoral, Sandimunne) given to transplant patients, and the high blood pressure medication nifedipine (Procardia). It competes for receptor sites and decreases the effectiveness of quinolone antibiotics, which include:

- ciprofloxacin (Cipro, Baycip, Cetraxal, Ciflox, Cifran, Ciplox, Cyprobay, Quintor)

- enoxacin (Penetrex)

- gatifloxacin (Tequin)

- gemifloxacin (a relatively new drug)

- grepafloxacin (Raxar)

- levofloxacin (Levaquin)

- lomefloxacin (Maxaquin)

- moxifloxacin (Avelox)

- norfloxacin (Amicrobin, Anquin, Baccidal, Barazan, Biofloxin, Floxenor, Fulgram, Janacin, Lexinor, Norofin, Noroxin, Norxacin, Orixacin, Oroflox, Urinox, Zoroxin)

- ofloxacin (Floxin)

- sparfloxacin (Zagam)

- temafloxacin (Omniflox)

- trovafloxacin (Trovan)

Vitamin A lowers the production of the inflammatory immunoglobulin IgE, which is overabundant in skin affected by poison ivy, oak, or sumac. Vitamin A's effects are most noticeable, however, when inflammation is minimal. That is, severe outbreaks are less responsive to vitamin A treatment.[7]

There is some recent laboratory evidence that vitamin E could be formulated in a way to prevent delayed hypersensitivity reactions, such as those that cause eczema.[8] This idea has not yet been clinically proven. Nonetheless, vitamin E is useful as a cofactor for vitamin A. In laboratory studies with animals, the amount of vitamin A in the bloodstream stays low regardless of intake until vitamin E levels are normal. Vitamin E supplementation is useful even if vitamin A is not taken, since it complements the vitamin A available from the diet.

Both hair[9] and blood[10] analyses find lower levels of zinc in children who have skin outbreaks than in healthy children. On the other hand, hair and blood analysis shows that copper and the blood protein that binds it are more abundant in children who have skin outbreaks than in healthy children. These findings support the frequent recommendation of zinc supplementation as a treatment for conditions such as poison ivy, oak, and sumac in children. Similar findings have not, however, been found for adults. Maintenance supplementation with zinc is useful since zinc, like vitamin E, is a cofactor for vitamin A.

Burdock is a rich source of inulin, which activates the alternate complement pathway (ACP).[11] This is a secondary means of immune defense against bacterial infection. The ACP is especially important in poison ivy, oak, and sumac, since constant scratching leaves the skin at risk of infection with *Staphylococcus aureus.*

Dandelion is also a useful source of inulin. If capsulated burdock or dandelion is unavailable, take 2–8 grams of dried root, 1–2 teaspoons of fluid extract, or 1–2 teaspoons of fresh juice of either herb, daily.

There is laboratory evidence that forskolin, the primary active chemical constituent of coleus, is highly antiallergenic.[12] Forskolin stimulates the production of greater quantities of cyclic adenosine monophosphate (cAMP). This substance acts as a "second messenger" for dozens of hormonal processes. When a hormone comes in contact with the outer membrane of a cell, cAMP is released to carry a message to the organelles within the cell to perform desired functions. The cAMP system is a second messenger for anti-inflammatory hormones, both those manufactured by the body itself and those provided by medication. Forskolin is especially helpful when used with steroids to control inflammation.

While coleus helps the body form second messengers for hormones, licorice keeps useful hormones from breaking down. The action of one of the components of licorice, glycyrrhetinic acid, potentiates the effects of hydrocortisone creams and conserves both the hormones produced by the body and those provided by medication. Licorice may be taken internally, most conveniently in capsule form (do not use DGL to treat poison ivy, oak, or sumac) or in a cream such as Simicort.

CONCEPTS FOR COPING WITH POISON IVY, POISON OAK, AND POISON SUMAC

Important steps in self-care:

○ Do not touch the skin or clothing of someone who has been exposed to poison ivy, oak, or sumac.

○ Avoid excessive washing of the skin. Washing the skin too often dries it out and leaves it vulnerable to inflammatory substances.

○ Avoid scratching when you itch. If you must relieve the itch, gently rubbing with the flat of your hand is less likely to do damage.

○ Avoid wool and polyester clothing when working around poison ivy, poison oak, and poison sumac. Wool scratches and leaves the skin more vulnerable to their volatile oils.

○ Take quick showers instead of long baths. The natural moisturizing agent of the skin, sodium pyrrolidine carboxylic acid (PCA), can leach out, especially in alkaline water. This slows the healing process and leaves the skin vulnerable to further inflammation.

○ See a doctor if itching cannot be controlled, if the rash affects the eyes, face, genitals, or lips, or if there are signs of infection, such as increased tenderness, odor, or pus.

○ Seek emergency medical attention if there is difficulty breathing, if the victim is coughing after exposure to burning plants, or if the rash covers more than one-quarter of the body.

Preeclampsia and Eclampsia

SYMPTOM SUMMARY

All symptoms occur during pregnancy.

Preeclampsia:

○ Elevated blood pressure, an increase of 15 mm Hg or more in the bottom number (diastolic) and 30 mm Hg or more in the top number (systolic)

○ Swollen face and hands when getting up in the morning (swollen ankles and feet are considered normal during pregnancy)

○ Weight gain of more than 2 pounds (1 kilogram) per week, may be very sudden (1 or 2 days)

○ May present no early symptoms

Eclampsia

○ Breathing stops for brief periods (apnea)

○ Bruises

○ Loss of consciousness

○ Muscle aches and pains after trauma

○ Seizures

○ Severe agitation

○ Doctor's exam may find slowed reflex when tendon struck with hammer and changes in the retina caused by high blood pressure

UNDERSTANDING THE DISEASE PROCESS

Preeclampsia is a toxic condition that sometimes occurs in the late second or third trimesters of pregnancy. In pregnancy, the kidneys are "reset" so that their output is greatly increases. The removal of large quantities of fluid normally lowers blood pressure. This compensates for the physical pressure placed on the veins by the developing baby.

In preeclampsia, the cells lining the filtration units of the kidney adhere to each other too strongly to allow the outflow of additional fluid into the bladder. Ordinarily, the body has a backup system for this problem. The blood vessels use vitamin C to produce nitric oxide (NO) from a chemical called S-nitrosoalbumin. The NO released from S-nitrosoalbumin is enough to prevent stress on the cardiovascular system. Women who get preeclampsia, however, tend to have oxidant stress[1] leading to low levels of vitamin C[2] and high levels of S-nitrosoalbumin in their blood.[3] These expectant mothers experience weight gain and elevated blood pressure. If the condition is untreated, it may cause seizures, caused eclampsia. Untreated preeclampsia can cause developmental problems in the baby. The mother's blood becomes "sticky" and tends to clot, there is a possibility of damage to the mother's kidney and liver, and there is severe stress on the mother's central nervous system. Because preeclampsia affects the blood supply to the uterus, babies can be smaller and are often born prematurely, or, in mothers who have diabetes or polycystic ovarian syndrome, have a very high birth weight.

Preeclampsia occurs in approximately 1 in 20 pregnancies. Eclampsia occurs in approximately 1 in 1,500 pregnancies. The risk of preeclampsia is greatest in first-time pregnancies, teenage pregnancies, pregnancies in women over the age of 40, African-American women, women with higher than average body fat, women with a family history of the disease, and in women with a history of diabetes, high blood pressure, kidney disease, lupus, rheumatoid arthritis, or polycystic ovarian syndrome.

TREATMENT SUMMARY

DIET

○ Avoid sodium in all forms, including:

• All drugs containing sodium, such as Alka-Seltzer and aspirin.

• Anchovies, canned salmon, sardines, and shellfish in general.

• Any "fizzy" drink not specifically labeled as low-sodium.

• Any kind of salted grilled meat, soup, or consommé.

• Bacon, ham, sausages, and all cured meats, pork or otherwise.

• Beer, carbonated beverages whether sweetened with sugar or aspartame, and mineral water.

• Beets, celery, and spinach.

• Breakfast cereals, bread, biscuits, pancakes, and waffles.

• Cheeses and other processed dairy products.

• Chocolate.

• Dried fruit and nuts.

• Egg *whites*. Egg yolks are permissible.

• Peanuts, whether salted or not.

• Popcorn.

• Prepared foods of all types, especially salad dressings.

○ Consume natural diuretic foods and beverages such as melons and cranberry juice in moderation.

NUTRITIONAL SUPPLEMENTS

○ Calcium: 2,000 milligrams daily. (A formula combining calcium citrate and magnesium is best.)

○ Folic acid: 800 micrograms daily (Especially important if you avoid processed grain products, which in the United States are fortified with folic acid).

○ Magnesium: 200 milligrams 3 times a day.

○ Vitamin C: 1,000 milligrams daily.

○ Vitamin E: 400 IU daily.

○ Zinc: 20–30 milligrams daily if zinc deficient.

○ Avoid iron supplements unless your doctor prescribes them.

HERBS

○ Avoid immunostimulant herbs, especially echinacea, and stimulant herbs, including ephedra, guaraná, and maté.

UNDERSTANDING THE HEALING PROCESS

Preeclampsia and eclampsia are usually cured when the baby is born, although preeclampsia sometimes occurs as late as 6 weeks after delivery. If seizures and vascular damage can be avoided, there are almost never any long-term consequences of the disease itself, although other health problems may be revealed during pregnancy. There is considerable evidence that nutritional supplementation can greatly reduce the risk of preeclampsia becoming eclampsia, which requires bed rest and constant medical attention until delivery and endangers the health and life of both mother and child.

The kidneys maintain a constant concentration of sodium in the blood plasma. In preeclampsia, the glomerular endothelial cells are inflamed or injured, so the ability of the kidneys to filter sodium out of plasma is compromised. The kidneys compensate by retaining fluid. Drastically reducing the consumption of dietary sodium gives the kidneys less work to do. This reduces swelling and lowers blood pressure.

Calcium and magnesium have been extensively researched as preventatives for preeclampsia. Nine clinical studies involving more than 6,000 women found that calcium is especially useful in preventing preeclampsia in women who are calcium deficient or who have a history of high blood pressure.[4] (A tenth study involving 4,589 pregnant women did not find statistically significant differences between groups of women given supplemental calcium and women who were not, although the calcium-treatment group did experience slightly lower rates of preeclampsia and high blood pressure. This study also confirmed that there are no potential side effects from taking modest dosages of supplemental calcium during pregnancy.[5]) Calcium supplementation has the additional benefit of counteracting the effects of exposure to toxic forms of lead.[6]

A study of magnesium supplementation in 189 pregnant women conducted by the University of Tennessee in Memphis found neither significant benefits nor side effects when women were given 365 milligrams daily.[7] However, this study focused on blood pressure control and length of pregnancy. Another study of 568 women at the University of Zurich in Switzerland, found that magnesium supplementation during pregnancy was associated with significantly fewer maternal hospitalizations, a reduction in preterm delivery, and less frequent referral of the newborn to the neonatal intensive care unit.[8] A study at the University of Copenhagen found that intravenous magnesium supplementation increased birth weight of first-born children and also lowered blood pressure in mothers during pregnancy.[9]

The evidence as a whole suggests magnesium supplementation may be helpful for mothers in their first pregnancy. Like milk of magnesia, magnesium taken in high dosages is likely to cause loose stools. In extreme cases, magnesium overdose can cause diarrhea resulting in dehydration. Do not take more than the recommended dosage, and be sure to drink 6–8 glasses of water daily. If diarrhea results, discontinue magnesium but continue with a Cal-Mag supplement.

Folic acid and zinc have no direct effect on preeclampsia, but are extremely important to the normal neurological development of the embryo, especially in the first month of pregnancy. Studies of folic acid consumption in Wales[10] and zinc consumption in California[11] have confirmed that mothers who are not deficient in these nutrients are much less likely to bear children who have neural tube defects, birth defects occurring in the brain or spinal cord, such as anencephaly or spina bifida.

Researchers at St. Thomas' Hospital in London gave 283 women who were found to be at high risk for eclampsia either 1,000 milligrams of vitamin C and 400 IU of vitamin E, or a placebo, during weeks 16 through 22 of pregnancy. Women who took the vitamins were less than half as likely to develop preeclampsia as those who took the placebo.[12]

Women who develop preeclampsia tend to have excessive levels of iron in their bloodstreams. One study found that the women being studied had bloodstream iron levels that were an average 48 percent higher than normal, although iron levels fell to normal within 1–2 days after giving birth. The same group of women had a 98 percent higher than normal rate of iron binding, reflecting a much greater need for antioxidants than in women who do not have preeclampsia.[13]

Iron is strong oxidant that depletes the antioxidants needed for the production of vessel-relaxant nitric oxide. Women who have preeclampsia or who have experienced preeclampsia during earlier pregnancies should avoid it unless the doctor recommends it for anemia after doing a blood test for ferritin.

The tissue injury in the kidney that causes preeclampsia and eclampsia is mediated by white blood cells. In preeclampsia, leukocytes are especially "adhesive." They tend to accumulate in the filtration tubules of the kidney, where they release inflammatory hormones and destroy kidney tissue. For this reason, it is important to avoid immunostimulant herbs, especially those that increase the production of white blood cells, such as echinacea. Stimulant herbs, including ephedra, guaraná, and maté, elevate blood pressure and also must be avoided.

CONCEPTS FOR COPING WITH PREECLAMPSIA AND ECLAMPSIA

○ If you are not already under a doctor's care for high blood pressure, take and record your blood pressure as soon as you become pregnant. Then take your blood pressure every day, in the same position and at the same time of day if possible. Keep a log or list of blood pressure readings to share with your healthcare provider. Seek immediate medical attention if your systolic pressure (top number) increases more than 30 points or if your diastolic pressure (bottom number) increases more than 15 points.

○ Excessive swelling, or pitting edema, can be detected by pressing a thumb into your skin. If an indentation remains for a few seconds, or if your skin changes color, seek medical attention.

○ To relieve edema, put your feet up every day but avoid sitting for extended periods.

○ Drink water to remain hydrated. Dark yellow urine is usually a sign of inadequate water intake. Urine that is reddish or the color of cola indicates serious dehydration.

○ Do not diet or try to lose weight. Do not attempt to disguise weight gain for a prenatal visit by skipping breakfast, using diet pills, or fasting. Accurate weight measurement is important for detecting preeclampsia.

○ If you have had preeclampsia before, consider purchasing test strips for protein in the urine (the strips are expensive and insurance may not cover them). The strips have markings for "trace," 1+, 2+, and so on. A reading of 2+ or higher indicates a need for urgent medical attention.

○ Nausea or vomiting is a significant symptom if it occurs in the second or third trimester of pregnancy. If you experience nausea or vomiting after your first trimester, seek medical attention and insist on having your blood pressure tested and urine checked for proteins.

○ A headache with sensitivity to light or changes in vision, such as seeing auras or flashing lights or blurry vision or spots, is a symptom of irritation of the central nervous system and should be taken seriously. See the doctor immediately if you experience these symptoms.

○ Anxiety, mental confusion, racing pulse, or trouble catching your breath are signs of high blood pressure.

○ Muscle strain is common in pregnancy. Shoulder pain that feels like someone is pinching you along your bra strap, pain when lying on your right side, or acute lower back pain may be a sign of a liver problem known as HELLP syndrome (hemolysis, elevated liver enzymes, and low platelet count).

○ Self-care does not substitute for prenatal visits. It is important to understand that home blood pressure monitors and the blood pressure monitoring machines in pharmacies are not as accurate as those in your doctor's or midwife's office.

Premenstrual Syndrome (PMS)

SYMPTOM SUMMARY

○ Anxiety (clumsiness, insomnia, irritability, mood swings, tension)

○ Cravings (cravings for salty or sweet foods, headache when these foods are not supplied)

○ Depression (anger or sadness for no apparent reason, poor concentration or memory)

○ Hydration (bloating, breast tenderness, fluid retention)

○ Other symptoms:
  • Acne
  • Constipation, Diarrhea
  • General aches and pains
  • Hot flashes, cold sweats

UNDERSTANDING THE DISEASE PROCESS

Premenstrual syndrome, or PMS, is a recurrent condition of discomfort before and during menstruation affecting approximately 1 in 3 women in the United States. PMS can begin in adolescence, but it is most severe for women in their forties. Symptoms disappear at menopause. There is no definitive explanation of the causes of the disease. It is *not* due to excessive estrogen levels, deficient estrogen levels, discontinuation of estrogen therapy, deficient progesterone, vitamin deficiency, insulin resistance, or electrolyte imbalances.

TREATMENT SUMMARY

NUTRITIONAL SUPPLEMENTS

○ Calcium: 1,000–1,200 milligrams per day, preferably in 2 or more doses.

○ Magnesium: 200 milligrams per day.

○ Vitamin B_6: 200 milligrams per day.

HERBS

○ Vitex: 200 milligrams per day.

UNDERSTANDING THE HEALING PROCESS

Modern medicine sometimes prescribes the "heavy artillery" of antipsychotic medication for PMS. While rare cases require antidepressants, the primary documented effect of low-dose antidepressants such as fluvoxamine (Luvox) in PMS is to increase the incidence of "caffeine craziness" in caffeine-sensitive women.[1] Progesterone, the principal component in birth control pills, is also frequently prescribed, but a study of 5,891 women found it to be of limited or no benefit.[2] Most women benefit from a natural, nutritional approach. Several supplements relieve PMS symptoms without risk of serious side effects.

Calcium is the simplest and least expensive intervention for PMS. A clinical study involving 497 women at St. Luke's-Roosevelt Hospital in New York found taking 1,200 milligrams of calcium carbonate daily led to a lessening of fluid retention, food cravings, and pain after

3 months. Calcium is effective without limitation by age, height, weight, use of oral contraceptives, or length of the menstrual period.[3]

Many women with PMS benefit from supplemental magnesium combined with vitamin B_6. These two supplements are particularly beneficial for anxiety. A study at the University of Reading in the United Kingdom found that supplementation with 200 milligrams of magnesium plus 50 milligrams of vitamin B_6 for just 1 month led to a reduction in anxiety, irritability, mood swings, and nervous tension.[4] Although these supplements help almost immediately, correcting magnesium deficiencies may take several months. Do not take magnesium if diarrhea is a problem.

The herb vitex has a long history in the treatment of PMS. Clinical trials in Germany have found that the herb does not relieve bloating and fluid retention, but has significant benefit in reducing anger, breast pain and breast enlargement, irritability, mood swings, and headache pain. The German researchers rejected the idea that vitex was completely safe, but nonetheless could not document any detrimental side effects among the 170 women who used it for 3 months.[5] Vitex should be discontinued, however, in pregnancy.

CONCEPTS FOR COPING WITH PMS

○ It is important to rule out other conditions that cause the same symptoms as PMS. Temporal lobe epilepsy can mimic PMS, but symptoms should not cluster around the menstrual period. Parents of teenaged daughters who display depression sometimes attribute severe sadness or speaking of suicide to PMS, when there is in fact mental disturbance requiring immediate professional attention.

Prostate Cancer

SYMPTOM SUMMARY

○ Difficulty starting or stopping stream of urine

○ Increased frequency of urination

○ Pain while urinating

○ Blood in urine (rare)

○ Impotence (rare as a result of the disease itself)

○ Usually no symptoms, condition discovered when a rectal exam is performed

UNDERSTANDING THE DISEASE PROCESS

The prostate surrounds the urethra, the channel that carries urine from the bladder. The prostate provides the seminal fluid for the transport of sperm, and almost all prostate cancers arise in the cells that secrete semen. In the United States, prostate cancer is the second most common cancer in men after lung cancer. In any given year, about 1 in 100,000 men under the age of 40 is diagnosed with prostate cancer, but about 1 in 100 men over the age of 80 is found to have the condition.

Prostate cancer occurs in men all over the world, but American men tend to have more invasive forms of the disease. The key factor in the severity of prostate cancer seems to be diet. Prostate cancer cells only metastasize from the prostate to other organs after a years- or decades-long process of inflammation. Fatty acids from beef, lard, and shortening are converted into the hormones that accelerate inflammation,[1] while fatty acids from fish, nuts, and seeds seem to prevent the formation of hormones responsible for inflammation.[2] Epidemiological studies reveal that men who eat high-fat diets are more than twice as likely to have prostate cancer spread to other organs than men who do not.[3]

Dietary antioxidants also play a role in preventing prostate cancer. The Clark Study, which tracked the effects on skin cancer of taking 200 micrograms of selenium a day, unexpectedly found that taking selenium reduced the number of cases of prostate cancer by 60 percent.[4] The antioxidant lycopene, found in tomatoes, is associated with a 30 to 40 percent reduction in prostate cancer, although its effects are greatest in the men with the very highest consumption of tomato products and seem to be greater in preventing the spread of prostate cancer than in preventing cancers in the prostate itself. Lycopene both prevents and treats advanced forms of the disease.[5]

Scientists have long observed that men who eat an Asian diet have lower levels of *treated* prostate cancer than men who eat a Western diet, that is, men who eat large quantities of soy develop prostate cancer but do not need radical treatment. Since soy contains estrogenlike chemicals, it has been supposed that they were responsible for this effect. The latest research, however, asserts that the protective effect of soy is not related to estrogen. Experiments with animals suggest that soy can protect against the most invasive forms of prostate cancer that are not affected by hormonal balances.[6]

TREATMENT SUMMARY

DIET

○ Limit consumption of fatty meats, fried foods, butter, lard, and margarine. Eat tomatoes, preferably cooked tomatoes, as often as possible.

NUTRITIONAL SUPPLEMENTS

○ Fish oil: 3 grams daily.

○ Lycopene: 5 milligrams per day.

○ Vitamin C: 2,000 milligrams daily.

○ Vitamin D: up to 2,000 IU daily, under medical supervision.

○ Vitamin E: 800 IU daily.

HERBS

○ PC-SPES: under medical supervision.

UNDERSTANDING THE HEALING PROCESS

While there are no studies that confirm that switching to a low-fat diet heals prostate cancer once it has been diagnosed, there are at least 9 studies confirming that n-3 fatty acids slow the proliferation of prostate cancer cells. Taking 3 grams of fish oil or eating 2 servings of baked or steamed cold-water fish daily can provide the essential fatty acids needed to slow the process of inflammation and the progress of the disease.

The antioxidant lycopene both prevents prostate cancer and is helpful in advanced prostate cancer. In laboratory tests, lycopene offered better protection against carcinogenic mutations than vitamin E, but mixtures of lycopene and vitamin E were more effective than either supplement alone.[7] The combination of lycopene and vitamin E shifts a biochemical pathway involving n-3 fatty acids to reduce the production of inflammatory hormones that the prostate cancer tumor needs to "burn out an escape route" to the rest of the body.[8] The combination activates enzymes that cause prostate cancer cells to enter a normal life cycle, rather than a self-perpetuating cycle of runaway growth.[9]

Cooked tomatoes are a better source of lycopene than raw tomatoes. Lycopene is absorbed better when tomatoes are cooked with olive oil.

Activated vitamin D is often helpful when prostate cancer has spread to the bones, reducing bone pain and preventing fractures.[10] A beneficial dosage of vitamin D is well below the amount that would cause anorexia, nausea, and vomiting, but since vitamin D can interfere with prescription medications, it should only be used for this purpose under the supervision of a physician.

The herbal formula PC-SPES is both effective and controversial in the treatment of prostate cancer. Laboratory studies show that it reduces the production of prostate-specific antigen (PSA) by testosterone-sensitive prostate cancer cells, but not through any process mimicking the action of estrogen.[11] On the other hand, in rare cases, PC-SPES has been associated with some of the same side effects as treatment with estrogen, specifically, formation of blood clots in the lung. If you choose to use PC-SPES, be sure to have a physician do blood work to ensure that you are not at risk for blood clots.

CONCEPTS FOR COPING WITH PROSTATE CANCER

○ Zinc is heavily concentrated in semen, but supplemental zinc is of questionable value in treating prostate cancer. There would be no detrimental effects from using 15–30 milligrams of a zinc supplement daily. Melatonin, shark cartilage, and coenzyme Q_{10} are similarly of only anecdotal benefit.

○ Back and hip pain are a warning sign that prostate cancer has spread to the spine. Weakness in the legs and difficulty walking, increased difficulty urinating, and decreased sensation in the legs are a sign of compression of the spine, which is a medical emergency.

○ PSA measures inflammation, not cancer. A high PSA usually but not always indicates prostate cancer. Drawing blood for the PSA test immediately after a rectal exam can cause a false positive PSA test.

Prostate Enlargement
See Benign Prostatic Hyperplasia (BPH).

Prostatitis

SYMPTOM SUMMARY

○ Difficulty starting or stopping stream of urine

○ Increased frequency of urination

○ Pain while urinating

○ Blood in urine (rare)

○ Impotence (rare as a result of the disease itself)

○ Pain during ejaculation

○ Fever and chills

○ Pain in the lower back, penis, scrotum, or testicles

○ Mild, general aches and pains

UNDERSTANDING THE DISEASE PROCESS

Prostatitis is a noncancerous inflammation of the prostate. Acute bacterial prostatitis (ABP) is typically an *E. coli* infection acquired from the urinary tract. ABP may be accompanied by fever and chills. Chronic nonbacterial prostatitis (NBP) is caused by infection with fungi, molds, or viruses, and usually follows a blockage of the urinary tract by benign prostate enlargement. Chlamydia and gonorrhea also cause similar symptoms.

TREATMENT SUMMARY

NUTRITIONAL SUPPLEMENTS

○ Bromelain and/or papain: 1,000 milligrams daily.

○ Flower (not bee) pollen: 120 milligrams 3 times a day.

○ Quercetin: 500 milligrams twice a day.

UNDERSTANDING THE HEALING PROCESS

The treatment program for acute bacterial prostatitis is the same as for urinary tract infections (see CYSTITIS). Chronic prostatitis is sometimes cured by ejaculation. During ejaculation, the prostate secretes prostatic antibacterial factor into the seminal fluid to fight infection. In one study, unmarried men who avoided sexual intercourse for religious reasons were encouraged to masturbate at least twice a week for 12 weeks. Of the 18 men participating in the study, 14 experienced total or substantial relief of symptoms.[1]

Bromelain and papain relax the muscles around the prostate and allow greater flow of urine. Use of a combination of the two enzymes minimizes even the remote likelihood of a mild allergic reaction.

Flower (primarily rye) pollen is anti-inflammatory and counteracts the stimulatory effect of testosterone on the prostate. A British study found that 13 of 15 men with NBP experienced marked-to-complete relief of symptoms after taking flower pollen extract for 4 weeks.[2] In rare cases, flower pollen extract can cause allergic reactions.

About 2 out of 3 men experience improvement in symptoms after taking 500 milligrams of quercetin twice a day for a month. Combining quercetin with bromelain or papain increases quercetin's absorption and accelerates relief of symptoms. The drawback to using quercetin is that it competes with and reduces the effectiveness of quinolone antibiotics, including:

- ciprofloxacin (Cipro, Baycip, Cetraxal, Ciflox, Cifran, Ciplox, Cyprobay, Quintor)
- enoxacin (Penetrex)
- gatifloxacin (Tequin)
- gemifloxacin (a relatively new drug)
- grepafloxacin (Raxar)
- levofloxacin (Levaquin)
- lomefloxacin (Maxaquin)
- moxifloxacin (Avelox)
- norfloxacin (Amicrobin, Anquin, Baccidal, Barazan, Biofloxin, Floxenor, Fulgram, Janacin, Lexinor, Norofin, Noroxin, Norxacin, Orixacin, Oroflox, Urinox, Zoroxin)
  - ofloxacin (Floxin)
  - sparfloxacin (Zagam)
  - temafloxacin (Omniflox)
  - trovafloxacin (Trovan)

CONCEPTS FOR COPING WITH PROSTATITIS

○ Prostate massage is frequently recommended for prostatitis. It should be avoided during acute infection and by men who have prostate stones. Only an experienced professional should perform prostate massage.

Psoriasis

SYMPTOM SUMMARY

○ Clearly defined red rash covered with overlapping silvery scales

○ Itch that comes and goes

○ Most common on ankles, back of the wrists, buttocks, elbows, and knees

○ Areas of thickening and depigmentation on the nails in a "tear drop" pattern

○ In about 10 percent of cases, arthritis of the joints in the fingers and toes, or occasionally, ankles, hips, knees, and wrists

○ Aggravated by stress, bacterial infections, and certain medications (beta-blockers for high blood pressure, lithium for bipolar disorder, and drugs for malaria)

UNDERSTANDING THE DISEASE PROCESS

Psoriasis is a common skin disorder, affecting between 1 and 2 percent of the world's population and between 2 and 4 percent of the population of the United States. It is a chronic condition manifesting itself in clearly defined red papules, that is, pores with ruptured walls. The papules merge to form rounded plaques, continuously covering an area of skin with a silvery scale.

Psoriatic lesions tend to break out symmetrically on the body. They remain unchanged for long periods of time. In certain locations, such as the scalp and buttocks, they tend to be weepy. Psoriasis usually begins in early adulthood. It is relatively rare in childhood, usually precipitated by strep throat.

Psoriasis is caused by the extremely rapid proliferation of cells in the skin. Cells in psoriatic lesions multiply at a rate 1,000 times faster than normal skin, even faster than cells in skin cancers. In people with psoriasis, even blemish-free skin replenishes itself at $2\frac{1}{2}$ times the normal rate.

Unlike eczema, in which the underlying problem is an allergic reaction, psoriasis is caused by a defect within the skin cells themselves. Psoriasis is the result of a disturbance in a delicate balance between two internal control compounds, cyclic adenosine monophosphate (cAMP) and cyclic guanine monophosphate (cGMP). Increased levels of cAMP favor the maturation of skin cells. Increased levels of cGMP favor the proliferation of skin cells.

These two cyclic nucleotides are intimately associated with the central nervous system. Stimulating the parasympathetic nervous system increases the production of cGMP. This is the same part of the central nervous system that causes the pupils of the eyes to constrict and enhances near vision, activates sweating on the palms of the hands but inhibits sweating elsewhere on the body, and slows the heart rate. Stimulating the production of cGMP in turn stimulates the growth of skin cells.

Stimulating the sympathetic nervous system increases the production of cAMP. This is the part of the central nervous system that causes the pupils of the eyes to dilate and enhances far vision, inhibits sweating on the palms of the hands but allows copious sweating elsewhere on the body, and increases the heart rate.[1] Stimulating the production of cAMP modulates the growth of skin cells.

The chemicals cGMP and cAMP are also intimately associated with the immune system. Cyclic GMP enhances the ability of white blood cells to kill infectious microorganisms. It also increases the production of white blood cells, and increases their responsiveness to infectious agents.[2] Activating the immune system increases the production of cGMP, which in turn stimulates the production of skin cells in psoriatic skin.

Cyclic AMP has the opposite effect on the immune system.[3] It keeps the immune system from overproducing white blood cells and keeps white blood cells from attacking healthy tissues. Cyclic AMP inhibits the production of skin cells in psoriatic skin.

These complex interactions link psoriasis and stress. They establish a connection between psoriasis and drugs that act on mood, emotions, and the central nervous system. They also establish a connection between psoriasis and infection. From the perspective of holistic care, controlling psoriasis is largely a matter of finding healthy responses to infection and stress with the help of diet, herbs, and nutritional supplements.

TREATMENT SUMMARY

DIET

○ Eat 3 servings of cold-water fish weekly.

○ Eliminate gluten (wheat and corn products).

○ Identify and correct food allergies.

○ Limit saturated fats and alcohol.

NUTRITIONAL SUPPLEMENTS

○ High-potency multivitamin and mineral formula.

○ Chromium: 400 micrograms per day.

○ Selenium: 200 micrograms per day.

○ Vitamin A: 50,000 IU per day. Women who are or who may become pregnant should strictly limit their intake of vitamin A to 5,000 IU per day or less.

○ Vitamin E: 400 IU per day.

○ Water-soluble fiber: 1 tablespoon at bedtime.

○ Zinc picolinate: 30 milligrams per day. Especially important in psoriatic arthritis.

HERBS

Apply topically:

○ Creams containing aloe, avocado oil, chamomile, capsaicin, or glycyrrhetinic acid (licorice), and/or vitamin B_{12}.

○ Creams containing barberry, coptis, goldenseal, or smilax are also helpful, but should not be used to the exclusion of aloe or capsaicin.

Take internally:

○ Goldenseal

• Dried root: 2–4 grams 3 times a day, *or*

• Fluid extract: 1/2–1 teaspoon 3 times a day, *or*

• Solid extract (standardized for 8–12% berberine content): 250–500 milligrams 3 times a day.

○ Milk thistle: 210–500 milligrams daily. Silymarin liposomes or phytosomes are better absorbed.

○ Smilax

• Dried root (may be taken as a tea): 2–4 grams 3 times a day, *or*

• Fluid extract: 2–4 teaspoons 3 times a day, *or*

• Solid extract: 250–500 milligrams 3 times a day.

UNDERSTANDING THE HEALING PROCESS

A frequently overlooked key to the process of healing psoriasis is avoiding infection. Simple infections activate the immune system and accelerate the disease process in the skin. Just avoiding everyday infections is of immeasurable benefit to controlling skin inflammation.

Chemically synthesized vitamin A has been used in the treatment of psoriasis since the early 1970s. The biologically active form of the vitamin, retinoic acid, is known to be a regulator of the genes that control cell division in the skin.[4] Psoriatic skin cells require unusually large amounts of retinoic acid due to immune imbalances (an excess of the chemical interferon) in the region of the skin forming a plaque.[5]

A preliminary study in Poland has found that selenium deficiency is most frequent in men who have had psoriasis for longer than 3 years.[6] While many nutritional experts hold that the combination of selenium and vitamin E is important to maintain healthful levels of the antioxidant glutathione peroxidase, there is some evidence that the glutathione peroxidase in psoriasis-affected skin cells is formed without selenium. Therefore, it is possible that selenium really does not help in psoriasis.[7] Moreover, at least one study found that taking selenium supplements did not cause selenium levels to increase in the skin.[8] However, since it is possible that selenium deficiency causes long-term psoriasis inflammation through an unknown mechanism, supplementation is recommended with the caveat that benefits may not appear immediately, and selenium may not help people who have not had psoriasis for very long.

The antioxidant action of zinc is especially important in psoriatic arthritis. It is especially important to avoid supplementation with copper. Elevated bloodstream concentrations of copper are associated with the disease.[9]

It is possible that there is no better single treatment for psoriasis, whether an over-the-counter remedy or a prescription drug, than aloe. The results of a double-blind, placebo-controlled clinical study at the Malmo University Hospital in Sweden showed that 25 out of 30 psoriasis patients who applied aloe to inflamed skin 5 times a week for 16 months were cured of the disease. There were no reports of any undesirable side effects.[10]

The most recent research into natural treatments for psoriasis involved a comparison of the synthetic vitamin D cream, calcipotriol, and an ointment made of avocado oil and vitamin B_{12}. Physicians at the Rühr University in Germany conducted a randomized, prospective trial involving 13 patients who were given one of the two test agents. Calcipotriol gave better results during the first week. The two treatments were equally effective in the second week. As the study progressed, however, the beneficial effects of calcipotriol peaked and then began to subside after 4 weeks, whereas the cream containing avocado oil and vitamin B_{12} continued to provide the same level of relief throughout the study.[11]

Capsaicin, the pungent chemical in cayenne pepper, is an ingredient in many creams to relieve inflammation of the skin and skeletal muscles. Researchers at the skin clinic of the Wilhelms University in Münster, Germany reported in 2000 that capsaicin creams completely stopped itching in *all* psoriasis patients. There was significant but less complete benefit in healing skin lesions.[12]

Chamomile, also known by its botanical name *Matricaria,* is widely used in Europe to treat both psoriasis and eczema. When chamomile is treated with hot water, it releases chamazulene, a potent antioxidant that absorbs free radicals needed for an allergic response.[13] Chamazulene also inhibits the formation of inflammatory leukotrienes.[14] The essential oil, which has to be extracted by a different process, stops the release of histamine by mast cells, further blunting any allergic reactions in the skin.[15]

Using the essential oil of chamomile as an aromatherapy has been shown, at least in animal studies, to lower stress,[16] and may be useful in preventing recurrences of psoriasis.

Glycyrrhetinic acid, found in licorice, is another common ingredient in European skin care products. The best-documented use of glycyrrhetinic acid creams in the treatment of psoriasis is as a complement to treatment with hydrocortisone, making hydrocortisone more effective in smaller doses.[17]

Naturopathic physicians frequently recommend goldenseal as a primary treatment for incomplete protein digestion, which is believed to be a contributing factor in psoriasis. Bacteria in the bowel can process the amino acids arginine and ornithine into toxic forms known as polyamines. These toxins inhibit the formation of cAMP and therefore contribute to the excessive proliferation of skin cells.[18] The resulting toxic proteins, cadaverine, putrescine, and spermidine, are highly concentrated in the gut in persons who have psoriasis. Lowered levels of polyamines are associated with improvement in psoriasis.[19]

Naturopathic physicians also recommend goldenseal in the treatment for bowel toxemia, also believed to be a contributing factor in psoriasis. Endotoxins (cell walls shed by bacteria in the colon), yeasts, and various metabolic products of *Streptococcus* in the bowel act on the immune system in a way that increases the production of cGMP in skin cells.[20] The increase in cGMP increases the rate at which skin cells multiply and exacerbates psoriasis.

Milk thistle complements goldenseal by stimulating the liver to produce bile. Bile emulsifies fatty acid by-products of bacterial digestion and hastens their excretion into the stool. The silibinin in milk thistle keeps the intestine from reabsorbing cholesterol[21] and, presumably, sterols in bacterial endotoxins.

Smilax (sarsaparilla) contains compounds that directly bind endotoxins and promote their excretion. A study reported in *The New England Journal of Medicine* in 1942 found that smilax was especially helpful in treating chronic, large plaques. This controlled study found that treatment with smilax eliminated psoriasis in 18 percent of people in the study and "greatly improved" psoriasis in another 62 percent of patients, that is, smilax helped 80 percent of patients who used it.[22]

CONCEPTS FOR COPING WITH PSORIASIS

O Sunlight has long been used in the treatment of psoriasis. The standard medical treatment of psoriasis involves the use of the drug psoralen (used in a synthetic version in prescription drugs but found in the Chinese herb psoralea, also known as scruffy pea). However, in psoriatic skin, the UVA component of sunlight increases the risk of a nonaggressive skin cancer, basal cell carcinoma.[23] For this reason, treatment with a UVB lamp for 3 minutes 3 times a week is preferable. UVB treatment is as effective in limiting proliferation of psoriatic skin cells as UVA without raising the risk of skin cancer.[24]

O For persons with psoriasis whose work or leisure activities require a great deal of time in the sun, research at the University of Graz in Austria published in 2001 suggests a helpful treatment. The increased risk of basal cell carcinoma in skin affected by psoriasis is due to a deactivation of a "cancer watchdog" gene, p53.[25] Certain foods greatly increase the activity of p53. Curries made with turmeric or supplementation with the antioxidant curcumin protects p53[26] and reduces the risk of cancer in sun-damaged skin.

O Ultrasound, 42–45°C for 20 minutes, 3 times per week. Ultrasound treats skin lesions by generating heat. At least two studies have found that using an ultrasound device 3 times a week is beneficial in psoriasis.[27,28] The exact way in which this "artificial fever" helps psoriasis is not known, but it is likely to involve the production or activation of an oxidation reaction that competes with inflammatory processes for free radicals.

Radon Exposure

SYMPTOM SUMMARY

O None, increased risk of emphysema, pulmonary fibrosis, and lung cancer

UNDERSTANDING THE DISEASE PROCESS

Radon is an invisible, odorless, and tasteless element that comes from the natural breakdown of uranium in soil, rocks, and water. Once uranium has broken down into radon, science has confirmed that it remains in a gaseous state for hundreds of years. For a few days before it is further transformed into the element polonium, however, it becomes an airborne particulate known as Radon-222 that can settle into the lungs.

Radon has been recognized as a cancer risk since A.D. 1556, when the German doctor Agricola theorized that an invisible gas was poisoning the copper miners of Schneeburg. In the twenty-first century, radon-222 is recognized as a special health risk factor for miners, anyone who works in tunnels, employees of radon health spas, and employees of fish hatcheries and hydroelectric plants, which capture large quantities of waterborne radon. Most North Americans, however, are exposed to radon in their own homes. Radon-222 gas enters the home from the soil through cracks in the home's foundation, loose-fitting pipe penetrations, sump openings, crawl spaces, and the open tops of block walls.

Numerous public health agencies rank residential radon-222 exposure as the second leading cause of lung cancer after cigarette smoking. Overall, exposure to radon increases the risk of developing lung cancer by about 15 percent.[1]

TREATMENT SUMMARY

O Treat iron deficiency.

UNDERSTANDING THE HEALING PROCESS

Not everyone has to worry about radon exposure. In vast stretches of the United States, especially in Texas and the deep South and the Pacific Coast, there is very little radon in soil or water. But for people who live in areas where radon is endemic, home testing is called for. Testing kits are available at most hardware stores. If your house has radon, or if you work in an occupation with a high risk of radon exposure, no single measure lowers your risk of radon exposure more than treating iron deficiency.

Laboratory experiments have found that animals with iron deficiency absorb up to 25 times more uranium isotopes than animals given supplemental iron.[2] While these experiments do not prove that people will be protected from radon exposure by taking supplemental iron, they certainly point out a value in preventing iron deficiency. People with blood types AB and B are the most likely to accumulate uranium isotopes.[3]

Not everyone is iron deficient, and some people should not take iron supplements. The relatively rare conditions hemochromatosis, hemosiderosis, and thalassemia are made worse by taking supplemental iron. The best indicator of iron deficiency is a blood test for ferritin, the protein that stores iron. (Other indicators, such as plasma iron levels, can vary from day to day too much to give an accurate test.) Ferritin levels of less than 12 micrograms per milliliter indicate deficiency. Always have a blood test for iron before taking iron supplements.

If your blood test indicates iron deficiency, then take 200–250 milligrams of ferrous sulphate or 500–650 milligrams of ferrous gluconate daily. Do not take iron with supplements containing calcium, inositol hexaphosphate, magnesium, vanadium, or vitamin E, since taking the supplements together may interfere with absorption of one supplement or the other. Do not take iron supplements with antacids, or if you have a history of gastritis, gastrointestinal bleeding, or peptic ulcer disease. You also should not take iron with L-dopa, penicillamine, thyroxine, or most antibiotics, since iron can interfere with the absorption of these prescription drugs.

Raynaud's Phenomenon

SYMPTOM SUMMARY

- Fingers or toes that change color when exposed to the cold or when pressed

- Pain in the fingers or toes when exposed to the cold

- Tingling or pain on warming

- Bluish skin discoloration

- Reddish skin discoloration

- Sclerodactyly, thickening and tightening of the subsurface layers of the skin of the fingers and toes

Recommendations for Raynaud's phenomenon are also helpful for Buerger's disease.

UNDERSTANDING THE DISEASE PROCESS

Raynaud's phenomenon is a condition in which the fingers and toes are unusually sensitive to pressure and cold. In slightly fewer than half of all cases, Raynaud's phenomenon is secondary to another illness, such as lupus or scleroderma. In slightly more than half of all cases, Raynaud's phenomenon is not caused by any other illness. In these cases the condition is called Raynaud's disease. An abnormality in the structure of the microscopic blood vessels serving the skin of the fingers and toes is responsible for symptoms.[1] There may also be an abnormality of white blood cells such that vibration causes them to emit inflammatory chemicals that reduce circulation, especially in cases in which there is some other systemic illness.[2]

Between 80 and 90 percent of people who have scleroderma experience Raynaud's phenomenon, as do about 20 percent of those with lupus. Raynaud's phenomenon in men over 50 frequently results from atherosclerosis. The phenomenon can be caused by blood dyscrasias, in which red blood cells tend to clump together when exposed to cold, or it can be the first sign of a very rare hyperviscosity (syrupy blood) syndrome known as Waldenström's macroglobulinemia. Raynaud's disease most frequently strikes pianists and typists. It may follow frostbite or electric shock to the hands.

The first attack of Raynaud's phenomenon usually affects only the tips of one or two fingers. Subsequent attacks may affect an entire finger or all the fingers. About 40 percent of people who endure Raynaud's phenomenon have similar circulatory problems in their toes, nose, or ear lobes. The condition increases the risk of losing a finger or toe to frostbite, but this occurs in less than 1 percent of patients.[3]

People who have a systemic problem (Raynaud's phenomenon) are likely to have attacks year-round, although not as frequently during the summer. People who have Raynaud's disease are more likely to have attacks just during cold weather.[4]

TREATMENT SUMMARY

NUTRITIONAL SUPPLEMENTS

- Inositol nicotinate: 4 grams (eight 500-milligram capsules) daily.

- GLA (gamma-linolenic acid): 10 grams per day.

- Vitamin E: 400 IU daily.

HERBS

○ Ginkgo is often recommended, but there is a potential side effect. See Understanding the Healing Process.

UNDERSTANDING THE HEALING PROCESS

Spontaneous healing is not unusual in Raynaud's phenomenon. About 1 in 6 people who have an attack never have another. On the other hand, about 1 in 3 gets progressively worse without treatment.

Inositol nicotinate is a special form of niacin (vitamin B₃) that does not usually cause the flushing reaction that can occur in those taking the immediate-release form of the vitamin. It may be labeled as inositol hexanicotinate or myo-inositol hexa-3-pyridinecarboxylic acid, among several other less commonly used epithets. In a double-blind, placebo-controlled trial, 23 patients with Raynaud's disease (not Raynaud's phenomenon) received either 4 grams of inositol nicotinate or a placebo daily during cold weather. Those who received inositol had fewer and shorter attacks than those who received the placebo. The effect of inositol on Raynaud's disease is probably due to the action of its metabolic byproduct nicotinic acid, which can cause dilation of blood vessels just below the skin.

Four grams is a relatively high daily dose of inositol. There is a remote possibility that taking substantially more than this level of the vitamin could result in flushing, itching, dizziness, palpitations, and a "sugar rush." Inositol nicotinate has only recently been introduced to the market in the United States. However, in the 30 years it has been used in Europe, adverse reactions have been very rare.

GLA, or gamma-linolenic acid, is a fatty acid found in plant seed oils such as evening primrose oil (EPO), borage seed oil, or blackcurrant seed oil. A small-scale study in Scotland found that taking EPO significantly reduced the frequency of attacks coming with cold weather.[5] Researchers at Albany Medical College in New York have found that fish oil offers similar benefits, but only to people whose Raynaud's symptoms are due to another systemic disease such as lupus or scleroderma.[6] Pregnant women, anyone taking a blood thinner such as Coumadin, and people with hemophilia should not use either EPO or fish oil, since they reduce the viscosity of the blood and increase the risk of bleeding. Neither should they take vitamin E, which is added to treatment programs to reduce the formation of harmful fatty acids from EPO or fish oil in the bloodstream.

The evidence that ginkgo extract can help in Raynaud's phenomenon is anecdotal, but makes good sense. At least one scientific study has found that ginkgo increases circulation to the fingertips. A dose of 40 to 80 milligrams of the extract 3 times a day should have this effect. However, ginkgo should be used with caution, especially by people who are susceptible to bleeding (pregnant women, users of blood thinning medication, and hemophiliacs), and by anyone taking the combination of GLA and vitamin E.

CONCEPTS FOR COPING WITH RAYNAUD'S PHENOMENON

○ Don't smoke. Smoking reduces circulation to the fingers.

○ Periodic episodes of laryngitis and "lump in the throat" can be due to attacks of the disease, especially if they come and go with exposure to cold.[7]

○ If you take the prescription drug nifedipine (Adalat) for Raynaud's symptoms, use echinacea with caution. *Echinacea angustifolia* can slow the rate at which the liver breaks down the drug and allow it to build up to levels that cause side effects.

Restless Legs Syndrome

SYMPTOM SUMMARY

○ Creepy-crawly sensations in the legs (and sometimes in other parts of the body), accompanied by a strong urge to move

○ Fidgeting or nervous movements of the toes, feet, or legs while awake during the evening

○ Involuntary leg jerks when awake

○ Symptoms lessened by moving the leg

○ Symptoms worse in the evening and night than during the day, especially when lying down

○ Trouble falling or staying asleep, daytime fatigue

People who have restless legs syndrome may be told by their bed partners that their legs or arms move involuntarily when they are asleep.

UNDERSTANDING THE DISEASE PROCESS

Restless legs syndrome (RLS) produces uncomfortable sensations, most commonly in the legs. These annoying feelings are described as being like an electric current, insects crawling, water moving, or as aching, grabbing, or tingling. Some of the more colorful descriptions of the phenomenon include "like soda water coursing through my veins, "Elvis legs," and "the gotta moves." From 20–30 percent of people who have RLS experience similar sensations in their arms as the disease progresses.[1] About 20 percent find the condition painful.[2]

The symptoms of RLS are worse at rest. Travel by train or plane or as a passenger in an automobile becomes extremely unpleasant, as does prolonged sitting while dining, watching a film or live performance, or reading a book.

Although some RLS sufferers obtain relief simply by standing in place, most RLS sufferers relieve the urge to move by walking around. They may obtain relief through a variety of other movements, such as bending, stretching, riding an exercise bicycle, marching in place, or rocking. All of the movements that relieve RLS are under voluntary control and can be suppressed at will.

RLS can begin at any age, even in early childhood, but most individuals will become symptomatic only when elderly.[3] Some patients will experience remissions in which their symptoms decrease significantly or disappear for a period of time. Usually, and unfortunately, symptoms remain and often become more severe over time. In general, the RLS patients who report RLS onset associated with another medical condition, such as Parkinson's disease or during chemotherapy for cancer, rapidly develop symptoms over a few years. In contrast, those patients whose RLS is not related to any other medical condition, and who report symptoms starting in childhood or young adult life, show a very slow progression of symptoms requiring many years before symptoms occur every day.[4]

People with RLS typically have normal reflexes and normal muscular control. The condition is caused by subtle differences in a portion of the brain known as the striatum to respond to the neurotransmitter dopamine.[5] Treatment with L-dopa produces nearly total relief of symptoms,[6] but is not without side effects.

There is a reversible form of RLS that is related to iron deficiencies. Pregnancy greatly depletes the body's store of iron, and 15–20 percent of women experience some degree of RLS during pregnancy. Bloodstream concentrations of ferritin, the primary storage unit for iron, have been found to inversely correlate with the severity of RLS symptoms.[7] An MRI study of iron content in the substantia nigra and putamen of the brain found that iron levels were significantly lower in RLS patients compared to controls and the degree of the abnormality related to the severity of the RLS symptoms.[8] In these cases, treatment with supplemental iron completely reverses symptoms. In other cases, treatment with iron may substantially reduce symptoms.

TREATMENT SUMMARY

DIET

○ Avoid alcohol and caffeine (as well as over-the-counter cold and sinus remedies). Unless you are of African or Mediterranean descent, add fava beans to your diet.

NUTRITIONAL SUPPLEMENTS

○ Folic acid: 800 micrograms daily. Although vitamin B_{12} deficiency is only a problem when folic acid is taken in a dosage greater than 1 milligram (1,000 micrograms per day), never take folic acid supplements without also taking vitamin B_{12}, to avoid vitamin B_{12} deficiency.

○ Magnesium: up to 350 milligrams daily.

○ Vitamin B_{12}: 800 micrograms daily.

○ Vitamin C: 500–1,000 milligrams 3 times daily.

○ See your healthcare provider about a blood test for ferritin, which measures iron deficiency. Do not take supplemental iron unless a blood test confirms iron deficiency. Take iron and magnesium supplements at different times of day, since magnesium supplements slow the absorption of iron.

UNDERSTANDING THE HEALING PROCESS

Many of the medically recommended nondrug treatments for RLS could be characterized as draconian. Physicians sometimes attempt to treat RLS with surgical procedures (sclerotherapy or "vein stripping") to eliminate incompetent veins in the legs, but a clinical study of the practice has found it to be ineffective.[9] The overwhelming majority of RLS sufferers are better off with nonsurgical, pharmaceutical, or self-administered treatments.

Fava beans are dopaminomimetics, that is, they contain chemicals which are precursors in the brain's production of dopamine, which is in relatively short supply in RLS. Some persons of Mediterranean descent, however, may be at risk for "favism" (glucose-6-phosphate dehydrogenase deficiency), a severe reaction to fava beans causing fever, sweating, and anemia.

Symptoms of RLS are often reduced with correction of nutritional deficiencies. With the exception of the studies of RLS treatment with iron, however, most of the research reported in the medical literature has been based on unblinded evaluations that could be reporting placebo effects. A 1977 study found that treatment with folic acid improved symptoms of the condition.[10] This study, however, only involved 16 people. Treatment of RLS with vitamins B$_{12}$, C, and E is largely speculative but there are anecdotal reports that it helps. Two studies have shown a correlation between magnesium deficiency and RLS symptoms.[11,12] Magnesium supplementation is especially helpful in improving quality of sleep.[13]

Iron supplements should be taken only after obtaining the advice of a doctor. Not all cases of RLS involve iron deficiency. In fact, some cases of RLS occur with hemochromatosis, a potentially fatal iron-surplus disease that can be made worse with iron supplementation.[14] RLS sufferers with ferritin levels less than 45–50 mcg/L are likely to have a positive response to oral iron supplementation. The lower the iron level and the more acute the onset of symptoms, the more likely the improvement in RLS symptoms with iron supplements. The benefit of raising the ferritin levels much above 50 mcg/L is doubtful.

CONCEPTS FOR COPING WITH RESTLESS LEGS SYNDROME

O The best nondrug treatments are always those activities that the individual has discovered help reduce the symptoms of RLS. Possibilities include:

- Any activity that is mentally engaging, such as computer programming, video games, or needlepoint.

- Moderate exercise. Moderate exercise tends to suppress symptoms, while the aftermath of either sustained inactivity or bursts of heightened exercise can increase symptoms in some people with RLS.

- Very hot or very cold baths.

Retinitis Pigmentosa

SYMPTOM SUMMARY

O Impaired vision at night or in low light, coupled with:

- Loss of peripheral vision
- Loss of central vision as the condition progresses

UNDERSTANDING THE DISEASE PROCESS

Retinitis pigmentosa (RP) is a group of ocular disorders with similar symptoms. In a healthy eye, the interior of the eyeball or *fundus* has an orange-red appearance due to the presence of cells containing pigment. In RP, the fundus is littered with star-shaped concentrations of pigment settling around the rods of the retina, the eye's sensors for low light.

Over a period of decades, the rods of the retina become darkly pigmented and lose their ability to respond to low light. A person with RP may have perfect vision in daylight but be almost totally blind at night. Later, the outer fringes of vision are lost, taking away the ability to "see form in the corner of the eye." Finally, central vision is affected, first causing an inability to distinguish color and ultimately, in many cases, total blindness. RP may also cause macular degeneration and cataracts.

Signs and symptoms of RP may first occur in childhood, but the serious loss of vision usually does not occur until early adulthood. RP is currently incurable, but the progress of the disease may be slowed by nutritional measures.

TREATMENT SUMMARY

NUTRITIONAL SUPPLEMENTS

O Coenzyme Q$_{10}$: 100 milligrams daily.

O Melatonin: 1 milligram daily.

O Taurine: 1,000 milligrams daily.

O Vitamin A: 15,000 IU daily. Women who are or who may become pregnant should strictly limit their intake of vitamin A to 5,000 IU per day or less.

O Vitamin B$_{12}$ (as methylcobalamin) and folic acid: 800 micrograms of each, daily.

○ Avoid supplements containing molybdenum and those providing more than 100 milligrams of vitamin B_6 per day.

UNDERSTANDING THE HEALING PROCESS

The degenerative processes of RP take place over a period of years, and the benefits of dietary supplementation are only evident over a period of years. Studies that are completed in a year or less usually find no benefits; studies that are conducted over a period of 5–12 years usually find significant benefits. Unfortunately, nutritional supplementation does not cure RP. However, it does slow its progression or helps the eye use its remaining capacity more effectively.

Coenzyme Q_{10} increases the energy-storage capacity of the retina. Supplementation with CoQ_{10} increases the retina's supply of phosphocreatine,[1] probably allowing it to adapt better to the stresses of impaired circulation caused by the deposit of pigment.

Among many factors in night blindness in RP is faulty secretion of melatonin. In some people with RP, the pineal gland releases melatonin so that it is more available to the retina during the day than at night. Melatonin supplementation may benefit in these cases. Vitamin B_{12} also helps restore normal secretion of melatonin. The active-enzyme form of vitamin B_{12}, methylcobalamin, has the greatest effect on retinal function.[2] People over the age of 50 may experience a vitamin B_{12} deficiency due to failures of the digestive tract to absorb it (see HYPOCHLORHYDRIA).

The amino acid taurine is found in high concentrations in the retina. The retina releases taurine when it is exposed to light, and the released taurine is transported away from the retina by the reddish orange pigmented epithelium, the portion of the eye distorted by RP. In studies of animals with experimentally induced RP, taurine supplementation improved retinal function.[3] Some but not all people with RP suffer a deficiency of taurine. Most people with RP have an impaired ability to absorb taurine.[4]

To date, no clinical studies have confirmed the benefit of taurine supplementation in treating RP, but taurine supplements are likely to help and will not hurt. Additionally, it is important to avoid excessive doses of supplements that interfere with the retina's ability to use taurine, including molybdenum and vitamin B_6 (the latter if taken in doses over about 100 milligrams per day).

A study at Harvard Medical School found that taking a relatively low dose (15,000 IU) of vitamin A every day for 5 years decreased the risk of a sudden loss of vision in RP. The same study found that taking vitamin E *accelerated* loss of vision in RP.[5] Short-term (6- and 12-month) studies have not confirmed the findings of the Harvard researchers, so the benefits of vitamin A therapy may be cumulative.

Retinopathy of Prematurity
(Retrolental Fibroplasia)

SYMPTOM SUMMARY

○ Growth of new blood vessels from the retina toward the center of the eyeball in infants born prematurely, detected in medical examination

UNDERSTANDING THE DISEASE PROCESS

Retinopathy of prematurity (ROP) is the leading cause of blindness among children. In babies who are born 40 weeks after conception, the last 12 weeks are especially active for the growth of the eye. The blood vessels supplying the retina gradually spread over its surface and stop their progression at about the time of birth.

In some babies who are born prematurely, a barrier to the growth of normal blood vessels encircles the eye. Abnormal blood vessels grow forward from the retina instead of across it and are gradually covered with scar tissue. This ring of scar tissue, in some cases, can pull on the retina. In a minority of cases, the retina becomes completely detached and blindness may result.

Premature children are at risk of developing ROP when they are exposed to high levels of oxygen, variations in light and temperature, and certain medications. Fortunately, most premature infants do not develop ROP, and most babies with ROP get better spontaneously. However, in the United States alone there are over 150,000 cases of the disease.[1]

TREATMENT SUMMARY

NUTRITIONAL SUPPLEMENTS

○ Vitamin E: high dosage, exact amount to be determined by the neonatologist.

UNDERSTANDING THE HEALING PROCESS

Between 1981 and 1984, six clinical studies confirmed the usefulness of vitamin E in preventing the progression of ROP to its most serious forms. One study of preterm infants supplemented with vitamin E found that none of the 99 surviving infants developed worse than stage 2 ROP (a stage from which the eyes recover on their own), while three infants in a control group who were not given vitamin E were blinded in both eyes.[2] Another study found that infants given vitamin E in the very first hours of their lives did not develop ROP at all.[3] Yet another study found that vitamin E preserved the embryonic character of spindle cells in babies delivered at least 28 weeks after conception, keeping these cells from triggering the development of misplaced, enlarged, and twisted blood vessels.[4]

Since infants born prematurely are placed in round-the-clock neonatal care, decisions about the administration of supplements have to be made by the physician. Parents are urged, however, to discuss vitamin E supplementation with their child's physician.

Retinopathy, Diabetic

SYMPTOM SUMMARY

○ "Fuzzy" vision

○ Decreased sensitivity to colors

UNDERSTANDING THE DISEASE CONDITION

Diabetic retinopathy is a condition of progressive damage to the retina at the back of the eye. It is caused by a combination of poorly controlled blood sugars in diabetes and high blood pressure. Usually developing 5 to 10 years after the onset of diabetes, diabetic retinopathy can go unnoticed for many years. A slight "fuzziness" in the field of vision can be mistaken for a need for new glasses. If the condition is allowed to progress untreated, however, blindness can result. Diabetic retinopathy occurs in both type 1 (insulin-dependent) and type 2 (non-insulin-dependent) diabetes. It is the leading cause of blindness in the United States.

There are two types of diabetic retinopathy. The more common and less serious type of the disease is called simple, nonproliferative or background retinopathy. This condition causes increased "leakiness" in the capillaries circulating blood in the retina, swelling, hemorrhages, microscopic aneurysms, and slowly growing areas of "oozing" proteins covering more and more of the retina. The less common and more serious type of the disease is called malignant or proliferative retinopathy. This condition causes the growth of new blood vessels extending forward from the retina into the vitreous humor. This form of diabetic retinopathy can cause scarring. The fibrous tissues supporting the new, misplaced blood vessels can cause the retina to detach from the back of the eye.

The underlying mechanism of both types of diabetic retinopathy is glycosylation, the attachment of sugars to blood proteins in the presence of high glucose levels. "Sticky" sugar-coated glycosylated proteins generate free radicals, oxidizing, that is, burning, the lipid linings of the cells that form the walls of blood vessels. Glycosylated proteins themselves can attach to the lipids in the cell membranes, stimulating the growth of new blood vessels.

Several other factors accelerate diabetic retinopathy. Although there are contradictory reports in the medical literature, diabetics with retinopathy tend to have high levels of homocysteine, which can directly and indirectly damage the cells lining capillaries. Homocysteine is a special risk factor for diabetics who have kidney damage. Type 1 diabetics tend to have "thick" blood. The red blood cells of type 1 diabetics are less able to bend and stretch to pass tiny blockages in the capillaries. High LDL cholesterol levels coupled with low HDL cholesterol levels compound this problem.

A risk factor for both retinopathy and cataracts in diabetics is the production of sorbitol. In non-diabetics and diabetics alike, sorbitol is a byproduct of the breakdown of glucose. In non-diabetics, once sorbitol is formed it is broken down into fructose and flows out of the cell. In diabetics with high blood sugars, sorbitol cannot be broken down and remains in the cell. This additional sugar draws water into the cell, causing it to swell. When the cells lining the capillaries in the retina swell, blood does not flow smoothly or regularly.

TREATMENT SUMMARY

DIET

○ In addition to ordinary diabetic restrictions, be especially careful to eliminate all prepared foods containing fructose sweeteners, usually labeled as "corn syrup."

NUTRITIONAL SUPPLEMENTS

○ Magnesium aspartate or magnesium citrate: 350–500 milligrams daily.

○ Pyridoxine (Vitamin B₆): 50 milligrams per day.

○ Oligomeric proanthocyanidins (OPCs): 150 milligrams daily.

○ Vitamin C: 2,000 milligrams daily.

○ Vitamin E: 800 IU per day.

HERBS

○ Bilberry: 150–160 milligrams of proanthocyanidins daily.

○ Ginkgo: 70 milligrams twice a day.

It is not necessary to take additional amounts of any supplement you are already taking for diabetes or any other eye condition.

See Part Three if you take prescription medication.

UNDERSTANDING THE HEALING PROCESS

The standard treatment for diabetic retinopathy is laser coagulation surgery. As its name suggests, laser coagulation therapy coagulates the proteins in selected blood vessels in the side of the eye. Many people with diabetic retinopathy have laser surgery, not realizing that the procedure destroys vision at the side of the eye to preserve vision at the center of the eye, and also reduces color perception and night vision.

A much better approach to treating diabetic retinopathy is "tight control" of blood sugars. The United Kingdom Prospective Diabetes Study was the largest, longest-running study of people with type 2 diabetes. It enrolled 5,200 participants and gathered data from 1977 to 1997. The researchers found that what was then considered "intense" blood-sugar control with either insulin or oral diabetes drugs reduced the risk of retinopathy and kidney disease each by 25 percent. However, "intense" control only kept blood sugars down to an average of 7.0 percent HbA1C, roughly corresponding to 165 mg/dl. Among diabetics who also had high blood pressure, keeping blood pressure down to an average 144/82 in addition to controlling blood sugars reduced the risk of retinopathy by 47 percent.[1] Most diabetes control programs today seek much lower levels of both blood sugars and blood pressure—and get much better results. See DIABETES for additional information on tight control.

In achieving diabetic control, it is especially important to avoid fructose (corn syrup) sweeteners. The latest laboratory research suggests that a complex interaction of stress hormones and high levels of fructose in the bloodstream can cause high blood pressure, high cholesterol, and high triglycerides, all of which are detrimental in diabetic retinopathy. Nothing in the research suggests that fructose from fresh fruit would be inherently less detrimental than fructose from corn sweeteners, but sugars from whole foods are absorbed more slowly and the body has greater opportunity to process them.[2] For this reason, fresh fruit, in moderation, is not harmful in diets for diabetic retinopathy.

Magnesium is an essential cofactor for the reactions that use glucose to store energy by converting ADP to ATP. Without magnesium, cells cannot use glucose. Magnesium may also help transmit the signals that allow cells to receive insulin. Medical studies have found that diabetics of European descent who have diabetic retinopathy are usually deficient in magnesium,[3] although diabetics of African descent who have diabetic retinopathy usually are not.[4] Supplementation with 350–500 milligrams of magnesium aspartate or magnesium citrate daily is enough to prevent deficiency, provided there is also an adequate supply of pyridoxine (Vitamin B₆). Without this B vitamin, magnesium is not carried into the cell.

Vitamin C is essential to the production of collagen. This protein is used to make the linings of the blood vessels in the retina in much the same way as sheet rock is hung over a wooden frame to make a wall. Since insulin "carries" vitamin C from the bloodstream into a cell, many diabetics, especially type 1 diabetics and type 2 diabetics who do not take insulin, are deficient in vitamin C despite adequate amounts of vitamin C in their diets.[5] Even a slight vitamin C deficiency can cause increased tendency of the retinal blood vessels to bleed and slow healing when they do.

Clinical studies have found that taking as little as 100 milligrams of vitamin C a day for 2 months reduces the production of sorbitol in the eye in insulin-dependent young adults, even if blood sugars are poorly controlled.[6] Lowered levels of sorbitol allow fructose to leave cells in the eye. This reduces swelling and breakage of blood vessels. Larger daily doses of vitamin C are helpful for enhancing the production of collagen.

A single study conducted by researchers at the Beetham Eye Institute, Joslin Diabetes Center, and Harvard Medical School has found that very high doses of vitamin E not only helped prevent diabetic retinopathy, but, in very mild cases, completely reversed it. Researchers gave 18 diabetics with minimal retinopathy 1,800 IU of vitamin E daily for 8 months. Blood flow through the retina increased an average of 25 percent, less in volunteers who were able to control their blood sugars well, more in volunteers who had poorly controlled blood sugars. Side effects from vitamin E treatment were minimal, and consisted of nine brief episodes of diarrhea, breast pain, dizziness, and headache among 45 patients over the course of 8 months.[7] No one who takes any kind of blood-thinning medication should take this level of vitamin E, and anyone having surgery needs to inform the doctor of vitamin E use. However, the lower dosage recommended here, 800 IU daily, will have similar effects.

OPCs (oligomeric proanthocyanidins) such as those found in grape seed extract protect collagen by stopping an enzyme that breaks it down.[8] Anthocyanosides, such as those found in high concentrations in bilberry, also strengthen fragile capillaries by protecting collagen. Additionally, anthocyanosides reduce capillary flow.[9] In a double-blind study, 14 patients with diabetic and/or hypertensive retinopathy were supplemented with bilberry extract in an amount equivalent to 115 milligrams anthocyanosides, daily for 1 month. Significant improvements in vision were observed in 11 volunteers receiving bilberry, and 12 patients were found to have improved retinal blood flow.[10]

Preliminary studies have found that 140 milligrams of ginkgo extract taken twice a day for 6 months improves color vision in diabetics with mild retinopathy.[11]

Rheumatoid Arthritis

SYMPTOM SUMMARY

- ○ Joint pain, stiffness, and swelling, usually on both sides of the body
- ○ Pain in ankles, knees, fingers, wrists, toes, elbows, and/or neck
- ○ Limited range of motion
- ○ Morning stiffness lasting more than 1 hour

- ○ Burning eyes with tearing and discharge
- ○ Deformities of hands and feet
- ○ General discomfort and fatigue
- ○ Numbness and/or tingling
- ○ Pallor between attacks, reddened skin during attacks
- ○ Round, painless nodules under the skin
- ○ Swollen glands

UNDERSTANDING THE DISEASE PROCESS

Rheumatoid arthritis (RA) is a condition of inflammation affecting the whole body that is most intense in the joints. No one knows precisely what causes RA, although there is general agreement that damage to the joints occurs as white blood cells thicken the linings of the joints. The joints themselves release enzymes that destroy collagen as well as inflammatory cytokines and prostaglandins, chemicals that the body makes more readily when certain kinds of fatty acids are in short supply.

Since prooxidants trigger inflammatory processes and antioxidants stop them, researchers have tried to determine whether RA might simply be the result of a shortage of antioxidants. Research results have been mixed. One study found that people with RA have normal levels of the antioxidant vitamin E,[1] while another study found that people with RA have deficient levels of several antioxidants including vitamin E.[2]

Later research found elements of truth in both findings. The immune systems of people who have RA are supersensitive, sending out floods of inflammatory chemicals and white blood cells in response to allergies or infection.[3] Put in everyday terms, their immune systems lack an "off switch." In the open bloodstream, massive amounts of antioxidants usually overcome the aberrant tendency of these white blood cells to cause inflammation. Within the confines of a joint, however, antioxidants do not reach the T cells and inflammation continues unchecked.[4] In especially severe cases of RA, the same process occurs even outside joints, resulting in fatigue, fever, and the formation of nodules.

TREATMENT SUMMARY

DIET

- ○ Rotation and elimination diet. If you are not sensitive

to dairy products, eat yogurt or other cultured milk products on a regular basis. If you cannot eat dairy products, take 1 or 2 capsules of *aqcidophilus* or *Lactobacillus* daily.

NUTRITIONAL SUPPLEMENTS

○ Antioxidants, including:

- Alpha-lipoic acid: 100 milligrams per day.
- Selenium: 100 micrograms per day.
- Vitamin E: at least 400 IU per day.

○ Glucosamine sulphate: 1,500 milligrams per day.

○ Chondroitin: 1,200 milligrams per day.

○ SAM-e: 400 milligrams 3 times a day.

○ Copper: 1 milligram every other day, or wear a copper bracelet.

○ Essential fatty acids (preferred form): borage seed oil, 1,000 milligrams twice a day.

○ Do not take more than 600 milligrams of vitamin C or 30 milligrams of zinc a day. Never take zinc when you are taking antibiotics.

Other potentially useful supplements:

○ Bromelain: 500 milligrams 3 times a day (preferably encapsulated).

○ Curcuminoids or boswellin with curcuminoids: 400–500 milligrams 3 times a day.

○ L-cysteine: 500 milligrams taken with a full glass of water 3 times a day.

○ L-histidine: 1,000–6,000 milligrams daily.

○ Niacin or nicotinamide: ask your doctor about an appropriate dosage.

HERBS

○ Capsaicin cream: apply to the back daily. If you are sensitive to capsaicin, substitute diluted essential oils of peppermint, eucalyptus, rosemary, or wintergreen.

Also choose from among:

○ Devil's claw: 405–520 milligrams up to 8 times a day.

○ Feverfew: 70–100 milligrams of dried extract daily.

○ Ginger (fresh): 2 tablespoons included in vegetable dishes, fruit salad, or used to make a tea.

○ Willow bark: 1 teaspoon in a cup of hot water or tea, as desired.

See Part Three if you take prescription medication.

UNDERSTANDING THE HEALING PROCESS

There are serious limitations to all kinds of treatment for RA. No conventional medication cures the disease, and all of them have serious side effects, although the newer COX-2 inhibitors for pain relief present notably fewer problems (and they are considerably more expensive). Natural treatments for RA have their own downside. Nothing recommended here is going to create a new set of problems for you, but no holistic intervention works for everyone who has RA, and most complementary treatments take 3–6 months to show results. Occasionally, however, people with RA experience dramatic and complete remissions as a result of dietary changes, herbs, or nutritional supplementation. Read carefully as you choose the therapies most likely to bring a remission of your symptoms.

Doctors seldom recommend dietary changes for the simple reason that most doctors don't believe in the theory of food allergy. Nonetheless, eliminating certain foods brings some RA sufferers considerable relief. One study found that eliminating beef, dairy products, eggs, nuts, and wheat flour brought drug-free relief to 23 out of 25 RA patients in 10–18 days.[5] Another found that eliminating gluten, meat, fish, eggs, dairy products, refined sugar, citrus fruits, preservatives, coffee, tea, alcohol, salt, and strong spices completely (although dairy and wheat products were allowed after 14 weeks if they did not cause resumption of symptoms) not only relieved pain, but decreased the number of tender joints and swollen joints, and improved pain score, duration of morning stiffness, grip strength, and range of motion. Benefits of the diet continued throughout the 2 years of the study.[6] Elimination diets are best suited for palindromic rheumatism, a form of arthritis primarily affecting people under age 45 that does not cause heat in the joints or damage to cartilage, and is clearly triggered by a specific food.[7] Vegan (meat-, fish-, egg-, and dairy-free) diets can be helpful when symptoms vary greatly from day to day.[8]

The problem with elimination diets is that patients beg the question, "If I eliminate all of these foods, what's left?" In the case of the 2-year elimination diet study, the answer was herbal teas, garlic, vegetable broth, a thin soup of potato and parsley, and juices from carrots, beets, and celery, at least during the first month of treatment. (The study notes that patients following the 2-year elimination diet lost weight.) Most RA sufferers who don't live alone would find following a severely restricted diet extremely difficult. Moreover, elimination diets are based on the principle that "one size fits all." In other words, the assumption is that everyone with RA has food allergies, and everyone who has food allergies is allergic to the same foods. This simply isn't true, and there is an easier way to get relief from RA through dietary restriction.

A study published in the British medical journal *The Lancet* reported the experience of 53 people with RA who either ate their regular diet or ate meals excluding common allergenic foods. (The following table lists allergenic foods and the percentages of people allergic to them.) After 1 week, foods with the potential to cause allergies were reintroduced one at a time. If the test participant experienced no change in symptoms, the food was restored to the diet plan. If the food made symptoms worse, it was permanently excluded. One-third of patients on dietary exclusion therapy remained well on diet alone, without any medication, for up to 7.5 years after starting treatment. Many participants in the study lost weight, but weight loss was not necessary for improvement in RA.[9]

COMMON FOOD ALLERGIES IN RHEUMATOID ARTHRITIS[10]

Food	Percentage of RA Patients
Corn	56%
Wheat	54%
Bacon or Pork	39%
Oranges	37%
Milk	37%
Rye	34%
Eggs	32%
Beef	32%
Coffee	32%
Malt	27%
Cheese	24%
Grapefruit	24%
Tomato	22%
Peanuts	20%
Cane sugar	20%
Butter	17%
Melons	17%
Lemon	17%
Soy	17%

Russian scientists report that rotation diets work best when there is a healthy balance of bacteria in the intestine.[11] You can encourage friendly bacteria by eating yogurt or similar dairy products on a regular basis. If you cannot eat dairy foods, take 1 or 2 capsules of *acidophilus* or *Lactobacillus* every day.

Fasting isn't a good way to control the symptoms of RA. Some RA sufferers don't benefit from fasting at all, and no clinical study has found fasting to reduce symptoms for more than 10 days. There is usually an improvement in pain and swelling on day 4 or 5 of a fast, and benefits continue as long as the fast is observed. However, other serious, even life-threatening health problems can arise during fasting, especially for people with RA who also have heart disease or diabetes, and symptoms always return when the fast is broken.

While dietary modification is your first and best treatment for RA, realistically, most of us have problems staying on a diet for a few weeks, much less for a lifetime. Nutritional supplements and herbs can also be extremely helpful, but the first thing to understand is that not all supplements that are helpful in osteoarthritis (OA) are necessarily helpful in RA.

Why not take the same supplements for both kinds of arthritis? The bottom line is that RA is a disease of excessive collagen being attacked by the immune system, while OA is a disease of deficient collagen that the immune system leaves alone. Taking too much vitamin C can interfere with the body's absorption of copper, another essential element, and increase requirements for zinc. Taking additional zinc, however, is also problematic in RA. If you are going to take zinc supplements, you need to avoid taking them with certain foods spared by most RA diets: foods rich in oxalic acid (beans, rhubarb, spinach, or sweet potatoes), and foods rich in phytic acid (matzo, nuts, or seeds), coffee, tea, or caffeinated soft drinks. These foods interfere with the absorption of zinc. No matter what your diet, you should never take zinc with quinolone antibiotics, such as:

- ciprofloxacin (Cipro, Baycip, Cetraxal, Ciflox, Cifran, Ciplox, Cyprobay, Quintor)
- enoxacin (Penetrex)
- gatifloxacin (Tequin)
- gemifloxacin (a relatively new drug)
- grepafloxacin (Raxar)
- levofloxacin (Levaquin)

- lomefloxacin (Maxaquin)
- moxifloxacin (Avelox)
- norfloxacin (Amicrobin, Anquin, Baccidal, Barazan, Biofloxin, Floxenor, Fulgram, Janacin, Lexinor, Norofin, Noroxin, Norxacin, Orixacin, Oroflox, Urinox, Zoroxin)
- ofloxacin (Floxin)
- sparfloxacin (Zagam)
- temafloxacin (Omniflox)
- trovafloxacin (Trovan)

Taking zinc and a quinolone together can reduce absorption of the antibiotic and set off an immune reaction that is destructive to cartilage.

Antioxidant supplements that are helpful in RA include alpha-lipoic acid, selenium, and vitamin E. Alpha-lipoic acid may stop destructive immune cells from "sticking" to the joint, and it interacts directly with the DNA of immune cells to stop them from making the inflammatory hormone NF-kappa B.[12] Clinical studies have found that taking 400 IU of vitamin E per day begins to relieve arthritis pain in about a month.[13] Laboratory studies suggest that it stops joint destruction by RA.[14]

People with the highest intakes of dietary selenium are 5 times less likely to develop RA than people with the lowest intakes of dietary selenium.[15]

Millions of RA sufferers have used glucosamine, chondroitin, and SAM-e successfully, but only recently has there been a scientific explanation of why these supplements, well known to be helpful in OA, should also be helpful in RA. The inflammatory hormones white blood cells send out in RA destroy cartilage but create bone.[16] SAM-e modulates this hormone so that it continues to stimulate growth of bone but stops destroying cartilage.[17] The joint then can use glucosamine and chondroitin to repair itself.

Glucosamine stimulates the production of glycosaminoglycans, the building blocks of the collagen lining the joints. There are indications that the joints lose their ability to make glucosamine as they age. Even joints under attack from the immune system need a basic level of glucosamine to maintain normal production of collagen.

Three studies confirm that glucosamine give better results than aspirin or other NSAIDs in the long-term relief of pain.[18,19,20] Glucosamine has no anti-inflammatory effect and does not affect the central nervous system. Glucosamine relieves symptoms of pain at rest, during exercise, on standing, and during stretching and passive movement.[21]

Probably the only drawback to using glucosamine is that people who are overweight may not respond as well to it. There are some indications that overweight people need a higher dose. Overweight people who have diabetes, however, should not take a higher than recommended dose, since glucosamine increase the need for insulin. Anyone who has diabetes and takes glucosamine should monitor blood sugars carefully to make sure they do not need additional insulin or diabetes medication.

Chondroitin is one of the glycosaminoglycans that glucosamine stimulates the body to make. Found in fish, shark, and human cartilage, chondroitin was long thought to be too large a molecule to be absorbed if taken orally. Recent research, however, has found that a large percentage of the chondroitin taken in supplements is actually absorbed into the body.

Like glucosamine, chondroitin relieves pain by helping heal joints. One study found that people with arthritis of the knee who took chondroitin were able to increase their maximum walking speed, and that pain relief was noticed in as little as one month. More important, at the end of 12 months, study participants who had been taking chondroitin were found to have no worsening of the joints.[22] Chondroitin seems to protect joints from damage, preventing wear and tear on joints already inflamed by RA.

SAM-e also relieves pain. Various studies have found SAM-e to be as good or better for pain relief as Advil, Motrin, Naprosyn, and Nuprin. A study involving 20,641 people with OA of the finger, hip, knee, and spine found that SAM-e alone was as effective as their ordinary pain relievers.[23] In RA, SAM-e directs the effects of the hormone interleukin-1 (IL-1) to the bones instead of the joints, building bone rather than destroying cartilage.

The advantage of SAM-e is that it very seldom causes side effects. In the longest-running study involving the supplement, various minor side effects occurred in 20 out of 97 patients from time to time during the first 18 months of the intervention. In the final 6 months of the study, however, no patients experienced any side effects from SAM-e. Patients received relief of morning stiffness, pain at rest, and pain on movement, as well as depression.[24]

Of all the nutritional supplements for RA, the best known is transdermal copper in the form of a copper bracelet. Often dismissed as a myth of folk medicine, copper bracelets apparently do have some therapeutic effect. A clinical study enlisted 160 volunteers who had arthritis, half of whom had previously worn a copper bracelet. The study participants were assigned to two groups. One group wore a copper bracelet for 1 month, and then a placebo bracelet (electroplated aluminum resembling copper) for a second month. The other group wore the bracelets in reverse order. Of the participants who noticed a difference between the two bracelets, significantly more preferred copper to placebo. Users of copper bracelets deteriorated significantly during the time they were wearing the placebo bracelet.[25]

The amount of copper entering circulation through the skin by wearing a bracelet is very small, equivalent to taking 1 milligram ($\frac{1}{2}$ of the smallest tablet) every other day. The secret to success with copper supplementation may be taking smaller, rather than larger doses. There is at least some evidence that the copper shortages that contribute to RA occur within the cartilage of the joints but not elsewhere in the body.[26] This shortage can be due to a defect in the carrier proteins for copper rather than insufficient copper in the diet. (This defect is worse when more vitamin C supplementation exceeds 600 milligrams per day. Eating too much molasses or leafy green vegetables on a regular basis can cause copper deficiency, as can taking a daily dose of more than 50 milligrams of supplemental zinc.) Therefore, take just enough copper to make sure you are not copper deficient, a 1-milligram tablet every other day. Alternatively, you can wear a copper bracelet.

Various sources of essential fatty acids are well known to reduce swelling and inflammation in RA. Of these, the most effective with the fewest side effects is borage seed oil. In a double-blind trial, 37 patients with active RA were randomly assigned to receive borage seed oil (providing 1.4 grams of GLA per day) or a placebo (cottonseed oil) for 6 months. Treatment with borage seed oil lowered tender-joint scores by 45 percent and swollen-joint scores by 41 percent. The study volunteers who took cottonseed oil experienced no change or a worsening of disease activity. There were no serious side effects, although some participants taking borage seed oil experienced minor stomach upset.[27] Recent research suggests that essential fatty acids cause the defective immune system cells that cause RA to "fade away," passing through their normal life cycle without being replaced.[28]

Black currant seed oil, evening primrose oil (EPO), and fish oil are also helpful, although the results of using these oils are not likely to be as dramatic as those from using borage seed oil. Any essential fatty acid supplement can cause bloating, burping, diarrhea, or flatulence, although these side effects are likely to be mild. People with a history of partial seizures (blanking out or unexplained loss of emotional control should use black currant oil rather than borage seed oil, since the latter can lower the amount of stress precipitating an attack. Hempseed oil will also relieve arthritis pain. It will not give you a marijuana high, but it can cause a false positive reading for marijuana use in some home testing kits.

Capsaicin is the chemical that gives hot peppers their heat. As anyone who has cooked with chiles knows, capsaicin can cause burning, redness, and inflammation, especially to the eyes and mouth. The first time it is applied in a cream to the skin over a painful area, capsaicin causes these symptoms, but the nerve fibers serving the area become insensitive to it—and to pain.[29]

Capsaicin works best when there is good circulation to the skin to which it is applied.[30] Do not apply capsaicin to your feet if you have diabetes and never apply capsaicin to ulcerated skin. It is also important to keep capsaicin out of your nose and eyes. Allergic reactions to the herb are rare but are not unknown, and there have been cases of hypothermia in people who used capsaicin in an especially cold room. It is theoretically possible that capsaicin absorbed into the bloodstream could reduce the bioavailability of aspirin; if you use capsaicin, use pain relievers other than aspirin.

There is a long list of additional supplements and herbs that will relieve RA—over a period of weeks or months. Bromelain can start relieving pain and swelling almost as soon as you start taking it, provided you take it in an enteric-coated form (unavailable in the United States). Allergies to bromelain are very rare but not unheard of. Allergic reactions to this supplement are most likely in people who are already allergic to pineapple, papaya, wheat flour, rye flour, or birch pollen. There has never been a report of an anaphylactic reaction to bromelain. There have been isolated reports of heavy periods, nausea, vomiting, and hives when bromelain is taken in very large doses (2,000 milligrams and higher).

Curcumin, an antioxidant found in turmeric (curry powder), is almost as effective as NSAIDs in relieving pain and swelling. Unfortunately, curcumin is like

NSAIDs in that it can cause stomach upset, especially in people who have chronic gastroesophageal reflux disease (GERD).

The amino acid L-cysteine may relieve arthritis pain, but can also cause stomach upset. Be sure to drink 6–8 glasses of water a day when you take L-cysteine, to avoid the formation of cysteine-crystal kidney stones. The amino acid L-histidine regulates suppressor T cells to put a brake on the process of inflammation in RA. L-histidine is a building block of histamine, so it should be used with caution by anyone who has allergies or peptic ulcer disease, although there are no reports of severe side effects in the medical literature. Some people benefit from as little as 1,000 milligrams of L-histidine daily, but people who have had RA for a number of years usually need to take 5,000–6,000 milligrams daily to notice a difference.

Niacin, nicotinic acid, and nicotinamide are forms of a B vitamin that can cause flushing, nausea, vomiting, diarrhea, headache, and dizziness, although they may improve joint mobility. Anyone who has diabetes, gastritis, gout, liver disease, or peptic ulcer disease should only use niaicin or nicotinamide under a doctor's supervision. Facial flushing is less likely if these supplements are taken with food and after use of an aspirin or NSAID.

Devil's claw relieves joint pain, but only if it is taken in an enteric-coated form that protects its analgesic compounds from being digested in the stomach. Do not use devil's claw with NSAIDs such as aspirin and Tylenol and avoid it entirely if you have duodenal or gastric ulcers.

Clinical trials with women who have RA found that taking 70–86 milligrams of feverfew every day for 6 weeks increased grip strength. Feverfew likewise can cause stomach irritation. Do not use it with NSAIDs and avoid it if you have ulcers.

Two tablespoons of fresh ginger every day is likely to relieve pain and swelling even when pain relievers are discontinued, but the effect takes 1–3 months.

Willow bark is a natural substitute for aspirin. It contains salicin, a less potent pain reliever than the salicylates found in aspirin that does not generally cause bleeding or stomach irritation. Do not use willow bark during pregnancy, if you have tinnitus (ringing in the ears), or if you are allergic to aspirin. Do not give willow bark or aspirin to children who have colds or flu.

Provided you do not have a disease for which these supplements are contraindicated, there is no reason you cannot take any one or more of the other potentially helpful supplements in moderation. Chances are, they will help. Be forewarned, however, that you probably will not notice improvements in your arthritis for weeks or months.

CONCEPTS FOR COPING WITH RHEUMATOID ARTHRITIS

❍ Moist heat relieves the pain of RA. Moist hot packs (a hot water bottle or a steaming hot towel wrapped in a second layer of cloth and placed over points of inflammation) and hot baths for 20–30 minutes 1–3 times a day are helpful. Sea salts added to the bath water afford additional relief. If hot water causes excessive drying of the skin, paraffin baths are an alternative.

❍ Joints must be exercised regularly to keep them from "freezing up." Gently bend and stretch affected joints as far as they will go without pain through 3–10 repetitions at least once a day. It is especially helpful to do these exercises in warm water, preferably at body temperature. Bicycles, elliptical trainers, and rowing ergometers also minimize stress on joints, but a gentle walk (not jog) through a park is also helpful. If your arthritis is so advanced that you cannot move your limbs on your own power, passive exercise (having your limbs gently lifted by another person) will help keep your condition from becoming even worse.

❍ Make every effort to maintain normal weight. Overweight deforms joints.

❍ Living well with RA requires a balance between rest and exercise. Rest is important when inflammation flares, but doing nothing results in lost vitality, weak muscles, reduced range of motion, and stiff joints. When your symptoms are worst, you still need to go through your daily range of motion exercises—gently.

❍ DMSO (dimethyl sulfoxide) applied to the skin can relieve arthritis pain, although weaker solutions (70%) offer greater pain relief than stronger solutions (the more usual 90%). With respect to the joints (and only with respect to the joints), DMSO works like a fast-acting vitamin C. In as little as 30 seconds after application, the bloodstream carries DMSO to the joints, where it protects hyaluronic acid from damage by free radicals. This possibly keeps cartilage from being destroyed or helps new cartilage form. Unfortunately, DMSO also can dissolve any toxin on the skin and send it into circulation throughout the body in under 30 seconds. Industrial-grade DMSO, the form most commonly sold in flea markets, can contain toxic byproducts of the manufacturing process and should not be applied to the skin. MSM (methylsulfonylmethane) is a byproduct of DMSO as it is metabolized by the body, that is also found in alfalfa sprouts, corn, most fruits, tomatoes, coffee, tea, and milk. MSM is also used to treat arthritic pain, and unlike DMSO, is almost completely nontoxic. Most naturopaths recommend 1,000–2,000 milligrams of MSM daily to prevent RA pain and 3,000–5,000 milligrams of MSM daily to treat RA pain.

❍ Homeopathic physicians typically recommend ledum for foot and ankle pain (200C for relief of acute pain, 6C to 30C for prevention), lycopodium for arthritis that is relieved by application of warmth and for joint pain on the right side of the body, and cell salts, especially calcarea sulphurica (Calc Sulf) for general relief of either OA or RA.

❍ Ice massage, moist heat, and transcutaneous electrical nerve stimulation (TENS) all help relieve the pain of RA.

Rickets

SYMPTOM SUMMARY

❍ Skeletal deformities

- "Bow legs" or bowing of the bones in the arms

- "Pigeon chest" (forward projection of the breastbone)

- "Rickets rosary" (bumps along rib cage)

- Asymmetry in skull

- Scoliosis

- Kyphosis

❍ Pain in the bones of the arms, legs, pelvis, and spine

❍ Dental problems

- Delayed formation of teeth

- Holes in the enamel of the teeth

- Increased incidence of cavities

- Painful teeth, especially after eating sweets or drinking hot or cold drinks

❍ Slow growth, may reach a height of 5 feet (150 centimeters) or less at maturity

❍ Fractures (more common in adults than children)

❍ Nighttime fevers

❍ Loss of muscle strength

❍ Delays in muscle development

UNDERSTANDING THE DISEASE PROCESS

Rickets is a failure of the bones to grow in childhood. The bones become flexible and are slowly molded by the weight-bearing forces placed on them. Rickets causes deformities of the long bones of the legs, the breast bone, and the rib cage. Children who have rickets tend to break bones easily, and develop slowly.

In the early twentieth century rickets was epidemic in the northeastern United States and Great Britain. In some areas, entire classrooms of school children were affected. Public information campaigns informed mothers of the virtues of sunlight and cod liver oil, and the condition became much less common.

In the early twenty-first century, rickets has become resurgent in the United States, especially in the Southeast,[1] and also on Long Island.[2] The new cases of rickets are concentrated among breastfed babies of mothers who are themselves vitamin D deficient, usually because of a lack of exposure to sunlight. Breastfed babies of mothers who wear veils are at a distinctly higher risk of rickets. Children of color are also at greater risk for rickets, since melanin in dark skin blocks the sunlight that skin needs to make vitamin D.[3] Fortunately, rickets is easily curable if nutritional treatment begins in time.

TREATMENT SUMMARY

NUTRITIONAL SUPPLEMENTS

❍ Calcium carbonate: 1 teaspoon of liquid powder suspension, daily.

❍ Vitamin D: 200 IU per day.

❍ Vitamin K: 5 milligrams every other week, especially if taking antibiotics.

UNDERSTANDING THE HEALING PROCESS

The first step in healing rickets is recognizing the condition. Rickets should be suspected in breastfed babies who fail to sit up, crawl, or walk as expected, especially if the mother is too busy to get sun. Bowed legs, knots along the rib cage, or a protruding breastbone are signs of the condition in older children. Diagnosis by a qualified healthcare practitioner is essential to rule out other conditions, and the doctor can offer some treatments beyond calcium and vitamin D to accelerate healing. Once rickets has been diagnosed, however, the primary treatment is nutritional supplementation, and the condition is usually completely healed in 6 months.

The two most important nutrients in treating rickets are calcium and vitamin D. Appropriate dosages vary by the contributing causes of the condition. When rickets occurs after deprivation of sunlight, such as after a long period of confinement indoors, it is usually necessary for the child to take 800–4,000 IU of the vitamin daily for 6 weeks, tapering off to a dosage of 200–600 IU a day thereafter to prevent deficiency. Healing of fractures, leading to reductions in pain, usually begins in 3–4 weeks. Complete healing can occur in 6 months. If the only cause of rickets is sunlight deprivation, calcium supplements are not necessary. In the overwhelming majority of cases, however, calcium deficiency contributes to the disease. Babies can be given a liquid formulation of calcium carbonate in addition to milk.

Vitamin K is necessary for the bones to make osteocalcin, a protein that controls the uptake of calcium. Deficiencies of osteocalcin result in increased risk of fractures, especially in the hips.[4] Vitamin K is synthesized by bacteria in the intestine, so vitamin K levels go down during antibiotic treatment. However, taking vitamin K supplements as infrequently as every other week is usually sufficient.[5]

CONCEPTS FOR COPING WITH RICKETS

❍ Rice milk is not a substitute for breast milk, cow's milk, or soy. Severe malnutrition can result if an infant is fed only rice milk.

❍ Egg yolks, butter, vitamin D-fortified milk, fish liver oils, sardines, canned salmon, green leafy vegetables, and tofu are good sources of vitamin D and are beneficial in the child's diet. Vegetarians may use supplements in lieu of eggs and dairy.

❍ Sunlight exposure—at least 20 minutes a day of direct exposure of sun to skin (hands, face, arms, and so on)—is beneficial to both mother and child. Sunlight allows the skin to make its own supply of vitamin D.

Ringworm

SYMPTOM SUMMARY

❍ Scales, vesicles, or pustules forming a ring-shaped rash

❍ Borders advance outward while the center heals

❍ Affected skin is lighter or darker than surrounding skin

❍ Kerions, inflamed plaques that irritate surrounding tissues, in severe infections

UNDERSTANDING THE DISEASE PROCESS

Ringworm is a chronic fungal infection of the skin forming a characteristic ring-shaped rash. Ringworm of the scalp usually begins as a small pimple that grows and leaves scaly patches of temporary baldness. Infected hairs will become brittle and break off easily. Ringworm elsewhere on the body appears as flat, spreading ring-shaped areas. The edge is reddish and may be either dry and scaly, or moist and crusted. As it spreads, the center area clears and appears normal.

In some instances, ringworm is caused by the same microorganisms that cause athlete's foot, *Epidermophyton floccosum, Trichophyton mentagrophytes,* and *Trichophyton rubrum,* These infections can spread from one part of the body to another. Other cases are caused by closely related microorganisms that have an affinity for the keratin of just one skin site, and do not spread from one part of the body to another.

While ringworm does not always spread from one site on the body to another, it often spreads from one person to another. Ringworm is primarily a disease of children, especially between 2 and 9 years old. It is frequently transmitted from pets to children or from child to child, and can be picked up from infected walls, floors, and shower stalls.

TREATMENT SUMMARY

HERBS

❍ Tea tree oil, in creams containing 8–20% tea tree oil or 40% solution, massaged into affected skin 2–3 times daily.

UNDERSTANDING THE HEALING PROCESS

Ringworm is a benign disease if it is treated quickly. Children who have ringworm without inflammation almost never lose their hair. About 25 percent of children who have the kerion form of ringworm, however, suffer permanent, cosmetically significant hair loss.[1] See a healthcare provider if symptoms last longer than 4 weeks or if you notice increased redness, drainage, or fever.

Tea tree oil is the most effective herbal treatment for ringworm. Clinical studies have compared it against the prescription drug tolnaftate in treating the group of microorganisms that cause ringworm. Tea tree oil is not as effective as tolnaftate in eliminating the fungus. In a clinical trial involving 104 patients with athlete's foot, only 30 percent of subjects applying tea tree oil were culture negative, compared to 85 percent in the tolnaftate group. However, more patients in the test achieved relief of scaling, inflammation, itching, and burning from tea tree oil than from tolnaftate.[2]

CONCEPTS FOR COPING WITH RINGWORM

○ Key to the healing process is avoiding reinfection. To prevent ringworm from reinfecting treated skin and to keep ringworm from spreading from one child to another, be sure to:

- Thoroughly clean brushes, combs, or headgear that may have been infected.
- Wash hands before and after examining your child.
- Keep your child's linens separate from the rest of the family's.

Rosacea

SYMPTOM SUMMARY

Rosacea is an acnelike skin condition without blackheads or whiteheads but characterized by:

○ Papules—pimples or small, rounded bumps rising from the skin that are each usually less than 5 millimeters (0.2 inch) in diameter and which may open when scratched and become crusty and infected

○ Pustules—little pimples full of pus, a mixture of inflammatory cells and liquid

○ Rhinophyma—growth of the nose, leading to a bulbous, enlarged red nose and puffy cheeks

○ Seborrhea—accumulation of scales of greasy skin

○ Telangiectasias—red spots caused by the widening of capillaries and arterioles (small arteries) under the skin

UNDERSTANDING THE DISEASE PROCESS

Rosacea (pronounced rose-ay-shah) is a chronic acnelike disease affecting both the skin of the face and the eyes. As many as 13 million people in North America alone may have the disease. Rosacea typically first appears when people reach their 30s and 40s as a flushing or subtle redness on the cheeks, nose, chin, or forehead. The symptoms of rosacea come and go and may be triggered by consumption of alcohol, hot beverages, or spicy foods.

If left untreated, rosacea tends to worsen over time. As the condition progresses, the redness becomes more persistent. Bumps and pimples called papules and pustules appear, and small, dilated blood vessels may become visible. By the age of 60 the eyes may also be affected, causing them to be irritated and bloodshot. In advanced cases, the nose may become red and swollen from excess tissue—the condition that gave the late comedian W. C. Fields his trademark bulbous nose. Rosacea is more frequently treated in women but occurs with equal frequency in men and women,[1] and in people of all races.[2] Symptoms are recognized at a later stage in persons of African descent. The eyes are affected in about 50 percent of people who have the disease.

Like acne, rosacea seems to be caused by multiple factors. A very large body of scientific research has attempted to link rosacea to the presence of the bacterium *Helicobacter pylori,* which is also implicated as a cause of peptic ulcers. A recent Japanese study found that the microorganism is found in 65 percent of rosacea patients, but in 70 percent of the population as a whole. Nonetheless, an antibody associated with eradication of *Helicobacter pylori* infection was found in 100 percent of patients who completely recovered from rosacea after antibiotic treatment.[3] These confusing results seem to suggest that the bacterium does not cause the disease, but killing the bacterium cures it.

Another large body of scientific investigation has linked rosacea to the house mite *Demodex folliculorum.* This microscopic relative of spiders normally inhabits healthy skin. It feeds on sebum, an oil secreted by the skin. (For a discussion of the function of sebum in healthy skin, see ACNE.) Infestations of *Demodex folliculorum* are probably found in only about 20 percent of people who have rosacea.[4] Eliminating the mite from the skin, however, often cures the disease.[5] Scientists testing laboratory animals in the late 1920s found that the mite only infects riboflavin-deficient skin.[6]

Yet another stream of research has attempted to explain rosacea in terms of facial flushing. The disease is more common in cold climates, where people get red faces from exposure to the weather.[7] Exposure to sun, however, is just as likely to cause rosacea as exposure to cold. Biopsies of rosacea-affected skin frequently show sun damage, in which connective tissues have broken down.[8] These loose tissues do not support the blood vessels of the skin, some scientists reason, and allow inflammatory agents from the immune system to accumulate and cause outbreaks.[9]

Two of the systemic processes that influence acne may be relevant to rosacea, although neither has a conclusive role in the disease. Stress causes microscopic packets in the ends of nerve cells controlling the muscles and skin to break open and release adrenaline and substance P, a chemical that helps nerve signals jump from cell to cell. Once in the bloodstream, substance P eventually reaches the skin and signals the cells that make oils to grow not only in numbers but also in productivity. Under conditions of stress, greatly increased numbers of sebum glands pour out greatly increased amounts of oily sebum into follicles.[10]

Another hormonal process that influences acne and is likely to influence rosacea is insulin resistance. Insulin moves sugar from the bloodstream into cells. When skin cells are unable to respond to insulin, sugar accumulates in the fluid between them and feeds bacteria. The insulin resistance that causes acne is localized to the skin. This condition is a kind of "skin diabetes" that does not result in other complications. People who have inflammatory skin conditions do not generally have systemic problems with blood sugars or full-blown diabetes.[11]

Standard care for rosacea outbreaks consists of round-the-clock antibiotic therapy. The mainstay of medical treatment is tetracycline. When tetracycline is not effective, doxycycline and minocycline are used.

Physicians also frequently recommend tretinoin (Retin-A) for inflammation, although it has no effect on the characteristic red spots (telangiectasias) of the disease and can cause eye irritation. Corticosteroids are also used to treat inflammation, but over a long period of use they also can cause atrophy of connective tissues, dilation of blood vessels in the nose, and telangiectasias. Similar complications result whether the treatments are used for the skin or eyes.

TREATMENT SUMMARY

DIET

○ Avoid alcohol, coffee, spicy foods, and any other food or beverage that causes a facial flush. As often as possible, include the "three Bs" of the rosacea diet: blackberries, blueberries, and buckwheat. Cherries, raspberries, and other dark blue or dark red fruits are also helpful.

NUTRITIONAL SUPPLEMENTS

○ Bioflavonoids with rutin: 500–1,000 milligrams twice a day.

○ Vitamin B complex: 100 milligrams once a day.

○ Vitamin C: 1,000 milligrams per day, if taking rutin.

HERBS

○ Deglycyrrhizinated licorice root (DGL): 380–760 milligrams 20 minutes before meals, 3 times per day.

Other helpful natural products:

○ Alpha hydroxy acids (lotions containing 5–10% glycolic acid).

○ Hydrochloric acid tablets: see "Hydrochloric Acid Supplementation" on page 487.

○ Pancreatic extract (8–10 x USP): 350–500 milligrams before meals.

UNDERSTANDING THE HEALING PROCESS

Facial skin damaged by rosacea requires gentle care. It is particularly important not to "dry out" oily skin. Drying the skin with alcohol or alcohol-based astringents or gels does not eliminate the pus "clogging" the skin follicle. It only tightens the skin and makes the natural elimination of sebum and dead skin cells more difficult. Dry skin ages more quickly and wrinkles at an earlier age.

Medical authorities agree that avoiding all foods and beverages that cause flushing of the face is essential in

Hydrochloric Acid Supplementation

Insufficient stomach acid produces a number of obvious symptoms. There may be:

- Adult acne
- Chronic intestinal parasites
- Chronic yeast infections
- Cracked, peeling, or weak fingernails
- Dilated capillaries in the cheeks and nose
- Frequent gas or bloating
- Iron deficiency
- Undigested food in stool

Supplementation with hydrochloric acid (HCl), however, should only be attempted after evaluation by a naturopathic physician. Most naturopaths test for hypochlorhydria with a Heidelberg pH capsule. In this method, the patient swallows a capsule (which may or may not be tethered with a long string for easy retrieval from the stomach) containing radio telemetry which is monitored through a receiver worn as a waistband. The capsule measures fasting pH and the stomach's ability to produce acid when the patient drinks an alkaline solution. Acidification of the stomach in 5 minutes or less after the patient drinks the alkaline solution indicates hyperchlorhydria (too much acid). Acidification of the stomach requiring 20 minutes or more indicates hypochlorhydria (too little acid). If there is no acidification of the stomach after 2 hours the diagnosis is achlorhydria (no acid). Hypochlorhydria (too little acid) and achlorhydria (no acid) are treated with HCl supplements.

HCl comes in 10-grain tablets. Take 1 tablet before a large meal, increasing the dosage by 1 tablet before meals until a dosage is reached that causes a warm sensation in the stomach. That dosage is increased by 1 capsule and taken with all large meals, reduced by 1 capsule with snacks.

The stomach usually recovers its ability to produce acid after a few weeks of supplementation. As acid production increases, the stomach begins to feel warm again.

The dosage of HCl should be reduced by 1 tablet per meal every 3 days, more rapidly if the warmth continues. If symptoms of poor digestion return, increase dosage by 1 capsule per meal until digestion improves again.

---

rosacea care. Coffee, "hot toddies," and chiles are especially likely to cause redness of the face. Repeated flushing over the face and chest by itself is enough to cause rosacea.[12]

The "three Bs," blackberries, blueberries, and buckwheat, as well as cherries and raspberries, contain biologically active pigments known as bioflavonoids. These compounds are extraordinarily useful in maintaining vascular health. Increasing the integrity of the walls of capillaries and arterioles reduces the risk of rhinophyma.

Blackberries, blueberries, and cherries are especially rich sources of anthocyanidins and proanthocyanidins, the bioflavonoids that give them their blue-red color.[13] Anthocyanidins and proanthocyanidins increase the integrity of the ground substance, the "cement" between blood vessels and soft tissues. They prevent the vasodilation, which causes facial flushes.[14]

Several flavonoids inhibit *Helicobacter pylori*.[15]

O The bioflavonoid prominent in buckwheat, rutin, is especially useful in preventing vasodilation. In one study, buckwheat tea standardized to yield 270 milligrams of rutin was given to 77 patients with varicose veins, a condition in which blood vessels break down in a manner similar to that in rosacea. After 12 weeks, most patients showed a significant reduction in the total volume of the leg, indicating that the veins had strengthened.[16]

Do not take rutin without vitamin C. Although rutin protects vitamin C from oxidation, it also slows the rate at which vitamin C is absorbed by cells. Rutin will interfere with the action of quinolone antibiotics (not to be confused with the anabolic steroid quinolone). Antibiotics that may interact with rutin includes:

- ciprofloxacin (Cipro, Baycip, Cetraxal, Ciflox, Cifran, Ciplox, Cyprobay, Quintor)

- enoxacin (Penetrex)

- gatifloxacin (Tequin)

- gemifloxacin (a relatively new drug)

- grepafloxacin (Raxar)

- levofloxacin (Levaquin)

- lomefloxacin (Maxaquin)

- moxifloxacin (Avelox)

- norfloxacin (Amicrobin, Anquin, Baccidal, Barazan, Biofloxin, Floxenor, Fulgram, Janacin, Lexinor, Norofin, Noroxin, Norxacin, Orixacin, Oroflox, Urinox, Zoroxin)

- ofloxacin (Floxin)

- sparfloxacin (Zagam)

- temafloxacin (Omniflox)

- trovafloxacin (Trovan)

Many naturopathic physicians recommend vitamin B supplements to rosacea patients on the basis of the 1920s study that found that, at least in lab rats, the mite *Demodex folliculorum* only infects riboflavin-deficient skin.[17] Complete vitamin B supplements provide riboflavin balanced with other B vitamins. It is especially important not to overdose, since one of the B vitamins, niacin, can actually cause skin outbreaks similar to rosacea when taken in a dosage exceeding 3,000 milligrams per day. This dosage, however, corresponds to taking more than 30 times the recommended amount of vitamin B complex.

Deglycyrrhizinated licorice root contains several flavonoids that inhibit the multiplication of *Helicobacter pylori* in the stomach.[18]

Alpha hydroxy acids are commonly found and isolated from fruits of all sorts. Exactly how they help control acne is not fully understood, but they function in at least two ways. First, they act as a humectant, increasing the water content of the skin and thus moisturizing the outer layer of the epidermis. This makes the skin softer and more flexible. The second method by which alpha hydroxy acids are thought to act is by reducing skin-cell adhesion and accelerating cell proliferation within the deeper basal layer of the skin. They encourage the growth of blood vessels to oxygenate the skin. They also activate an internal clock at the surface of skin cells reminding them of the time to die and be sloughed off, providing room for the growth of new healthy skin. The growth of skin underneath the follicle forces it open and allows the release of dead skin cells and irritants.[19]

Recognizing which products contain alpha hydroxy acids requires reading the label. Alpha hydroxy acid ingredients may be listed as:

- alpha hydroxy and botanical complex

- alpha hydroxycaprylic acid

- alpha hydroxyethanoic acid + ammonium alpha hydroxyethanoate

- alpha hydroxyoctanoic acid

- citric acid

- glycolic acid

- glycolic acid + ammonium glycolate

- glycomer in cross-linked fatty acids alpha nutrium (3 AHAs).

- hydroxycaprylic acid

- lactic acid

- L-alpha hydroxy acid

- malic acid

- mixed fruit acid

- sugarcane extract

- tri-alpha hydroxy fruit acids

- triple fruit acid

Of these, the most frequently used in cosmetics are glycolic acid and lactic acid.

Naturopathic physicians frequently prescribe hydrochloric acid tablets and pancreas extract for difficult cases of rosacea. The theory behind the use of hydrochloric acid supplementation in rosacea stems from a research finding in 1920 that rosacea patients frequently have low concentrations of hydrochloric acid in the stomach. Stomach acid is depleted in conditions of constant emotional stress. Hydrochloric acid supplementation was found to be helpful to patients who have low concentrations of stomach acid.[20]

Much later research found that rosacea patients tend to lack the pancreatic enzyme lipase.[21] Supplementing with pancreas extracts frequently relieves symptoms. Pancreatic extracts at 8–10 times the strength specified in the USP (US Pharmacopeia) do not have the milk sugars or salt used as fillers in lower-strength products.

Rotator Cuff Tendonitis

SYMPTOM SUMMARY

○ Aching in the top and front of the shoulder or outer side of the upper arm (deltoid muscle)

○ Pain worse when the arm is lifted overhead

○ Pain worse at night

○ Interrupted sleep

○ Arm cannot be lifted forward or outward

○ Weakness in the arm

UNDERSTANDING THE DISEASE PROCESS

The rotator cuff is a group of tendons merged together to encase the front, back, and top of the shoulder joint like a cuff on a shirt sleeve. These tendons are connected individually to muscles that originate from the scapula. When the muscles contract, they pull on the rotator cuff tendon, causing the shoulder to rotate inward, upward, or outward.

Tendinitis is commonly misunderstood to be an inflammatory condition, but the modern understanding of the biology of the disease is that its principal cause is not inflammation.[1] Instead, tendinitis results from the fraying and tangling of fibers of collagen forming the framework of the tendon, and only when the collagen itself is healed does pain stop.[2] Anti-inflammatory treatments such as cortisone and other steroids may relieve pain in surrounding tissues, but they have no effect on the underlying cause of the condition.

Rotator cuff tendinitis commonly results from a breakdown of collagen caused by repetitive throwing, overhead racquet sports, or swimming. As the rotator cuff stretches, the fibers of collagen that make up the tendons tear first and then the tendons as a whole tear. There may be a looseness in the front of the shoulder. There will almost always be pain in the top and front of the shoulder and outside of the upper arm.

TREATMENT SUMMARY

HERBS

For pain relief without aspirin, ibuprofen, or similar medications, select from:

○ Bromelain: 250–500 milligrams 3 times a day.

○ Capsaicin cream: apply to affected area.

○ Devil's claw: 405–520 milligrams up to 8 times a day.

○ Feverfew: 70–100 milligrams of dried extract daily.

○ Ginger (fresh): 2 tablespoons included in vegetable dishes, fruit salad, or used to make a tea.

○ Willow bark: 1 teaspoon in a cup of hot water or tea, as desired.

NUTRITIONAL SUPPLEMENTS

To encourage healing:

○ Vitamin B_6: 200 milligrams daily.

○ Do *not* take supplemental vitamin C unless you also take vitamin B_6.

If swelling is a problem:

○ Pycnogenol creams or lotions: apply to the skin according to label directions, or 200 milligrams of Pycnogenol in capsule form daily.

If you take steroid injections:

○ Glycyrrhizin: 250–500 milligrams daily for up to 6 weeks at a time.

If you take aspirin or NSAIDs on a regular basis:

○ Any B-vitamin supplement: 1 tablet daily.

See Part Three if you take prescription medication.

UNDERSTANDING THE HEALING PROCESS

For most people with rotator cuff tendinitis, the first priority in treatment is relieving pain. There are a number of natural products that offer pain relief. Several other supplements encourage healing. Bromelain can start relieving pain and swelling almost as soon as you start taking it, provided you take it in an enteric-coated form (unavailable in the United States).[3] For those of us who have to take uncoated bromelain tablets, it is best to experiment with the smallest dose and increase by 250 milligrams a day until you reach the highest recommended dose. It may be necessary to take the highest recommended dose of uncoated bromelain for a week before obtaining relief.

Allergies to bromelain are very rare but not unheard of. Allergic reactions to this supplement are most likely in people who are already allergic to pineapple, papaya, wheat flour, rye flour, or birch pollen. There has never been a report of an anaphylactic reaction to bromelain.

There have been isolated reports of heavy periods, nausea, vomiting, and hives when bromelain is taken in very large doses (2,000 milligrams and higher).

Capsaicin is the chemical that gives hot peppers their heat. As anyone who has cooked with chiles knows, capsaicin can cause burning, redness, and inflammation, especially to the eyes and mouth. The first time it is applied in a cream to the skin over a painful shoulder, capsaicin causes these symptoms, but the nerve fibers serving the shoulder become insensitive to it—and to pain.[4]

Capsaicin works best when there is good circulation to the skin to which it is applied.[5] Never apply capsaicin to ulcerated skin. It is also important to keep capsaicin out of your nose and eyes. Allergic reactions to capsaicin are rare but are not unknown, and there have been cases of hypothermia in people who used capsaicin in an especially cold room. It is theoretically possible that capsaicin absorbed into the bloodstream could reduce the bioavailability of aspirin; if you use capsaicin, use pain relievers other than aspirin. If you are sensitive to capsaicin, diluted essential oils of peppermint, eucalyptus, rosemary, or wintergreen may be used instead. Never take essential oils internally.

Devil's claw relieves tendon pain, but only if it is taken in an enteric-coated form that protects its analgesic compounds from being digested in the stomach. Do not use devil's claw with NSAIDs such as aspirin and Tylenol, and avoid it entirely if you have duodenal or gastric ulcers.

Like other herbs to relieve pain, feverfew can cause stomach irritation. Do not use it with NSAIDs and avoid it if you have ulcers.

Two tablespoons of fresh ginger every day is likely to relieve pain and swelling even when pain relievers are discontinued, but the effect takes 1–3 months.

Willow bark is a natural substitute for aspirin. It contains salicin, a less potent pain reliever than the salicylates found in aspirin and one that does not generally cause bleeding or stomach irritation. Do not use willow bark during pregnancy, if you have tinnitus (ringing in the ears), or if you are allergic to aspirin. Do not give willow bark or aspirin to children who have colds or flu.

The only nutritional supplement with a probable effect on the disease process of rotator cuff tendinitis itself is vitamin B_6. This vitamin has little effect on the function of the tendon, but is useful in relieving pain.[6] The *balance* between vitamin B_6 and vitamin C in the bloodstream may be more important in a similar condition, carpal tunnel syndrome (CTS). In a study of 441 adults with CTS, higher ratios of vitamin C to vitamin B_6 (such as might occur when taking supplemental vitamin C without vitamin B_6) were associated with the severity of pain and the frequency of pain, tingling, and waking up at night.[7]

Most of the research studies involving vitamin B_6 used a dosage of 200 milligrams daily. This dosage is too much for pregnant women and nursing mothers, who should limit intake to 100 milligrams per day. There have been only a few cases in which taking 100–200 milligrams of B_6 a day aggravated existing nerve damage. Diabetics also should only use more than 100 milligrams per day if they do not suffer sensory neuropathy, that is, nerve damage to the hands and feet. Men who use sildenafil citrate (Viagra) should avoid high doses of this vitamin for the same reason.

Vitamin B_6 requirements are affected by many medications. The use of oral contraceptives increases vitamin B_6 requirements. The vitamin is depleted during treatment with carbamazepine for bipolar disorder; cycloserine or ethionamide for tuberculosis; hydralazine for high blood pressure; penicillamine for arthritis, Wilson's disease, and certain skin conditions; and phenelzine for cocaine addiction, eating disorders, headaches, and panic attacks. If you take any of these prescription drugs and have rotator cuff tendinitis, you should take supplemental vitamin B_6. On the other hand, if you take levodopa for Parkinson's disease, theophylline for asthma, or phenytoin or valproic acid for seizures, you should not take vitamin B_6 supplements, since the vitamin can deactivate these medications. Regardless of the medications you take, if you experience abdominal pain, loss of appetite, nausea, vomiting, breast pain, or unexplained sensitivity to the sun, discontinue use of the vitamin.

While Pycnogenol has no effect on the underlying disease process, it may help relieve swelling. Pycnogenol contains oligomeric procyanidins and oligomericproanthocyanidins (OPCs) that stop inflammation secondary to an immune process triggered by the destruction of collagen.[8] These chemicals also help the walls of capillaries retain their strength and elasticity, making it less likely that they will leak fluids into the muscles and cause swelling.

Because Pycnogenol helps the body retain vitamin C, and an imbalance between vitamin C and vitamin B_6 is an underling cause of this condition, you should not take both Pycnogenol and supplemental vitamin C.

Also, if you are a smoker taking an anticoagulant drug such as Coumadin (warfarin) or any drug for frostbite, do not take Pycnogenol. Aside from these rare instances, Pycnogenol is generally safe and free of side effects.

If you are taking injections of steroids to relieve pain, a licorice derivative called glycyrrhizin can help make them more effective. It increases the half-life of cortisol and other steroids, making them work longer to undo the damage done to your joints.[9] The downside of using glycyrrhizin for this purpose is that it *will* increase any side effects you experience from cortisone. When you take both glycyrrhizin and any corticosteroid drug, you are more likely to experience weight gain, puffiness, and elevated blood pressure. Do not take glycyrrhizin for more than 6 weeks at a time. Preferably, take it during your peak allergy season. Do not take glycyrrhizin if you have high blood pressure. DGL is another licorice derivative that does not aggravate side effects of steroid treatment, but it will not help rotator cuff tendinitis.

The B vitamins thiamine, pyridoxine, and cobalamin (B_1, B_6, and B_{12}) make it possible to use lower doses of aspirin and other nonsteroidal anti-inflammatory agents for the same degree of pain relief.[10] Lowering doses of aspirin or NSAIDs reduces stomach upset. Vitamin B supplements may be especially useful for sufferers of back pain who take the diuretic furosemide (Lasix) or who are heavy drinkers of coffee or tea. The drawback to using B vitamins is that they reduce, rather than elimini-ate, the need for pain relievers. B vitamins enhance nerve function so that if the vitamins are taken for 3 days and the aspirin or NSAIDs are eliminated entirely, pain worsens.[11] Do not discontinue aspirin or NSAIDs without also discontinuing vitamin B.

CONCEPTS FOR COPING WITH ROTATOR CUFF TENDINITIS

O During an acute attack of rotator cuff pain, a cold pack can reduce inflammation by constricting blood vessels and bringing swelling down. A flexible gel pack available from pharmacies, a plastic bag filled with ice, or even a package of frozen vegetables can be placed against your wrist for 10 minutes at a time to stop pain. Wrapping the cold pack in a towel can minimize dis-comfort to your skin.

O Many people get relief of pain from acupuncture. One to 2 weeks before beginning acupuncture for back pain, start taking 500 milligrams of DL-phenylalanine 2– 3 times a day. DL-phenylalanine increases the analgesic effect of acupuncture in both laboratory tests with ani-mals and in clinical trials.[12]

O DMSO (dimethyl sulfoxide) applied to the skin can relieve pain, although it is important to note that weak-er solutions (70%) offer greater pain relief than stronger solutions (the more usual 90%). DMSO works like a fast-acting vitamin C. In as little as 30 seconds after applica-tion, the bloodstream carries DMSO to the joints, where it protects hyaluronic acid, one of the components of collagen, from damage by free radicals.[13] This possibly keeps cartilage from being destroyed or helps new car-tilage form.[14] DMSO can dissolve any toxin on the skin and send it into circulation throughout the body in under 30 seconds. Industrial-grade DMSO, the form most commonly sold in flea markets, can contain toxic byproducts of the manufacturing process and should not be applied to the skin. MSM (methylsulfonylmeth-ane) is a byproduct of DMSO as it is metabolized by the body, that is also found in alfalfa sprouts, corn, most fruits, tomatoes, coffee, tea, and milk. MSM is also used to treat arthritic pain, and unlike DMSO, is almost com-pletely nontoxic. Most naturopaths recommend 1,000–2,000 milligrams of MSM daily to prevent osteoarthritis pain and 3,000–5,000 milligrams of MSM daily to treat osteoarthritis pain.

O Gentle exercise can relieve pain and prevent further injury to your rotator cuff. Here are four key examples and the movements that can help you visualize them:

• This exercise imitates catching a baseball, only you are lying face down. Stretch out on your stomach on a table or a bed. Put your left arm out at shoulder lev-el with your elbow bent to 90 degrees and your hand down. Keeping your elbow bent, slowly raise your left hand. Stop when your hand is level with your shoul-der. Lower your hand slowly. Repeat the exercise until your left arm is tired. Then do the whole exercise again with your right arm.

• This exercise imitates the backhand swing in ten-nis. Lie on your right side and place a rolled-up tow-el under your right armpit. Stretch your right arm above your head. Put your left arm at your side with your elbow bent to 90 degrees. Then roll your left shoulder out, raising the left forearm until it is level with your shoulder. Lower the arm slowly. Repeat the exercise until your arm is tired. Then do the whole exercise again with your right arm.

• This exercise imitates the forehand swing in tennis. Lie down on your right side. Keep your left arm along the upper side of your body. Bend your right elbow to 90 degrees. Keep the right forearm resting on the table. Then roll your right shoulder in, raising your right forearm up to your chest. Lower the forearm slowly. Repeat the exercise until your arm is tired. Then do the whole exercise again with your left arm.

• This exercise imitates emptying a trash can. In a standing position, start with your right arm halfway between the front and the side of your body, thumb down. Raise your right arm until almost level (about a 45-degree angle). *Don't lift beyond the point of pain.* Slowly lower your arm. Repeat the exercise until your arm is tired. Then do the whole exercise again with your left arm.

❍ Keep repeating each exercise until your arm is tired. Use a light enough weight that you don't get tired until you've done the exercise about 20–30 times, beginning with a weight of 2 ounces (50–60 grams) the first week, 4 ounces (110–120 grams) the second week, and so on. Each time you complete a set of all 4 exercises, place an ice pack on your shoulder for 20 minutes. A "lumpy" ice pack such as a plastic baggie filled with ice cubes or a package of frozen peas is more effective than a gel pack. Doing all 4 exercises 3–5 times a week will help your shoulder gain strength as it forms new collagen, and enable you to regain strength over a period of months.

❍ Daily use of TENS (transcutaneous electrical nerve stimulation) for 1–2 weeks reduces or eliminates pain in patients with tendinitis. TENS is widely available in the United States from physical therapists and massage therapists, and at some sports clubs.

❍ Ultrasound therapy is widely and successfully used as a nonsurgical treatment for tendon pain. Extracorporeal sound wave therapy (ESWT), involves focusing sound blasts to the area of pain. The treatment is being used in Canada and Europe to treat chronic pain or pain over a small area, particularly near a bone. The joint pain treated by this system includes the shoulder, elbow, ankle, and, knee. ESWT or Sonocur is not approved for use in the United States or Japan.

SAD
See **Seasonal Affective Disorder (SAD)**.

Sarcoidosis

SYMPTOM SUMMARY

❍ Shortness of breath

❍ Cough

❍ Generalized joint pain

❍ Rashes

UNDERSTANDING THE DISEASE PROCESS

Sarcoidosis is a condition of joint and lung inflammation caused by overactive T cells, white blood cells orchestrating the immune system's response to disease. Immune-mediated inflammation causes fibrosis and the formation of small tumors known as granulomas in various organs, most typically the lungs, but sometimes the joints.

In the United States, sarcoidosis is most frequent in two ethnic groups, African-Americans and Swedish-Americans. It is most commonly diagnosed in men aged 25–35, although the second most frequently diagnosed group is women aged 55–65. In general, sarcoidosis appears briefly and heals naturally in 70 percent of the cases, often without the patient knowing or doing anything about it. In a minority of cases, sarcoidosis may cause permanent lung damage. Symptoms may disappear and reappear.

TREATMENT SUMMARY

NUTRITIONAL SUPPLEMENTS

❍ Iodine: 300 milligrams per day.

UNDERSTANDING THE HEALING PROCESS

There is a clinical study in which 300 milligrams of iodine in the form of potassium iodide, 3 times a day, offered patients with sarcoidosis rapid (48-hour) relief from swelling and skin inflammation association with the disease.[1] This dosage of iodine is not likely to have any detrimental side effects, but should be avoided by anyone with any form of hyperthyroidism.

CONCEPTS FOR COPING WITH SARCOIDOSIS

❍ Since sarcoidosis is caused by overactive T cells, herbs that stimulate the activity of T cells, especially echinacea and baptisia, must be avoided.

○ Try avoiding Brussels sprouts, broccoli, cabbage, cauliflower, rutabaga, and soy in your diet. These vegetables contain compounds that interfere with the metabolism of iodine, and could aggravate symptoms of the disease.

Schizophrenia

SYMPTOM SUMMARY

○ Delusions (beliefs held despite evidence to the contrary)

○ Hallucinations (usually hearing, sometimes seeing, things that do not physically exist)

○ Loss of appetite

○ Social withdrawal

○ Loss of hygiene

○ Sense of being controlled from the outside

UNDERSTANDING THE DISEASE PROCESS

Schizophrenia is a collection of illnesses that cause similar symptoms: delusions, hallucinations, loss of a sense of control, and their corresponding behaviors, withdrawal from family and friends, loss of hygiene, and loss of appetite. People with schizophrenia vary greatly in their conduct as they struggle to deal with the disease. Catatonic schizophrenics experience disorders of movement, keeping themselves perfectly still or moving around aimlessly, saying nothing or repeating nonsense sentences. Disorganized schizophrenics tend to be disconnected from events around them, as evidenced by laughing inappropriately at, for instance, a blinking VCR light or at a serious comment in conversation. They may lose their ability to maintain personal hygiene, dress, and eat regularly. Paranoid schizophrenics may believe themselves to be extraordinarily significant or extraordinarily insignificant in society, and tend to hear and see events and objects others do not. Paranoid schizophrenics are frequently angry, aloof, or anxious. Undifferentiated schizophrenics may exhibit tendencies of all the other types.

TREATMENT SUMMARY

DIET

○ Dairy- and gluten-free diet, if indicated.

NUTRITIONAL SUPPLEMENTS

○ Fish oil: 2 grams per day.

UNDERSTANDING THE HEALING PROCESS

Because schizophrenia is a collection of diseases, responses to nutritional interventions vary greatly. Clinical studies tell us that simply identifying a nutritional deficiency and treating it with megadoses of vitamins almost never works.[1] When nutritional changes do help, however, the results are sometimes spectacular. Here are a few interventions that have resulted in success.

Some psychiatrists theorize that at least some cases of schizophrenia result from an interaction of genetic factors and an overload of peptides from the digestion of proteins in casein and gluten, that is, primarily dairy products and wheat.[2] When schizophrenic symptoms are associated with chronic diarrhea and weight loss, there is at least a possibility that they signal a complication of celiac disease. In at least some cases, removing dairy products and all sources of gluten results in complete remission of symptoms.[3] A simple saliva test can tell you whether a dairy- and gluten-free diet would help. If a schizophrenic's saliva tests positive for antibodies to gliadin, a dairy- and gluten-free diet is likely to effect drastic improvement in symptoms. For information, ask your physician to contact Great Smokies Diagnostic Laboratory in Asheville, North Carolina, 1-800-252-9303. (Also see CELIAC DISEASE.)

Another promising nutritional intervention for schizophrenia is fish oil. Most of the current research focuses on giving fish oil to schizophrenics who take conventional antipsychotic medications. Among schizophrenics treated with clozapine, the most effective dose for relief of symptoms is 2 grams per day—higher doses are not helpful. In a British clinical trial, taking 2 grams of fish oil per day with clozapine resulted in improvement in all psychiatric measures for the severity of the disease.[4]

For schizophrenics not treated with antipsychotic medication, a dose of 3 grams a day is not effective.[5] However, a large dosage, 10 grams a day, has helped some schizophrenics who do not respond to other medications.

Other sources of essential fatty acids, such as evening primrose oil, do not have a beneficial effect.[6] A daily dose of 2 grams of fish oil is not likely to cause side effects, but 10 grams can cause fishy burps and diarrhea. This effect is eliminated by using highly refined fish oils. Fish oils are especially useful for schizophrenic women who are pregnant.

CONCEPTS FOR COPING WITH SCHIZOPHRENIA

○ There are reports of individual recoveries after taking large doses (up to 100 times the RDA) of B vitamins, vitamin C, glycine, and serine. If a desirable response to fish oil is not achieved, test any one of these supplements for 1 month, continuing if symptoms improve:

• Folic acid: 15 milligrams per day. Schizophrenic symptoms due to folic acid deficiency are most likely to occur in the elderly, especially those maintained on diuretic medications such as furosemide (Lasix). Folic acid should not be taken at this dosage with SSRIs for depression, that is, Luvox, Paxil, Prozac, or Zoloft. Theoretically, "manic" symptoms could result.

• Glycine: 10 grams per day. The problem with using glycine is that the clinical studies that got the best results used very large dosages, roughly 1 gram per pound of body weight, that could cause nerve damage over a period of months of years. The 10-gram dosage will not cause nerve damage and is the lowest that has produced benefits in treating schizophrenia. Overdoses of glycine will produce drastic reductions in pulse rate before causing other symptoms.

• Serine: Up to 3 grams per day. Serine modulates the brain's use of glycine. Several small-scale trials have found that supplementation with serine reduces symptoms of schizophrenia, especially hyperactivity, but schizophrenics who respond to clozapine are not likely to respond to serine.

• Vitamin B_6: 100 milligrams per day. Responses to vitamin B_6 range from nothing to complete remission. It is most likely to be helpful for schizophrenics who have alcohol abuse problems.

• Vitamin C: 6–8 grams per day. One small trial found that schizophrenics on other medications experienced reduction in hallucinations and paranoid delusions when given 8 grams of vitamin C per day. A dosage of 6 grams combined with 400 IU of vitamin E produced similar results. However, this high dose of vitamin C can cause diarrhea in which case it must be discontinued gradually, reducing the dosage of vitamin C to 7 grams a day the first week, 6 grams a day the second week, and so on, to avoid vitamin C deficiency symptoms.

○ When a person with schizophrenia tells you he or she wants to kill himself or herself or some other person, take the statement literally and seek emergency help.

○ Facial tics and twisting muscles are often the result of tardive dyskinesia, a complication of drug treatment for schizophrenia. Fortunately, tardive dyskinesia often responds to nutritional intervention. See TARDIVE DYSKINESIA.

Scleroderma

SYMPTOM SUMMARY

○ "Puffiness" or "salt and pepper" coloration in the skin of the hands, followed by:

• Hardening
• Inability to make a skin fold
• Loss of hair
• Loss of sweat glands
• Shiny appearance
• Swelling
• Tightness
• Similar symptoms on forearms, elbows, knees, and face

○ General joint pain

○ Morning stiffness

○ Loss of lung capacity

○ Heartburn due to decreased pressure on the esophagus

○ Fecal incontinence

○ Renal crisis

UNDERSTANDING THE DISEASE PROCESS

The term scleroderma is derived from two Greek words meaning "hard skin." Scleroderma causes the thickening, hardening, and cracking of the skin of the fingers and sometimes the face, neck, and trunk. As the disease progresses, hardened collagen is deposited throughout the body, causing particular distress in the lungs and kidneys. The underlying cause of scleroderma is autoimmunity, misdirected activity of the immune system.

TREATMENT SUMMARY

NUTRITIONAL SUPPLEMENTS

○ Para-aminobenzoic acid (PABA): used under medical supervision.

UNDERSTANDING THE HEALING PROCESS

In a clinical study, 90 percent of 224 patients treated with 12 grams of para-aminobenzoic acid (PABA) a day developed mild, moderate, or marked skin softening. In the study, no side effects were observed.[1] Since this dosage of PABA can cause anorexia, nausea, or vomiting, consult your physician before taking the supplement. Your physician may recommend a salt of PABA, potassium para-aminobenzoate, as a prescription medication covered by insurance. As a side effect, graying hair may regain its normal color.

CONCEPTS FOR COPING WITH SCLERODERMA

○ Skin hardened by scleroderma sometimes responds to DMSO. Be forewarned that skin irritation and a strong, garliclike taste in the mouth are common complications. Using DMSO when you are taking the arthritis drug sulindac (Clinoril in the United States, Apo-Sulin or Nu-Sulindac in Canada) can result in permanent nerve damage to the hands.

Seasonal Affective Disorder (SAD)

SYMPTOM SUMMARY

○ Depression beginning in autumn or winter and lifting in the spring

○ Decreased interest in work or significant personal activities

○ Increased sleep, need to sleep during the day

○ Lack of energy

○ Slow, sluggish, languid movement

○ Slumps in the afternoon with decreased energy and concentration

○ Social withdrawal

○ Sugar cravings

○ Weight gain

UNDERSTANDING THE DISEASE PROCESS

Seasonal affective disorder (SAD) is a condition in which a natural tendency to "hibernate" during the winter becomes disruptive to daily activities and well-being. Especially at locations north or south of 45° latitude, susceptible individuals feel depressed, slow down, oversleep, overeat, and crave carbohydrates. In the summer, the same individuals feel active, energetic, and elated.

Generally winter depression is not as severe a disorder as nonseasonal depression. Nonetheless, some people will become totally unable to function, and suicide is not unknown. Most people with SAD continue to be able to work, just not as creatively or efficiently. They are still able to interact socially. They just prefer not to.

The obvious cause of SAD is deprivation of light. Simply exposing the skin to light greatly relieves symptoms. The mediating factors in the condition, however, are highly complex.

One of the contributing causes of the condition is low levels of thyroid hormone. Studies of scientists spending the winter in Antarctica found that falling levels of the thyroid hormones T_3 and T_4 preceded the onset of anger, confusion, and depression. Mental disturbance itself caused a lowering of thyroid hormone levels, establishing a vicious feedback loop.[1] The fluctuations in thyroid hormone levels that contribute to SAD take place in the brain itself, and are not easily detected by blood tests.[2]

The relationship between mood and food intake in SAD is also complex. Contrary to expectation, studies at the National Institute of Mental Health in Bethesda, Maryland have found that people with SAD have unusually high metabolic rates rather than unusually low metabolic rates.[3] Moreover, sugar cravings in SAD do not fill the same role as sugar cravings in nonseasonal depression. Most forms of depression are related to a deficiency of the brain chemical serotonin, a renewable hormone that makes it possible for electrical messages to jump from one neuron to another in the brain. The more serotonin, the more brain activity, and the better the mood. The brain (and the digestive tract) make serotonin from the amino acid tryptophan, which enters the brain more readily when blood sugar levels are high. In this way, sugar is a self-medication for depression. However, in SAD, there is no shortage of tryptophan in the brain.[4]

What some scientists think triggers "the munchies" in SAD is an abnormality peculiar to SAD patients in the hormonal regulation of the production of a brain chemical known as neuropeptide Y. This chemical stimulates appetite. Neuropeptide Y is in part regulated by stress hormones such as norepinephrine. In both men and women with SAD, the body produces relatively little norepinephrine but relatively large amounts of insulin. Insulin moves sugar out of the bloodstream and into cells. If there are high levels of insulin in the bloodstream, the body's first response is to produce stress hormones that release sugars from storage in the liver. This response is blunted in people with SAD. The body's second response to high levels of insulin is to stimulate the appetite for carbohydrates so that sugar levels are maintained. To do this, the brain produces massive amounts of neuropeptide Y and sugar cravings follow. The effect is even greater in women who have low levels of available estrogen.[5]

TREATMENT SUMMARY

DIET

❍ Avoid dietary fats as much as possible. Substitute whole grains for white breads and fructose for white sugar whenever possible. Avoid corn, potatoes, raisins, and puffed rice, as well as sugar-sweetened foods.

NUTRITIONAL SUPPLEMENTS

❍ Chromium: 200–400 micrograms per day.

❍ Vitamin B_{12}: 1.5 milligrams per day.

❍ Melatonin may be helpful if insomnia is a problem. *Do not take melatonin during daytime hours.*

HERBS

❍ St. John's wort: 300 milligrams of solid extract containing 0.3% hypericin, 3 times daily.

UNDERSTANDING THE HEALING PROCESS

The good news about the weight gain caused by SAD is that there is more than one way to correct it. Clinical researchers in the Siberian city of Novosibirsk have determined that either exercise or exposure to sunlight will cause weight loss. The Russian physicians recommended either 1 hour of aerobic exercise or 2 hours of high-intensity light therapy daily in the afternoon; both approaches reduce symptoms.[6] A craving for sweets in the afternoon, however, may indicate that light therapy will produce a rapid and lasting improvement in symptoms.[7] The best treatment for SAD, however, is exercise outdoors in morning light. A unique study undertaken by Swiss researchers found that daily 1-hour morning walks were twice as effective as low-dose artificial light therapy in relieving the symptoms of SAD.[8]

In most people, eating fatty foods activates pathways in the brain that give a feeling of satiety. In people with SAD, eating fatty foods stimulates production of neuropeptide Y and actually increases appetite.[9] Avoiding simple sugars and emphasizing complex carbohydrates and fructose reduces blood sugar levels which in turn lowers insulin levels, reducing food cravings, at least in people with type 2 diabetes, and probably in general.[10]

Supplemental chromium increases insulin sensitivity.[11] This in turn lowers the production of the appetite stimulant neuropeptide Y. Chromium supplementation is especially beneficial in elderly persons.[12]

Vitamin B_{12} has been shown to influence melatonin secretion.[13] Melatonin supplements of as little as 0.1–0.3 gram per day, taken at bedtime, will be helpful if insomnia is a problem.[14]

The benefits of St. John's wort are enhanced by light therapy. A double-blind study in which patients with SAD were given 900 milligrams of standardized St. John's wort and either bright (3,000 lux) or low-intensity (300 lux) light therapy found that both groups of patients improved, although the effects were greater in the high-intensity light treatment group.[15]

St. John's wort does not act on the biochemical pathways specifically involved in SAD, but instead works on general pathways associated with depression. Combining St. John's wort with drugs in the Prozac family (SSRIs) might raise serotonin too much and cause a number of serious problems.[16,17] Wait at least 4 weeks after taking Prozac, Paxil, or Zoloft before taking St. John's wort.

St. John's wort decreases the effectiveness of amitriptyline (for depression and diabetic neuropathy), coumarin or warfarin (given to patients after heart attack or stroke), cyclosporine (for transplant patients), digoxin (for congestive heart failure), oral contraceptives, and protease inhibitors used to treat HIV. It may react badly with some of the newer medications for schizophrenia, including clozapine and olanzapine. If you take St. John's wort and Feldene, Prevacid, Prilosec, or any of the sulfa drugs, exercise caution using light therapies, since the combination of any of these drugs with St. John's wort increases the sensitivity of the skin to light. There is a case report of severe and unexpected burning in an individual who used St. John's wort and then received ultraviolet therapy for psoriasis.[18]

Do not rely on St. John's wort to treat severe depression. If you experience thoughts of suicide, or are unable to continue work or personal activities, seek professional help.

CONCEPTS FOR COPING WITH SEASONAL AFFECTIVE DISORDER

O Exercise, 1 hour per day for 4 weeks, at a pace elevating the pulse to 50 percent of maximum, if your doctor approves. Shorter periods of less vigorous exercise will have lesser effect. *Avoid exercise during nighttime hours.*

O Replace standard light bulbs with full-spectrum light bulbs.

O Sit 3 feet away for a full-spectrum light therapy device (such as Vitalite) for up to 6 hours a day, preferably in session in the early morning and late afternoon, coinciding with the times of *summer* sunrise and sunset. Glance at the light as frequently as possible. Do *not* use light therapy during the hours corresponding to nighttime in the summer months, generally before 5 A.M. or after 9 P.M. in the northern United States.

O Exposure to artificial light, especially the green band of wavelengths of approximately 540 nanometers, at any time during the night reduces the body's production of melatonin. Since the body expects winter nights to be 14 hours long or longer, almost everyone experiences melatonin deprivation during the winter months.[19] Exposure to bright light tricks the body into acting as if it is summer, expecting the nights to be short, and reducing the period in which melatonin breaks down. Glancing at the light from time to time, as often as once a minute, intensifies the effect.

O The antidepressant effect of light therapy is probably due to restoring the proper balance of synthesis and secretion of melatonin in the pineal gland.[20]

O About 80 percent of people with SAD are "phase-delayed," that is, they do not feel sleepy until late at night and then have trouble getting up in the morning. SAD sufferers in this group benefit most from light therapy in the morning hours, between 5 and 8 A.M. About 20 percent of people with SAD are "phase-advanced," that is, they feel energetic in the morning but their energy levels steadily decline after noon. SAD sufferers in this second group benefit from light therapy between 3 and 7 P.M.

O Avoid the use of electric blankets. Research with laboratory animals indicates that the electromagnetic field generated by an electric blanket is sufficient to reduce production of melatonin.[21]

O Exercise is clinically proven to relieve SAD, but patients who crave sweets in the afternoon and evening hours should also receive light therapy. Best results are obtained when exercise periods are at least 1 hour per day, but lesser amounts of exercise will also be beneficial.

Seborrheic Dermatitis

SYMPTOM SUMMARY

O Absence of itching

O Erythema (abnormal redness caused by capillary congestion) and scaly eruptions on the scalp and neck

O Intertrigo (chafing) on the groin and neck

O Oily skin and/or skin flakes resembling dandruff

O Worse in winter

UNDERSTANDING THE DISEASE PROCESS

Seborrheic dermatitis is a chronic inflammation of the upper layers of the skin. It causes scales on the scalp, face, and neck and chafing elsewhere on the body. It may be associated with either oily or dry skin, or both. The scales may be yellowish and either oily or dry, and they may coalesce to form large patches with distinct borders.

The condition occurs either in infancy, usually in babies between 2 and 12 weeks old, or in middle age, and recurs throughout life. In newborns the condition is known as cradle cap. Skin chafed by seborrheic dermatitis in both infants and adults is especially vulnerable to yeast infection.

Newborns with cradle cap might get a persistent diaper rash, scales behind their ears, or red bumps on their faces. Older children with seborrheic dermatitis usually develop a patchy rash producing skin flakes. In adults, the condition starts gradually. The first symptom may be flaking similar to dandruff, except the flakes are yellow rather than white. There is inflammation, itch, and burning on the scalp, and hair loss may ensue. There may be oily or inflamed skin on the bridge of the nose, around the nose, on the eyebrows, on the skin behind the years, or on the chest and back.

Seborrheic dermatitis is usually worse in the winter. The cause of the condition is unknown. Nutrient deficiencies, stress, hormones, and yeast infection are all likely factors in the disease, but no one factor is known to be the single cause of the condition. The observation that about 40 percent of AIDS patients suffer seborrheic dermatitis,[1] however, suggests that yeast infection is a common cause of the condition.

TREATMENT SUMMARY

DIET

○ Avoid excessive protein intake (more than 6 servings of protein foods daily). In addition, eat 3 ounces of cold-water fish 3 times weekly, or take 1 tablespoon per day of flaxseed or hempseed oil.

NUTRITIONAL SUPPLEMENTS

○ Biotin: 3 milligrams 2 times a day.

○ Folic acid: 4–5 milligrams per day.

○ Vitamin B complex: 100 milligrams daily.

○ Zinc picolinate: 25 milligrams per day while taking folic acid.

HERBS

○ Aloe: apply any *Aloe vera* gel liberally once a day.

○ Dandelion (*Taraxacum officinale*): any of the following 3 forms and dosages, 3 times a day:

- Dried extract (4:1): 250–500 milligrams.
- Dried root: 4 grams.
- Fluid extract (1:1): 4–8 milliliters.

○ *Kami-shoyo-san:* take the dosage recommended on the label of any these products based on this Kampo formula.

- Bupleurum & Peony Formula (Lotus Classics, Qualiherb, Sun Ten)
- Free and Easy Wanderer Plus (Golden Flower)
- Jia Wei Xiao Yao San (Lotus Classics, Qualiherb, Sun Ten)

- Kami-shoyo-san (Tsumura)
- Kampo4WomenMindEase (Honso)

OTHER HELPFUL NATURAL TREATMENTS

○ Honey: crude honey diluted with a small amount of warm water, left on seborrheic skin for 3 hours at a time, applied daily.

○ Pyridoxine ointment: can be prepared by any pharmacy, 50 milligrams of pyridoxine per gram of ointment in a water-soluble base.

UNDERSTANDING THE HEALING PROCESS

Seborrheic dermatitis is a condition in which the skin craves normal moisture. Applying a moisturizing cream of any kind, whether medicated or not, usually helps the condition.[2] It is particularly important not to attempt to "dry out" oily skin. Drying the skin with alcohol or alcohol-based astringents or gels does not eliminate the pus "clogging" the skin follicle. It only tightens the skin and makes the natural elimination of sebum and dead skin cells more difficult. Dry skin ages more quickly and wrinkles at an earlier age.

Many medications cause seborrheic dermatitis as a side effect. These include dopamine for Parkinson's disease, hydralazine for congestive heart failure and high blood pressure, isoniazid (INH) for tuberculosis, penicillamine for kidney stones, rheumatoid arthritis, and Wilson's disease, and oral contraceptives.

There is long-held belief in naturopathic medicine that excessive protein consumption, especially of fatty meats and eggs, aggravates skin conditions. It is possible that incomplete digestion of proteins or poor intestinal absorption of protein breakdown products results in elevated levels of certain amino acids in the bowels. Bacteria in the bowel metabolize these amino acids into cadaverine, putrescine, and spermidine. These compounds enter the bloodstream and remove a biochemical "brake" on skin-cell growth.[3] Multiplying, unchecked, affected skin cells coalesce into rashes and produce excessive amounts of sebum.

While this theory is unproved in the case of seborrheic dermatitis, limiting the consumption of fatty meats and eggs is of general benefit to health. Supplementing the diet with cold-water fish 3 times a week or taking a tablespoon of flaxseed or hempseed oil daily counteracts another effect of excessive protein consumption, the inflammatory arachidonic acid cascade.[4]

Seborrheic dermatitis in infants is greatly influenced by supplementation with biotin. A large part of the body's supply of this vitamin is produced by bacteria in the colon, which have not had a chance to be established in very young children. Supplemental biotin given to infants or taken by nursing mothers is effective against cradle cap.[5] In adults, however, biotin by itself is of no value in treating the condition.

Adults are more responsive to vitamin B supplements. Experimentally induced vitamin B_2 (riboflavin) deficiency produces drying and flaking of the skin and dandruff.[6] Supplementation with vitamin B_{12} (cyanocobalamin) is helpful in oily seborrheic dermatitis, although oral vitamin B_{12} supplements do not relieve drying and flaking. (Injections of vitamin B_{12}, available from your doctor, may be helpful.)

Folic acid supplementation is helpful for oily seborrhea. It is of little value in preventing dandruff.[7] Since folic acid may interfere with the absorption of *zinc,* take 25 milligrams of zinc picolinate daily while taking folic acid.

The gel from the leaves of the aloe (*Aloe vera*) plant is a proven remedy for skin damage of all kinds. In a 1999 study, 44 adults with seborrheic dermatitis applied either an aloe ointment or a placebo cream to affected areas twice daily for 4–6 weeks. A majority of those who used aloe reported that their symptoms improved significantly (62 percent versus 25 in the placebo group). Researchers determined that those using aloe had a significant decrease in scaliness, itching, and number of affected areas.[8]

Dandelion (*Taraxacum officinale*) is a rich source of choline, an important nutrient for the liver and an important cofactor for vitamin B_{12}.

The traditional Japanese herbal remedy *kami-shoyo-san* is frequently recommended for women who experience seborrhea after menopause. Traditional East Asian medicine teaches that the formula is best suited for women who experience fatigue, painful tension of the shoulder and neck muscles, anxiety, insomnia, constipation, and/or missed or scanty periods.

CONCEPTS FOR COPING WITH SEBORRHEIC DERMATITIS

O In the treatment of seborrheic dermatitis, honey is an ointment rather than a food. Honey has antifungal, antibacterial, and antioxidant properties. A study of the use honey in the treatment of seborrheic dermatitis conducted in the United Arab Emirates involved 30 patients with chronic lesions on the scalp, face, and chest. Twenty patients were male and 10 were female. All the participants in the study suffered itching and hair loss as well as scaling and dry white plaques with crusts and fissures.

Half of the patients were asked to apply diluted crude honey (90% honey diluted in warm water) every other day on the lesions with gentle rubbing for 2–3 minutes. The honey was left for 3 hours before gentle rinsing with warm water. Patients were followed for 4 weeks. They were examined daily for itching, scaling, hair loss, and lesions. All of the patients who used honey showed a significant response. Itching was relieved and scaling had disappeared within 1 week. Skin lesions had healed and disappeared completely within 2 weeks. In addition, patients who used honey reported reversal of hair loss.

After the end of the 4-week test period, all of the patients were instructed to use honey for 6 months. Fifteen complied. None of the patients who continued to use honey relapsed, while 12 out of 15 patients who did not continue to use honey experienced a return of the lesions 2–4 months after stopping treatment.[9]

O Treatment with pyridoxine (vitamin B_6) creams is helpful in treating seborrhea that causes greasy scales on the face. In one study, all patients with these symptoms who took a pyridoxine cream cleared completely within 10 days. The creams were not helpful, however, for seborrheic dermatitis complicated by infection, and did not clear lesions on the neck, chest, or groin.[10]

Senile Dementia
See **Alzheimer's Disease**.

Shingles

SYMPTOM SUMMARY

O Initially causes tingling, itchiness, or shooting pain, within the dermatome, a nerve cell of the face, neck, or trunk infected by the virus, *followed 48–72 hours later by:*

○ Eruption of maculopapular lesions (rashes in which some bumps are filled with pus and others are not) tracing the path of the nerve, *which quickly develop into*

○ Vesicles filled with eosinophils (white blood cells containing granules of inflammatory chemicals) and cloudy pus

○ In severe cases eosinophil-filled vesicles surrounded by locally infected bleeding capillaries and accompanied by *zoster-associated pain* ranging from mild itching to intense pain at the height of inflammation

○ Complications, such as postherpetic neuralgia, possible in persons over the age of 40.

UNDERSTANDING THE DISEASE PROCESS

Shingles (herpes zoster) is an acute and painful infection with the varicella-zoster virus (VZV), the organism that causes chicken pox. Nearly everyone in temperate climates is exposed to the virus by the age of 15, although in many cases it does not cause symptoms.[1] After infection, the virus hides in the ganglion, or "root," of sensory nerves for the face, trunk, and neck. It stays dormant for years, or, more often, decades, until a disturbance to the nerve reactivates the virus.

When the virus is awakened in the nerve, the first symptom is usually a tingling or an itch. Within 48–72 hours the itch becomes persistent deep aching, burning pain, and itch along the course of the affected nerve. The skin over the nerve is covered with rash. In persons with normal immune systems, the skin lesions usually clear up within 7–10 days, although complete healing can take up to 4 weeks. In persons with immune deficiency, the rash covers a much larger area, and healing can take weeks or never be fully achieved.

The bad news about shingles is that the disease can sometimes present devastating complications. The most common complication of shingles is postherpetic neuralgia, persistent pain at the site of inflammation lasting for a month or longer. Studies associated with drug testing claim that up to 50 percent of people who suffer shingles after the age of 60 might develop this complication.[2] One of the most serious complications of shingles occurs when the virus is activated in the trigeminal nerve, lying over the corner of the cheekbone and near the nose. When herpes spreads along this nerve, vascular inflammation and infection affect the eye and can even cause blindness. Open skin can be superinfected with *Streptococcus* and/or *Staphylococcus* bacteria causing cellullitis, bone infections, and lingering wounds.

The good news about shingles is the bad news about shingles is probably overstated. A long-term study of 421 herpes zoster patients reported in the *British Medical Journal* reported that the risk of developing postherpetic neuralgia was slight. Only 2 percent of patients under the age of 60 had pain associated with shingles 3 months after the first outbreak, which was mild in all cases. About 7 percent of patients over the age of 60 had moderate to severe pain 3 months after the first appearance of a rash, but in all cases the pain had abated within a year. In this study, only 1 in 25 patients received any antiviral drugs.[3]

The antiviral drugs used to treat shingles are acyclovir, vancyclovir, famciclovir, and foscarnet. The more strongly antiviral the medication, the worse the side effects. Foscarnet stops replication of all known strains of the herpesvirus (under laboratory test conditions), but can cause kidney failure, destruction of the heart muscles, and seizures.[4] Nutritional measures can ease side effects when these drugs are medically required.

Older patients sometimes are given relatively high doses of steroids such as prednisone to control pain, although only one of several studies indicated that this class of drugs leads to shorter dependency on pain medications and better sleep.[5] Interestingly, the only drug approved by the FDA for treating the pain of postherpetic neuralgia, capsaicin, is herbal.

TREATMENT SUMMARY

DIET

○ Eliminate all polyunsaturated vegetable oils, margarines, vegetable shortenings, and products made with partially hydrogenated oils.

○ Increase your consumption of omega-3 fatty acids by eating oily fish (salmon, sardines, and herring) or flaxseeds.

NUTRITIONAL SUPPLEMENTS

○ Bromelain *or* papain *or* chymotrypsin, in dosages recommended on the product label, taken with a glass of water. Be sure to use an enteric-coated form.

○ Vitamin B complex: 100 milligrams daily.

○ Vitamin E: 400 IU daily.

HERBS

○ Capsaicin (Zostrix) cream: apply sparingly to the affected area 3–4 times daily. Use after blisters have healed. *Never apply to broken skin. Do not get the cream into eyes or mouth.*

UNDERSTANDING THE HEALING PROCESS

Nutritional supplements are as effective as antiviral drugs in most cases of shingles. However, persons who take corticosteroids or who have diabetes or HIV, and anyone experiencing an outbreak affecting the eyes, should consult a physician about necessary medical treatment.

There is some scientific evidence that shingles can be relieved by proteolytic enzymes, the chemicals that help digest the proteins in food. The two richest plant sources of these enzymes are pineapple and papaya, which produce bromelain and papain, respectively. The proteolytic enzymes in these fruits have long been recognized for their use as "natural tenderizers" for meat. Chymotrypsin is produced by the body itself and extracted from the pancreases of various animals.

Proteolytic enzymes were compared to the standard antiviral drug acyclovir in a double-blind study involving 192 people. The participants in the test were given either the natural enzymes or the drug and evaluated on the seventh and fourteenth days of the study. Both groups had similar pain relief, although reddening of the skin was reduced more by acyclovir.[6] Similar results were found in a study involving 90 people.[7]

Proteolytic enzymes can be broken down by stomach acid. For this reason, most brands are enteric-coated, meaning they are covered with cellulose so that the tablet does not dissolve until it reaches the intestine. Make sure the brand you use is coated. Chymotrypsin is usually a pork product, so vegetarians and other persons who do not eat pork may prefer bromelain or papain. Holding the pill in the mouth can dissolve soft tissues, so always take proteolytic enzymes with water.

Digestive enzymes are safe for almost everyone. However, enteric-coated pancreatic enzymes given to children with cystic fibrosis have been known to cause a serious complication known as fibrosing colonopathy, probably due to an interaction between the enzymes and the coating of the tablet.[8] Frequent use of proteolytic enzymes can cause pale or pungent stools, and occasionally allergic reactions, such as sneezing, wheezing, or tearing.

Hypersensitivity reactions to the enzyme preparations are usually caused by allergies to the pineapple, papaya, or pork from which the product was derived.

Physicians have been reporting for 50 years that vitamin B_{12} and vitamin E help relieve the pain of postherpetic neuralgia.[9,10,11] While no systematic studies have confirmed that these vitamins help outbreaks of shingles (herpes zoster), laboratory experiments have shown that vitamin E, sodium pyruvate (a sports supplement), and membrane-stabilizing free fatty acids work together to stop lesions in herpes simplex.[12] It is possible that vitamins B_{12} and E act as antioxidants to similar benefit in shingles. For this reason, eliminating saturated fats and fortifying the diet with sources of omega-3 fatty acids may be helpful in treating the aftereffects of shingles.

Capsaicin is a prominent chemical constituent of cayenne peppers, the hot kitchen spice that flavors chili and curry. Capsaicin creams "distract" sensory nerves from the pain of postherpetic neuralgia. The stinging and burning caused by capsaicin acts as a "second source" of pain that depletes stores of a substance involved in pain called substance P. When regular application of capsaicin uses up the supply of substance P in a given area, pain levels decrease.

The greater the patient's ability to perceive pain, the greater the probability of relief by capsaicin.[13] Capsaicin works best when there has been minimal damage to sensory nerves. About half of shingles patients who use capsaicin creams report substantial benefit. About 10 percent of the shingles patients who try capsaicin creams discontinue them because of inflammation of the breasts or excessive pain immediately after the cream is applied.[14] The people who are most likely to benefit from capsaicin creams are those whose ability to perceive warm and cold is not impaired by the outbreak.[15]

CONCEPTS FOR COPING WITH SHINGLES

○ Acupuncture tends to be disappointing in the treatment of postherpetic neuralgia.

○ Cold packs, applied frequently with a towel separating the cold pack from the skin may help relieve pain. Shingles sufferers whose pain is activated by exposure to cold cannot use this method.

○ In TENS, or transcutaneous electrical nerve stimulation, a gentle electrical current is applied to the skin. This helps some people find pain relief. Home TENS units are available by prescription and from some chiropractors and massage therapists.

Sickle-Cell Anemia

SYMPTOM SUMMARY

○ Delayed development in childhood

○ Anemia

○ Increased numbers of infections

○ Leg ulcers

○ Yellow eyes or jaundice

○ Chronic obstruction to breathing

○ Excessive urination

○ Gallstones at early age

○ In men, priapism (painful erections)

UNDERSTANDING THE DISEASE PROCESS

Sickle-cell anemia is a hereditary condition causing red blood cells to be misformed. Healthy red blood cells have a contour roughly resembling a doughnut. They are flexible and can pass through narrow passageways in the bloodstream. Sickle cells develop an elongated, bent shape like a sickle. They are fragile and are easily broken. They fail to deliver adequate amounts of oxygen, and the kidneys are severely strained by the need to clear proteins from broken blood cells out of the bloodstream. Sickle-cell anemia begins before birth and causes numerous health complications throughout life.

Persons of African descent are most likely to have sickle-cell anemia, but it is also relatively common among people of Mediterranean, Arab, and South Asian ancestry, and it is not unknown among Caucasians. Inheriting a gene for sickle-cell anemia from both parents results in full expression of the disease. Inheriting a gene for sickle-cell anemia from only one parent causes changes in hemoglobin that are identifiable by blood tests, but does not cause symptoms.

TREATMENT SUMMARY

NUTRITIONAL SUPPLEMENTS

For children:

○ Zinc: 10 milligrams per day.

For adults:

○ Mixed carotenoids: 25,000 IU per day.

○ Vitamin C: 1,000 milligrams per day.

○ Vitamin E: 400 IU per day.

UNDERSTANDING THE HEALING PROCESS

Children with sickle-cell anemia have a relatively fast metabolism that can require up to 30 percent more calories just to meet the body's basic needs.[1] Acute illnesses such as colds, fevers, and infections only increase the child's need for energy by about 50 calories a day, but many children with sickle-cell anemia suffer developmental setbacks because they are not fed enough when they are sick.[2] Medically prescribed hyroxyurea treatment can reduce, but not eliminate, a child's need for extra calories and encourage growth.[3]

Zinc deficiency is another common cause of delayed development in children with sickle-cell anemia. Without zinc, the immune system cannot activate natural killer cells and macrophages to fight infection, and other immune cells tend to mature and die early.[4] Reduced resistance to infection diverts nutrients needed for growth. Children who receive supplemental zinc grow taller and have stronger knees and arms. The difference between receiving adequate zinc and zinc deficiency amounts to only a fraction of an inch of growth per year, but the benefits of zinc supplementation throughout childhood and adolescence can be substantial.[5]

Since zinc is critical to the child's development but it has an unpleasant taste, it is usually best to give this supplement in the form of a fruit-flavored syrup. Cherry-flavored zinc syrups are available from sickle-cell treatment specialists and compounding pharmacies. Be sure the child receives at least 10 milligrams of zinc per day, but do not overdose.

Very little research has been done concerning the nutritional needs of adults with sickle-cell anemia, although a study in the late 1980s found that most people with the disease suffer various antioxidant deficiencies.[6] Moderate amounts of antioxidant supplementation may reduce the severity of some symptoms of sickle-cell anemia.

CONCEPTS FOR COPING WITH SICKLE-CELL ANEMIA

○ Maintaining body fluids is a special problem for people with sickle-cell anemia. Be sure to drink 8–10 glasses of water a day in hot weather, and to avoid heat as much as possible.

○ Teenagers with sickle-cell anemia usually need more calories than other teens even when they get less exercise.[7] Although vigorous physical exercise by itself does not aggravate sickle-cell anemia,[8] confounding factors such as heat stress, dehydration, viral illness, and poor physical conditioning can cause serious complications or even sudden death in young people with sickle-cell anemia who are engaged in vigorous physical activity.[9]

○ People with sickle-cell anemia are more likely to get cavities and gum disease.[10] Regular dental care improves quality of life.

○ Some complications of sickle-cell anemia require immediate medical attention. Among them are:

- Abdominal swelling
- Any sudden weakness or loss of feeling
- Chest pain
- Fever
- Increasing tiredness
- Pain that will not go away with home treatment
- Priapism (painful erection that will not go down)
- Shortness of breath
- Sudden vision change
- Unusual headache

SIDS, Lowering Risk of

SYMPTOM SUMMARY

Sudden death of infants tends to affect babies who are:

○ Part of a multiple birth (twins, triplets, quadruplets)

○ Of low birth weight

○ Recently recovering from a respiratory infection

UNDERSTANDING THE DISEASE PROCESS

Sudden infant death syndrome, better known as crib death or SIDS, is the sudden, unexplainable death of an infant before his or her first birthday. SIDS typically occurs between the hours of midnight and 8 A.M., with no apparent suffering by the baby. Boys are slightly more at risk than girls, and the greatest number of crib deaths occur among children aged 2–4 months.

PREVENTION SUMMARY

NUTRITIONAL SUPPLEMENTS

During pregnancy, the mother should take:

○ L-carnitine: at least 500 milligrams per day.

○ Magnesium: at least 200 milligrams per day.

○ Selenium: 100 milligrams every other day.

○ Vitamin E: no more than 100 IU per day.

During nursing, the mother should take:

○ Vitamin C: 1,000 milligrams per day.

UNDERSTANDING THE PREVENTION PROCESS

SIDS has been tied to several nutritional deficiencies. Infants of vegetarian mothers are at highest risk of SIDS during the first few days of life. While the mother's vegetarian diet is not usually a risk factor for the child, babies born with carnitine transfer enzyme deficiencies may develop unexpected respiratory failure.[1] There are no studies that prove that L-carnitine supplementation reduces rates of SIDS in infants born to vegetarian mothers, but taking 1 capsule of L-carnitine every day during pregnancy and nursing is a prudent and possibly preventive measure.

Rates of SIDS are higher among Native Americans and urban African-Americans, who tend to have a magnesium-deficient diet.[2] The role of magnesium deficiency in SIDS is unproven, but avoiding deficiency is prudent. Similarly, there is a theoretical link between urinary tract infections in the mother, selenium deficiencies in the fetus, reduced thyroid function in the baby, reduced oxygenation of the baby's blood, and SIDS.[3] Modest supplementation with selenium, vitamin C, and vitamin E during pregnancy and nursing counteracts this deficiency. High doses of vitamin E should be avoided before delivery to avoid creating imbalances in blood-clotting factors.

CONCEPTS FOR PREVENTING SIDS

○ SIDS deaths are less frequent when the baby:

- Is not put to bed in a soft blanket.
- Sleeps in a warm, but not hot, room.
- Sleeps in a smoke-free environment.

Sinusitis

SYMPTOM SUMMARY

○ Bad breath

○ Chills

○ Fever

○ Frontal headache

○ Nasal congestion with thick discharge

○ Nosebleed

○ Pain, redness, swelling, and tenderness over affected sinuses

○ Sore throat

In especially severe cases one or both eyes may be fixed in a "down and out" position and there may be what the medical literature terms "Pott's puffy tumor" across the forehead.

UNDERSTANDING THE DISEASE PROCESS

Sinusitis is an inflammation of the sinuses, air-filled cavities in the bones of the face that are fully formed after age 7. The linings of the sinuses are filled with mucus-producing cells. The blanket of mucus they form is carried toward the openings of the sinuses by the rhythmic beating of tiny hairs known as cilia. The openings of the sinuses into the nose are very narrow, only 1–2 millimeters (0.04–0.08 of an inch) across. When the openings of the sinuses are clogged, the sinuses swell and become inflamed.

Almost all acute (short-term) cases of sinusitis are caused by colds viruses. Sinus inflammation caused by a cold usually resolves when the cold goes away. Longer-term sinus infections, those lasting 7–10 days or more, are usually caused by bacteria. *Streptococcus pneumoniae* and *Haemophilus influenzae* are the most common causes of bacterial sinusitis, although the hospital-borne bacteria *Staphylococcus aureus* and *Pseudomonas* cause the most persistent cases. Dental infections may cause 5–10 percent of all infections involving the maxillary sinuses behind the nose. Other causes of sinusitis include barotraumas from deep-sea diving or air travel, mucus abnormalities such as cystic fibrosis, and chemical irritants.[1]

Antibiotics cannot help sinus infections caused by viruses. (Despite the fact that antibiotics do not help,

survey data show that doctors prescribe them in 24.2 percent of cases overall, and to almost all smokers who come in with colds.[2]) Doctors usually prescribe a short-term course of antibiotic treatment when sinus inflammation has persisted for more than 10 days. When the patient does not respond to antibiotics, CT (computed tomography) scans are ordered to rule out tumors and other serious conditions.

TREATMENT SUMMARY

NUTRITIONAL SUPPLEMENTS

○ Bioflavonoids: 1,000 milligrams per day.

○ Thymus extract: 500 milligrams of crude polypeptides daily.

○ Vitamin A: 5,000 IU per day.

○ Vitamin C: 500 milligrams 3–4 times a day.

○ Zinc picolinate: 30 milligrams per day.

HERBS

○ Echinacea: 150–300 milligrams of solid extract (3.5% echinacosides) 3 times a day, or dried root, freeze-dried plant, juice, fluid extract, or tincture, as recommended on the label.

○ Goldenseal: as recommended on the label.

UNDERSTANDING THE HEALING PROCESS

The most recent understanding of how antibiotics work in treating sinusitis would surprise many patients who take them—as well as many doctors who prescribe them. Antibiotics in the class including erythromycin (macrolide antibiotics) act not by reducing infection, since reinfection reestablishes the bacteria almost as quickly as the antibiotics kill them, but by reducing inflammation. Antibiotics reduce inflammation by killing immune cells, specifically neutrophils, by simultaneously reducing the vigor of the immune response and the vigor of bacteria, and by increasing the rate at which mucus is propelled out of the sinuses. Macrolide antibiotics are effective in 60–80 percent of cases.[3] The combination of natural treatments recommended here also relieves inflammation, but not at the expense of immune function.

Although there are no studies that directly confirm the usefulness of thymus extract in treating sinus infections, there is considerable evidence that thymus extracts correct low immune function. In particular, research has shown that thymus extract normalizes the ratio of T-helper cells to T suppressor cells, maintaining a healthy immune response that neither destroys healthy tissue nor allows infectious microorganisms to flourish.[4]

Relatively low doses of vitamin A are sufficient to prevent "burnout" due to stress on the immune output of the thymus.[5] Vitamin A also enhances antibody response, increases the rate at which macrophages destroy bacteria, and stimulates natural killer cells.[6]

Vitamin C levels are quickly depleted during the stress of an infection.[7] In combination with bioflavonoids, it helps increase the stability of the ground substance, the "glue" between the mucous membrane and the tissues below it.[8]

Zinc is an important cofactor for vitamin A. When zinc is deficient, the immune system's ability to produce white blood cells in response to infection is reduced, thymic hormone levels are lower, the immune response in the skin is especially reduced, and phagocytosis, the process in which bacteria are engulfed and digested, is slowed. When zinc is deficient, all of these processes can be corrected by taking zinc supplements.[9]

A quick method for detecting zinc deficiency is a taste test. Powder a tablet of any zinc-based supplement or cold medication and mix with $1/4$ cup (50 milliliters) of water. Slosh the mixture in the mouth. People who notice no taste at all or who notice a "dry," "mineral," or "sweet" taste are likely to be zinc deficient. Anyone who notices a definite strong and unpleasant taste that intensifies over time is not likely to be zinc deficient.

Zinc picolinate is the most readily absorbed form of zinc. Do not take more than 50 milligrams of any zinc supplement daily. In rare cases, excessive intake of zinc depletes copper to cause anemia, that is, a deficiency of red blood cells, and neutropenia, a serious deficiency of white blood cells.

Echinacea relieves inflammation as effectively as antibiotics do, but instead of blunting the body's immune response, it enhances it. This herb is especially useful in stimulating phagocytosis. A study of oral administration of an *Echinacea purpurea* root extract (30 drops 3 times per day) to healthy men for 5 days resulted in a 120 percent increase in phagocytosis.[10] In laboratory tests, caffeic acid and echinacoside, two important chemical constituents of the herb, have been found to have specific antibacterial action against *Staphylococcus aureus*.[11]

Goldenseal contains berberine. This alkaloid kills *Helicobacter pylori,* a bacterium implicated in ulcers and chronic gastritis as well as chronic sinusitis.[12] One study of 275 patients with peptic ulcers found that sinusitis and hives were more common among those who tested positive for *Helicobacter pylori.* Treatment of the bacterial infection not only relieved ulcers but reduced sinusitis symptoms.[13]

People's Pharmacy authors Joe and Teresa Graedon warn that goldenseal reportedly limits the effectiveness of the anticoagulants heparin and warfarin (Coumadin). Do not take goldenseal with these medications. Avoid supplements containing vitamin B_6 or L-histidine if you take goldenseal, since they can interfere with goldenseal's antibacterial action.

CONCEPTS FOR COPING WITH SINUSITIS

❍ Breathe in steam from a vaporizer to relieve inflammation. Breathing vapors from water to which you have added $1/2$ teaspoon of eucalyptus stimulates the secretion of fluids in the sinuses to loosen mucus.

❍ Apply moist heat to the face by applying moist hot packs or by sitting in a steam room as often as possible, unless you experience facial pain.

❍ Drink 8 glasses of water daily, especially if you live in a dry climate or travel by air frequently. Adequate hydration ensures fluid mucus that drains more easily.

❍ Eliminate allergies by installing an air cleaner with an HEPA (High Energy Particulate Air) filter, keeping air dry (with a dehumidifier, if necessary) so humidity stays under 50 percent, and by washing bed linens in hot water heated to at least 135°F (58°C).

❍ If both sinusitis and frequent heartburn, indigestion, or gastroesophageal reflux disease (GERD) are a problem, try sleeping on your left side rather than the right. The esophagus curves slightly to the left as it connects with the stomach. During sleep when the right side of the body is against the bed, gravity straightens out the curve, causing stomach acids to spill into the esophagus.

❍ "Snort" a nasal douche made with $1/2$ teaspoon of salt or $1/4$ teaspoon of goldenseal powder in 1 cup of warm water. To apply the douche, pour the liquid into your cupped hand and inhale in into one nostril at a time, while closing the other nostril with your index finger. Alternatively, use a net pot, a ceramic container with a curved spout that allows you to pour water directly into the nose.

○ Swab the nasal passages with oil of bitter orange to relieve inflammation.

Sjögren's Syndrome

SYMPTOM SUMMARY

○ Dry eyes

○ Dry mouth

○ Swollen lymph glands

○ Fatigue

○ Joint pain and swelling

UNDERSTANDING THE DISEASE PROCESS

Sjögren's syndrome (SS) is a chronic condition in which secretions from the immune system clog the exocrine glands, especially the tear ducts and the salivary glands. The condition is usually first noticed as a set of complications from dry mouth, such as inability to eat dry food, unusually large numbers of caries and cavities in the teeth, and altered sense of taste. The condition can also cause a gritty sensation in the eyes and sometimes severe eye inflammation.

SS is caused by overactivity of the immune system. It typically occurs in people who already have rheumatoid arthritis, lupus, or scleroderma. SS is a surprisingly common condition, afflicting up to 9 million people in the United States, 90 percent of them women.[1]

TREATMENT SUMMARY

NUTRITIONAL SUPPLEMENTS

○ Evening primrose oil: 1,500 milligrams daily, preferably in 2–3 doses.

UNDERSTANDING THE HEALING PROCESS

Evening primrose oil (EPO) is a rich source of gamma-linolenic acid, a natural anti-inflammatory. At least one study has found that taking 1,500 milligrams of EPO daily relieves eye irritation, dry mouth, and dry skin, although the effects are modest.[2] Interestingly, recent research has found that higher doses are ineffective.[3]

EPO can cause mild diarrhea when it is first used. If this occurs, reduce the dose. Schizophrenics treated with chlorpromazine should not take EPO, borage seed oil, blackcurrant seed oil, hempseed oil, or GLA. The combination can cause seizures.

CONCEPTS FOR COPING WITH SJÖGREN'S SYNDROME

○ Make liberal use of artificial tears. Need for artificial tears is greater in dry environments, for example, heated or air-conditioned rooms, airplanes, or desert environments. If you use artificial tears more than once every 4 hours, make sure that the brand you use does not contain preservatives that can cause eye irritation. Lacri-Lube applied at bedtime can prevent matting of the eyes in the morning, but excessive use can cause blepharitis.

○ Glasses fitted with moisture shields can reduce dryness.

○ Use of humidifiers helps both dry eyes and dry mouth.

○ Avoid antihistamines. These increase dryness of the eyes and mouth.

○ Sugar-free lemon drops stimulate salivation. If this does not work, try artificial saliva products such as MouthKote, Saliment, Salivart, and Xero-Lube.

○ See your dentist regularly. The dentist may recommend special toothpastes for dry mouth, such as Biotene, Dental Care, or Oral Balance.

○ Be sure to disinfect dentures.

○ Dry skin can be treated with moisturizers such as Eucerin and Lubriderm. Replens relieves vaginal dryness.

Skin Tags

SYMPTOM SUMMARY

○ Soft, fleshy growths of excess tissue each with a narrow base that hang from the skin of the:

• Armpits

• Eyelids

• Groin

• Neck

• Creases between "love handles"

UNDERSTANDING THE DISEASE PROCESS

Skin tags, known in the medical literature as acrochordons, are benign tumors of the skin that occur in nearly half of the population. These growths are typically tiny, less than 2 millimeters ($1/10$ of an inch) in diameter, but occasionally skin tags grow as large as 5 centimeters (2 inches) around.[1] Taking on the color of the skin, skin tags almost never become malignant and are primarily a cosmetic concern, unless they are repeatedly caught in folds of clothing or zippers.

Unlike other kinds of warts, skin tags are an outward manifestation of insulin resistance, an inability of cells throughout the body to process sugar. Skin tags form on areas of skin that get the least circulation of blood. The combination of poor circulation and insulin resistance deprives these skin cells of adequate insulin, so they are never able to "climb" to the surface of the skin and complete a normal life cycle.[2] Diabetes is 4 times as common in people who have skin tags as it is in people who have clear skin.

TREATMENT SUMMARY

To prevent skin tags:

❍ Alpha-lipoic acid: 200 milligrams daily.

❍ Chromium (from brewer's yeast): 1,000 micrograms daily.

❍ Niacin (a cofactor for chromium): at least 20 milligrams but no more than 100 milligrams, daily.

To treat skin tags:

❍ Bloodroot: Alpha Omega Bloodroot Ointment, used as directed on the label.

See Part Three if you take prescription medication.

UNDERSTANDING THE HEALING PROCESS

In the long run, preventing future formation of skin tags is a matter of reducing insulin resistance, or in diabetics, controlling blood sugars. Alpha-lipoic acid reduces the concentration of a blood sugar byproduct known as fructosamine.[3] This chemical attaches to proteins in the skin, interfering with normal shedding of the skin, and is a contributing factor in diabetic kidney disease. The supplement also stops the process that robs fat cells underlying the skin of their sensitivity to insulin during the earlier stages of diabetes.[4] Laboratory experiments with animals have found that alpha-lipoic acid lowers blood

pressure[5] and helps muscle tissues absorb glucose from the bloodstream,[6] although it is of limited benefit once insulin sensitivity has been established through exercise.[7] Alpha-lipoic acid does not interfere with medications commonly prescribed for diabetes, and can be taken in dosages of up 1,200 milligrams per day without side effects.

People who have insulin resistance serious enough to cause skin tags tend to excrete chromium into their urine.[8] Experiments with animals have found that supplemental chromium is particularly helpful when blood sugars are especially high, so high that the body has begun to break down proteins inside cells because it cannot use insulin to transport glucose into cells. These experiments have also shown that chromium helps insulin resistance and high blood sugars caused by stress.[9]

Chromium that is derived from brewer's yeast is more beneficial than inorganic chromium,[10] although neither form has an immediate effect on skin tags. The key to successful use of chromium may be making sure that the body has an adequate supply of its cofactor niacin. At least one study found that taking chromium by itself had no discernible effect on diabetes, but taking both chromium and niacin lowered fasting blood sugars by 7 percent and reduced overall blood sugars (the total amount of glucose in the bloodstream over a 28-day period) by 15 percent—an enormous benefit.[11] No scientific study has directly confirmed the benefits of this combination on diabetic skin, although many diabetics who have skin tags report that taking both supplements seems to help. Since high dosages of niacin can cause increased sensitivity to sunlight and sunburn and aggravate hot flashes or rosacea, be sure not to take more than 100 milligrams per day.

The advantage of using alpha-lipoic acid, chromium, and niacin in treating skin tags is that, over a period of 2–3 months, they keep new skin tags from forming. The drawback of using alpha-lipoic acid, chromium, and niacin in treating skin tags is that they do not remove existing skin tags. The potent herbal skin treatment bloodroot is useful for this purpose.

Bloodroot contains an orange-red latex that oxidizes to a dark brown or black when exposed to the air. This sap is used as a "black salve" to treat skin growths of various kinds. Bloodroot pastes will remove skin tags, but left on the skin too long, they will also remove healthy skin. In a few cases, inappropriate use of bloodroot has caused permanent scarring. Never use bloodroot around the eyes, mouth, nose, ears, anus, or genitals, and never take bloodroot internally. The maximum area of skin that should be treated with bloodroot is a 2-inch square (4 square inches, or 25 square centimeters). As little as 1 gram ($\frac{1}{30}$ of an ounce) of bloodroot taken by mouth can cause vomiting.

A safe formulation of bloodroot called Alpha Omega Bloodroot Ointment is manufactured by Alpha Omega Labs. Follow the label directions, and keep the skin tag covered with a bandage until you wash off the ointment.

CONCEPTS FOR COPING WITH SKIN TAGS

❍ Skin tags are the same color as surrounding skin or slightly darker. If a skin growth you believe to be a skin tag begins bleeding, changes color rapidly, or hurts, see a physician for a proper diagnosis.

❍ Doctors may remove skin tags with sharp scissors, a sharp blade, or less commonly by freezing or burning off at the stalk. Bleeding is usually stopped by cauterizing the skin with an electrical needle or by packing the wound in aluminum chloride. Healing after this procedure usually takes 3–4 weeks.

Spina Bifida, Prevention of

SYMPTOM SUMMARY

❍ Exposure of the spinal cord to the outside of the body at birth

UNDERSTANDING THE DISEASE PROCESS

Spina bifida is a congenital deformity resulting in the exposure of the central nervous system to the outside of the body. Universally fatal before the advent of antibiotics and advanced surgical techniques, spina bifida is now considered the most difficult of the treatable birth defects.

For reasons that are not understood, spina bifida is most common among persons of English, Scottish, or Welsh descent. There is general agreement in the scientific community that the condition is influenced by deficiency of the B vitamin folic acid. This may be caused by poor diet, or exposure to compounds that deplete the vitamin. Folic acid deficiency is induced by treatment with valproic acid (Depakote) for epilepsy or methotrexate (Methotrex) for cancer, rheumatoid arthritis, and other inflammatory conditions. Folic acid deficiency can also be caused by eating green peels of Irish potatoes.

PREVENTION SUMMARY

NUTRITIONAL SUPPLEMENTS

❍ Folic acid: 400 milligrams per day.

UNDERSTANDING THE PREVENTION PROCESS

In September of 1992, the United States Public Health Service made the following strong recommendation: All women of childbearing age in the United States who are capable of becoming pregnant should consume 0.4 milligrams of folic acid per day for the purpose of reducing the risk of having a pregnancy affected with spina bifida and other neural tube defects. Because the effects of high intakes are not well known, but include complicating the diagnosis of vitamin B_{12} deficiency, care should be taken to keep total consumption to less than 1 milligram per day, except under the supervision of a physician.

Folic acid replacement is especially important for women who take drugs for seizure disorders or arthritis. Taking folic acid does not provide a guarantee against spina bifida, but the incidence of this defect is reduced by up to 75 percent in children of mothers who take needed nutritional supplements.[1]

CONCEPTS FOR PREVENTING SPINA BIFIDA

❍ If you are a woman treated with valproic acid or methotrexate, see your physician about a prescription for high-dose folic acid. A daily dose of 4,000 milligrams of folic acid is believed adequate for mothers taking folate-depleting medications.

Sprue
See **Celiac Disease.**

Strep Throat

SYMPTOM SUMMARY

❍ Rapid onset of throat pain

❍ Tender lymph nodes on the sides of the neck

❍ Deep, red inflammation of the throat

❍ No cough

UNDERSTANDING THE DISEASE PROCESS

Slightly more than half of all cases of sore throat are caused by colds viruses. Over 100 other microorganisms also cause sore throat; the most significant among them is the bacterium *Streptococcus pyrogenes,* the organism causing strep throat. Approximately 1 in 6 cases of sore throat is due to strep throat.

Strep infections can strike at any age, but they are most common in children aged 4–7. The hallmark of a strep infection is the sudden onset of symptoms. Sore throats caused by colds usually are not accompanied by fever, but strep infection can cause fevers as high as 106°F (41.2°C). Pain upon swallowing often leads to dehydration. Complications of strep throat are rare but potentially serious; the bright red streptococcal rash called scarlet fever was once a leading cause of heart disease.

TREATMENT SUMMARY

To support antibiotic therapy:

○ *Lactobacillus:* 1 capsule daily.

To combat the disease:

○ *Echinacea angustifolia:* juice (preferred), 20 drops every 2 hours you are awake for the first day, then 3 times a day for 10 days.

UNDERSTANDING THE HEALING PROCESS

Doctors usually prescribe antibiotics for strep throat to shorten the duration of the disease and to prevent the complications. Penicillin G benzathine (Bicillin) is the only antibiotic that prevents scarlet and rheumatic fevers, although other medications may be more effective when the bacterium is rapidly multiplying. Antibiotics should only be dispensed when a throat swab proves the presence of the *Streptococcus* bacterium. It is important not to demand antibiotic treatment for sore throat due to viral infections, distinguishable by slow onset of symptoms and the absence of fever or fever below 101.5°F (42°C). Antibiotics have no effect on viral infections and the overuse of antibiotics helps create strains of bacteria that are resistant to future antibiotic treatment. The absorption of penicillin is increased if the antibiotic is taken with pineapple (not apple, grape, orange, or other) juice. Giving a child 1 capsule of *Lactobacillus* or a serving of yogurt daily reduces the chances of developing yeast infections as a complication of antibiotic treatment.

Echinacea angustifolia counteracts an enzyme *Streptococcus* needs to attach itself to the lining of the throat.[1] Other forms of echinacea may also have an immunostimulant effect, but *Echinacea angustifolia* is preferred.

There is laboratory evidence that *Echinacea angustifolia* contains chemicals that deactivate CYP3A4. This is a liver enzyme that breaks down a wide range of medications, including anabolic steroids, the chemotherapy drug methotrexate used in treating cancer and lupus, astemizole (Hismanal) for allergies, nifedipine (Adalat) and captopril (Capoten) for high blood pressure, and sildenafil (Viagra) for impotence, as well as many others. *Echinacea angustifolia* might help maintain levels of these drugs in the bloodstream and make them more effective, or it might also cause them to accumulate to levels at which they cause side effects. Switch to a brand of echinacea that does not contain *Echinacea angustifolia* if you experience unexpected side effects while taking any of these drugs.[2]

Echinacea stimulates immune function, but it also slightly increases production of T cells.[3] These are the immune cells attacked by HIV. When there are more T cells, the virus has more cells to infect. This gives it more opportunities to mutate into a drug-resistant form. The authoritative reference work *The Complete German Commission E Monographs* counsels against the use of echinacea for treating upper respiratory infections by people who have HIV or autoimmune diseases such as multiple sclerosis. Later communications between the senior editor of the *Monographs* and the German Food and Drug Administration revealed that the warning in the reference book was based on theoretical speculation rather than practical experience.[4] Still, as a precaution, people with HIV should only use echinacea for *treating* strep throat rather than preventing it.

CONCEPTS FOR COPING WITH STREP THROAT

○ There are a number of homeopathic remedies for strep throat. Usually it is best to start with a single dose of the lowest strength (6C, 6X, or 12C) of the remedy matching the symptoms to be treated, and then wait for a response. If there is an improvement in symptoms, let the remedy continue to work until there is no more improvement, then take another dose. If there is no improvement, try a different potency (30X or 30C). Sometimes homeopathic medicines work for a few minutes, and sometimes they work for an entire day before another dose is needed.

- Aconitum napellus is recommended when symptoms come on suddenly, especially after a stressful or traumatic experience. Symptoms relieved by this homeopathic formula include scratchy throat, choking cough, tightness across the chest, and dry, stuffy nose.

- Arsenicum album is recommended for people who have frequent colds and sore throat. Most effective when symptoms are worse at night and when there is thick, burning mucus.

- Baryta carbonica treats runny nose, swollen lips, swollen tonsils, and adenoids.

- Euphrasia relieves red eyes and frequent sneezing with a clear discharge. Helpful when symptoms interrupt sleep and when the person feels better after eating.

- Gelsemium treats fatigue, headache, fever, and chills. Especially recommended when the person with the cold feels shaky. Treats colds occurring in hot weather.

- Kali bichromicum helps break up thick, stringy mucus in the nose and throat.

- Mercurius solubilis treats colds in people who wake up sweaty. Also treats bad breath, swollen lymph nodes, and earache.

- Natrum muriaticum treats sore throat with a white (not clear) discharge, sneezing that is worse early in the morning, and chapped lips.

- Rhus toxicodendron treats sore throat occuring with stiffness and body aches before sneezing, tearing, and cough occur.

Stretch Marks

SYMPTOM SUMMARY

❍ Fine lines in the skin that appear reddish or purple but lighten with time

❍ Most common on the abdomen and hips

❍ Tend to dissipate over time

UNDERSTANDING THE DISEASE PROCESS

Stretch marks, a condition known in the medical literature as striae gravidarum, are a buildup of collagen by skin that has to grow too fast. While stretch marks look like fine scars, they are anatomically the opposite phenomenon. In stretch marks, the skin lacks fibrillin microfibrils, the specialized cells that give the skin its resilience, and the microfibrils that exist are looser. This allows collagen to accumulate and form striae, or stretch marks.[1]

Stretch marks tend to lighten over time. They are especially common in adolescent girls and in women who use steroid creams (such as hydrocortisone) on their skin for more than a few weeks.

TREATMENT SUMMARY

For treating stretch marks:

❍ Any cream containing alpha hydroxy acids plus vitamin C.

For preventing stretch marks:

❍ Any cream containing gotu kola *(Centella asiatica)* extract and vitamin E.

UNDERSTANDING THE HEALING PROCESS

Physicians commonly treat stretch marks with pulsed laser surgery or a chemical derivative of vitamin A known as tretinoin (Renova). This cream typically shortens a stretch mark by about 20 percent after 3 months of use.[2] In many cases, however, tretinoin treatment causes redness and scaling.

There are at least two effective alternatives to tretinoin. A study at the Naval Medical Center in Portsmouth, Virginia found that women with stretch marks on their abdomens and thighs responded equally well to Renova and a safer cream containing alpha hydroxy acids and vitamin C (MD Forté). Both products took about 12 weeks to produce results. Other products containing the same active ingredients as MD Forté may be labeled as:

- alpha hydroxy and botanical complex
- alpha hydroxycaprylic acid
- alpha hydroxyethanoic acid + ammonium alpha hydroxyethanoate
- alpha hydroxyoctanoic acid
- citric acid
- glycolic acid

- glycolic acid + ammonium glycolate
- glycomer in cross-linked fatty acids alpha nutrium (three AHAs).
- hydroxycaprylic acid
- lactic acid
- L-alpha hydroxy acid
- malic acid
- mixed fruit acid
- sugarcane extract
- tri-alpha hydroxy fruit acids
- triple fruit acid

Of these, the most frequently used in cosmetics are glycolic acid and lactic acid.

A cream for *preventing* stretch marks contains the herb gotu kola. A study involving 100 women found that the combination of gotu kola extract, vitamin E, and collagen prevented the formation of new stretch marks during pregnancy, although the study only examined women who had had stretch marks during a previous pregnancy. Women who are still trying to get pregnant should not take gotu kola, since it can interfere with ovulation.

Stroke

SYMPTOM SUMMARY

- Difficulty speaking or understanding speech
- Dizziness
- Sudden loss of vision, especially in one eye
- Sudden weakness or numbness, especially on one side of the body
- If any of these symptoms occurs, seek immediate medical care.

UNDERSTANDING THE DISEASE PROCESS

A stroke occurs when the blood supply to the part of the brain is suddenly interrupted (ischemic stroke) or when a blood vessel in the brain bursts, spilling blood into the spaces surrounding the brain cells (hemorrhagic stroke). Some brain cells die when they no longer receive oxygen and nutrients from the blood or when they are damaged by sudden bleeding into or around the brain, but some of the most severe damage of stroke occurs when the flow of blood within the brain is reestablished, flooding resting blood cells with oxygen and free radicals.

The most important risk factor for stroke is uncontrolled high blood pressure. Smoking cigarettes, diabetes, heavy consumption of alcohol, high cholesterol, use of illicit drugs, and surgery are other important contributing causes of stroke. Thrombolytic ("clot-busting") therapy sometimes greatly reduces the damage caused by a stroke, provided the treatment is initiated in the emergency room, but in the United States, fewer than 2 percent of stroke victims receive thrombolytic agents. The majority of stroke victims suffer long-term disability.

TREATMENT SUMMARY

To lower risk of stroke:

DIET

○ Eat 5 or more servings of fruit and vegetables daily, preferably at every meal.

○ Eat fish at least once a week.

○ Avoid salty foods.

After stroke has occurred:

DIET

○ Follow dietary guidelines for stroke prevention.

NUTRITIONAL SUPPLEMENTS

○ Vitamin C: dosage chosen in consultation with physician.

○ Avoid alpha-lipoic acid.

UNDERSTANDING THE HEALING PROCESS

There is mounting evidence that antioxidants, fiber, folic acid, micronutrients, potassium, and phytochemicals in fruits and vegetables protect against stroke. This view is supported by a 19-year study of 9,608 men and women aged 25–74 by the Department of Epidemiology of Tulane University in New Orleans. The research team at Tulane reported:

- Adult men and women of all ages whose diets provide a high amount of folic acid (400 micrograms per day) are 21 percent less likely to have strokes than those who consume the lowest amounts of folic acid (100 micrograms per day).[1]

• Over the 19-year period, men and women who consumed the lowest amounts of dietary potassium were 28 percent more likely to have a stroke.2

• Over the same period, men and women who consumed fruits and vegetables 3 or more times a day were 27 percent less likely to have a stroke and 42 percent less likely to die of a stroke than men and women who consumed fruits and vegetables once a day or less.3 They were also 24 percent less likely to die of heart attack.

• People who consumed beans, peas, soy, or other legumes 4 times a week were 11 percent less likely to have a stroke.4

• Consuming more than 6,500 milligrams of salt per day (probably by eating salted foods at most meals) corresponded to a 32 percent increased risk of having a stroke and an 89 percent increased risk of dying from stroke.5

Researchers at Brigham and Women's Hospital and Harvard Medical School have found that women who consumed the highest amounts of fiber (more than 26 grams a day) are 35 percent less likely to have a stroke and 54 percent less likely to have a heart attack than women who consume half as much fiber.6 This research team also found that the consumption of whole grains is associated with lesser incidence of stroke in women, even among women who consumed high-fat foods or smoked.7 The Framingham Study, also administered by Harvard, found that men enjoy roughly a 15 percent reduction in rates of cardiovascular disease for every 100 calorie reduction of total fat in their diets.8 A study by the Centers for Disease Control and Prevention found that eating fish is associated with lower rates of stroke. White women aged 45–74 years who consumed fish more than once a week had an age-adjusted risk of stroke only about half that of women who never consumed fish. For black men and women the reduction was even greater, and for white men, eating fish once a week corresponds to a reduction in risk of stroke of 15 percent.9

There are many limitations in the studies. They look at only one factor at a time, and they cannot estimate the benefits of increasing consumption of fish, folic acid, potassium, legumes, fruits, whole grains, and vegetables, while simultaneously reducing fat and salt. Their data are derived from interviews with participants, usually relying on the interviewee's memory of what they ate. Most important, they do not tell what happens when people *change* their diets, and they tell nothing about the use of supplements to replace foods rich in folic acid. They only report the relationship between nutrition and disease in the past. Nonetheless, these studies are the best available guidance for the nutritional prevention of stroke.

Once a stroke has occurred, the nutritional key to recovery is maintaining high levels of antioxidants. When the flow of blood is reestablished around a clot, the return of oxygen generates free radicals in many areas of the brain. Free radicals of oxygen attack all parts of the brain and all parts of brain cells, their effect most noticeable on cells that have been deprived of nutrients and oxygen for the longest time. Antioxidants in the bloodstream soak up free radicals and protect brain tissue.

Ironically, taking antioxidant supplements can in some cases lower the amount of antioxidants in the brain rather than raise it. Vitamin C is very important for reestablishing the flexibility of the blood vessels leading to the brain and restoring normal circulation. However, it is poorly absorbed by the brain in its primary form. An oxidized form of vitamin C known as dehydroascorbic acid crosses into the brain much more readily and is available to protect brain tissues from the surge of free radicals when circulation is restored. Taking vitamin C increases the body's supply of both vitamin C and dehydroascorbic acid. Taking alpha-lipoic acid recycles dehydroascorbic acid back into vitamin C, a form less readily absorbed by the brain.10

Clinical research has not yet determined an appropriate dose of vitamin C to be taken after stroke, and the most effective dose for any individual is best determined in consultation with a physician familiar with the complete health picture of the person recovering from stroke.

CONCEPTS FOR COPING WITH STROKE

○ People who have had strokes (and people who have not) should avoid pressure on the back of the neck. Be careful not to "crunch" the back of the neck when having hair washed in a barbershop or hairdressing salon. The head should be guided down gently and supported with towels laid over the porcelain surface of the sink.

○ Traditional Chinese Medicine frequently treats stroke patients with an herbal formula based on coptis, Huang Lian Jie Du Tang (Japanese: *oren-gedoku-to*). A clinical study of 20 stroke patients and 20 healthy volunteers in Japan found that the formula slowed the rate at which blood clots formed. Moreover, this blood-thinning effect was more pronounced in stroke patients than in the volunteers, leading researchers to speculate that long-term use of the formula would reduce the risk of a second stroke.[11] Subsequent studies of the formula found that it slowed the rate at which free radicals of oxygen attacked the cholesterol-rich linings of brain cells when flow of oxygenated blood was restored to them after stroke.[12] Brands of this formula available in the United States and Canada include:

- CoptiDetox (Kan Traditionals)

- Coptis & Scute Combination (Lotus Classics, Sun Ten)

- Coptis & Scute Formula (Chinese Classics)

- Coptis & Scutellaria (Qualiherb)

- Huang Lian Jie Du Tang (Chinese Classics, Kan Traditionals, Lotus Classics, Qualiherb, Sun Ten)

- Oregedokuto Formula 016 (Kampo Institute)

- Oren-gedoku-to (Honso, Tsumura)

○ The latest studies support the use of warfarin (Coumadin) in addition to aspirin after stroke.[13] Since Coumadin interacts with many herbs and nutritional supplements, be sure to consult the interactions guide before beginning any new supplement.

Stuffy Nose

SYMPTOM SUMMARY

○ Difficulty breathing through, or sensation of pressure in, the nose

UNDERSTANDING THE DISEASE PROCESS

Nasal congestion is one of the most common of all health complaints. This breathing blockage may result from swelling or inflammation of the nasal tissues, secretion of mucus, or deviated septum, obstruction by one of the small bones of the nose. Short-term sinus congestion is usually caused by the common cold, but a chronic problem with stuffy nose can be related to allergies, foreign bodies in the nose, dust, or tobacco smoke. Interestingly, an Australian study of nasal congestion in

the workplace found that stuffy nose is related not only to dust and mold, but also to workplace noise.[1] A stuffy nose can also be a complication of heartburn or gastroesophageal reflux disease (GERD).[2]

TREATMENT SUMMARY

HERBS

○ Anise

- Aromatherapy (if you can breathe through your nose): 10–20 drops of essential oil in a basin of hot water, vapors inhaled for several minutes once or twice a day. *Never drink essential oils of anise.*

- Tea: bagged anise tea brewed in 1 cup of hot, but not boiling, water.

○ Eucalyptus

- Cough lozenges containing eucalyptus, as desired.

○ Horehound (also known as marrubio)

- Cough lozenges containing horehound: As often as desired.

- Tea (from the chopped herb available in hierberías): 1 teaspoon brewed in a cup of hot, but not boiling, water for 10 minutes, strained before drinking, 2–3 times a day.

○ Horseradish, hot peppers, or wasabi

- Eat as much as you can stand several times a day.

○ Mullein

- Tincture: $1/4$ – $3/4$ teaspoon up to 4 times a day.

AROMATHERAPY

○ Add 5–10 drops of eucalyptus oil to the water in a vaporizer operated in your bedroom as you sleep.

UNDERSTANDING THE HEALING PROCESS

When a colds virus establishes itself in the lining of the nose, it causes release of histamine, which dramatically increases the blood flow to the nose, causing swelling and congestion of nasal tissues, and stimulating the nasal membranes to produce excessive amounts of mucus. Since the nose has a limited blood supply, it has poor resistance against bacterial infections, and bacterial infections of the nose and sinuses often follow a cold. When the nasal mucus turns from clear to yellow or green, it usually means that a bacterial infection has taken over and a physician should be consulted. Only time will cure a stuffy nose, but many natural products will relieve symptoms.

Anise and the related herb star anise contain an antimicrobial chemical, anethole.[3] The essential oil is especially deadly to molds and yeast infections.[4] Since anise stimulates production of secretions, it should not be used when the primary cause of congestion is deviated septum or a foreign body in the nose.

Horehound, also known as marrubio, is a traditional remedy for stuffy nose in the southwestern United States and Mexico. It is also widely used in the Arab world. Unlike over-the-counter remedies for nasal congestion, it lowers blood pressure[5] (and is nonaddictive). It also relieves the pain of sore throat.[6] Complications from using horehound are rare, but since it is a bitter and bitters stimulate production of stomach acids, people with gastroesophageal reflux disease (GERD), chronic heartburn, or peptic ulcers should use the herb in moderation.

Horseradish, hot peppers, and wasabi contain volatile oils that have antibacterial properties. They also open nasal and bronchial passages. Hot peppers clear the nose by acting directly on the nerves controlling flow through the nose and tear ducts. Capsaicin creams applied directly to the lining of the nose can shrink nasal polyps,[7] although extreme care must be exercised to keep capsaicin out of the eyes.

Mullein contains chemicals that kill bacteria and stop pain.[8] Taken at the same time as a flu treatment such as amatadine (Symmetrel), it greatly increases the probability that the flu treatment will work.[9] The combination of mullein and zanamivir (Relenza) has not yet been tested. Mullein does not generally cause any side effects, although some people may be allergic to it.

Eucalyptus is a common ingredient in lozenges and vaporizer additives for coughs and colds. A study of 246 people with chronic bronchitis found that eucalyptus oils stop the worsening of cough and congestion that commonly occurs in the winter (in wet climates where heaters are used) or summer (in desert climates).[10] Other essential oils can also be helpful in the vaporizer, or breathed in during a steaming bath. Chamomile, elderberry, and lemon balm relieve pain in the nostrils. Yarrow stops inflammation in the nose and throat.

CONCEPTS FOR COPING WITH STUFFY NOSE

❍ Using decongestant sprays for more than 2–3 days

can cause vasomotor rhinitis, an inflammation of the nose not associated with allergies, colds, or infections. In this condition—which can also be caused by psychological stress, inadequate thyroid function, pregnancy, certain anti–high blood pressure drugs, or prolonged exposure to irritants such as perfumes and tobacco smoke—the blood vessels in the nose enlarge like varicose veins. They fill with excess blood and block the passage of air through the nose. They expand when the person lies down and turns to one side, the lower side becoming congested. This congestion often interferes with sleep. Vasomotor rhinitis can become permanent if decongestants are used over a period of months or years. To relieve stuffy nose caused by vasomotor rhinitis at night, elevate the head of the bed by placing a brick under the castors at the head of the bed, lifting the head of the bed 2–4 inches (5–10 centimeters). Propping yourself up with pillows is not effective.

❍ Ephedra is effective but has fallen out of favor for treating stuffy nose. Safe and effective herbal formulas that contain small, reliably measured quantities of ephedra buffered with other herbs include:

• Ge Gen Tang, a Chinese herbal remedy combining kudzu, ephedra, and other herbs to treat stuffy nose accompanying ear infections and allergies (especially those with tension headaches) in adults. This formula is sold under a variety of trade names:

  • Ge Gen Tang (Chinese Classics, Golden Flower Chinese Herbs, Honso, Kan Traditionals, Lotus Classics, ProBotanixx, Qualiherb, Sun Ten)

  • Kakkon-to (Tsumura)

  • Kakkonto Formula 026 (Kampo Institute)

  • Kampo4Cold/Flu Pueraria Formula (Honso)

  • Kudzu Releasing Formula (Kan Traditionals)

  • Pueraria Combination (Lotus Classics, Qualiherb, Sun Ten)

  • Pueraria Formula (Golden Flower Chinese Herbs)

  • Pueraria Plus Formula (Chinese Classics)

  • Shu Jin 1 (ProBotanixx)

• Ma Huang Tang, a Chinese herbal remedy containing ephedra, peach seed, cinnamon, and licorice, used to treat stuffy nose occurring in conditions that do not cause fever. This formula is made by several companies marketing it as Ma Huang Combination.

○ Due to circadian variations in the activity of the immune system, stuffy noses caused by allergies are usually worst early in the morning, especially in children.[11] In these cases, vaporizers are very helpful.

○ If you have heartburn or GERD and stuffy nose is a recurrent problem, avoid eating for 3 or 4 hours before going to bed. Elevating the head of the bed as for vasomotor rhinitis is also helpful.

Sunburn

SYMPTOM SUMMARY

○ Skin marked by:

- Pain

- Redness

- Inflammation

○ Occurs 15 minutes to 12 hours after exposure to bright sun

UNDERSTANDING THE DISEASE PROCESS

Sunburn is a very common affliction of the skin caused by exposure to ultraviolet rays. Generally speaking, the severity of sunburn is inversely proportional to the amount of the skin pigment melanin. Melanin is a giant molecule formed by linking together smaller molecules of the amino acid tyrosine. It is made in specialized skin cells known as melanocytes, where it is packaged into tiny spheres known as melanosomes, which are absorbed by the outer layers of the skin.

Melanin absorbs sunlight, and sunlight stimulates the production of melanin. When the skin is exposed to so much ultraviolet radiation that melanin cannot absorb it all, however, excess radiation goes into the DNA of outer layers of skin cells known as keratinocytes. When the DNA is these cells is disrupted, they become "sunburn cells," programmed to die. Inflammatory processes clear these cells away for the renewal of healthy skin. The process of clearing the skin causes pain, redness, and inflammation. The destruction of skin cell DNA continues for up to 24 hours after exposure to sunlight and then diminishes. The immune systems of older persons are usually less active and cause a less severe inflammatory reaction to sunburn.

TREATMENT SUMMARY

DIET

○ Eat orange vegetables (such as carrots or sweet potatoes) daily. Include hearts of palm or palm oil in the diet when other nutritional concerns permit. Avoid celeriac (celery root).

NUTRITIONAL SUPPLEMENTS

○ Mixed carotenoids: 25 milligrams per day. The alga *Dunaliella salina* is a particularly rich source of carotenoids. Start taking mixed carotenoids 8–10 weeks before summer sun exposure.

○ Vitamin C: 2,000 milligrams per day.

○ Vitamin E: 800 IU per day.

Vitamins C and E must be taken together for a protective effect.

HERBS

○ Red clover: 40–160 milligrams of isoflavones daily.

Apply liberally to sunburned skin:

○ Any Aloe vera gel, *or*

○ Any cream containing EGCG (a potent antioxidant found in green tea).

Use with Caution:

○ Dong quai, khella, psoralea, and St. John's wort.

UNDERSTANDING THE HEALING PROCESS

The most effective approach to healing sunburn is prevention. Stay out of the sun, wear protective clothing, or use sunblock with an SPF rating of 15 or more. The SPF number gives you a rough idea of how long you can stay out in the sun without burning. For instance, if you ordinarily burn in 10 minutes when you do not use sunscreen, you would be protected for 150 minutes by using a sunscreen with an SPF of 15. People who have fair skin, work or play outdoors most of the day, live at high altitudes, or perspire heavily should use a sunscreen with an SPF higher than 15. Swimming or perspiring heavily reduces the SPF effect of any sunscreen.

In hereditary diseases causing severe sun sensitivity, beta-carotene slightly raises the minimum level of UV exposure that causes tissue damage, so that people taking beta-carotene are more likely to tan than to burn.[1] Orange vegetables such as carrots and sweet potatoes are an excellent source of beta-carotene. While synthetic beta-carotene is better absorbed, natural sources of this vitamin have a greater positive effect on the immune system.[2] The carotenes in palm oil are 4–10 times better absorbed that synthetic *trans*-beta carotene.[3,4]

Eating very large quantities of carrots, in the range of 450–1,000 grams (1–2 pounds) per day can cause a condition known as carotenodermia, in which the skin turns yellow and then orange. The condition is reversible when carrots are discontinued. Eating large quantities of carrots daily for several years can cause depletion of white blood cells (neutropenia)[5] and menstrual disorders.[6]

Severe sunburn has been noted in people who eat large quantities (500 grams, or more than 1 pound) of the vegetable celeriac in a single meal.

Mixed carotenoids, a group of vegetable pigments found in orange and yellow vegetables and the alga *Dunaliella salina,* have been tested in several clinical trials as a preventative for sunburn. In one study, 20 young women took 30 milligrams daily of beta-carotene or a placebo for 10 weeks before a 13-day stretch of controlled sun exposure at a resort on the shores of the Red Sea. Participants taking beta-carotene before and during the sun exposure experienced less skin redness than those taking a placebo, even when both groups used sunscreen.[7] Two other studies conducted without a control group reported similar results. One study involving 20 participants and one study involving 22 participants found that supplementation with mixed carotenoids for 12–24 weeks increased tolerance for summer sun.[8,9] The evidence shows that it is necessary to take mixed carotenoids for several months to gain any benefit. A study lasting 23 days[10] and another study lasting 4 weeks[11] did not find any benefit of taking mixed carotenoids over taking a placebo in reducing sensitivity to sun.

Experiments with animals have confirmed that applying vitamin C and vitamin E directly to the skin protects against UV damage. One study found that topical vitamin C protected more against UVA rays, topical vitamin E protected more against UVB rays, and that applying vitamins C and E together worked better than either by itself.[12] The sun-protective value of the vitamins was even greater when they were applied with sunscreen.[13]

It is important to note that the recommendations here call for the use of mixed carotenoids, not beta-carotene. A controversial study in Finland reported in 1995 that taking beta-carotene could increase the risk of lung cancer among smokers (from approximately 0.4 percent per year to approximately 0.5 percent per year),[14] and the Carotene and Retinol Efficacy Trial in the United States was halted prematurely when it was found that it also increased the risk of lung cancer among smokers and asbestos workers (from 0.5 percent to 0.6 percent).[15] The reason for these menacing findings likely has to do with the fact that beta-carotene, without other nutrients, is an oxidant rather than an antioxidant.[16] Beta-carotene is protected from oxidation by the presence of other nutrients, such as those provided by mixed carotenoids.[17]

Recent research points to red clover as a source of potent antioxidants that stop the breakdown of tyrosine in the melanin in the skin and also stop the immune reactions that cause swelling of sunburned skin. Although experiments have been limited to animals, scientists at the University of Sydney in Australia have found that both red clover in the diet and red clover ointments offer protection against moderate sun exposure. The most potent phytochemical in red clover for sun protection is equol, which is best applied in the form of a skin cream formulated by a compounding pharmacist. The red clover component genistein, which is contained in red clover isoflavone tablets, also protects against the sun.[18]

Aloe vera gels have been tested in 13 studies as a remedy for burns, but have not been scientifically tested as a treatment for sunburn. The vast body of practical experience suggests aloe will relieve pain and inflammation, although a small clinical study found that it does not relieve redness.[19] Jojoba and poplar bud may also be helpful.

Dr. Steven Stratton at the Arizona Cancer Center in Tucson is developing sun-care creams from the green tea derivative epigallocatechin gallate (EGCG), one of which was approved by the FDA for investigational use and is in early clinical development. The center's ultimate goal is to develop "super sunscreens" that will reverse or inhibit cancers in sun-damaged skin. According to two studies, mice given green tea in their drinking water or receiving skin creams containing green tea catechins were protected against as much as 90 percent of the immune system's response to sunburn causing inflammation, as well as swelling induced by the migration of white blood cells into the skin.[20] Scientists speculated that EGCG could prevent carcinogenesis caused by exposure to UVB[21] Studies at the Medical School at

Case Western Reserve University involving human test subjects found that EGCG prevented damage to skin cell DNA by sunlight, the pain and redness of sunburn,[22] and also the formation of sunburn cells, skin cells in which the DNA has been disrupted causing them to be programmed to die.[23]

Most of the commercial sunburn creams that contain EGCG mix the green tea catechin with other ingredients, such as bovine colostrum. While other ingredients do not usually offer protection against the sun and are of no direct benefit in healing sunburn, they may aid the general health of the skin by fighting infection.

CONCEPTS FOR COPING WITH SUNBURN

○ Many medications make the skin more sensitive to the sun or aggravate rashes. Dong quai and St. John's wort may make the skin more sensitive to sun, especially if you also take oral contraceptives, sulfa drugs, tetracycline, the blood pressure medication lisinopril (Prinivil or Zestril), or the arthritis drug piroxicam (Feldene).

○ Sun-protective clothes differ from typical summer clothes by having a tighter weave. They usually come in dark colors. The UPF (Ultraviolet Protection Factor) rating indicates how much of the sun's damaging rays are blocked by the fabric. A garment with a UPF rating of 20 only allows $1/20$ of the sun's ultraviolet radiation to pass through. All garments with a UPF of over 50 are rated as 50+. All garments with a UPF of 50+ block at least 98 percent of the sun's radiation.

○ Children are especially susceptible to sunburn. It is important to apply a sunblock with an SPF of 15 or higher at least 30 minutes before children go outdoors. Reapply sunscreens after they swim, towel off, or play hard. Infants under the age of 6 months should be kept out of the sun altogether, since sunblock can irritate babies' skin.

Syphilis

SYMPTOM SUMMARY

○ Chancres—painless ulcers forming on the genitalia, anus, fingers, lips, tongue, tonsils or eyelids, or on the wall of the vagina and cervix in women—beginning a few days after infection and healing after 3–6 weeks

○ Headache, nausea, vomiting, fatigue, hair loss, and a highly infectious oozing rash beginning a few days after infection and lasting up to 8 weeks

○ Periodic recurrences of infectious rash

○ Gummas—disfiguring scar tissue of the skin that can also occur in the bones, several years after infection

○ Chronic headache, psychosis, and damage to heart and kidneys many years after infection

UNDERSTANDING THE DISEASE PROCESS

Syphilis is a highly contagious sexually transmitted disease caused by the microbe *Treponema pallidum*. In the United States, syphilis is the third most commonly reported venereal disease, after chlamydia and gonorrhea.

The symptoms of syphilis occur in four stages. During the first or primary stage, painless ulcers called chancres appear on the genitals, anus, fingers, lips, tongue, tonsils, or eyelids of both sexes and on the wall of the vagina and cervix in women. Even if the infection is not treated, chancres usually disappear after 3–6 weeks. A few days to a few weeks after infection, syphilis causes symptoms of the secondary stage, including headache, nausea, vomiting, fatigue, hair loss, and an oozing rash consisting of small, red, scaly bumps. During this stage syphilis is highly contagious through the secretions released by the rash. There may also be fever or swelling of the lymph nodes in the armpits or groin.

During the latent stage of syphilis, there are no symptoms, although the rash may periodically reappear. During the fourth stage of syphilis, men may become impotent, and infected persons of both sexes may experience shooting pains in the legs, loss of balance, mental deterioration, and heart or kidney disease.

TREATMENT SUMMARY

NUTRITIONAL SUPPLEMENTS

○ Vitamin B$_6$: 100–200 milligrams daily.

○ Avoid 5-HTP.

HERBS

○ Copaiba cream: apply to rash.

UNDERSTANDING THE HEALING PROCESS

Antibiotics are essential in the treatment of syphilis. During antibiotic therapy, it is important to avoid foods and nutritional supplements containing quercetin or rutin, including supplemental quercetin and rutin as well as buckwheat, grapefruit juice, and onions. Quercetin and rutin counteract ciprofloxacin antibiotics used to treat the disease. Antibiotics are better absorbed when taken with bromelain. A single tablet of bromelain with each dose of antibiotic is sufficient.

Drug therapy usually eradicates syphilis in 3 months, but about 10 percent of treated people reacquire the disease within a year. It is responsible to avoid sexual intercourse during the first 3 months of treatment, and to use barriers (condoms or dams) for sexual intercourse even after treatment. If you experience fever, sore throat, or joint pain (especially in the knee) after treatment for syphilis, you should seek medical attention to make sure the disease has not returned. It is also important to make sure sexual partner(s) get treatment, to avoid reinfection.

The neurological damage caused by late-stage syphilis is made worse by excessive supplies of the amino acid tryptophan, a byproduct of 5-HTP. Chronic syphilis causes the nervous system to convert tryptophan into kynurenine, a nerve toxin. The production of kynurenine is greatest when vitamin B_6 is deficient,[1] so it is helpful to take 100–200 milligrams of vitamin B_6 daily and avoid 5-HTP.

Tropical herbal medicine expert Leslie Taylor advises that copaiba cream can form a protective layer over the rash caused by syphilis. Relief from inflammation is usually almost instantaneous. It is likely that copaiba reduces infectivity of the rash, but use of the cream is not a substitute for appropriate hygiene.

CONCEPTS FOR COPING WITH SYPHILIS

❍ Syphilis is similar to chancroid, a sexually transmitted disease caused by *Haemophilus ducreyi,* one of the most common causes of genital ulcer disease worldwide. In developed countries, chancroid is most frequently acquired in urban areas where crack cocaine use and prostitution are prominent. Chancroid causes swellings of the lymphatic system known as buboes, and chancroid infection greatly increases the risk of acquiring HIV.[2]

Systemic Lupus Erythematosus (SLE)
See **Lupus**.

Tardive Dyskinesia

SYMPTOM SUMMARY

❍ Uncontrollable, repetitive movements after prolonged use of medications for schizophrenia

UNDERSTANDING THE DISEASE PROCESS

"Tardive" means late, and "dyskinesia" means abnormal movement. Tardive dyskinesia (TD) is a debilitating side effect of prolonged treatment with the antipsychotic drugs chlorpromazine (Thorazine), thioridazine (Mellaril), and trifluoperazine (Stelazine). People with tardive dyskinesia may display repetitive blinking, grimaces, hunching, sucking, slow twisting of the hands, or tics. Discontinuing medication that causes TD usually does not help and may even make the symptoms of TD worse, as well as aggravate the underlying schizophrenia.

TREATMENT SUMMARY

NUTRITIONAL SUPPLEMENTS

❍ Branched-chain amino acids: see Understanding the Healing Process.

❍ Vitamin E: 1,600 IU per day.

UNDERSTANDING THE HEALING PROCESS

Medications for TD are only about 35 percent effective, so researchers have actively sought other forms of treatment. One theory of the causes of TD is that antipsychotic drugs generate free radicals that damage brain tissue.[1] Numerous clinical trials have attempted to relieve TD by providing supplemental antioxidants that counteract free radicals.

The best results have been obtained with branched-chain amino acids (a combination of isoleucine, leucine, and valine). A small clinical trial sponsored by the New York State Office of Mental Health found that *every* patient taking branched-chain amino acids for just 2 weeks experienced at least a 38 percent decrease in dyskinetic motion, that is, twitches, tics, and uncontrollable movements. Two-thirds of patients in the small study had decreases of 58 percent, a dramatic improvement in quality of life.[2]

The branched-chain amino acid study gave patients

150–229 milligrams of amino acid supplements for every kilogram (2.2 pounds) of body weight. A person weighing 150 pounds (70 kilograms), for example, would receive 150 x 70 or 10,500 milligrams of the supplement daily. Up to 229 x 70 or 16,030 milligrams of the supplement may be helpful. Do not use amino acid combination products that contain phenylalanine. This amino acid, also found in eggs, fish, legumes, meat, nuts, and soy, may interact with medications to cause release of free radicals that damage brain tissue.

Vitamin E is the least expensive treatment for TD. Several studies have found that taking vitamin E for just a few weeks has little effect. However, a clinical trial sponsored by the Veteran Administration found that TD patients on high doses of vitamin E for at least 10 weeks experienced gradual improvement in symptoms from the tenth week and continuing for another 6–7 months.[3]

CONCEPTS FOR COPING WITH TARDIVE DYSKINESIA

O Doctors at North Nassau Mental Health Center in New York report they are able to *prevent* TD by providing their patients with megadoses of common vitamins: up to 4,000 milligrams of vitamin C daily, up to 4,000 milligrams of niacin daily, up to 800 milligrams of vitamin B_6, and up to 1,200 IU of vitamin E. During a 10-year period, no patient treated for schizophrenia at the center developed TD.[4] Since the combination of niacin and schizophrenia medications can cause liver damage, high-dose therapy should be attempted only under a doctor's supervision.

Tennis Elbow

SYMPTOM SUMMARY

O Elbow pain worsening over a period of several weeks to several months

O Pain shooting from the elbow to the forearm and back of the hand

O Difficulty grasping objects

O Pain when the tendon attached to the upper arm is touched

UNDERSTANDING THE DISEASE PROCESS

In tennis elbow, identified in the medical literature as lateral epicondylitis, the outer part of the elbow becomes painful and tender, usually as a result of a specific strain, overuse, or a hard blow. The condition is also known as golfer's elbow, and is common among people who do mechanic work, painting, or plastering for a living. The most common cause of tennis elbow is overuse of the muscles which are attached to the bone at the outside of the elbow, that is, the wrist extensors, the muscles that pull the hand backward.

Tennis elbow is commonly misunderstood to be an inflammatory condition, but the modern understanding of the biology of the disease is that its principal cause is not inflammation.[1] Instead, tennis elbow results from the fraying and tangling of fibers of collagen that form the framework of the tendon, and only when the collagen itself is healed does pain stop.[2] Anti-inflammatory treatments such as cortisone and other steroids may relieve pain in surrounding tissues, but they have no effect on the underlying cause of the condition.

TREATMENT SUMMARY

HERBS

For pain relief without aspirin, ibuprofen, or similar medications, select from:

O Bromelain: 250–500 milligrams 3 times a day.

O Capsaicin cream: apply to affected area.

O Devil's claw: 405–520 milligrams up to 8 times a day.

O Feverfew: 70–100 milligrams of dried extract daily.

O Ginger (fresh): 2 tablespoons included in vegetable dishes, fruit salad, or used to make a tea.

O Willow bark: 1 teaspoon in a cup of hot water or tea, as desired.

NUTRITIONAL SUPPLEMENTS

To encourage healing:

O Vitamin B_6: 200 milligrams daily.

O Do *not* take supplemental vitamin C unless you also take vitamin B_6.

If swelling is a problem:

O Pycnogenol creams or lotions: apply to the skin according to label directions, or 200 milligrams of Pycnogenol in capsule form, daily.

If you take steroid injections:

❍ Glycyrrhizin: 250–500 milligrams daily for up to 6 weeks at a time.

If you take aspirin or NSAIDs on a regular basis:

❍ Any B-vitamin supplement: 1 tablet daily.

See Part Three if you take prescription medication.

UNDERSTANDING THE HEALING PROCESS

For most people with tennis elbow, the first priority in treatment is relieving pain. There are a number of natural products and supplements that offer pain relief. Bromelain can start relieving pain and swelling almost as soon as you start taking it, provided you take it in an enteric-coated form (unavailable in the United States).[3] For those of us who have to take uncoated bromelain tablets, it is best to experiment with the smallest dose and increase by 250 milligrams a day until you reach the highest recommended dose. It may be necessary to take the highest recommended dose of uncoated bromelain for a week before obtaining relief.

Allergies to bromelain are very rare but not unheard of. Allergic reactions to this supplement are most likely in people who are already allergic to pineapple, papaya, wheat flour, rye flour, or birch pollen. There has never been a report of an anaphylactic reaction to bromelain. There have been isolated reports of heavy periods, nausea, vomiting, and hives when bromelain is taken in very large doses (2,000 milligrams and higher).

Capsaicin is the chemical that gives hot peppers their heat. As anyone who has cooked with chiles knows, capsaicin can cause burning, redness, and inflammation, especially to the eyes and mouth. The first time it is applied in a cream to the skin over a painful joint, capsaicin causes these symptoms, but the nerve fibers serving the joint become insensitive to it—and to pain.[4]

Capsaicin works best when there is good circulation to the skin to which it is applied.[5] Never apply capsaicin to ulcerated skin. It is also important to keep capsaicin out of your nose and eyes. Allergic reactions to capsaicin are rare but are not unknown, and there have been cases of hypothermia in people who used capsaicin in an especially cold room. It is theoretically possible that capsaicin absorbed into the bloodstream could reduce the bioavailability of aspirin; if you use capsaicin, use pain relievers other than aspirin. If you are sensitive to capsaicin, diluted essential oils of peppermint, eucalyptus,

rosemary, or wintergreen may be used instead. Never take essential oils internally.

Devil's claw relieves the pain of tennis elbow, but only if it is taken in an enteric-coated form that protects its analgesic compounds from being digested in the stomach. Do not use devil's claw with NSAIDs such as aspirin and Tylenol, and avoid it entirely if you have duodenal or gastric ulcers.

Like other herbs to relieve pain, feverfew can cause stomach irritation. Do not use it with NSAIDs and avoid it if you have ulcers.

Two tablespoons of fresh ginger every day is likely to relieve pain and swelling even when pain relievers are discontinued, but the effect takes 1–3 months.

Willow bark is a natural substitute for aspirin. It contains salicin, a less potent pain reliever than the salicylates found in aspirin and one that does not generally cause bleeding or stomach irritation. Do not use willow bark during pregnancy, if you have tinnitus (ringing in the ears), or if you are allergic to aspirin. Do not give willow bark or aspirin to children who have colds or flu.

The only nutritional supplement with a probable effect on the disease process of tennis elbow itself is vitamin B_6. This vitamin has little effect on the function of the tendon, but is useful in relieving pain.[6] The *balance* between vitamin B_6 and vitamin C in the bloodstream may be more important in a similar condition, carpal tunnel syndrome (CTS). In a study of 441 adults with CTS, higher ratios of vitamin C to vitamin B_6 (such as might occur when taking supplemental vitamin C without vitamin B_6) were associated with the severity of pain and the frequency of pain, tingling, and waking up at night.[7]

Most of the research studies involving vitamin B_6 used a dosage of 200 milligrams daily. This dosage is too much for pregnant women and nursing mothers, who should limit intake to 100 milligrams per day. There have been only a few cases in which taking 100–200 milligrams of B_6 a day aggravated existing nerve damage. Diabetics also should only use more than 100 milligrams per day if they do not suffer sensory neuropathy, that is, nerve damage to the hands and feet. Men who use sildenafil citrate (Viagra) should avoid high doses of this vitamin for the same reason.

Vitamin B_6 requirements are affected by many medications. The use of oral contraceptives increases vitamin B_6 requirements. The vitamin is depleted during treatment with carbamazepine for bipolar disorder; cycloserine or ethionamide for tuberculosis; hydralazine for high blood pressure; penicillamine for arthritis, Wilson's disease, and certain skin conditions; and phenelzine for cocaine addiction, eating disorders, headaches, and panic attacks. If you take any of these prescription drugs and have tennis elbow, you should take supplemental vitamin B_6. On the other hand, if you take levodopa for Parkinson's disease, theophylline for asthma, or phenytoin or valproic acid for seizures, you should not take vitamin B_6 supplements, since the vitamin can deactivate these medications. Regardless of the medications you take, if you experience abdominal pain, loss of appetite, nausea, vomiting, breast pain, or unexplained sensitivity to the sun, discontinue use of the vitamin.

While Pycnogenol has no effect on the underlying disease process, it may help relieve swelling. Pycnogenol contains oligomeric procyanidins and oligomeric proanthocyanidins (OPCs) that stop inflammation secondary to an immune process triggered by the destruction of collagen.[8] These chemicals also help the walls of capillaries retain their strength and elasticity, making it less likely that they will leak fluids into the muscles and cause swelling.

Because Pycnogenol helps the body retain vitamin C, and an imbalance between vitamin C and vitamin B_6 is an underling cause of this condition, you should not take both Pycnogenol and supplemental vitamin C. Also, if you are a smoker taking an anticoagulant drug such as Coumadin (warfarin) or any drug for frostbite, do not take Pycnogenol. Aside from these rare instances, Pycnogenol is generally safe and free of side effects.

If you are taking injections of steroids to relieve pain, a licorice derivative called glycyrrhizin can help make them more effective. It increases the half-life of cortisol and other steroids, making them work longer to undo the damage done to your joints.[9] The downside of using glycyrrhizin for this purpose is that it *will* increase any side effects you experience from cortisone. When you take both glycyrrhizin and any corticosteroid drug, you are more likely to experience weight gain, puffiness, and elevated blood pressure. Do not take glycyrrhizin for more than 6 weeks at a time. Preferably, use it during your peak allergy season. Do not take glycyrrhizin if you have high blood pressure. DGL is another licorice derivative that does not aggravate side effects of steroid treatment, but it will not help tennis elbow.

The B vitamins thiamine, pyridoxine, and cobalamin (B_1, B_6, and B_{12}) make it possible to use lower doses of aspirin and other nonsteroidal anti-inflammatory agents for the same degree of pain relief.[10] Lowering doses of aspirin or NSAIDs reduces stomach upset. Vitamin B supplements may be especially useful for sufferers of tennis elbow who take the diuretic furosemide (Lasix) or who are heavy drinkers of coffee or tea. The drawback to using B vitamins is that they reduce, rather than eliminate, the need for pain relievers. B vitamins enhance nerve function so that if the vitamins are taken for 3 days and the aspirin or NSAIDs are eliminated entirely, pain worsens.[11] Do not discontinue aspirin or NSAIDs without also discontinuing vitamin B.

CONCEPTS FOR COPING WITH TENNIS ELBOW

O Many people get relief of pain from acupuncture. One to 2 weeks before beginning acupuncture for tennis elbow, start taking 500 milligrams of DL-phenylalanine 2–3 times a day. DL-phenylalanine increases the analgesic effect of acupuncture in both laboratory tests with animals and in clinical trials.[12]

O DMSO (dimethyl sulfoxide) applied to the skin can relieve pain, although it is important to note that weaker solutions (70%) offer greater pain relief than stronger solutions (the more usual 90%). DMSO works like a fast-acting vitamin C. In as little as 30 seconds after application, the bloodstream carries DMSO to the joints, where it protects hyaluronic acid, one of the components of collagen, from damage by free radicals.[13] This possibly keeps cartilage from being destroyed or helps new cartilage form.[14]

DMSO can dissolve any toxin on the skin and send it into circulation throughout the body in under 30 seconds. Industrial-grade DMSO, the form most commonly sold in flea markets, can contain toxic byproducts of the manufacturing process and should not be applied to the skin. MSM (methylsulfonylmethane) is a byproduct of DMSO as it is metabolized by the body, that is also found in alfalfa sprouts, corn, most fruits, tomatoes, coffee, tea, and milk. MSM is also used to treat arthritic pain, and unlike DMSO, is almost completely nontoxic. Most naturopaths recommend 1,000–2,000 milligrams of MSM daily to prevent tennis elbow pain and 3,000–5,000 milligrams of MSM daily to treat tennis elbow pain.

O Daily use of TENS (transcutaneous electrical nerve stimulation) for 1–2 weeks reduces or eliminates pain in patients with tennis elbow. TENS is widely available in the United States from physical therapists and massage therapists, and at some sports clubs.

○ Ultrasound therapy is widely and successfully used as a nonsurgical treatment for tendon pain. Extracorporeal sound wave therapy (ESWT), involves focusing sound blasts to the area of pain. The treatment is being used in Canada and Europe to treat chronic pain or pain over a small area, particularly near a bone. The joint pain treated by this system includes the shoulder, elbow, ankle, and, as in Jackson's case, the knee. ESWT or Sonocur is not approved for use in the United States or Japan.

Tension Headaches

SYMPTOM SUMMARY

○ Dull pain and pressure on both sides of the head

○ No sense of pulsation

○ Sensitivity to light or sound but not both

○ May last from 30 minutes to a week

○ No nausea or vomiting

○ Not aggravated by physical activity

○ Not associated with a prodrome in which "you can feel it coming on"

UNDERSTANDING THE DISEASE PROCESS

Tension headaches are the most common type of headache. Nearly 90 percent of women and 70 percent of men develop a tension headache at some point in their lives. Although this kind of headache is most commonly triggered by tension, stress, eyestrain, lack of sleep, or missing meals, its true cause seems to be an imbalance in the production of the neurotransmitters dopamine, norepinephrine, and serotonin in the brain.[1]

TREATMENT SUMMARY

NUTRITIONAL SUPPLEMENTS

○ 5-HTP: 100 milligrams per day.

○ Vitamin B_6: 100 milligrams per day.

HERBS

○ Peppermint oil: dab a few drops on the forehead when headache begins, repeat every 15 minutes.

UNDERSTANDING THE HEALING PROCESS

To avoid tension headaches, minimize your exposure to stressful situations, get regular exercise, go to bed early, eat balanced meals, avoid eyestrain, and sit up straight. If your routine does not permit these changes in lifestyle, two supplements may be helpful.

The brain converts 5-hydroxytrytophan (5-HTP) into the neurotransmitter serotonin. Various clinical trials have found that taking 5-HTP reduces anxiety and depression. European research confirms that people who take 5-HTP on a regular basis need fewer pain relievers to control headache pain.[2] Taking vitamin B_6 enhances the brain's use of 5-HTP to make serotonin.

Do not overdose 5-HTP. There is a long list of medications that preclude use of 5-HTP. Consult Part Three.

Peppermint oil applied to the forehead or scalp is a traditional remedy for headache. Clinical study in Germany has confirmed its use as a pain reliever. Using both acetaminophen (Tylenol) and peppermint oil has an additive analgesic effect.[3]

CONCEPTS FOR COPING WITH TENSION HEADACHES

○ If you feel you are experiencing "the worst headache of your life," seek emergency medical attention. Extreme headache pain without a history of cluster headaches or migraine may indicate bleeding in the brain.

○ When headache comes on with fever or rash, see a physician to rule out encephalitis, Lyme disease, or meningitis.

○ At least one study found that chiropractic manipulation has lasting benefits in preventing tension headaches, and chiropractic care is more effective than simple massage.[4] If tension headaches with cramping in the neck and shoulders is a persistent problem, consider asking a chiropractor or physician about TENS (transcutaneous electroneural stimulation). Many people also benefit from reflexology (foot massage).

Testicular Inflammation
See **Epididymitis**.

Tinea Barbasae
See **Barber's Itch**.

Tinea Pedis

See **Athlete's Foot**.

Tinnitus

SYMPTOM SUMMARY

○ Ringing, buzzing, or other sounds in the ears when no external sound is present

UNDERSTANDING THE DISEASE PROCESS

Tinnitus (tin-night'-is *or* tin'-it-is, either pronunciation is correct) is the perception of ringing, hissing, or other sound in the ears or head when no external sound is present. For some people, tinnitus is just a nuisance. For others, it is a life-altering condition. According to the American Tinnitus Association, 12 million people in the United States have tinnitus severe enough to disrupt their daily (and nightly) activities.

The sounds of tinnitus include ringing, buzzing, hissing, whistling, roaring, blowing, pulsating, high- or low-pitched sounds, gunshots, and others. The mechanism that causes the perception of sounds where there is no outside source of the noise is not known, but tinnitus is a common complication of ear infections, wax in the ear, Ménière's disease, and acoustic trauma. It is also a symptom of age-related hearing loss, hardening of the carotid arteries, aneurysm, brain tumors, and anemia.

TREATMENT SUMMARY

NUTRITIONAL SUPPLEMENTS

○ Vitamin A: 300,000 IU *weekly* for 6 weeks. Women who are or who may become pregnant should strictly limit their intake of vitamin A to 5,000 IU per day or less.

○ Vitamin B$_{12}$: 250 milligrams daily for 6 weeks.

○ Vitamin E: 100 IU daily for 6 weeks.

HERBS

○ Ginkgo: 80 milligrams of an extract containing 24% ginkgo flavonglycosides taken 3 times a day for 3 months.

UNDERSTANDING THE HEALING PROCESS

The primary rule of thumb in treating tinnitus is the sooner, the better. The very best way to deal with acous-tic trauma is to wear hearing protection so that it never occurs. If you can't avoid exposure to loud noise, then you must take immediate steps to treat it. Ideally, treatment should begin within 12 hours of trauma. Vitamins A, B$_{12}$, and E are helpful in the early stages of tinnitus. Both acute and chronic tinnitus may be treated with ginkgo.

Vitamin A in very high doses for very short periods can sometimes greatly improve hearing loss. A Swiss study in 1952 found that survivors of explosions sometimes regained hearing after treatment with 300,000 IU of vitamin A per *week* for 6 weeks. The effect of the vitamin was greatest for people whose acoustic trauma was the most recent. Vitamin A helped recover the ability to hear high pitches more than it helped recover the ability to hear low-intensity sounds, such as whispers.[1]

The drawback to using vitamin A as a supplement is that a dose that is big enough to help heal acoustic trauma is big enough to cause side effects. Problems from using even up to 300,000 IU of vitamin A per *day* (nearly 7 times as much as was used in the Swiss study) are rare, but they are significant. The first signs of vitamin A overdose are dry skin and chapped lips, especially in dry weather. Later signs of toxicity are headache, mood swings, and pain in muscles and joints. In massive doses, vitamin A can cause liver damage. In the first 3 months of pregnancy, it can cause birth defects. Women who are or who could become pregnant should strictly limit their intake of vitamin A to 5,000 IU per day or less. Discontinue vitamin A at the first sign of toxicity, and do not use it for longer than the recommended 6 weeks.

A study by the Israeli Army found that about half of the 86 soldiers in the study who suffered hearing loss related to acoustic trauma also suffered vitamin B$_{12}$ deficiency. (The study also found that about a quarter of soldiers who do *not* have hearing loss suffer vitamin B$_{12}$ deficiency.) The researchers concluded that there is a relationship between vitamin B$_{12}$ deficiency and dysfunction of the auditory pathway. Some of the soldiers given vitamin B$_{12}$ supplements regained some of their hearing.[2]

The people who are most likely to be deficient in vitamin B$_{12}$ are vegetarians or those who take either antibiotics or any kind of medication for gastroesophageal reflux disease (GERD) on a regular basis. Vitamin B$_{12}$ is nontoxic even when it is taken in a dosage 1,000 times greater than the RDA.

Vitamin E is an important cofactor for vitamin A. In

laboratory studies with animals, the amount of vitamin A in the bloodstream stays low regardless of intake until vitamin E levels are normalized. Vitamin E supplementation is useful even if you don't take vitamin A, since it complements the vitamin A available from the diet. The very low dosage of vitamin E recommended here is just enough to activate the vitamin A needed for treating acoustic trauma. It will not hurt you to take more, but you should be careful to watch for bruising and bleeding if you take any amount of vitamin E with the blood thinners warfarin (Coumadin), clopidogrel (Plavix), or aspirin. If bruising or bleeding occurs, stop taking vitamin E immediately.

There is some ambivalence in the medical literature concerning the efficacy of ginkgo in treating acoustic trauma. An often-cited experiment with guinea pigs found that ginkgo reduces noise-related hearing loss only when it is given intravenously, but this study only tracked ginkgo's effects on the animals for $3\frac{1}{2}$ hours.[3] Another study found positive benefits of ginkgo in treating laboratory rats.[4] A clinical study with human volunteers in Switzerland found considerable benefit in the emergency treatment of acoustic trauma with *injections* of ginkgo, but this treatment program also used repeated treatments in a hyperbaric (high pressure) oxygen chamber, and prednisone shots.[5] Low doses of ginkgo do not help problems related to acoustic trauma.[6] In treating tinnitus caused by acoustic trauma, you probably need to take 240 milligrams of ginkgo a day to get any benefit at all.

Recent research in Germany confirms that ginkgo can be used to treat chronic tinnitus, although it is not likely to be a complete cure. Patients with chronic tinnitus were given a daily injection of either 200 milligrams of ginkgo extract or a placebo for 10 days and then 160 milligrams of ginkgo tablets or a placebo for 3 months. At the 4 weeks, 8 weeks, and at the end of the trial, patients treated with ginkgo experienced significant relief over patients treated with the placebo, and there were no side effects.[7] It is likely that a slightly higher dosage of ginkgo taken by mouth, 240 milligrams per day, will be safe and effective in treating tinnitus in lieu of ginkgo injections.

Like vitamin E, ginkgo also can increase the risk of bleeding or bruising if you take the blood thinners wafarin (Coumadin), clopidogrel (Plavix), or aspirin, although this side effect is highly unlikely if you take only 100 IU of ginkgo per day. If bruising or bleeding occur, stop taking ginkgo immediately. Don't take more than 240 milligrams a day, because high dosages of ginkgo can cause nausea, diarrhea, stomach cramps, or headaches in some individuals.

CONCEPTS FOR COPING WITH TINNITUS

❍ When tinnitus cannot be treated by natural supplements, masking may help. Masking is the technique of producing external "white noise" to make sounds within the ear less distracting. Masking machines come in both in-the-ear and portable models that produce sounds ranging from random white noise to waterfalls and crickets, plus random auxillary sounds such as fog horns, buoy bells, and birds. Units are available at prices ranging from $150–$300 from retailers such as Sharper Image (1-800-344-4444). Hearing aids can also function as maskers by amplifying external sounds. When using a hearing aid to mask tinnitus, it is extremely important to have the hearing aid properly adjusted.

❍ In clinical studies, most tinnitus sufferers benefit from masking, but a small number find that masking actually makes symptoms worse.[8] Many people who do not care for commercial white-noise generators find that tuning a regular FM radio to an empty frequency and listening to the static is beneficial. Another popular method is to run an electric fan. If you have an audio CD player, consider putting on a nature sounds (ocean, jungle, whales, and so on) CD in auto-repeat mode before going to bed.

❍ Since 1990, only 2 of 18 studies testing acupuncture as a treatment for tinnitus found that it reduces symptoms in the ears, but a majority found that it improves sleep, decreases muscle tension, and improves blood circulation. In other words, acupuncture does not reduce tinnitus but makes it easier to cope with the stress of tinnitus. Many months of treatment may be necessary to achieve a noticeable result.

❍ About 50 percent of people who have fibromyalgia have some degree of tinnitus caused by fibromyalgia itself rather than the nerve damage usually associated with tinnitus.[9] Treating fibromyalgia treats hearing loss in these cases.

❍ In one of the few scientific studies of the use of homeopathy in the treatment of tinnitus, researchers at the Medical School of the University of Birmingham in England noted that test participants preferred the homeopathic remedy over placebo, but audiologists could not find a measurable difference between the homeopathic treatment group and the placebo group.[10] This is probably because both the discomfort of tinnitus and the practice of homeopathy are highly subjective. Substantial relief from tinnitus may occur because of changes in the sensory apparatus in the ear, or emotional changes leading to lesser irritation by sound; these effects are thought to be produced by classical homeopathy. Homeopathic remedies frequently used in the treatment of tinnitus include the following.

- Calcarea carbonica treats tinnitus compounded by dizziness. The individual who benefits from calcarea carbonica may have cracking and throbbing sensations in the ears or may be hard of hearing. People who benefit from this remedy usually have a "sweet tooth" and are sensitive to cold drafts.

- Carbo vegetabilis is recommended for nausea occurring at the same time as ringing in the ears. It is also useful for tinnitus occurring during recovery from the flu, especially if recovery is slow.

- Cinchona officinalis was originally used to treat malaria. As a homeopathic remedy, it is used to treat tinnitus that occurs with some of the same symptoms as malaria, such as chills and dizziness causing buzzing and ringing sounds to seem louder.

- Chininum sulphuricum relieves ringing and roaring sounds that are loud enough to interfere with normal hearing. Like cinchona officinalis, it treats chills and dizziness that make sounds seem louder.

- Cimicifuga (black cohosh) was used in Traditional Chinese Medicine to treat neck pain and is used in modern herbal medicine to treat menstrual irregularities. It is also used in homeopathy to treat tinnitus occurring with pain or tightness in the neck and/or shoulder muscles, or during the menstrual period. Women who benefit from this remedy tend to be naturally outgoing but moody when they do not feel well.

- Coffea cruda treats tinnitus occurring with symptoms that could be caused by overconsumption of coffee, such as a "buzz" in the back of the head and insomnia. People who respond well to this remedy tend to be excitable and nervous.

- Graphites treats symptoms that need "lubrication," such as crackling or creaking sounds, gunshot sounds, or hissing with accompanying deafness. People who respond well to this remedy tend to be constipated and have poor concentration.

- Kali carbonicum is a chemical fertilizer applied to "sour" soils. In homeopathy, it treats tinnitus accompanied by "sour" symptoms, such as rigid conservatism, tension in the stomach, and dizziness when turning.

- Lycopodium relieves echoes and hums. People who respond well to this remedy tend to have urinary tract ailments.

- Natrum salicylicum and salicylicum acidum treat tinnitus occurring with Ménière's disease. As a form of aspirin, salicylicum acidum is used under the principle of "like treats like" to relieve tinnitus occurring after overconsumption of acetylsalicylic acid (aspirin).

Tooth Decay, Baby Bottle

SYMPTOM SUMMARY

○ Visible brown or black spots

UNDERSTANDING THE DISEASE PROCESS

Baby bottle tooth decay is a dental condition occurring in children aged 18–36 months. It is the result of babies falling asleep with a bottle in their mouths. When the baby teeth are continually bathed in milk or juice, they are exposed to the bacteria that cause tooth decay. The lactic acid produced by the bacteria erodes the enamel of the teeth and leads to brown or black spots. The longer sugar stays on the teeth, the more lactic acid the bacteria produce, and the worse the tooth decay. The upper front teeth are the most susceptible to decay.

A similar condition occurs in children aged 3–5 who are given "sippy cups," cups with a lid and a raised slit with a narrow opening through which the child sucks sweet liquids. While sippy cups prevent drips, drools, and spills, they can also contribute to tooth decay. The American Dental Association estimates that 15 percent of all children under the age of 5 have serious tooth decay resulting from improper use of bottles and cups.

TREATMENT SUMMARY

DIET

○ If your child needs the comfort of a bottle in order to fall asleep, make sure it is filled with water rather than milk or juice.

○ Make sure your child eats a serving of a dark green, yellow, or orange fruit or vegetable 5 days a week.

○ Children over the age of 3 should be given chewable vitamins containing *at least* folic acid, vitamins C and E, and zinc.

UNDERSTANDING THE HEALING PROCESS

Once baby bottle tooth decay has begun, it requires dental treatment. Just because the affected teeth are "baby teeth" does not mean they can be allowed literally to rot in your child's mouth. Untreated cavities in baby teeth can cause deformities in the jaw and serious misalignment—requiring braces—when permanent teeth come in later.

Prevention is preferable to expensive dental treatment. Tooth decay can be avoided by making sure the baby does not fall asleep with a bottle of milk, formula, or juice in his or her mouth, and, later, by avoiding the use of "sippy cups" that stop drips and drools. The best preventative strategy for a 1-year-old is to dilute milk with water. If the baby ordinarily gets 8 ounces of milk at bedtime, fill the bottle with 7 ounces of milk and one ounce of water on the first night. Each night, add more water and less milk until eventually the bottle contains only water. To meet your child's nutritional needs, be sure to offer additional milk, juice, or formula during the day. The flavor of the milk, juice, or formula will make the diluted nighttime drink less appealing, and eventually, probably after some fuss, your child will give up his or her nighttime bottle.

If you have not taken these steps with your infant or toddler, dental treatment may be unavoidable, but there are nutritional measures you can take to minimize the damage and accelerate healing.

Dentists frequently recommend fluoride treatment. Fluoride stimulates bone production and a healthy calcium balance within the tooth. Finding the right dose of fluoride, however, can be problematic. Too little fluoride has no effect, and too much fluoride can cause mottling and brown spots on permanent teeth, also requiring dental treatment.

CONCEPTS FOR COPING WITH BABY BOTTLE TOOTH DECAY

○ Baby bottle tooth decay begins *behind* the front teeth and spreads to other teeth. To catch the condition when it is easiest to treat, check your child's teeth, front and back, every time you brush.

○ Gently wipe your baby's teeth with a clean cloth or gauze every day and every evening as soon as they begin to come in, usually at 7 months. Begin flossing as soon as all the primary teeth have come in.

○ Give juice from a cup or a spoon. If your child becomes thirsty between feedings, offer clear water.

○ Never give punch, gelatin, or soft drinks by bottle.

○ Avoid teething biscuits, even if they do not contain sugar.

○ Avoid pacifiers and never put honey or syrup on a pacifier. Avoid giving young children medications on a sugar cube.

○ Babies who fall asleep while breastfeeding should be removed from the breast. Tooth decay sometimes occurs after prolonged exposure to breast milk.

○ If you see brown or black spots on your child's teeth, visit your dentist. Early treatment is less expensive and less painful for your child.

Tooth Grinding
See **Bruxism**.

Tourette's Syndrome

SYMPTOM SUMMARY

○ Simple motor tics:

- Snapping jaw
- Twitching eyelid
- Trembling lip

○ Complex motor tics:

- Repeatedly undoing and redoing the same action (putting a chair into just the right position, writing over a letter, and so on)
- Lip biting
- Eye poking
- Nose picking

○ Simple vocal tics:

  • Barking

  • Hissing

  • Whistling

○ Complex vocal tics:

  • Inappropriate utterances such as "Boy, that's it," "Oh, yeah," and so on

  • Profanity (a well-known symptom affecting no more than 40 percent of people with Tourette's)

○ Echopraxia (imitating what has just been seen)

○ Echolalia (mimicking what has just been heard)

○ Palilalia (repeating what has just been said)

UNDERSTANDING THE DISEASE PROCESS

An estimated 100,000 Americans suffer from Tourette's syndrome, characterized by uncontrollable verbal and physical tics. About 40 percent experience coprolalia, the obsessive use of obscene language. The syndrome was named by French physician Gilles de la Tourette in 1884, who attributed it to unknown neurological causes. Even in the twenty-first century, the causes of the syndrome are unknown.

TREATMENT SUMMARY

NUTRITIONAL SUPPLEMENTS

○ Calcium: 1,000 milligrams per day.

○ Magnesium: 500 milligrams per day.

○ Vitamin B_6: 40–60 milligrams per day for children, 100 milligrams per day for adults.

UNDERSTANDING THE HEALING PROCESS

Some scientists speculate that at least some of the symptoms of Tourette's syndrome are caused by deficiencies of calcium, magnesium, and vitamin B_6. According to Dr. B. L. Grimaldi, the astonishing range of symptoms associated with deficiencies in these nutrients includes allergy, asthma, autism, attention deficit hyperactivity disorder, obsessive-compulsive disorder, unusual tongue movement,, anxiety, depression, restless legs syndrome, migraine, self-injurious behavior, autoimmunity, rage, bruxism, seizure, heart arrhythmia, heightened sensitivity to sensory stimuli, and an exaggerated startle response.[1] There are no reports that megadoses of the supplements will help (and excessive amounts of magnesium will cause diarrhea), but preventing deficiency is a prudent and inexpensive step in maintaining health.

CONCEPTS FOR COPING WITH TOURETTE'S SYNDROME

○ Many people with Tourette's syndrome learn to redirect their tics for a positive outcome. The Denver Nuggets basketball player Chris Jackson, for instance, used Tourette's to improve his basketball shots. In the American South, where both friends and strangers are offered social greetings, some sufferers of Tourette's develop a "Howdy, y'all" tic, which is socially acceptable.

○ See also ADD/ADHD, and OBSESSIVE-COMPULSIVE DISORDER.

Trachoma

SYMPTOM SUMMARY

○ Cloudy cornea

○ Conjunctivitis (inflamed eyelids)

○ Puslike discharge from the eye

○ Swollen eyelids

○ Swollen lymph nodes just in front of the ears

UNDERSTANDING THE DISEASE PROCESS

Trachoma is a chlamydia infection of the eye. Among natives of the United States, trachoma most frequently results from the transfer of the infection from genital secretions to the eyes. The disease may persist for 6 weeks to 2 years, causing bloodshot eyes and discrete areas of cloudiness in the lens of the eye. Patients who are treated for long periods with glucocorticoid drugs may develop a contraction or eversion (turning inside out) of the eyelids.

Some immigrants to the United States arrive from regions of the world in which trachoma is so widespread that it is not only spread by sexual contact. In Africa, the Middle East, some parts of Asia, and in the Mexican migrant worker community, trachoma is spread from person to person through eye-to-eye contact via infected clothes and washcloths. Older immigrants sometimes experience a relapse of trachoma when they are given cortisone eye ointments for other conditions.

TREATMENT SUMMARY

NUTRITIONAL SUPPLEMENTS

❍ *Acidophilus:* 1,000 milligrams daily while taking erythromycin.

❍ Bioflavonoids: 1,000 milligrams per day.

❍ Thymus extract: 500 milligrams of crude polypeptides daily.

❍ Vitamin A: 5,000 IU per day.

❍ Vitamin C: 500 milligrams 3–4 times a day.

❍ Vitamin E: 400 IU per day for the first 2 months.

❍ Zinc picolinate: 30 milligrams per day.

HERBS

❍ Echinacea: 150–300 milligrams of solid extract (3.5% echinacosides) 3 times a day, or dried root, freeze-dried plant, juice, fluid extract, or tincture, as recommended on the label.

❍ Goldenseal: as recommended on the label.

UNDERSTANDING THE HEALING PROCESS

Oral erythromycin is the doctor's drug of choice for trachoma. It is very important to take all the erythromycin or tetracycline tablets or ointments the doctor prescribes. Discontinuation of antibiotic therapy before the prescription is completely used can leave only the most virulent bacteria to reinfect the eye.

Although *acidophilus* has no direct effect on the course of trachoma, it helps restore friendly bacteria of the digestive tract that may be destroyed by antibiotic treatment. The first day you take *acidophilus* you may experience an unusual amount of flatulence and gas, but the effect usually goes away quickly.

Bioflavonoids are especially important to eye health. They help stabilize the connective tissues supporting the eyelids[1] and strengthen the microscopic blood vessels serving the eyes.[2] It is theoretically possible that bioflavonoids would interact with medications prescribed to thin the blood, such as Coumadin or warfarin. Consult your physician before taking bioflavonoids if you take these or closely related medications.

There are no studies that directly confirm the usefulness of thymus extract in treating trachoma, but there is considerable evidence that thymus extracts correct low immune function. In particular, research has shown that thymus extract normalizes the ratio of T-helper cells to T suppressor cells, maintaining a healthy immune response that neither destroys healthy tissue nor allows infectious microorganisms to flourish.[3]

Relatively low doses of vitamin A are sufficient to prevent "burnout" due to stress on the immune output of the thymus.[4] Vitamin A also enhances antibody response, increases the rate at which macrophages destroy bacteria, and stimulates natural killer cells.[5]

Vitamin C levels are quickly depleted during the stress of an infection.[6] In combination with bioflavonoids, it helps increase the stability of the collagen matrix of the connective tissues, the "glue" between the inner layer of the eyelid and the tissues supporting it.[7]

Zinc is an important cofactor for vitamin A. When zinc is deficient, the immune system's ability to produce white blood cells in response to infection is reduced, thymic hormone levels are lower, the immune response in the lining of the eyelids is especially reduced, and phagocytosis, the process in which bacteria are engulfed and digested, is slowed. When zinc is deficient, all of these processes can be corrected by taking zinc supplements.[8]

A quick method for detecting zinc deficiency is a taste test. Powder a tablet of any zinc-based supplement or cold medication and mix with $1/4$ cup (50 milliliters) of water. Slosh the mixture in the mouth. People who notice no taste at all or who notice a "dry," "mineral," or "sweet" taste are likely to be zinc deficient. Anyone who notices a definite strong and unpleasant taste that intensifies over time is not likely to be zinc deficient.

Zinc picolinate is the most readily absorbed form of zinc. Do not take more than 50 milligrams of any zinc supplement daily. In rare cases, excessive intake of zinc depletes copper to cause anemia, that is, a deficiency of red blood cells, and neutropenia, a serious deficiency of white blood cells.

Echinacea relieves inflammation. One study found that a teaspoon of *Echinacea purpurea* juice is as effective in relieving pain and swelling as 100 milligrams of cortisone.[9] Echinacea also enhances the immune system's response to bacterial infections. It is especially useful in stimulating phagocytosis. A study of oral administration of an *Echinacea purpurea* root extract

(30 drops 3 times per day) to healthy men for 5 days resulted in a 120 percent increase in phagocytosis.[10]

Women who are trying to get pregnant should avoid *Echinacea purpurea.* It contains caffeoyl esters that can interfere with the action of hyaluronidase, an enzyme essential to the release of unfertilized eggs into the fallopian tube.[11]

There is laboratory evidence that *Echinacea angustifolia* contains chemicals that deactivate CYP3A4. This is a liver enzyme that breaks down a wide range of medications, including anabolic steroids, the chemotherapy drug methotrexate used in treating cancer and lupus, astemizole (Hismanal) for allergies, nifedipine (Adalat) and captopril (Capoten) for high blood pressure, and sildenafil (Viagra) for impotence, as well as many others. *Echinacea angustifolia* might help maintain levels of these drugs in the bloodstream and make them more effective, or it might cause them to accumulate to levels at which they cause side effects. Switch to a brand of echinacea that does not contain *Echinacea angustifolia* if you experience unexpected side effects while taking any of these drugs.[12]

Avoid all forms of echinacea for treating trachoma if you have HIV. (Short-term use for treating other conditions is acceptable.) Echinacea stimulates immune function, but it also slightly increases production of T cells.[13] These are the immune cells attacked by HIV. When there are more T cells, the virus has more cells to infect. This gives it more opportunities to mutate into a drug-resistant form. This effect also makes echinacea inadvisable in autoimmune conditions, such as lupus, rheumatoid arthritis, and Sjögren's syndrome.

The combination of echinacea and goldenseal is especially useful in treating conditions that involve drainage. A 1999 study reported that the combination of the two herbs stimulates the production of the immunoglobulins IgG and IgM, infection fighters that "remember" specific infections.[14] Goldenseal contains the general antibacterial compound berberine. This alkaloid kills a wide range of bacteria, including those in the same family as *Chlamydia.*

People's Pharmacy authors Joe and Teresa Graedon warn that goldenseal reportedly limits the effectiveness of the anticoagulants heparin and warfarin (Coumadin). Do not take goldenseal with these medications. Avoid supplements containing vitamin B_6 or L-histidine if you take goldenseal, since they can interfere with goldenseal's antibacterial action.

CONCEPTS FOR COPING WITH TRACHOMA

○ Apply a warm compress to the affected area several times a day. The *Chlamydia* bacterium does not grow well under conditions of excessive heat.

○ Do not share bath towels or washcloths.

○ The Mexican folk remedy for trachoma, the chopped root of the madeira vine, available at *hierberías* in the southwestern United States, is being studied as a treatment for trachoma at the Pharmaceutical Institute of the University of Bonn in Germany. Anecdotal reports state that it is very helpful in relieving pain.

Trench Mouth

SYMPTOM SUMMARY

○ "Craters" between the teeth on the gums

○ Bad breath

○ Foul taste in the mouth

○ Grayish film on the gums

○ Painful, red, and swollen gums

○ Profuse bleeding from the gums in response to irritation or pressure

○ Symptoms may appear very suddenly

UNDERSTANDING THE DISEASE PROCESS

Trench mouth is an especially painful form of gum irritation or gingivitis. Also known as acute necrotizing ulcerating gingivitis or Vincent's stomatitis, its name is derived from a popular term for the condition originating when it was especially common among soldiers in trenches in World War I.

Trench mouth is essentially an overgrowth of bacteria that normally reside in the mouth. The mass of bacteria secretes toxic enzymes that dissolve the collagen of the gums and overwhelm the ability of the gums to repair themselves. Trench mouth is almost never seen in people who have access to good oral hygiene. It is most common in men aged 15–35.

TREATMENT SUMMARY

DIET

○ Avoid sugar.

○ Drink black *tea* (without sugar) as often as desired.

NUTRITIONAL SUPPLEMENTS

○ Quercetin: 500 milligrams 3 times a day.

○ Selenium: 400 micrograms per day.

○ Vitamin A: 15,000 IU per day. Women who are or who may become pregnant should strictly limit their intake of vitamin A to 5,000 IU per day or less.

○ Vitamin C: 1,000 milligrams 3 times a day with meals.

○ Vitamin E: 400 IU per day.

○ Zinc picolinate: 30 milligrams a day.

HERBS

○ Chamomile tea can be used as a soothing beverage or even as a mouthwash.

UNDERSTANDING THE HEALING PROCESS

Trench mouth can be quite painful until it is treated. If trench mouth is untreated or treatment is delayed, the infection can spread to the cheeks, lips, or jawbone. Bacterial infection can destroy these tissues. The objectives in treating trench mouth are decreasing inflammation, increasing immune resistance, decreasing the time the gums take to heal, and enhancing the integrity of the membranes lining the gums. The recommendations in the treatment summary are discussed as they contribute to these objectives.

Sugar feeds the bacteria that cause plaque. It draws fluid out of the gums and interferes with their absorption of vitamin C. It also weakens immune resistance by interfering with the chemical signals that the gums send to the immune system to attract polymorphonuclear leukocytes, large white blood cells that are the first line of defense against excessive accumulations of bacteria. The effects of sugar on the gums are most severe in people with chronic diseases that already depress the activity of polymorphonuclear leukocytes, such as diabetes, Crohn's disease, Down syndrome, Chediak-Higashi syndrome, and juvenile periodontitis.[3]

In much of East Asia even today, green tea is used as a toothpaste. Green and black teas contain two chemical compounds, (-)-epigallocatechin gallate and (-)-epicatechin gallate, which together prevent the transfer of sugar from the saliva to bacteria.[4] Deprived of sugar, bacteria do not grow and cannot cause inflammation.

Quercetin, a chemical found in green tea, onions, red wine, and St. John's wort, belongs to a family of compounds that stabilize collagen in the gums by preventing the release of histamine. Quercetin may be especially valuable for treating trench mouth in people who have food allergies.

Vitamin A stimulates the production of keratin, the protein that "toughens" the gums. It is also necessary for the production of collagen to heal wounds made by bacterial infection.[5] Vitamin A is especially important in treating trench mouth in people who have hepatitis C, Crohn's disease, ulcerative colitis, short bowel syndrome, pancreatic disease, cystic fibrosis, or Whipple's disease.

Side effects from accidental overdosing of vitamin A are rare, but they are significant. The first signs of vitamin A overdose are dry skin and chapped lips, especially in dry weather. Later signs of toxicity are headache, mood swings, and pain in muscles and joints. In massive doses, vitamin A can cause liver damage. In the first 3 months of pregnancy, it can cause birth defects. Women who are or who could become pregnant should strictly limit their intake of vitamin A to 5,000 IU per day or less. Discontinue vitamin A at the first sign of toxicity.

Gum disease may be a sign of vitamin C deficiency. It is possible to take considerably more than the RDA of vitamin C and still be deficient, if the body has become accustomed to high doses. That is, someone who drinks large quantities of fruit juices and stops, or who takes high doses of vitamin C and stops, may become vitamin C deficient even while eating a healthy diet. If trench mouth occurs, it is best to assume that there is a functional deficiency of the vitamin and take the supplement.

Vitamin E speeds up the healing of wounds. It is especially important if mercury amalgams are present. Mercury depletes the gums of the antioxidant enzymes catalase, glutathione peroxidase, and superoxide dismutase. At least in animal studies, this toxic effect of mercury is counteracted by vitamin E.[6] Selenium is an important cofactor for vitamin E.

Zinc is essential to dozens of enzymatic processes, including those that send a signal to polymorphonuclear leukocytes to fight bacterial infection. Zinc is also needed for the gums to make enzymes that slow down the process of tissue destruction initiated by endotoxins released by bacteria.[7] Gum disease is especially severe when there is a deficiency of zinc coupled with an excess of copper.[8]

While it is important to take zinc in treating trench mouth, it is equally important not to take too much. Except where otherwise directed, do not take more than 50 milligrams of any zinc supplement daily. In rare cases, excessive intake of zinc depletes copper to cause anemia, that is, a deficiency of red blood cells, and neutropenia, a serious deficiency of white blood cells.

Chamomile tea (and actually, teas made of several related plants, such as calendula, chrysanthemum, cosmos, and the flower but not the oil of safflower) contains triterpenes that stop inflammation.

CONCEPTS FOR COPING WITH TRENCH MOUTH

○ Hydrogen peroxide, used to rinse or irrigate the gums, is often recommended to remove decayed gum tissue. *Do not swallow hydrogen peroxide.*

○ To prevent recurrences of trench mouth, floss after every meal and at bedtime.

○ Regular cleanings by a dentist remove bacteria-laden plaque that may develop even with diligent brushing and flossing. Most dentists recommend having the teeth cleaned once or twice a year, and every 3 months if trench mouth is a problem.

○ Don't bite your nails or pick your teeth. Both practices can damage tender gums.

○ The active ingredient in Listerine mouthwash is thymol, a compound found in the herb thyme. Thymol is a potent antibacterial agent.

○ Faulty fillings create a breeding ground for the bacteria that cause trench mouth. Overhanging margins accumulate plaque and offer a shelter for bacteria. Mercury amalgams deplete antioxidant enzymes in small areas of the gums, exposing the glycosaminoglycans and proteoglycans that make up the collagen matrix of the gums to bacterial attack.[1]

○ The herb bloodroot is the source of mouthwashes and toothpastes labeled as containing benzophenanthridine alkaloids or sanguinarine. These compounds cause bacteria to "clump" so that they cannot form colonies on the gums. Some studies indicate they are not as effective in controlling plaque as the synthetic chemical chlorhexidine,[2] but alternating mouthwashes containing sanguinarine and mouthwashes that do not offers maximum benefit.

○ If you smoke, stop.

○ Electric toothbrushes are recommended for persons who have problems with manual strength or dexterity.

○ Consider using a tongue cleaner as a final step in oral hygiene. Cleaning the soft plaque from the back of the tongue removes most of the bacteria and other debris that are the primary source of plaque—and frequently are the cause of halitosis. A tongue cleaner should have smooth, well-rounded cleaning edges. Unbreakable stainless steel is preferable to potentially breakable plastic. Avoid cleaners that have holes that can trap the plaque you are trying to remove.

Tuberculosis

SYMPTOM SUMMARY

Initially:

○ Minor cough

○ Mild fever

After infection has become established:

○ Chest pain

○ Coughing up blood

○ Difficulty breathing

○ Fatigue

○ Fever

○ Heavy phlegm

○ Night sweats or excessive sweating

○ Weight loss

○ Wheezing

○ Positive skin (PPD) test, and spots and shadows visible on x-ray of infected lungs

UNDERSTANDING THE DISEASE PROCESS

Tuberculosis (TB) is a global problem. Epidemiologists estimate that 1.7–2.0 billion people are infected with *Mycobacterium tuberculosis,* the causative organism of TB. Approximately 8.8 million new TB cases occur each year.[1] This translates into 1,000 new cases every hour of every day.

TREATMENT SUMMARY

NUTRITIONAL SUPPLEMENTS

○ Vitamin A: 5,000 IU per day.

○ Vitamin B$_6$: 100 milligrams per day.

○ Zinc: 15 milligrams per day.

UNDERSTANDING THE HEALING PROCESS

Antibiotics are essential in treating TB. Usually, after a week or more of taking effective medication, most patients with TB will stop spreading the disease. The antibiotic isoniazid (a component of the medication rifampin), however, can cause nerve damage unless supplemental vitamin B$_6$ is taken. TB patients receiving rifampin do not develop nerve damage if they take at least 100 milligrams of vitamin B$_6$ a day.

Clinical trials have shown that very small doses of vitamin A and zinc enhance response to antibiotic drugs. Taking these supplements accelerates recovery and shortens the time it takes to achieve a normal chest x-ray.[2] It is important *not* to take more than the recommended dose of these supplements while recovering from TB. Taking more than 5,000 IU of vitamin A is not safe in women who are or who could become pregnant, and very high doses of zinc can slow the immune system's response to bacterial infection.

CONCEPTS FOR COPING WITH TUBERCULOSIS

○ During antibiotic therapy, it is important to avoid foods and nutritional supplements containing quercetin or rutin, including supplemental quercetin and rutin as well as buckwheat, grapefruit juice, and onions. Quercetin and rutin counteract ciprofloxacin and levofloxacin, the antibiotics most often used to treat the disease. Antibiotics are better absorbed when taken with bromelain. A single tablet of bromelain with each dose of antibiotic is sufficient.

Ulcer
See **Peptic Ulcer Disease.**

Ulcerative Colitis
See **Inflammatory Bowel Disease (IBD).**

Uncombable Hair Syndrome

SYMPTOM SUMMARY

○ Hair that will not lay flat and cannot be combed, usually blond or straw-colored

UNDERSTANDING THE DISEASE PROCESS

Uncombable hair syndrome is, as its name suggests, a condition in which the hair cannot be combed. In uncombable hair syndrome, there is an excessively ordered arrangement of the protein bundles from which individual hairs are formed. The keratin proteins of the hair are forced to form a long, inflexible tube that breaks easily. Uncombable hair syndrome is a genetic trait, expressed when a child has a single dominant gene inherited from either parent, one of whom would have had the condition in childhood.[1]

Most cases of uncombable hair syndrome are noticeable when the child is about 3 months old. The hair becomes dry, glossy, lighter in color, and progressively uncombable. Only the hair of the scalp is affected. While uncombable hair syndrome may occur in genetic syndromes causing mental retardation, most children with uncombable hair are developmentally normal.

TREATMENT SUMMARY

NUTRITIONAL SUPPLEMENTS

○ Biotin: 300 micrograms 3 times a day.

○ Avoid high doses of pantothenic acid (vitamin B$_5$).

UNDERSTANDING THE HEALING PROCESS

The good news about uncombable hair syndrome is that it typically corrects itself as the child grows older, usually in about 5 years. In at least one case, however, biotin treatment corrected the condition in 4 months.[2] When uncombable hair syndrome occurs later in childhood, after a child is put on medications for seizures, biotin treatment is especially likely to help.

CONCEPTS FOR COPING WITH UNCOMBABLE HAIR SYNDROME

○ Do not try to force uncombable hair to lie down by

combing it. The hair is not always anchored in the hair follicle properly, and the defects in the structure of the hair can make it easy to break off.

Vaginal Dryness

SYMPTOM SUMMARY

❍ Burning itching, or irritation of the vagina and/or vulva

❍ Pain during sexual intercourse

❍ Patchy irritation in the lining of the vagina

UNDERSTANDING THE DISEASE PROCESS

Vaginal dryness is among the most common health complaints in women who are going through or who have gone through menopause. Decreased estrogen levels lead to slowed growth of the lining of the vagina. Older cells are not replaced rapidly enough to prevent dryness and inflammation. In some cases the thinning of the wall becomes obvious. A similar condition results after removal of the ovaries.

Dryness after menopause makes the vagina more prone to infection, despite the scarcity of the usual organisms found in women of childbearing age (for example, *Gardnerella* species, *Trichomonas* species, and yeast). The pH of the vagina rises, the energy stored as glycogen in the cells lining the vagina decreases, and protective *Lactobacillus* becomes less abundant.[1]

TREATMENT SUMMARY

DIET

❍ Eat soy products on a regular basis.

NUTRITIONAL SUPPLEMENTS

❍ *Lactobacillus:* 1 capsule daily, used as a vaginal suppository.

UNDERSTANDING THE HEALING PROCESS

It is generally accepted that phytoestrogens from soy and flaxseed reduce vaginal dryness and limit vaginal irritation. Tofu, roasted soy nuts, boiled soy beans, soy milk, tempeh, and miso used on a regular basis provide these helpful chemicals. Japanese, but not Chinese or American, brands of soy sauce also provide phytoestrogens.

Lactobacillus bacteria preserve a healthy microbial ecosystem in the vagina. They produce peroxides, lactic acid, and other antibacterial agents that prevent the overgrowth of less desirable species. They compete with yeast by using glucose. Clinical studies have found that microbial cultures of this strain of bacteria are fully as effective in preventing recurrences of vaginal infections as standard antifungal drugs.[2]

There are two methods of *Lactobacillus* treatment: insertion of live yogurt cultures, or placement of 1 capsule of *Lactobacillus* into the vagina twice daily for 1–2 weeks.

CONCEPTS FOR COPING WITH VAGINITIS

❍ Natural progesterone relieves vaginal dryness. Be forewarned, however, that the progesterone content of over-the-counter creams varies widely. Many women find creams containing progesterone plus dioscorea most helpful.

❍ Wearing cotton panties allows greater air circulation and encourages growth of *Lactobacillus* bacteria.

❍ Douching increases rather than decreases the risk of developing vaginitis. One study found that women who had used douches in the 2 months prior to the survey were 2.9 times more likely to develop vaginitis than women who had not used douches.[3]

❍ Decreased sexual activity leads to increased vaginal dryness. On the other hand, it is important to avoid sexually transmitted diseases. Vaginitis increases the risk of contracting HIV, even among women who are past childbearing age.[4] *Trichomonas* is emerging as one of the most important cofactors in amplifying HIV transmission, particularly in African-American communities of the United States.[5]

Vaginosis

SYMPTOM SUMMARY

❍ Abnormal color, consistency, or odor of vaginal secretions

❍ Odor may only be noticeable after sexual intercourse

❍ Increased volume of vaginal secretions

UNDERSTANDING THE DISEASE PROCESS

Vaginosis is an overgrowth of anaerobic bacteria, bacteria that do not require oxygen from the air, in the vagina. Vaginosis is not an infection and is not a sexually transmitted disease. It typically occurs after antibiotic treatment has destroyed the oxygen-loving *Lactobacillus* bacteria that ordinarily inhabit the vagina and keep other kinds of bacteria in check by secreting minute quantities of hydrogen peroxide. When *Gardnerella, Mycoplasma,* and *Peptostreptococcus* are allowed to multiply unchecked, they produce the aptly named amino acids cadaverine and putrescine, causing an unpleasant odor in the vaginal secretions variously described as fishy, foul, or rotten. These bacteria reduce the acidity of the vagina so that vaginal secretions are less easily dissolved, becoming grey, pasty, or sometimes frothy. When overgrowth of these bacteria is relatively light, their odor may only be noticeable after sexual intercourse. Contact of semen with the vagina intensifies the odor of the vaginal discharge. Some women mistakenly believe that this odor is characteristic of sexual relations or due to infection of their male partner.

Bacterial vaginosis causes a number of serious medical complications in women, including:

❍ Miscarriage

❍ Preterm labor and preterm delivery

❍ Severe tubal infections or pelvic inflammatory disease

❍ Uterine infections following cesarean-section surgery

❍ Uterine infections following surgical abortions

Vaginosis also increases the risk of contracting HIV.[1] Bacterial vaginal infection is emerging as one of the most important cofactors in amplifying HIV transmission, particularly in African-American communities of the United States.[2]

Douching increases rather than decreases the risk of developing vaginosis. One study found that women who had used douches in the 2 months prior to the survey were 2.9 times more likely to develop vaginosis than women who had not used douches.[3] Vaginosis can be caused by yeast infection, but true overgrowth of *Candida* is sufficiently rare that the Centers for Disease Control advises doctors to do an AIDS test in young women who experience repeated, verified vaginal yeast infections. Women with healthy immune systems who get yeast infections tend to be college-aged or younger, to employ condoms rather than other contraceptive methods during vaginal intercourse, or to have completed treatment with an oral antibiotic within the previous 15–30 days. Diabetic women and women having to take oral steroid medication for conditions as severe as asthma are particularly susceptible to yeast infections of the vagina. Women who regularly use over-the-counter medications such as Gyne-Lotrimin and Monistat to treat supposed "yeast" infections kill the protective *Lactobacillus* bacteria and set themselves up for repeated episodes of vaginosis.

TREATMENT SUMMARY

NUTRITONAL SUPPLEMENTS

❍ *Lactobacillus:* as directed in Understanding the Healing Process.

UNDERSTANDING THE HEALING PROCESS

The doctor's prescription of choice for bacterial vaginosis is oral metronidazole (Flagyl). At $1 a dose, this oral medication is relatively cheap as a generic drug. It costs about one-third as much as Cleocin vaginal suppositories of and one-fifth as much as Cleocin or MetroGel-Vaginal lotion. (Some doctors still prescribe amoxicillin or Triple Sulfa vaginal cream, but these medications are not very effective.) The downside of metronidazole is that the tablet has an extremely bitter metallic taste and a bitter aftertaste that can last all day, and if it is taken with alcohol, it can cause severe nausea and vomiting. Metronidazole, Cleocin, and MetroGel lotion are all effective in about 5 out of 6 cases with 1 week of treatment. Four weeks later, however, 1 in 6 women using any of the medications will find vaginosis has returned, and almost all women taking these medications will eventually experience a relapse.

The reason these medications are a short-term remedy is that they kill the *Lactobacillus* bacteria needed to keep the bacteria that cause vaginosis in check. Cleocin kills not only the bacterial anaerobes that cause bacterial vaginosis, but also healthy *Lactobacillus* bacteria surviving in the vagina. MetroGel does not kill *Lactobacillus* species, but it does not replace the Lactobacillus bacteria killed by competing bacteria or other drug treatments. The key to avoiding recurring vaginosis is to reestablish the healthy bacteria that normally reside in the vagina.

Lactobacilli bacteria preserve a healthy microbial ecosystem in the vagina. They produce peroxides, lactic acid, and other antibacterial agents that prevent the overgrowth of less desirable species. They compete with yeast by using glucose. Every case of vaginosis benefits from the use of *Lactobacillus.* Clinical studies have found that microbial cultures of this strain of bacteria are fully as effective in preventing recurrences of vaginosis as standard antifungal drugs.[4]

There are two methods of *Lactobacillus* treatment: insertion of live yogurt cultures, or placement of 1 capsule of *Lactobacillus* into the vagina twice daily for 1–2 weeks.

CONCEPTS FOR COPING WITH VAGINOSIS

○ Wearing cotton panties allows greater air circulation and encourages growth of *Lactobacillus* bacteria.

○ A variety of douches and soaks for tampons are appropriate for *short-term* use, to control vaginosis once symptoms have become noticeable, but none should be used for more than 2 weeks and they must be followed with *Lactobacillus* replacement. Possible treatments include the following:

• Betadine is iodine that does not sting or burn (although it may stain undergarments). One-quarter of a teaspoon in 1 pint of water used in a retention douche kills most microorganisms in less than 1 minute.

• Goldenseal, barberry, or Oregon grape root mixed in a ratio of 2 teaspoons per cup of hot water makes a suitable douche. However, the herb is not effective against vaginosis in women who take supplemental B vitamins (which are absorbed by bacteria as well as the body).

• Lithium succinate (8% solution, available from compounding pharmacists) is especially helpful for women who also have had herpes infections. Lithium stops the replication of the herpesvirus without damaging cells in the vagina.

• Tea tree oil (a 1% solution, no stronger) can be used to soak a tampon, changed daily.

• White vinegar (1–2 tablespoons) by itself or mixed with 2 tablespoons of green clay (available from health food suppliers) in 1 pint (500 milliliters) of water.

○ Boric acid and garlic are not recommended because they frequently cause irritation.

○ If vaginal inflammation, burning, and itching, or pain after sexual intercourse are problems, the condition may be a vaginal infection such as chlamydia, gonorrhea, or most frequently, trichomoniasas. Unlike bacterial vaginosis, these conditions cause green, yellow, sticky, or no vaginal secretion.

Varicose Veins

SYMPTOM SUMMARY

○ Dilated, twisting blue veins near the surface of the skin on the feet and legs

○ Dull pain, itch, or feeling of heaviness in the legs

○ In advanced cases, swollen ankles or ulcerated skin on the legs

UNDERSTANDING THE DISEASE PROCESS

Varicose veins are enlarged blood vessels near the surface of the skin on the feet and legs. Varicose veins are a very common problem. According to some estimates, at any given time approximately 15 percent of men and 25 percent of women have varicose veins.[1] At some point in their lifetimes, 58 percent of men and 48 percent of women will develop the condition.[2] The group most frequently seeking treatment for varicose veins is women aged 30–50. The men most likely to get varicose veins have high cholesterol.[3]

Varicose veins are caused by "blown" valves in the vessels carrying blood away from the feet and legs. The circulatory system contains valves to make sure that blood flows against the pull of gravity to the tissues where it is needed and then back to the heart and lungs. When valves in the veins of the legs and feet fail, blood tends to pool in the feet. Veins gradually stretch to accommodate the stagnant circulation and become elongated, pouched, thickened, and tortuous.

Even small veins can pose cosmetic problems, but swelling, itching, tenderness, and pain tend to worsen as the veins grow larger. Varicose veins are complicated by any factor that reduces circulation, such as high systolic blood pressure (elevation of the upper number with or without elevation of the lower number), lack of exercise, smoking, liver disease, abdominal masses, or occupations that cause prolonged standing.

TREATMENT SUMMARY

HERBS

○ Gotu kola (*Centella asiatica*) extract taken orally: 30 milligrams 2–4 times per day, *or*

○ Grape leaf (red vine leaf) extract: 360–720 milligrams per day, *or*

○ Grape seed or pine bark OPCs (Pycnogenol): 100 milligrams 3 times per day, *or*

○ Horse chestnut (aescin with bioflavonoids): 10 milligrams 2–3 times daily.

Additional treatments include:

○ *Collinsonia* (stone root): As directed on label.

○ Calendula creams: Apply as desired to relieve inflammation.

○ Buckwheat teas: As desired.

UNDERSTANDING THE HEALING PROCESS

The simplest and least expensive treatment for varicose veins is compression stockings, or, for women, support hose. Compression stockings are hard to put on and uncomfortable to wear, but they reduce the diameter of varicose veins by an average of 20 percent after use for 3 months.[4] Elastic bandages are often prescribed for the most severe cases. It is important to avoid making the bandage so tight that it acts as a tourniquet.

Sclerotherapy (injecting the vein with a salt solution) or surgery (stripping out the vein by making an incision above and below and pulling the vein out with a wire) may be required when varicose veins become ulcerated, but neither procedure keeps varicose veins from coming back. The bruises caused by sclerotherapy may take up to 3 months to heal.

Generally speaking, herbal treatments are about as effective as compression stockings (and can be used by people who are using compression stockings). Some herbs act more quickly than others. The herb gotu kola (sometimes sold under its botanical name *Centella*) contains chemicals that stop the breakdown of ground substance, the mixture of proteins that give veins the ability to spring back to their original dimensions when they are stressed by high blood pressure.[5] It stimulates the production of glycosaminoglycans, the building blocks for collagen, from which connective tissues are formed. It increases the oxygen supply delivered through the capillaries.[6] It elevates antioxidant levels to make the walls of blood vessels more permeable, allowing fluid to drain off into interstitial tissues rather than to pool in the vessel itself.[7] Clinical studies have found that gotu kola reduces the diameter of varicose veins and limits swelling in the ankles and feet.[8] Gotu kola creams treat swollen ankles.

It is usually necessary to take gotu kola for 2–3 months before noticing results. A daily dose of 60 milligrams may be effective, but clinical studies have found that 120 milligrams is likely to be more effective.

Grape seed and pine bark (as well as bilberries, blueberries, cranberries, and hawthorn) contain oligomeric proanthocyanidins (OPCs), compounds that are well documented for their ability to strengthen veins. A double-blind study comparing grape seed OPCs against a placebo in 71 individuals with varicose veins showed improvement in 75 percent of the treated group, as compared to 41 percent in the control group.[9] A 60-day controlled clinical trial of 40 individuals with chronic venous insufficiency found that taking 100 milligrams of Pycnogenol 3 times a day significantly reduced edema, pain, and the sensation of heaviness in the leg.[10] Another placebo-controlled study of 20 individuals also found OPCs from pine bark effective.

Another effective but little-used herbal remedy for varicose veins is grape leaf extract (also known as red vine leaf extract). In 2000 a research team at the Institut für Transfusionsmedizin und Immunhaematologie in Berlin gave 260 patients with varicose veins either 360 or 720 milligrams of grape leaf extract every day for 3 months. In the 219 patients who completed the study, taking the higher dose of the herb resulted in reduced swelling in the calves and ankles (about 1.5 centimeters, or $\frac{3}{5}$ of an inch in circumference, slightly more than would be expected from using compression stockings). Side effects from the herb were mild, mostly stomach upset or headache.[11]

The most popular of all treatments for varicose veins in Europe is horse chestnut (sometimes identified by its key chemical component, aescin or escin). The escin component of the herb escin plugs leaking capillaries and prevents the release of enzymes that break down collagen and open holes in capillary walls. There have been at least 8 clinical trials of horse chestnut extract in the treatment of varicose veins. The largest study, involving 212 people found that the herb reduced pain, swelling, and sensation of heaviness when used for 20 days.[12]

Horse chestnut is the herb of choice for varicose veins in people who have congestive heart failure or orthostatic hypotension (periodic dizziness when standing from a seated position). Most horse chestnut products combine the herb with citrus bioflavonoids, which also increase venous strength. Diosmin, hesperidin, and other citrus bioflavonoids have been clinically demonstrated to heal hemorrhoids, which are essentially varicose veins in the rectum (see HEMORRHOIDS).

None of these herbs is recommended for internal use by women who are trying to get pregnant. There is no risk, however, to using topical creams containing these herbs, as directed on the label, while trying to get pregnant or during pregnancy or nursing.

The herb butcher's broom is a traditional remedy for varicose veins, as are calendula and *Collinsonia* root (stone root). Buckwheat teas (and possibly buckwheat kasha or buckwheat pancakes eaten daily) also have a positive effect.[13] Any of these herbs is likely to be effective, but do not use butcher's broom or buckwheat if you take antibiotics, especially Cipro.

CONCEPTS FOR COPING WITH VARICOSE VEINS

○ Taking regular walks improves circulation in varicose veins. If you cannot leave your home or office to take a walk, try rotating your feet at the ankles, alternating clockwise and counterclockwise motion. Lift your legs parallel to the floor and point your toes up and then down. Repeat these exercises at least once an hour.

○ If you have to remain in a standing position for long periods, lean on one leg and then the other from time to time.

○ When traveling by plane, reserve an aisle seat so you can stretch your legs as often as possible.

○ Pain in the calf can be caused by a blood clot, and requires medical attention. Women who take estrogen replacement therapy are at higher risk for blood clots if they also have varicose veins. A cold feeling in the feet coupled with heat in the legs is also a warning sign of a clot. Chest pain after surgery to "strip" varicose veins is a medical emergency.

○ There are a number of homeopathic remedies for varicose veins. Usually it is best to start with a single dose of the lowest strength (6C, 6X, or 12C) of the remedy matching the symptoms to be treated, and then wait for a response. If there is an improvement in symptoms, let the remedy continue to work until there is no more improvement, then take another dose. If there is no improvement, try a different potency (30X or 30C). Sometimes homeopathic medicines work for a few minutes, and sometimes they work for an entire day before another dose is needed.

• Arnica Montana is a widely-available homeopathic remedy for bruises and sports injuries that is also appropriate when varicose veins make legs look black and blue or feel sore to the touch.

• Calcarea carbonia treats varicose veins in people who have poor circulation and who are easily chilled. It is appropriate for varicose veins that hurt when the person is standing or walking, and for varicose veins in people who are overweight.

• Carbo vegetabilis is homeopathic charcoal, used to "color" mottled skin characterized by distended veins and a "marbled" look. This remedy is recommended for older people or for anyone in a prolonged recovery from a serious illness.

• Hamamelis is homeopathic witch hazel, recommended when varicose veins are easily injured and prone to bleeding. People who benefit from hamamelis may also develop varicose veins on the genitals or hemorrhoids.

• Lycopodium is used to treat varicose veins that are surrounded by numbness or varicose veins that cause tearing pains. People who most benefit from lycopodium tend to have leg cramps at night.

• Pulsatilla treats hot and painful varicose veins that cause discomfort at night, and varicose veins that develop in pregnancy.

• Zincum metallicum treats large varicose veins that are tender to the touch. People who benefit from this remedy may have crawling sensations on the skin or a tendency to fidget. Alcohol worsens symptoms.

Vitiligo

SYMPTOM SUMMARY

○ Loss of pigment in irregular patches of skin, most frequently on the hands, feet, arms, face, and lips

> ○ Loss of pigment sometimes also affects skin around the mouth, nose, eyes, and genitals
>
> *Hair growing from areas of skin affected by vitiligo may turn white.*

UNDERSTANDING THE DISEASE PROCESS

Depigmentation, also known as vitiligo, is a physiological process causing patches of skin to lose their color. In this process the immune system attacks melanocytes, the cells in the skin that contain the pigment melanin. This pigment absorbs harmful ultraviolet radiation that might otherwise damage skin cell DNA. Melanin is most abundant in naturally dark skin, and vitiligo is most prominent in persons of naturally dark skin.

The exact cause of the condition is not known. Until recently, vitiligo was believed to be exclusively an autoimmune disease, in which improperly programmed cells of the immune system attack healthy tissues. The scientific data fail to confirm this theory. Some scientific studies have found that vitiligo-affected skin contains more of the immune cells known as T cells than normal skin.[1] Other scientific studies have found vitiligo-affected skin contains fewer T cells than normal skin.[2] Some of the most recent research suggests that the condition results from an imbalance in the various kinds of cytokines, the inflammatory hormones produced by these cells.[3]

In some cases, vitiligo is a sign of a defensive reaction against melanoma. The depigmentation of the skin caused by vitiligo occurs through a reversal of the physiological steps that cause this form of skin cancer.[4] Depigmentation is also associated with various autoimmune diseases, although the relationship does not hold true in every case or even in most cases. Fewer than 10 percent of people who have vitiligo show active symptoms of autoimmune diseases such as pernicious anemia, Graves' disease (hypothyroidism),[5] type 1 diabetes,[6] or alopecia areata (sudden hair loss other than male-pattern baldness),[7] but as many as 50 percent have antibodies characteristic of these diseases.[8]

Some of the most recent research reconnects the biochemical understanding of vitiligo with the traditional idea that it is a disease caused by stress. Researchers at the University of Pavia in Italy have determined that skin tissues in the early stages of vitiligo contain unusually high concentrations of the metabolic byproducts of the stress hormones epinephrine (adrenaline), norepinephrine, and dopamine.[9]

Other recent research confirms a nutritional view of the disease. British scientists have found that skin cells affected by vitiligo lack an enzyme to convert the amino acid L-phenylalanine into its byproduct tyrosine.[10] Concentrations of L-phenylalanine build up in the cell, but at the same time the cell is deficient in L-phenylalanine. The cell is less able to derive energy from glucose through the citric acid cycle, and essentially becomes so "tired" that it is subject to autoimmune attack.

While the disease process of vitiligo is very poorly understood, it is treated with relative success. Especially in children, treatment is more likely to be successful when started early.

TREATMENT SUMMARY

NUTRITIONAL SUPPLEMENTS

○ L-phenylalanine: one 500-milligram capsule for every 20 pounds of body weight daily. For example, a person weighing 200 pounds should take ten 500-milligram capsules daily.

○ Vitamin B_{12} and folic acid: 800 micrograms of each, daily.

HERBS

○ Khellin: 100 milligrams daily.

See Part Three if you take prescription medication.

UNDERSTANDING THE HEALING PROCESS

Both prescription medications and natural medications for vitiligo are activated by sunlight. Get at least 20 minutes exposure to natural sunlight or a sunlamp daily, and take L-phenylalanine and khellin 45 minutes before light therapy. Sunlight is especially important for restoring pigmentation to the face.

The longest-running clinical trial of L-phenylalanine for the treatment of vitiligo found that about 85 percent of patients regain pigment to at least 25 percent of vitiligo-affected skin after taking the supplement for 6 months. About 60 percent of all patients who take L-phenylalanine experience repigmentation of 75 percent of affected skin after taking the supplement for 6 months. Eight-five percent of patients taking the supplement for 6 *years* experienced 100 percent restoration of skin color to the face, although complete restoration of skin color to the hands and trunk is relatively rare. Researchers have found that more is not better when it comes to using L-phenylalanine; doubling the dosage had no effect on rates of cure.[11]

A 2-year study of 100 patients at the Department of Dermatology of University Hospital in Uppsala, Sweden found that giving vitiligo patients vitamin B_{12} and folic acid supplements and directing them to get exposure to sunlight or a sunlamp was more effect than either treatment alone. Fifty-two of 100 patients in this study experienced some degree of repigmentation after 2 years, but only six had complete restoration of skin color. It is important to note that these two vitamins plus sun exposure were the only treatments given to patients in this study.[12]

The latest study of the use of khellin with sunlight in the treatment of vitiligo found that the combination can greatly restore pigmentation in as little as 6 months. Scientists at the University of Graz in Australia found that, the longer people took the combination of khellin and sunlight treatments, the greater the degree of improvement. About 40 percent of patients experienced restoration of 70 percent of affected skin in 6 months. Even when treatment was continued for as long as 11 years, the physicians conducting the study noted no skin cancers or sun damage in any patient.[13]

Khellin can cause nausea and stomach upset, but this side effect usually subsides after the first week of treatment. About two-thirds of people who take the herb experience no unpleasant side effects of any kind.

CONCEPTS FOR COPING WITH VITILIGO

○ Cosmetics in a variety of shades are available for covering up vitiligo. Many are designed for use by children as well as by adults, and by boys as well as girls. Chromelin, Clinique, Dermablend, and Lydia O'Leary's Covermark are leading brands.

○ Tattooing is often used to restore color to skin around the lips, especially in people who have dark skin. It is difficult for the doctor to match perfectly the color of the skin surrounding the area of depigmentation, and it is important to consider that tattoos fade with time. Tattooing may reactivate herpes in people who have had prior infection.

○ Even though some exposure to sun is necessary to make most medications for repigmentation work, people with vitiligo should use sunscreen to avoid sunburn and long-term skin damage. Sunscreen also lessens tanning, making the contrast between normal and depigmented skin less noticeable.

Wasting

SYMPTOM SUMMARY

○ Severe weight loss

○ Wasting of muscles

○ Altered taste perception

○ Anorexia

○ Constipation

○ Depression

○ Diarrhea

○ Nausea

○ Pain

○ Severe fatigue

○ Shortness of breath

○ Sleep disturbances

○ Vomiting

UNDERSTANDING THE DISEASE PROCESS

Wasting, also known by the medical term cachexia, is a condition of severe malnutrition causing anorexia, destruction of muscle, and weight loss. Its symptoms also include fatigue, gastrointestinal distress, shortness of breath, depression, and pain. In cachexia, appetite may be satisfied with small portions of food, or food becomes altogether unappetizing and eating may become painful. The condition is not unusual in the later stages of AIDS, Alzheimer's disease, cancer, cerebral palsy, congestive heart failure, cystic fibrosis, emphysema, cirrhosis of the liver, and degenerative neurological conditions. Various studies describe cachexia as the immediate cause of death in 20–50 percent of cases of cancer and AIDS.

Cachexia is also a common problem in the elderly. One survey found that 1 in 5 nursing home residents lost 6 pounds (3 kilograms) during the first 6 months of their stay.[1] Weight loss even of this magnitude is associated with increased risk of bedsores and increased numbers of infections.[2] Malnutrition can exacerbate cognitive disorders such as Alzheimer's disease,[3] and people over 65 who have the lowest levels of body fat are twice as likely to die as those who have normal amounts of body fat.[4]

Cachexia is not starvation. In starvation, the body's metabolism slows down to conserve energy. In cachexia, energy is burned and proteins are recycled at an unusually high rate. One study found that people with rheumatoid arthritis, for instance, burned calories at an average rate 12 percent higher than people without the disease, even though their average body mass was an average of 13 percent lower.[5] For reasons that are still poorly understood, cancer can cause the release of lipid-mobilizing factors, releasing fatty acids from fat cells into the bloodstream in concentrations greater than the body can use,[6] and protein mobilizing factors, taking amino acids away from healthy muscle cells.[7]

Cachexia also is not due to cancer or a virus consuming nutrients intended for the human body. Cachexia is caused by many different illnesses. The common feature of all of these diseases is that they induce the release of inflammatory mediators known as cytokines. Scientists have identified specific cytokines associated with cachexia in AIDS, rheumatoid arthritis,[8] and cancer.[9]

These chemicals attack injured, infected, or cancerous tissue. They also accelerate metabolism, the rate at which the body burns calories at rest as well as the rate at which proteins are recycled in cells. They trigger the release of serotonin, which causes nausea, vomiting, and constipation even while it lifts mood and relieves depression.[10]

The best understood of the cytokines involved in cachexia is interleukin-6 (IL-6). The body has redundant systems for making IL-6. This hormone is elevated by emotional stress, physical trauma, severe inflammatory disease, and during withdrawal from steroid treatments to prevent cachexia.[11] Experiments with animals have found that injecting antibodies to IL-6 can reverse cachexia.[12] One of the most common treatments for cachexia in South American rain forest medicine, cat's claw, also neutralizes IL-6.[13]

TREATMENT SUMMARY

DIET

○ Use supplemental nutrition drinks (such as Boost or Ensure) as often as possible.

NUTRITIONAL SUPPLEMENTS

○ Essential fatty acids: 10 grams per day (or as much as can be tolerated) of black currant seed oil, flaxseed oil, evening primrose seed oil, or fish oil.

○ Magnesium chloride (extended release): 500–600 milligrams daily.

○ Melatonin: 20 milligrams, *taken in the evening.*

○ Vitamin E: 200 IU per day.

Avoid or use with caution:

○ Creatine.

○ L-glutamine.

○ Ornithine alpha-ketoglutarate.

HERBS

○ Cat's claw: Tincture, 1 dropper taken in a cup of water with 1 teaspoon of lemon juice, 2–3 times daily.

See Part Three if you take prescription medication.

UNDERSTANDING THE HEALING PROCESS

Far too often, cachexia is considered only as an inevitable symptom of the end stages of terminal disease rather than as a condition that can be ameliorated. Many healthcare professionals treat cachexia as a signal of death rather than as a cause of death and ignore potential treatments. Diligent attention to loss of appetite and weight in the early stages of cachexia can extend life and prevent suffering. If cachexia is ignored, however, there is a point of no return. In AIDS patients, death is usually imminent if one-third of body weight has been lost.[14] In the elderly, loss of as little as 4 percent of body weight is associated with an increased rate of death.

Nothing in this book is intended to discourage you from seeking medical intervention to stop your body from wasting away. In AIDS, there are initial reports of good results from anabolic steroids. Speakers at international AIDS conferences have reported that oxandrolone (Oxandrin) prevents wasting in women who have AIDS. Dr. Marc Hellerstein of the University of California at Berkeley reports that a medically administered combination of oxandrolone, testosterone, and exercise can enable recovery of 2 pounds (1 kilogram) of body mass a week in men in the earlier stages of AIDS. The FDA-approved marijuana derivative dronabinol has been found to increase weight in Alzheimer's patients[15] (although it can cause changes in mental state that are more severe than those induced by marijuana). Growth hormone, a very expensive therapy, can lead to weight gain in the elderly with other conditions.[16] The recommendations here can be used with medical therapies, or, if medical intervention is not available, in place of them.

High-protein dietary supplement drinks are a mainstay in treating cachexia. The advantage of these drinks is that they are easily digested, conserving part of the 5–10 percent of total calories the body burns just to digest food. Various brands tend to be of equal value. However, if ornithine alpha-ketoglutarate (which lowers blood sugars as part of the process of stimulating the growth of muscle) is part of the supplementation plan, it is better to use a formula that prevents hypoglycemia, such as Glucerna.

As this book is being written, there are two large-scale studies in progress concerning the use of essential fatty acids plus vitamin E in the treatment of cachexia in cancer patients. Four preliminary studies found that fish oil plus nutritional supplement drinks greatly reduces weight loss in advanced pancreatic cancer.[17] The anti-inflammatory activity of essential fatty acids and vitamin E is likely to be beneficial in other forms of cancer and most other conditions that cause cachexia.

Fish oil, in particular, can cause burping. Reduce dosage if there is diarrhea or heartburn. People at risk for seizures should not use seed oil.

Magnesium is essential to the synthesis of fat, protein, and nucleic acids. Deficiencies of magnesium cause irregular heartbeats, muscle weakness, seizures, and loss of appetite. They may play a role in the production of the cytokines that cause cachexia.[18] Magnesium deficiency is very common in the elderly.[19]

The best form of magnesium for cachexia is a slow-release formulation of magnesium chloride. Magnesium is the active ingredient in the laxative milk of magnesia, so don't take magnesium supplements if diarrhea is a problem.

There have been reports in the medical literature for a number years that melatonin can prevent wasting. A study of 86 cancer patients in Italy found that giving 20 milligrams of melatonin every evening prevented weight loss without requiring additional consumption of food.[20] The same group of scientists also found that melatonin appeared to slow the process of angiogenesis, the growth of new blood vessels to supply solid tumors.[21]

Large-scale studies of melatonin in the treatment of cachexia in cancer patients have been only recently reported, also from Italy. The San Gerardo Hospital in Milan has used high doses of melatonin in the care of 1,640 cancer patients. Taking 20 milligrams of melatonin in the evening lowers the frequency not only of cachexia, but also of fatigue, thrombocytopenia (red blood cell destruction), and lymphocytopenia (white blood cell destruction). Among patients who continued chemotherapy, melatonin reduced the frequency of heart damage, mouth sores, and neurological side effects.[22]

Melatonin supplements should not be taken by people who have melanoma. People who have seizures should also avoid melatonin. The only other significant precaution in the use of this supplement is that it must be taken in the evening, rather than during the day, to assist nighttime sleep.

Mexican clinics treating as many as 3,000 AIDS patients anecdotally report prevention of cachexia after treatment with cat's claw. These results have not been scientifically documented, but recent research confirms that the herb inhibits production of the cytokines IL-6 and TNF-alpha.[23] This may be the mode of its healing action.

Tropical herb expert Leslie Taylor advises using tinctures rather than solid forms for most applications of cat's claw. Active tannins in the tinctures are released in the presence of citric acid, easily provided by lemon juice. If you use a brand of cat's claw made with vinegar, you do not need to add lemon juice. There is one report of an adverse reaction to cat's claw in lupus (although the authenticity of the product as cat's claw was not confirmed). As a precaution, do not use cat's claw in the treatment of cachexia associated with advanced lupus or rheumatoid arthritis.

There are some supplements that should be avoided by people who are experiencing wasting or who have diseases that cause wasting. It would seem logical to treat cachexia with creatine, since it is well known to stimulate muscle growth. In younger persons in the early stages of cancer or HIV, creatine supplementation might help. By the time muscle wasting has begun to occur, however, creatine will only add water weight.

Glutamine is the most abundant amino acid in the body. It helps maintain the immune system, it protects the lining of the gastrointestinal system, and it is critical to building healthy tissues. But it is also an essential element for cell division, and the cytokines that cause cachexia are triggered by cell division.[24] It is also possible that glutamine supplements could stimulate the growth of cancers.

Ornithine alpha-ketoglutarate (which is not the same as L-ornithine) stimulates the production of growth hormone by stimulating the production of arginine. One study has found it can stimulate appetite and weight gain in the elderly.[25] Part of its mode of action, however, is the production of insulin. Use of the amino acid can cause hypoglycemia, which is especially dangerous for people who have conditions of intellectual impairment.

CONCEPTS FOR COPING WITH WASTING

○ People in various stages of wasting often fear being a burden on family and friends and allow themselves to become isolated. Even if eating becomes impossible, it is important to provide the person with cachexia with opportunities for social interaction at mealtimes.

○ For every 1°C (1.8°F) increase in body temperature, resting calorie consumption goes up 17 percent.[26] Early treatment of fevers is very important in stopping weight loss.

○ Wasting is a frequent complication of uncontrolled diabetes. Blood sugar control through the use of insulin, however, reverses the process.

○ Weight loss in people with Alzheimer's is often associated with the calories expended in pacing back and forth. Loss of weight can lead to loss of muscle and incapacitating falls. Early intervention to prevent weight loss can make caring for an Alzheimer's patient much easier over the long run.

○ Wasting is frequently a complication of gastric or pancreatic cancer. It is seldom a complication of leukemia or breast or prostate cancer.

Weight Control

OBJECTIVE

○ Maintaining current weight in the face of changes in diet, lifestyle, or health status.

UNDERSTANDING THE DISEASE PROCESS

Weight control is the leading health concern of most North Americans. Although losing weight, or at least lim-

iting weight gain, really is a matter of exercising more or eating less, the fact is that all diets, much less all dieters, are not equal. Under scientifically controlled conditions, dieters beginning at the same weight, eating exactly the same amount of food, and performing exactly the same amount of exercise lose weight at rates differing by up to 50 percent.[1] A meta-analysis of diet studies performed by a researcher at the prestigious Harvard School of Public Health recently found that reducing the amount of fat in the diet, even drastically, has no relationship to the amount of fat in the body.[2] Low-fat, low-carbohydrate, and even dangerous low-protein diets have all been touted as the ideal path to permanent weight loss, but the fact is that people do not stay on reduced-calorie diets of any kind long enough to do scientific tests.[3]

Overweight is generally recognized as a major risk factor for heart disease and diabetes. Scientists are coming to realize, however, that "catch-up" fat regained after weight loss diets is an even bigger risk factor for heart disease and diabetes, largely due to derangements in thermogenesis, the basal metabolism of the body, caused by dieting.[4]

TREATMENT SUMMARY

NUTRITIONAL SUPPLEMENTS

○ Hydroxycitric acid (HCA): 1,500 milligrams daily.

HERBS

○ Cayenne: 10 grams (1 tablespoon) at most meals.

UNDERSTANDING THE HEALING PROCESS

The best approach for most of us is to avoid gaining weight—without disturbing other aspects of health. Out of dozens of products that have demonstrable effect on weight loss, only 2 prevent weight gain without creating other imbalances.

Laboratory experiments with animals (but not yet clinical studies with people) have shown that hydroxycitric acid (HCA), extracted from the *Garcinia cambogia* fruit, interferes with enzymes that convert stored carbohydrates into fat.[5] Since HCA acts on carbohydrates, it naturally is of limited value in low-carbohydrate diets. A study published in the *Journal of the American Medical Association* found no benefit when HCA was used as an adjunct to high-protein, reduced-calorie diets.[6] The real value of HCA is for people who *aren't* dieting, pursuing normal diets containing carbohydrates.

The other natural product that encourages weight stability is cayenne. For the simple reason that hot peppers sting the lining of the mouth, using a tablespoon of cayenne in preparing a meal reduces average consumption by 200 calories.[7] If you don't want to gain weight from fatty foods, make them spicy.

CONCEPTS FOR ACHIEVING WEIGHT CONTROL

❍ Sugar cravings are frequently the body's attempt to treat depression. For additional information, see DEPRESSION and SEASONAL AFFECTIVE DISORDER (SAD).

West Syndrome

SYMPTOM SUMMARY

❍ Spasms in which an infant assumes a "jack-knife" position

UNDERSTANDING THE DISEASE PROCESS

West syndrome is a neurological disease of infants slowing motor development and causing seizures in which the infant bends over and assumes a folded position. The spasms are different in different children, but usually they start suddenly and last for only 1–2 seconds. The infant's arms stretch out, the head nods forward, and the eyes look upward. In the beginning, a baby may experience only 1 or 2 spasms at a time when waking up or falling asleep, but usually over a period of days or weeks they build up to 20–30 throughout the day. The spasm may upset the baby, or may be followed by a brief smile.

This disease is identified by a grossly disorganized brainwave pattern on an electroencephalograph (EEG) known as hypsarrhythmia. The EEG in a baby with infantile spasms does not have regular "quiet" rhythms. Instead there are frequent, sudden bursts of high-voltage electrical activity, making the recording appear chaotic. EEG changes are most marked as the child wakes up or falls asleep.

TREATMENT SUMMARY

NUTRITIONAL SUPPLEMENTS

❍ Vitamin B$_6$: dosage selected in consultation with a physician.

UNDERSTANDING THE HEALING PROCESS

West syndrome is difficult to control with conventional medications, but 10 to 30 percent of babies with West syndrome respond to high doses of vitamin B$_6$. The response to vitamin therapy is rapid, seizures disappearing within the first 2 weeks of treatment when the therapy works. Since high-dose vitamin B$_6$ therapy can cause diarrhea, vomiting, and liver dysfunction in the baby, monitoring by a doctor is essential.

CONCEPTS FOR COPING WITH WEST SYNDROME

❍ Vitamin B$_6$ therapy can be extremely helpful in West syndrome but can actually cause seizures in other forms of epilepsy. Do not use vitamin B$_6$ unless the diagnosis has been confirmed by a physician.

Wilson's Disease

SYMPTOM SUMMARY

❍ Clumsiness

❍ Drooling

❍ Fatigue

❍ Headaches

❍ In women, missed menstrual periods

❍ Joint pain

❍ Tremor

UNDERSTANDING THE DISEASE PROCESS

Wilson's disease is a hereditary disease causing copper to accumulate in the liver and other tissues. The effects of Wilson's disease are not usually noticed until adulthood. Absent menstrual periods and miscarriage may occur in women with the disease, and both sexes may experience fatigue, headaches, and joint pain, leading over a period of years to loss of muscular coordination. Wilson's disease is easily treated by medical means, but when left untreated, it usually results in death.

TREATMENT SUMMARY

NUTRITIONAL SUPPLEMENTS

When on medication:

○ Vitamin B_6: 100 milligrams per day.

When not on medication:

○ Zinc: dosage prescribed by a physician.

UNDERSTANDING THE HEALING PROCESS

Treating Wilson's disease is a lifelong process that requires prescription medications to remove excess copper from tissues. The most common agent prescribed for this purpose is penicillamine (not to be confused with penicillin). This drug should not be combined with zinc supplements. Taking 100 milligrams of vitamin B_6 daily greatly reduces the risk of complications, especially nerve damage, that might otherwise result from penicillamine treatment.

When not on medication, most people with Wilson's disease take high doses of zinc supplements to counteract the tendency of the tissues to accumulate copper. Since the correct dosage depends on improvement in copper load that can only be measured by blood tests, the amount of zinc to be taken should be decided in consultation with a physician.[1]

CONCEPTS FOR COPING WITH WILSON'S DISEASE

○ Certain foods are high in copper, notably nuts, seeds, kidney, liver, oysters, and wheat and other kinds of bran. These foods must be eliminated from the diet. Never take copper supplements for relief of joint pain if you have Wilson's disease.

Wrinkles

SYMPTOM SUMMARY

○ Furrows, creases, sags, and areas of lusterless skin

○ Regions of dark pigmentation

UNDERSTANDING THE DISEASE PROCESS

The processes that cause wrinkles, age spots, folds, creases, crow's feet, and sagging or sallow skin can be understood at a molecular level. Essentially, for many of us, the skin slowly becomes "tired" as we age. UV radiation from excessive sun exposure, air pollution, microbial colonization, prescription medications, inflammatory disorders, and nutritional stress team together to generate massive quantities of free radicals. Free radicals are essential to the process of respiration, but these free radicals accumulate on the surfaces of skin cells, locking sodium inside. The cell membrane loses its electrical charge so that nutrients are kept out. The caustic action of sodium ions within the cell on lipids, proteins, and DNA creates wrinkles, age spots, and other manifestations of aging skin.[1]

Of all the natural processes that damage the skin, the most destructive is excessive exposure to sunlight. Sun damage occurs even when there is not enough exposure to sun to cause sunburn. Doctors report that it is common in clinical practice to see patients with major wrinkling who systematically apply a sufficient quantity of sunscreen before exposing themselves to the sun.

The problem is that sunscreens with SPF values of 15–30 allow UVA rays to reach the skin. At least 95 percent of all the solar radiation reaching the earth consists of UVA. And UVA is present from sunrise to sunset, unlike UVB which only reaches significant levels between 10 A.M. and 3 P.M. The amount of UVA radiation and sunlight does change according to the season; there is just as much UVA in winter sun as in summer sun.

Exposure to UVA for even 1 hour a day 5 days a week for 5 weeks can cause substantial damage to the skin. Eighty-five percent of UVA radiation penetrates to the dermis, compared to only 15 percent of UVB. UVA exposure activates a system of enzymes known as the metalloproteinases. These enzymes break down connective proteins in the skin. As the metalloproteinases do their work, the stratum corneum thickens and the skin's outer layers dry out and become more fragile. Tiny cracks develop. Portions of the outermost layers of skin detach and flake off easily.

Wrinkles and the appearance or deepening of lines are major signs of photoaging, but heavy sun exposure may also cause the skin to take on a yellowish tint. Skin that is forced to produce massive amounts of protective pigments develops freckles and age spots. Spots on the skin that are strictly related to aging are rare—the number of pigment-producing cells in the skin across the entire surface of the body actually drops by 10–20 percent every 10 years. Sun-related age spots, or lentigos, are the result of the overproduction of protective pigments in the bottommost layer of the epidermis in skin that is exposed to UVA over a period of years.

The aging process is especially acute in the skin of

smokers. Tobacco smoke interferes with the ability of fibroblasts to use the genetic coding of RNA to make collagen, the structural material of the skin. Laboratory studies have found that exposure to tobacco smoke reduces the production of collagen within fibroblasts by as much as 40 percent.[2] Without this vital material for the scaffolding of the skin, wrinkles are inevitable.

Nutritional deficiencies cause the same skin problems in nonsmokers. Inadequate skin levels of vitamin C, vitamin E, and coenzyme Q_{10}, combined with exposure to ultraviolet radiation, cause a cascade of oxidative processes. These chemical changes activate the production of pigments and damage DNA. Over time, poor nutrition produces many of the same defects in the skin as smoking.

TREATMENT SUMMARY

DIET

○ Avoid sugar.

○ Drink six to eight 8-ounce glasses of water daily.

○ Eat 2–3 servings of yellow or orange vegetables daily.

○ Eat three 3-ounce servings of cold-water fish (such as herring, mackerel, sardines, tuna, or wild salmon) weekly, *or* take DHA and EPA supplements *or* 1 tablespoon of flaxseed oil daily.

NUTRITIONAL SUPPLEMENTS

○ Alpha-lipoic acid: 100 milligrams daily.

○ Mixed carotenoids: 25 milligrams per day. The alga *Dunaliella salina* is a particularly rich source of carotenoids. It is especially important to take mixed carotenoids every day beginning 8–10 weeks before exposure to summer sun.

○ Vitamin C: 2,000 milligrams per day.

○ Vitamin E: 800 IU per day.

Vitamins C and E must be taken together for a protective effect.

OTHER HELPFUL NATURAL PRODUCTS

○ Alpha hydroxy acids (lotions containing 5–10% glycolic acid).

○ DMAE (dimethylaminoethanol) creams and supplements.

○ Vitamin C ester (ascorbyl palmitate) creams.

UNDERSTANDING THE HEALING PROCESS

Aging skin is most readily treated with topical applications of alpha-lipoic acid, DMAE, and vitamin C esters. These relatively expensive treatments sometimes produce visible results within a few days, whereas oral supplementation may not yield improvements for several weeks. If expense is a concern, however, oral supplementation will work, only more slowly. Whatever treatments you choose, diet, smoking cessation, and use of sunscreens greatly increase the rate at which your skin is rejuvenated.

Sugar is the enemy of circulation in the skin. Excessive levels of sugar in the bloodstream "sugar-coat" cells in a process known as glycation. In the skin, sugar forms cross-links in the collagen, making the skin less supple and impeding circulation. Drinking adequate amounts of water lowers the concentration of sugar in the bloodstream and reduces glycation.

Orange and yellow vegetables make the skin less sensitive to the sun. In hereditary diseases causing severe sun sensitivity, beta-carotene slightly raises the minimum level of UV exposure that causes tissue damage, so that people taking beta-carotene are more likely to tan than to burn.[3] Orange vegetables such as carrots and sweet potatoes are an excellent source of beta-carotene. While synthetic beta-carotene is better absorbed, natural sources of this vitamin have a greater positive effect on the immune system.[4] The carotenes in palm oil are 4–10 times better absorbed that synthetic *trans*-beta carotene.[5]

Eating very large quantities of carrots, in the range of 450–1,000 grams (1–2 pounds) per day can cause a condition known as carotenodermia, in which the skin turns yellow and then orange. The condition is reversible when carrots are discontinued. Eating large quantities of carrots daily for several years can cause depletion of white blood cells (neutropenia)[6] and menstrual disorders.[7]

Omega-3 fatty acids from cold-water fish moderate the skin's susceptibility to inflammation. Fatty acid deficiency increases the rate at which skin cells multiply,[8] makes them more permeable to water, induces the formation of abnormal keratinocytes,[9] and accelerates the production of natural steroid hormones in the skin.[10]

Alpha-lipoic acid counteracts the damage done by excessive sugar in the diet. In a study of diabetics with a condition called peripheral diabetic neuropathy (damage to the sensory nerves of the skin caused by poor circulation), German researchers found that a relatively large dose (600 milligrams) of alpha-lipoic acid given by injection increased blood circulation in the skin by approximately 70 percent.[11] Although this clinical trial and similar studies do not conclusively establish that alpha-lipoic acid is useful in treating aging skin, many dermatologists use the supplement to treat bags under the eyes, enlarged pores, and sallow or dull skin.

Mixed carotenoids, a group of vegetable pigments found in orange and yellow vegetables and the alga *Dunaliella salina,* have been tested in several clinical trials as a preventative for sunburn. In one study, 20 young women took 30 milligrams daily of beta-carotene or a placebo for 10 weeks before a 13-day stretch of controlled sun exposure at a resort on the shores of the Red Sea. Participants taking beta-carotene before and during the sun exposure experienced less skin redness than those taking a placebo, even when both groups used sunscreen. Two other studies conducted without a control group reported similar results. One study involving 20 participants and one study involving 22 participants found that supplementation with mixed carotenoids for 12–24 weeks increased tolerance for summer sun. The evidence shows that it is necessary to take mixed carotenoids for several months to gain any benefit. A study lasting 23 days and another study lasting 4 weeks did not find any benefit of taking mixed carotenoids over taking a placebo in reducing sensitivity to sun.

It is important to note that the recommendations here call for the use of mixed carotenoids, not beta-carotene. A controversial study in Finland reported in 1995 that taking beta-carotene could increase the risk of lung cancer among smokers (from approximately 0.4 percent per year to approximately 0.5 percent per year), and the Carotene and Retinol Efficacy Trial in the United States was halted prematurely when it was found that it also increased the risk of lung cancer among smokers and asbestos workers (from 0.5 percent to 0.6 percent). The reason for these menacing findings likely has to do with the fact that beta-carotene, without other nutrients, is an oxidant rather than an antioxidant. Beta-carotene is protected from oxidation by the presence of other nutrients, such as those provided by mixed carotenoids.

Experiments with animals have confirmed that applying vitamin C and vitamin E directly to the skin protects against UV damage. One study found that topical vitamin C protected more against UVA rays, topical vitamin E protected more against UVB rays, and that applying vitamins C and E together worked better than applying either by itself. The sun-protective value of the vitamins was even greater when they were applied with sunscreen. Dr. Steve Bratman reports a study in which 20 women aged 55–60 with sun-damaged skin on the neck were given either 5 percent vitamin C or a placebo. The results at 3 and 6 months, according to Dr. Bratman, showed that use of vitamin C improves cosmetic appearance, especially wrinkles, and the general health of the skin as evaluated under a microscope.[12] It is important to note that these studies focused on the use of topical vitamin C rather than vitamin C supplements.

Japanese scientists have made extensive study of the efficacy of alpha hydroxy acids in the treatment of wrinkles. They found, not unexpectedly, that the best results of treatment were in middle-aged adults. People under 30 years old and people over 70 years old experienced few changes after treatment. The scientists believe that the lack of response in subjects over 70 years of age might be due to their wrinkles being mainly coarse wrinkles rather than fine ones. Even in people aged between 30 and 70, the effect of treatment with alpha hydroxy acids was primarily to shorten wrinkles rather than eliminate them. In some cases, the number of wrinkles appeared to increase as long, deep wrinkles divided into multiple smaller wrinkles during their improvement.[13]

Exactly how alpha hydroxy acids reduce wrinkles is not fully understood, but they function in at least two ways. First, they act as a humectant, increasing the water content of the skin and thus moisturizing the outer layer of the epidermis. This makes the skin softer and more flexible. They also reduce skin cell adhesion and accelerate cell proliferation within the deeper basal layer of the skin. They encourage the growth of blood vessels to oxygenate the skin. They also activate an internal clock inside skin cells at the surface reminding them of the time to die and be sloughed off, providing room for the growth of new, healthy skin. The growth of skin underneath the follicle forces it open and allows the release of dead skin cells and irritants.

Recognizing which products contain alpha hydroxy acids requires reading the label. Alpha hydroxy acid ingredients may be listed as:

- alpha hydroxy and botanical complex
- alpha hydroxycaprylic acid

- alpha hydroxyethanoic acid + ammonium alpha hydroxyethanoate
- alpha hydroxyoctanoic acid
- citric acid
- glycolic acid
- glycolic acid + ammonium glycolate
- glycomer in cross-linked fatty acids alpha nutrium (3 AHAs)
- hydroxycaprylic acid
- lactic acid
- L-alpha hydroxy acid
- malic acid
- mixed fruit acid
- sugarcane extract
- tri-alpha hydroxy fruit acids
- Triple fruit acid

Of these, the most frequently used in cosmetics are glycolic acid and lactic acid.

DMAE (dimethylaminoethanol) is frequently used by dermatologists to treat sagging skin around the eyes, at the tip of the nose, and around the lips. Hollywood makeup artists use DMAE to give actors and actresses plumper lips. Scientific research confirming this use of DMAE is in a very preliminary stage.

Vitamin C esters (ascorbyl palmitate) stimulate collagen synthesis in the fibroblasts. The advantage of the vitamin C ester over ordinary vitamin C is that it is readily absorbed. Ascorbyl palmitate is about 10 times as active in the skin as vitamin C.[14]

CONCEPTS FOR COPING WITH WRINKLES

If you have dry skin:

O Don't fail to apply an SPF-30 sunscreen to exposed skin every day.

O Don't use buffing pads or granular cleaning products.

O Don't wash skin with hard soap.

O Choose moisturizers formulated with dimethicone, glycerin, or hyaluronic acid.

O Just splash your face with warm water in the morning, and use a "superfatted" cleansing bar (a "beauty bar" with lanolin or olive oil) or a mild, soap-free liquid cleanser to wash your skin at night.

O Lock in skin moisture with moisturizers while your face and body are still damp.

O Protect sun-exposed skin with a sunblock with an SPF of at least 30.

O Soften fine lines and wrinkles with oil-based foundations and cream or cream-powder blushers.

If you have oily skin:

O Don't scrub your skin. Removing oils deprives your skin of its protective layer.

O Don't use astringents more than twice a week.

O Don't use moisturizers if you don't need them.

O Don't wash your skin more than twice a day, unless you exercise.

O Cleanse your face twice a day with a mild liquid cleanser.

O Protect sun-exposed skin with a sunblock with an SPF of at least 30.

O Use Clinac O.C. rather than an astringent to soak up excessive oil.

O Use oil-free or oil-blotting foundation and powder.

Yellow Nail Syndrome

SYMPTOM SUMMARY

O Slow-growing, yellow nails

O Swollen lymph glands, especially in the lower half of the body

O Breathing difficulties

UNDERSTANDING THE DISEASE PROCESS

Yellow nail syndrome is a respiratory condition heralded by the appearance of yellow, slow-growing nails, followed by swellings in the lymph glands and drainage within the lungs. The swelling is worse in the lower half of the body. Pleural effusions, or "oozing" in the lungs, may require surgical treatment.

TREATMENT SUMMARY

NUTRITIONAL SUPPLEMENTS

O Vitamin E: 800 IU per day.

UNDERSTANDING THE HEALING PROCESS

Supplemental vitamin E gradually restores normal color to the nails. Its value in treating other aspects of yellow nail syndrome has not been established.[1]

CONCEPTS FOR COPING WITH YELLOW NAIL SYNDROME

O Many people with advanced yellow nail syndrome benefit from postural drainage. For more information, see PNEUMONIA.

Zinc Deficiency

SYMPTOM SUMMARY

O Sticky eyelids

O Scaly patches of inflammation on and around the fingernails, eyes, and mouth, and on the genitals

O Hair loss

O Diarrhea

O Mood swings and confusion

O Photophobia (pain in the eyes in bright light or sunlight)

O Low zinc levels measured by blood test

O Rapid improvement in symptoms after taking supplemental zinc

UNDERSTANDING THE DISEASE PROCESS

Skin inflammation caused by zinc deficiency is known in the medical literature as acrodermatitis enteropathica. Although zinc deficiency severe enough to produce the range of symptoms associated with this disease can be caused by poor diet, very recent research has identified defects in a single gene responsible for making a zinc-transporting protein as the usual cause of the disease.[1] This relatively rare condition causes swelling and redness around the fingernails, and psoriasis-like inflammation on other parts of the skin. In people who do not receive treatment for zinc deficiency until adulthood, there may be bone deformities caused by a failure of the zinc-dependent enzyme alkaline phosphatase. Mood swings are a diagnostic key to distinguishing this condition from other malabsorption syndromes. While most people find zinc supplements unpleasantly bitter, people with acrodermatitis enteropathica usually find them sweet or cannot taste them at all.

Acrodermatitis enteropathica also occurs in babies born prematurely. Most of the infant's supply of zinc is accumulated during the third trimester of pregnancy, so premature babies are frequently zinc deficient.

TREATMENT SUMMARY

DIET

O Eat oysters, beef, pecans, and Brazil nuts often.

NUTRITIONAL SUPPLEMENTS

O Zinc: 30–150 milligrams per day, with bloodstream levels measured by the doctor several times a year to ensure adequate supply.

O Copper: 1–3 milligrams per day.

UNDERSTANDING THE HEALING PROCESS

Once a proper diagnosis is made, treating zinc deficiency is extremely simple and very fast. Two or 3 days of taking 30–150 milligrams of zinc usually reverses symptoms. The initial dosage of zinc should be chosen by a doctor familiar with the disease, and bloodstream levels of zinc should be monitored regularly. It is also important to take supplemental copper. High levels of zinc sometimes deplete the body's stores of copper. Eating oysters, beef, pecans, and Brazil nuts will provide additional zinc, although not enough to replace the need for zinc supplements, as well as copper supplements.

CONCEPTS FOR COPING WITH ZINC DEFICIENCY

O Symptoms resembling zinc deficiency are sometimes caused by infection with the Epstein-Barr virus[2] or by Lyme disease,[3] particularly if symptoms appear for the first time in adulthood.

O Infants who are given measles and hepatitis B vaccines at the same time sometimes develop Gianotti-Crosti syndrome, a condition with symptoms similar to those of zinc deficiency.[4]

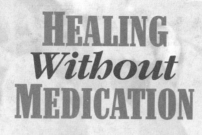

HEALING
Without
MEDICATION

Part Two

Healing Tools

Healing Tools

Sometimes improving health is as simple as taking a pill. Prescription medications are the mainstay of conventional medicine, and nutritional supplements are an important part of natural healing. Healing Tools offers brief summaries of essential information on the scientific and reliable use of vitamins, minerals, amino acids, phytochemicals, enzymes, aromatherapies, homeopathics, and standardized herbs. In these summaries, you will find a brief description of the product and how it works in the human body, important applications, dosages, and precautions for use with prescription medications.

5-HTP

Used to treat depression, overweight, fibromyalgia, and headache, **5-Hydroxytryptophan (5-HTP)** is a naturally occurring amino acid commercially extracted from a plant related to carob and found in trace amounts in avocados, bananas, eggplant, pineapples, tomatoes, and walnuts. 5-HTP was brought onto the market in the early 1990s as a substitute for L-tryptophan supplements, after a contaminant in a batch of the supplement made with a genetically modified bacterium caused several deaths.

5-HTP is converted by the brain in a single step to 5-HT, more commonly known as serotonin, a key regulator of mood. 5-HTP also increases the production of endorphins and enkephalins that relieve pain. Its effects on appetite are not clearly understood, but scientists believe that 5-HTP increases the production of leptin. Deficiencies of leptin are implicated in a number of obesity-related disorders.

As of August 2002, only two clinical trials involving 64 volunteers have tested 5-HTP as a treatment for depression under scientifically controlled conditions. Both studies, however, showed marked superiority of 5-HTP over the placebo. A less rigorous study found that 5-HTP was slightly superior to fluvoxamine (Luvox). Clinical study has found that 5-HTP relieves anxiety, fatigue, and quality of sleep and lessens reactivity at trigger points in fibromyalgia. The best results from 5-HTP in promoting weight loss are found in type 2 (non-insulin dependent) diabetics.

Generally speaking, the minimum dosage of 5-HTP needed to have a noticeable effect is 100 milligrams per day, and benefits may not be obvious until the supplement has been taken for 90 days. The body uses 5-HTP more effectively if there are adequate supplies of vitamin B_6. Do not take 5-HTP if you have taken drugs for depression or migraine at any time within the last 4 weeks and do not take 5-HTP at all if you have Parkinson's disease. Most authorities recommend against taking 5-HTP with St. John's wort.

7-Oxo-Dehydroepiandrosterone

7-Oxo-dehydroepiandrosterone (7-Oxo-DHEA) is a form of DHEA that does not have an effect on the production of sex hormones. Naturally produced in the adrenal glands, brain, ovaries, and testicles, this hormone is believed to stimulate thermogenesis, the burning of food to maintain body temperature. Laboratory studies with animals find that 7-Oxo-DHEA can stimulate weight loss without reduction of food intake by stimulating thermogenesis, but the dosage for this effect in humans, if any, is unknown. Laboratory studies also find that 7-Oxo-DHEA reverses memory impairment in both young and old mice. There are some indications that this supplement can increase the immune system's production of T cells, but since it increases the production of both CD4+ (helper T cells) and CD8+ (suppressor T cells), it is of unknown benefit in HIV.

Typical dosages of 7-Oxo-DHEA are 50–100 milligrams per day, although a study at the Chicago Center for Clinical Research found no ill effects from taking 200 milligrams per day for a prolonged period. Since the supplement has a half-life of only 2 hours, several smaller doses are likely to be more effective than 1 large dose. Pregnant women and nursing mothers should not take this supplement.

19-Norandrostenedione

Primarily used by bodybuilders, **19-norandrostenedione** (also known as **Andro**) is a chemical building block for the male sex hormone testosterone in both men and women. Although a single dose of 19-norandrostenedione can be detected in blood and urine tests for up to 10 days, scientists do not know conclusively whether short-term use of the supplement can stimulate the growth of muscle. Studies at the University of Nebraska have found no side effects—and no significant benefits—when the supplement is used by previously trained weight lifters for up to 8 weeks. Some users report that benefits are limited to improvement in ability to leg press.

However, there is considerable evidence that long-term use of the supplement can cause acne, breast enlargement, testicle shrinkage, and sudden anger syndrome in men, and acne, male-pattern baldness, clitoral thickening, missed menstruation, thickening of the skin, and deepening of the voice in women. Teenagers who have not finished growing can stop growing upward if they take the supplement. This supplement should not be taken by anyone who has any hormone-sensitive form of cancer (cancers of the breast, ovaries, prostate, or uterus, or cancers of any organ secondary to cancers in the breast, ovaries, prostate, or uterus). It should be completely avoided by any woman who is or who could become pregnant. People who choose to use 19-norandrostenedione typically take 100 milligrams per day.

Acetyl-L-Carnitine

Acetyl-L-carnitine is a chemically modified form of L-carnitine that is readily absorbed by the brain. L-carnitine transports the long-chain fatty acids used in the mitochondrial energy production centers of brain cells, and also protects the linings of brain cells by acting as an antioxidant. Use of the supplement often enhances attention, logical reasoning, and verbal memory in people under the age of 55 with Alzheimer's disease; older Alzheimer's patients decline less rapidly when on the supplement. There are preliminary indications that the supplement may help preserve memory in aging people who do not have Alzheimer's or other senile dementias.

Acetyl-L-carnitine is also used to enhance attention and visual memory in Down syndrome. Scientists at Umea University in Sweden are investigating its use in restoring nerve function in the hands and feet after accidents.

There are generally no side effects from acetyl-L-carnitine, although people who have seizure disorders should only use it under medical advisement. It is theoretically possible that the supplement could increase activity in the brain and lower the threshold for a seizure; epilepsy treatment with valproic acid (Depakene, Depakote), however, creates a deficiency of L-carnitine. AIDS patients taking didanosine (ddI), stavudine (d4T), and/or zalcitabine (ddC) also may become deficient in L-carnitine and should consult with their healthcare providers about taking acetyl-L-carnitine supplements if neurological symptoms or memory loss occur.

Activated Charcoal

Activated charcoal absorbs offensive odors released in flatulence and the "purple burps" caused by giardiasis. Doses of 500–1,000 milligrams 2–4 times a day are sufficient for this purpose. Higher doses of activated charcoal bind to the cholesterol in food and may lower cholesterol levels, but the amount of charcoal needed for this purpose (5–8 grams at every meal) may cause constipation.

Never take charcoal within 2 hours of taking any other medication, supplement, or herb. Always take charcoal with a large glass of water.

Alkoxyglycerols

Alkoxyglycerols are fatty acids extracted from shark liver oil. While they are sometimes recommended for treatment of cancer, the only, slightly positive evidence for their use comes from Denmark, where researchers found that akloxyglycerols sometimes reduced side effects of radiation treatment for cervical cancer. No one should rely on alkoxyglycerols as a sole treatment for cancer. Since the concentration of alkoxyglycerols varies among brands, take the dosage recommended on the product label. Overdoses may cause flatulence or diarrhea.

Alpha-Galactosidase

Alpha-galactosidase is an enzyme derived from the fungus *Aspergillus niger*. In the human body, alpha-galactosidase dissolves complex polysaccharides in beans, peas, broccoli, brussels sprouts, and cabbage that otherwise would be digested by gas-producing bacteria in the intestine. Since alpha-galactosidase changes these polysaccharides into sugars, it slightly increases the caloric content of these foods.

The most common alpha-galactosidase product in the United States is Bean-o. If used, follow label directions. Cramping, diarrhea, and itch occur in rare instances.

Alpha-Glycerylphosphorylcholine

L-alpha-glycerylphosphorylcholine or **alpha-GPC** is a soy extract found in a single European study in the early 1990s to stimulate the release of growth hormone. This study found that alpha-GPC had a more pronounced effect on elderly users, but did not establish a therapeutic range for effective dosing. It is possible that some persons with Alzheimer's disease may benefit from supplemental alpha-GPC, but caution should be taken to make sure increased activity does not lead to increased accidents.

Alpha-Lipoic Acid

Once thought to be a vitamin, **alpha-lipoic acid** is a potent antioxidant and a cofactor in energy production throughout the body. The primary use of alpha-lipoic acid is treating pain, numbness, and burning caused by nerve damage in type 2 diabetes. Clinical studies have found that doses of 600–1,200 milligrams per day reverse the symptoms in about 3 weeks. Some men suffering erectile dysfunction due to nerve damage from diabetes also benefit from alpha-lipoic acid. There are preliminary studies indicating benefit of alpha-lipoic acid in treating Alzheimer's disease, amyotrophic lateral scle-

rosis (Lou Gehrig's disease), Huntington's disease, and Parkinson's disease. Antioxidant effects of the supplement improve blood flow through arteries, especially after a heart attack.

Do not use more than 600 milligrams of alpha-lipoic acid a day for more than a month. Alpha-lipoic acid can lower blood sugar levels, so diabetics should monitor blood sugar levels when taking this supplement.

Alpha-Tocopherol Nicotinate

Alpha-tocopherol nicotinate is a chemically modified form of vitamin E used to treat high cholesterol and high triglycerides. It is found in multiple vitamin products manufactured in Europe and Japan. Used in accordance with directions on the label in the dosages provided in these products, side effects and drug interactions are highly unlikely.

Alpha-Tocopherol Polyethylene Glycol Succinate

Alpha-tocopherol polyethylene glycol succinate (TPGS), is a form of vitamin E that enters the bloodstream without the help of bile salts. This is especially important for children who have chronic gallbladder problems, and possibly for people with Crohn's disease, ulcerative colitis, or cystic fibrosis. In children with chronic gallbladder problems, treatment with TPGS largely prevents worsening of neurological symptoms. TPGS also greatly increases absorption and availability of the HIV drug amprenavir (Agenerase).

TPGS greatly increases the body's absorption of vitamins A, D, and K, as well as flavonoids such as quercetin and resveratrol. Taking a vitamin C supplement enhances the antioxidant effect of TPGS. It is important not to use TPGS with garlic or ginkgo, especially if you take any blood-thinning medication.

Aluminum

Aluminum is a metal entering the diet from sodium aluminum phosphate in cake mixes, frozen cookie dough, processed cheese, and self-rising flour, and from sodium aluminum sulfate in baking powder. It is also found in trace amounts in many brands of tea, and in large amounts in some over-the-counter antacids. Toxic effects of aluminum are most evident in people with kidney failure, and the element has not been ruled out as a cause of Alzheimer's disease. Products containing aluminum should be avoided by people with Alzheimer's disease or kidney disorders, and by low-birth-weight infants.

Androstenediol and Androstenedione

Androstenediol refers to 2 chemicals that are marketed as dietary supplements for bodybuilders, both of them highly similar to androstenedione. Studies at Iowa State University confirm that male volunteers taking androstenediol experience an immediate surge in androstenedione and the male hormone testosterone, as well as the female hormone estrogen. The problem with using androstenediol as a bodybuilding aid is that increased testosterone may not stay in the bloodstream long enough to encourage muscle growth, although time-released formulations of the supplement may eventually overcome this problem. Since the boost to testosterone is temporary, testosterone-related side effects (acne, breast enlargement, shrinkage of testicles, and sudden anger syndrome in men; acne, male-pattern baldness, clitoral thickening, missed menstruation, thickening of the skin, and deepening of the voice in women) should also be limited. However, no woman with a history of cancer of the breast, ovaries, or uterus and no man with a history of prostate cancer should take androstenediol. There are some indications that a single dose of androstenediol might boost the immune system's response to infection under conditions of emotional stress, and there is current medical research focusing on the use of androstenediol as a protective agent against the effects of radiation exposure.

Androstenedione is also marketed as a bodybuilding aid, but taking the recommended dosage of androstenedione does not cause a surge in testosterone —except in women. It does, however, increase bloodstream concentrations of estrogen in men. Very high doses of androstenedione may increase testosterone levels, but there is no conclusive evidence that they enhance athletic performance. There is no indication that androstenedione burns fat or builds muscle, certainly not among beginning exercisers. Since increased estrogen levels raise the risk of breast cancer in women and pancreatic cancer in men, prolonged use of androstenediol or androstenedione cannot be recommended.

Arginine Pyroglutamate

European studies have shown that **arginine pyroglutamate**, also known as **pyroglutamate**, may help restore memory defects caused by alcohol abuse and may help improve memory in people with Alzheimer's disease and mental retardation. The supplement seems to make the membranes of brain cells more permeable to nutrients and correspondingly more active. A typical dose of the supplement is 500–1,000 milligrams per day. Diarrhea and nausea occasionally occur as a result of taking this supplement. Its safety during pregnancy and nursing has not been established.

Aromatherapy

The term **aromatherapy** was coined in 1937 by the French chemist Rene-Maurice Gattefosse, who burned his hand while working in a perfume laboratory. Knowing lavender was used in medicine for treating burns and inflammation, he immersed his hand in a container of essence of lavender. The burns healed quickly and completely, and the experience inspired Gattefosse to research the healing properties of other aromatic oils.

The essential oils used in aromatherapy are applied through diffusers, floral waters, nose cones, and steam tents, and applied directly to the skin. Essential oils may also be added to baths and massage oils, but it is important to shower after using them so that the skin does not absorb any toxins. Anise, lavender, peppermint, sage, and thyme may be taken internally. One only needs to place 1 or 2 drops of the essential oil on a sugar cube, in a teaspoon of honey, or in a small amount ($1/4$ cup, or approximately 50 milliliters) of warm water to use essential oils as a lozenge, carminative, or mouthwash.

- A drop of **anise** on a sugar cube or in a spoon of honey is used to relieve abdominal cramping.

- **Bergamot**, especially when mixed with geranium or vetivert, is used as a calmative. Bergamot contributes a distinctive flavor to Earl Grey tea.

- **Black spruce** is used to give a "shot of adrenaline" in periods of fatigue.

- **Cedarwood**, lavender, rosemary, and thyme together have been used to grow hair lost to alopecia areata. Applied directly to the scalp daily, they may produce visible results in 3–7 months.

- **Cinnamon**, clove, and thyme are often combined in massage oils to relieve pain of arthritis.

- **Clary sage**, lavender, and Roman chamomile are combined in massage oils to relieve muscle spasms.

- **Eucalyptus** is the world's most widely used aromatherapeutic agent. Inhaled through a diffuser or vaporizer, applied topically as a chest rub, or taken in lozenges, eucalyptus is antibacterial and antiviral and relieves respiratory congestion.

- **Everlast** is applied to the skin to prevent bruising and swelling after sports injuries. It is also used to soften scars. Never take everlast by mouth.

- **Geranium** adds fragrance to bath oils, and treats fungal infections of the skin.

- **German chamomile** is used in baths and massage oils. A disinfectant, it can in rare instances cause mild allergic reactions.

- **Ginger** is a common remedy for diarrhea, gas, and motion sickness, but when used for this purpose it should be taken in the form of chopped fresh ginger or encapsulated dried ginger. Essential oils of ginger can be added to water used to make a warm compress, which can be applied to the abdomen to relieve cramping and stomach ache.

- **Helichrysum** is applied to the skin to relieve nerve pain in the feet and pain from athletic injuries in the knees. It may be combined with oil of cloves, ginger, and/or rosemary.

- **Klosterfrau Melissengeist** or **KMG** is a German formula combining angelica, cloves, elecampane, gentian, ginger, galangal, melissa, and black pepper oil for various conditions of nervous excess. German physicians use it to treat blushing, excitability, headaches, heart palpitations, hot flashes, migraines, and vertigo.

- **Lavender** is the most extensively studied essential oil used in aromatherapy. Studies in Japan have shown that it acts on the autonomic nervous system to increase the flow of blood to the skin to which it is applied, without increasing heart rate or blood pressure. Improved circulation allows the bloodstream to carry away inflammatory hormones and accelerates the healing of burns, cuts, and scrapes.

- **Mandarin** is a calmative, usually dispersed into a room with a vaporizer. It is most commonly used to calm overactive children.

- **Psychiatric** facilities have conducted controlled clinical trials of the use of aromatherapy with **melissa** as a calmative. Physicians at the Newcastle General Hospital in Newcastle-on-Tyne in the United Kingdom report a 30 percent reduction in agitation and a significant improvement in socialization among psychiatric patients given melissa oil rubs on their hands and faces twice a day for 4 weeks. Melissa is also used to relieve pain of herpes.

- **Neroli** is used in perfumes to relieve premenstrual tension.

- **Niaouli** is used to revitalize oily skin, and also as an analgesic agent for external hemorrhoids.

- **Oil of cloves** is a traditional and scientifically proven remedy for toothache. Apply directly to the affected tooth.

- **Palmarosa** is used to add a pleasant fragrance and additional antiviral power to mixtures of oils used to treat herpes.

- **Peppermint** is taken by mouth for irritable bowel syndrome. Scientists at the Cedars-Sinai Medical Center Burns and Allen Research Institute in Los Angeles have made extensive tests of the usefulness of peppermint oil in treating esophageal spasms, the uncoordinated muscle movements that make belches possible. Using a pressure gauge called a manometer, the research team measured pressure at the bottom and at the top of the esophagus before and after taking peppermint oil. The scientists found that peppermint oil eliminated simultaneous contractions—muscle movements that force the escape of air through the mouth—in all patients. Peppermint oil made contractions of the esophageal muscles more uniform and relieved chest pain in 2 of 8 patients in the test. Peppermint is the best-documented natural remedy for belching, but not everyone should take peppermint. Peppermint stimulates the release of bile, so it should be avoided by people who have gallstones, gallbladder inflammation, or severe liver damage. Anyone who has an allergy to menthol should avoid peppermint. If you cannot take peppermint, try increasing your use of other carminative herbs.

- **Ravensara** is also known as **camphor**, a traditional remedy for childhood bronchitis and other respiratory infections. It can be applied topically to shingles in an advanced stage of healing to help relieve pain.

- **Roman chamomile** is used with eucalyptus and ravensura in disinfectant air sprays.

- Tibetan medicine teaches that **spikenard oil** embodies the prana, or vital energy, of the plant. For this reason, spikenard is used to enhance psychic energy.

- **Tarragon** stimulates digestion and calms both irritable bowel and irritable bladder.

- **Tea tree oil** is added to footbaths to treat fungal infections of the skin.

- **Thyme** is a well-known antifungal oil, useful in douches to treat yeast infections, but it should not be used more than once a month.

Ascorbyl Palmitate

Ascorbyl palmitate is a form of vitamin C used as a food preservative. Since it is fat-soluble, it is better absorbed by cell membranes than ascorbic acid, the more common form of the vitamin. A little less than half of ascorbyl palmitate is vitamin C, so a little more than twice the dose is required. For more information on uses and precautions, see Vitamin C.

Bach Flower Remedies

The **Bach flower remedies** are well-established in natural medicine's repertoire for treating anxiety. Researchers conducting a double-blind, placebo-controlled, randomized clinical study in Germany concluded that these widely used treatments are (1) a placebo but (2) nonetheless effective, in as much as both patients who received a "placebo" flower remedy and patients who received a Bach flower remedy enjoyed lowered anxiety. One way of interpreting the results is that all flower remedies help lessen anxiety, or that the remedies' effectiveness is not limited to their traditional categories.

TRADITIONAL USES OF BACH FLOWER REMEDIES

Flower Remedy	Emotional Theme
Agrimony	Unreleased grief
Aspen	Anxiety compounded by fear
Beech	Critical of others
Centaury	Dependent on praise of others
Cerato	Lacking self-confidence
Cherry Plum	Need to control
Chestnut Bud	Stuck in old patterns
Chicory	Manipulative of others
Clematis	Lack of concentration or motivation
Crab Apple	Poor self-image
Elm	Overwhelmed by circumstances
Gentian	Discouragement
Gorse	Hopelessness
Heather	Loneliness
Holly	Negative feelings
Honeysuckle	Posttraumatic stress
Hornbeam	Fatigue
Impatiens	Impatience
Larch	Lack of self-confidence
Mustard	Crying spells
Oak	Struggling against the odds
Olive	Exhaustion
Pine	Dissatisfaction
Red Chestnut	Anxiety for other's well-being
Rock Rose	Nightmares
Rock Water	Pinned in by responsibility
Scleranthus	Indecision
Star of Bethlehem	Emotional trauma
Sweet Chestnut	Despair
Vervain	Argumentative
Walnut	Need to make emotional adjustments
Wild Oat	Unfulfilled ambitions
Wild Rose	Ennui
Willow	Bitterness

Bee Pollen

Bee pollen is a mixture of plant pollens and nectars collected by worker bees and bee saliva. It is sometimes recommended for hay fever. It is best to start with a small dose of bee pollen, to make sure it does not contain any pollen to which you may be intensely allergic. Use bee pollen for no more than 2 weeks at a time to avoid developing an allergy to the preparation. Typical doses are 1,000–1,500 milligrams per day. Bee pollen is available in capsules, chewable tablets, granules, liquids, powders, and tablets. The safety of bee pollen for children, pregnant women, and nursing mothers has not been established.

Bentonite

Bentonite is a type of clay used to absorb toxins, notably those from small doses of poorly chosen herbs. It is also used to coat the skin over outbreaks of poison ivy, poison oak, and poison sumac, to keep irritants from spreading. If you use bentonite as a "colon cleanser," never take more than 1 teaspoon per day, and always take the mineral with 2 glasses of water. Failure to drink water with bentonite can cause intestinal obstruction, although bentonite taken with water is laxative. Bentonite should not be taken within 2 hours of taking any other nutritional supplement or medication.

Beta-Carotene

Beta-carotene is a member of a class of healing plant pigments known as carotenoids. Scientists consider beta-carotene to be a conditionally essential nutrient. That is, consuming beta-carotene is essential to health when vitamin A is deficient. The supposition that high doses of beta-carotene can substitute for high doses of vitamin A, however, does not necessarily follow. Beta-carotene is usually an antioxidant; however, in the lungs of smokers, high concentrations of oxygen make beta-carotene a tissue-destructive pro-oxidant.

Low levels of beta-carotene have been associated with ovarian cysts, vaginal yeast infections, macular degeneration, cataracts, and skin cancer. Supplementing with beta-carotene alone, however, does not lower the risk of contracting or accelerate the process of healing these conditions. An important exception is erythropoietic protoporphyria (EPP), a rare skin condition in which exposure to visible light causes hives. Taking 25,000–300,000 IU of beta-carotene daily for 4–6 weeks reduces symptoms of EPP. For other conditions, it is best to take mixed carotenoids, including alpha- and gamma-carotene in addition to beta-carotene, and also lutein, lycopene, and zeaxanthin. Mixed carotenoids are most effective when taken with other antioxidants, notably selenium and vitamins C and E.

Pregnant women and nursing mothers should get beta-carotene by eating 5 or more servings of fruits and vegetables daily. Smokers need to know that taking more than 20 milligrams of beta-carotene per day is associated with a higher risk of lung cancer. Beta-carotene and mixed carotenes are not completely absorbed if they are taken at the same time as the cholesterol medications cholestyramine or colestipol, or if they are taken after eating foods made with Olestra.

Beta-Hydroxy-Beta-Methylbutyrate

Beta-hydroxy-beta-methylbutyrate (HMB), is a natural byproduct of the body's use of the amino acid leucine. HMB stimulates protein synthesis in muscle and stops the breakdown of tissue. It may be useful in treating people with severe burns, sepsis, or surgical trauma. A Polish study published in 2001 found that HMB stops the breakdown of muscle tissue after weight lifting, and that weight lifters using the supplement gained muscle at a faster rate. The effects of HMB are additive to creatine since the 2 supplements work on different biochemical pathways. In the Polish study, weight lifters who used HMB alone gained an average of 390 grams ($\frac{3}{4}$ pound) of muscle mass in 3 weeks. Athletes who used creatine gained an average of 920 grams (nearly 2 pounds) of muscle mass, but those who used both HMB and creatine gained an average of 1,540 grams (over 3 pounds) of muscle during the 3-week test period.

Some athletes use 3,000 milligrams of HMB daily. There are no side effects and no drug interactions, but HMB has not been proven safe for use by pregnant women or nursing mothers.

Beta-Sitosterol

Beta-sitosterol is a chemical cousin of cholesterol that is found in plants, especially concentrated in pumpkin seeds, pygeum, and saw palmetto. Laboratory tests with animals have found that supplemental beta-sitosterol shrinks (but does not eliminate) prostate tumors, and 3 clinical studies have shown that it improves flow of urine in men with enlarged prostates. A small-scale study published in 2002 found that giving men a combination of beta-sitosterol and saw palmetto partially reversed male pattern baldness.

When beta-sitosterol is first taken for prostate problems, an appropriate dosage is 300–400 milligrams per day. Once flow or urine has improved, 10–65 milligrams 3 times a day is sufficient. Beta-sitosterol is better absorbed if it is taken with food. This supplement has not been proven safe for pregnant women or nursing mothers.

Betaine Hydrochloride

Betaine hydrochloride, also known as **betaine** or **betaine HCl**, is an ammonia compound found in sugar beets. Betaine has two very different uses. As a source of for hydrochloric acid, it replaces stomach acid and aids the digestion of protein. As a source of betaine, it provides trimethylglycine, which works with folic acid to lower levels of homocysteine, involved in coronary artery disease.

A typical dosage of betaine hydrochloride is 600–650 milligrams, usually taken in the form of a combination product containing pepsin after a meal. A warm feeling in the stomach after taking betaine hydrochloride is a warning signal of overdose. Since betaine hydrochloride increases the acidity of the stomach, it must be avoided by anyone who has gastritis, gastroesophageal reflux disease (GERD), heartburn, or peptic or duodenal ulcers. If betaine hydrochloride is used to treat high homocysteine levels, folic acid, vitamin B_6, vitamin B_{12}, and zinc should also be taken (see HIGH HOMOCYSTEINE in Part One).

Bilberry

Bilberry is the primary herbal treatment for eye problems. Bilberry has been used as a remedy for poor night vision at least since World War II, when pilots in the Royal Air Force reported that an extra serving of bilberry jam with breakfast dramatically improved their night vision. French physicians examined the RAF pilots and found that administration of bilberry extract resulted in improved nighttime visual acuity, faster adjustment to darkness, and faster restoration of visual acuity after exposure to glare. In the 1960s and 1970s, French scientists attempted to demonstrate the benefits of bilberry in noncombat conditions. A study involving 14 air traffic controllers found that the 5 who had poor night vision had better night vision after taking bilberry for 8 days.

Bilberry is also used to treat diabetic retinopathy. Anthocyanosides, found in high concentrations in bilberry, strengthen fragile capillaries by protecting collagen. Additionally, anthocyanosides reduce capillary flow. In a double-blind clinical study, 14 patients with diabetic and/or hypertensive retinopathy were given a dosage of bilberry extract equivalent to 115 milligrams of anthocyanosides daily (or placebo) for 1 month. Sig-

nificant improvements in vision were observed in 11 volunteers receiving bilberry, and 12 patients were found to have improved retinal blood flow.

Many bilberry products combine the herb extract with lutein, which also improves night vision. Bilberry extracts are extremely nontoxic and difficult to overdose, although no added benefit can be expected from taking more than 540 milligrams per day.

Biochanin A

Biochanin A is an estrogenlike compound extracted from red clover, which also contains daidzein, formononetin, and genistein, the same phytoestrogens found in soy. Biochanin counteracts 17-beta-hydroxysteroid dehydrogenase type 5, an enzyme that breaks down estrogen. By conserving estrogen, biochanin reduces the frequency of hot flashes and relieves vaginal dryness.

Biochanin is typically included in a mixture of red clover isoflavones. Women who have estrogen receptor-positive breast cancer tumors should not take biochanin A or any other isoflavone product.

Biotin

Biotin is a B vitamin used by the body to release sugar from loaded carbohydrates, make energy from fat, and to form proteins from the branched-chain amino acids, L-isoleucine, L-leucine, and L-valine. Severe biotin deficiency causes graying and loss of hair. Biotin supplements are helpful in treating brittle fingernails in women, cradle cap in infants, and seborrheic dermatitis in children and adults.

Although some studies suggest biotin deficiencies may cause birth defects, the Food and Nutrition Board suggests that pregnant women take no more than 30 micrograms of biotin daily. Antibiotics, anticonvulsants, and high doses of the B vitamin pantothenic acid deplete biotin and call for biotin supplementation.

Bitter Orange Extracts

Bitter orange extracts appear in some sports supplements as a "thermogenic" aid, purportedly increasing metabolic rate and decreasing deposit of fats. Scientific evidence of this effect is preliminary, but the use of bitter orange oil (applied with a cotton swab) in the treatment of nasal inflammation and the use of chopped bitter orange in various Kampo formulas is well established.

There is no standard dosage of bitter orange extracts or oils. People who have pancreatitis, gastroesophageal reflux disease, or peptic ulcers should not take bitter orange products by mouth.

Black Cohosh

No herb is more useful in treating uterine fibroids than **black cohosh**. This widely used women's herb contains chemicals that keep estrogen from stimulating the proliferation of cells, stopping the growth of fibroid tissue. Laboratory studies specifically confirm that black cohosh, unlike so many other hormone-related products, absolutely does not stimulate the growth of cancerous cells. Unlike medications for uterine fibroids, black cohosh does not block the *beneficial* actions of estrogen.

Three classes of compounds in black cohosh bind to receptor sites in the reproductive tract, the brain, and other organs that otherwise would receive estrogen. This reduces overall estrogen activity when estrogen levels are high. Other compounds in black cohosh compounds block the formation of luteinizing hormone (LH), which stimulates a surge of estrogen production in the first 14 days of the menstrual period. This stimulates estrogen production when estrogen levels are low. The dual action of the herb allows it to stabilize the body's estrogen usage.

There is general agreement in the scientific literature that black cohosh can stop hot flashes in women who have not had breast cancer. It is also a useful treatment for vaginal dryness in menopause for women who cannot or who choose not to take estrogen replacement therapy. Supplemental black cohosh may minimize discomforts of menopause in women who are discontinuing estrogen replacement therapy. The herb is also a traditional remedy for menstrual discomforts.

Typical dosages of black cohosh are 500–1,000 milligrams a day. Taking more than 3,000 milligrams of black cohosh a day may cause abdominal pain, nausea, headaches, and dizziness. Women who are pregnant or breastfeeding should not use black cohosh.

Blackcurrant Seed Oil (BSO)

Blackcurrant seed oil (BSO) is a rich source of the essential fatty acids alpha-linolenic acid (ALA) and gamma-linolenic acid (GLA). A typical dose is two 500-milligram capsules, 3 times a day. For more information about the benefits of blackcurrant seed oil, see Gamma-Linolenic Acid.

Bone Meal

Bone meal is the finely crushed, processed bone of cattle and horses. It is a natural source of calcium, but it is also frequently contaminated with lead. The use of bone meal is not recommended.

Borage Oil

Borage oil—also known as **borage seed oil** and **starflower oil**—is, like blackcurrant seed oil, evening primrose oil, and hempseed oil, a rich source of gamma-linolenic acid (GLA).

People with rheumatoid arthritis may use from 300–3,000 milligrams of borage oil daily, preferably taken in 4 or 5 doses. Up to 2,000 milligrams a daily is helpful in lowering high triglycerides. Generally speaking, borage seed oil does not produce side effects. However, contaminants in borage seed oil can increase the risk of seizures in people who have temporal lobe epilepsy and in schizophrenics treated with chlorpromazine (Thorazine). There are also warnings that contaminants in borage oil can reduce immune function in HIV. For these reasons, it is important to use only products that are certified as free of pyrrolizidine alkaloids. Borage oil can also cause easy bruising in people taking prescription anticoagulants. For information about the health benefits of borage oil, see Gamma-Linolenic Acid.

Boron

Boron is a trace mineral that helps the body conserve calcium and magnesium, critical elements for bone health. At least one clinical study has found that boron supplementation helps prevent osteoporosis in women, and another has found that supplemental boron relieves pain of osteoarthritis. There are preliminary indications that boron supplements may improve memory and alertness.

Boron is contained in fruits and vegetables. An optimal level of supplementation to prevent boron deficiency is 3 milligrams per day, although up to 18 milligrams per day may be helpful in osteoarthritis. Boron asparate, boron citrate, boron glycinate, and sodium borate are all equally absorbed by the body. Boron is included in many combination products for arthritis and joint health.

Boswellin

Boswellin is a standardized form of the Ayurvedic herb boswellia, also known as mukul or Indian frankincense. In the treatment of asthma, it acts in the body in a way that complements zafirkulast (Accolate) and montelukast (Singulair). Bronchial constriction is caused by leukotrienes, which are made from n-6 fatty acids. Accolate and Singulair make cells insensitive to leukotrienes. Boswellin deactivates an enzyme so that leukotrienes are never made in the first place. And if enough of the enzyme 5-lipoxygenase is active so that leukotrienes are made, boswellin keeps them from being attracted after the release of histamine.

Physicians conducting a double-blind, placebo-controlled clinical study gave 40 asthmatics 300 milligrams of boswellin 3 times a day for 6 weeks. Seventy percent experienced improvement in lung capacity and fewer incidents of wheezing, compared with 27 percent in the control group. Boswellin is not known to interact with any prescription drugs, but it should be used with caution by people who have peptic ulcer disease. For this reason, boswellin is not an herb of choice for people who have rheumatoid arthritis, since it can compound stomach irritation caused by regular use of aspirin and other anti-inflammatory medications.

Bovine Cartilage

Bovine cartilage is collagen extracted from the cartilage of cows. Bovine cartilage was studied as a preventative treatment for angiogenesis, the growth of new blood vessels by a cancerous tumor, before shark cartilage became more popular. Proof of its usefulness in treating cancer, however, is lacking.

Bovine Colostrum

Bovine colostrum is the first "milk" a mother cow provides a newborn calf. It contains a variety of immunostimulant proteins that are especially useful in combating yeast infections and diarrhea caused by *Cryptosporidium* in AIDS patients. Since it also contains growth factors that activate certain forms of cancer, it

must be avoided by premenopausal women with breast cancer, by men with colorectal or prostate cancer, and by anyone who has lung cancer. A typical dosage is 10 grams taken 4 times a day for 21 days under a doctor's supervision.

Branched-Chain Amino Acids

The **branched-chain amino acids**, L-isoleucine, L-leucine, and L-valine, are so named because of their chemical structure. They are found in small amounts in vegetables and fruit juices, and in yogurt and miso. They have some usefulness in treating late-stage complications of cirrhosis of the liver, early stages of Lou Gehrig's disease, and phenylketonuria (PKU), but there is no reliable evidence that they enhance athletic performance. Their greatest usefulness is in treating the complication of drug treatment for schizophrenia known as tardive dyskinesia (see TARDIVE DYSKINESIA in Part One).

Branched chain amino acids are best used under medical supervision. They have not been proven safe for use by pregnant women or nursing mothers.

Brewer's Yeast

Brewer's yeast is a natural source of chromium, selenium, and B vitamins. It is *not* a probiotic, that is, a source of "friendly" bacteria. One study has found that taking selenium from brewer's yeast lowers the risk of colorectal, lung, and prostate cancer. Chromium that is derived from brewer's yeast is more beneficial than inorganic chromium in treating diabetes. Brewer's yeast has a bitter taste and can cause flatulence. Do not use brewer's yeast if you are taking monoamine oxidase inhibitors (MAOIs) for depression. Typical dosage is 486 or 500 milligrams, with meals 3 times a day.

Bromelain

Bromelain is a proteolytic or protein-dissolving enzyme found in pineapple. In the human body, it seems to short-circuit one of the chemical steps in making blood clots and it also seems to make white blood cells more "magnetic" to allergens and microorganisms, taking them out of circulation faster. Bromelain is useful in treating a variety of conditions in which enhanced circulation is desirable, including bruising, swelling, nasal congestion, and recovery from surgery, especially dental procedures, episiotomy (incision to widen the cervix, usually during childbirth), and vasectomy. It also relieves menstrual cramps by relaxing the smooth muscles lining the uterus. Used with another proteolytic enzyme found in a fruit, papain, it improves the body's digestion of protein foods.

The concentration varies from product to product. Follow the manufacture's instructions. Bromelain improves the absorption of amoxicillin and tetracycline. While bromelain is used to accelerate the healing of bruises, it can lead to easier bruising in people who take aspirin or anticoagulant drugs. In rare cases, bromelain can cause allergic reactions in people who are also allergic to pineapple.

Calcium

Calcium is an essential element for healthy bones. Supplemental calcium with adequate supplies of magnesium, phosphorus, selenium, and vitamin D reduces bone pain and risk of fracture in osteoporosis. Calcium reduces the risk of colorectal cancer. Women who consume the highest amounts of calcium have a lower risk of strokes. Supplemental calcium reduces the severity of menstrual pain. There has even been a study to suggest that consuming adequate amounts of calcium slows weight gain by accelerating the use of fatty acids within fat cells for energy.

A number of studies have found that calcium citrate is better absorbed than other forms of calcium. Typical dosage is 1,000 milligrams per day. Calcium is better absorbed if it is taken in 2 or 3 small doses rather than a single large dose. Do not take calcium at the same time you take supplemental inositol hexaphosphate or biphosphonates prescribed for osteoporosis or osteomalacia. Taking calcium supplements at the same time as medications for heartburn minimizes the absorption of calcium, and taking calcium at the same time as taking thyroid hormone reduces the absorption of thyroid hormone. Calcium supplements increase the absorption of the antibiotic tetracycline but decrease the absorption of antibiotics in the same class as Cipro.

Sufferers of kidney stones are traditionally told to avoid calcium supplements; however, this effect does not occur with the use of calcium citrate, and it is minimized in the use of other forms of calcium by avoiding orange and grapefruit juice (lemon juice is acceptable). People who have cancer should not take supplemental calcium, nor should anyone with hyperparathyroidism, hypervitaminosis D, or sarcoidosis.

Caprylic Acid

Caprylic acid is found in butterfat. Some studies in the 1940s found that it controls yeast infections, and some naturopaths use it as an infusion to flush the gallbladder. When taken by mouth as a nutritional supplement, typical dosage is 300–1,200 milligrams daily. Caprylic acid should be avoided by pregnant women and during diarrhea. Its primary use is as a carrier for specialized medications for osteoporosis.

Capsaicin

Capsaicin is the chemical that gives hot peppers their heat. As anyone who has cooked with chiles knows, capsaicin can cause burning, redness, and inflammation, especially to the eyes and mouth. The first time it is applied in a cream to the skin over a painful back, capsaicin causes these symptoms, but the nerve fibers serving the back become insensitive to it—and to back pain.

Capsaicin works best when there is good circulation to the skin to which it is applied. Do not apply it to your feet if you have diabetes and never apply it to ulcerated skin. It is also important to keep capsaicin out of your nose and eyes. Allergic reactions to capsaicin are rare but are not unknown, and there have been cases of hypothermia in people who used capsaicin in an especially cold room. It is theoretically possible that capsaicin absorbed into the bloodstream could reduce the bioavailability of aspirin; if you use capsaicin, use pain relievers other than aspirin. If you are sensitive to capsaicin, substitute diluted essential oils of peppermint, eucalyptus, rosemary, or wintergreen.

CDP-Choline

CDP-choline is a chemical the body makes in the process of synthesizing phosphatidylcholine, a major component in the membranes lining every cell. In red blood cells, phosphatidylcholine is essential for making the cells flexible enough to travel around tight corners or blockages. In nerve cells and brain cells, phosphatidylcholine protects the interior of the cell from trauma, toxins, infections, and oxidation.

The most extensively studied application of CDP-choline is the treatment of amblyopia in children. It is not a substitute for wearing an eye patch, but it will accelerate improvement. CDP-choline is also used to treat double vision caused by stroke or Parkinson's disease. It is used to treat memory loss in Alzheimer's disease, with better results earlier in the disease. Current research focuses on using CDP-choline to treat transient ischemic attacks and stroke.

Among the newer applications of CDP-choline is to reduce cravings for cocaine, heroin, and methamphetamines. Brain tissue in chronic users of these drugs becomes less efficient at producing phosphatidylcholine, and compensates by breaking down tissues that make the pleasure chemical dopamine. Taking the drugs stimulates the production of dopamine, but taking CDP-choline preserves the tissues that make dopamine, with the same effect on mood. CDP-choline may also protect brain tissue from damage by a combination of recreational drug use and HIV.

Daily doses of CDP-choline range from 500 milligrams for children to 2,000 milligrams for adults. Overdoses may cause burping, belching, nausea, headache, or rash. If these occur, cut back the dosage or discontinue the supplement. The safety of CDP-choline for pregnant women and nursing mothers has not been established.

Cellulase

Cellulase is a digestive enzyme extracted from the fungi *Aspergillus niger* and *Trichoderma longbrachiatum*. Cellulase digests cellulose, an indigestible polysaccharide found in plant fibers. The primary use of cellulose innatural health is in controlling flatulence after eating meals or taking supplements high in fiber. Dosage is variable. Follow the manufacturer's directions or consult your physician.

Cetyl Myristoleate

Cetyl myristoleate is a fatty acid originally identified in whale blubber, and is also found in the musk glands of certain beavers. Claims that research found that it makes laboratory mice "immune" to arthritis are overstated, although it greatly reduced inflammation caused by injection of a bacterial toxin. There are also claims that it is a "fast-acting" essential fatty acid, but these are likewise overstated. There are numerous anecdotal reports that supplemental cetyl myristoleate relieves pain in chronic

fatigue syndrome, fibromyalgia, and both osteoarthritis and rheumatoid arthritis.

Typical dosage of cetyl myristoleate is 300–400 milligrams per day. Overdoses may cause diarrhea. The safety of cetyl myristoleate for pregnant women and nursing mothers has not been established.

Chelated Minerals

Chelated minerals are minerals manufactured as artificial complexes with amino acids or cholesterol. There is some evidence that chelated chromium and zinc are better absorbed by the body. See listings for individual minerals for further information.

Chicken Collagen

Chicken collagen is a protein extracted from the breastbone of chickens. The type of collagen extracted for use in nutritional supplements, chicken collagen II, is similar to type II collagen in humans. The rationale for using chicken collagen is that since rheumatoid arthritis is a disease in which the immune system attacks collagen that lines joints, "distracting" the immune system with chicken collagen might lower inflammation. Interestingly, clinical trials have found that only the very *lowest* doses of chicken collagen have a beneficial effect.

If you want to use chicken collagen, consult with a holistically oriented physician first. If you are hypersensitive to collagen from meats, use of chicken collagen could aggravate symptoms rather than relieve them. Clinical trials have found that doses of 20 micrograms per day are mildly beneficial, but doses of 100 and 500 micrograms per day are not. There is one case report of a child who developed hot flashes and facial redness from taking chicken collagen; both symptoms went away when the collagen was discontinued.

Chitin and Chitosan

Chitin and **chitosan** are tough protein polymers found in the shells of crabs, shrimp, and other shellfish as well as in some fungi. Chitin is the material from which glucosamine is extracted. The primary use of supplemental chitin is to absorb nutrients from food that may be in excess. In very high doses in tests with animals, chitin produces a dramatic lowering of cholesterol levels. In clinical tests of doses humans find tolerable, chitin lowers LDL cholesterol without lowering HDL cholesterol, although triglycerides may be slightly raised. Chitin binds cholesterol by complexing with the bile salts the gallbladder releases to carry cholesterol into the body. The benefits of chitin are variable. Total cholesterol may be lowered 5 to 40 percent and LDL cholesterol may be lowered 15 to 35 percent, provided dietary cholesterol is kept in moderation. A recent clinical trial at the University of California at Davis found that chitosan is not effective for people eating high-fat diets (1,000 calories of fat or more per day).

A more important but less widely known use of chitin is to treat people with chronic kidney failure. When the kidneys fail, even small excesses of dietary protein can lead to toxic buildup of urea. In a clinical trial in which dialysis patients took 4,050 milligrams of chitin a day, 4 weeks of treatment dramatically lowered the amounts of urea and creatine in the bloodstream. Twelve weeks of treatment improved appetite, sleep patterns, and physical strength.

Supplemental chitosan produces dramatic reductions in obesity in lab rats, but minimal effects in obese humans. Chitin breaks down into positively charged ions that attract negatively charged fat molecules, but in humans, "sloshing" through the digestive tract seems to break up the chitin-bound fat so that much of it is absorbed.

The German research journal *Arzneimittelforschung* reports that between 2 and 5 percent of users of chitin or chitosan will experience mild allergies. People who are allergic to shellfish should not use the product. Typical dosage is 1,000–1,200 milligrams per day, taken before or after meals with a glass of water. Do not take chitosan within 2 hours of taking supplemental zinc or vitamins A, D, E, or K. Be sure to use brands that are certified as free of heavy metals.

Chlorella

Chlorella is a popular "green food" in the United States and Japan. A clinical trial at the Virginia Commonwealth University found that daily dietary supplementation with chlorella may reduce high blood pressure, lower serum cholesterol levels, accelerate wound healing, and enhance immune functions. A pilot study also conducted at the Virginia Commonwealth University found that taking 10 grams of Sun Chlorella tablets and 100 milliliters of liquid Wakasa Gold daily significantly lowered

the intensity of pain for fibromyalgia patients, but a few participants in the trial reported that their pain got worse. Effects on chlorella on pain may not be noticeable for up to 2 months.

There is no standard dosage for chlorella, as it is typically combined with other green foods such as barley, grass, wheat grass, and spirulina. The safety of chlorella for pregnant women and nursing mothers has not been established. Some formulations of chlorella contain enough vitamin K that they increase blood-clotting factors and counteract warfarin (Coumadin).

Chlorophyll

Chlorophyll is the familiar green pigment of plants. It captures sunlight to power the reaction by which plants make carbohydrates from carbon dioxide and release oxygen. The primary use of chlorophyll and its water-soluble chemical derivative chlorophyllin is to absorb odors. Chlorophyllin absorbs odors after colostomy or ileostomy and reduces odors due to severe constipation or incontinence. Taking chlorophyllin can reduce urinary odors, notably in diabetics taking very high dosages of insulin. Chlorophyll is also sometimes used in douches (see PELVIC INFLAMMATORY DISEASE in Part One).

A typical dosage of chlorophyllin for reducing various body odors is 100 milligrams per day, taken by mouth. Using the supplement can cause green urine or green feces, and in rare cases, it can leave a green or black stain on the tongue. The safety of chlorophyllin for pregnant women and nursing mothers has not been established.

Choline

The human body uses **choline** to make phosphatidylcholine, a major component in the membranes lining every cell. In red blood cells, phosphatidylcholine is essential for making the cells flexible enough to travel around tight corners or blockages. In nerve cells and brain cells, phosphatidylcholine protects the interior of the cell from trauma, toxins, infections, and oxidation. Choline is the primary nutrient in iceberg lettuce. It is also found in beef liver, cauliflower, egg yolks, peanuts, and soy. For information about choline's uses in health, see Phosphatidylcholine.

Typical dosages of choline range from 300–1,200 milligrams per day. Supplemental choline may be helpful for people who have been treated for cancer or arthritis with methotrexate (Methotrex), which depletes choline in the liver. Approximately 1 in 500 people will develop a rotten-fish odor in the breath, sweat, and urine when taking supplemental choline. This distressing side effect stops when the supplement is discontinued. Taking more than 3,000 milligrams of choline a day can cause diarrhea, nausea, or loose stools.

Chondroitin Sulfate

Chondroitin sulfate is a complex protein found in the cartilage of fish and humans. Before the 1990s, chondroitin was long thought to be such a large molecule that it could not be absorbed if taken orally. Recent research, however, has found that a large percentage of the chondroitin taken in supplements is actually absorbed into the body.

Like glucosamine, chondroitin relieves pain by helping to heal joints. One study found that people with arthritis of the knee who took chondroitin were able to increase their maximum walking speed, and that pain relief was noticed in as little as 1 month. More important, at the end of 12 months, study participants who had been taking chondroitin were found to have no worsening of the joints. Chondroitin seems to protect joints from damage, perhaps halting the course of the disease.

One small-scale clinical trial found that use of chondroitin also protects against heart attack in patients with severe coronary artery disease.

A typical dosage of chondroitin is 1,200 milligrams per day, preferably taken in 2 or more doses. Do not take chondroitin with chitosan; chondroitin, like cholesterol, chemically binds to chitosan and is excreted. Benefits from taking chondroitin may not be noticeable for 4–6 weeks. In rare cases, chondroitin can cause mild stomach upset. If this occurs, reduce dosage of the supplement. The safety of chondroitin for pregnant women and nursing mothers has not been established.

Chromium

Chromium is an essential trace element used by the body to make a glucose tolerance factor. The exact way chromium acts in the body is not known, but it is thought to increase the number of insulin receptors on the linings of muscle cells, making them more receptive to both sugars and free fatty acids. Diabetes seems to cause the body to excrete needed chromium into the urine. Experiments with animals have found that supplemental chromium is particulary helpful when blood sugars are especially high, so high that the body has begun to break down proteins inside cells because it cannot use insulin to transport glucose to the cells. These experiments have also shown that chromium helps insulin resistance and high blood sugars caused by stress.

Studies of the use of chromium in treating diabetes, hypoglycemia, and high cholesterol have been promising. A dosage of up to 1,600 micrograms per day has been found to be helpful in controlling gestational diabetes, that is, diabetes induced by pregnancy. Lower blood sugar levels are found in diabetics treated with 200–1,000 micrograms per day for at least 6 months, higher doses bringing about faster decreases in blood sugar levels. Chromium causes significant reductions in total and LDL cholesterol and slight reduction in HDL cholesterol in athletes, but no study has found similar results in people who do not exercise.

Studies of chromium as a weight-loss aid have been disappointing. A clinical trial at the University of Massachusetts failed to find that women taking 400 micrograms of supplemental chromium a day during a 12-week walking and diet weight-loss program lost more weight or more fat or experienced significant benefits in fasting blood sugars or insulin production. A clinical trial at Purdue University failed to find that supplemental chromium enhanced weight loss in women in a strength-training program for weight loss.

A typical maintenance dosage of chromium is 200 micrograms per day, although some experts believe that in diabetes it is better to use 1,000 micrograms a day for the first 6 months. Chromium that is derived from brewer's yeast is more beneficial than inorganic chromium, and chelated chromium is more effective than non-chelated chromium. Chromium is attracted to phytates found in seeds, nuts, miso, and matzo. Eating foods containing phytates at the same time as taking chromium supplements binds chromium so that it is not absorbed. Toxic side effects of chromium probably do not exist, but at least one person reported "feeling funny," disrupted thinking, and difficulty driving after taking a chromium product combined with yeast. Symptoms subsided in a few hours. Three other suspected cases of chromium toxicity can be explained by taking massive doses of prescription drugs in addition to supplemental chromium.

Only about 2 out of 3 diabetics benefit from taking chromium, and the supplement may prevent the production of harmful byproducts from blood sugars rather than lowering blood sugars in a way that will be noticed in blood tests. The key to successful use of chromium may be making sure that the body has an adequate supply of its cofactor niacin. At least one study found that taking chromium by itself had no discernible benefit for diabetes, but taking both chromium and niacin lowered fasting blood sugars by 7 percent and reduced overall blood sugars (the total amount of glucose in the bloodstream over a 28-day period) by 15 percent—an enormous benefit. Since high dosages of niacin can cause increased sensitivity to sunlight and sunburn and aggravate hot flashes or rosacea, be sure not to take more than 100 milligrams of niacin per day as an adjunct to chromium.

Chrysin

Chrysin is a passionflower extract that probably slows but does not prevent the conversion of androstenedione and testosterone into estrogen in a man's body. More important, it inhibits excess production of the stress hormone cortisol, encouraging mental relaxation and muscle repair. It is used as a stand-alone supplement and in combination with androstenedione to encourage muscle formation in weight lifters and to restore sexual desire in both men and women. Since chrysin does not increase the production of testosterone, it does not carry the same risk of side effects as the better-known androstenedione.

Chrysin has been studied as a sports supplement in several recent clinical trials at Iowa State University, but only in combination with androstenedione and an herbal product also containing saw palmetto and *Tribulus terrestris*. These studies did not find that herbal products including chrysin prevented the conversion of testosterone into estrogen; however, they did not control for changes in cortisol.

Typical dosage of chrysin is 1,000 milligrams per day. Pregnant women and nursing mothers should not take the drug, nor should women with a history of estrogen-dependent malignancy of the breast, ovaries, or uterus. Women in the United Kingdom treated with the breast cancer drug anastrazole (Femara) should be aware that use of any product containing chrysin can increase the side effects of Femara.

Chymotrypsin

Chymotrypsin is a digestive enzyme derived from ox pancreas. Used to assist the digestion of proteins, chymotrypsin liberates the amino acids arginine and lysine from food and it is especially helpful in assisting the digestion of amino acids in fatty meats. Supplemental chymotrypsin is medically prescribed to treat pancreatitis. Dosages should be chosen in consultation with a health professional.

Cocoa Flavonoids

Cocoa flavonoids are being researched as a means of reducing the oxidation of LDL cholesterol and preventing the formation of atherosclerotic plaques. Dosage has not been established. Avoid cocoa flavonoids if you are allergic to chocolate.

Coenzyme Q_{10} (CoQ_{10})

Coenzyme Q_{10} (CoQ_{10}) is synthesized by every cell in the body to capture electrons released as the mitochondria release the energy by combining sugar with oxygen. A solid, waxlike substance, CoQ_{10} is made by the same chemical process that makes cholesterol, and, like cholesterol, CoQ_{10} is especially abundant in the healthy heart. Since the heart muscle makes and uses energy 24 hours a day, it needs a large quantity of CoQ_{10}. Heart tissue biopsies of people with various heart diseases show a deficiency of CoQ_{10} of 50 to 75 percent compared to normal.

As people age, the heart makes less CoQ_{10}. Certain cholesterol-lowering drugs also reduce the heart's supply of this vital enzyme. Replacing CoQ_{10} is important in treating angina. In one study, 12 patients with angina were given 150 milligrams of CoQ_{10} daily for 4 weeks. Taking CoQ_{10} reduced the average frequency of angina attacks by 53 percent. CoQ_{10} treatment also allowed the angina patients to last longer on a treadmill before experiencing chest pain or abnormal EKGs. A review of more than 100 research studies conducted between 1974 and 2000 finds consistent benefit from CoQ_{10} for angina sufferers.

Even heart patients with severe heart damage benefit from CoQ_{10}. A Danish study found that treatment with the supplement for 12 weeks increased the output of the heart at rest and during exercise. The supplement is similarly useful in treating hereditary hypertrophic cardiomyopathy, more commonly known as "enlarged heart." Doctors at the Langsjoen Clinic in Tyler, Texas, found that giving patients 200 milligrams of CoQ$_{10}$ for 3 months reduced the thickness of the septum dividing the heart muscle by an average of 24 percent and the thickness of the posterior wall by 26 percent.

European studies have found preliminary indications of a role for CoQ$_{10}$ in preventing the spread of breast cancer (see BREAST CANCER in Part One). A number of studies with animals have confirmed that CoQ$_{10}$ reduces the risk of heart damage during chemotherapy with doxorubicin (Adriamycin). One study with humans found that taking 50–100 milligrams of the supplement per day reduces the risk of heart damage by 20 percent and also prevents diarrhea and mouth sores.

Animal studies have shown that CoQ$_{10}$ greatly increases survival time after infection with *Pseudomonas aeruginosa*, a frequent complication of cystic fibrosis. It increases the activity of the bacteria-eating cells known as macrophages, and spares antioxidant vitamin E, reducing inflammation. Used with alpha-lipoic acid and other antioxidants, the supplement may prevent nerve damage in chronic fatigue syndrome.

CoQ$_{10}$ may be helpful in treating high blood pressure when only systolic (upper number) pressures are elevated. A study by the Veterans Health Administration found that men with isolated systolic hypertension who took 60 milligrams of CoQ$_{10}$ daily for 3 months had decreases in systolic pressure of 8–25 points without decreases in diastolic (lower number) pressures. The advantage of CoQ$_{10}$ over other treatments is that it avoids the complication of orthostatic hypotension, feeling faint (or actually passing out) when moving from a seated to a standing position, which could be caused by drugs that lower both systolic and diastolic pressures.

CoQ$_{10}$ reduces the side effects beta-blockers used to treat high blood pressure and glaucoma have on the cardiovascular system. It prevents reduction in the output of the heart and hastens the restoration of normal pulse rates after each dose of medication. A Japanese study of 16 patients found that taking the supplement to relieve side effects of treatment with Timoptic (timolol) did not interfere with the medication's beneficial effects on glaucoma.

Effective doses of CoQ$_{10}$ range from 50–200 milligrams per day. There are very few precautions to take in the use of CoQ$_{10}$. The medical literature contains one report of CoQ$_{10}$ decreasing the effectiveness of warfarin (Coumadin). It may improve sugar control in some cases of diabetes. If you are diabetic, check your blood sugars regularly when you take CoQ$_{10}$. Black pepper increases bloodstream levels of CoQ$_{10}$ and seasoning your food with pepper would be helpful when you take CoQ$_{10}$. If you are taking heparin, clopidogrel (Plavix), or warfarin (Coumadin), you need to let your doctor know you are taking CoQ$_{10}$, since the combination can make these anticlotting drugs less effective.

Colloidal Minerals

Colloidal minerals are formulations of humic acids, more commonly used as fertilizers, for humans. They have been popularized as natural sources of boron, calcium, copper, iodine, manganese, magnesium, selenium, and zinc and are reported to be more completely absorbed than their manufactured counterparts. However, colloidal minerals may also contain aluminum, arsenic, lead, mercury, and strontium. Liquid mineral is a distinct product extracted from sea salts.

The problem with using colloidal minerals is that their mineral content varies from batch to batch. People with copper or iron overload diseases (Wilson's disease or hemochromatosis) should not use colloidal minerals under any circumstances. If you choose to use colloidal minerals, be sure to refrigerate the bottle after opening.

Colloidal Silver

Colloidal silver is highly toxic to bacteria. It is safely used as a topical disinfectant in liquids and creams. It is also prescribed by some naturopathic physicians for internal use to treat infection, especially diarrhea in AIDS, but an appropriate dosage is 1 teaspoon of a solution containing 1 part per *million* of silver once a day. Never take any colloidal silver product internally except under the supervision of an experienced naturopathic physician. Overdose of colloidal silver can cause permanent and irreversible discoloration of the skin, leaving a black tinge where skin is exposed to sunlight.

Colosolic Acid

Colosolic acid is extract from the Filipino herb banaba (*Lagerstroemia speciosa*). It is sometimes referred to as corosolic acid, 2-alpha-hydroxyursolic acid, and as a "plant insulin," although it contains no human insulin. (Analogs of human insulin are found in some African fungi and a few South American rainforest herbs.) Laboratory experiments confirm that it does, however, increase the transport of sugar into cells. In the United States, colosolic acid is most commonly available in 160-milligram capsules. Dosage depends on its effects on blood sugar. These effects are only known by blood test (finger prick for home testing). The safety of colosolic acid for pregnant women and nursing mothers has not been established.

Conjugated Linolenic Acid (CLA)

Conjugated linolenic acid (CLA) is a naturally occurring fatty acid found in red meat, cheese, and safflower and sunflower oil. Scientists believe that it could activate a gene known as peroxisome proliferator-activated receptor gamma (PPAR-gamma), giving it a variety of as yet unproven anticancer, anticholesterol, and antidiabetic effects. In the laboratory, CLA has stopped growth of breast, colorectal, lung, and prostate cancer cells as well as melanoma. A specific isomer of CLA, tans-10, cis-12 linolenic acid, may be helpful in reducing body fat, effectively shrinking fat cells and making them stay that way. CLA may eventually prove helpful for diabetics experiencing weight gain after treatment with pioglitazone (Actos) and rosiglitazone (Avandia).

Typical daily dosage of CLA is up to 2,000 milligrams. Overdosage of the supplement may cause nausea. The safety of CLA for pregnant women, nursing mothers, and children has not been proven.

Copper

Copper is an essential trace element in human nutrition. The richest dietary sources of copper are beans, bran, nuts, seeds, shellfish, and beef liver and kidney. Deficiency of copper can cause anemia not responsive to iron supplementation, high cholesterol, loss of skin pigmentation, diabetes, an immune deficiency condition known as neutropenia, and osteoporosis. Mild copper deficiency may be an important contributing factor in heart disease. Eating too much molasses or leafy greens on a regular basis can cause copper deficiency, as can taking a daily dose of more than 50 milligrams of supplemental zinc.

Of all the nutritional supplements for rheumatoid arthritis, the best known is transdermal copper in the form of a copper bracelet. Often dismissed as a myth of folk medicine, copper bracelets apparently do have some therapeutic effect. A clinical study enlisted 160 volunteers who had arthritis, half of whom had previously worn a copper bracelet. The study participants were assigned to 2 groups. One group wore a copper bracelet for 1 month, and then a placebo bracelet (electroplated aluminum resembling copper) for a second month. The other group wore the bracelets in reverse order. Of the participants who noticed a difference between the 2 bracelets, significantly more preferred copper to placebo. Users of copper bracelets deteriorated significantly during the time they were wearing the placebo bracelet.

The amount of copper entering circulation through the skin by wearing a bracelet is very small, equivalent to taking 1 milligram ($\frac{1}{2}$ of the smallest tablet) every other day. The secret to success with copper supplementation may be taking smaller doses. There is at least some evidence that the copper shortages that contribute to rheumatiod arthritis occur within the cartilage of the joints but not elsewhere in the body. This shortage can be due to a defect in the carrier proteins for copper rather than insufficient copper in the diet. (This defect is worse when vitamin C supplementation exceeds 600 milligrams per day.) Therefore, take just enough copper to make sure you are not copper deficient (a 1 milligram tablet every other day). Alternatively, you can wear a copper bracelet.

Copper is also sometimes recommended for treating irregular heartbeats. This recommendation is based on the experience of just 3 patients, and should be considered premature.

Limit supplemental copper to at most 3 milligrams a day. Taking too much copper can cause stomach ache, nausea, diarrhea, and vomiting. Copper is poorly absorbed when supplements are taken within 2 hours of eating a meal including raw green beans, pumpkin or other seeds, nuts, or matzo.

Copper supplements should be avoided by women who have cervical dysplasia. Recent studies have found that copper levels are positively associated with the severity of cervical dysplasia. No one with Wilson's disease should take any supplement containing copper except on the advice of a physician.

Cranberry Juice

Cranberry juice is a familiar remedy for urinary tract infections. The *Journal of the American Medical Association* reports that blueberry juice may work just as well at keeping 19 different strains of antibiotic-resistant bacteria from taking root in the lining of the urinary tract, enabling the kidneys to flush them away. Since the effect of cranberry or blueberry juice tannins only lasts 8 hours and takes 2 hours to start, it is important to drink a cup of juice 3 times a day. If the calories from 3 cups of juice a day would put a strain on your diet, cranberry juice extracts are also available. Just be sure to take at least two 1,000 milligram capsules 3 times a day.

Don't give cranberry juice or cranberry juice extracts to infants. The medical literature reports a case of cranberry juice intoxication in a 4-month old baby given ¾ cup of cranberry juice who developed diarrhea severe enough to cause dehydration. The cranberry juice acidified not only the urine but the child's entire system. The child recovered after being put on a lactose-free formula.

Creatine

Creatine is an amino acid the body uses to store energy rather than to make proteins. Supplemental creatine makes it possible to move faster during a sprint, but the effect is cumulative. That is, it is not possible to load up on creatine to increase speed in a single athletic event. Weight gain after taking creatine for a few days to a few weeks is common, but the weight is more likely to be fluid than muscle. Wrestlers, in particular, frequently note weight gains of 1.1–3.5 pounds (0.5–1.5 kilograms) after taking creatine for 1 week.

Preliminary studies suggest that creatine may prolong survival in Lou Gehrig's disease and improve muscle strength in muscular dystrophy. There are also indications creatine could protect against further brain damage in Parkinson's disease.

Most athletes take 20 grams of creatine 4 times a day. Caffeine in coffee, tea, and colas seems to interfere with the beneficial effects of creatine supplementation. Overdosing commonly causes diarrhea.

The body's needs for fluid are not increased by the use of creatine, but athletes using creatine are cautioned not to attempt to limit weight gain by cutting back on water intake. Fatal dehydration and renal failure, not caused by the use of creatine, has been known to result. Do not take creatine if you have any kind of nephritis or chronic kidney failure.

Curcuminoids

Curcuminoids are potent antioxidant pigments found in turmeric. In one clinical trial, taking 1,200 milligrams of curcuminoids a day for 2 weeks reduced morning stiffness and joint swelling caused by rheumatoid arthritis, although the supplement had no effect on objective laboratory measures of the severity of the disease. Another clinical trial found that curcuminoids were as effective as prescription steroids in treating chronic uveitis, without side effects. Various preliminary studies hint that curcuminoids may also be beneficial in treating hepatitis C and HIV. It is worth noting that rates of breast cancer are extremely low in cultures where curries are a major part of the diet, curry being a rich source of curcumin. There are also laboratory studies that have found that curcuminoids enhance the anticancer effects of cisplatin (Platinol).

Effective doses of curcuminoids range from 500–4,000 milligrams a day. Taking curcuminoids on an empty stomach may cause heartburn. People with chronic heartburn should not take this supplement. Cancer patients should only use curcuminoids supplements under medical supervision, since the combination of curcuminoids and various anticancer drugs can have drastic effects on blood-clotting factors.

Daidzein

Daidzein is a plant estrogen found in soy, kudzu, and red clover. Taken with other soy flavones, daidzein has a number of benefits for women in menopause. Soy products do not offer relief as quickly as hormone replacement, but the body of clinical research considered as a whole indicates that most women will experience relief from hot flashes by taking 100 milligrams of soy isoflavones (daidzein + genistein) daily.

Daidzein is found in various formulas containing soy isoflavones. The safety of daidzein for pregnant women and nursing mothers has not been established. Men with prostate cancer and women with estrogen receptor-positive cancers of the breast, ovaries, or uterus should only use a formula containing daidzein if they are recommended and monitored by a physician.

Deanol (DMAE)

Deanol, also known as **demithylaminoethanol** or **DMAE**, is turned into the neurotransmitter acetylcholine in the brain. There are numerous anecdotal reports of its helpfulness in ADD and ADHD, Alzheimer's disease, amnesia, age-related memory loss, tardive dyskinesia, and Tourette's syndrome, but clinical trials have failed to prove a clear benefit. The supplement is frequently used by dermatologists to treat sagging skin around the eyes, at the tip of the nose, and around the lips. Hollywood makeup artists use DMAE to give actors and actresses plumper lips. Scientific research confirming this use of DMAE is in a very preliminary stage.

A typical dosage of oral DMAE is 100 milligrams. The supplement is also available as a liquid and in skin creams. DMAE must be avoided by anyone who has high homocysteine levels, and its safety has not been established for pregnant women, nursing mothers, or children. Oral DMAE in rare instances has caused headache, cramps, constipation, sleep disturbances, and lucid dreams. In an isolated case, a man taking DMAE for 10 years for essential tremor developed a severe facial tic that was only partially resolved by discontinuing DMAE.

Deglycyrrhizinated Licorice (DGL)

Deglycyrrhizinated licorice (DGL) is licorice treated to remove potentially hazardous glycyrrhizin. Glycyrrhizin inhibits the breakdown of stress hormones such as cortisol and can cause hypertension, water retention, and low potassium levels. DGL does not have this side effect.

At least one study has found that a mixture of DGL and water applied to the inside of the mouth can shorten the healing time for canker sores, with complete healing typically occurring on the third day. DGL reduces stomach irritation caused by regular use of aspirin and NSAID pain relievers for arthritis. DGL treats peptic ulcer and other forms of chronic stomach irritation through the action of flavonoid compounds that inhibit the growth of *Helicobacter pylori*. Licorice flavonoids stimulate the production of mucus to coat and protect the stomach. DGL also increases the life span of intestinal cells and improves blood flow to the intestinal lining.

A typical dosage of DGL is 1–4 380-milligram tablets or wafers chewed thoroughly for a few minutes before each meal. Chewing and mixing DGL with saliva is essential for releasing its therapeutic flavonoids. DGL increases the excretion of the antibiotic nitrofurantoin (Macrobid) and may make it less effective.

Dehydroepiandrosterone (DHEA)

Dehydroepiandrosterone, more commonly known as **DHEA**, is a steroid hormone produced from cholesterol in the adrenal glands, sex organs, and brain. DHEA supplementation in adrenal insufficiency, a state of pathological loss of dehydroepiandrosterone production, improves well-being, mood, and sexuality. For reasons that are not completely understood, low levels of DHEA are associated with especially severe symptoms of lupus. The latest clinical research finds that about half of women with lupus who take 100 or 200 milligrams of DHEA per day for 9 months can reduce their dosage of steroid medications for relief of joint pain—but nearly as many women got better on placebo. Several recent studies have failed to find benefit for DHEA replacement in men over 55. Under medical supervision, DHEA may be used to treat lipodystrophy caused by drug treatment for HIV.

DHEA should be used only under medical supervision. It is usually dosed at 25–50 milligrams per day. Acne, male pattern hair loss, growth of facial and body hair, and deepening of the voice have been reported in women who use DHEA. The anxiety medication alprazolam (Xanax) and the blood pressure medication diltiazem (Norvasc) increase side effects of DHEA. Contrary to some publications, DHEA increases rather than decreases risk of breast and prostate cancer. Use of DHEA can enhance adverse effects of the sports supplements 4-androstenedione, 4-androstenediol, 5-androstenedione, 19-4-norandrostenedione, and 19-15-norandrostenediol. DHEA is banned in the United Kingdom and Canada.

Devil's Claw

Devil's claw relieves joint pain, but only if it is taken in an enteric-coated form that protects its analgesic compounds from being digested in the stomach. Typical dosage is 405–520 milligrams up to 8 times a day. Do not use devil's claw with NSAID pain relievers such as aspirin and Tylenol and avoid it entirely if you have duodenal or gastric ulcers.

Dimethylglycine (DMG)

Dimethylglycine (DMG), not to be confused with tri-methylglycine (also known as betaine), is an amino acid occurring naturally in the body, produced as an intermediate step of the transformation of choline into glycine. There are some indications DMG may be helpful in reducing free-radical stress on the brain in autism and Down syndrome, although no clinical trials have been conducted. There are numerous reports DMG reduces muscle fatigue and enhances oxygen capacity in runners, but the clinical evidence for this claimed benefit is sketchy.

Typical dosage of DMG is 125 milligrams a day, taken with meals. People with a rare hereditary enzyme deficiency may develop a fishy odor when taking DMG supplements. The safety of DMG for pregnant women and nursing mothers has not been established.

Dimethyl Sulfoxide (DMSO)

Dimethyl sulfoxide or **DMSO** is a colorless liquid with a faint scent of sulfur that is rapidly absorbed through the skin. In the United Kingdom, creams made of DMSO and idoxuridine are used to treat shingles. In the United States, DMSO is an FDA-approved treatment for cystitis and a common remedy for joint pain.

DMSO applied to the skin can relieve arthritis pain, although weaker solutions (70 percent) offer greater pain relief than stronger solutions (the more usual 90 percent). With respect to the joints (and only with respect to the joints), DMSO works like a fast-acting vitamin C. In as little as 30 seconds after application, the bloodstream carries DMSO to the joints, where it protects hyaluronic acid from damage by free radicals. Unfortunately, DMSO also can dissolve any toxin on the skin and send it into circulation throughout the body in under 30 seconds. Industrial grade DMSO, the form most commonly sold in flea markets, can contain toxic byproducts of the manufacturing process and should not be applied to the skin. DMSO is not recommended.

An acceptable alternative to DMSO is MSM (methyl-sulfonylmethane). See Methylsulfonylmethane.

DL-Phenylalanine

DL-phenylalanine is a mixture of the amino acids D-phenylalanine and L-phenylalanine, both found in trace amounts in some foods. A German study in the late 1970s found that the amino acids act as a mild antidepressant as effective as the most readily available prescription at that time, imipramine (Tofranil). The L-phenylalanine component of the mixture is converted into the mood-enhancing reward chemicals norepinephrine and dopamine in the brain. DL-phenylalanine may also be helpful in dealing with alcohol problems. Some scientists believe it decreases alcohol craving by increasing the production of the reward chemical enkephalin in the brain.

Typical dosage of DL-phenylalanine is 375–2,250 milligrams daily. People with phenylketonuria must avoid this supplement. Use of supplemental DL-phenylalanine may worsen tardive dyskinesia in schizophrenics and cause high blood pressure in people being treated for depression with MAOIs. It is also not recommended for people taking selegiline (Eldepryl) for Parkinson's disease. The combination can cause elation or giddiness.

Docahexaenoic Acid (DHA)

Docahexaenoic acid (DHA) is an essential component of human cell membranes, especially in the brain and retina. It is necessary for development of the brain and vision in early childhood. Human breast milk contains DHA, but American-made baby formulas do not contain significant amounts of DHA unless they are specifically fortified with this important nutrient.

The most dramatic effects of DHA supplementation are found in the treatment of Zellweger syndrome. Zellweger patients given 100–500 milligrams of DHA a day improve their vision, liver function, social skills, and muscle tone, and normalization of brain tissue sometimes occurs. DHA may also be helpful in treating dyslexia. A scientific study has concluded that boys with better reading and math skills have higher bloodstream concentrations of DHA than boys with poorer reading and math skills. Small-scale clinical studies have confirmed that taking DHA improves athletic skills and night vision in children with dyslexia.

DHA in fish oil is helpful for lowering high triglycerides, especially in diabetes. Supplemental DHA may reduce heavy menstrual periods. DHA may also ameliorate the symptoms of multiple sclerosis. A study published in the *New England Journal of Medicine* suggests that smokers are protected from the development of bronchitis, emphysema, and pneumonia when their diets include DHA from fish oils, coldwater fish, or eggs from chickens that are fed fish meal.

Doses of DHA for high triglycerides range from 1,000–4,000 milligrams daily. DHA occasionally causes belches with a fishy odor, but this effect is minimized if the supplement is taken with meals. Due to increased risk of bleeding, pregnant women should not take more than 1,000 milligrams of DHA daily.

Dolomite

Dolomite was once a popular source of calcium and magnesium. Since contamination with aluminum, arsenic, cadmium, lead, and zinc is common, dolomite is not generally available as a nutritional supplement today.

D-Ribose

D-ribose is a sugar found in the energy molecule ATP and in the nucleic acids that make up RNA in every cell of every living thing on earth. It is very useful in treating exercise-induced muscle pain and stiffness caused by a relatively rare enzyme deficiency, but for most athletes it is more helpful in increasing the growth of "fast-twitch" muscles. A preliminary clinical trial found that the supplement relieves angina in men over 45 who have a history of heart disease.

D-ribose is usually used in very high doses, up to 60 grams per day. It should not be used by diabetics, and, since it increases the production of uric acid, by people who have gout. The safety of D-ribose for pregnant women and nursing women has not been established.

Echinacea

Echinacea is the most commonly used herbal treatment for infection. The best way to take echinacea to stop a cold is as a liquid extract or tincture (alcohol-free versions are available for children and for adults who are sensitive to alcohol), although other forms of echinacea also work. In a study reported in the *European Journal of Clinical Research*, 120 people were given either *Echinacea purpurea* juice (prepared by the German company that makes the American product Echinagard) or a placebo, as soon as they started showing symptoms of a cold. The volunteers took 20 drops of echinacea or the placebo, every 2 hours for 1 day, then 20 drops 3 times

a day for a total of 10 days. Only 40 percent of those taking echinacea developed "real colds," compared to 60 percent of those taking the placebo. Among the volunteers who did develop colds, those taking echinacea started getting better in an average of 4 days compared to an average of 8 days for those who took the placebo.

Other studies of echinacea have found similar results. The benefits of echinacea in treating colds seem to be greatest in people who have low T-cell counts, such as people on chemotherapy or who use corticosteroids for lupus, multiple sclerosis, rheumatoid arthritis, or Sjögren's syndrome, or people with HIV or AIDS. Some people shouldn't use echinacea. Women who are trying to get pregnant should avoid *Echinacea purpurea*. It contains caffeoyl esters that can interfere with the action of hyaluronidase, an enzyme essential to the release of unfertilized eggs into the fallopian tube.

There is laboratory evidence that *Echinacea angustifolia* contains chemicals that deactivate CYP3A4. This liver enzyme breaks down a wide range of medications, including anabolic steroids, the chemotherapy drug methotrexate used in treating cancer and lupus, astemizole (Hismanal) for allergies, nifedipine (Adalat) and captopril (Capoten) for high blood pressure, and sildenafil (Viagra) for impotence, as well as many others. *Echinacea angustifolia* might help maintain levels of these drugs in the bloodstream and make them more effective, or it might also cause them to accumulate to levels at which they cause side effects. Switch to a brand of echinacea that does not contain *Echinacea angustifolia* if you experience unexpected side effects while taking any of these drugs.

Echinacea stimulates immune function, but it also slightly increases production of T cells. These are the immune cells attacked by HIV. When there are more T cells, the virus has more cells to infect. This gives it more opportunities to mutate into a drug-resistant form. The authoritative reference work *The Complete German Commission E Monographs* counsels against the use of echinacea for treating colds by people who have HIV or autoimmune diseases such as multiple sclerosis. Later communications between the senior editor of the *Monographs* and the German Food and Drug Administration revealed that the warning in the reference book was based on theoretical speculation rather than practical experience. Still, as a precaution, people with HIV should only use echinacea for *treating* colds rather than for preventing them.

Eicosapentaenoic Acid (EPA)

Eicosapentaenoic acid (EPA) is a fatty acid found in fish oil. A natural anti-inflammatory, it reduces lung damage in cystic fibrosis and kidney damage in diabetes. (For more information, see Fish Oils.) Doses up to 15 grams a day are well tolerated, although they may cause fishy belches. Hemophiliacs and persons treated with warfarin (Coumadin) after a heart attack should not take EPA because of increased risk of bleeding. Pregnant women and people anticipating surgery should inform their doctors if they are taking EPA.

Elderberry Extracts

Elderberry extracts serve as a preventative and treatment for the flu. Dr. Madeleine Mumcuouglu, a virologist in Israel, discovered that elderberry contains a protein that prevents hemagluttin, the "spikes" of the flu virus, from attaching to cells. This action effectively confines the flu virus and limits the duration of symptoms. Clinical studies at Hebrew University in Jerusalem found that taking elderberry extract reduces the duration of flu symptoms from an average of 6 days to 2–3 days. Elderberry is effective against both influenza A and influenza B.

The best way to use elderberry is as a preventative. Beginning in October and continuing through March, give 1–2 teaspoons of extract daily to children and 2–4 teaspoons of extract daily for adults. There are no known adverse reactions to the use of the herb, although the possibility of an individual allergic reaction can never be discounted. Children may respond best to an elderberry formula made with glycerin or sugar syrup, rather than with alcohol.

Enzyme Therapy

Enzyme therapy restores health by correcting digestive problems that allow allergens and toxins to enter the body through the intestines. The enzymes available from food are greatest in raw plant foods and lowest in cooked meats and fried foods. Devotees of fast food, in particular, can benefit from enzyme supplementation. Certain conditions, including cystic fibrosis, pancreatitis, and intestinal malabsorption, cannot be managed without supplemental digestive enzymes. See **Alphagalactosidase, Bromelain, Cellulase, Chymotrypsin,** **Lactaid, Pancrelipase, Papain, Pepsin, Trypsin, Wobe-Mugos and Wobenzyme.**

Evening Primrose Oil (EPO)

Evening primrose oil (EPO) is, like blackcurrant seed oil, borage oil, and hempseed oil, a rich source of gamma-linolenic acid (GLA). For more information about the benefits of borage oil, see Gamma-Linolenic Acid.

People with inflammatory conditions may use from 300–3,000 milligrams of EPO daily, preferably taken in 4 or 5 doses. Up to 2,000 milligrams daily is helpful in lowering high triglycerides. Generally speaking, EPO does not produce side effects; however, it is important to buy brands including vitamin E as a preservative. Contaminants in EPO can increase the risk of seizures in people who have temporal lobe epilepsy and in schizophrenics treated with chlorpromazine (Thorazine).

Feverfew

Feverfew is an herb used to prevent attacks of migraine and rheumatoid arthritis. Three clinical studies have found that regular use of the herb reduces the frequency and severity of migraine attacks. Results may not be noticeable until the herb has been taken for 4–6 weeks. Clinical trials with women who have rheumatoid arthritis found that taking 70–86 milligrams of feverfew every day for 6 weeks increased grip strength.

The standard dosage of feverfew is 250 micrograms of parthenolide per day. Feverfew can cause stomach irritation. Do not use it with NSAID pain relievers and avoid it if you have ulcers.

Fish Oils

Fish oils are the best natural source of DHA and EPA. The applications of fish oil are numerous and growing. Fish oil has a protective role in asthma. Several studies from Australia suggest that asthmatics who eat fresh cold-water fish several times a week gain relief from wheezing and increased lung capacity. One study found that children who ate fish more than once per week had lower rates of airway hyperresponsiveness than children who ate fish less often. Another study found that consumption of fresh fish, and particularly oily fish, was protective against wheezing. It should be noted that at least one study reports contrary findings: in Japan, where fish is a staple food, eating fish is associated with increased asthma in children, although the difference may be that Japanese children who eat fish more frequently tend to eat salted fish.

Another promising application for fish oil is in treating schizophrenia. Most of the current research focuses on giving fish oil to schizophrenics who take conventional antipsychotic medications. Among schizophrenics treated with clozapine, the most effective dose for relief of symptoms is 2 grams per day—higher doses are not helpful. In a British clinical trial, taking 2 grams of fish oil per day with clozapine resulted in improvement in all psychiatric measures for the severity of the disease. For schizophrenics not treated with antipsychotic medication, a dose of 3 grams a day is not effective. However, a large dosage, 10 grams a day, has helped some schizophrenics who do not respond to other medications.

Fish oil is the newest and most promising natural treatment for bipolar disorder. In 1999, Andrew Stoll, an assistant professor of psychiatry at Harvard Medical School, and his colleagues announced the results of a 4-month double-blind clinical trial involving 30 men and women aged 18–65 with bipolar disorder. Half of the patients were given fish oil, and half of the patients were given an olive oil placebo. Eight patients in the study received no medication other than fish oil or a placebo.

The researchers attempted to measure changes in mood in the different groups. Patients ended their participation in the study and treatment was considered to have failed if the mood symptoms emerged or continued for more than 30 days. Patients were also evaluated on Young Mania Rating Scale, Hamilton Rating Scale for Depression, Clinical Global Impression Scale and Global Assessment Scale ratings, taken before and after treatment.

Overall, 9 of the 14 patients who received fish oil reported relief of mood swings, while only 3 out of 16 patients who received the placebo experienced improvement. Of the 8 patients who received no other medications at all, the 4 patients who received fish oil remained in remission for a significantly longer time than the 4 patients who received the placebo.

The researchers interpret their results as reason to recommend quitting other medications and taking fish oil. Patients who were given only fish oil had not responded to prescription medications offered to them before the study.

Four preliminary studies have found that fish oil plus nutritional supplement drinks greatly reduces weight loss in advanced pancreatic cancer. There is some research confirming that limiting simple sugars and consuming essential fatty acids on a regular basis could be useful in preventing menstrual cramps. Taking fish oil when dieting reduces the risk of developing gallstones.

Appropriate dosage of fish oil varies by indication. For inflammatory conditions such as Crohn's disease, rheumatoid arthritis, scleroderma, and ulcerative colitis, take 3–4 grams daily. To prevent closing of arteries opened by angioplasty or coronary bypass surgery or to lower high triglycerides, take 5 grams daily. Up to 15 grams of fish oil a day causes no side effects other than belching or diarrhea, both of which are minimized by taking fish oil with meals. Do not use cod liver oil as a substitute for fish oil; cod liver oil can contain excessive amounts of vitamin A, causing chapped lips, cracked skin, or headache.

Flaxseed Oil

Flaxseed oil is a rich source of alpha-linolenic acid (ALA), which the body converts into eicosapentaenoic acid (EPA). Studies suggest that flaxseed oil can lower cholesterol (but not triglycerides) and blood pressure and relieve inflammation caused by rheumatoid arthritis. Current research focuses on the use of flaxseed lignans as a means of blocking the carcinogenic effects of estrogen in the breasts, ovaries, and uterus.

Since it takes 10 grams of ALA to make 1 gram of EPA, it is easier to use fish oil or microalgae as a source of essential fatty acids. The easiest way to use flaxseed oil is in salad dressing and in functional foods, such as eggs from hens fed flaxseed. If you prefer to use flaxseed oil as your source of EPA, 3 tablespoons of oil provides 2 grams of essential fatty acids, a mimimum daily dose for controlling inflammation.

Flower Pollen

Flower pollen is, as its name suggests, pollen collected directly from flowering plants. Unlike bee pollen, it contains no insect secretions. A British study found that 13 of 15 men with nonbacterial prostatitis experienced marked to complete relief of symptoms after taking flower pollen extract for 4 weeks. Flower pollen can also relieve symptoms of enlarged prostate.

Typical dosage of flower pollen is 360 milligrams a day, taken in 2 or 3 doses. Allergic reactions to flower pollen are possible, especially if there is an allergy to rye.

Folic Acid

Folic acid is a synthetic B vitamin used interchangeably with 6 chemically similar naturally occurring *folates* found in dark green, leafy vegetables (arugula, beet greens, bok choi, dandelion greens, escarole, kale, mache, mustard greens, radicchio, rapini, spinach, Swiss chard, and turnip greens), asparagus, cauliflower, garbanzo beans, liver, orange juice, and yeast. Folates are poorly absorbed in Crohn's disease, and increased demand for folates in eczema, psoriasis, and sickle cell anemia and during dialysis can cause shortages of the vitamin. Folate deficiencies are associated with a plethora of disease conditions including Alzheimer's disease, birth defects, depression, high homocysteine, and pernicious anemia. Folic acid is used as a supplement because it is absorbed more readily by the body than naturally occurring folates.

The Nurses' Health Study, involving 88,756 women, found a 75 percent reduction in the rate of colorectal cancer among women who take at least 400 micrograms of supplemental folic acid for 15 or more years. One clinical study found that colon cancer patients given a milligram of folic acid (roughly a year's supply) in a single dose had a 50 percent lower rate of recurrences. There are studies that suggest that folic acid prevents cancers of the brain, esophagus, and stomach.

A typical daily dose of folic acid is 400 micrograms, although 1,000 micrograms may offer better protection against cancer. Very large doses of folic acid, in the range of 15 milligrams a day, can cause sleep disturbances and other mental changes, but even these are rare. Taking supplemental folic acid reduces homocysteine levels in diabetics who take metformin (Glucophage) and in arthritis sufferers who take large amounts of aspirin, Tylenol, and other NSAIDs. Men and women who have ulcerative colitis and who take sulfasalazine (Azulfidine) should take supplements containing folic acid to prevent deficiency. Supplemental folic acid also increases the efficacy of fluoxetine (Prozac) for depression and lithium for bipolar disorder. High-dose folic acid may reduce side effects of methotrexate (Methotrex) for rheumatoid arthritis; consult with your physician about the exact dosage. The epilepsy drug phenytoin (Dilantin) depletes folic acid, but high-dosage folic acid supplements interfere with the action of the drug. Consult with your physician before taking folic acid if you are taking drugs for cancer or parasitic infections.

Forskolin

Forskolin is a chemical extract from the leaf of the coleus. Its primary use is in preventing scars from minor burns, cuts, and scrapes. Forskolin stops a chemical signaling system by which inflammatory hormones shut down fibroblasts, the cells that generate the extracellular connective tissue matrix. Keeping fibroblasts at the site of the wound encourages the production of collagen and connective tissues across the region of damaged skin. This action is also helpful in the treatment of eczema.

Forskolin has several other applications. Coleus extracts lower blood pressure while strengthening the heartbeat and lowering the pulse rate. It is likely that taking forskolin can offset some of the symptoms of Lyme disease associated with nerve cell irritation, such as headache, tingling, burning, numbness, stabbing sensations, tremor, unexplained lactation, or severe hangover. And forskolin is used to increase lean body mass and decrease fat mass in athletic training.

A typical dosage of forskolin is 5–10 milligrams 3 times a day (or 50 milligrams of 18 percent forskolin extract 3 times a day). People who have unusually low blood pressure or who have peptic ulcers should not take forskolin. Forskolin also should be used with caution by people who take the asthma medication theophylline (Theo-Dur), since it increases the medication's effects on the lungs.

Fructo-Oligosaccharides (FOS)

Fructo-oligosaccharides, better known as **FOS**, serve as a probiotic nutrient for healthy bacteria in the intestine. The fermentation of FOS by bacteria in the intestine produces butyric acid, which is believed to have significant antitumor acid in colon cancer. FOS seems to bind calcium and magnesium in the intestine, reducing the risk of colon cancer and helping prevent osteoporosis. Through biochemical mechanisms that are poorly understood, FOS lowers blood sugars, cholesterol, and triglycerides.

Dosages of FOS vary from 4–10 grams per day. People who experience gassiness after taking fiber supplements should avoid FOS, as should those with irritable bowel syndrome and those receiving radiation treatment in the colon.

Gamma-Linolenic Acid (GLA)

Gamma-linolenic acid (GLA) is a polyunsaturated fatty acid found in blackcurrant, borage, evening primrose, flaxseed, and hempseed oils. The usefulness of GLA in controlling eczema has been recognized for more than 60 years. It provides relief in a variety of inflammatory conditions, including ulcerative colitis, respiratory distress syndrome, rheumatoid arthritis, and Sjögren's syndrome. GLA is helpful for dialysis patients suffering skin inflammation. The primary drawback to the use of GLA is that it exerts its anti-inflammatory effect by serving as a substrate for hormones that diminish, rather than increase, the activity of the immune system.

Doses of GLA range from 300–3,000 milligrams a day. It may be necessary to experiment with dosages to find the smallest amount needed for relief of symptoms. Bruising and nosebleeds may occur with very high doses. If these are a problem, reduce the dose. The safety of GLA for pregnant women and nursing mothers has not been established. Be sure to inform your physician if you have been taking GLA before any surgery.

Gamma-Tocopherol

Gamma-tocopherol is one of four chemicals collectively referred to as vitamin E. Gamma-tocopherol is an especially potent antioxidant, more effective in preventing the oxidation of LDL cholesterol than the better-known alpha-tocopherol. Recent studies suggest that gamma-tocopherol may be more effective than alpha-tocopherol in preventing the growth of prostate cancer cells, at least under laboratory conditions.

Supplements emphasizing gamma-tocopherol usually contain other forms of vitamin E as well. Typical daily dosage is specified in milligrams rather than in international units (IU); 200 milligrams of gamma-tocopherol is typical. One study suggests that high levels of gamma-tocopherol may increase incidence of arthritis of the knee, especially in African-Americans. People who have bleeding disorders or who take prescription anticoagulants should not take gamma-tocopherol. Some medications for high cholesterol, fungal infections, and stomach ulcers interfere with the absorption of gamma-tocopherol. Taking gamma-tocopherol at the same time as iron supplements reduces the vitamin's antioxidant capacity. The effects of gamma-tocopherol may be enhanced by taking supplemental vitamin C and selenium.

Garlic

More than 300 scientific studies, most of them conducted in Germany, confirm that **garlic** and onions are helpful in lowering blood pressure. If you are concerned about bad breath, consider taking a garlic supplement such as Kwai. Recent research has found that taking 600 milligrams of Kwai garlic extract daily lowered systolic (upper number) blood pressures 8–11 mm/Hg and diastolic (lower number) blood pressures an average of 6 mm/Hg. More is not better—taking more than 600 milligrams of Kwai daily did not lower blood pressures further. Limiting your use of supplemental garlic to this dosage makes drug interactions and side effects extremely unlikely, although increased bleeding and bruising may occur with the concurrent use of garlic and prescription anticoagulants.

Genistein

Genistein is a plant estrogen found in soy, kudzu, and red clover. Taken with other soy flavones, genistein has a number of benefits for women in menopause. Soy products do not offer relief as quickly as hormone replacement, but the body of clinical research considered as a whole indicates that most women will experience relief from hot flashes by taking 100 milligrams of soy isoflavones (genistein + daidzein) daily.

Genistein is found in various formulas containing soy isoflavones. The safety of genistein for pregnant women and nursing mothers has not been established. Men with prostate cancer and women with estrogen receptor-positive cancers of the breast, ovaries, or uterus should only use formula containing genistein if they are recommended and monitored by a physician.

Ginkgo

Ginkgo is the world's most widely used herbal treatment for failing memory. A controversy concerning the use of ginkgo as a memory aid arose in August 2002 through a highly publicized article published in the *Journal of the American Medical Association*. Researchers at Williams College in Williamstown, Massachusetts, tested healthy older adults for changes in learning, memory, attention, concentration, and verbal fluency after taking a dose of 120 milligrams of ginkgo extract per day for 6 weeks. The authors concluded that ginkgo did not help.

In all likelihood, the conclusions of this study were correct. However, the researchers used a dosage of ginkgo much smaller than the 360 milligrams a day used as a memory aid in young adults. In a study published the same year in *Human Psychopharmacology* using a similar design with a higher dosage (180 milligrams per day), researchers observed clinically significant cognitive benefits in healthy individuals. An optimal dosage of ginkgo for benign memory loss is probably 180–240 milligrams per day in most adults.

Never take a whole-leaf preparation of ginkgo. The whole leaf of the herb can contain toxins that can be especially detrimental to Alzheimer's disease patients. Instead, always take ginkgo extract. Do not take ginkgo with high dosages of vitamin E, since the combination can increase the risk of bleeding.

Ginsana

Testing the well-known herbal formula **Ginsana**, scientists at the University of Milan found that taking ginseng every day beginning a month before getting a flu shot and for 3 months thereafter reduces the incidence of both colds and flu by two-thirds. Ginsana increased antibody levels by more than 50 percent and nearly doubled the number of natural killer (NK) cells by the eighth week of the study. There were very few adverse reactions to the herb, primarily insomnia.

Ginseng

Ginseng extracts are widely used as an energy supplement. Taken in moderate doses, they boost energy by encouraging restful sleep. There are a number of studies which indicate that ginseng is effective in treating insomnia in both men and women. A Japanese clinical study involving 12 postmenopausal women suffering emotional disturbance with menopause and 8 postmenopausal women without any symptoms of menopause tested the efficacy of the herb as a treatment for insomnia. The sci-

entists found that the ratio of the stress hormone cortisol to bloodstream concentrations of DHEA was significantly higher in women who suffered insomnia than in women who did not. Taking ginseng for 30 days lowered the cortisol/DHEA ratio in the women who had insomnia (although not to the levels of the women who did not have insomnia) and relieved depression, fatigue, and insomnia.

Since concentrations of ginseng in over-the-counter products vary greatly, follow label instructions. Do not take ginseng if you are also taking estrogen replacement therapy (ERT). Animal studies indicate that the herb stimulates estrogen production by the ovaries, and the combination of ERT and ginseng may be excessive.

Glandulars

Glandulars are dried extracts from beef and pork adrenal glands, brain, ovaries, heart, lung, pancreas, pituitary, prostate, thymus, thyroid, or testes. Adrenal extracts are now used to treat fatigue, but their traditional application was the treatment of morning sickness. Side effects from a single dose may be caused by allergic reactions to beef or pork. Constant use may lead to fluid retention, anxiety, insomnia, or irritability.

Spleen extracts were traditionally used to treat malaria and typhus. Some naturopathic physicians use them today to relieve side effects of chemotherapy.

There is considerable evidence that thymus extracts correct low immune function. Research has shown that the thymus extract Thymomodulin normalizes the ratio of T-helper cells to T-suppressor cells, maintaining a healthy immune response that neither destroys healthy tissue nor allows infectious microorganisms to flourish. This is critical in AIDS and helpful in acute hepatitis, eczema, food allergies, hay fever, and recurrent upper respiratory tract infections.

Some doctors use desiccated thyroid, also called thyroid extract (for example, Armour Thyroid) as an alternative to synthetic thyroid hormones. Dessicated thyroid extract contains 2 biologically active hormones, thyroxine and triiodothyronine, whereas the most commonly prescribed thyroid-hormone preparations contain only thyroxine. One study showed that the combination of the 2 hormones contained in desiccated thyroid is more effective than thyroxine alone, especially in fighting depression and improving mental acuity. This combination is also especially effective for women who have to take thyroid hormone replacement after surgery for thyroid cancer. Dried thyroid products sold in health food stores have had most of the thyroid hormone removed and are not effective for people with hypothyroidism. Intact desiccated thyroid is available only by prescription.

There are no standard dosages for glandular extracts. They are not acceptable substitutes for medically prescribed estrogen or testosterone replacement. Ovary extracts should not be used by women with a history of breast, ovarian, or uterine cancer. Testis extracts should not be used by men with prostate enlargement or prostate cancer.

Glucomannan

Glucomannan is a soluble fiber extracted from the konjac plant. Since the fiber is largely indigestible, it absorbs water and makes the stool bulkier and easier to pass, relieving constipation. Clinical trials have found that glucomannan supplementes are especially helpful in helping children lose weight, and they also function as "fat blockers" in adults.

Dosages of glucomannan range from 1–4 grams a day. Use glucomannan powder or capsules; tablets can cause blockages. Never take glucomannan without water, and avoid taking the supplement just before going to bed. Do not take glucomannan at the same time as supplemental vitamin A, D, E, or K. Since glucomannan interferes with the absorption of sugars as well as fats, diabetics taking glucomannan may have to adjust their medications.

Glucosamine

Glucosamine relieves arthritis as it stimulates the production of glycosaminoglycans, the building blocks of the collagen lining the joints. There are indications that the joints lose their ability to make glucosamine as they age. There is wide agreement that a lack of glucosamine may be one of the most important contributing factors to the development of osteoarthritis.

Three studies confirm that glucosamine gives better long-term pain relief than aspirin or other NSAIDs. Glucosamine has no anti-inflammatory effect and does not affect the central nervous system. Instead, it corrects the underlying problem and thereby relieves pain. One study found glucosamine is more effective than piroxi-cam (Feldene) or even a combination of glucosamine and piroxicam. Glucosamine relieves symptoms of pain at rest, during exercise, on standing, and during stretching and passive movement.

The usual dosage of glucosamine is three 500-milligram capsules a day. Probably the only drawback to using glucosamine is that people who are overweight may not respond as well to it. There are some indications that overweight people need a higher dose. Overweight people who have diabetes, however, should not take a higher than recommended dose, since glucosamine increases the need for insulin. Anyone who has diabetes and takes glucosamine should monitor blood sugars carefully to make sure they do not need additional insulin or diabetes medication.

Glutathione

Glutathione is a potent antioxidant found in all plants and animals. It is essential to the processes that make proteins following the code recorded in DNA. It is involved in uncounted numbers of metabolic processes and is critical to the regulation of the life cycle of cells.

Glutathione occurs in food, but with adequate supplies of vitamin C and selenium, the body synthesizes most of the glutathione it needs. Deficiencies of glutathione are both the cause and effect of cancer, HIV, and some parasitic diseases. Supplemental glutathione is used in only a few, relatively unusual applications: prevention of wasting in AIDS, improvement of male fertility when the main problem is the motility of sperm, protection of lung tissue in pulmonary fibrosis and cystic fibrosis, and protection against hearing loss after exposure to loud noises. Glutathione is used in an injected form to protect against side effects of chemotherapy with cis-platin (Platinol).

Glutathione is best used under supervision of a holistically oriented physician. Typical dosage is 600 milligrams per day. The safety of glutathione for pregnant women and nursing mothers has not been established.

Glycerol

Glycerol is an alcohol used to make water "wetter." Water combined with glycerol is more hydrating to the body than water alone. For this reason, glycerol is included in some sports supplements. At least one clinical trial has found that long-distance cyclists who take glycerol before working out have greater endurance and achieve higher speeds at a lower heart rate. Glycerol supplements have also been used to prevent hearing loss in childhood meningitis. Intravenous glycerol has been used to minimize neurological damage after a stroke.

Some athletes use 2–4 tablespoons of glycerol in water, orange juice, or a sports drink. Type 2 diabetics should avoid glycerol, since it can cause extremely high blood sugars. Elderly persons sometimes experience amnesia, confusion, dizziness, or headache after taking glycerol. Glycerol must be stored separately from chemical agents; the combination of glycerol and chromium trioxide, potassium chlorate, or potassium permanganate (none of which occur in the body) can produce a violent explosion.

Glycine

Glycine is a nonessential amino acid that the body synthesizes and uses to make proteins, DNA and RNA, hemoglobin, glutathione, creatine, bile salts, and glucose, among many other substances. The primary use of glycine supplements is in treating spasticity. A small-scale clinical trial found that supplemental glycine prevented leg spasms in multiple sclerosis. High doses of glycine may reduce symptoms of schizophrenia. Some makers of sports supplements claim that glycine has the same potential as creatine; at least one study has found that supplementing with both glycine and arginine increased muscle performance in weight lifting by delaying muscle fatigue.

A typical dosage of glycine is 4 grams a day, although up to 90 grams a day have been used with no ill effects in clinical trials of glycine as a treatment for schizophrenia. Since the body breaks down glycine into ammonia, no one with advanced liver disease should take the supplement. Mental confusion would result. Supplemental glycine will increase the sedative effects of prescription drugs used to control spasticity. The safety of glycine for pregnant women and nursing mothers has not been established.

Glycitein

Glycitein is a plant estrogen found in soy and kudzu, in the same class as daidzein and genistein. It is believed to relieve hot flashes, vaginal dryness, loss of libido, and excessive growth of facial hair in menopause, although its use as a separate supplement has not been investigated.

Grape Seed Proanthocyanidins

Grape seed proanthocyanidins are a subset of the oligomeric proanthocyanidins, a group of plant chemicals found in pine bark, chocolate, apples, blueberries, cranberries, peanuts, and almonds. These chemicals are potent antioxidants, anticarcinogens, and antiatherosclerotics, at least in laboratory studies. Most commercial formulations of oligomeric proanthocyanidins are primarily composed of grape seed extracts.

Grape seed proanthocyanidins stop bruising by protecting the collagen that stabilizes the lining of blood vessels. They reduce internal bleeding and nosebleeds due to loss of clotting factors in cirrhosis and hepatitis C. They improve circulation in the retina and may retard macular degeneration. They are also a standard supplement for varicose veins. In laboratory tests, they have protected brain and heart tissue from the toxic effects of reoxygenation as circulation is restored after a heart attack or a stroke. Laboratory studies have found that grape seed proanthocyanidins stop proliferation of breast, lung, and stomach cancer cells.

Typical dosages of grape seed proanthocyanidins are 50–100 milligrams per day. The safety of grape seed proanthocyanidins for pregnant women and nursing mothers has not been established.

Green Tea Catechins

Green tea catechins make up nearly 30 percent of the dry weight of green tea. They are used in the management of a number of health conditions. Green tea catechins comprise a group of 4 major plant chemicals in tea, epicatechin (EC), (-)-epigallocatechin (EGC), (-)-epicatechin gallate (ECG), and (-)-epigallocatechin gallate (EGCG). Some supplements emphasize 1 of these 4 chemicals.

Laboratory tests have found that EGCG stops the growth of bladder, breast, colon, leukemia, liver, lung, ovarian, pancreatic, skin, and stomach cancers. Epidemiological studies in Japan have found that women who consume more than 10 cups of green tea daily have exceptionally low rates of breast cancer. Supplementation with a *combination* of EGCG and caffeine increases the metabolic rate, the rate at which the body burns calories at rest, by an average of 4 percent in men. Green tea supplements are also widely used in oral hygiene.

Green tea catechins are used in daily doses of 125–250 milligrams per day. If you choose to drink green tea, at least 10 cups a day are needed for significant protective benefits. Adding milk or sugar to green tea does not affect absorption of green tea catechins. Use beverage green tea rather than green tea catechins if you take anticoagulant drugs such as warfarin (Coumadin) or pentoxifylline (Trental).

Hawthorn

Hawthorn is both extraordinarily safe and extraordinarily effective in treating angina. This herb contains a variety of flavonoids. Some increase blood flow through the coronary arteries. Some increase left ventricular pressure, making each heart beat stronger. Some accelerate the heart rate—and some decelerate it. But the most important property of hawthorn is its ability to protect the heart from the effects of oxygen deprivation.

Heart cells, like many other tissues, are able to adapt to oxygen deprivation. They shift their energy production from pathways requiring the use of oxygen to pathways requiring the use of fatty acids. However, when their oxygen supply is restored, as it is when an angina attack ends, they are sometimes damaged and sometimes destroyed.

At the end of an angina attack, the neutrophils of the immune system release a compound known as human neutrophil elastase (HNE), allowing the arteries to stretch back to a more normal size. The process of relaxing the artery, however, releases massive quantities of free radicals that disrupt the cholesterol coats of heart cells and interfere with the action of L-carnitine. At least one of the flavonoid compounds in hawthorn counteracts HNE.

Hawthorn has several other beneficial effects. Animal studies have found that hawthorn stimulates the liver to use LDL cholesterol to make bile salts, cholesterol salts that are flushed out of the liver into the stool. Other studies with laboratory animals have found that the hawthorn compound monoacetyl-vitexin rhamnoside relaxes the linings of the arteries, permitting greater blood flow, through a complicated chemical process. And at least one animal study suggests that hawthorn can prevent irreversible tissue damage during heart attack.

Hawthorn is taken in any 1 of the following forms, 3 times a day:

- Solid extract (standardized to contain 1.8 percent vitexin-4'-rhamnoside): 100–250 milligrams

- Leaf and flowers as a tea: 1–2 teaspoons (3–5 grams)

- Fluid extract: 1-2 milliliters ($\frac{1}{2}$–1 teaspoon)

There are very few precautions for the use of hawthorn. It is almost completely nontoxic. Like many other natural treatments for angina, however, it can cause diarrhea the first few days you take it.

Hempseed Oil

Hempseed oil is a rich source alpha-linolenic acid (ALA) and one of a very few plant oils containing significant amounts of gamma-linolenic acid (GLA). United States laws written in 1937 protected the use of sterile hempseed and hempseed oils, but the current legal status of hempseed in the United States is in question. Use of hempseed oils does not always but can occasionally cause positive tests for THC.

Hesperidin

Hesperidin is a plant chemical found in the membrane and peel of lemons and oranges. It is also found in the pulp sometimes included with orange juice. Together with the plant chemical diosmin, hesperidin is used to treat problems with weak blood vessels such as bruising, nosebleeds, varicose veins, and hemorrhoids. Hesperidin and diosmin have been clinically tested in France as a treatment for varicose veins.

The easiest way to get hesperidin is to drink orange juice with pulp. In the United States, hesperidin and diosmin are marketed as citrus bioflavonoids. To get an adequate dose of hesperidin for treating weak veins, you should take at least 500 milligrams and preferably 2,000 milligrams of citrus bioflavonoids daily. Pregnant women, however, should limit their intake of citrus bioflavonoids to 500 milligrams per day.

Scientists are unsure of the interaction between citrus bioflavonoids and vitamin C. Citrus bioflavonoids and vitamin C were once thought to be synergistic, but some recent studies suggest that diosmin and hesperidin may actually interfere with the body's ability to absorb this vitamin. To be sure vitamin C requirements are met, take at least a small dose (500 milligrams) of vitamin C when taking citrus bioflavonoids.

If you are taking tamoxifen (Nolvadex) for breast cancer, you should avoid both citrus bioflavonoids and citrus juices. Although citrus bioflavonoids have been used to treat hemorrhoids during pregnancy, most authorities recommend that pregnant women and nursing mothers take no more than 20 milligrams of diosmin and hesperidin daily.

Hexacosanol

Hexacosanol is a naturally occurring alcohol found in wheat bran oil and rice bran oil. Current research focuses on using hexacosanol to protect brain tissue in exicotox-in-related diseases such as amyotrophic lateral sclerosis (Lou Gehrig's disease) and Huntington's disease. Studies with animals have found that it may be useful in repairing nerve damage in sciatica. There are also indications it may retard the physiological processes that turn excess dietary sugars into fat

Homeopathy

Homeopathy is often misunderstood as a method of treating illnesses with vanishingly small quantities of biologically derived substances. While homeopathy does involve the use of homeopathics, greatly diluted quantities of compounds thought to cause "suffering" similar to the patient's disease, the practice of homeopathy is more comprehensive. It requires identifying patterns, or "delusions," in the whole person that resolve as suffering is relieved. Since homeopathy treats persons rather than diseases, the choice of remedies in terms of "suffering" does not exactly match illnesses as they are defined in conventional medicine. Nonetheless, homeopathic remedies, even without the benefit of understanding "delusions" and the "suffering" that must be relieved to eliminate them, offer scientifically verifiable cures as understood in mainstream medicine.

Patterns of disease are best identified with the help of a trained homeopathic physician, but homeopathic remedies can produce results even when they are self-administered. Usually it is best to start with a single dose of the lowest strength (6C, 6X, or 12C) of the remedy matching the symptoms to be treated, and then wait for a response. If there is an improvement in symptoms, let the remedy continue to work until there is no more improvement,

then take another dose. If there is no improvement, try a different potency (30X or 30C). Sometimes homeopathic medicines work for a few minutes, sometimes they work for an entire day before another dose is needed.

Some disease patterns than can help you choose homeopathic remedies follow:

- **Aconitum napellus** is used to treat illnesses when symptoms come on suddenly, especially after a stressful or traumatic experience.

- **Actae racemosa**, also known as **Cimicifuga**, treats diseases causing pain or prominent symptoms in the neck.

- **Apis mellifica** is a remedy for skin irritations that resemble bee stings, such as pink and puffy blisters that itch a lot and hurt when touched. If ice helps relieve some pain, apis mellifica should give complete relief. If the skin does not feel better when ice is applied to it, apis mellifica may not help.

- **Argentum nitricum** is a remedy for "stage fright" or anticipatory stress causing high blood pressure and other symptoms. It also relieves bloating, flatulence, diarrhea, dizziness, headache, and racing pulse. Those who benefit most from this remedy are people who have strong cravings for sugar and salt.

- **Aurum metallicum** is a treatment for conditions associated with ongoing stress, especially in people who relieve stress with alcohol. An important indication for this preparation is symptoms becoming worse at night.

- **Belladonna** is the homeopathic remedy for symptoms caused by overdoses of the herb belladonna, redness in the face and neck, dilated pupils, throbbing headache, sensation of racing pulse so strong it can be felt not just in the heart but throughout the body. Another indication for this treatment is cold hands and feet.

- **Bryonia** is used for pain that is relieved by pressure and aggravated by warmth.

- **Calcarea carbonica** relieves symptoms in people who tend to get cold and clammy. They are easily tired by exertion, but can also have a racing pulse when lying down. People who benefit from calcarea carbonic tend to like sweets and to have problems with weight control.

- **Colcynthis** is recommended when symptoms are worsened by personal loss or emotional upset. Homeopathic physicians often recommend this remedy when pain is relieved by leaning forward or bending over.

• **Dulcamara** is used when symptoms accompany a cold, particularly during cold, rainy weather.

• **Euphrasia** is indicated in any condition causing red eyes and frequent sneezing with a clear discharge. It is helpful when symptoms interrupt sleep and when the person feels better after eating.

• **Glonoinum** is the homeopathic remedy for "being out of it," in addition to a pounding heartbeat, especially in hot weather or after drinking alcohol or taking drugs.

• **Ipecacuanha** is a homeopathic preparation of ipecac, the medication used to treat certain kinds of poisoning by inducing vomiting. In homeopathic doses, ipecac stops vomiting as well as diarrhea accompanying it.

• **Lachesis** is used when symptoms "come too soon." It treats logorrhea, a tendency to spew out words while experiencing constriction in the chest. Symptoms treated by this remedy are typically worse after sleeping.

• **Mercurius solubilis** treats diseases of people who wake up sweaty. It also treats bad breath, swollen lymph nodes, and earache.

• **Natrum muriaticum** treats conditions of people who keep their emotions inside. A craving for salt and symptoms that get worse as the day progresses are other indications for this remedy.

• **Nux vomica** relieves stress disorders in people who take offense easily, allowing them to "spit up" the emotions that are bothering them. Constipation and hemorrhoids are also common in the personality type treated by this remedy, as are sugar cravings and a tendency to drink a lot of coffee.

• **Plumbum**, the homeopathic remedy made from minute amounts of lead, treats the symptoms that lead causes, including degeneration of the nerves, hardening of the arteries, tics, twitches, and paralysis. Homeopaths also recommend plumbum for people who develop high blood pressure while "living in the fast lane," and then become fatigued or depressed when symptoms develop.

• **Rhus toxicodendron** treats conditions that cause stiffness and pain that is worst in the morning. It is used to treat diseases at the first sign of an outbreak.

• **Sanguinaria** treats illnesses occurring with "red" symptoms: red cheeks, red neck, heartburn, reddened skin from allergies, burning pains of the skin, sunburn, and migraine. Symptoms are usually worse on the right side of the body.

Human Growth Hormone (HGH)

Synthetic **human growth hormone** (**HGH**) is used in medicine to treat short stature in children with chronic kidney disease or Turner's syndrome, and also to treat AIDS-related wasting. It has been used experimentally to treat cardiomyopathy and Crohn's disease.

The body's production of HGH declines with age. When researchers injected HGH into men aged 61–81, they found significant improvements in muscle mass, muscle tone, skin thickness, and bone density, as well as loss of fat. However, side effects also occurred, including joint pain, higher blood sugars, swollen ankles, carpal tunnel syndrome, headaches, and breast enlargement.

The problem with HGH supplements taken orally is that they are too poorly absorbed to be of reliable benefit. Some athletes take arginine, lysine, and ornithine to stimulate the body's production of HGH, and there is some evidence that the net result is increased muscle mass after exercise. Amino acids are of no benefit in stimulating HGH without exercise. Pregnant women, children, and teenagers should not take HGH of any kind without close medical supervision, as unintended effects may occur.

Huperzine A

Huperzine A is a neuroactive enzyme extracted from club moss. This Chinese plant is also a source of huperzine B, which has much less activity in the nerve tissue. Numerous laboratory studies confirm that huperzine A prevents the breakdown of the neurotransmitter acetylcholine, conserving the chemical and improving transmission of electrical signals in the brain. In late 2002, the Chinese Academy of Medical Sciences published a report of a clinical study involving 202 Alzheimer's patients. Researchers found that supplementation with 400 micrograms of huperzine A daily (twice the dose used in other studies) reduced behavioral problems and enabled patients to participate more fully in daily activities. There were no reports of increased rates of falls and other accidents as patients gained increased mobility, but 3 patients experienced swollen ankles or insomnia for a short time. Other tests have found huperzine A as helpful in managing Alzheimer's disease as the prescription medication tacrine, but without the risk of potential liver damage. Unlike tacrine, huperzine A dosages can be increased to meet the patient's needs.

The new recommended dosage of huperzine A is 400 micrograms daily, used under medical supervision. Cramping, drooling, diarrhea, sweating, blurred vision, and dizziness have been known to occur with the use of this supplement. Using huperzine with choline, CDP-choline, phosphatidylcholine, or other prescription medications for Alzheimer's disease may amplify both benefits and side effects.

Hydrolized Collagen

Hydrolized collagen is extracted from cow or pig bone. Theoretically, the amino acids of hydrolized collagen contribute to the synthesis of new cartilage in arthritic joints, although this assertion has not been proven by clinical study. Hydrolized collagen is sometimes included in supplements also containing glucosamine and chondroitin.

Typical daily dosage of hydrolyzed collagen is 10 grams a day. Be sure to use only products certified as carrying no detectable infections. Spine and skull bones of cows may carry prions for bovine spongiform encephalopathy (BSE), better know as mad cow disease.

Hydroxycitric Acid (HCA)

Laboratory experiments with animals (but not yet clinical studies with people) have shown that **hydroxycitric acid (HCA)**, extracted from the *Garcinia cambogia* fruit, interferes with enzymes that convert stored carbohydrates into fat. Since HCA acts on carbohydrates, it naturally is of limited value in low-carbohydrate diets. A study published in the *Journal of the American Medical Association* in which HCA was used as an adjunct to high-protein, reduced-calorie diets found no benefit. The real value of HCA is for people who *aren't* dieting, but are pursuing normal diets containing carbohydrates.

Typical dosage of HCA is 1,500 milligrams per day. Products labeled as not containing lactones are preferable. The safety of HCA for pregnant women and nursing mothers has not been established. People with Alzheimer's disease should avoid HCA, since it may interfere with the brain's production of acetylcholine.

Hydroxyethylrutosides (HR)

Hydroxyethylrutosides (HR) are a mixture of chemically modified forms of rutin, a popular remedy for varicose veins in Latin America. They are also useful for treating Ménière's disease. A clinical study found that using hydroxyethylrutosides for 3 months reduced hearing loss at all frequencies and also reduced attacks of vertigo.

Typical dosages are 500–2,000 milligrams per day. Hydroxyethylrutosides cause no side effects in themselves, although most authorities advise that they should not be used during pregnancy. The drawback to using hydroxyethylrutosides is that they are incompatible with many antibiotics, including:

- ciprofloxacin (Cipro, Baycip, Cetraxal, Ciflox, Cifran, Ciplox, Cyprobay, Quintor)

- enoxacin (Penetrex)

- gatifloxacin (Tequin)

- gemifloxacin (a relatively new drug)

- grepafloxacin (Raxar)

- levofloxacin (Levaquin)

- lomefloxacin (Maxaquin)

- moxifloxacin (Avelox)

- norfloxacin (Noroxin Amicrobin, Anquin, Baccidal, Barazan, Biofloxin, Floxenor, Fulgram, Janacin, Lexinor, Norofin, Norxacin, Orixacin, Oroflo, Urinox, Zoroxin)

- ofloxacin (Floxin)

- sparfloxacin (Zagam)

- temafloxacin (Omniflox) and

- trovafloxacin (Trovan)

Indole-3-Carbinol

Indole-3-carbinol is a medically active chemical found in bok choi, broccoli and especially broccoli sprouts, Brussels sprouts, cabbage, cauliflower, and kale. This plant chemical is particularly important for women, since it reduces the carcinogenic activity of estrogen in breast tissue. Laboratory experiments with animals have found that it blocks some of the carcinogenic effects of tobacco smoke. Research to date neither proves nor disproves the assertion that indole-3-carbinol increases muscle growth during weight training.

When indole-3-carbinol is taken by itself, typical daily dosages range from 200–800 milligrams a day. This supplement is also included in combination products for use by athletes. Do not take indole-3-carbinol within 2 hours of taking an antacid or any product to stop heartburn.

Inosine

Inosine is an energy storage compound in both plants and animals. In Europe, inosine is widely used to treat cardiomyopathy and irregular heartbeats, and in the United States it is an orphan drug for the treatment of some forms of encephalitis and for spinal cord injury. Inosine is also marketed as a sports supplement. Use of inosine may prolong the time it takes distance runners to become exhausted, but it does not increase power and it may increase lactic acid, causing more of a "burn" and increasing the time it takes to recover.

Athletes typically use 5–10 grams of inosine a day. People who have any history of gout or kidney disease should not use this supplement. The safety of inosine for pregnant women or nursing mothers has not been established.

Inositol Hexaphosphate (IP6)

Inositol hexaphosphate (IP6) is an energy source for germinating seeds that is found in substantial amounts in whole grains, beans, nuts, and seeds. In the human body, it is theoretically possible that supplemental IP6 influences several disease processes by binding excess calcium, iron, magnesium, and zinc. Laboratory tests have found that IP6 slows the growth of breast, colon, liver, and soft tissue (rhabdomyosarcoma) cells. Clinical trials indicate that IP6 slows the formation of calcium oxalate kidney stones.

Typical dosage of IP6 is 8–10 grams per day. The safety of IP6 for pregnant women and nursing mothers has not been established.

Inositol Nicotinate

Inositol nicotinate, also known as **inositol hexaniacinate** and **inositol hexanicotinate**, is a slow-release form of niacin used by physicians in Europe and Japan to treat Buerger's disease, gangrene, intermittent claudication, leg ulcers (necrobiosis lipoidica), peripheral vascular disease, Raynaud's phenomenon, and restless legs syndrome. Inositol nicotinate treats these conditions by dilating arteries and increasing the flow of oxygen. The advantage of inositol nicotinate over niacin is that at recommended dosages it does not cause redness in the face.

Dosages of inositol nicotinate range from 500–4,000 milligrams a day. People with liver problems should not use this supplement, nor should anyone who has unstable angina, diabetes, gastritis, gout, or peptic ulcer disease. Overdoses of inositol nicotinate may cause itching, dizziness, and flushing in the face (although these symptoms are not as severe as those caused by equivalent doses of niacin). If you take inositol nicotinate for any vascular condition and your doctor advises you to switch to fast-acting forms of niacin after you develop a liver problem, be sure to use very small doses until you know you will not have flushing and headaches. The safety of inositol nicotinate for pregnant women and nursing mothers has not been established.

Insulin-like Growth Factor 1 (IGF-1)

Insulin-like growth factor 1 (IGF-1) is a chemical messenger for human growth factor. It appears to preserve nerve cell function and to promote nerve growth, and is being investigated as a treatment for amyotrophic lateral sclerosis (Lou Gehrig's disease). Since IGF-1 also stimulates growth of muscle tissue, it is being tested as a treatment for muscle wasting in AIDS, and as a treatment for children who have suffered injury to the growth plates in bones.

Naturally high levels of IGF-1 are found in the heart muscle of elite athletes. For this reason, IGF-1 is marketed as a muscle-building aid, but it cannot be recommended for this purpose. IGF-1 taken by mouth is poorly absorbed by the body, so it must be injected or used as a nose spray. In addition to stimulating the growth of nerve and muscle, IGF-1 stimulates the multiplication of cancer cells, especially prostate cancer.

Inulins

Inulins, not to be confused with insulins, are complex sugars found in plants, notably in Jerusalem artichokes.

At least one clinical study found that the use of a nutritional supplement containing inulin and chromium picolinate, capsicum, and L-phenylalanine increased loss of body fat during short-term diet and exercise programs. Inulins are also used to encourage the activity of beneficial bacteria in the intestine. They enhance the absorption of calcium and magnesium from foods, and may help reduce the risk of colon cancer.

Typical dosages of inulins are 4–10 grams a day. Taking more 30 grams in any single day may cause cramping, bloating, gas, and diarrhea. Taking inulins at the same time as calcium and magnesium supplements increases mineral absorption.

Iodine

Iodine is a trace element vital to the function of the thyroid gland. Since the introduction of iodized salt, iodine deficiency is a relatively rare condition, at least in the United States. People who choose not to use iodized salt can get adequate amounts of iodine from seaweeds.

Supplemental iodine is used as an expectorant in asthma, bronchitis, and emphysema. It is also sometimes helpful in fibrocystic breast disease and rapidly reduces leg irritation in sarcoidosis. Potassium iodide reduces the thyroid's uptake of radioactive iodine from fallout, but does not protect against other radioactive substances.

Typical dosages of potassium iodide are 300–1,000 micrograms daily. Pregnant women, however, should not use more than 175 micrograms a day, and nursing mothers should not use more than 200 micrograms a day, to avoid thyroid suppression in the infant. Excessive iodine can cause goiter. Children with cystic fibrosis are unusually susceptible to this effect.

Never take iodine if you take lithium (Lithobid). The combination can result in hypothyroidism. Taking high doses of iodine can counteract the anticoagulant effect of warfarin (Coumadin).

Ipriflavone

Ipriflavone is a synthetic derivative of the soy flavonoid genistein. This supplement ameliorates degenerative diseases of the bone by blocking a chemical signal that attracts the recycling cells, known as osteoclasts, to the bone. It is significantly helpful in Paget's disease. In one study in Italy, all the Paget's disease patients taking 1,200 milligrams of ipriflavone daily experienced a reduction in bone pain within 3 months. This supplement is also used to treat osteoporosis in women and bone loss after prostate cancer treatment in men.

Effective dosages of ipriflavone range from 600–1,200 milligrams a day, preferably in at least 3 doses.

Women who take the estrogen-sequestering drug leuprolide (Lupron) for uterine fibroids are at risk for bone loss. Taking supplemental ipriflavone can reduce the risk of bone loss and also keep LDL cholesterol levels during treatment with this drug.

Ipriflavone also enhances the effects of bisphosphonates, boron, calcitonin, calcium, estrogen, fluoride, and vitamins D and K in preventing bone loss. It counteracts and should not be taken with nifedipine for blood pressure, theophylline for asthma, or tolbutamide for diabetes.

Iron

Iron is an essential element involved in the production of hemoglobin, the oxygen-transport protein in the blood. Iron deficiency is associated with anemia and Plummer-Vinson syndrome, an abnormal growth in the esophagus. Iron supplementation has the interesting application of reducing breath-holding spells in small children. Iron excess, however, is associated with the potentially fatal disease hemachromatosis.

For specific dosing information, see ANEMIA, IRON-DEFICIENCY in Part One. Never take iron supplements unless a blood test has confirmed iron deficiency. Iron supplements are only effective for iron-deficiency anemia, not pernicious anemia or anemia induced by chemotherapy. Supplemental iron can accelerate the growth of bacterial infections, parasites, and yeast. Iron supplements should be used with extreme caution by anyone with alcoholic cirrhosis of the liver, chronic liver failure, or pancreatic insufficiency.

Taking antacids, acid pump inhibitors (lansoprazole, omeprazole, pantoprazole, or rabeprazole for gastroesophageal reflux disease), H2 blockers (cimetidine, famotidine, nizatidine, or ranitidine for heartburn), beta-carotene, calcium supplements, inositol hexaphosphate, magnesium supplements, N-acetyl cysteine, vanadium, or zinc reduces absorption of iron. Carbonyl iron, in particular, cannot be absorbed if it is taken at the same time as antacids. Taking iron at the same time as biphosphonates for osteoporosis and other bone conditions (alendronate, etidronate, risedronate), L-dopa, thyroid hormone, most antibiotics including Cipro and tetracycline, or copper reduces absorption of the drug or supplement. Iron supplements will create free radicals and reduce the effectiveness of tocotrienols and vitamin E. Eating meat increases the absorption of iron, as does drinking fruit juices or taking vitamin C. Eating raw green beans, seeds, nuts, soy, matzo, rhubarb, spinach, or sweet potatoes or drinking tea will reduce absorption of iron.

Kava

Kava plays the same role in treating anxiety in Polynesian culture that alcohol plays in European and North American culture. In Polynesian society, numerous health benefits are attributed to this herb. Recent research even suggests that people who use kava are less likely to develop cancer.

Kavalactones bind to the same receptor sites in the brain as benzodiazepam tranquilizers such as Librium and Valium. They also modify the brain's responses to GABA, dopamine, histamine, and endorphins, as well as to the stress hormone norepinephrine. They release tension in the skeletal muscles, and, in laboratory experiments with animals, prevent epileptic seizures.

One clinical test found that, over a period of 6 months, kava offered about the same degree of relief as using the benzodiazepam tranquilizers bromazepam (Xanax) and oxazepam (Ox-Pam). A small clinical study at a gynecological hospital in Germany found that 1 month's treatment with kava was effective in relieving anxiety associated with menopause. A later clinical study at the University of Jena in Germany involved 101 outpatients suffering from agoraphobia, specific phobias, adjustment disorders, and/or generalized anxiety disorder. The participants in the study were given kava or a placebo for 25 weeks. The researchers concluded that kava was as effective as either tricyclic antidepressants, such as amitriptyline (Elavil, Limbitriol), imipramine (Tofranil), or doxepin (Adapin, Sinequan), or benzodiazepine tranquilizers (such as Librium, Valium, or Xanax) with "none" of the side effects associated with the commonly prescribed drugs. More recent research has found that kava is especially useful in controlling racing pulse associated with anxiety. Researchers at Duke University believe that controlling racing pulse may reduce the risk of heart attack associated with generalized anxiety disorder.

Do not take kava in addition to prescription tranquilizers, especially Xanax. Taking kava with antipsychotic medications can cause abnormal movements, called a dystonic reaction. Kava reduces the effectiveness of L-dopa in the treatment of Parkinson's disease. See the inset "Kava Ban" on page 77 in Part One.

Kombucha

Kombucha is a mixture of several bacteria and yeasts. Laboratory studies with animals indicate that it is generally nontoxic and that it protects against stress and protects the liver from toxic exposure. However, extensive claims that kombucha cures human diseases are not substantiated. People with HIV, in particular, should avoid kombucha teas, to avoid yeast infections.

Lactaid

Lactaid is an over-the-counter product that may reduce belching caused by eating or drinking dairy foods and other products containing milk sugars, including convenience foods and medications. It treats an enzyme deficiency for milk sugar rather than an allergy to milk. To determine if Lactaid may be helpful to you, eat a normal breakfast and include a large, 12-ounce glass of milk of any kind. Over the next 6 hours, keep track of any discomfort you may have (if you experience any kind of severe reaction, consult a physician). The next day, prepare an identical breakfast with another 12-ounce glass of milk. Swallow a Lactaid tablet with your first sip of milk. If your symptoms are not as bad on the second day, Lactaid may be beneficial for you.

Lactoferrin

Lactoferrin is a protein found in whey. Its primary role in nature is as a source of iron for the suckling infant, but it also has antibacterial, antifungal, anti-inflammatory, antioxidant, and antiviral properties. Laboratory tests have found that lactoferrin stops the growth of *E. coli, Proteus, Staphylococcus,* herpesvirus, hepatitis C virus, cytomegalovirus, and HIV. Its primary use in natural medicine is in controlling fungal and yeast infections.

Lactoferrin from cow's milk is termed bovine lactoferrin or bLF. Typical dosage is 250 milligrams per day. The safety of lactoferrin supplements for pregnant women and nursing mothers has not been established.

Lactulose

Lactulose is a synthetic sugar that can be digested by bacteria but not by the human intestine. By feeding beneficial bacteria, lactulose helps protect against salmonella and a number of other intestinal pathogens. The increased mass of bacteria softens stool, and makes lactulose useful in treating chronic constipation. Beneficial bacteria keep ammonia from entering the hepatic portal vein, and make lactulose useful in treating hepatic encephalopathy in late-stage cirrhosis of the liver. Laboratory studies indicate that lactulose fed bacteria increase the concentrations of calcium and magnesium in the colon, probably reducing risk of colon cancer. Clinical study has found that supplemental lactulose reduces recurrence of colon polyps.

In the United States, lactulose is available by prescription only. Doses higher than 10 grams a day are likely to cause bloating, cramping, diarrhea, and gas, but 40–120 grams a day of lactulose may be needed for hepatic encephalopathy. Taking probiotics such as *Bifidobacterium longum* with lactulose makes it more effective.

Larch Arabinogalactan

Larch arabinogalactan is a complex, indigestible sugar extracted from larch wood. Clinical studies have found that using larch arabinogalactan in combination with *Echinacea angustifolia* and *Echinacea purpurea* increases the immune system's production of complement (proteins that carry out immune reactions) for fighting infection.

Typical dosage of larch arabinogalactan is 1–3 grams a day. Doses of up to 10 grams a day are well tolerated, but taking more than 30 grams a day will cause bloating, cramping, diarrhea, and flatulence. Avoid this supplement if you are on a galactose-restricted diet. The safety of larch arabinogalactan for pregnant women and nursing mothers has not been established.

L-Arginine

L-arginine is not an essential amino acid inasmuch as it can be synthesized by the human body, but it is vital to good health. L-arginine is the chemical precursor to nitric oxide (NO), which regulates the contraction and dilation of blood vessels. NO regulates blood pressure, helps the blood vessels compensate for excess cholesterol, activates the immune system's natural killer cells, and makes erection possible in men.

The potential indications for supplemental L-arginine are numerous: angina, cystitis, diabetic kidney disease, chronic renal failure, HIV, low sperm counts, migraine, nasal congestion, sepsis, and trauma. L-arginine is frequently recommended for erectile dysfunction, and may increase the effectiveness of sildenafil (Viagra).

L-arginine is also very useful in lowering blood pressure. Survey studies have found that women who consume more protein (about 25 percent of their total calories), and therefore more L-arginine, are significantly less likely to develop coronary heart disease. High doses of supplemental L-arginine can produce dramatic increases in arterial blood flow. A clinical trial involving participants with high cholesterol levels found that taking 21 grams of L-arginine a day for 4 weeks increased blood flow by 3.9 percent. Another clinical trial involving participants with confirmed coronary disease found that taking 21 grams of L-arginine a day for 4 weeks increased arterial blood flow by 4.7 percent. These percentages sound like small improvements, but they correspond to a 6–8 point drop in blood pressure without side effects, comparable to a low dose of most prescription blood pressure medications.

Appropriate doses of L-arginine vary by disease condition. Clinical studies of L-arginine for erectile dysfunction have used relatively small doses, no more than 3,000 milligrams per day; using more than 5,000 milligrams of L-arginine may make erectile dysfunction worse. On the other hand, 10,000–20,000 milligrams a day are needed for male infertility. Most other indications benefit from 8,000–10,000 milligrams per day. Taking more than 30,000 milligrams a day can cause cramping, diarrhea, and nausea. Sports supplements that include L-arginine usually emphasize branched-chain amino acids.

Pregnant women and nursing mothers must avoid L-arginine, since it interfere with the metabolism of growth hormone in the child's body. L-arginine also should be avoided by people who have herpes infections, shingles, or cold sores. Supplemental L-arginine increases the effectiveness of nitrates for angina, yohimbe and sildenafil (Viagra) for erectile dysfunction, and ibuprofen for pain relief (although it will not help if the drugs are inappropriately prescribed). It may help normalize urination in people who take cyclosporine to prevent transplant rejection.

L-Aspartate

L-aspartate is an amino acid found in all life forms, and in the dietary sweetener aspartame (Nutrasweet). Supplemental L-asparate has been used with ipriflavone in successful treatment of osteoporosis occurring as a complication of Sjögren's disease. L-aspartate is used as a sports supplement, but it has only been found to increase muscle endurance when taken on a long-term basis with L-asparagine and L-carnitine.

Dosages of L-aspartate begin at 600 milligrams per day. Up to 2,000 milligrams will have no side effects. The safety of supplemental L-aspartate has not been established for pregnant women or nursing mothers.

L-Carnitine

L-carnitine is an amino acid derivative that helps muscle cells release energy from fatty acids. It is found in most meats, avocados, and tempeh. Most of the body's supply of L-carnitine is made in the kidneys and the liver. Stresses on these organs (such as diabetes or chronic alcohol abuse) diminish the supply of L-carnitine for the heart. When the heart has an inadequate oxygen supply, it quickly uses up its supply of L-carnitine and is then less able to produce energy.

Supplemental L-carnitine increases the heart's energy supply. Administering massive doses of L-carnitine, 2,000 milligrams for every 100 pounds (45 kilograms) of body weight, after a heart attack has been shown to reduce heart damage. A Japanese study found that taking 900 milligrams of L-carnitine daily allowed heart patients to last 2.4 minutes longer in their stress tests. An Italian study in which men with angina were given 1,000 milligrams of L-carnitine daily found they not only could last longer under stress, but also work harder, as measured by a bicycle ergometer.

L-carnitine increases endurance in athletes, but its effects are only measurable when it is taken at the same time as caffeine.

Doses of L-carnitine range from 500–2,000 milligrams per day. The safety of supplemental L-carnitine for pregnant women and nursing mothers has not been established. People who have seizure disorders should only take L-carnitine after checking with their physicians. People who have adrenal insufficiency, AIDS, hypopituitarism, or liver damage caused by treatment with valproic acid (Depakote) may become deficient in L-car-

nitine and should consult a nutritionally oriented health practitioner about appropriate dosages for L-carnitine replacement.

L-Cysteine

L-cysteine, not to be confused with N-acetyl cysteine (NAC), is a sulfur-containing amino acid found in all life forms but is especially abundant in garlic. The presence of L-cysteine explains the therapeutic effect of garlic in treating bacterial infections. Supplemental L-cysteine is sometimes used to treat stomach inflammation occurring in persons who use large quantities of aspirin and similar pain relievers, but most supplements today contain the chemical derivative of this amino acid, NAC.

Typical dosages of L-cysteine are 500–1,500 milligrams daily. To prevent formation of kidney stones, always drink at least 6–8 glasses of water a day when taking this supplement. Taking supplemental L-cysteine can produce a false positive result when using test strips to measure urinary ketones in diabetes. The safety of supplemental L-cysteine for pregnant women and nursing mothers has not been established.

L-Glutamine

L-glutamine is the most abundant amino acid in the human body. Although L-glutamine is synthesized in the skeletal muscles, the body's ability to make this amino acid cannot keep up with the demands of muscle injury or stress. Additional L-glutamine is often required from plant or animal protein foods or from nutritional supplements.

Several studies have found that L-glutamine helps prevent infection after surgery to the intestine. Colon cancer patients have shorter stays in the hospital if they receive supplemental L-glutamine after surgery. Very-low-birth-weight babies are less likely to acquire infections if they receive glutamine supplementation during the first few days of life.

There is evidence that taking L-glutamine can help prevent upper respiratory infections in athletes who "overtrain." There is no clearly defined benefit of taking L-glutamine for overall athletic performance, but laboratory studies with animals suggest that the supplement can increase blood flow to the heart during stress.

For most people, doses of L-glutamine up to 21 grams a day cause no ill effects. Some persons with bipolar disorder have been known to enter the manic phase of their illness after taking 2–4 grams of L-glutamine a day, and the effect stopped when the supplement was withdrawn. L-glutamine enhances nutrient absorption in short bowel syndrome. It helps prevent "leaky gut" and food sensitivities occurring during regular use of the pain reliever indomethacin. There is at least one report of L-glutamine reversing oral and sinus inflammation caused by chemotherapy with methotrexate, and there is another report that taking 30 grams of L-glutamine a day prevents join and muscle pain after chemotherapy with paclitaxel.

L-Histidine

L-histidine is an amino acid the body uses to make histamine, the initiator of allergic inflammation. There are some reports that people with rheumatoid arthritis have unusually low bloodstream concentrations of L-histidine, and one study found that taking 6 grams of supplemental histidine a day improved symptoms, especially in those taking prescription gold, steroids, or aspirin for rheumatoid arthritis on a regular basis. Supplemental histidine increases the absorption of zinc.

Take up to 6,000 milligrams a day. A minimum dosage for therapeutic benefit is 1,000 milligrams a day. Do not take L-histidine if you have peptic ulcer disease, as the supplement might increase the production of irritant histamine in the stomach. Avoid supplements containing vitamin B_6 or L-histidine if you take goldenseal, since they can interfere with goldenseal's antibacterial action.

Lithium

Lithium is a trace element in the diet. It is best known as a treatment for bipolar disorder. Interestingly, El Paso, Texas, where the municipal water supply has a content of lithium, has a very low rate of bipolar disorder. Since serious intoxication regularly occurs after even a slight overdose of this element, its use as a nutritional supplement is not recommended.

Lithium Gamma-Linolenic Acid (Li-GLA)

Lithium gamma-linolenic acid (Li-GLA) is a lithium salt of the fatty acid GLA, which is manufactured in this form to increase its absorption into the bloodstream. Labora-tory studies report that Li-GLA inhibits the growth of pancreatic cancer cells, and a preliminary trial has found that supplemental Li-GLA extends life in people who have pancreatic cancer.

No standard dosage of Li-GLA has been established. If bruising or nosebleeds occur when taking this supplement, it should be immediately discontinued.

Liver Supplements

Dessicated **liver supplements** are prepared by freeze-drying raw beef liver, retaining fat and cholesterol. It is used as a source of heme-iron, which the body absorbs almost as easily as mineral iron.

There are no typical doses of liver supplements. Anyone who frequently receives blood transfusions should avoid the use of dessicated liver and other iron supplements, as should people with hemochromatosis and thalassemia. The safety of dessicated liver supplements for pregnant women, nursing mothers, and children has not been established.

L-Lysine

L-lysine is an essential amino acid found in meat, poultry, milk, and wheat germ. Eating foods rich in the amino acid lysine and avoiding foods rich in the amino acid arginine is of proven value in controlling herpes infections. The presence of arginine has long been thought to "trigger" the virus to replicate itself. Lysine has a chemical structure that is similar to that of arginine. It competes with and blocks arginine from entering the nerve tissues that harbor the herpesvirus between outbreaks. Lysine more recently has been found to be essential to "coding" the virus so that it is recognized and destroyed by antibodies.

In a study conducted in the mid-1980s, herpes patients were given lysine in a large dosage (3,000 milligrams per day), and chocolate, gelatin, and nuts were restricted. After 6 months, herpes outbreaks were 25 percent less frequent among patients treated with lysine than among patients in the placebo group. Apparently a high dosage is necessary for successful treatment. A clinical test using a lower dosage of lysine (1,200 milligrams) failed to show that lysine supplementation helps control herpes outbreaks.

The maximum daily dosage of L-lysine is 15,000

milligrams a day. Since supplemental lysine is extracted from milk casein, persons with milk allergies or casein sensitivity should choose L-lysine supplements with care. Supplemental L-lysine is not recommended for persons with chronic kidney or liver disease. Pregnant women should only use L-lysine if they eat a strictly vegetarian diet.

L-Methionine

L-methionine is the amino acid the body uses to make s-adenosyl-L-methionine, better known as SAM-e. The primary use of supplemental L-methionine is to prevent hearing loss during treatment with the antibiotic gentamycin. It is also used to help repair liver damage after overdoses with acetaminophen (Tylenol) or methotrexate.

A typical dosage of L-methionine is 250 milligrams a day. Taking high doses of L-methionine can deplete folic acid and elevate homocysteine levels, contributing to cardiovascular disease. High doses of L-methionine also cause excretion of calcium.

There is some evidence that various kinds of cancer tumors feed on L-methionine, and that the supplement is particularly detrimental in stomach cancer. Schizophrenics and persons with advanced kidney or liver disease must avoid this supplement.

L-Ornithine

L-ornithine is a nonprotein amino acid the body uses to make L-arginine. A clinical trial in France found that supplemental L-ornithine improves several measures of quality of life in elderly persons recovering from serious illnesses, and the supplement is also used to prevent muscle wasting caused by AIDS or cancer.

Typical dosage of L-ornithine is 500 milligrams taken on an empty stomach before bedtime. If ornithine alpha-ketoglutarate (which lowers blood sugars as part of the process of stimulating the growth of muscle) is part of the supplementation plan, it is better to use a formula that prevents hypoglycemia, such as Glucerna. Bodybuilders should use L-ornithine *in combination* with L-arginine to promote muscle growth; taking more than 10 grams of either supplement a day can cause bloating, diarrhea, and gas. The only study that found that supplementation with L-ornithine stimulated production of human growth hormone used a dosage of 13 grams a day, causing numerous digestive upsets.

L-Phenylalanine

L-phenylalanine is an essential amino acid used by the human body to make various proteins. Some studies have found it to be helpful in treating unipolar depression (bipolar disorder without the manic phase). The primary application of supplemental L-phenylalanine, however, is the treatment of vitiligo.

The longest-running clinical trial of L-phenylalanine for the treatment of vitiligo found that about 85 percent of patients regain pigment to at least 25 percent of vitiligo-affected skin after taking the supplement for 6 months. About 60 percent of all patients who take L-phenylalanine experience repigmentation of 75 percent of affected skin after taking the supplement for 6 months. Eight-five percent of patients taking the supplement for six *years* experienced 100 percent restoration of skin color to the face, although complete restoration of skin color to the hands and trunk is relatively rare. Researchers have found that more is not better when it comes to using L-phenylalanine for skin problems; doubling the dosage had no effect on rates of cure.

Typical dosages of L-phenylalanine range from 500–1,500 milligrams per day. This supplement absolutely must be avoided by persons with phenylketonuria (PKU). Supplemental L-phenylalanine can cause elation and giddiness in Parkinson's disease patients taking selegiline (Eldepryl). It should not be combined with drugs for depression or schizophrenia. The safety of L-phenylalanine supplements for pregnant women and nursing mothers has not been established.

L-Theanine

L-theanine is an amino acid found in green tea. Laboratory studies with animals suggest that it might be used to greatly increase the efficacy and reduce the side effects of doxorubicin (Adriamycin) in the treatment of leukemia and ovarian cancer. A clinical study in Japan found that L-theanine reduces anxiety as objectively measured by an electroencephalograph (EEG).

A dosage of 200 milligrams a day is optimal for reducing anxiety. The safety of L-theanine for pregnant women and nursing mothers has not been established.

L-Tyrosine

L-tyrosine is an amino acid used by the brain to make

the neurotransmitters dopamine and norepinephrine, both of which are associated with lifting depression and elevating mood. Preliminary clinical studies have found that supplemental L-tyrosine increases resistance to stress, and one small-scale study found limited benefit in the prevention of narcolepsy. The primary research application of supplementation L-tyrosine is for improving intellectual performance in phenylketonuria (PKU).

All applications of L-tyrosine are experimental, and dosages are best determined in consultation with a healthcare professional knowledgeable about nutrition. L-tyrosine should not be taken by anyone who has melanoma, and it should be used with caution by people who have high blood pressure. If you have high blood pressure, be sure to take blood pressure readings daily for the first 2 weeks you take supplemental L-tyrosine. The antidepressants pargyline HCl and tranylcypromine sulfate may cause high blood pressure when taken with L-tyrosine.

Lutein and Zeaxanthin

Lutein and zeaxanthin are yellowish pigments closely related to beta-carotene. Lutein is found in carrots, corn, greens, potatoes, tomatoes, and most fruits. Zeaxanthin is abundant in corn, fruit, paprika, and spinach. Both compounds are strong antioxidants. Along with 3 other antioxidants, vitamins A, C, and E, they are found in relatively high concentrations in the retina. Lutein and zeaxanthin give the macula its characteristic yellow color, lutein tending to accumulate around the edges of the eye, and zeaxanthin accumulating in the center of the eye.

A dosage of 5–15 milligrams of supplemental lutein and zeaxanthin, taken with vitamins C and E (see MACULAR DEGENERATION in Part One) affords protection against cataracts and macular degeneration. The higher dosage is desirable when the diet contains relatively few red or yellow vegetables. Cholesterol-lowering medications and mineral oil interfere with absorption of lutein and zeaxanthin, as does supplemental beta-carotene. Dietary oils and medium-chain triglycerides increase the absorption of these supplements.

Lycopene

Lycopene is a red pigment found in tomatoes, watermelon, pink grapefruit, pink guava, and papaya. Like lutein and zeaxanthin, it is closely related to beta-carotene. This antioxidant is associated with a 30–40 percent reduction in prostate cancer, although its effects are greatest in men with the very highest consumption of tomato products and seem to be greater in preventing the spread of prostate cancer rather than cancers in the prostate itself. Lycopene both prevents and treats advanced forms of the disease.

In laboratory tests, lycopene offered better protection against carcinogenic mutations than vitamin E, but mixtures of lycopene and vitamin E were more effective than either supplement alone. The combination of lycopene and vitamin E shifts a biochemical pathway involving n-3 fatty acids to reduce the production of inflammatory hormones that the prostate cancer tumor needs in order to "burn out an escape route" to the rest of the body. The combination activates enzymes that cause prostate cancer cells to enter a normal lifecycle, rather than a self-perpetuating cycle of runaway growth.

Cooked tomatoes are a better source of lycopene than raw tomatoes. Lycopene is absorbed better when tomatoes are cooked with olive oil.

A typical dosage of supplemental lycopene is 5 milligrams per day. Up to 15 milligrams is appropriate if tomatoes and other plant sources of lycopene are not included in the diet. Cholesterol-lowering medications and mineral oil interfere with absorption of lycopene, as does supplemental beta-carotene. Dietary oils and medium-chain triglycerides increase the absorption of this supplement.

Magnesium

Magnesium is an essential mineral involved in more than 300 physiological processes in the human body. The applications of magnesium in promoting human health are also numerous. Magnesium may be helpful for children who have tics and twitches due to ADD, ADHD, or Tourette's syndrome. Some researchers believe that magnesium deficiencies cause the alcohol withdrawal symptom known as delirium tremens, a terrifying combination of uncontrollable shaking and hallucinations. Magnesium deficiency is likely to be the major reason heavy drinkers are a high risk for heart disease.

Intravenous magnesium sulfate is part of standard treatment for severe asthma in the emergency room, and often begins to relieve symptoms as soon as it is administered, although it is preferable to take magnesium before emergencies arise. A large British study of dietary magnesium intake and asthma symptoms in 2,633 people found that asthmatics who had a greater dietary intake of magnesium had a significantly greater lung capacity and significantly less airway hyperreactivity. Taking magnesium for just a few weeks will not reduce the need for inhalers, because the body pools magnesium very slowly.

Magnesium deficiency plays a major role in spasms of the coronary arteries, the source of chest pain in Prinzmetal's variant angina. A series of studies have found that magnesium and vitamin B$_6$ *used together* are of considerable benefit in treating autism, considerably more than either supplement used by itself.

Magnesium supplementation reduces anxiety. A double-blind study involving 80 healthy male volunteers given a multivitamin and multimineral supplement including calcium, magnesium, and zinc for 28 days found that treatment reduced anxiety and perception of stress.

Various studies and anecdotal reports support the use of trace amounts of magnesium, boron, silicon, strontium, and B vitamins in the prevention and treatment of fractures.

These are only a few of the more than 100 health conditions that can be treated with supplemental magnesium. Dosages of supplemental magnesium range from 100 to more than 1,000 milligrams per day, but the use of magnesium for any application requiring more than 250 milligrams per day in children under the age of 9 or more than 750 milligrams per day in adults should be medically monitored.

Magnesium is the principle element in milk of magnesia, and magnesium overdoses usually cause diarrhea. Extreme overdoses can cause dehydration and irregular heartbeat.

Bisphosphonate drugs for osteoporosis, osteomalacia, or Paget's disease should not be taken as magnesium, and magnesium supplements should not be taken at the same time as supplemental inositol hexaphosphate, iron, manganese, phosphate, or calcium, despite the fact that calcium and magnesium are frequently included in the same tablet. Taking more than 2,000 milligrams of calcium supplements a day can decrease the absorption of magnesium. Magnesium supplements interfere with absorption of tetracycline and quinolone antibiotics such as:

- ciprofloxacin (Cipro, Baycip, Cetraxal, Ciflox, Cifran, Ciplox, Cyprobay, Quintor)
- enoxacin (Penetrex)
- gatifloxacin (Tequin)
- gemifloxacin (a relatively new drug)
- grepafloxacin (Raxar)
- levofloxacin (Levaquin)
- lomefloxacin (Maxaquin)
- moxifloxacin (Avelox)
- norfloxacin (Noroxin, Amicrobin, Anquin, Baccidal, Barazan, Biofloxin, Floxenor, Fulgram, Janacin, Lexinor, Norofin, Norxacin, Orixacin, Oroflox, Urinox, Zoroxin)
- ofloxacin (Floxin)
- sparfloxacin (Zagam)
- temafloxacin (Omniflox) and
- trovafloxacin (Trovan)

Maitake-D Polysaccharides

Maitake-D polysaccharides are used as an immunostimulant in the treatment of liver and lung cancers and leukemia. A series of case studies in Japan found that maitake-D helped 23 out of a total 36 cancer patients treated with it. The most notable effect of treatment with maitake is improvement of prothrombin activation, making additional clotting factors for the blood. Maitake-D is also immunostimulant; for 9 patients for whom measurements were recorded, maitake-D treatment increased interleukin-2 production by 29 percent and increased CD4+ (T-cell) counts by 42 percent. In the Japanese study, there was 1 complete remission, and some patients previously classified as stage III (a tumor more than 4 centimeters in diameter, not metastasized to another organ) were classified as stage I (tumor no more than 2 centimeters in diameter) after maitake-D treatment.

Effective dosages of maitake-D range from 4,000–10,000 milligrams daily. No side effects have been recorded in the medical literature.

Malic Acid

Malic acid is found in abundance in apples but is also produced by the human body. Supplementation with a combination of malic acid and magnesium called Super Malic has been found in studies at the University of Texas at San Antonio to reduce the severity of pain and tenderness in fibromyalgia.

The fibromyalgia studies used 1,200–2,400 milligrams of malic acid daily combined with 300–600 milligrams of magnesium daily. No side effects from the use of malic acid have been reported, but its safety for pregnant women and nursing mothers has not been established.

Manganese

Manganese is an essential trace mineral. It is an important cofactor in the body's production of glycosaminoglycans, the proteins made from glucosamine, and it is essential for the production of antioxidant enzymes active in the heart and nerves. The richest dietary sources of manganese are dark green, leafy vegetables, whole grains, nuts, and tea. Vegetarians tend to have higher manganese levels than people who eat meat.

Researchers have found that manganese complements calcium in the treatment of PMS. Taking calcium without taking manganese will not control premenstrual pain and mood swings, although supplemental calcium alone is enough to reduce fluid retention. Manganese along with calcium, copper, and zinc slows bone loss in osteoporosis in women. Manganese ascorbate, in combination with glucosamine and chondroitin, has been shown in clinical trials to reduce knee pain caused by arthritis.

Typical dosages of supplemental manganese range from 2–5 milligrams daily. Persons with chronic liver disease should avoid manganese supplements; they may experience Parkinson's-like symptoms when taking the supplement. Antacids, laxatives and tetracycline reduce the absorption of supplemental manganese, as do calcium supplements and all kinds of iron supplements except desiccated liver.

Medium-Chain Triglycerides (MCTs)

Medium-chain triglycerides (MCTs) are fatty acids found in coconut and palm oils. Supplementation with MCTs causes the body to use fat rather than glycogen during prolonged exercise. This keeps bloodstream concentrations of sugars from falling during races. While race times measured in tests on treadmills are not lowered by use of MCTs, the athlete's ability to maintain

mental focus in an actual athletic event may be improved.

MCTs have also been used with success in the treatment of drug-resistant epilepsy in children, and to relieve nutritional deficiencies caused by chronic diarrhea in AIDS and colon cancer. Interestingly, there are a number of scientific studies that suggest that these fats can be used in weight *loss* programs, because they induce a feeling of satiety after consuming a relatively small amount of fat and they increase the burning of fat. A study of women in a weight-loss program at McGill University in Montreal found that the effects of MCTs on the rate of weight loss are measurable after they have been taken for about 2 weeks.

A typical dosage of MCTs for athletic training or weight loss is 1–3 tablespoons (15–45 grams) per day, the lower dosage used in dieting. Taking more than 5 tablespoons (80 grams) a day can cause abdominal cramping and gas. People with chronic liver disease should not take MCTs, since they can cause accumulation of free fatty acids and glycerol in the bloodstream if they are not processed by the liver. Diabetics should avoid MCTs because they reduce the response of blood sugars to insulin. Use of MCTs in cancer, epilepsy, and AIDS should be supervised by a physician.

Melatonin

Melatonin is the hormone the body uses to regulate its biological clock. Produced in the pineal gland in the brain during darkness, melatonin helps the brain produce moods and behaviors appropriate for times of day and times of year.

Melatonin is especially useful in treating insomnia in adults over 50. A study at the Massachusetts Institute of Technology (MIT) found dosages of melatonin from 0.1–3 grams all improved sleep in insomniacs, although they had no effect on people who did not have insomnia. Melatonin has its greatest effect on the third and fourth hours of sleep. The MIT researchers found that the most effective dose was 0.3 grams. A 0.1-gram dose improved sleep but did not bring melatonin levels to normal. A 3-gram dose also improved sleep but could cause shakes and chills.

Dutch researchers have tested melatonin in the treatment of insomnia in children aged 6–12. They found that a relatively high (5 milligram) dose for a week helped children fall asleep an average of a half-hour earlier and sleep for as much as 1 hour longer each night. The only side effect noted was mild headache in 2 of the 33 children in the study, and only 1 of the 33 children in the study was not helped by the supplement. The researchers noted that 1 child developed a mild seizure disorder during the trial, but they did not believe that melatonin caused the condition.

Melatonin has been investigated as a treatment for autism. A recent study at the San Gerardo Hospital in Milan found that none of the autistic children studied had a normal day-night sleep rhythm. A study published in Japan found that restoring normal sleep patterns with melatonin greatly reduced "excitability," although it had no effect on compulsive behaviors or "obstinacy." In older children, giving the melatonin as late as possible (for instance, at 11 P.M. rather than at 9 P.M.) may prolong morning sleep and reduce sleep disruptions.

Melatonin also has been clinically tested for treating jet lag. A 1986 study of 17 travelers flying from San Francisco to London (8 time zones away) found that the 8 subjects who took 5 milligrams of melatonin experienced essentially no symptoms while the 9 travelers given a placebo experienced noteworthy symptoms. Most people sleep well with melatonin, and wake up the next morning with few symptoms of jet lag, although most will have some fatigue from the flight itself. More recently, the U.S. Army conducted studies in the use of melatonin in preventing jet lag in aviation personnel in rapid deployments overseas, and confirmed that melatonin greatly reduces sleep disturbance and increases proficiency in task performance. The Army study used a relatively high dosage of melatonin, 10 milligrams. At least 10 other studies report similar results.

With melatonin and other drugs for reestablishing body rhythms, timing is critical. The pineal gland produces melatonin at night. Taking melatonin is a signal to the pineal gland that it is night; taking melatonin during the day can induce artificial jet lag. Early clinical studies rejected melatonin as a sleep aid, noting that users were less alert, more sleepy, and had more sluggish reaction times because test subjects were given the supplement during the day.

Typical doses of melatonin range up to 5 milligrams a day. Melatonin should be taken only in the hour before going to bed. Generally speaking, it is best not to use melatonin for more than 2 weeks at a time. Melatonin can accumulate in body fat to be released unpredictably. Always let your physician know you are being treated with melatonin if you seek other medications, especially for insomnia.

High doses of melatonin can inhibit ovulation and decreases fertility in women, particularly in women who take progesterone. Melatonin should not be taken with kava, valerian, or 5-HTP, since the combination can cause severe drowsiness the next morning. People who have taken the antidepressant drugs fluoxetine (Prozac) and fluvoxamine (Luvox) in the last 6 weeks should not take melatonin, since these drugs decrease the clearance of melatonin from the bloodstream and increase daytime drowsiness. People who take benzodiazepine tranquilizers, such as Librium, Valium, or Xanax, should also avoid melatonin to avoid excessive daytime sedation.

Methylsulfonylmethane (MSM)

Methylsulfonylmethane (MSM) is a byproduct of dimethyl sulfoxide (DMSO) as it is metabolized by the body. MSM is also found in alfalfa sprouts, corn, most fruits, tomatoes, coffee, tea, and milk. MSM is used to treat arthritic pain, and unlike DMSO, is almost completely nontoxic. Most naturopaths recommend 1,000–2,000 milligrams of MSM daily to prevent arthritis pain and 3,000–5,000 milligrams of MSM daily to treat arthritis pain.

Molybdenum

Molybdenum is an essential trace mineral that the body uses to form molybdenum cofactor or Moco. This cofactor assists enzymes that break down DNA from food and from recycled cells. Deficiencies of molybdenum increase the risk of stomach cancer, since the enzyme that enables the stomach to process potentially carcinogenic nitrosamines from grilled and cured meats depends on Moco.

Molybdenum supplements are taken to avoid molybdenum deficiency. Typical dosages range up to 250 micrograms per day, but 75 micrograms a day is sufficient.

Avoid overdosing molybdenum. In one case, a man taking 300–800 micrograms of molybdenum a day for 18 days experienced visual and auditory hallucinations and a series of seizures. Chelation therapy to remove molybdenum from his body corrected the symptoms, although he experienced major depression and a learning disability for a year after the molybdenum was discontinued. Molybdenum surplus more commonly causes a condition very similar to gout. It is also important to avoid overdoses of molybdenum in phenylketonuria (PKU) and retinitis pigmentosa.

Avoid taking molybdenum supplements after eating garlic. Molybdenum is essential to the process of sulfoxidation, the metabolic step in which the sulfur found in foods such as garlic is metabolized. Molybdenum activates the enzyme sulfite oxidase. Bad breath is a more common problem in countries in which the diet contains high amounts of molybdenum.

Myo-Inositol

Myo-inositol is a form of inositol hexanicotinate found in food. Beginning to appear in some nutritional supplement mixtures, myo-inositol has been used in small-scale clinical trials as a successful treatment for agoraphobia, bipolar disorder, treatment-resistant obsessive-compulsive disorder, and panic attacks.

Since available nutritional supplements typically supply 12 milligrams of myo-inositol per dose and the clinical trials used 12,000 milligrams per day, therapeutic use of myo-inositol is not yet practical unless formulas are specially prepared by a compounding pharmacist. There are reports that myo-inositol can aggravate symptoms of ADD and ADHD in children. Persons with bipolar disorder should not use this supplement without the supervision of a physician, as it potentially could trigger manic episodes. Myo-inositol stimulates uterine contractions and must be avoided during pregnancy. The safety of myo-inositol for nursing mothers has not been established.

N-Acetyl Cysteine (NAC)

N-acetyl cysteine (NAC) is both an over-the-counter nutritional supplement and a prescription drug for treating overdose of acetaminophen (Tylenol) and poisoning with the mushroom *Amanita phalloides*. (Infants who may have been given toxic overdoses of acetaminophen and anyone who may have eaten a poisonous mushroom should receive immediate medical care.) NAC is a form of the amino acid L-cysteine that is more rapidly absorbed throughout the digestive tract and more easily distributed throughout the body.

NAC reacts with the sulfur atoms critical to forming a "glue" in mucus. Regular use of NAC is beneficial in conditions of respiratory congestion, including bronchi-

tis, black lung, asbestosis, cystic fibrosis, and emphysema. There are some indications that NAC may stop the progression of adult-onset diabetes, lowering blood sugar levels and protecting the insulin-producing beta cells of the pancreas from the toxic effects of high blood sugars. Taken with vitamins C and E, NAC seems to enhance recovery from nonmalignant forms of skin cancer such actinic keratosis and basal cell carcinoma.

NAC will reverse tolerance of nitroglycerin in people who use nitroglycerin to control angina, and it is important to note that it will also increase side effects of nitroglycerin, such as headache. People who take carbamazepine (Carbatrol) for bipolar disorder or seizures should not take NAC, since the combination lowers carbamazepine levels in the bloodstream. Some authorities counsel avoidance of NAC by people who have leukemia. Smokers should not use NAC on a long-term basis (see COUGH, SMOKER'S in Part One). Cysteine is a component of kidney stones, but drinking 8 glasses of water a day when taking NAC eliminates the risk of this side effect.

Niacin

Niacin is a B vitamin sometimes referred to as vitamin B_3 and also known as nicotinic acid. Physicians typically recommend niacin as a second line of treatment for lowering cholesterol after they have placed the patient on a statin drug such as atorvastatin (Lipitor), lovastatin (Mevacor), pravastatin (Pravachol), or simvastatin (Zocor), but niacin can be used to lower cholesterol with or without other medications. The problem with using niacin as a primary treatment for high cholesterol is that doses exceeding 1,000 milligrams can cause high homocysteine levels. Niacin complements the cholesterol-lowering effects of red yeast rice, but overdosing the 2 supplements can, in rare cases, cause muscle damage.

The key to using niacin is moderation. Unless you are under medical supervision, limit your intake of supplemental niacin to 100 milligrams per day, and be sure also to take at least 400 micrograms of folic acid daily to keep homocysteine levels down. Never take niacin within 30 minutes of drinking hot beverages or alcohol. The combination can cause noticeable redness in the face.

Your physician may approve use of up to 2,000 milligrams of extended-release niacin or 3,000 milligrams of immediate-release niacin daily. Immediate-release niacin is more likely to cause facial flushing, although taking an aspirin or Tylenol just before taking the niacin supplement will minimize this effect. You should not take niacin at the same time as prescription drugs for lowering cholesterol, as they may interfere with the absorption of niacin.

People who have rosacea or chronic liver disease should not take supplemental niacin. Dosages of up to 500 milligrams a day are not likely to interact with prescription drugs, but medically prescribed dosages of 1,000 milligrams a day and up may interfere with the action of almost all prescription medications for diabetes, aggravate the side effects of calcium channel blockers, such as amlopidine (Norvasc) for high blood pressure, and increase the side effects of nitroglycerin and other nitrates used for angina. Taking niacin while wearing a nicotine patch may cause an especially severe flushing reaction.

Nicotinamide

Nicotinamide is a B vitamin that has the same effects on high cholesterol as niacin. Nicotinamide, however, has very different side effects. Unlike niacin, nicotinamide does not cause flushing and does not raise blood sugars. In fact, nicotinamide is being investigated as a means of extending the "honeymoon" period in which newly diagnosed type 1 diabetics do not need regular injections of insulin. There are also studies that suggest that nicotinamide might be used as a diabetes drug by type 2 diabetics who are not overweight.

Recommended dosages of nicotinamide range from 20–100 milligrams a day. Nicotinamide is tolerated by people who have liver disease, although enormous overdoses, more than 10,000 milligrams a day, may cause liver injury. People who take carbamazepine (Tegretol) may find that taking nicotinamide increases both benefits and side effects of this prescription medication.

Nicotinamide Adenine Dinculeotide (NADH)

Nicotinamide adenine dinucleotide (NADH) is synthesized by the body to be used in energy production inside every living cell. Supplemental NADH has been shown to increase the production of dopamine in the brain in Parkinson's patients, but researchers have not yet proven or disproven that it improves symptoms of the disease.

NADH should be taken in an enteric-coated form. Typical dosages are 5–10 milligrams a day. This supplement can sometimes cause mild stomach upset. The safety of NADH for pregnant women and nursing mothers has not been established.

Nucleic Acids

Nucleic acids occur in every living cell and are provided by all kinds of food. Dietary nucleotides provide DNA and RNA as a nutritional supplement. Studies with pre-term infants at the University of South Florida have found that dietary nucleotides increase blood flow to the intestine, enhancing the absorption of other nutrients. Doctors in Spain report that adding dietary nucleotides to infant formula decreases the incidence of infectious diarrhea. In older children and adults, dietary nucleotides have been used to help restore immune function after bowel injury or bowel surgery and prolonged infections complicated by malnutrition.

Typical dosages of DNA and RNA supplements range from 500–1,500 milligrams daily. The safety of nucleic acid supplements for pregnant women and nursing mothers has not been established.

Oat Bran

Oat bran (oat beta-d-glucans) is a popular supplement for lowering cholesterol. Finnish studies have found that pure oat bran is more effective than oatmeal and oat muffins by virtue of its better dispersal in the intestine. Typical dosages of oat bran range from 3,000–6,000 milligrams per day. The product is safe for pregnant women, nursing mothers, and children and does not interfere with the action of prescription medications, although overdosing causes flatulence.

Octacosanol

Octacosanol is an alcohol found in sugar cane, the waxy skins of fruits and vegetables, beeswax, and wheat germ oil. Most of the research concerning this supplement has focused on its use to counteract some effects of simulated weightlessness on rats hung by their tails in laboratory centrifuges. Not surprisingly, clinical trials with humans showed that use of supplemental octacosanol improved grip strength and balance.

Dosages of octacosanol for athletes range from 1–8

grams a day, taken with food. People who have Parkinson's disease should not take this supplement, because it may interfere with the action of L-dopa. The safety of octacosanol for pregnant women and nursing mothers has not been established.

Ornithine Alpha-Ketoglutarate (OKG)

Ornithine alpha-ketoglutarate or **OKG** is a synthetic amino acid. It increases the body's production of both growth hormone and insulin. OKG's primary use is in treating muscle loss after burns, surgery, trauma, or starvation. Athletes need to know that OKG by itself increases muscle mass but not muscle activity. No clinical study has proven that OKG enhances athletic performance.

People who are generally healthy do not need to take more than 10,000 milligrams of OKG a day. OKG is typically taken before and after exercise to stimulate muscle growth, and in the morning and before bedtime. Higher dosages are given by IV to bowel transplant, colon surgery, and burn patients during hospitalization. Dieters should avoid OKG, since increased insulin production can lead to low blood sugars.

Pancreatin

Pancreatin is a mixture of enzymes extracted from hog pancreas. It contains amylase, which helps digest starches, lipases, which helps digest triglycerides, and trypsin, which helps digest proteins. It is medically prescribed for treatment of pancreatitis. Initial dosages should be chosen in consultation with a physician knowledgeable about nutrition. People who have gout should not use pancreatin.

Pancrelipase

Pancrelipase is a variation of pancreatin with a higher dosage of lipase. It is indicated as a supplement in diseases of chronic malabsorption of fats, such as cystic fibrosis and alcoholic cirrhosis of the liver, to increase absorption of fats and fat-soluble vitamins, and to control steatorrhea (high concentrations of fat in stool, causing odor and difficulties in disposal). Initial dosages of pancrelipase should be chosen in consultation with a knowledgeable healthcare professional. Overdosing can cause fibrous degeneration of the colon in cystic fibrosis patients. People who have gout should not use pancrelipase.

Pantethine

Pantethine is the biologically active form of pantothenic acid, also known as vitamin B_5. Pantethine helps transport useful fatty acids into cells. It lowers total cholesterol, LDL, and triglycerides, and raises HDL without interfering with the production of L-carnitine. In one study involving diabetics, taking 600 milligrams of pantethine daily lowered triglyceride levels by 37 percent. Generally, pantethine lowers total cholesterol by 15 to 25 percent and triglycerides by 25 to 40 percent.

Clinical trials of pantethine have used doses of 600–1,200 milligrams a day, but taking much more than 600 milligrams per day can increase your susceptibility to sunburn, especially if you take the blood pressure medication lisinopril (Prinivil or Zestril). Use of supplemental pantethine enhances the cholesterol-lowering effects of atorvastatin (Lipitor), lovastatin (Mevacor), pravastatin (Pravachol), simvastatin (Zocor), and nicotinamide. The safety of pantethine supplementation for pregnant women and nursing mothers has not been established.

Pantothenic Acid

Pantothenic acid is synonymous with vitamin B_5. The term pantothenic is derived from the Greek word *pantos*, meaning everywhere. Pantothenic acid occurs in avocados, broccoli, cashews, egg yolks, organ meats, brown rice, and milk and in especially high concentrations of brewer's yeast and royal jelly. The discoverer of pantothenic acid, Dr. Roger Williams, noted that bloodstream concentrations of the vitamin are significantly reduced in persons who have rheumatoid arthritis. Supplementation with pantothenic acid increases levels of the vitamin in the blood and relieves morning stiffness, disability, and pain, especially in vegetarians who take a combination of pantothenic acid and royal jelly.

Rheumatoid arthritis is the only form of arthritis that supplemental pantothenic acid helps. Studies have found that pantothenic acid concentrations in the blood of trained athletes falls during competition, and studies with animals suggest that supplementation with pantothenic acid could improve muscles' use of glycogen (loaded carbohydrates). However, only one clinical trial has found that taking supplemental pantothenic acid improves athletic performance (of long-distance runners), and that study used an enormous dosage of the vitamin, 2,000 milligrams a day, or approximately 280 times the RDA.

Limit use of supplemental pantothenic acid to 500 milligrams per day. Higher doses of the supplement may interfere with the body's absorption of biotin. Pregnant women and nursing mothers should not take more than 10 milligrams of pantothenic acid a day unless a higher dosage is medically prescribed.

Papain

Papain is a digestive enzyme extracted from papaya. It breaks down gluten protein in wheat and other grains. Mild celiac disease is sometimes controlled with the regular use of this enzyme, although observing dietary restrictions is still required. German physicians use papain as a treatment for herpes, at least one clinical trial finding it as effective as acyclovir. Dosages vary by the strength of the product.

Para-Aminobenzoic Acid (PABA)

Para-aminobenzoic acid (PABA) is an amino acid sometimes referred to as vitamin B_x, although it is neither a vitamin nor an essential nutrient for humans. The 2 health conditions most commonly treated with PABA are an unusual angularity of the penis known as Peyronnie's disease and the skin condition scleroderma.

A fast-acting potassium salt of PABA known as POTABA is available by prescription. A typical dosage of PABA is 12 grams a day. Loss of appetite, nausea, vomiting, fever, and rashes occasionally occur when PABA is taken at this dosage. The side effects stop when the supplement is discontinued. PABA is not appropriate for pregnant women, nursing mothers, children, or athletes, and it should not be taken by anyone being treated with sulfonamide antibiotics.

Passionflower

Passionflower consists of the dried flowering and fruit-bearing top of a perennial climbing vine native to north-eastern Mexico and Texas. It contains a number of flavonoid compounds, one of which, chrysin, acts on the same sites in the brain as the benzodiazepine drugs Librium and Valium, but without causing daytime drowsiness.

Take passionflower in any of the following forms:

- Dried herb in tea: 4–8 grams

- Dry powdered extract containing 2.6 percent flavonoids: 300–400 milligrams

- Fluid extract: 1/2–1 teaspoon

- Tincture: 1 1/2–2 teaspoons

Since passionflower is used in folk medicine as a stimulant for childbirth, pregnant women should not take it.

PC-SPES

The herbal formula **PC-SPES** is both effective and controversial in the treatment of prostate cancer. Laboratory studies show that it reduces the production of prostate specific antigen (PSA) by testosterone-sensitive prostate cancer cells, but not through any process mimicking the action of estrogen. On the other hand, in rare cases, PC-SPES has been associated with some of the same side effects as treatment with estrogen, specifically formation of blood clots in the lung. If you choose to use PC-SPES, be sure to have a physician do blood work to ensure that you are not at risk for blood clots. Consult with your physician regarding dosage.

Pectin

Pectin is a soluble fiber extracted from apples, mixed citrus, and grapefruit. Using pectin supplements for 3–4 months typically lowers LDL cholesterol levels by approximately 10 percent.

Always taken pectin with plenty of fluid. Doses of pectin used in clinical trials for lowering cholesterol average 15 grams a day. Pectin can cause bloating, cramps, diarrhea, and gas, and it should not be taken at the same time as supplements containing beta-carotene, calcium, copper, iron, magnesium, or zinc. Although pectin is used to lower cholesterol, it counteracts the absorption of lovastatin (Mevacor) and red yeast rice and makes these agents less effective in the treatment of high cholesterol. Combinations of pectin and kaolin used to treat diarrhea interfere with the absorption of the heart medication digoxin (Lanoxin) and tetracycline antibiotics.

Pepsin

Pepsin is a digestive enzyme secreted by the stomach for the digestion of proteins. Supplemental pepsin is sometimes used with betaine in the treatment of hypochlorhydria. Initial dosage should be chosen in consultation with a knowledgeable healthcare professional.

Perilla Oil

Perilla oil is extracted from the seed of the Japanese vegetable beefsteak plant. Rich in alpha-linolenic acid (ALA), it is used by people with ulcerative colitis who find the taste of fish oil unpleasant.

Typical dosage of perilla oil is 6 grams a day, although up to 15 grams a day may be helpful. Hemophiliacs, pregnant women, small children, and people taking prescription anticoagulants should not use perilla oil, since it may increase bleeding.

Phosphatidylcholine

Phosphatidylcholine, known in chemistry but not in commerce as **lecithin**, is an important building block for cell membranes. (Commercial lecithin preparations contain a mixture of nutrients closely related to phosphatidylcholine.) The use of phosphatidylcholine in the treatment of cirrhosis of the liver caused by alcoholism or chronic hepatitis is backed by long-term studies of alcohol-indulgent baboons. Heavy-drinking baboons given soy-derived phosphatidylcholine did not develop cirrhosis even after 8 years of heavy alcohol consumption, equivalent to 50 percent of their total calories. Researchers believe that lecithin protects the liver by encouraging the breakdown of collagen in fibrous tissue.

Typical dosages are 1–3 teaspoons (3–9 grams) a day. Phosphatidylcholine is used when supplemental choline causes diarrhea, nausea, or increased salivation. People with absorption problems, especially those with cystic fibrosis or pancreatitis, should avoid phosphatidylcholine.

Phosphatidylserine (PS)

Phosphatidylserine (PS) is a major component of the membranes lining nerve cells, particularly at their junctures with other nerve cells. Experiments with animals indicate that PS somehow encourages the regrowth of nerve networks within the brain. At its peak performance state, usually around the age of 30, the human brain may have up to 10,000 connections per each of its approximately 100 billion nerve cells, yielding as many as 1,000 trillion cell-to-cell connections, that is, a quadrillion nerve pathways. In Alzheimer's disease up to 90 percent of these connections are lost. By the end of life, an Alzheimer's disease patient may have virtually nothing remaining of the CA₁ region of the hippocampus, the region of the brain in which memories are formed.

PS seems to stimulate nerve growth factor in the cerebral cortex and the hippocampus, the 2 regions of the brain most affected by Alzheimer's disease. Loosely controlled clinical testing in the United States has found that it helps sufferers of age-associated memory loss recover their abilities of verbal association and recall. It helps restore hormone rhythms that help Alzheimer's disease patients deal with emotional stress. In advanced Alzheimer's disease or advanced dementia, PS will often improve sociability, attention to personal welfare, and cooperation with caregivers.

A dosage of 300 milligrams per day helps memory and a dosage of 600 milligrams per day lowers anxiety. PS is completely nontoxic and does not interfere with medications. Since European brands of PS are extracted from cow brain, there has been concern about mad cow disease, but functionally equivalent formulations made from soy are also available.

Phosphorus

Phosphorus is an essential mineral used to make bone. Some nutritional supplements are designed to provide phosphorus that accelerates the formation of bone in osteoporosis, but phosphorus (phosphate) supplements have to be used with caution since they cause the excretion of calcium. Controlled clinical trials have found that use of phosphate supplements by athletes can increase oxygen uptake by muscle and reduce the lactic acid-induced "burn" after anaerobic exercise, but these products cannot be used for more than 7 days in a month without risk of calcium depletion.

The recommended supplement for phosphorus-deficient individuals is milk. Athletes "load" phosphates by taking 1,000 milligrams of calcium or sodium phosphate 3 times a day for up to 7 days in any month. For bone health, take 4,000 milligrams of *calcium* phosphate for up to 7 days in any month. Pregnant women and nursing mothers should not take sodium phosphate, and should not take more than 4,000 milligrams of *calcium* phosphate per day, and should not use phosphorus supplements for more than 1 week without medical supervision.

Phytostanols and Phytosterols

Phytostanols and **phytosterols** are cholesterol-like compounds found in plants. Used as an additive in margarine, they block cholesterol from food from being absorbed and bind cholesterol salts in stool. Use of cholesterol-lowering margarines may lower absorption of beta-carotene and vitamin E (but not vitamins A and D) from supplements and food. Pregnant women and nursing mothers should limit their use of products containing phytostanols or phytosterols.

Piperine

Piperine is the chemical that gives black pepper its distinctive taste. Taking piperine or eating foods seasoned with black pepper at the same time as taking supplemental beta-carotene, coenzyme Q_{10}, curcuminoids, vitamin B_6, vitamin C, or organic selenium increases their absorption. Piperine is added to nutritional supplements for this purpose, or one may take 5–15 milligrams of piperine with the supplements. Higher doses of piperine (over 20 milligrams) interfere with the body's use and excretion of more than 20 medications. (See Part Three for information about specific drugs.)

Policosanol

Policosanol is a plant alcohol usually found with octacosanol (see Octacosanol). Clinical trials in Germany and Cuba have shown that daily doses of 10 milligrams of policosanol are equally effective in lowering total or LDL cholesterol as the same dose of simvastatin (Zocor) or pravastatin (Pravachol)—without their toxic side effects.

Typical daily dosage of policosanol is 10 milligrams. Higher doses may be more effective, but 20 milligrams a day is the maximum recommended dose. The safety of supplemental policosanol for pregnant women and nursing mothers has not been established, and it should

be avoided by hemophiliacs and anyone who is taking a prescription anticoagulant. Inform your physician if you have been taking policosanol before any surgical procedure.

Potassium

Potassium is an essential mineral that maintains electrostatic balance between the contents of a cell and the fluids surrounding it. Supplemental potassium causes small but lasting reductions in blood pressure. Diets high in potassium, magnesium, and fiber are associated with lower risk of stroke. Potassium supplementation was once important in treating cardiac arrhythmias, but nowadays relatively few people with arrhythmias benefit from supplemental potassium—because modern prescription drugs have been specifically designed to help the body retain potassium. If you take hydrochlorothiazide (the active ingredient in Dyazide, HCTZ, hydro-DIURIL, Maxzide, and Moduretic) as your *only* heart medication, you can benefit by increasing your consumption of fruits and vegetables, valuable sources of potassium, and by taking a supplemental source of potassium such as Slo-K. Large-scale surveys have found that potassium deficiencies are associated with cardiac arrhythmias, and at least for people who take hydrochlorothiazide, supplemental potassium can prevent arrhythmias.

Consult your physician about an appropriate dosage of potassium. Overdosing can cause serious and potentially deadly side effects.

Pregnenolone

Pregnenolone is a steroid hormone the body uses to make DHEA. Experiments with lab rats have found that it increases memory capacity and relieves stress, and pregnenolone levels are lower in humans diagnosed with depression. Supplemental pregnenolone, however, does not reliably lift mood, improve memory, or treat depression, at least in people who receive prescription medications. Some recent research suggests that pregnenolone may be useful in treating postpartum depression.

Typical doses of pregnenolone range from 5–50 milligrams per day, but the safety of the supplement is not established. Persons with seizure disorders should avoid pregnenolone completely.

Probiotics and Prebiotics

Probiotics are microorganisms resident in the intestine that are beneficial to human health. **Prebiotics** are food sources for probiotics. By colonizing on the surface of the intestine, probiotics reinforce its function as a natural barrier against infection. They also compete with infectious bacteria for nutrients, keeping the numbers of pathogenic microorganisms in check.

Lactobacillus and *Saccharomyces boulardii* help prevent diarrhea after use of antibiotics. *Lactobacillus acidophilus* and *Bifidobacterium* greatly reduce the risk of recurrence of "pouchitis," an inflammatory condition that commonly occurs after surgery for inflammatory bowel disease. *Lactobacillus* is also useful in treating the various kinds of infections that cause vaginosis.

Typical dosage of probiotics is 1–2 capsules several times a week. If constipation or flatulence occurs, cut back on the dose. Taking prebiotics such as inulin or lactulose make probiotics more effective. Probiotics should be avoided by diabetics with poor sugar control and by persons recovering from surgery.

Propolis

Propolis is the "glue" bees use to make honeycombs. Hundreds of scientific studies have confirmed the antihepatotoxic, antitumor, antioxidative, antimicrobial and anti-inflammatory properties of this supplement. Propolis, bioflavonoids, and vitamin C act synergistically to control herpes outbreaks. In a study in which women were given 3,000 milligrams of water-soluble bioflavonoids and 3,000 milligrams of vitamin C beginning at the onset of symptoms, blisters healed in an average of 4.4 days in the treatment group compared with 10 days in the placebo group.

In a study in Ukraine, women with cervical herpes were treated with either propolis or the commonly prescribed medication acyclovir. Women given propolis were twice as likely to have crusted lesions rather than open lesions on the third day of treatment. They were slightly less than twice as likely to have complete healing of the outbreak on the tenth day. Moreover, only women in the propolis group showed improvement in yeast infections during the course of treatment.

Cuban studies have found that propolis is more effective than the medication tinidazole against giardia-

sis. In a study of school children, propolis extracts prevented runny nose and sore throat.

Typical dosages of propolis are 50–250 grains (1–5 lozenges) or 500–2,000 milligrams (1–4 tablets) daily. Allergies to propolis are possible. The safety of propolis for pregnant women and nursing mothers has not been established.

Psyllium

Psyllium is a fiber supplement most commonly used to treat constipation. By absorbing water, psyllium adds bulk to stool and makes bowel movement possible with less straining. Eight clinical trials confirm that regular use of psyllium powder lowers total cholesterol by an average of 8–10 mg/dl and lowers LDL cholesterol by an average of 10–12 mg/dl.

Psyllium comes in powder, wafers, and "cookies." Follow the dosage recommendations of the manufacturer. Never take psyllium without drinking a full glass of water. Failure to take adequate fluid with psyllium powders can result in choking, and failure to take adequate fluid with any form of psyllium can result in intestinal blockage. Always take medications and other nutritional supplements at least 2 hours before or 2 hours after taking psyllium.

Pycnogenol

Pycnogenol is a mixture of oligomeric procyanidines extracted from the bark of a French pine. There are preliminary reports of exciting applications of Pycnogenol as an antioxidant. Laboratory experiments with animals have found that Pycnogenol protects against oxidation by NKK, a carcinogenic chemical found in tobacco smoke. Clinical trials have found that Pycnogenol reduces the risk of phlebitis and blood clots in smokers. One study has found that Pycnogenol increases the effectiveness of dextroamphetamine (Adderall) in treating ADD.

The primary use of supplemental Pycnogenol, however, is in treating varicose veins. A 60-day controlled clinical trial of 40 individuals with chronic venous insufficiency found that taking 100 milligrams of Pycnogenol 3 times a day significantly reduced edema, pain, and the sensation of heaviness in the leg. Pycnogenol may also be helpful in reducing pain and swelling in Achilles and rotator cuff tendonitis.

Typical daily dosage of Pycnogenol is 200 milligrams, although sometimes doses as small as 25 milligrams a day provide symptomatic relief. The safety of Pycnogenol for pregnant women and nursing mothers has not been established.

Pyruvate

Pyruvate is a biological fuel. It is especially abundant in red apples, red wine, and dark beer. Clinical studies have found that women who take high doses (30 grams a day) of pyruvate while dieting lose more overall weight and more weight from fat. Even higher doses (36–53 grams a day) lower diastolic blood pressure and resting heart rate in persons with high cholesterol. Two studies have found that supplemental pyruvate increases muscular endurance of the arms and legs, although a study with football players found it does not reduce the "burn" caused by anaerobic exercise unless it is complemented by supplemental creatine. Some studies suggest that the effects of pyruvate in persons over the age of 50 are greater when supplemental acetyl-L-carnitine is also taken.

Despite the high doses used in clinical trials, most authorities recommend a daily dosage of 5–6 grams for weight loss or during athletic training. Higher doses can cause bloating, cramping, and gas. The safety of supplemental pyruvate for pregnant women and nursing mothers has not been established.

Quercetin

Quercetin is a plant chemical found in barks and rinds. Taken as a supplement, it blocks the action of enzymes that trigger the release of allergy-causing histamine. Japanese scientists studied mast cells taken from the nasal passages of volunteers who had yearly bouts of hay fever. Quercetin significantly reduced allergen-stimulated release of histamine, twice as effectively as the placebo. Quercetin's effect was almost twice that of sodium cromoglycate (Nalcrom) at the same concentration.

About 2 out of 3 men with prostate inflammation experience improvement in symptoms after taking 500 milligrams of quercetin twice a day for a month.

Dosages of quercetin range from 200–1,200 milligrams per day. For best results, take bromelain and quercetin together 5–10 minutes before meals. Taking bromelain or papain supplements at the same time as quercetin increases the absorption of quercetin. Overdoses of quercetin can cause nausea, headache, or mild tingling in the fingers and toes. The safety of quercetin for pregnant women and nursing mothers has not been established.

A significant drawback to using quercetin is that it competes with and may reduce the effectiveness of quinolone antibiotics, including:

- ciprofloxacin (Cipro, Baycip, Cetraxal, Ciflox, Cifran, Ciplox, Cyprobay, Quintor)

- enoxacin (Penetrex)

- gatifloxacin (Tequin)

- gemifloxacin (a relatively new drug)

- grepafloxacin (Raxar)

- levofloxacin (Levaquin)

- lomefloxacin (Maxaquin)

- moxifloxacin (Avelox)

- norfloxacin (Noroxin, Amicrobin, Anquin, Baccidal, Barazan, Biofloxin, Floxenor, Fulgram, Janacin, Lexinor, Norofin, Norxacin, Orixacin, Oroflox, Urinox, Zoroxin)

- ofloxacin (Floxin)

- sparfloxacin (Zagam)

- temafloxacin (Omniflox) and

- trovafloxacin (Trovan)

Quercetin is also often recommended during cancer treatment. People who take Adriamycin, however, should not take quercetin. Laboratory studies have shown that quercetin makes Adriamycin more effective in treating multidrug-resistant breast cancer, but less effective in treating breast cancer that is not multi-drug resistant. If you have cancer and you do not know whether you have a drug-resistant cancer, you definitely should not take quercetin.

Red Yeast Rice

Red yeast rice is a fermented rice product used in food and medicine in China at least since the Tang Dynasty in A.D. 800. It has been used to make rice wine, as a food preservative for maintaining the color and taste of fish and meat. The medicinal properties of red yeast rice are described in detail in the Chinese pharmacopoeia, *Ben*

Cao Gang Mu-Dan Shi Bu Yi, published during the Ming Dynasty (A.D. 1368–1644).

Red yeast rice (Cholestin) contains a naturally occurring form of lovastatin (Mevacor), a commonly prescribed cholesterol-lowering medication. The first clinical study of red yeast was conducted in China. Physicians gave 324 people with high cholesterol (average total cholesterol, 230 mg/dl, average LDL, 130 mg/dl, average HDL, under 40 mg/dl either red yeast or a placebo for 8 weeks. Total cholesterol dropped by 23 percent, LDL cholesterol by 31 percent, and triglycerides by 34 percent. Serum HDL cholesterol levels increased by 20 percent.

A second study gave 65 adults with high cholesterol either 2.4 grams of red yeast rice daily or a placebo. Participants in this study were asked to follow a 30-percent fat, 10-percent saturated fat diet with no more than 300 milligrams of cholesterol daily. After 8 weeks, the participants in the study who had been given red yeast rice had an average 18 percent reduction in total cholesterol, 23 percent reduction in LDL cholesterol, and 16 percent reduction in triglycerides. In this study, there were no changes in HDL cholesterol levels.

Follow dosage instructions on the product label.

Unlike lovastatin (Mevacor), red yeast rice (Cholestin) has never been known to cause serious side effects. Red yeast rice products have only caused headaches and stomach upset. Some precautions, however, are prudent. Like lovastatin, red yeast rice should be avoided by women who are or who may become pregnant, by nursing mothers, and by anyone with kidney or liver disease. It should not be taken with antibiotics, cyclosporine (a medication for preventing rejection of transplants), niacin, or protease inhibitors.

If you have been prescribed any of the statin drugs atorvastatin (Lipitor), lovastatin (Mevacor), pravastatin (Pravachol), or simvastatin (Zocor), ask you doctor about using red yeast rice. Treatment with this natural supplement costs $20–30 per month, compared to $120–300 for the prescription drug.

Resveratrol

Resveratrol is a chemical that plants make to heal tissues injured by fungal infections and other injuries. It is especially abundant in red wine. A potent antioxidant, resveratrol has been found in laboratory studies to be highly effective in stopping the biochemical processes that cause atherosclerosis and malignancy, but it has never been clinically tested. Scientists do not know conclusively whether low rates of heart disease in drinkers of red wine and purple grape juice are due to resveratrol or to some other component.

There is no standard dosage of resveratrol. Pregnant women and nursing mothers should drink purple grape juice in preference to taking supplemental resveratrol.

Riboflavin

Riboflavin, also known as vitamin B_2, is a key element in the body's production of energy. Supplemental riboflavin is extremely useful in controlling migraines. One clinical trial found that taking large doses of riboflavin for 2 months led to at least a 50 percent reduction in the number of migraine attacks in 59 percent of people taking it. Riboflavin is most useful for controlling migraines in women who take birth control pills and in both men and women on cholesterol-lowering medications.

Standard dosage of riboflavin used for preventing migraines is 400 milligrams per day. Riboflavin deficiency is most common in alcoholics and people with sickle cell anemia. Mild riboflavin deficiencies are common in women who take oral contraceptives, and in people who take excessive amounts of supplements containing boron. Persons at risk for mild riboflavin deficiency should take any complete B-vitamin supplement containing at least 5 milligrams of riboflavin daily. Severe riboflavin deficiencies can occur during treatment for HIV with didanosine, lamivudine, stavudine, or zidovudine. HIV patients taking these drugs should consult with their physicians about adequate supplementation with riboflavin. Use of riboflavin supplements can cause a harmless bright yellow or orange discoloration of the urine.

Royal Jelly

Royal jelly is a secretion from worker bees that stimulates growth and development of the queen. Without royal jelly, the queen bee would be no different from worker bees and would only live 7–8 weeks. With royal jelly, the queen bee may live 5–7 years.

Use of royal jelly as a nutritional supplement frequently lowers total cholesterol levels by 20–30 mg/dl. There are isolated reports of the successful use of royal jelly in treating foot ulcers caused by diabetes and other slow-to-heal wounds. Laboratory testing with white mice has found that it offers complete protection against experimentally induced leukemia, but no clinical trials have proven the usefulness of royal jelly in treating any form of cancer in humans.

Typical doses of royal jelly range from 50–100 milligrams per day. Asthma, eczema, hives, and nasal irritation can occur in persons allergic to any component of royal jelly. The safety of supplemental royal jelly for pregnant women and nursing mothers has not been established.

Rutin

Rutin is a flavonoid closely related to quercetin and found in abundance in buckwheat, black tea, and apple peels. The primary use of rutin supplements is to treat conditions caused by fragile capillaries, such as easy bruising and swollen ankles in peripheral venous insufficiency. Some experiments with laboratory animals have found that rutin prevents oxidation of LDL cholesterol by "recharging" vitamin C, but these findings are only preliminary.

A typical dosage of rutin is 500 milligrams twice a day. It is theoretically possible that rutin could interact with nitrosamines found in cured and smoked meats to form a carcinogenic compound, so it is advisable to avoid consumption of cured and smoked meats while taking rutin supplements. Use of rutin is incompatible with many antibiotics, including:

- ciprofloxacin (Cipro, Baycip, Cetraxal, Ciflox, Cifran, Ciplox, Cyprobay, Quintor)

- enoxacin (Penetrex)

- gatifloxacin (Tequin)

- gemifloxacin (a relatively new drug)

- grepafloxacin (Raxar)

- levofloxacin (Levaquin)

- lomefloxacin (Maxaquin)

- moxifloxacin (Avelox)

- norfloxacin (Noroxin, Amicrobin, Anquin, Baccidal, Barazan, Biofloxin, Floxenor, Fulgram, Janacin, Lexinor, Norofin, Norxacin, Orixacin, Oroflox, Urinox, Zoroxin)

- ofloxacin (Floxin)

- sparfloxacin (Zagam)

- temafloxacin (Omniflox) and

- trovafloxacin (Trovan)

S-Adenosyl-L-Methionine (SAM-e)

S-adenosyl-L-methionine, more commonly known as **SAM-e**, plays a critical role in the body's synthesis of DNA and RNA, lecithin, proteins, epinephrine, melatonin, and creatine. A number of studies support the use of SAM-e in the treatment of cirrhosis. A double-blind clinical trial found that 1,200 milligrams of SAM-e per day for 2 years decreased the overall death rate and the need for liver transplantation with alcohol liver cirrhosis. Later trials have found that doses as low as 180 milligrams per day may be helpful, especially for persons in earlier stages of cirrhosis. The most important benefit of SAM-e in alcoholic cirrhosis is that it regulates the biochemical pathways so that alcohol has a greater effect on the central nervous system, and less has to be drunk for its drug effect. SAM-e also acts in part by protecting the liver's supply of vitamin E, so best results are likely to be obtained when there are adequate supplies of the vitamin.

Clinical studies have found SAM-e to be effective in treating depression, the most recent study finding it to be as effective in relieving mild depression as imipramine (Tofranil). SAM-e also relieves pain of arthritis. Various studies have found SAM-e as good or better for pain relief as Advil, Motrin, Naprosyn, and Nuprin. A study involving 20,641 people with osteoarthritis of the finger, hip, knee, and spine found that SAM-e alone was as effective as their ordinary pain relievers. Another study involving 734 subjects found that it was more effective than Naprosyn (naproxen sodium).

The advantage of SAM-e is that it very seldom causes side effects. In the longest-running study involving the supplement, various minor side effects occurred in 20 out of 97 patients from time to time during the first 18 months of the intervention. In the final 6 months of the study, however, no patients experienced any side effects from SAM-e. Patients received relief of morning stiffness, pain at rest, and pain on movement, and depression as well.

The disadvantage of SAM-e is that it is expensive. Occasionally people improve while taking as little as 20 milligrams of SAM-e a day, but scientists believe that the 200-milligram doses offered as an "affordable" supplement are too small to be effective. Effective treatment of depression with SAM-e requires a dosage of 1,600 milligrams a day. Start with a small dose and gradually increase over a period of 3 weeks to avoid stomach upset.

SAM-e may interfere with the Parkinson's disease drug L-dopa. Do not combine SAM-e with L-dopa or prescription antidepressants except under the supervision of a physician who knows you are taking SAM-e. Taking both SAM-e and prescription antidepressants may cause excessive production of serotonin, leading to anxiety, elevated blood pressure, and mania. People with bipolar disorder or subject to panic attacks should not take SAM-e.

SAM-e is better absorbed when it is taken on an empty stomach. SAM-e works in tandem with vitamin B_{12}, so avoiding B_{12} deficiency by taking a complete B supplement daily may increase the effectiveness of SAM-e.

Saw Palmetto

The most widely used herbal remedy for benign prostate enlargement (benign prostatic hyperplasia, or BPH) is **saw palmetto**. There is abundant clinical evidence that taking saw palmetto relieves the symptoms of prostate enlargement. Saw palmetto is fully as effective as Proscar. Clinical studies in Germany have found that a combination of saw palmetto and stinging nettle improved urine flow just as much as Proscar and had fewer adverse effects on sexual performance. Like Proscar, saw palmetto changes the metabolism of testosterone and stops the unchecked multiplication of cells in the fibrous sheath around the prostate. Clinical studies published in 2002 confirm that it is more effective than another medication often prescribed for the condition, tamsulosin (Flomax). Saw palmetto is more likely to shrink the prostate, and men treated with saw palmetto are less likely to experience problems with ejaculation. There are even reports that balding men who take saw palmetto begin to regrow their hair (see HAIR LOSS, MALE-PATTERN in Part One). Roughly 90 percent of men with mild to moderate BPH experience some improvement in symptoms during the first 4–6 weeks of taking saw palmetto.

Typical daily dosage of saw palmetto is 160 milligrams twice a day. (Combinations of saw palmetto and stinging nettle offer additional relief.) The problem with saw palmetto is that it frequently interferes with erectile function. If you have erectile dysfunction (ED), you should not take saw palmetto, and you should make sure any supplement you take for BPH does not contain saw palmetto. Stinging nettle acts on the prostate through the same mechanism as saw palmetto, and also should be avoided in treating ED.

The herbal alternatives for BPH when ED is a problem are pollen and pygeum. In Germany, where saw palmetto is very commonly prescribed for BPH, pollen is described by a medical association as providing "half the pain and twice the sexual pleasure" for men with the condition. Pollen especially reduces dribbling and decreases urgency of urination in about 75 percent of men who take it. There are no side effects from pollen, although some men may be allergic to it. Tested in 18 clinical studies involving 1,562 men, pygeum is somewhat less effective than saw palmetto in increasing urine flow and stopping nighttime urination, but still helpful to a majority of men taking it. Side effects of pygeum are rare, although it can cause diarrhea, constipation, dizziness, gastric pain, and visual disturbances.

Secoisolariciresinol Diglycoside (SDG)

Secoisolariciresinol diglycoside (SDG) is a plant estrogen found in flaxseed. Laboratory experiments with animals hint at applications for preventing hardening of the arteries, preventing type 1 diabetes, and protecting against breast cancer and the spread of melanoma, but no study has confirmed any of these benefits in humans. Standard dosages of SDG have not been established, and it should not be used by pregnant women, nursing women, or women who have estrogen-sensitive cancers of the breast, ovaries, or uterus.

Selenium

Selenium is an essential trace element first described by the explorer Marco Polo, who noticed that horses lost their hooves when they ate grasses grown in ground covered with a salt now known to be selenium. In small amounts, selenium is a necessary and therapeutic antioxidant. Dietary deficiencies of selenium are associated with increased risk of colorectal, gastric, lung, prostate, and skin cancers, viral infections, cardiomyopathy, hardening of the arteries, heart attack, and stroke. In excessive amounts, selenium is toxic, causing sudden hair loss, blackening, streaking, and loss of the nails, garliclike breath odor, fatigue, rashes, irritability, nausea, and vomiting.

The therapeutic benefits of limited amounts of selenium in combination with other antioxidant supplements are numerous. Selenium is an important cofactor for vitamin E in the treatment of acne. Adult male acne patients have low levels of the antioxidant glutathione peroxidase, which normalizes with vitamin E and selenium treatment. Glutathione peroxidase puts a brake on inflammatory reactions throughout the body, especially in the skin. Selenium depresses the parts of the immune system that cause allergic reactions, but encourages the parts of the immune system that respond to bacterial infection. There is also evidence that selenium compounds control the breakdown of thyroid hormones into forms that do not aggravate acne.

Laboratory experiments with skin cells have found that providing the cells with selenium, vitamin C, and vitamin E *before* exposure to ultraviolet light greatly reduces the amount of DNA damage. Even after exposure to sunlight, selenium and vitamin E help the skin make glutathione, which in turn stops the process through which sunlight causes apoptosis, the initiation of skin cell death.

Only the most preliminary clinical study supports the use of selenium in treating cirrhosis of the liver, but these laboratory experiments suggest that it could be very important. Selenium participates in a series of biochemical steps that make liver cells insensitive to tumor necrosis factor, a hormone the immune system ordinarily uses to destroy tumors that also destroys healthy tissues in the presence of alcohol. Cirrhosis patients with higher bloodstream concentrations of selenium have less severe liver damage.

The antioxidant selenium has long been considered cancer-protective for the colon. For reasons that are not yet understood, selenium in foods, such as broccoli, offers greater protection against colon cancer than selenium supplements.

Immigrants from China sometimes suffer from Keshan disease, a form of cardiomyopathy related to selenium deficiency. Known only among people who have eaten a "one-sided diet," a limited variety of local foods in certain areas of northeastern China and Taiwan, this condition usually results from an inability of the heart to respond to viral infection after many years of eating foods grown on soil that lacks selenium. In rare cases, people with an inability to absorb selenium can also develop the disease. Although taking a modest amount of supplemental selenium (100 micrograms a day) might help prevent disease in people who have recently immigrated from areas where it is common, once Keshan cardiomyopathy occurs, it cannot be treated with selenium supplementation alone.

People who have cataracts have lower levels of selenium than people who do not. Alpha-lipoic acid, N-acetyl cysteine, and selenium increase the body's supply of glutathione, a vital antioxidant that protects nerve cells against additional damage in chronic fatigue syndrome.

These are only a few of the uses of this mineral. Selenium from yeast is the best form for most applications. Taking selenium at the same time you take vitamin C reduces the absorption of selenium, and you should never take more than 1,000 milligrams of selenium a day. The first sign you have overdosed on selenium is usually is a garlicky breath odor. Excessive use of selenium also can cause hair loss, fatigue, irritability, and hyperreflexia or "jumpiness." Horizontal streaking, blackening, and fragility of the nails when you take selenium is a sure sign you are taking too much or you are taking a product that has been improperly standardized.

Silymarin

Silymarin, a group of chemicals extracted from milk thistle, is the most commonly used herbal remedy for various liver conditions. Relatively high doses of milk thistle, preferably taken as a phytosome (the active ingredient silymarin chemically joined to phosphatidylcholine), reduce liver damage in alcoholic cirrhosis. At molecular level, silibinin, one of the components of silymarin, prevents damage to the outer membranes of liver cells from free radicals of oxygen. It helps liver cells use oxygen more efficiently and assists in the formation of proteins. Most important, it increases synthesis of proteins needed by the liver to repair itself.

Silymarin from milk thistle has been associated with a single case of complete remission from liver cancer. At the time of this report, there had been only 9 cases of liver cancer ever known to go into remission, so the finding about silymarin electrified the herbal community. Later laboratory research failed to yield an easy explanation of how silymarin works in liver cancer—in fact, milk thistle was found to be a prooxidant, accelerating destruction of DNA in liver cells and presumably in liver cancer cells.

Typical dosage of silymarin is 360 milligrams a day. Silymarin phytosomes are more completely absorbed than other forms of milk thistle. In some cases, silymarin can cause mild diarrhea. Reduce the dosage if diarrhea occurs. Some people with cirrhosis may not benefit from taking silymarin. One study found that milk thistle is not helpful when there is a complication of cirrhosis known as portal hypertension.

Sodium Alginates

Sodium alginates are salts extracted from seaweeds. In Japan, they are used to treat "ouch-ouch" disease, a condition of severe join inflammation in children caused by exposure to cadmium in drinking water contaminated by smelting operations. Sodium alginates absorb cadmium, barium, and radium so that they are excreted in stool. There are preliminary reports that extracts from Irish seaweeds may exert an antiviral effect on herpes and HIV. Extracts of the Japanese brown seaweed hijiki may stimulate the activity of B cells, although not T cells, in the immune system and increase immune defenses in AIDS.

Sodium alginate supplements are offered as products made from arame, brown seaweed, red seaweed, Irish moss, aga or agar-agar, dulse, hijiki, kombu, nori, and wakame. There is no standard dosage. Avoid seaweed products if you have Crohn's disease or ulcerative colitis. The safety of sodium alginates for pregnant women and nursing mothers has not been established.

Soy Isoflavones

Soy isoflavones are mixtures of the phytoestrogens daidzein, genistein, and glycitein extracted from soy. They are beneficial for treating acute distress occurring in women in menopause. Soy products do not offer relief as quickly as hormone replacement, but the body of clinical research considered as a whole indicates that most women will experience relief from hot flashes by taking soy isoflavones daily. Soy isoflavones are not used to treat osteoporosis, but a closely related product, ipriflavone, is.

A recent study in *The Journal of Nutrition* reported that soy milk corrects mild high blood pressure in both men and women, but it is not known if the effect is due to isoflavones or some other component of soy. Soy isoflavones, however, have a definite protective effect against cancer. A study in the journal *Metabolism* reported that consuming soy isoflavones from soy

or soy isoflavone supplements stimulated the production of cancer-fighting interleukin-6 (IL-6), involved in the immune response to almost all cancers. High consumption of soy products in childhood and early adulthood is specifically linked to low rates of breast cancer after menopause in women, although is not yet known whether soy isoflavone supplements have the same protective effect against breast cancer as eating soy foods.

A typical dosage of soy isoflavones is 125 milligrams a day. The safety of soy isoflavones for pregnant women and nursing mothers has not been established. Men with prostate cancer and women with estrogen receptor-positive cancers of the breast, ovaries, or uterus should use soy isoflavones only if they are recommended and monitored by a physician, since the use of soy isoflavones may make it difficult to gauge responses to other hormonal therapies. Soy isoflavones should be avoided in hyperthyroidism and by women who have goiter.

Soy Protein

Soy protein is FDA approved as a treatment for lowering the risk of heart disease. A series of studies confirm that consumption of as little as 20 grams of soy protein a day lowers total cholesterol, LDL cholesterol, triglycerides, and the cardiac risk marker apo-lipoprotein B in men and women without lowering levels of the protective HDL cholesterol. A study sponsored by the National Academy of Sciences (U.S.), however, cautions against the use of soy protein supplements in children, since animal studies find that soy proteins reduce the production of T cells to fight infection.

Intake of 25–50 grams of soy protein a day is beneficial for heart health. Soy shakes should not be taken with 2 hours of taking supplemental calcium, copper, iron, magnesium, manganese, or zinc, since the phytic acid in soy binds minerals and causes them to be excreted with stool. The safety of soy protein for pregnant women and nursing mothers has not been established. Men with prostate cancer and women with estrogen receptor-positive cancers of the breast, ovaries, or uterus should use soy products only if they are recommended and monitored by a physician, since the use of soy may make it difficult to gauge responses to other hormonal therapies. Soy products of all kinds should be avoided in hyperthyroidism and by women who have goiter.

Spirulina

Spirulina is a blue-green algae classed with barley grass, wheat grass, and chlorella as a green food. Spirulina is a rich source of protein, chlorophyll, carotenoids, minerals, GLA, and several pigments. Spirulina is a useful immune modulator, increasing the activity of natural killer (NK) cells in response to infection but reducing the activity of mast cells in causing allergy and inflammation. Laboratory experiments with animals suggest spirulina may contain chemicals protective against herpes and HIV.

Doses of green foods range from 250 milligrams to 5 grams a day. It is important to choose products from reputable dealers that are certified as free of heavy metal contaminants. Allergies to spirulina are rare but occasionally do occur. The safety of spirulina for pregnant women and nursing mothers has not been established.

Sports and Weight-Loss Supplements

Sports and weight-loss supplements sometimes give a winning edge to dedicated athletes who devote regular attention to training for their sport. They also give a winning edge to dieters—provided they exercise. Carefully consider all potential side effects before adding any sports or weight-loss supplement to your health routine.

See **19-norandrostenedione, Androstenediol, Androstenedione, Beta-hydroxy-beta-methylbutyrate (HMB), Bitter orange extracts, Chrysin, Creatine, D-ribose, Forskolin, Glycerol, human growth hormone (HGH), Inosine, Insulin-like growth factor 1 (IGF-1), L-glutamine, Medium-chain triglycerides (MCTs), Octacosanol, Ornithine alpha-ketoglutarate (OKG), Phosphorus, Pyruvate, Whey protein**.

Squalene

Squalene is a fat found in olive and shark liver oils. Squalene should not be confused with squalamine, a natural antibiotic found in the dogfish shark. Very preliminary studies suggest that supplemental squalene may lower cholesterol and have some cancer-fighting properties, but recommendations for its use as a supplement are premature.

Safe doses of squalene fall within the range of 500–4,000 milligrams a day. Excessive doses may cause bloating, cramping, diarrhea, and flatulence. A peculiarity of squalene is that it should not be carried out of doors. Squalene is also found in human skin, and squalene exposed to open air is a long-distance tick and mosquito attractant.

St. John's Wort

St. John's wort is an extraordinarily well-researched herb. Nearly 180 studies document the efficacy of St. John's wort in treating anxiety, anorexia, depression, and sleep disturbances. In the European Union, St. John's wort is a prescription antidepressant prescribed by doctors and paid for by health insurance companies.

Various clinical studies have compared St. John's wort with the tricyclic antidepressants Elavil (amitriptyline) and Tofranil (imipramine) and with the selective serotonin reuptake inhibitors (SSRIs) Paxil (fluoxetine) and Zoloft (sertraline). Clinical studies repeatedly find that St. John's wort is as effective as mainstream antidepressant drugs with fewer side effects and a lower cost.

A psychiatric clinic in Darmstadt, Germany, conducted a double-blind comparison trial of St. John's wort and Elavil. The 135 depressed patients were given either the herb or the prescription medication for 6 weeks. At the end of the trial, patients who had been taking St. John's wort had an average score on the Hamilton Depression Rating Scale of 8.8, compared to an average score of 10.7 for the patients treated with Elavil (that is, the patients taking St. John's wort were less depressed). The St. John's wort also had fewer and milder side effects.

A randomized, double-blind clinical comparison trial of St. John's wort and Tofranil conducted by the Remotiv-Imipramine Study Group in Germany involved 324 outpatients with mild to moderate depression at 40 outpatient clinics. After 6 weeks of treatment with either St. John's wort or Tofranil, the average score on the Hamilton Depression Rating Scale was 12.00 for patients taking St. John's wort and 12.75 for patients taking Tofranil. Adverse reactions such as agitation, anxiety, dizziness, retching, tiredness, and erectile dysfunction occurred in 39 percent of participants taking St. John's wort, but in 63 percent of patients taking Tofranil. The most important difference between St. John's wort and Tofranil, however, was the patient's experience of anxiety while in treatment. The mean score on the anxiety-somatization subscale of the Hamilton measurement system was 3.79 in the St. John's wort group and 4.26 in the Tofranil group. Patients who took St. John's wort were significantly less likely to experience anxiety than patients who took Tofranil.

Another German study compared St. John's wort with Prozac. Researchers enrolled 240 mildly to moderately depressed individuals into a randomized, double-blind, parallel group comparison in which 114 patients received Prozac and 126 patients received St. John's wort. After 6 weeks of treatment, the mean Hamilton Depression Rating Scale rating decreased to 11.54 in the group taking St. John's wort and to 12.20 in the group taking Prozac. Eight percent of patients experienced adverse events, compared to 23 percent of patients on Prozac. The researchers concluded that St. John's wort and Prozac were equally effective in treating mild to moderate depression but that St. John's wort was a safer choice.

A double-blind clinical study at St. John's Episcopal Hospital in Far Rockaway, New York, tested the comparative benefit of St. John's wort and Zoloft. Thirty outpatients were given a low dose of either St. John's wort or Zoloft for a week, and then a standard dose of either St. John's wort or Zoloft for 6 weeks. A clinical response defined as a 50 percent reduction in scores on the Hamilton Depression Rating Scale was noted in 47 percent of patients receiving St. John's wort and 40 percent of patients receiving Zoloft. The difference between the 2 drugs was too small to say with statistical confidence which was more effective.

Exactly how St. John's wort works is not known. The most recent research suggests that the chemical hyperforin in the herb modifies the expression of genes in parts of the brain that are physically changed by stress, specifically the hippocampus, locus coeruleus, and striatum. These parts of the brain respond to adrenaline released in states of stress, excitement, and joy; restoring them to normal function may counteract other processes that cause depression.

Although the clinical evidence for St. John's wort is impressive, critics of herbal medicine correctly point out that it will not reliably treat severe depression. A well-publicized study published in the *Journal of the American Medical* Association in 2001 reported that only 24 percent of severely depressed patients given a relatively high dose of St. John's wort (1,200 milligrams of hypericin per day) went into remission during an 8-week trial, compared to 19 percent of patients who were given a placebo. A similar controversy arose after reports of a clinical study in 2002. However, the news reports did not clarify that a response rate of less than 50 percent is typical for aggressive drug treatment of major depression, nor did the news reports compare side effects of standard medical treatments for major depression with side effects of St. John's wort. Nonetheless, anytime there is a risk of suicide, reliance on St. John's wort is inappropriate.

Effective dosages of St. John's wort range from 900–1,200 milligrams a day. Do not take St. John's wort unless you have been off prescription antidepressants for at least 4 weeks. Prescription antidepressants linger in the bloodstream for a long time, and there have been several reports of "serotonin syndrome" (anxiety, elevated blood pressure, and mania) occurring when St. John's wort and medications such as Prozac were taken together. Natural medicine specialist Dr. Steve Bratman notes that the antimigraine drug sumatriptan (Imitrex) and the painkilling drug tramadol (Ultram) also raise serotonin levels and might interact similarly with the herb. St. John's wort may make the skin more sensitive to sun, especially if you also take oral contraceptives, sulfa drugs, tetracycline, the blood pressure medication lisinopril (Prinivil or Zestril), or the arthritis drug piroxicam (Feldene.)

Most important, St. John's wort may reduce the effectiveness of chemotherapy drugs, clozapine (Clozaril) or olanzapine (Zyprexa) for schizophrenia, cyclosporine (Neoral, Sandimmune, Sangcya) for organ transplants, digoxin (Lanoxin) for heart disease, oral contraceptives, protease inhibitors for HIV, theophylline (Theo-Dur) for asthma, and warfarin (Coumadin), used as a blood thinner. If you are taking St. John's wort and one of these medications at the same time and then stop taking the herb, blood levels of the drug may rise. Increasing bloodstream concentrations of the drug may be dangerous in some circumstances.

Sulforophanes

Sulforophanes are the source of indole-3-carbinol found in bok choi, broccoli and especially broccoli sprouts, Brussels sprouts, cabbage, cauliflower, and kale. This plant chemical is especially important for women, since it reduces the carcinogenic activity of estrogen in breast tissue. Laboratory experiments with animals have found that it blocks some of the carcinogenic effects of tobacco smoke. Research to date neither proves nor disproves the assertion that sulforophanes or indole-3-carbinol increase muscle growth during weight training.

Sulforophanes are found in commercial products made from broccoli sprouts. When indole-3-carbinol is taken by itself, typical daily dosages range from 200–800 milligrams a day. They are also included in combination products for use by athletes. Do not take sulforophanes within 2 hours of taking an antacid or any product to stop heartburn.

Superoxide Dismutase (SOD)

Superoxide dismutase (SOD) is an enzyme produced throughout the body to protect cells from antioxidant damage. A copper/zinc SOD isolated from beef liver sometimes relieves arthritic inflammation.

Synbiotics

Synbiotics are combinations of symbiotic bacteria, or probiotics, plus the materials that feed them, or prebiotics. Synbiotics are used for the same purposes as probiotics, although they have the added benefit of increasing intestinal absorption of calcium, magnesium, and trace minerals.

Taurine

Taurine is an amino acid that is essential for the development of the nervous system before and immediately after birth. The role of taurine in the function of the nervous system was first discovered by veterinarians seeking to explain cardiomyopathy, retinopathy, and blood-clotting abnormalities in cats. Understanding taurine deficiency diseases in cats led to understanding the role of taurine in humans.

Two clinical studies have found benefits of taurine supplementation in treating cystic fibrosis in children. Supplemental taurine improves the absorption of fats and reduces diarrhea and fat in the stool. Clinical trials have found that taurine can be beneficial in treating congestive heart failure after heart attack in adults. There are also studies that suggest it can help lower blood sugars levels and reduce the frequency of seizures.

Children with cystic fibrosis are given 15 milligrams of taurine per day for every pound of body weight (approximately 30 milligrams per kilogram). For instance,

a child weighing 33 pounds (15 kilograms) would receive 500 milligrams of taurine a day. Initial dosage of taurine for children should be chosen in consultation with a knowledgeable natural healthcare professional. Standard dosage of taurine for adults is 3,000 milligrams per day, but initial dosage should be chosen in consultation with a physician. Expectant mothers should use supplemental taurine with caution, since it can cause blood sugar levels to fluctuate during pregnancy.

Thiamine

Thiamine, also known as vitamin B_1, was thought to have been isolated in 1911 from rice bran extracts by the Polish chemist Casimir Funk. Because he believed he had discovered a vital substance for life in the form of an amine, Funk coined the term "vitamin." It turned out that Funk had not extracted the substance later identified as thiamine or vitamin B_1, but the term "vitamin" and the concept of essential nutrients became a foundation of modern nutrition.

Thiamine's historical use was as a treatment for beri-beri, a sudden and often fatal neurological disease causing confusion, staggering, visual disturbances, and heart failure. Today, supplemental thiamine is used to prevent symptoms similar to those of beri-beri in diseases associated with chronic deprivation of thiamine, such as alcoholic cirrhosis of the liver, anorexia, and HIV. Supplemental thiamine is also often helpful in treating congestive heart failure, especially in people who take furosemide (Lasix), a diuretic that depletes the vitamin. Trainers report that supplemental thiamine can reduce fatigue after prolonged exercise, a finding supported by preliminary clinical trials. Regular exercise depletes thiamine, riboflavin, and vitamin B_6.

Dosages of thiamine range up to 200 milligrams per day. Anyone who takes furosemide should take at least 50 milligrams of supplemental thiamine daily. Coffee and tea taken within 2 hours of taking supplemental thiamine deactivate the vitamin. Avoid supplemental thiamine if you have cancer. There is some evidence that certain cancers "feed" on thiamine.

Transgalacto-Oligosaccharides (TOS)

Transgalacto-oligosaccharides (TOS) are polymers of galactose and glucose produced by the fermentation of milk sugars. TOS are not digested by humans, but they serve as a food for symbiotic bacteria in the intestine. There is strong experimental evidence that TOS can stop the multiplication of *Clostridium*, *E. coli*, *Listeria*, *Salmonella*, and *Shigella*. Some experiments suggest that TOS increase the activity of bacteria that increase the intestine's absorption of calcium and may reduce the risk of, or even treat, colon cancer.

Typical dosage of TOS is 2,500 milligrams 4 times a day. Overdosage may cause bloating, diarrhea, or flatulence, particularly in persons who are lactose intolerant.

Trypsin

Trypsin is a digestive enzyme included in pancreatin. Sometimes offered as a stand-alone supplement, trypsin is especially effective for releasing arginine and lysine and may be helpful for people with herpes. It also relieves some cases of arthritic inflammation. Dosages vary by brand.

Tylophora Asthmatica

Tylophora asthmatica is an Ayurvedic medicine for asthma, bronchitis, and rheumatoid arthritis. Taken in large doses, it induces vomiting. Taken in small doses, it seems to increase the body's production of anti-inflammatory steroids. The unique advantage of *Tylophora* is that its benefits continue even after its use is discontinued. Indian researchers had 110 asthmatics chew and swallow 1 *Tylophora* leaf per day for 6 days. At 1 week, 62 percent of individuals taking *Tylophora* had moderate to complete symptom relief. Relief from asthma continued for 4 weeks after the trial.

Standard dosage of *Tylophora* is 400 milligrams of dried leaf or two 40-milligram capsules daily. The drawback to using *Tylophora* is that, for it to be effective, you have to experience a little discomfort. A significant percentage of participants in the Indian study complained of nausea, although there was a positive correlation between nausea and degree of improvement.

Valerian

Valerian has been used as a sleep aid for more than 1,000 years. It contains valepotriates, valerenic acid, and other water-soluble chemicals that contribute to its sedative properties.

Valerian is a clinically effective source of GABA, a chemical that blocks extraneous nerve impulses in the brain. A clinical trial with 128 volunteers given 400 milligrams of valerian extract at bedtime found that the herb improved sleep quality, decreased the time needed to fall asleep, and reduced the number of awakenings during the night. A study in which participants were given 135 milligrams of a dry extract of valerian 3 times a day found that the herb improved slow-wave sleep and decreased the amount of time spent in stage 1 sleep.

Take valerian in any of the following forms:

- Dried root as a tea: 2–3 grams
- Dry powdered extract containing 0.8 percent valerenic acid: 150–300 milligrams
- Fluid extract: 1/2–1 teaspoon
- Tincture: 1 1/2–2 teaspoons

Small-scale clinical studies suggest that kava may be a better choice than valerian for people who are troubled by vivid dreams, but passionflower and valerian may be better choices for people who have diseases affecting balance or causing dizziness.

Valerian is generally a very safe herb, although there have been reports of withdrawal symptoms in persons who quit using it abruptly after taking higher-than-recommended dosages for a period of several years. Valerian has an additive effect when used with barbiturates or benzodiazepine tranquilizers such as Librium and Valium. Do not use both the herb and these prescription medications.

A pilot study conducted by an herbal products company in Switzerland found that the combination of valerian and hops is also helpful in treating mild insomnia. Thirty patients were given a combination of 250 milligrams of valerian extract and 60 milligrams of hops extract. After 2 weeks of treatment, polysomnography showed a decline in sleep latency, that is, the time required to go to sleep, and also in the time required to wake up. More important, the combination of the 2 herbs increased slow-wave sleep, the period in which the body replenishes interleukin-6, growth hormone, and melatonin. There were no side effects from the herbal treatment.

Vanadium

Vanadium is a metallic element found in ores of striking, varied colors. For this reason, vanadium was first named panchromium. In human nutrition, vanadium performs some of the same functions as chromium, making skeletal muscles more sensitive to glucose and lowering fasting blood sugars. Vanadium may also help prevent hypoglycemia.

If you choose to use vanadium to help you manage blood sugar levels, use doses measured in micrograms rather than in milligrams. Vanadium is available in 10-milligram tablets, but this dosage often causes cramping, diarrhea, nausea, vomiting, and a long-lasting green polychromatic stain on the tongue. Since as little as 30 micrograms a day (30,000 times smaller than a 10-milligram dose) may be helpful, restrict intake of vanadium to 500 micrograms a day.

Vinpocetine

Vinpocetine is a product manufactured from an extract of the leaf of the periwinkle plant. Vinpocetine prevents the accumulation of sodium in cells in the brain, lowering their overall "charge" and preventing tissue-destructive reactions of sodium and oxygen when circulation to brain tissue is reestablished after a stroke. Use of vinpocetine for this application, however, is still being investigated. Vinpocetine is better documented as a treatment for hearing loss after acoustic trauma, improving hearing acuity in 79 percent of patients and improving tinnitus in 66 percent of patients. There are also reports of successful use of vinpocetine in treating Ménière's disease and loss of vision caused by hardening of the arteries.

A typical daily dosage of vinpocetine is 10 milligrams. Up to 20 milligrams is generally safe, although reductions in blood pressure, dizziness, drowsiness, dry mouth, facial flushing, tension headaches, and insomnia have been known to occur in rare instances after using the supplement. Use of vinpocetine may intensify a side effect of blood pressure medications causing dizziness when moving from a seated to a standing position. No one who has an allergy to periwinkle or vinca should take vinpocetine. The safety of vinpocetine supplements for pregnant women and nursing mothers has not been established.

Vitamin A

Vitamin A is a group of fat-soluble substances that play a key role in vision, development of bone and skin, and production of red blood cells. They are also important to the establishment of patterns in the human embryo. The applications of carefully limited doses of supplemental vitamin A in maintaining health are numerous.

Vitamin A seems to prevent the progression of cervical dysplasia to cervical cancer. A Japanese study found that women with the lowest bloodstream concentrations of vitamin A were 4.5 times more likely to develop cervical cancer than women with the highest bloodstream levels of the vitamin.

The problem with vitamin A is that there is a possibility of birth defects if it is accidentally overdosed during the first 3 months of pregnancy. Unless otherwise indicated for special health conditions, women of reproductive age should limit consumption of supplemental vitamin A to 5,000 IU per day. Very high doses of the vitamin (more than 300,000 IU) have, on rare occasions (approximately 1 in 5 million births in the United States), caused birth defects. A daily dose of 5,000 IU per day can be used safely during pregnancy but may not prevent in cervical cancer.

Vitamin A and zinc deficiency produce the major complications of alcohol abuse: poor night vision, slow healing of wounds to the skin, depressed production of testosterone and estrogen, and poor immune function. Alcohol interferes with the intestines' ability to absorb vitamin A and zinc, and the liver's constant need to manufacture the detoxifying enzymes alcohol dehydrogenase and acetylaldehyde dehydrogenase depletes the vitamin A and zinc that make it through the intestines. Tissue damage makes it impossible for the liver to store these nutrients or to process them in large quantities. Only consistent, low-dose supplementation can correct this problem as long as you consume alcohol.

Night blindness is a serious health problem in societies in which women, in particular, are chronically deficient in vitamin A. Vitamin A supplementation greatly reduces but does not eliminate the problem. Zinc supplements added to vitamin A, however, nearly completely eliminate night blindness when the underlying cause is nutritional deficiency.

Relatively low doses of vitamin A are sufficient to prevent immune "burn-out" due to stress on the thymus during various kinds of infections. Vitamin A also makes antibodies more responsive to various kinds of infections, increases the rate at which macrophages engulf and destroy bacteria, and stimulates natural killer (NK) cells.

The first signs of vitamin A overdose are dry skin and

chapped lips, especially in dry weather. Later signs of toxicity are headache, mood swings, and pain in muscles and joints. In massive doses, vitamin A itself can cause liver damage. Discontinue vitamin A at the first sign of toxicity.

Vitamin B$_6$

Vitamin B$_6$ is a term for a group of related compounds including pyridoxal-5´-phosphate, pyridoxine-5´-phosphate, and pyridoxiamine-5´-phosphate, which are absorbed by tissues at slightly different rates. Deficiencies of vitamin B$_6$ are associated with a number of diseases.

Vitamin B$_6$ (pyridoxine) deficiencies cause increased sensitivity to testosterone in the skin. Women who have flare-ups of acne along with PMS often improve after taking vitamin B$_6$. Women who develop acne during testosterone treatment usually benefit from taking B$_6$.

Vitamin B$_6$ is useful in treating ADD and ADHD, preferably in its active form, pyridoxal-5´-phosphate (PLP). A very small-scale, preliminary study found that vitamin B$_6$ was as effective as Ritalin in controlling "hyper" behaviors, and that the benefits of vitamin B$_6$ supplementation continued for nearly a month after its daily use was discontinued. Vitamin B$_6$ had an additional advantage in that it increased bloodstream levels of the hormone serotonin, associated with improved social orientation in ADHD.

Supplementation with vitamin B$_6$ can help treat amenorrhea in women who have high levels of the hormone prolactin. This is the hormone that enables milk production, so vitamin B$_6$ is most likely to help women who develop amenorrhea while nursing. It may also help amenorrheic women whose stores of the vitamin have been depleted as a side effect of using oral contraceptives or prescription drugs for asthma or epilepsy.

Vitamin B$_6$ is important for children with asthma and for adults who take theophylline (Theo-Dur). In a study of 76 children with asthma, taking 100 milligrams of vitamin B$_6$ twice a day resulted in fewer attacks, less wheezing, coughing, and chest tightness, and less frequent use of inhalers. In adults, vitamin B$_6$ does not necessarily improve lung capacity, but taking the vitamin results in decreased wheezing. Asthma patients of all ages who use theophylline have lower levels of PLP, and benefit from taking vitamin B$_6$ in the form of PLP.

A series of studies have found that magnesium and vitamin B$_6$ *used together* are of considerable benefit in treating autism, considerably more than either supplement used by itself. Supplementation with magnesium and vitamin B$_6$ reduces the excretion of homovanillic acid, which is a rough measure of the presence of the stress hormones epinephrine and norepinephrine in the brain. Presumably the combination of supplements reduces stress. Approximately 35 percent of children will respond to this combination within 2 weeks.

Treatment with pyridoxine creams is helpful in treating seborrhea causing greasy scales on the face. In one study, all patients with these symptoms who took a pyridoxine cream cleared up completely within 10 days. The creams were not helpful, however, for seborrheic dermatitis complicated by infection, and did not clear lesions on the neck, chest, or groin.

These are only a few of the applications of vitamin B$_6$. Dosages range up to 500 milligrams per day, but taking more than this amount may cause tingling, numbness, or burning in the fingers or toes.

Women who use oral contraceptives and people who take prescription medications for bipolar disorder, unipolar depression, tuberculosis, or seizures are at risk for vitamin B$_6$ deficiency. If you take theophylline (Theo-Dur) for asthma and have any history of seizure disorder or unexplained loss of consciousness, you should not take vitamin B$_6$.

Vitamin B$_{12}$

Vitamin B$_{12}$ or cobalamin is a collective term for a group of B vitamins containing cobalt. Deficiency of this vitamin is associated with pernicious anemia, a particularly destructive form of vitamin B$_{12}$ deficiency that causes blood cells to be broken down faster than they can be replaced. This form of anemia is called "pernicious" because it develops slowly over a period of at least 3–6 years and the damage it causes is well advanced before symptoms occur.

If you have pernicious anemia, your treatment should begin with an injection of vitamin B$_{12}$ by a healthcare professional. Once your symptoms begin to improve, you need to take only 1,000–2,000 micrograms (1 or 2 milligrams) of vitamin B$_{12}$ a day to prevent recurrences of deficiency. Even if your body can no longer produce intrinsic factor, the 1 to 2 percent of the B$_{12}$ supplement actually absorbed is enough to prevent future problems. Lifetime injections are not necessary.

You should consider taking supplemental vitamin

B_{12} in a dosage of 3–30 micrograms a day if you take antibiotics, colchicine for gout, metformin for diabetes, or any medication for gastroesophageal reflux disease. Postmenopausal women who have breast cancer, children on macrobiotic diets, and people with HIV also benefit from supplemental B_{12} to prevent deficiency.

Vitamin C

Vitamin C is the best known and most widely used nutritional supplement. The Hungarian scientist Albert Szent-Györgi isolated a combination of vitamin C and "vitamin P," a collection of citrus bioflavonoids, he called anti-scurvy factors, and the American scientist Glen King later isolated the individual compound vitamin C. Szent-Györgi's Nobel Prize–winning discovery was not the discovery of vitamin C, but rather the discovery that vitamin C together with other plant cofactors correct the bleeding, dry eyes and mouth, muscle weakness, muscle pain, diarrhea, anorexia, frequent infections, and pulmonary problems associated with scurvy.

Vitamin C supports the healing process in conditions too numerous to mention. (See specific disease conditions throughout Part One of this book.)

It is important not to neglect fruit and vegetables when taking vitamin C to treat various health complaints. There is probably no upper limit to a safe dosage of vitamin C except for people who have hemochromatosis. But most people will experience diarrhea or nausea when taking more than 5,000 milligrams a day. With relatively few exceptions, 2,000 milligrams a day is enough vitamin C to influence the healing process.

Take vitamin C with caution if you take certain prescription drugs. Vitamin C taken in the form of vitamin C with bioflavonoids can interfere with the liver's ability to process statin drugs for controlling cholesterol, calcium channel blockers for hypertension such as nifedipine (Procardia), or cyclosporine for preventing transplant rejection. Rose hip vitamin C should not be taken by people with any allergy or sensitivity to rose hips.

People who take vitamin C for colds need to disregard the adage "Starve a fever, feed a cold," at least with regard to carbohydrates. Vitamin C is most effective in an alkaline environment. Diets high in carbohydrates and refined sugars produce acidity, so if you are going to take vitamin C, your best results will come if you also restrict sugars and refined carbohydrates.

Vitamin D

Vitamin D is a group of chemicals synthesized in the skin from cholesterol with the help of sunlight, and also found in food. Deficiencies of vitamin D can result from failure to get enough sun. Mild vitamin D deficiencies are common in active elderly persons who avoid the sun because of concerns about wrinkles or skin cancer. Severe vitamin D deficiencies are common among persons confined to nursing homes. Mild vitamin D deficiency can also result from being overweight. Subcutaneous fat absorbs the vitamin D made by the skin and keeps it from entering circulation.

Vitamin D increases calcium absorption and strengthens bone. Vitamin D supplements are important for people who have diseases of absorption, such as celiac disease, cystic fibrosis, and pancreatitis. Activated vitamin D is often helpful when prostate cancer has spread to the bones, as it reduces bone pain and preventing fractures. However, it can interfere with prescription medications for the condition and should be used under the supervision of a physician.

Whether the bacterium that causes Lyme disease is trapped or escapes, causing an infection, after the skin is broken by a tick bite depends in part on whether the skin has an adequate supply of vitamin D. Skin cells that have an adequate supply of vitamin D are better able to secrete an immune hormone known as interleukin-8 (IL-8), which signals to white blood cells that a bacterium has invaded the skin. Vitamin D continues to be important in fighting Lyme disease as the infection spreads beyond the skin, enabling cells in other tissues to send out an alarm to the immune system.

For most conditions, vitamin D is dosed at 400–1,000 IU per day, although treatment of fractures sometimes requires 2,000 IU per day or even more for a short time. Use of ketoconazole (the active ingredient in the antifungal drug Nizoral), phenytoin (Dilantin) for epilepsy, phenobarbitol for anxiety or insomnia, or colestipol or cholestyramine for high cholesterol reduce absorption of vitamin D and may call for supplementation.

Vitamin E

Vitamin E refers to a group of 8 antioxidants known as tocopherols. Low levels of vitamin E are associated with an increased risk of cardiovascular disease, and supplemental vitamin E is used to stop inflammatory processes contributing to dozens of diseases too numerous to mention here. (See specific disease conditions throughout Part One of this book.)

Effective daily doses of vitamin E range from 100–1,000 IU per day (1 milligram of vitamin E corresponds to 1½ international units, or IU). Vitamin E should not be taken at the same time as iron supplements, since iron can oxidize and deactivate the vitamin. Any fatty food or supplemental essential fatty acid taken at the same time as vitamin E increases absorption of the vitamin, and most medications used to lower cholesterol taken at the same time as vitamin E decreases absorption of the vitamin. In combination with prescription blood thinners such as Coumadin (warfarin), heparin, Plavix (clopidogrel), Ticlid (ticlopidine), Trental (pentoxifylline), or aspirin, vitamin E increases risk of bleeding. Always tell your doctor that you are taking vitamin E if you are prescribed any blood-thinning medication. Since vitamin E reduces clotting factors in the blood, be sure to inform your doctor that you take vitamin E before any surgical procedure.

Vitamin K

Vitamin K is essential to the body's production of clotting factors and also to the formation of bone. Since vitamin K is dissolved in fats in food, supplemental vitamin K is essential in any condition impairing the body's ability to absorb fats, such as celiac disease, cystic fibrosis, or pancreatitis. Supplemental vitamin K is also helpful in treating heavy periods and osteoporosis. Vitamin K is synthesized by bacteria in the intestine, so vitamin K levels go down during antibiotic treatment. However, taking vitamin K supplements as infrequently as every other week is usually sufficient.

A typical dosage of vitamin K is 5–10 milligrams, no more than twice a week except under medical advice. The Japanese soybean product natto is an excellent source of vitamin K for periods when vitamin tablets are not used. You should consider taking vitamin K supplements if you take more than 1,000 IU of vitamin E a day or if you take any medication for lowering cholesterol.

Vitex Agnus-Castus

Vitex agnus-castus, also known as chasteberry or chaste tree fruit, is a common herbal remedy for amenorrhea. The herb corrects "luteal phase defect," a condition in which the endometrium of the uterus fails to regrow after it is sloughed off. It also corrects abnormally high levels of prolactin. A small-scale clinical trial found that 10 out of 15 women began having normal periods after taking vitex for 6 months.

Typical dosages of vitex range from 40–100 milligrams per day. In rare cases, vitex can cause itching. Pregnant women should never take vitex, since it can cause miscarriage. Men should never take vitex, since it can cause testicular atrophy.

Whey Protein

Whey protein increases muscle mass and muscle strength when combined with resistance training. A study recently reported in the *International Journal of Sports Nutrition & Exercise Metabolism* found that use of whey supplements increases knee torsion, making the ligaments of the knee resistant to tearing. Dr. Marcus Elliot of the New England Patriots staff states that he believes that use of whey protein encourages the body's production of anabolic, muscle-building hormones.

There is no standard dosage of whey protein. Since whey protein is a food, the only limitations on its use are limitations on total calorie and protein intake and, in some individuals, lactose intolerance.

Willow Bark

Willow bark is a natural substitute for aspirin. It contains silicon, a less potent pain reliever than the salicylates found in aspirin that does not generally cause bleeding or stomach irritation. Use 1 teaspoon of willow bark in herbal teas or take capsules according to directions on the label. Do not use willow bark during pregnancy, if you have tinnitus (ringing in the ears), or if you are allergic to aspirin. Do not give willow bark or aspirin to children who have colds or flu.

Wobe-Mugos and Wobenzyme

Wobe-Mugos and **Wobenzyme** are proprietary products made with chymotrypsin and trypsin extracted from beef pancreas and papain derived from papaya. Wobenzyme also contains bromelain from pineapple and pancreatin from pork pancreas. Several clinical trials have found these products helpful in relieving arthritis pain and inflammation, particularly arthritis of the knee and periarthritis of the shoulder. Wobe-Mugos has also been used to relieve pain caused by shingles. Dosages vary by product. Overdoses may cause abdominal pain, diarrhea, nausea, or vomiting.

Zinc

Zinc is an essential element in human nutrition involved in more than 200 enzymes. Adequate levels of zinc are essential for fighting infection, but excessive use of supplemental zinc can actually weaken the immune system's response to bacterial infections.

Do not take more than 50 milligrams of any zinc supplement daily. The best-absorbed form of zinc is zinc picolinate. If you take tetracycline antibiotics for skin infections, chances are you are deficient in zinc. Taking tetracycline interferes with the body's absorption of zinc (and taking zinc interferes with the body's absorption of tetracycline).

A quick method for detecting zinc deficiency is a taste test. Crush a tablet to powder of any zinc-based supplement or cold medication and mix with ¼ cup (50 milliliters) of water. Slosh the mixture around in the mouth. People who notice no taste at all or who notice a "dry," "mineral," or "sweet" taste are likely to be zinc-deficient. Anyone who notices a definite strong and unpleasant taste that intensifies over time is not likely to be zinc deficient.

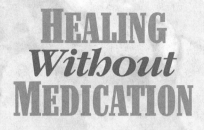

HEALING
Without
MEDICATION

Part Three

Healing Partners

INTERACTION GUIDE

Healing without medication is possible for many conditions, but an overwhelming majority of people in the developed world choose to take both prescription medications and natural supplements. In this part, you will find a partial summary of known and potential interactions between herbs, vitamins, minerals, and other nutritional supplements and commonly prescribed prescription drugs.

The study of interactions between prescription drugs and nutritional supplements is far from an exact science. When multiple medications and/or multiple supplements are taken, multiple interactions—sometimes offsetting one another—are possible. Relatively few interactions between medications and supplements are known to a high degree of certainty:

• Taking St. John's wort while taking the antirejection drug cyclosporine can lead to tissue rejection.

• Chewing betel nut when taking the schizophrenia drug fluphenazine greatly increases the side effects of the drug.

• Kava increases the number and duration of "off periods" for people with Parkinson's disease taking L-dopa.

• Siberian ginseng increases the toxicity of digoxin (Lanoxin), and either dan shen or dong quai can increase the risk of bleeding when taken with warfarin (Coumadin).

These are the best-documented interactions in the medical literature. Other detrimental interactions are more or less speculative, but it is always best to err on the side of caution.

In many cases, prescription drugs deplete the body's supply of specific nutrients. These nutrients can be replaced by taking supplements. If you see the word "depletes" after the name of a medication in the following table, you can benefit from taking the nutrient in supplemental form. In some cases, taking a specific mineral, vitamin, herb, or other nutritional supplement can interfere with the action of a prescription drug. In these cases, you should take either the prescription medication or the supplement, but not both. In a few cases, a prescription drug can increase the body's supply of a nutrient. Most important, many drugs work better if you take specific herbs, vitamins, minerals, or other supplements. For more than 100 medications, supplements can help you heal faster while you take the drugs your doctor prescribes.

Note: This chart does not represent an exhaustive list of available medications. When taking medication, prescription or otherwise, always check with your pharmacist or heathcare practitioner for possible side effects and interactions with other substances.

Medication	Interaction(s)
3TC	See lamivudine.
5-FU	See fluorouracil.
Abciximab	Asian ginseng, arnica, astragalus, bilberry, coleus, dan shen, devil's claw, dong quai, feverfew, garlic, ginger, ginkgo, green tea, horse chestnut, and quinine may increase risk of bruising, bleeding, or hemorrhage if taken with this drug.
	High doses (more than 500 milligrams daily) of the form of vitamin E known as alpha-tocopherol polyethylene glycol succinate (TPGS) may increase risk of bleeding.
	Borage seed oil, especially if taken with fish oil, may increase risk of bleeding or bruising if taken with this drug.
	Bromelain may increase anticlotting effect. Taking this drug with bromelain may increase risk of bleeding and brusing.
	Tiratricol (TRIAC) may interfere with accurate blood tests for PT (prothrombin time) when taken with this drug.
	Curcuminoids may increase anticlotting effect.
	Gamma-tocopherol may increase anticlotting effect.
	Ganoderma mushroom may increase anticlotting effect.
	Green catechins (although not beverage green tea) may increase anticlotting effect.
acarbose	Amylase, pancreatin, and pancrelipase (digestive enzymes) may make this drug less effective.
	Inositol nicotinate may make this drug less effective.
	Niacin may make this drug less effective.
Accupril	See ACE inhibitors.
Accutane	See isotretinoin.
ACE Inhibitors	These blood pressure medications may deplete zinc. If you take an ACE inhibitor, take 15 milligrams of zinc gluconate or 25 milligrams of zinc picolinate daily, preferably in a formula that also contains copper.
	Do not take ACE inhibitors with potassium supplements or salt substitutes that contain potassium (CardiaSalt, Morton's); potentially life-threatening hyperkalemia may result.
	All ACE inhibitors increase risk of sunburn when they are first used. Taking European angelica, dong quai, psoralea, or St. John's wort with an ACE inhibitor increases risk of sunburn caused by the herb.
acebutolol	Pleurisy root may unpredictably enhance effects of this drug.
Aceon	Taking European angelica, psoralea, or St. John's wort with this drug increases risk of sunburn.
	Taking supplemental potassium with this drug can cause potentially life-threatening hyperkalemia (excessive potassium in the bloodstream).
Acephen	See acetaminophen.
Acetamin	See acetaminophen.
acetaminophen	Do not take L-methionine or molybdenum with this pain reliever if you have liver disease or if you take any prescription drug that can cause liver problems, especially seizure medications and statin drugs for lowering cholesterol.
	Milk thistle, N-acetyl cysteine (NAC), or schisandra may prevent toxic effects of acetaminophen to the liver, especially in children.
	Vitamin C increases the length of time acetaminophen stays in the body, enhancing both its analgesic and toxic effects.

Medication	Interaction(s)
	Also see NSAIDs.
acetohexamide	Doses of niacin in excess of 20 milligrams per day may make this drug ineffective.
acitretin	Taking this drug with vitamin A may cause toxic side effects.
Aclovate topical	See topical corticosteroids.
Actimmune	See interferon.
Actos	Doses of niacin in excess of 20 milligrams per day may make this drug ineffective.
	Glucosamine may make any diabetes drug less effective by increasing insulin resistance.
Acutrim	Regular (not decaf) coffee and tea, yohimbe, ephedra, or guaraná taken with this drug may cause high blood pressure.
Adalat	Ipriflavone can cause buildup of this drug in the bloodstream resulting in unusually low blood pressure (dizziness, fainting, light-headedness).
	Pleurisy root or tobacco reduces the effectiveness of this drug in treating angina.
	This drug makes aloe, buckthorn, cascara sagrada, frangula, rhubarb root, and senna less effective in relieving constipation.
Adapin	See doxepin and tricyclic antidepressants.
Adderall	See dextroamphetamine.
adrenaline (epinephrine)	Caffeine or ephedra may cause excessively high blood pressure when used with this drug.
	Coleus may add to the effects of adrenaline in opening airways unpredictably. Do not take coleus or forskolin if you carry adrenaline for emergency treatments of allergies.
Adriamycin	See doxorubicin.
Adrucil	See fluorouracil.
Advil	See NSAIDs.
Advil Children's	See NSAIDs.
Aeroseb-Dex topical	See topical corticosteroids.
Ala-Tet	See tetracycline antibiotics.
alclometasone topical	See topical corticosteroids.
alcoholic beverages	Inositol nicotinate and niacin increase redness in the face after drinking alcohol.
	Soy isoflavones, especially daidzein, increase absorption of alcohol into the bloodstream and may increase blood alcohol levels above what would be ordinarily expected.
alendronate	Calcium supplements, iron supplements, and magnesium supplements reduce absorption of this drug if taken within 2 hours of taking this drug.
	Ipriflavone increases effectiveness of this drug.
Alesse	See oral contraceptives.
Alferon N	See interferon.
alprazolam	Chamomile, kava, or melatonin increases sedative effect of this drug.
Altace	See ACE inhibitors.
Alti-Desipramine	See tricyclic antidepressants.
Alti-Doxepin	See tricyclic antidepressants.
Amaryl	Doses of niacin in excess of 20 milligrams per day may make this drug ineffective.
	Glucosamine may make any diabetes drug less effective by increasing insulin resistance.
Ambien	See zolpidem.
Amerge	Taking this drug with 5-HTP may cause headaches and/or excitement.
Amficot	See ampicillin.
Amicrobin	See norfloxacin.

Medication	Interaction(s)
amiodarone	Arnica may cause irregular heartbeat when taken with this drug (prolonged QT interval). Side effects may be worsened by homeopathic arnica.
	Vitamin B_6 may increase sensitivity to sunburn when taken with this drug.
	Vitamin E may relieve side effects of this drug on lung tissue.
	Grapefruit juice, quercetin, or rutin (as well as herbs containing rutin, such as barley leaf and Scotch broom) increase the concentration of this drug in the bloodstream and may make its side effects much worse.
amitriptyline	5-HTP may increase side effects of this drug.
	B vitamins may help elderly people think more clearly while taking this drug.
	Brewer's yeast, ephedra, and Scotch broom increase blood pressure when taken with this drug.
	Ginseng may cause headaches or mania when taken with this drug.
	Black and green tea may interfere with the body's absorption of this drug.
	Coenzyme Q_{10} may reduce detrimental effects of this drug on heart function.
	SAM-e helps this drug bring relief from depression sooner.
	St. John's wort may cause excessive accumulation of this drug in the bloodstream. St. John's wort should not be taken with this drug.
	Side effects may be worsened by homeopathic arnica.
amlodipine	Grapefruit juice, quercetin, or rutin (as well as herbs containing rutin, such as barley leaf and Scotch broom) may increase the body's retention of this drug and cause unusually low blood pressure.
	Pleurisy root may increase the effects of this drug in unpredictable ways.
Amnivent	See theophylline.
amoxapine	See tricyclic antidepressants.
amoxicillin	Bromelain increases concentration of this antibiotic in the bloodstream. Also see penicillins.
amoxil	See penicillins.
ampicillin	Depletes vitamin C and vitamin K.
	Probiotics such as *Acidophilus* and *Lactobacillus* stop diarrhea caused by using this antibiotic.
	Khat (an herb that is chewed, available in some Middle Eastern speciality shops) interferes with the body's absorption of this antibiotic.
	Also see penicillins.
Anaguard	See adrenaline.
anastrozole	Chrysin may enhance the effectiveness of this drug and its side effects.
Anquin	See norfloxacin.
Ansaid	See NSAIDs.
antacids (general)	Do not take calcium citrate (other calcium supplements are OK) within 2 hours of taking this drug; increases absorption of aluminum.
	Do not drink more than 8 ounces (1 cup) of any citrus juice within 2 hours of taking this drug.
	This drug may interfere with calcium absorption
	Use Milk of Magnesia or Tums instead of Di-Gel, Maalox, or Riopan if you have osteoporosis.
Anthra-derm	See anthralin.
Anthraforte	See anthralin.
anthralin	Vitamin E reduces skin irritation caused by this drug.
Anthranol	See anthralin.
Anthrascalp	See anthralin.

Medication	Interaction(s)
antibiotics (general)	Decrease availability of vitamin K. Supplementing the vitamin once or twice a week is sufficient.
anticonvulsants	Deplete biotin, calcium, L-carnitine, and vitamins A, B_{12}, B_6, D, and K.
	Depletes folic acid, but supplemental folic acid can either increase or decrease number of seizures.
	Evening primrose oil (EPO) may lower the threshold for seizures; that is, smaller environmental triggers may result in seizures if EPO is taken.
antihistamines (general)	L-histidine may decrease effectiveness of antihistamine.
	Melatonin may increase daytime drowsiness if taken with these drugs.
Apacet	See acetaminophen.
Apo-Amitriptyline	See tricyclic antidepressants.
Apo-Ampi	See ampicillin.
Apo-Carbamazepine	See anticonvulsants.
Apo-Chlorthalidone	See hydrochlorothiazide.
Apo-Doxepin	See tricyclic antidepressants.
Apo-Gemfibrozil	See gemfibrozil.
Apo-Hydralazine	See hydralazine.
Apo-Hydro	See hydrochlorothiazide.
Apo-Primidone	See anticonvulsants.
Apo-Theo	See theophylline.
Apresoline	See hydralazine.
Aricept	See donepezil HCl.
Arimidex	See anastrozole.
Aristocort topical	See topical corticosteroids.
Asendin	See tricyclic antidepressants.
aspirin	Asian ginseng, arnica, astragalus, bilberry, coleus, dan shen, devil's claw, dong quai, feverfew, garlic, ginger, ginkgo, green tea, horse chestnut, and quinine may increase risk of bruising, bleeding, or hemorrhage if taken by people who use this drug daily.
	High doses (more than 500 milligrams daily) of the form of vitamin E known as alpha-tocopherol polyethylene glycol succinate (TPGS) may increase risk of bleeding if taken with this drug.
	Borage seed oil, especially if taken with fish oil, may increase risk of bleeding or bruising if taken with this drug.
	Bromelain may increase anticlotting effect. Taking this drug with bromelain may increase risk of bleeding and bruising.
	Tiratricol (TRIAC) may interfere with accurate blood tests for PT (prothrombin time) if taken by people who use this drug daily.
	Cayenne decreases analgesic effect of this drug.
	Curcuminoids may increase anticlotting effect.
	DGL (deglycyrrhizinated licorice) may reduce stomach irritation caused by this drug.
	Gamma-tocopherol may increase anticlotting effect.
	Ganoderma mushroom may increase anticlotting effect.
	Green catechins (although not beverage green tea) may increase anticlotting effect.
	Glycol succinate may increase risk of bleeding.
	Evening primrose oil (EPO) may increase risk of bleeding.
	Hempseed oil may increase susceptibility to bruising.
	Reduces risk of redness in the face (flushing) after taking inositol.

Medication	Interaction(s)
	Perilla oil may increase risk of bleeding.
	Large doses of aspirin may cause vitamin C deficiency.
	May deplete melatonin.
Aspirin Free Anacin	See acetaminophen.
Aspirin Free Pain Relief Children's Pain Reliever	See acetaminophen.
asthmahaler	See adrenaline.
asthma inhalers (general)	If the dose of medication from the inhaler is mostly swallowed rather than inhaled, calcium deficiency may result over time. Calcium supplementation counteracts deficiency.
Asthmolase	See atropine.
atenolol	May deplete melatonin.
	Taking chromium from brewer's yeast may raise HDL ("good") cholesterol levels in people who take this drug.
Ativan	Chamomile, kava, or melatonin may increase sedative effect of this drug.
atorvastatin	Magnesium supplements and antacids containing magnesium should not be taken within 2 hours of taking this drug.
	Depletes CoQ_{10}.
	Increases vitamin A levels in the bloodstream. If you take vitamin A and this medication, have a doctor monitor vitamin A levels for you to prevent toxicity.
	Inositol nicotinate may increase effectiveness of this drug and also increase risk of muscle damage.
Atretol	See carbamazepine.
atropine	Black tea, green tea, raspberry leaf, uva ursi, and witch hazel interfere with absorption of this drug if taken by mouth.
Avandia	Doses of niacin in excess of 20 milligrams per day may make this drug ineffective.
	Glucosamine may make any diabetes drug less effective by increasing insulin resistance.
Avelox	See moxifloxacin.
Avonex	See interferon.
Axid	Reduces body's absorption of calcium.
AZT	Depletes vitamin B_{12}.
	L-carnitine may reduce muscle damage caused by this drug.
	N-acetyl cysteine (NAC) may reduce toxicity of this drug.
	Riboflavin may reverse fatty liver or lactic acidosis caused by this drug.
	Zinc may increase body weight, increase CD4+ levels, and help prevent *Pneumocystis carinii* pneumonia if taken with this drug.
Azulfidine	See sulfasalazine.
bacampicillin	See penicillins.
Baccidal	See norfloxacin.
baclofen	Glycine may increase relaxant effect of this drug.
Bactocil	See penicillins.
Barazan	See norfloxacin.
Baycip	See ciprofloxacin.
Bayer Select Pain Relief Formula	See NSAIDs.
Beepen-VK	See penicillins.

Medication	Interaction(s)
benazepril	See ACE inhibitors.
Betaferon	See interferon.
betamethasone topical	See topical corticosteroids.
Betaseron	See interferon.
betaxolol	May deplete melatonin.
	Taking chromium from brewer's yeast may raise HDL ("good") cholesterol levels in people who take this drug.
Bicillin C-R	See penicillins.
Biofloxin	See norfloxacin.
Bio-Tab	See tetracycline antibiotics.
bismuth subsalicylate	Sarsaparilla may cause toxic side effects when taken with this drug.
bleomycin	Taurine may reduce toxicity to the lungs.
Brevicon	See oral contraceptives.
Bronkaid	See adrenaline.
Brontin	See adrenaline.
bumetanide	Depletes thiamine.
bupropion	Yohimbe may increase effects of this drug.
Cafcit	See caffeine.
Caffedrine	See caffeine.
caffeine	May deplete calcium.
	Ephedra and guraná may cause nervous agitation when taken with this drug.
Calciparine	See heparin.
Capoten	See ACE inhibitors.
captopril	See ACE inhibitors.
carbamazepine	Acetyl-L-carnitine, ascorbyl palmitate, or citrus bioflavonoids may increase concentration of this drug in the bloodstream.
	Depletes biotin, especially in women.
	Depletes folic acid and raises homocysteine levels (factor in heart disease).
	Depletes useful form of vitamin B_6 known as pyridoxal-5'-phosphate.
	Use of psyllium fiber products reduces absorption of this drug.
	N-acetyl cysteine (NAC) interferes with the action of this drug.
	Also see anticonvulsants.
Carbatrol	See carbamazepine.
carbenicillin	See penicillins.
Carbex	See selegiline.
carbidopa	Iron supplements interfere with this drug.
	Octacosanol reduces effectiveness of this drug in treating Parkinson's disease.
	Taking this drug with 5-HTP may cause headaches and/or excitement.
Cardura	Taking inositol, niacin, or saw palmetto may cause unusually low blood pressure.
carvedilol	May deplete melatonin.
	Taking chromium from brewer's yeast may raise HDL ("good") cholesterol levels in people who take this drug.
Catapres	Taking inositol, niacin, or saw palmetto may cause unusually low blood pressure.

Medication	Interaction(s)
Celebrex	See celecoxib.
celecoxib	Willow bark taken with this drug may cause stomach upset or aggravate peptic ulcer disease.
Cerebrovase	Asian ginseng, arnica, astragalus, bilberry, dan shen, devil's claw, dong quai, feverfew, garlic, ginger, ginkgo, green tea, horse chestnut, and quinine may increase risk of bruising, bleeding, or hemorrhage if taken with this drug.
	High doses (more than 500 milligrams daily) of the form of vitamin E known as alpha-tocopherol polyethylene glycol succinate (TPGS) may increase risk of bleeding.
Cerebyx	See Fosphenytoin.
Cetraxal	See Ciprofloxacin.
chlordiazepoxide	Chamomile, kava, or melatonin increases the sedative effect of this drug.
chlorothiazide	See hydrochlorothiazide.
chlorpromazine	Side effects may be worsened by homeopathic arnica.
	Taking borage seed oil may cause various kinds of seizures, including partial seizures mimicking mental illness.
chlorpropamide	Doses of niacin in excess of 20 milligrams per day may make this drug ineffective.
chlorthalidone	See hydrochlorothiazide.
chlorzoxazone	Garlic taken as a supplement or eaten as a food, broccoli, Brussels sprouts, cabbage, and kale interfere with the body's ability to break down this drug.
	Coffee, tea, and guaraná are more likely to cause insomnia or nervousness when taking this drug.
cholestyramine	Reduces body's absorption of beta-carotene, folic acid, gamma-tocopherol, inositol, lutein, lycopene, niacin, riboflavin, vitamin A, vitamin B_{12}, vitamin D, vitamin E, and vitamin K.
	Taking this drug at same time as beta-carotene reduces absorption of beta-carotene.
Ciflox	See ciprofloxacin.
Cifran	See ciprofloxacin.
Cimetidine	DGL (deglycyrrhizinated licorice) increases effectiveness of this drug in relieving stomach upset caused by aspirin.
	Reduces vitamin B_{12} absorption from food.
	Reduces body's absorption of calcium.
	Taking magnesium supplements within 2 hours of taking this drug reduces absorption of this drug.
	Taking this drug at the same time as calcium supplements may reduce absorption of calcium.
Ciplox	See ciprofloxacin.
Cipro	See ciprofloxacin.
ciprofloxacin	Calcium, iron, magnesium, quercetin, or rutin (as well as herbs containing rutin, such as barley leaf and Scotch broom) interfere with the body's absorption of this antibiotic.
	Slows the body's elimination of caffeine; increases detrimental effects of caffeine.
	Taking this drug at same time as calcium supplements may reduce absorption of this drug.
cisapride	Menthol and peppermint interfere with the action of this drug.
cisplatin	Citrus bioflavonoids, beverage grapefruit juice, and quercetin may cause genetic damage in non-cancerous tissues if taken with this drug.
	Milk thistle may reduce toxicity and increase effectiveness of this form of chemotherapy.
	Very high doses of melatonin (20 milligrams, an amount that should be taken only under a doctor's supervision) have reduced the toxicity of chemotherapy with cisplatin plus fluorouracil.
	Very high doses of selenium (4,000 micrograms per day, an amount that should be taken only under a doctor's supervision) have prevented kidney damage by this drug.

Medication	Interaction(s)
cisplatin (cont.)	Vitamin E applied to sores in the mouth caused by this form of chemotherapy helps them heal more rapidly.
clavulanate	See penicillins.
Clobetasol topical	See topical cortisteroids.
Clocortolone pivalate topical	See topical corticosteroids.
Cloderm topical	See topical corticosteroids.
clonazepam	Chamomile, kava, or melatonin increases sedative effect of this drug.
clonidine	Taking inositol or niacin with this drug may cause unusually low blood pressure.
clopidogrel	Asian ginseng, arnica, astragalus, bilberry, coleus, dan shen, devil's claw, dong quai, feverfew, garlic, ginger, ginkgo, green tea, horse chestnut, and quinine may increase risk of bruising, bleeding, or hemorrhage if taken with this drug.
	High doses (more than 500 milligrams daily) of the form of vitamin E known as alpha-tocopherol polyethylene glycol succinate (TPGS) may increase risk of bleeding.
	Borage seed oil, especially if taken with fish oil, may increase risk of bleeding or bruising if taken with this drug.
	Bromelain may increase anticlotting effect of this drug.
	Tiratricol may interfere with accurate blood tests for PT (prothrombin time).
	Curcuminoids may increase anticlotting effect of this drug.
	Gamma-tocopherol may increase anticlotting effect of this drug.
	Ganoderma mushroom may increase anticlotting effect of this drug.
	Green catechins (although not beverage green tea) may increase anticlotting effect of this drug.
Clopra	Depletes riboflavin.
clorazepate dipotassium	Chamomile, kava, or melatonin increases sedative effects of this drug.
clotrimazole	In rare cases, taking this drug with red yeast rice can cause muscle damage.
Cloxapen	See penicillins.
codeine	Black tea, green tea, raspberry leaf, and uva ursi interfere with absorption of this drug.
Cognex	See tacrine HCl.
colchicine	Reduces body's absorption of folic acid and vitamin B_{12}.
colestipol, Colestid	Reduces body's absorption of beta-carotene, folic acid, gamma-tocopherol, inositol, lutein, lycopene, niacin, riboflavin, vitamin A, vitamin B_{12}, vitamin D, vitamin E, and vitamin K.
	Taking this drug at same time as beta-carotene reduces absorption of beta-carotene.
conjugated estrogens	Deplete vitamin B_6.
	Calcium, ipriflavone, and vitamin D enhance benefits of this drug.
	Red clover and soy isoflavones interfere with absorption of this drug.
Cordarone	See amiodarone.
Coreg	Taking chromium from brewer's yeast may raise HDL ("good") cholesterol levels in people who take this drug.
Cortef topical	See topical corticosteroids.
Cortizone topical	See topical corticosteroids.
Cortone topical	See topical corticosteroids.
Coumadin	Asian ginseng, arnica, astragalus, bilberry, coleus, dan shen, devil's claw, dong quai, feverfew, garlic, ginger, ginkgo, green tea, horse chestnut, and quinine may increase risk of bruising, bleeding, or hemorrhage if taken with this drug.

Medication	Interaction(s)
Coumadin (cont.)	Broccoli, Brussels sprouts, cabbage, kale, onions, parsley, soy, and spinach may increase risk of bruising, bleeding, or hemorrhage if eaten in unusually large quantities when taking this drug.
	Reishi and St. John's wort decrease the effectiveness of this drug.
	Taking more than 500 milligrams a day of the form of vitamin E known as alpha-tocopherol polyethylene glycol succinate (TPGS) may increase risk of bleeding.
	This drug interferes with the absorption of iron, magnesium, and zinc. Do not take supplements of these minerals within 2 hours of taking this drug.
	Borage seed oil, especially if taken with fish oil, may increase risk of bleeding or bruising if taken with this drug.
	Niacin may increase risk of bleeding and bruising.
	Taking this drug with bromelain may increase risk of bleeding and bruising.
	Vitamin K in chlorella may increase risk of bleeding or bruising.
cream of magnesia	See magnesium hydroxide.
Crixivan	St. John's wort lowers bloodstream concentrations of this drug.
Cutivate topical	See topical corticosteroids.
Cycloserine	Interferes with absorption of B vitamins, calcium, and magnesium.
cyclosporine	Ascorbyl palmitate or citrus bioflavonoids may increase concentration of this drug in the bloodstream.
	Astragalus and *Echinacea angustifolia* (although not *Echinacea purpurea*) may make this drug less effective.
	Borage seed oil, especially if taken with fish oil, may increase risk of bleeding or bruising if taken with this drug.
	Coleus or ginkgo may increase risk of bleeding, bruising, and internal hemorrhage when taken with this drug.
	Grapefruit juice, but not other citrus juices, interferes with the body's elimination of this drug.
	L-arginine may counteract bloating and fluid retention.
	Red yeast rice may increase risk of muscle damage.
	St. John's wort lowers the amount of available cyclosporine in the bloodstream.
	Vitamin E may protect kidneys from side effects of this drug.
	Taking this drug with bromelain may increase risk of bleeding and bruising.
	The form of vitamin E known as alpha-tocopherol polyethylene glycol succinate (TPGS) may decrease absorption if taken at the same time.
Cyprobay	See ciprofloxacin.
cyproheptadine HCl	5-HTP may make this drug less effective.
d4T	Depletes vitamin B_{12}.
	L-carnitine may reduce muscle damage caused by this drug.
	N-acetyl cysteine (NAC) may reduce toxicity of this drug.
	Riboflavin may reverse fatty liver or lactic acidosis caused by this drug.
	Zinc may increase body weight, increase CD4+ levels, and help prevent *Pneumocystis carinii* pneumonia if taken with this drug.
Daktarin	In rare cases, taking this drug with red yeast rice can cause muscle damage.
Dalmane	Chamomile, kava, or melatonin may increase sedative effect of this drug.
dantrolene sodium	Glycine may make this drug less effective.
Dapacin	See acetaminophen.
Dapsone	Black pepper or piperine may inhibit body's use and excretion of this drug.

Medication	Interaction(s)
DayQuil	See phenylpropanolamine.
ddI (didanosine)	Depletes vitamin B_{12}.
	L-carnitine may reduce muscle damage caused by this drug.
	N-acetyl cysteine (NAC) may reduce toxicity of this drug.
	Riboflavin may reverse fatty liver or lactic acidosis caused by this drug.
	Zinc may increase body weight, increase CD4+ levels, and help prevent *Pneumocystis carinii* pneumonia if taken with this drug.
Decadron topical	See topical corticosteroids.
Decaspray topical	See topical corticosteroids.
Demeclocycline	See tetracycline antibiotics.
Demulen (various)	See oral contraceptives.
Depakene, Depakote	Depletes carnitine. Supplemental *acetyl-L-*carnitine is recommended.
Deponit	See nitrates, nitroglycerin.
Derma-Smoothe/FS topical	See topical corticosteroids.
Deseryl	Artemisia and wormwood increase risk of seizures when taken with this drug.
desipramine	See tricyclic antidepressants.
Desogen	See oral contraceptives.
desoximetasone topical	See topical corticosteroids.
dexamethasone topical	See topical corticosteroids.
Dexatrim	Regular (not decaf) coffee and tea, yohimbe, ephedra, or guraná taken with this drug may cause high blood pressure.
dextroamphetamine	Alcohol makes the heart work harder when taken with this drug. People who have heart problems should not drink alcohol if taking dextroamphetamine.
	Magnesium may prolong the circulation of this drug through the bloodstream, making it more effective in treating ADD and ADHD but also increasing its side effects.
	Lithium (found in some mineral supplements) interferes with the brain's use of this drug.
	L-tyrosine deficiency may make this drug less effective.
	Pycnogenol may increase effectiveness of this drug in treating ADD and ADHD.
	Taking vitamin C or drinking fruit juices within 2 hours of taking this drug may interfere with its absorption into the body.
	Vitamin B_6 may help reduce obsessive-compulsive behaviors in people on this drug.
Diabeta	Doses of niacin in excess of 20 milligrams per day may make this drug ineffective.
	Glucosamine may make any diabetes drug less effective by increasing insulin resistance.
diabetes drugs (general)	Glucosamine may make any diabetes drug less effective by increasing insulin resistance.
Diabinese	Doses of niacin in excess of 20 milligrams per day may make this drug ineffective.
	Glucosamine may make any diabetes drug less effective by increasing insulin resistance.
diazepam	Glycine may increase effects of this drug.
	Chamomile, kava, or melatonin may increase sedative effect of this drug.
Dicloxacillin	See penicillins.
didanosine	Depletes L-carnitine.
	Riboflavin may reverse lactic acidosis caused by this drug.
	Depletes vitamin B_{12}.

Medication	Interaction(s)
didanosine (cont.)	L-carnitine may reduce muscle damage caused by this drug.
	N-acetyl cysteine (NAC) may reduce toxicity of this drug.
	Riboflavin may reverse fatty liver or lactic acidosis caused by this drug.
	Zinc may help increase body weight, increase CD4+ levels, and prevent *Pneumocystis carinii* pneumonia if taken with this drug.
Di-Gel	See antacids.
digoxin, digitalis	Aloe used as a laxative, buckthorn, cascara sagrada, frangula, guaraná, licorice, rhubarb root, and senna (Senekot) deplete potassium when used with this drug. The combination can cause fatigue and irregular heartbeats.
	Extreme low-salt diets can cause toxicity of this drug.
	Rauwolfia can cause severely slowed heartbeat when taken with this drug.
	Siberian ginseng (eleuthero) increses toxicity of this drug.
	Uzara increases the toxicity of this drug.
dihydrochlorothiazide	See hydrochlorothiazide.
Dilantin	See anticonvulsants.
Dimetapp	See phenylpropanolamine.
Diprolene topical	See topical corticosteroids.
dipyridamide	Borage seed oil, especially if taken with fish oil, may increase risk of bleeding or bruising if taken with this drug.
	Bromelain may increase anticlotting effect.
	Tiratricol may interfere with accurate blood tests for PT (prothrombin time).
	Coleus or ginkgo may increase risk of bleeding, bruising, and internal hemorrhage when taken with this drug.
	Curcuminoids may increase anticlotting effect.
	Gamma-tocopherol may increase anticlotting effect.
	Ganoderma mushroom may increase anticlotting effect.
	Green catechins (although not beverage green tea) may increase anticlotting effect.
	Taking this drug with bromelain may increase risk of bleeding and bruising.
dipyridamole	Asian ginseng, arnica, astragalus, bilberry, dan shen, devil's claw, dong quai, feverfew, garlic, ginger, ginkgo, green tea, horse chestnut, and quinine may increase risk of bruising, bleeding, or hemorrhage if taken with this drug.
	High doses (more than 500 milligrams daily) of the form of vitamin E known as alpha-tocopherol polyethylene glycol succinate (TPGS) may increase risk of bleeding.
disopyramide	Side effects of this drug may be worsened by homeopathic arnica.
dithranol	See anthralin.
Diuril	See hydrochlorothiazide.
DMSO (dimethyl sulfoxide)	Sulindac may increase side effects of DMSO
Domical	See tricyclic antidepressants.
Donepezil HCl	Huperzine A may increase both the effectiveness of this drug and the severity of its side effects.
Doral	Grapefruit juice, quercetin, or rutin (as well as herbs containing rutin, such as barley leaf and Scotch broom) drastically increase concentration of this drug in the bloodstream and intensify its side effects.
	Chamomile, kava, or melatonin increases sedative effects of this drug.
Doryx	See tetracycline antibiotics.

628

Medication	Interaction(s)
Doxepin	Side effects may be worsened by homeopathic arnica.
	5-HTP may increase side effects of this drug.
	B vitamins may help elderly people think more clearly while taking this drug.
	Brewer's yeast, ephedra, and Scotch broom increase blood pressure when taken with this drug.
	Ginseng may cause headaches or mania when taken with this drug.
	Black and green tea may interfere with the body's absorption of this drug.
	Coenzyme Q$_{10}$ may reduce detrimental effects of this drug on heart function.
	SAM-e helps this drug bring relief from depression sooner.
	St. John's wort may cause excessive accumulation of this drug in the bloodstream. St. John's wort should not be taken with this drug.
doxorubicin	Ascorbyl palmitate, citrus bioflavonoids, or vitamin C may increase effect against cancer.
	L-carnitine may prevent toxic effects of this drug.
	Taking coenzyme Q$_{10}$ before taking this drug may reduce risk of heart damage.
	High doses of melatonin (20 milligrams per day) and vitamin E (1,600 IU per day) have decreased toxicity and increased cancer-fighting ability of this drug. Some people have found that vitamin E helps prevent hair loss while on this form of chemotherapy.
	Depletes riboflavin.
	Animal studies suggest taking vitamin C may help prevent damage to the heart caused by this drug.
	Milk thistle may reduce toxicity and increase effectiveness of this form of chemotherapy.
Doxychel Hyclate	See tetracycline antibiotics.
doxycycline	See tetracycline antibiotics.
Doxy-Tabs	See tetracycline antibiotics.
drithocreme	See anthralin.
Drixoral	Black tea, black walnut, green tea, oak bark, raspberry leaf, uva ursi, and witch hazel contain tannins that interfere with the body's absorption of this drug.
	Coleus and ephedra may cause unpredictable side effects of this drug.
Dymelor	Doses of niacin in excess of 20 milligrams per day may make this drug ineffective.
Dynacin	See tetracycline antibiotics.
Dynafed	See acetaminophen.
Eco-Derm	In rare cases, taking this drug with red yeast rice can cause muscle damage.
econazole	In rare cases, taking this drug with red yeast rice can cause muscle damage.
Efudex	See fluorouracil.
Elavil	5-HTP may increase side effects of this drug.
	B vitamins may help elderly people think more clearly while taking this drug.
	Brewer's yeast, ephedra, and Scotch broom increase blood pressure when taken with this drug.
	Ginseng may cause headaches or mania when taken with this drug.
	Black and green tea may interfere with the body's absorption of this drug.
	Coenzyme Q$_{10}$ may reduce detrimental effects of this drug on heart function.
	SAM-e helps this drug bring relief from depression sooner.
	St. John's wort may cause excessive accumulation of this drug in the bloodstream. St. John's wort should not be taken with this drug.
Eldepryl	See selegiline.
Elocon topical	See topical corticosteroids.
Eltroxin	Calcium and iron supplements decrease body's absorption of this drug.

Medication	Interaction(s)
Emfib	See gemfibrozil.
Enalapril	See ACE inhibitors.
Enerjets	See caffeine.
enoxacin	Calcium, iron, magnesium, quercetin, or rutin (as well as herbs containing rutin, such as barley leaf and Scotch broom) interfere with the body's absorption of this antibiotic.
Epanutin	See anticonvulsants.
ephedrine *and* pseudoephedrine	Black tea, black walnut, green tea, oak bark, raspberry leaf, uva ursi, and witch hazel contain tannins that interfere with the body's absorption of this drug.
	Coleus and ephedra may cause unpredictable side effects of this drug.
eptifibatide	Asian ginseng, arnica, astragalus, bilberry, coleus, dan shen, devil's claw, dong quai, feverfew, garlic, ginger, ginkgo, green tea, horse chestnut, and quinine may increase risk of bruising, bleeding, or hemorrhage if taken with this drug.
	High doses (more than 500 milligrams daily) of the form of vitamin E known as alpha-tocopherol polyethylene glycol succinate (TPGS) may increase risk of bleeding.
	Borage seed oil, especially if taken with fish oil, may increase risk of bleeding or bruising if taken with this drug.
	Bromelain may increase anticlotting effect. Taking this drug with bromelain may increase risk of bleeding and bruising.
	Tiratricol may interfere with accurate blood tests for PT (prothrombin time).
	Curcuminoids may increase anticlotting effect.
	Gamma-tocopherol may increase anticlotting effect.
	Ganoderma mushroom may increase anticlotting effect.
	Green catechins (although not beverage green tea) may increase anticlotting effect.
Epifrin	See adrenaline.
Epitol	See anticonvulsants.
Epitrol	See carbamazepine.
Epivir	See lamivudine.
Eppy/N	See adrenaline.
Esidrix	See hydrochlorothiazide.
Eskalith	See lithium.
estazolam	Chamomile and melatonin both increase sedative effects of this drug.
estrogen replacement therapies	Ascorbyl palmitate may further lower LDL ("bad") cholesterol.
	Ipriflavone increases effectiveness of estrogen in preventing bone loss.
	Vitamin C may further lower LDL ("bad") cholesterol.
	Senna (Senekot) decreases estrogen levels when taken with these drugs.
Estrostep	See oral contraceptives.
etidronate	Taking this drug at the same time as calcium supplements may reduce absorption of this drug
Evista	See raloxifene.
famotidine	Taking this drug at the same time as calcium supplements may reduce absorption of calcium.
felodipine	Ascorbyl palmitate or citrus bioflavonoids may increase concentration of this drug in the bloodstream. Do not drink grapefruit juice if you take this drug.
Feverall	See acetaminophen.
Florone topical	See topical corticosteroids.
Floxenor	See norfloxacin.

Medication	Interaction(s)
Floxin	See ofloxacin.
flu vaccine	Taking Asian ginseng (*Panax ginseng*) continuously 4 weeks before and 8 weeks after vaccination may increase effectiveness of the vaccine.
	Taking eleuthero (Siberian ginseng) 2–3 days before vaccination may reduce swelling, fever, and other allergic reactions.
flunitrazepam	Chamomile, kava, or melatonin may increase sedative effects of this drug.
fluocinolone topical	See topical corticosteroids.
Fluonid topical	See topical corticosteroids.
Fluoroplex	See fluorouracil.
fluorouracil	A combination of N-acetyl cysteine (NAC) and vitamins C and E may prevent heart damage from this drug without interfering with its action against cancer.
	Very high doses of melatonin (20 milligrams, an amount that should be taken only under a doctor's supervision) have reduced the toxicity of chemotherapy with fluorouracil plus cisplatin and fluorouracil plus folinic acid.
	Vitamin E applied to sores in the mouth caused by this form of chemotherapy helps them heal more rapidly.
fluoxetine	5-HTP may increase side effects of this drug.
	Folic acid is necessary for this drug to be effective. Take 200 micrograms of folic acid daily while taking this drug.
	Ginkgo (240 milligrams daily) may counteract sexual dysfunction caused by this drug.
	Do not take this drug within 10 days of taking St. John's wort.
	Taking this drug with melatonin has been known to produce psychotic episodes.
fluphenazine (Permitil, Prolixin)	Betel nut increases side effects of this drug.
flurazepam	Chamomile, kava, or melatonin may increase sedative effects of this drug.
flurbiprofen	See NSAIDs.
fluticasone topical	See topical corticosteroids.
fluvoxamine	5-HTP may increase side effects of this drug.
	Decreases rate at which brain absorbs melatonin.
Fortovase	Ascorbyl palmitate or citrus bioflavonoids may increase concentration of this drug in the bloodstream. Do not drink grapefruit juice if you take this drug.
Fosamax	See alendronate.
fosinopril	See ACE inhibitors.
fosphenytoin	Depletes folic acid and raises homocysteine levels (factor in heart disease).
	Vitamin B_6 may make this drug less available to the body.
FS Shampoo	See topical corticosteroids.
Fulgram	See norfloxacin.
Furadantin	See nitrofurantoin.
furosemide	May cause magnesium, potassium, thiamine, or vitamin B_1 deficiency.
	Do not take this drug with diuretic herbs including buchu, cleavers, dandelion, gravel root, horsetail, juniper berries, and uva ursi.
	Ginseng and uva ursi make this drug less effective.
	Licorice increases blood pressure and counteracts this drug.
	Taking aloe, buckthorn, cascara sagrada, rhubarb root, or senna with this drug for more than 10 days can cause potassium deficiency.

Medication	Interaction(s)
gabapentin	See anticonvulsants.
Garamycin	See gentamycin.
gatifloxacin	Calcium, iron, magnesium, quercetin, or rutin (as well as herbs containing rutin, such as barley leaf and Scotch broom) interfere with the body's absorption of this antibiotic.
gemfibrozil	Red yeast rice may increase risk of muscle damage.
Gemifloxacin	Calcium, iron, magnesium, quercetin, or rutin (as well as herbs containing rutin, such as barley leaf and Scotch broom) interfere with the body's absorption of this antibiotic.
Genapap	See acetaminophen.
GenCept 0.5/35, GenCept 1/35	See oral contraceptives.
Genebs	See acetaminophen.
Genora 1/35	See oral contraceptives.
Genora 1/50	See oral contraceptives.
gentamycin	May deplete calcium, magnesium, and vitamin B_6.
glimepiride	Doses of niacin in excess of 20 milligrams per day may make this drug ineffective.
	Glucosamine may make any diabetes drug less effective by increasing insulin resistance.
glipizide	Doses of niacin in excess of 20 milligrams per day may make this drug ineffective.
	Glucosamine may make any diabetes drug less effective by increasing insulin resistance.
Glucophage	See metformin.
Glucotrol	Doses of niacin in excess of 20 milligrams per day may make this drug ineffective.
	Glucosamine may make any diabetes drug less effective by increasing insulin resistance.
glyburide	Doses of niacin in excess of 20 milligrams per day may make this drug ineffective.
	Glucosamine may make any diabetes drug less effective by increasing insulin resistance.
Glynase Prestab	Doses of niacin in excess of 20 milligrams per day may make this drug ineffective.
	Glucosamine may make any diabetes drug less effective by increasing insulin resistance.
grepafloxacin	Calcium, iron, magnesium, quercetin, or rutin (as well as herbs containing rutin, such as barley leaf and Scotch broom) interfere with the body's absorption of this antibiotic.
guanabenz	Taking inositol, niacin, or saw palmetto may cause unusually low blood pressure.
guanfacine	Taking inositol, niacin, or saw palmetto may cause unusually low blood pressure.
Gyne-Lotrimin	In rare cases, taking this drug with red yeast rice can cause muscle damage.
Halcion	Grapefruit juice, quercetin, or rutin (as well as herbs containing rutin, such as barley leaf and Scotch broom) drastically increase concentration of this drug in the bloodstream and intensify its side effects.
	Chamomile or melatonin increase sedative effects of this drug.
Haldol	See haloperidol.
Halenol	See acetaminophen.
haloperidol	Side effects of this drug may be worsened by homeopathic arnica.
	Arnica may cause irregular heart rhythms (prolonged QT interval).
	Vitamin E (1,600 IU) per day may relieve tardive dyskinesia caused by this drug.
	Extreme low-sodium diets should be avoided when taking this drug.
	High doses of glycerine, up to 30 grams per day, may enhance the effectiveness of this drug.
Haltran	See NSAIDs.
HCTZ	See hydrochlorothiazide.
Hepalean	See heparin.

Medication	Interaction(s)
heparin	Depletes vitamin D.
	Dong quai, fenugreek, ginger, ginkgo, horse chestnut, red clover, sweet clover, and sweet woodruff may unpredictably increase the effectiveness of this drug, causing bleeding, bruising, or hemorrhage.
	Potassium supplements may cause potentially life-threatening hyperkalemia (exessive potassium in the bloodstream) when taken with this drug.
	Reishi reduces the effectiveness of this drug.
Heparin Leo	See heparin.
Hexit	See lindane.
Hivid	See zalcitabine.
hydralazine	Depletes vitamin B_6.
hydrochlorothiazide	Depletes folic acid, magnesium, and potassium.
	Helps the kidneys conserve calcium, so calcium supplements may not be as important for people who take this drug.
	Adonis, aloe used as a laxative, buckthorn, cascara sagrada, frangula, lily of the valley, oleander, rhubarb root, senna, squill, and strophanthus increase side effects of this drug.
hydrocortisone topical	See topical corticosteroids.
HydroDIURIL	See hydrochlorothiazide.
HydroSaluric	See hydrochlorothiazide.
hydroxychloroquine	Magnesium supplements reduce the concentration of this drug in the bloodstream and make it less available and less effective.
	Taking vitamin B_6 with this drug greatly increases its effectiveness.
Hygroton	See hydrochlorothiazide.
Hytone topical	See topical corticosteroids.
Hytrin	Taking inositol, niacin, or saw palmetto may cause unusually low blood pressure.
IBU	See NSAIDs.
Ibuprin	See NSAIDs.
ibuprofen	See NSAIDs.
Ibuprohm	See NSAIDs.
imipramine	5-HTP may increase side effects of this drug.
	B vitamins may help elderly people think more clearly while taking this drug.
	Brewer's yeast, ephedra, and Scotch broom increase blood pressure when taken with this drug.
	Ginseng may cause headaches or mania when taken with this drug.
	Black and green tea may interfere with the body's absorption of this drug.
	Coenzyme Q_{10} may reduce detrimental effects of this drug on heart function.
	SAM-e helps this drug bring relief from depression sooner.
	St. John's wort may cause excessive accumulation of this drug in the bloodstream. St. John's wort should not be taken with this drug.
Imitrex	Taking this drug with 5-HTP may cause headaches and/or excitement.
Immukin	See interferon.
Inderal	Magnesium supplements and antacids containing magnesium should not be taken within 2 hours of taking this drug.
	Depletes CoQ_{10}.
	Increases vitamin A levels in the bloodstream. If you take vitamin A and this medication, have a doctor monitor vitamin A levels for you to prevent toxicity.

Medication	Interaction(s)
indinavir	St. John's wort lowers bloodstream concentrations of this drug.
Indocin	See indomethacin.
indomethacin	Cascara sagrada, senna, and wild yam decrease the pain relief offered by this drug.
Infant's Pain Reliever	See acetaminophen.
Infergen	See interferon.
insulin (all forms)	Fenugreek and gymnema sylvestre may reduce amount of insulin required to control blood sugars.
	Daily use of insulin may lower bloodstream DHEA levels.
	Glucosamine may make any diabetes drug less effective by increasing insulin resistance.
interferon	Preliminary studies suggest that N-acetyl cysteine (NAC) or thymus peptides may increase effectiveness of this drug against hepatitis.
	The Chinese herbal formula Xiao Chai Hu Tang has caused approximately 80 cases of interstitial pneumonia, some of them fatal, when used with interferon. Do not use this herbal product with interferon. Xiao Chai Hu Tang is sold as: • Liver Kampo (Honso) • Minor Bupleurum Combination (Lotus Classics, Qualiherb, Sun Ten) • Minor Bupleurum Formula (Chinese Classics, Golden Flower Chinese Herbs) • Minor Bupleurum Formulation (Kan Traditionals) • Sho-saiko-to (Tsumura) • Xiao Chai Hu Tang (Lotus Classics, Qualiherb, Sun Ten)
interleukin-2	Possible augmentation of antitumor effect when taken with melatonin.
Intron	See Interferon.
Invirase	Ascorbyl palmitate or citrus bioflavonoids may increase concentration of this drug in the bloodstream.
Isoptin	See amlodipine.
isotretinoin	Toxic side effects made worse by taking vitamin A with this drug.
	Vitamin E may prevent toxic side effects caused by this drug.
Janacin	See norfloxacin.
Janimine	See tricyclic antidepressants.
Jenest-28	See oral contraceptives.
Keep Alert	See caffeine.
Kenalog topical	See topical corticosteroids.
Kerlone	Taking chromium from brewer's yeast may raise HDL ("good") cholesterol levels in people who take this drug.
ketoconazole	In rare cases, taking this drug with red yeast rice can cause muscle damage.
	May deplete vitamin D.
ketoprofen	See NSAIDs.
Klonopin	Chamomile and melatonin both increase sedative effect of this drug.
Kwell	See lindane.
lamivudine	Riboflavin may reverse lactic acidosis caused by this drug.
Lanoxin	See digoxin.
lansoprazole	Taking this drug at same time as calcium supplements may reduce absorption of calcium.
	This drug interferes with absorption of beta-carotene and vitamin B_{12}. Sipping cranberry juice with meals prevents the drug from interfering with vitamin B_{12} absorption.
Lasix	May cause magnesium, potassium, thiamine, or vitamin B_1 deficiency.
	Do not take this drug with diuretic herbs including buchu, cleavers, dandelion, gravel root, horsetail, juniper berries, and uva ursi.

Medication	Interaction(s)
Lasix (cont.)	Do not take this drug with laxative herbs that deplete potassium, including aloe, buckthorn, cascara sagrada, frangula, or rhubarb root.
	Ginseng and uva ursa make this drug less effective.
	Licorice increases blood pressure and counteracts this drug.
	Taking buckthorn, cascara sagrada, rhubarb root, or senna with this drug for more than 10 days can cause potassium deficiency.
Lasma	See theophylline.
L-dopa	See levodopa.
Levaquin	See levofloxacin.
Levlen	See oral contraceptives.
Levlite	See oral contraceptives.
levodopa	Iron, octacosanol, and vitamin B_6 reduce effectiveness of this drug.
	Rauwolfia increases neck tension and facial paralysis when taken with this drug.
levofloxacin	Calcium, iron, magnesium, quercetin, or rutin (as well as herbs containing rutin, such as barley leaf and Scotch broom) interfere with the body's absorption of this antibiotic.
Levora	See oral contraceptives.
Levo-T	Calcium and iron supplements decrease body's absorption of this drug.
Levothroid	Calcium and iron supplements decrease body's absorption of this drug.
Levothyroxine, Levoxine, Levoxyl	Taking calcium supplements at same time as this drug may reduce absorption of this drug.
	Using 7-Oxo-DHEA or 7-KETO can raise thyroid hormone concentrations to levels that can harm the bones or heart.
Lexinor	See norfloxacin.
Librium	Chamomile, kava, or melatonin increases sedative effect of this drug.
Limbitrol	See amitriptyline.
lindane	Vitamin E may prevent damage and future tumors in the scalp after use of this shampoo.
Lioresal	See baclofen.
Lipitor	Magnesium supplements and antacids containing magnesium should not be taken within 2 hours of taking this drug.
	Depletes CoQ_{10}.
	Increases vitamin A levels in the bloodstream. If you take vitamin A with this medication, have a doctor monitor your vitamin A levels to prevent toxicity.
Liquiprin	See acetaminophen.
lisinopril	See ACE inhibitors.
lithium	Folic acid, inositol, and L-tryptophan may reduce side effects of this drug.
	Do not go on a low-sodium diet without doctor's approval.
	Fiber laxatives and psyllium interfere with lithium absorption.
Locoid topical	See topical corticosteroids.
Loestrin 1.5/30	See oral contraceptives.
lomefloxacin	Calcium, iron, magnesium, quercetin, or rutin (as well as herbs containing rutin, such as barley leaf and Scotch broom) interfere with the body's absorption of this antibiotic.
Lomotil, Lonox	Black tea, black walnut, green tea, oak bark, raspberry leaf, uva ursi, and witch hazel contain tannins that interfere with the body's absorption of this drug.
Lo/Ovral	See oral contraceptives.
Lopid	See gemfibrozil.

Medication	Interaction(s)
Lopressor	Taking chromium from brewer's yeast may raise HDL ("good") cholesterol levels in people who take this drug.
lorazepam	Chamomile and melatonin both increase sedative effects of this drug.
Lotensin	See ACE inhibitors.
Lotrisone	In rare cases, taking this drug with red yeast rice can cause muscle damage.
lovastatin	Ascorbyl palmitate or citrus bioflavonoids may increase concentration of this drug in the bloodstream.
	Inositol nicotinate may increase effectiveness of this drug and also increase risk of muscle damage.
	Magnesium supplements and antacids containing magnesium should not be taken within 2 hours of taking this drug.
	Depletes CoQ_{10}.
	Increases vitamin A levels in the bloodstream. If you take vitamin A with this medication, have a doctor monitor your vitamin A levels to prevent toxicity.
Lustra	See sertraline.
Luvox	5-HTP may increase side effects of this drug.
	Decreases rate at which brain absorbs melatonin.
Luxiq topical	See topical corticosteroids.
Maalox	See antacids.
Macrobid	See nitrofurantoin.
Macrodantin	See nitrofurantoin.
Mapap	See acetaminophen.
Maranox	See acetaminophen.
Marevan	Asian ginseng, arnica, astragalus, bilberry, dan shen, devil's claw, dong quai, feverfew, garlic, ginger, ginkgo, green tea, horse chestnut, and quinine may increase risk of bruising, bleeding, or hemorrhage if taken with this drug.
	Broccoli, Brussels sprouts, cabbage, kale, onions, parsley, soy, and spinach may increase risk of bruising, bleeding, or hemorrhage if eaten in unusually large quantities when taking this drug.
	Reishi and St. John's wort decrease the effectiveness of this drug.
	Taking more than 500 milligrams a day of the form of vitamin E known as alpha-tocopherol polyethylene glycol succinate (TPGS) may increase risk of bleeding.
	This drug interferes with the absorption of iron, magnesium, and zinc. Do not take supplements of these minerals within 2 hours of taking it.
Mavik	See ACE inhibitors.
Maxalt	Taking this drug with 5-HTP may cause headaches and/or excitement.
Maxaquin	See Lomefloxacin.
Maxivate topical	See topical corticosteroids.
Maxolon	Depletes riboflavin.
Meclan	See tetracycline antibiotics.
meclocycline sulfosalicylate	See tetracycline antibiotics.
Meda Cap/Tab	See acetaminophen.
Medihaler	See adrenaline.
Menadol	See NSAIDs.
Metenix 5	See hydrochlorothiazide.
metformin	Depletes folic acid and increases bloodstream levels of homocysteine, a risk factor in heart disease.

Medication	Interaction(s)
metformin (cont.)	Decreases absorption of vitamin B_{12}.
	Glucosamine may make any diabetes drug less effective by increasing insulin resistance.
	Doses of niacin in excess of 20 milligrams per day may make this drug ineffective.
methotrexate	Choline may reverse fatty liver, a side effect of this drug.
	L-methionine may reduce risk of liver damage by this drug.
	Folic acid may reduce toxic side effects of this drug.
methysergide	5-HTP may make this drug less effective.
metoclopramide HCl	Depletes riboflavin.
Metolazone	See hydrochlorothiazide.
metoprolol	This drug may deplete melatonin.
	Taking chromium from brewer's yeast may raise HDL ("good") cholesterol levels in people who take this drug.
Mevacor	Magnesium supplements and antacids containing magnesium should not be taken within 2 hours of taking this drug.
	Depletes CoQ_{10}.
	Increases vitamin A levels in the bloodstream. If you take vitamin A with this medication, have a doctor monitor your vitamin A levels to prevent toxicity.
Mezlin	See penicillins.
Micanol creme	See anthralin.
miconazole	In rare cases, taking this drug with red yeast rice can cause muscle damage.
Micronase	Doses of niacin in excess of 20 milligrams per day may make this drug ineffective.
	Glucosamine may make any diabetes drug less effective by increasing insulin resistance.
Micronor	See oral contraceptives.
midazolam	Chamomile, kava, or melatonin may increase sedative effects of this drug.
Midol IB	See NSAIDs.
Mifeprex	See mifepristone.
mifepristone	The Chinese herbal formula Shenghua Tang (available from practitioners of traditional Chinese medicine) reduces vaginal bleeding after administration of this drug.
miglitol	Doses of niacin in excess of 20 milligrams per day may make this drug ineffective.
milk of magnesia	See magnesium hydroxide.
Minihep Calcium	See heparin.
Minipress	Taking inositol, niacin, or saw palmetto with this drug may cause unusually low blood pressure.
Minitram	See nitrates, nitroglycerin.
Minocin	See tetracycline antibiotics.
Minocycline	Taking this antibiotic at same time as calcium supplements may reduce absorption of this antibiotic.
mizatidine	Taking this drug at same time as calcium supplements may reduce absorption of calcium.
Modaplate	Asian ginseng, arnica, astragalus, bilberry, dan shen, devil's claw, dong quai, feverfew, garlic, ginger, ginkgo, green tea, horse chestnut, and quinine may increase risk of bruising, bleeding, or hemorrhage if taken with this drug.
	High doses (more than 500 milligrams daily) of the form of vitamin E known as alpha-tocopherol polyethylene glycol succinate (TPGS) may increase risk of bleeding.
Modicon	See oral contraceptives
moexipril	See ACE inhibitors.
MOM (milk of magnesia)	See magnesium hydroxide.

Medication	Interaction(s)
mometasone topical	See topical corticosteroids.
Monodox	See tetracycline antibiotics.
Monoparin Calcium	See heparin.
Monopril	See ACE inhibitors.
morphine	Yohimbe increases sedative effect of morphine.
Motrin, Children's	See NSAIDs.
Motrin IB	See NSAIDs.
moxifloxacin	Calcium, iron, magnesium, quercetin, or rutin (as well as herbs containing rutin, such as barley leaf and Scotch broom) interfere with the body's absorption of this antibiotic.
	Taking this antibiotic at same time as calcium supplements may reduce absorption of this antibiotic.
Multiparin	See heparin.
Mycifradin	See neomycin.
Myciguent	See neomycin.
Mykrox	See hydrochlorothiazide.
Mylanta	See magnesium hydroxide.
nafcillin	See penicillins.
naltrexone	Increases side effects of yohimbe.
naratriptan	Taking this drug with 5-HTP may cause headaches and/or excitement.
Necon (various)	See oral contraceptives.
Nelova (various)	See oral contraceptives.
Nelulen (various)	See oral contraceptives.
neomycin	If taken by mouth, reduces effectiveness of gamma-tocopherol and vitamin E.
	Probiotics such as *acidophilus* and *Lactobacillus* reduce diarrhea caused by this drug.
	Depletes vitamin B_6 and K.
Neopap	See acetaminophen.
Neoral	See cyclosporine.
Neosporin	See neomycin.
NeoTab	See neomycin.
nicotine patches	This drug in combination with niacin may cause redness in the face, especially around the nose.
nifedipine	Grapefruit juice, but not other citrus juices, increases side effects of this drug.
	Ipriflavone can cause buildup of this drug in bloodstream resulting in unusually low blood pressure (dizziness, fainting, light-headedness).
	Pleurisy root or tobacco reduces the effectiveness of this drug in treating angina.
	This drug makes aloe, buckthorn, cascara sagrada, frangula, rhubarb root, and senna less effective in relieving constipation.
nisoldipine	Ascorbyl palmitate or citrus bioflavonoids may increase concentration of this drug in the bloodstream.
nitrates, nitroglycerin	Cause headaches if taken with N-acetyl cysteine (NAC).
Nitro-bid	See nitrates, nitroglycerin.
Nitrodisc	See nitrates, nitroglycerin.
Nitro-Dur	See nitrates, nitroglycerin.
nitrofurantoin	DGL (deglycyrrhizinated licorice) increases the rate at which the body excretes this drug and may make it less effective against urinary tract infection.
Nitrogard	See nitrates, nitroglycerin.

Medication	Interaction(s)
Nitrolingual	See nitrates, nitroglycerin.
Nitrostat	See nitrates, nitroglycerin.
Nivemycin	See neomycin.
nizatidine	Reduces body's absorption of calcium.
Nizoral	In rare cases, taking this drug with red yeast rice can cause muscle damage.
NoDoz	See caffeine.
Nordette	See oral contraceptives.
Norethin 1/50	See oral contraceptives.
norfloxacin	Calcium, iron, magnesium, quercetin, or rutin (as well as herbs containing rutin, such as barley leaf and Scotch broom) interfere with the body's absorption of this antibiotic.
norgestrel	See oral contraceptives.
Norinyl 1+35	See oral contraceptives.
Normodyne	Taking chromium from brewer's yeast may raise HDL ("good") cholesterol levels in people who take this drug.
Norofin	See norfloxacin.
Noroxin	See norfloxacin.
Norpace	See disopyramide.
Norphyllin	See theophylline.
Norpramin	See tricyclic antidepressants.
Nor-Tet	See tetracycline antibiotics.
Nortriptyline	See tricyclic antidepressants.
Norvasc	See amlodipine.
Norxacin	See norfloxacin.
Novo-Carbamaz	See anticonvulsants.
Novo-Doxepin	See tricyclic antidepressants.
Novo-Gemfibrozil	See gemfibrozil.
Novo-Hylazin	See hydralazine.
Novo-Theophyl	See theophylline.
NSAIDs (nonsteroidal anti-inflammatory drugs)	Taking copper with NSAIDs may increase their ability to reduce inflammation and stomach upset.
	Taking evening primrose oil, hempseed oil, or perilla oil with NSAIDs may increase brusing and bleeding.
	Deplete folic acid.
	May lower melatonin levels.
	Uva ursi reduces pain relief by these drugs.
	DGL (deglycyrrhizinated licorice) may counteract stomach irritation caused by NSAIDs.
	Taking NSAIDs long term can lead to iron deficiency. Do not take iron supplements unless a blood test confirms iron deficiency.
Nu-Carbamazepine	See anticonvulsants
Nuelin	See theophylline.
Nuelin SA	See theophylline.
Nu-Gemfibrozil	See gemfibrozil.
Nu-Hydral	See Hydralazine
Nuprin	See NSAIDs.
Octamide	Depletes riboflavin.

Medication	Interaction(s)
ofloxacin	Calcium, iron, magnesium, quercetin, or rutin (as well as herbs containing rutin, such as barley leaf and Scotch broom) interfere with the body's absorption of this antibiotic.
omeprazole	Taking this drug at the same time as calcium supplements may reduce absorption of calcium.
	Interferes with body's absorption of vitamin B_{12}. Sipping cranberry juice with meals compensates for this effect of the drug.
Omniflox	See temafloxacin.
Omnipen	See ampicillin.
Oracin	See norfloxacin.
oral contraceptives	May deplete folic acid, magnesium, riboflavin, and vitamin B_6. Deficiency of vitamin B_6 may contribute to depression.
	Do not take iron supplements if you are on the Pill unless a doctor confirms you are iron-deficient.
	Melatonin may increase effectiveness of oral contraceptives.
	St. John's wort may cause bleeding between periods if taken with oral contraceptives.
Oraphen-PD	See acetaminophen.
Oretic	See hydrochlorothiazide.
Orinase	Doses of niacin in excess of 20 milligrams per day may make this drug ineffective.
	Glucosamine may make any diabetes drug less effective by increasing insulin resistance.
orlistat	May deplete beta-carotene and vitamins A, D, E, and K.
	Taking this drug at the same time as beta-carotene reduces absorption of beta-carotene.
Oroflox	See norfloxacin
Ortho-Novum (various)	See oral contraceptives.
Ortho Tri-cyclen	See oral contraceptives.
Orudis	See NSAIDs.
Orvette	See oral contraceptives.
Ovcon (various)	See oral contraceptives.
Ovral	See oral contraceptives.
oxazepam	Chamomile and melatonin both increase sedative effects of this drug.
oxytetracycline	See tetracycline antibiotics.
oxytocin	Ephedra can cause high blood pressure when taken with this drug.
Pacerone	See amiodarone.
paclitaxel	Ascorbyl palmitate, citrus bioflavonoids, or vitamin C may increase this drug's effect against cancer.
	L-glutamine may reduce side effects of this drug.
Panadol	See acetaminophen.
Pandel topical	See topical corticosteroids.
Panmycin	See tetracycline antibiotics.
Paraflex	See chlorzoxazone.
Parafon Forte DSC	See chlorzoxazone.
pargyline HCl	Taking this drug with brewer's yeast may raise blood pressure.
Parnate	See tranylcypromine sulfate.
paroxetine, Paxil	5-HTP may increase side effects of this drug.
	Ginkgo (240 milligrams daily) may counteract sexual dysfunction caused by this drug.
	Do not take this drug within 10 days of taking St. John's wort.
	Do not go on a severe low-sodium diet while taking this drug.

Medication	Interaction(s)
Pediacare Fever	See NSAIDs.
Penetrex	See enoxacin.
penicillins	Probiotics such as *acidophilus* and *Lactobacillus* reduce diarrhea caused by penicillins.
	Deplete vitamin K.
pentamidine	Side effects of this drug may be worsened by homeopathic arnica.
Pepcid	Reduces body's absorption of calcium.
Pepto-Bismol	See bismuth subsalicylate.
Perindopril	Taking European angelica, psoralea, or St. John's wort with this drug increases risk of sunburn.
	Taking supplemental potassium with this drug can cause potentially life-threatening hyperkalemia (excessive potassium in the bloodstream).
Periostat	See tetracycline antibiotics.
Permole, Persantin, Persantine	Asian ginseng, arnica, astragalus, bilberry, dan shen, devil's claw, dong quai, feverfew, garlic, ginger, ginkgo, green tea, horse chestnut, and quinine may increase risk of bruising, bleeding, or hemorrhage if taken with this drug.
	High doses (more than 500 milligrams daily) of the form of vitamin E known as alpha-tocopherol polyethylene glycol succinate (TPGS) may increase risk of bleeding.
phenelzine	May cause vitamin B_6 deficiency.
	Taking this drug with brewer's yeast, L-phenylalanine, or L-tyrosine may raise blood pressure.
phenldrine	See phenylpropanolamine.
phenobarbital	Depletes biotin, especially in women. Also see Anticonvulsants.
Phenoxine	See phenylpropanolamine.
phenylpropanolamine	Regular (not decaf) coffee and tea, yohimbe, ephedra, or guaraná taken with this drug may cause high blood pressure.
phenytoin	Black pepper or piperine may inhibit body's use and excretion of this drug.
	Depletes biotin, especially in women.
	Also see anticonvulsants.
pioglitazone HCl	Doses of niacin in excess of 20 milligrams per day may make this drug ineffective.
	Glucosamine may make any diabetes drug less effective by increasing insulin resistance.
Plan B	See oral contraceptives.
Plaquenil	See hydroxychloroquine.
Plavix	Asian ginseng, arnica, astragalus, bilberry, coleus, dan shen, devil's claw, dong quai, feverfew, garlic, ginger, ginkgo, green tea, horse chestnut, and quinine may increase risk of bruising, bleeding, or hemorrhage if taken with this drug.
	High doses (more than 500 milligrams daily) of the form of vitamin E known as alpha-tocopherol polyethylene glycol succinate (TPGS) may increase risk of bleeding.
	Borage seed oil, especially if taken with fish oil, may increase risk of bleeding or bruising if taken with this drug.
	Bromelain may increase anticlotting effect of this drug.
	Tiratricol (TRIAC) may interfere with accurate blood tests for PT (prothrombin time) when taken with this drug.
	Curcuminoids may increase anticlotting effect of this drug.
	Gamma-tocopherol may increase anticlotting effect of this drug.
	Ganoderma mushroom may increase anticlotting effect of this drug.
	Green catechins (although not beverage green tea) may increase anticlotting effect of this drug.
Plendil	See felodipine.

Medication	Interaction(s)
PMS-Desipramine	See tricyclic antidepressants.
PMS-Gemfibrozil	See gemfibrozil.
PMS-Lindane	See lindane.
Prandin	See repaglinide.
Pravachol	Magnesium supplements and antacids containing magnesium should not be taken within 2 hours of taking this drug.
	Depletes CoQ_{10}.
	Increases vitamin A levels in the bloodstream. If you take vitamin A and this medication, have a doctor monitor your vitamin A levels to prevent toxicity.
Pravastatin	Inositol nicotinate may increase effectiveness of this drug and also increase risk of muscle damage.
	Magnesium supplements and antacids containing magnesium should not be taken within 2 hours of taking this drug.
	Depletes CoQ_{10}.
	Increases vitamin A levels in the bloodstream. If you take vitamin A with this medication, have a doctor monitor your vitamin A levels to prevent toxicity.
Prazosin	Taking inositol, niacin, or saw palmetto with this drug may cause unusually low blood pressure.
Precose	Amylase, pancreatin, and pancrelipase (digestive enzymes), as well as inositol nicotinate, niacin, and glucosamine may make this drug less effective.
Premarin, Prempro	See conjugated estrogens.
Preven	See oral contraceptives.
Prilosec	See omeprazole.
Primatene Mist	See adrenaline.
primidone	Depletes biotin, especially in women.
Principen	See ampicillin.
Prinivil	See ACE inhibitors.
procainamide	Side effects may be worsened by homeopathic arnica.
Procardia	Ipriflavone can cause buildup of this drug in bloodstream resulting in unusually low blood pressure (dizziness, fainting, light-headedness).
	Pleurisy root or tobacco reduces the effectiveness of this drug in treating angina.
	This drug makes aloe, buckthorn, cascara sagrada, frangula, rhubarb root, and senna less effective in relieving constipation.
prochlorperazine	Side effects of this drug may be worsened by homeopathic arnica.
Proctocort topical	See topical corticosteroids.
Propagest	See phenylpropanolamine.
propanolol	Black pepper or piperine may inhibit body's use and excretion of this drug.
	This drug may deplete melatonin.
	Taking chromium from brewer's yeast may raise HDL ("good") cholesterol levels in people who take this drug.
Propulsid	See cisapride.
ProSom	Grapefruit juice, quercetin, or rutin (as well as herbs containing rutin, such as barley leaf and Scotch broom) drastically increase concentration of this drug in the bloodstream and intensify its side effects.
	Chamomile, kava, or melatonin may increase sedative effects of this drug.
protriptyline	See tricyclic antidepressants.
Prozac	5-HTP may increase side effects of this drug.

Medication	Interaction(s)
Prozac (cont.)	Folic acid enhances antidepressant effects.
	Taking this drug with melatonin has been known to produce a psychotic episode.
Psorcon topical	See topical corticosteroids.
Psorin ointment	See anthralin.
Pump-Hep	See heparin.
pyrazinamide	Black pepper or piperine may inhibit body's use and excretion of this drug.
quazepam	Chamomile, kava, or melatonin may increase sedative effects of this drug.
Questran	Reduces body's absorption of beta-carotene, folic acid, gamma-tocopherol, inositol, lutein, lycopene, niacin, riboflavin, vitamin A, vitamin B_{12}, vitamin D, vitamin E, and vitamin K.
	Taking this drug at same time as beta-carotene reduces absorption of beta-carotene.
Quick Pep	See caffeine.
quinapril	See ACE inhibitors.
quinidine	Side effects of this drug may be worsened by homeopathic arnica and non-homeopathic adonis, belladonna, digitalis, henbane, Indian squill, kombé seed, lily of the valley, oleander, scopolia, squill, or strophanthus.
	Taking arnica with this drug may cause irregular heartbeats.
Quintor	See ciprofloxacin.
rabeprazole sodium	Taking this drug at same time as calcium supplements may reduce absorption of calcium.
raloxifene	May counteract soy isoflavones.
ramipril	See ACE inhibitors.
ranitidine	Reduces body's absorption of calcium.
	Taking this drug at the same time as calcium supplements may reduce absorption of calcium.
Rebif	See interferon.
Reclomide	Depletes riboflavin.
Redutemp	See acetaminophen.
Reglan	Depletes riboflavin.
repaglinide	Doses of niacin in excess of 20 milligrams per day may make this drug ineffective.
reserpine	St. John's wort counteracts this drug.
Restoril	Chamomile, kava, or melatonin may increase sedative effects of this drug.
Rhindecon	See phenylpropanolamine.
Ridenol	See acetaminophen.
rifampin	Melatonin may increase the effectiveness of this drug.
	Black pepper or piperine may interfere with the body's metabolism of this drug.
	Depletes gamma-tocopherol, vitamin B_6, and vitamin E.
Rifater	See pyrazinamide.
Rimacillin	See ampicillin.
risendronate	Taking this drug at the same time as calcium supplements may reduce absorption of this drug.
rizatriptan	Taking this drug with 5-HTP may cause headaches and/or excitement.
Robitussin-CF	See phenylpropanolamine.
rofecoxib	See tricyclic antidepressants.
Roferon	See interferon.
Rohypnol	See flunitrazepam.
Rolaids	See magnesium hydroxide.

Medication	Interaction(s)
rosiglitazone maleate	Doses of niacin in excess of 20 milligrams per day may make this drug ineffective.
	Glucosamine may make any diabetes drug less effective by increasing insulin resistance.
RU-486	See mifepristone.
Saleto	See NSAIDs.
Saluric	See hydrochlorothiazide.
Sandimmune	See cyclosporine.
SangCya	See cyclosporine.
Sansert	See methysergide.
saquinavir	Ascorbyl palmitate or citrus bioflavonoids may increase concentration of this drug in the bloodstream.
Sectral	Pleurisy root may unpredictably enhance effects of this drug.
selegiline	5-HTP may produce unpredictable effects when taken with this drug.
	Avocado, chocolate, eggplant, fava beans, and red wine may cause sudden and severe changes in blood pressure when eaten by people who take this drug.
	Ephedra can cause severe high blood pressure when taken with this drug.
Serax	Chamomile and melatonin both increase sedative effect of drug.
Seromycin	See cycloserine.
sertraline	Chromium may increase effectiveness of this drug in certain kinds of depression (dysthymic disorder, depression occurring on more days than not for more than 2 years).
	5-HTP may increase side effects of this drug.
Silapap	See acetaminophen.
sildenafil	L-arginine may make this drug more effective.
	Taking N-acetyl cysteine (NAC) with this drug may cause headaches.
	Taking more than 20 milligrams of niacin the same day as taking this drug may cause unusually low blood pressure (dizziness, fainting, light-headedness).
simvastatin	Inositol nicotinate may increase effectiveness of this drug and also increase risk of muscle damage.
	Magnesium supplements and antacids containing magnesium should not be taken within 2 hours of taking this drug.
	Depletes CoQ_{10}.
	Increases vitamin A levels in the bloodstream. If you take vitamin A with this medication, have a doctor monitor your vitamin A levels to prevent toxicity.
	Ascorbyl palmitate or citrus bioflavonoids may increase concentration of this drug in the bloodstream.
Sinemet	See carbidopa.
Sinequan	See doxepin.
Slo-Bid	See theophylline.
Slo-Phyllin	See theophylline.
Snap Back	See caffeine.
Soriatane	See acitretin.
Sotalol	Side effects may be worsened by homeopathic arnica.
Sparfloxacin	Calcium, iron, magnesium, quercetin, or rutin (as well as herbs containing rutin, such as barley leaf and Scotch broom) interfere with the body's absorption of this antibiotic.
Stavudine	Depletes vitamin B_{12}.
	L-carnitine may reduce muscle damage caused by this drug.

Medication	Interaction(s)
Stavudine (cont.)	N-acetyl cysteine (NAC) may reduce toxicity of this drug.
	Riboflavin may reverse fatty liver or lactic acidosis caused by this drug.
	Zinc may help increase body weight, increase CD4+ levels, and prevent *Pneumocystis carinii* pneumonia if taken with this drug.
Stay Alert	See caffeine.
Strifon Fort	See chlorzoxazone.
Sudafed	Black tea, black walnut, green tea, oak bark, raspberry leaf, uva ursi, and witch hazel contain tannins that interfere with the body's absorption of this drug.
	Coleus and ephedra may cause unpredictable side effects of this drug.
Sular	See nisoldipine.
sulfadiazine	Black pepper or piperine may inhibit body's use and excretion of this drug.
sulfasalazine	Interferes with body's absorption of folic acid.
sumatriptan	Taking this drug with 5-HTP may cause headaches and/or excitement.
Sus-Phrine	See adrenaline.
Synalar topical	See topical corticosteroids.
Synemol topical	See topical corticosteroids.
Synthroid	Calcium and iron supplements decrease body's absorption of this drug.
tacrine HCl	Huperzine A may increase both the effectiveness of this drug and the severity of its side effects.
Tagamet	Reduces body's absorption of calcium.
	See also cimetidine.
Tapanol	See acetaminophen.
Tavist-D	See phenylpropanolamine.
Taxol	Ascorbyl palmitate, citrus bioflavonoids, or vitamin C may increase this drug's effect against cancer.
Tegretol	See carbamazepine.
temafloxacin	Calcium, iron, magnesium, quercetin, or rutin (as well as herbs containing rutin, such as barley leaf and Scotch broom) interfere with the body's absorption of this antibiotic.
temazepam	Chamomile, kava, or melatonin may increase sedative effects of this drug.
Temovate topical	See topical corticosteroids.
Tempo tablets	See magnesium hydroxide.
Tempra	See acetaminophen.
Tenex	Taking inositol, niacin, or saw palmetto may cause unusually low blood pressure.
Tenormin	Taking chromium from brewer's yeast may raise HDL ("good") cholesterol levels in people who take this drug.
Tequin	See gatifloxacin.
terazosin	Taking inositol, niacin, or saw palmetto may cause unusually low blood pressure.
Teril	See anticonvulsants.
Terramycin	See tetracycline antibiotics.
testosterone	Can increase detrimental effects of DHEA.
	Saw palmetto counteracts this drug.
Tetracap	See tetracycline antibiotics.
tetracycline antibiotics	Calcium, iron, and magnesium supplements interfere with the body's absorption of the antibiotic.
	Bromelain helps the body retain the antibiotic.
	Tetracycline antibiotics interfere with body's ability to absorb manganese.

Medication	Interaction(s)
tetracycline antibiotics (cont.)	Vitamin C prevents "blue smile" (staining of lips and teeth) from occurring with repeated use of the antibiotic.
Tetracyn	See tetracycline antibiotics.
Tetralan	See tetracycline antibiotics.
Theo-24	See theophylline.
Theo-Bid	See theophylline.
Theocron	See theophylline.
Theo-Dur	See theophylline.
Theolair	See theophylline.
theophylline (and also asthma drugs containing aminophylline)	Black pepper or piperine may inhibit body's use and excretion of this drug.
	Black tea, black walnut, green tea, oak bark, raspberry leaf, uva ursi, and witch hazel contain tannins that interfere with the body's absorption of this drug.
	Depletes magnesium, potassium, and vitamin B_6.
	Guraná increases side effects of this drug.
	St. John's wort may cause the body to eliminate this drug too quickly and worsen asthma symptoms.
theophylline ethylenediamine	See theophylline.
Theo-SR	See theophylline.
Ticar	See penicillins.
ticarcillin	See penicillins.
Ticlid	See ticlopidine.
ticlopidine	Asian ginseng, arnica, astragalus, bilberry, coleus, dan shen, devil's claw, dong quai, feverfew, garlic, ginger, ginkgo, green tea, horse chestnut, and quinine may increase risk of bruising, bleeding, or hemorrhage if taken with this drug.
	High doses (more than 500 milligrams daily) of the form of vitamin E known as alpha-tocopherol polyethylene glycol succinate (TPGS) may increase risk of bleeding.
	Borage seed oil, especially if taken with fish oil, may increase risk of bleeding or bruising if taken with this drug.
	Bromelain may increase anticlotting effect of this drug. Taking this drug with bromelain may increase risk of bleeding and bruising.
	Tiratricol (TRIAC) may interfere with accurate blood tests for PT (prothrombin time) when taken with this drug.
	Curcuminoids may increase anticlotting effect of this drug.
	Gamma-tocopherol may increase anticlotting effect of this drug.
	Ganoderma mushroom may increase anticlotting effect of this drug.
	Green catechins (although not beverage green tea) may increase anticlotting effect of this drug.
Timentin	See penicillins.
Timonil	See anticonvulsants.
tirofiban	Asian ginseng, arnica, astragalus, bilberry, coleus, dan shen, devil's claw, dong quai, feverfew, garlic, ginger, ginkgo, green tea, horse chestnut, and quinine may increase risk of bruising, bleeding, or hemorrhage if taken with this drug.
	High doses (more than 500 milligrams daily) of the form of vitamin E known as alpha-tocopherol polyethylene glycol succinate (TPGS) may increase risk of bleeding.
	Borage seed oil, especially if taken with fish oil, may increase risk of bleeding or bruising if taken with this drug.

Medication	Interaction(s)
tirofiban (cont.)	Bromelain may increase anticlotting effect. Taking this drug with bromelain may increase risk of bleeding and bruising.
	Tiratricol (TRIAC) may interfere with accurate blood tests for PT (prothrombin time) when taken with this drug.
	Curcuminoids may increase anticlotting effect of this drug.
	Gamma-tocopherol may increase anticlotting effect of this drug.
	Ganoderma mushroom may increase anticlotting effect of this drug.
	Green catechins (although not beverage green tea) may increase anticlotting effect of this drug.
tizanidine	Glycine may make this drug more effective.
Tofranil	5-HTP may increase side effects of this drug.
	B vitamins may help elderly people think more clearly while taking this drug.
	Brewer's yeast, ephedra, and Scotch broom increase blood pressure when taken with this drug.
	Ginseng may cause headaches or mania when taken with this drug.
	Black and green tea may interfere with the body's absorption of this drug.
	Coenzyme Q_{10} may reduce detrimental effects of this drug on heart function.
	SAM-e helps this drug bring relief from depression sooner.
	St. John's wort may cause excessive accumulation of this drug in the bloodstream. St. John's wort should not be taken with this drug.
tolazamide	Doses of niacin in excess of 20 milligrams per day may make this drug ineffective.
tolbutamide	Doses of niacin in excess of 20 milligrams per day may make this drug ineffective.
	Glucosamine may make any diabetes drug less effective by increasing insulin resistance.
	Ipriflavone may increase concentrations of this drug in the bloodstream and cause unexpectedly low blood sugars.
Tolinase	Doses of niacin in excess of 20 milligrams per day may make this drug ineffective.
	Glucosamine may make any diabetes drug less effective by increasing insulin resistance.
	Ipriflavone may increase concentrations of this drug in the bloodstream and cause unexpectedly low blood sugars.
topical corticosteroids	Aloe or a cream containing glycyrrhetinic acid (such as Simicort) may increase the anti-inflammatory potency of this drug.
	Biotin and zinc may make topical corticosteroids more effective in the treatment of alopecia areata.
	Taking any of these drugs with adonis, licorice, lily of the valley, oleander, squill, or strophanthus may produce variable side effects.
Topicort tTopical	See topical corticosteroids.
Topicycline	See tetracycline antibiotics.
Toprol-XL	Taking chromium from brewer's yeast may raise HDL ("good") cholesterol levels in people who take this drug.
Totacillin	See ampicillin.
Trandate	Taking chromium from brewer's yeast may raise HDL ("good") cholesterol levels in people who take this drug.
trandolapril	See ACE inhibitors.
Transderm-Nitro	See nitrates, nitroglycerin.
Tranxene	Grapefruit juice, quercetin, or rutin (as well as herbs containing rutin, such as barley leaf and Scotch broom) drastically increase concentration of this drug in the bloodstream and intensify its side effects.
	Chamomile, kava, or melatonin may increase sedative effects of this drug.

Medication	Interaction(s)
tranylcypromine sulfate	Brewer's yeast, L-phenylalanine, or L-tyrosine can cause high blood pressure when taken with this drug.
Trazodone HCl	Artemisia and wormwood increase risk of seizures when taken with this drug.
triamcinolone topical	See topical corticosteroids.
Triaminic-12	See phenylpropanolamine.
triazolam	Grapefruit juice, quercetin, or rutin (as well as herbs containing rutin, such as barley leaf and Scotch broom) drastically increase concentration of this drug in the bloodstream and intensify its side effects.
	Chamomile, kava, or melatonin may increase sedative effects of this drug.
tricyclic antidepressants	5-HTP may increase side effects of this drug.
	Artemisia and wormwood increase risk of seizures when taking this drug.
	B vitamins may help elderly people think more clearly while taking this drug.
	Belladonna, henbane, and scopolia increase side effects of this drug.
	Brewer's yeast, ephedra, and Scotch broom increase blood pressure when taken with this drug.
	Ginseng may cause headaches or mania when taken with this drug.
	Black and green tea may interfere with the body's absorption of this drug.
	Coenzyme Q_{10} may reduce detrimental effects of this drug on heart function.
	SAM-e helps this drug bring relief from depression sooner.
	St. John's wort may cause excessive accumulation of this drug in the bloodstream. St. John's wort should not be taken with this drug.
Tri-Levlen	See oral contraceptives.
Trimox	See penicillins.
Tri-Norinyl	See oral contraceptives.
Triphasil	See oral contraceptives.
Trivora	See oral contraceptives.
trovafloxacin	Calcium, iron, magnesium, quercetin, or rutin (as well as herbs containing rutin, such as barley leaf and Scotch broom) interfere with the body's absorption of this antibiotic.
Trovan	See trovafloxacin.
Truphylline	See theophylline.
Tryptizol	See tricyclic antidepressants.
Tylenol	See acetaminophen.
Uni-Ace	See acetaminophen.
Uni-Dur	See theophylline.
Unihep	See heparin.
Uniparin Calcium	See heparin.
Uniparin Forte	See heparin.
Uniphyl	See theophylline.
Uniphyllin Continuous	See theophylline.
Unitrol	See phenylpropanolamine.
Univasc	See ACE inhibitors.
Urinox	See norfloxacin.
Uri-Tet	See tetracycline antibiotics.
Valium	Chamomile, kava, or melatonin may increase sedative effect of this drug.
valproic acid	Depletes carnitine.

Medication	Interaction(s)
Vasotec	Taking European angelica, psoralea, or St. John's wort with this drug increases risk of sunburn.
	Taking supplemental potassium with this drug can cause potentially life-threatening hyperkalemia (excessive potassium in the bloodstream).
Vectrin	See tetracycline antibiotics.
Versed	Chamomile, kava, or melatonin increases sedative effect of this drug.
Viagra	L-arginine may make this drug more effective.
	Taking N-acetyl cysteine (NAC) with this drug may cause headaches.
	Taking more than 20 milligrams of niacin the same day as taking this drug may cause unusually low blood pressure (dizziness, fainting, light-headedness).
Vibramycin	See tetracycline antibiotics.
Vibra-Tabs	See tetracycline antibiotics.
Videx	See ddI.
Vidopen	See ampicillin.
Viraferon	See interferon.
Vivactil	See tricyclic antidepressants.
Vivarin	See caffeine.
warfarin	Asian ginseng, arnica, astragalus, bilberry, dan shen, devil's claw, dong quai, feverfew, garlic, ginger, ginkgo, green tea, horse chestnut, and quinine may increase risk of bruising, bleeding, or hemorrhage if taken with this drug.
	Broccoli, Brussels sprouts, cabbage, kale, onions, parsley, soy, and spinach may increase risk of bruising, bleeding, or hemorrhage if eaten in unusually large quantities when taking this drug.
	Reishi and St. John's wort decrease the effectiveness of this drug.
	Taking more than 500 milligrams a day of the form of vitamin E known as alpha-tocopherol polyethylene glycol succinate (TPGS) may increase risk of bleeding.
	This drug interferes with the absorption of iron, magnesium, and zinc. Do not take supplements of these minerals within 2 hours of taking this drug.
	Borage seed oil, especially if taken with fish oil, may increase risk of bleeding or bruising if taken with this drug.
	Coleus or ginkgo may increase risk of bleeding, bruising, and internal hemorrhage when taken with this drug.
	Niacin may increase risk of bleeding and bruising.
	Taking this drug with bromelain may increase risk of bleeding and bruising.
	Vitamin K in chlorella may increase risk of bleeding or bruising.
Warfilone	Asian ginseng, arnica, astragalus, bilberry, dan shen, devil's claw, dong quai, feverfew, garlic, ginger, ginkgo, green tea, horse chestnut, and quinine may increase risk of bruising, bleeding, or hemorrhage if taken with this drug.
	Broccoli, Brussels sprouts, cabbage, kale, onions, parsley, soy, and spinach may increase risk of bruising, bleeding, or hemorrhage if eaten in unusually large quantities when taking this drug.
	Reishi and St. John's wort decrease the effectiveness of this drug.
	Taking more than 500 milligrams a day of the form of vitamin E known as alpha-tocopherol polyethylene glycol succinate (TPGS) may increase risk of bleeding.
	This drug interferes with the absorption of iron, magnesium, and zinc. Do not take supplements of these minerals within 2 hours of taking this drug.
Wellbutrin	See bupropion.
Wellferon	See interferon.
Westcort topical	See topical corticosteroids.

Medication	Interaction(s)
Wytensin	Taking inositol, niacin, or saw palmetto may cause unusually low blood pressure.
Xanax	Chamomile and melatonin both increase sedative effect of this drug.
Xenical	See orlistat.
yohimbine	L-arginine may make this drug more effective.
	Milk thistle (silymarin) makes this drug less effective.
Zagam	See Sparfloxacin.
zalcitabine	Depletes L-carnitine.
Zanaflex	See tizanidine HCl.
Zantac	Reduces body's absorption of calcium.
Zaroxolyn	See hydrochlorothiazide.
Zerit	Depletes vitamin B_{12}.
	L-carnitine may reduce muscle damage caused by this drug.
	N-acetyl cysteine (NAC) may reduce toxicity of this drug.
	Riboflavin may reverse fatty liver or lactic acidosis caused by this drug.
	Zinc may increase body weight, increase CD4+ levels, and help prevent *Pneumocystis carinii* pneumonia if taken with this drug.
Zestoretic	See hydrochlorothiazide *and* ACE inhibitors.
Zestril	See ACE inhibitors.
Zidovudine	Depletes vitamin B_{12}.
	L-carnitine may reduce muscle damage caused by this drug.
	N-acetyl cysteine (NAC) may reduce toxicity of this drug.
	Riboflavin may reverse fatty liver or lactic acidosis caused by this drug.
	Zinc may increase body weight, increase CD4+ levels, and help prevent *Pneumocystis carinii* pneumonia if taken with this drug.
	Vitamin E may lessen side effects of this drug.
Zocor	Magnesium supplements and antacids containing magnesium should not be taken within 2 hours of taking this drug.
	Depletes CoQ_{10}.
	Increases vitamin A levels in the bloodstream. If you take vitamin A with this medication, have a doctor monitor your vitamin A levels to prevent toxicity.
zolmitriptan	Taking this drug with 5-HTP may cause headaches and/or excitement.
Zoloft	Chromium may increase effectiveness of this drug in certain kinds of depression (dysthymic disorder, depression occurring on more days than not for more than 2 years).
	5-HTP may increase side effects of this drug.
	Ginkgo (240 milligrams daily) may offset sexual dysfunction induced by this drug.
	Do not take this drug within 10 days of taking St. John's wort.
	Do not go on an extreme low-sodium diet while taking this drug.
zolpidem	Taking 5-HTP with this drug may cause lucid dreaming or nightmares.
Zomig	Taking this drug with 5-HTP may cause headaches and/or excitement.
Zoroxin	See norfloxacin.
Zovia	See oral contraceptives.
Zyban	See buproprion.

NOTES

ABNORMAL PAP SMEAR

1. Yuan, F., Auborn, K., James, C., "Altered growth and viral gene expression in human papillomavirus type 16-containing cancer cell liens treated with progesterone," *Cancer Investigation,* 17(1), 19–29 (1999).

2. Ludicke, F., Stalberg, A., Vassilakos, P., Major, A.L, Campana, A., "High- and intermediate-risk human papillomavirus infection in sexually active adolescent females," *Journal of Pediatric and Adolescent Gynecology,* 14(4), 171–174 (November 2001).

3. Kahn, J.A., Rosenthal, S.L., Succop, P.A., Ho, G.Y., Burk, R.D., "Mediators of the association between age of first sexual intercourse and subsequent human papillomavirus infection," *Pediatrics,* 109(1), E5 (January 2002).

4. Butterworth, C.E., Jr., Hatch, K.D., Gore, H., Mueller, H., Krumdieck, C.L., "Improvement in cervical dysplasia associated with folic acid therapy in users of oral contraceptives," *American Journal of Clinical Nutrition,* 35, 73–82 (1982).

5. Zarcone, R., Bellini, P., Carfora, E., Vicinanza, G., Raucci, F., "Folic acid and cervical dysplasia," *Minerva Ginecologica,* 48, 397–400 (1996).

6. Goodman, M.T., Mcduffie, K., Hernandez, B., Wilkens, L.R., Bertram, C.C., Killeen, J., Le Marchand, L., Selhub, J., Murphy, S. Donlon, T.A., "Association of methylenetetrahydrofolate reductase polymorphism C677T and dietary folate with the risk of cervical dysplasia," *Cancer Epidemiology, Biomarkers, and Prevention,* 10(12), 1275–1280 (December 2001).

7. Kelly, G.S., "Folates: supplemental forms and therapeutic applications," *Alternative Medicine Review,* 3(3), 208–220 (June 1999).

8. Goodman, M.T., Mcduffie, K., Hernandez, B., Wilkens, L.R., Bertram, C.C., Killeen, J., Le Marchand, L., Selhub, J., Murphy, S. Donlon, T.A., ibid.

9. Romney, S.I., Palan, B.R., Basu, J., Mikhail, M., "Nutrient antioxidants in the pathogenesis and prevention of cervical dysplasias and cancer," *Journal of Cellular Biochemistry,* 23 (Suppl), 96–103 (1995).

10. Bendich, A., "Beta-carotene and the immune response," *Proceedings of the Nutrition Society,* 50, 263–274 (1991).

11. Mackerras, D., Irwig, L., Simpson, J.M., Weisberg, E., Cardona, M., Webster, F., Walton, L., Ghersi, D., "Randomized double-blind trial of beta-carotene and vitamin C in women with minor cervical abnormalities," *British Journal of Cancer,* 79(9–10), 1448–1453 (March 1999).

12. Nagata, C., Shimizu, H., Yoshikawa, H. Noda, K., Nozawa, S., Yamima, A., Sekiya, S., Sugimori, H., Hirai, Y., Kanazawa, K., Sugase, M., Kawana, T., "Serum carotenoids and vitamins and risk of cervical dysplasia froma case-control study in Japan," *British Journal of Cancer,* 81(7), 1234–1237 (December 1999).

13. Goodman, M.T., Kiviat, N., Mcduffie, K., Hankin, J.H., Hernandez, B., Wilkens, L.R., Franke, A., Kupyers, J., Kolonel, L.N., Nakamura, J., Ing, G., Branch, B., Bertram, C.C., Kamemoto, L., Sharma, S., Killeen, J., "The association of plasma micronutrients with the risk of cervical dysplasia in Hawaii," *Cancer Epidemiology, Biomarkers, and Prevention,* 7(6), 537–544 (June 1998).

14. Kanetsky, P.A., Gammon, M.D., Mandelblatt, J., Zhang, Z.F., Ramsey, E., Dnistrian, A., Norku, E.P., Wright, T.C., Jr., "Dietary intake and blood levels of lycopene: association with cervical dysplasia among non-Hispanic, black women," *Nutrition and Cancer,* 31(1), 31–40 (1998).

15. Nagata, C., Shimizu, H., Higashiiwai, H., Sugahara, N., Morita, N., Komatsu, S., Hisamichi, S., "Serum retinol level and risk of subsequent cervical cancer in cases with cervical dysplasia," *Cancer Investigation,* 17(4), 253–258 (1999).

16. Yeo, A.S., Schiff, M.A., Montoya, G., Masuk, M., van Asselt-King, L., Becker, T.M., "Serum micronutrients and cervical dysplasia in Southwestern American Indian women," *Nutrition and Cancer,* 38(2), 141–150 (2000).

17. Thomson, S.W., Heimburger, D.C., Cornwell, P.E., Turner, M.E., Superrich, H.L., Fox, L.H., Butterworth, C.E., "Correlates of total plasma homocysteine: folic acid, copper, and cervical dysplasia," *Nutrition,* 16(6), 411–416 (June 2000).

18. Linden, S.I., Hurwitz, C.A., Larson, C.J., Stanley, M.E., "Abnormal cervicovaginal smears due to endometriosis: a continuing problem," *Diagnostic Cytopathology,* 26(1), 35–40 (January 2002).

19. Cerqueira, E.M., Santotor, C.L., Donozo, N.F., Freitas, B.A., Pereira, C.A., Vebilacqua, R.G., Machado, Santelli, G.M., "Genetic damage in exfoliated cells of the uterine cervix: Association and interaction between cigarette smoking and progression to malignant transformation," *Acta Cytologica,* 42(3), 639–649 (May–June 1998).

20. de Vet, H.C.W., Stumran, F., "Risk factors for cervical dysplasia: implications for prevention," *Public Health,* 108, 241–249 (1994).

21. Sawaya, G.F., Grady, D., Kerlikowske, K., Valleur, J.L., Barnabei, V.M., Bass, K., Snyder, T.E., Pickar, J.H., Agarwal, S.K., Mandelblatt, J., "The positive predictive value of cervical smears in previously screened postmenopausal women: the heart and estrogen/progestin replacement study (HERS)," *Annals of Internal Medicine,* 133 (12), 942–950 (19 December 2000).

ABSESSES OF THE SKIN

1. Payne, M.C., Wood, H.F., Karakawa, W., Gluck, L., "A prospective study of staphylococcal colonization and infections in newborns and their families," *American Journal of Epidemiology,* 82, 305–316 (1966).

2. Wadlvogel, F.A., *Staphylococcus aureus* (including staphylococcal toxic shock). In: Mandell, G.L., Bennett, J.E., Dolin, R., editors. *Principles and Practice of Infectious Diseases,* Fifth Edition (Philadelphia: Churchill Livingstone, 2000), pp. 2072–2073.

3. Ross, S., Rodriguez, W., Controni, G., Khan, W., "Staphylococcal susceptibility to penicillin G: The changing pattern among community isolates," *Journal of the American Medical Association,* 2229, 1075–1077 (1974).

4. Sanford, M.D., Widmer, A.F., Bale, M.J., Jones, R.N., Wenzel, R.P., "Efficient detection and long-term persistence of the carriage of methicillin-resistant *Staphylococcus aureus,*" *Clinical Infectious Disease,* 19, 1123–1128 (1994).

5. Havsteen, B., "Flavonoids, a class of natural products of high pharmacological potency," *Biochemical Pharmacology,* 32, 1141–1148 (1983).

6. Rimoldi, R., Ginesu, F., Giura, R., "The use of bromelain in pneumological therapy," *Drugs in Experimental Clinical Research,* 4, 55–66 (1978).

7. Ako, H., Cheung, A., Matsura, P., "Isolation of a fibrinolysis enzyme activator from commercial bromelain," *Archives of International Pharmacodynamics,* 254, 157–167 (1981).

8. Bliznakov, E., Casey, A., Kishi, T., "Coenzyme Q deficiency in mice following infection with Friend leukemia virus," *International Journal of Vitamin and Nutrition Research,* 45, 388–395 (1975).

9. Cazzola, P., Mazzanti, P., Bossi, G., "In vivo modulating effect of a calf thymus acid lysate on human T lymphocyte subsets and CD4+/CD8+ ratio in the course of difference diseases," *Current Therapies Research,* 42, 1011–1017 (1987).

10. Seifter, E., Rettura, G., Seiter, J., "Thymotrophic action of vitamin A," *Federal Proceedings,* 32, 947 (1973).

11. Semba, R.D., "Vitamin A, immunity, and infection," *Clinical Infectious Disease,* 19, 489–499 (1994).

12. Ginter, E., "Optimum intake of vitamin C for the human organisms," *Nutrition and Health,* 1, 66–77 (1982).

13. Gabor, M., "Pharmacologic effects of flavonoids on blood vessels," *Angiologica,* 9, 355–374 (1972).

14. Prasad, A., "Clinical, biochemical and nutritional spectrum of zinc deficiency in human subjects. An update," *Nutrition Review,* 41, 197–208 (1983).

15. Porea, T.J., Belmont, J.W., Mahoney, D.H., Jr., "Zinc induced anemia and neutropenia in an adolescent," *Journal of Pediatrics,* 136(5), 688–690.

16. Klein, A.D., Penneys, N.S., "Aloe vera," *Journal of the American Academy of Dermatology,* 18, 714–719 (1988).

17. Chu, D.T., Wong, W.L., Mavlight, G.M., "Immunotherapy with Chinese medicinal herbs," *Journal of Clinical and Laboratory Immunology,* 25, 119–129 (1988).

18. Zhao, K.S., Mancini, C., Doria, G., "Enhancement of the immune response in mice by *Astragalus membranaceus,*" *Immunopharmacology,* 20, 225–233 (1990).

19. Wildfeuer, A., Mayerhofer, D., "The effects of plant preparations on cellular functions in body defense," *Arzneimittel-Forschung,* 44(3), 361–366 (March 1994).

20. Kuhn, O., untitled article, *Arzneimittel-Forschung,* 3, 194–200 (1953).

21. Facino, R.M., Carini, M., Aldini, G., Marinello, C., Arlandini, E., Franzoi, L., Colombo, M., Pietta, P., Mauri, P., "Direct characterization of caffeoyl esters with antihyaluronidase activity in crude extracts from *Echinacea angustifolia* roots by fast atom bombardment tandem mass spectrometry," *Farmaco,* 48(10), 1447–1461 (October 1993).

22. Murray, M., Pizzorno, J., *Encyclopedia of Natural Medicine* (Rocklin, California: 1998), p. 223.

ACHILLES TENDONITIS

1. Langberg, H., Bjorn, C., Boushel, R., Hellsten, Y., Kjaer, M., "Exercise-induced increase in interstitial bradykinin and adenosine concentrations in skeletal muscle and peritendinous tissue in humans," *Journal of Physiology,* 542(Pt 3), 977–983 (1 August 2002).

2. Langberg, H., Olesen, J.L., Gemmer, C., Kjaer, M., "Substantial elevation of interleukin-6 concentration in peritendinous tissue, in contrast to muscle, following prolonged exercise in humans," *Journal of Physiology,* 542(Pt 3), 985–990 (1 August 2002).

3. Vazquez, B., Ortiz, C., San Roman, J., Plasencia, M.A., Lopez-Bravo, A., "Hydrophilic polymers derived from vitamin E," *Journal of Biomaterials Applications,* 15(2), 118–139 (October 2000).

4. Berger, R., Nowak, H., "A new medical approach to the treatment of osteoarthritis. Report of an open phase IV study with ademetionine (Gumbaral)," *American Journal of Medicine,* 83, 84–88 (1987).

5. Konig, B., "A long term (two years) clinical trial with S-adenosylmethionine

for the treatment of osteoarthritis," *American Journal of Medicine,* 83, 89–94 (1987).

6. Singh, B.G., Atal, C.K., "Pharmacology of an extract of Sali guggal ex-*Boswellia serrata,* a new non-steroidal anti-inflammatory agent," *Agents and Actions,* 18, 407–412 (1986).

7. Beg, M., Singhal, K.C., Afzaal, S., "A study of effect of guggulsterone of hyperlipidemia of secondary glomerulopathy," *Indian Journal of Physiology and Pharmacology,* 40(3), 237–240 (July 1996).

8. Schnitzer, T.J., "Non-NSAID pharmacologic treatment options for the management of chronic pain," *American Journal of Medicine,* 105(1B), 45S-52S (27 July 1998).

9. McCleane, G., "The analgesic efficacy of topical capsaicin is enhanced by glyceryl trinitrate in painful osteoarthritis: a randomized, double blind, placebo controlled study," *European Journal of Pain,* 4(4), 355–360 (2000).

10. Murray, M., Pizzorno, J., *Encyclopedia of Natural Medicine* (London: Churchill-Livingstone, 1999), p. 1448.

ACNE

1. White, G.M. "Recent findings in the epidemiologic evidence, classification, and subtypes of acne vulgaris," *Journal of the American Academy of Dermatology,* 39, S34–S47 (1998).

2. Cunliffe, W.J., Gould, D.J., "Prevalence of facial acne vulgaris in late adolescence and in adults," *British Medical Journal,* 166, 1109–1110 (1979).

3. Toyoda, M., Morohashi, M., "Pathogenesis of acne," *Medical Electron Microscopy,* 34(1), 29–40 (March 2001).

4. Abdel, K.M., El Mofty, A., Ismail, A., Bassili, F., "Glucose tolerance in blood and skin of patients with acne vulgaris. I.," *Journal of Investigational Dermatology,* 40, 259–261 (1963).

5. DeCherney, A.H., "Hormone receptors and sexuality in the human female," *Journal of Women's Health and Gender Base Medicine,* 9 Supl 1, S9–S13 (2000).

6. Takayasu, S., Wakimoto, H., Itami, S., Sano, S., "Activity of testosterone 5-alpha-reductase in various tissues of human skin," *Journal of Investigational Dermatology,* 74, 187–191 (1980).

7. Sansone, G., Reisner, R., "Differential rates of conversion of testosterone to dihydrotestosterone in acne and normal human skin—a possible pathogenic factor in acne," *Journal of Investigational Dermatology,* 56, 366–372 (1971).

8. Sheretz, E.F., "Acneiform eruption due to 'megadose' vitamins B_6 and B_{12}," *Cutis,* 48(2), 119–120 (August 1991).

9. Kappas, A., Anderson, K.F., Conney, A.H., Pantuck, E.J., Fishman, J., Bradlow, H.L, "Nutrition-endocrine interactions: induction of reciprocal changes in the delta 4–5 alpha reduction of testosterone and the cytochrome P-450-dependent oxidation of estrodiol by dietary macronutrients in man," *Proceedings of the National Academy of Sciences of the USA,* 80 (24), 7646–7649 (December 1983).

10. Offenbach, E., Pistunyer, F., "Beneficial effect of chromium-rich yeast on glucose tolerance and blood lipids in elderly patients," *Diabetes,* 29, 919–925 (1980).

11. McCarty, M., "High chromium yeast for acne," *Medical Hypotheses,* 14, 307–310 (1984).

12. Williams, D.D., Mueller, A., Browder, W., "Glucan-based macrophage stimulators: a review of their anti-infective potential," *Clinical Immunotherapy,* 5, 392–399 (1996).

13. Kohrle, J., "The deiodinase family: selenoenzymes regulating thyroid hormone availability and action," *Cellular and Molecular Life Sciences,* 57(13–14), 1853–1863 (December 2000).

14. Michaelsson, G., Edqvist, I., "Erythrocyte glutathione peroxidase activity in acne vulgaris and the effect of selenium and vitamin E. treatment," *Acta Dermatologica et Venerologica* (Stockholm), 64, 9–14 (1984).

15. Basak, P.Y., Gultekin, F., Klinc, I., "The role of the antioxidative defense system in papulopustular acne," *Journal of Dermatology,* 28(3), 123–127 (March 2001).

16. Hamilton, I.M., Gilmore, W.S., Benzie, I.F., Mulholland, C.W., Strain, J.J.,

"Interactions between vitamins C and E in human subjects," *British Journal of Nutrition,* 84(3), 261–267 (September 2000).

17. Bowles, W.H., "Protection against minocycline pigment formation by ascorbic acid (vitamin C)," *Journal of Esthetic Dentistry,* 10(4), 182–186 (1998).

18. Dreno, B., Amblard, P., Agache, P., "Low doses of zinc gluconate for inflammatory acne," *Acta Dermatologica et Venereologica,* 69, 541–543 (1989).

19. Dreno, B., Moyse, D., Alirezai, M., Amblard, P., Auffret, N., Beylot, C., Bodokh, I., Chivot, M., Daniel, F., Humbert, P., Meynadier, J., Polie, F., "Multicenter randomized comparative double-blind controlled clinical trial of the safety and efficacy of zinc of gluconate versus minocycline hydrochloride in the treatment of inflammatory acne vulgaris," *Dermatology,* 203(2), 135–140 (2001).

20. Porea, T.J., Belmont, J.W., Mahoney, D.H., Jr., "Zinc induced anemia and neutropenia in an adolescent," *Journal of Pediatrics,* 136(5), 688–690 (1980).

21. Khanna, S., Atalay, M., Laaksonen, D.E., Gul, M., Sashwati, R., Sen, C.K., "(-Lipoic acid supplementation: tissue glutathione homeostasis at rest and after exercise," *Journal of Applied Physiology,* 86(4), 1191–1196 (1999).

22. Symes, E., Bender, D., Bowen, J., Coulson, W., "Increased target tissue uptake of, and sensitivity to, testosterone in the vitamin B$_6$ deficient state," *Journal of Steroid Biochemistry,* 20, 1089–1093 (1984).

23. Snider, B., Dieteman, D., "Pyridoxine therapy for premenstrual acne flare," *Archives of Dermatology,* 110, 130–131 (1974).

24. Bassett, I.B., Pannowitz, D.I., Barnetson, R.S.C., "A comparative study of tea-tree oil versus benzoyl peroxide in the treatment of acne," *Medical Journal of Australia,* 153, 455–458 (1990).

25. Carson, C.F., Riley, T.V., "The antimicrobial activity of tea tree oil," *Medical Hypotheses,* 44, 490–491 (1995).

26. Dumenil, G., Chemli, R., Balansard, C., Guiraud, H., Lallemand, M., "Evaluation of antibacterial properties of marigold flowers (*Calendula officinalis* L.) and other homeopathic tinctures of *C. officinalis* L. and *C. arvensis* L.," *Ann. Pharm. Franç,* 38, 493 (1980).

27. Zitterl-Eglseer, K., Sosa, S., Jurentisch, J., Schubert-Zsilavecz, M., Della Loggia, R., Tubaro, A., Bertoldi, M., Franz, C. "Anti-oedematous activities of the main triterpendiol esters of Marigold (*Calendula officinalis* L.)," *Journal of Ethnopharmacology,* 57, 139–144 (1997).

28. Rendi, M., Mayer, C., Weniger, W., Tschachler, E., "Topically applied lactic acid increases spontaneous secretion of vascular endothelial growth factor by human reconstructed epidermis," *British Journal of Dermatology,* 145(1), 3–9 (July 2001).

29. Oh, C. W., Myung, K.B., "An ultrastructural study of the retention hyperkeratosis of experimentally induced comedones in rabbits: the effects of three comedololytics," *Journal of Dermatology,* 23(3), 169–180 (1996).

30. Bojra, R. A., Holland, K.T., Cunliffe, W.J., "The in-vitro-antimicrobial effects of azelaic acid upon *Propionibacterium acnes* strain P37," *Journal of Antimicrobial Chemotherapy,* 28(6), 843–853 (1991).

31. Nguyen, Q.H., Bui, T.P., "Azelaic acid: Pharmacokinetic and pharmacodynamic properties and its therapeutic role in hyperpigmentary disorders and acne," *International Journal of Dermatology,* 34, 75–84 (1995).

32. Anonymous, "Azelaic acid–a new topical treatment for acne," *Drug Therapy Bulletin,* 3, 5052 (1993).

33. Leung, L.H., "Pantothenic acid deficiency as the pathogenesis of acne vulgaris," *Medical Hypotheses,* 44, 490–492 (1995).

ACOUSTIC TRAUMA

1. Rüedi, L., "Vitamin A und schwerhörigkeit," *Wissenschäftlicher Dienst Roche,* 1952.

2. Shemesh, Z., Attias, J., Ornan, M., Shapira, N., Shahar, A., "Vitamin B$_{12}$ deficiency in patients with chronic-tinnitus and noise-induced hearing loss," *American Journal of Otolaryngology,* 14(2), 94–99 (March–April 1993).

3. Lamm, K., Arnold, W., "The effect of blood flow promoting drugs on cochlear blood flow, perilymphatic pO(2) and auditory function in the normal and noise-damaged hypoxic and ischemic guinea pig inner ear," *Hearing Research,* 141(1–2), 199–219 (March 2000).

4. Stange, G., Benning, C.D., "The influence on sound damages by an extract of *Ginkgo biloba,*" *Archiv der Otorhinolaryngolie,* 209(3), 203–215 (8 July 1975).

5. Vavrina, J., Müller, W., "Therapeutic effect of hyperbaric oxygenation in acute acoustic trauma physiological mechanisms of HBO responsible for the clinical success in AAT," *Revue de Laryngologie-Otologie-Rhinologie* (Bordeaux),116(5), 377–380 (1995).

6. Drew, S., Davies, E., 'Effectiveness of *Ginkgo biloba* in treating tinnitus: double blind, placebo controlled trial," *British Medical Journal,* 322(7278), 73 (13 January 2001).

ACTINIC KERATOSIS

1. Ziegler, A., Leffell, D.J., Kunala, S., et al., "Mutation hotspots due to sunlight in the p53 gene of nonmelanoma skin cancers," *Proceedings of the National Academy of Sciences of the U.S.A.,* 90, 4216 (1993).

2. Miller, J.H., "Mutagenic specificity of ultraviolet light," *Journal of Molecular Biology,* 182, 45–68 (1985).

3. Michalovitz, D., Halvey, O., Oren, M., "Conditional inhibition of transformation and of cell proliferation by a temperature-sensitive mutant of p53," *Cell,* 62, 671–680 (1990).

4. Stewart, M.S., Cameron, G.S., Pence, B.C., "Antioxidant nutrients protect against UVB-induced oxidative damage to DNA of mouse keratinocytes in culture," *Journal of Investigational Dermatology,* 106, 1086–1089 (1996).

5. Miyachi, Horio, T., Imamura, S., "Sunburn cell formation is prevented by scavenging oxygen intermediates," *Clinical and Experimental Dermatology,* 8, 305–310 (1983).

6. Hanada, K., Gange, R.W., Connor, M.J., "Effect of glutathione depletion on sunburn cell formation in the hairless mouse," *Journal of Investigational Dermatology,* 96, 838–840 (1991).

7. Sansone, G., Reisner, R., "Differential rates of conversion of testosterone to dihydrotestosterone in acne and normal human skin—a possible pathogenic factor in acne," *Journal of Investigational Dermatology,* 56, 366–372 (1971).

ADD/ADHD

1. Kidd, P.M., "Attention deficit/hyperactivity disorder (ADHD) in children: rationale for its integrative management," *Alternative Medicine Review,* 5(5), 402–428 (October 2000).

2. Langseth, L., Dowd, J., "Glucose tolerance and hyperkinesi," *Food and Cosmetic Toxicology,* 16, 129–133 (1978).

3. Retz, W., Thome, J., Blocher, D., Baader, M., Rosler, M., "Association of attention deficit hyperactivity disorder-related psychopathology and personality traits with the serotonin transporter promoter region polymorphism," *Neuroscience Letters,* 22, 319(3), 133–136 (February 2002).

4. Swain, A., Soutter, V., Loblay, R., Truswell, A.S., "Salicylates, oligoantigenic diets, and behaviour," *Lancet,* ii, 41–42 (1985).

5. Schulte-Korne, G., Deimel, W., Gutenbrunner, C., Hennighausen, K., Blank, R., Rieger, C., Remschmidt, H., "Effect of an oligo-antigen diet on the behavior of hyperkinetic children," *Zeitschrift für Kinder- und Jugend- Psychiatrie und Psychotherapie,* 24(3), 176–183 (September 1996).

6. Colquhoun, I., Bunday, S., "A lack of essential fatty acids as a possible cause of hyperactivity in children," *Medical Hypotheses,* 7, 673–679 (1981).

7. Stevens, L.J., Zentall, S.S., Abate, M.L., Watkins, B.A., Lipp, S.R., Burgess, J.R., "Omega-3 fatty acids in boys with behavior, learning, and health problems," *Physiology and Behavior,* 59, 915–920 (1996).

8. Aman, M.G., Mitchell, E.A., Turbot, S.H., "The effects of essential fatty acid supplementation by Efamol in hyperactive children," *Journal of Abnormal Child Psychology,* 15, 75–90 (1987).

9. Arnold, L.E., Kleykamp, D., Votolato, N.A., Taylor, W.A., Kontras, S.B., Tobin, K., "Gamma-linolenic acid for attention deficit hyperactivity disorder: placebo-controlled comparison to D-amphetamine," *Biological Psychiatry,* 25, 222–228 (1989).

10. Arnold, L.E., Pinkham, S.M., Votolato, N., "Does zinc moderate essential fatty acid and amphetamine treatment of attention-deficit/hyperactivity disorder," *Journal of Child and Adolescent Psychopharmacology,* 10(2), 111–117 (Summer 2000).

11. Coleman, M., Steinberg, G., Tippett, J., Bhagavan, H.N., Coursin, D.B., Gross, M., Lewis, C., DeVeau, L., "A preliminary study of the effect of pyridoxine administration in a subgroup of hyperkinetic children: a double-blind crossover comparison with methylphenidate," *Biological Psychiatry,* 14(5), 741–51 (October 1979).

12. Abikoff, H., Courtney, M.E., Szeibel, P.J., Koplewicz, H.S., "The effects of auditory stimulation on the arithmetic performance of children with ADHD and nondisabled children," *Journal of Learning Disabilities,* 29(3), 238–246 (May 1996).

13. Mehta, S.K., "Oral flower essences for ADHD," Journal of the American Academy of Child and Adolescent Psychiatry," 41(8), 895 (August 2002).

ADDISON'S DISEASE (ADRENOCORTICAL INSUFFICIENCY)

1. Oelkers, W., "Adrenal insufficiency," *New England Journal of Medicine,* 335, 1206–1212 (1996).

2. Arlt, W., Callies, F., van Vlijmen, J.C., Koehler, I., Reincke, M., Bidlingmaier, M., Huebler, D., Oettel, M., Ernst, M., Schulte, H.M., Allolio, B., "Dehydroepiandrosterone replacement in women with adrenal insufficiency," *New England Journal of Medicine,* 341, 1013–1020 (1999).

3. Oelkers, W., "Dehydroepiandrosterone for adrenal insufficiency (editorial)," *New England Journal of Medicine,* 341(14), 1073–1074 (30 September 1999).

AGE SPOTS

1. Cross. E., van der Vliet, A., Louie, S., Thiele, J.J., Halliwell, B., "Oxidative stress and antioxidants at biosurfaces: plants, skin and respiratory tract surfaces," *Environmental Health Perspectives,* 106, 1241–1251 (1998).

2. Yin, L., Morita, A., Tsuji, T., "Alterations of extracellular matrix induced by tobacco smoke extract," *Archives of Dermatological Research,* 292(4), 188–194 (April 2000).

3. Clausen, W.W., "Carotinemia and resistance to infection," *Transactions of the American Pediatric Society,* 43, 27–30 (1931).

4. Carughim, A., Hooper, P. G., "Plasma carotenoid concentrations before and after supplementation with a carotenoid mixture," *American Journal of Clinical Nutrition,* 59, 896–899 (1994).

5. Ben-Amotz, A., Mokadya, S., Edelstein S, Avron, M., "Bioavailability of a natural isomer mixture as compared with synthetic all-trans-beta-carotene in rats and chicks," *Journal of Nutrition,* 119(7), 1013–1019 (July 1989).

6. Stampfer, M.J., Willett, W., Hennekens, C.H., "Carotene, carrots, and neutropenia," *Lancet,* ii, 615 (1982).

7. Kemmann, E., Pasquale, S.A., Skaf, R., "Amenorrhea associated with carotenemia," *Journal of the American Medical Association,* 249, 926–929 (1983).

8. Lowe, N.J., DeQuoy, P.R., "Linoleic acid effects on epidermal DNA synthesis and cutaneous prostaglandin levels in essential fatty acids deficiency," *Journal of Investigational Dermatology,* 70, 200–203 (1978).

9. Prottey, C., "Investigation of functions of essential fatty acids in the skin," *British Journal of Dermatology,* 9, 29–38 (1977).

10. Ziboh, V.A., "Biochemical abnormalities in essential fatty acid deficiency," *Models in Dermatology,* 3, 106–111 (1987).

11. Haak, E., Usadel, K.H., Kusterer, K., Amini, P., Frommeyer, R., Tritschler, H.J., Haak, T., "Effect of alpha-lipoic acid on microcirculation in patients with peripheral diabetic neuropathy," *Experimental and Clinical Endocrinology and Diabetes,* 108(3), 168–174 (2000).

12. Bratman, S., "Vitamin C for Nicer Skin," TNP.com (06 April 2001).

ALCOHOL WITHDRAWAL

1. Brown, R.J., Blum, K., Trachtenberg, M.C., "Neurodynamics of relapse prevention: a neuronutrient approach to outpatient DUI offenders," *Journal of Psychoactive Drugs,* 22(2), 173–187 (April–June 1990).

2. Blum, K., Trachtenberg, M.C., Ramsay, J.C., "Improvement of inpatient treatment of the alcoholic as a function of neurotransmitter restoration: a pilot study," *International Journal of Addiction,* 23(9), 991–998 (September 1988).

3. Ferenci, P., Dragosics, B., Dittrich, H., "Randomized controlled trial of silymarin treatment in patients with cirrhosis of the liver," *Journal of Hepatology,* 9, 105–113 (1989).

4. Deak, G., Muzes, G., Lang, I., "Immunomodulator effect of silymarin therapy in chornic alcoholic liver diseases [abstract]," *Orvosi Hetilap,* 131, 1291–1292, 1295–1296 (1990).

5. Moohouse, M., Loh, E., Lockett, D., Grymala, J., Chudzik, G., Wilson, A., "Carbohydrate craving by alcohol-dependent men during sobriety: relationship to nutrition and serotonergic function," *Alcoholism in Clinical and Experimental Research,* 24(5), 635–643 (May 2000).

6. Townshen, J.M., Duka, T., "Attentional bias associated with alcohol cues: differences between heavy and occasional social drinkers," *Psychopharmacology* (Berlin), 157(1), 67–74 (August 2001).

7. Scott, N.R., Stambuk, D., Chakraborty, J., Marks, V., Morgan, M.Y., "Caffeine clearance and biotransformation in patients with chronic liver disease," *Clinical Science* (London), 74(4), 377–384 (April 1988).

8. Sayette, M.A., Monti, P.M., Rohsenow, D.J., Gulliver, S.B., Colby, S.M., Sirota, A.D., Niaura, R., Abrams, D.B., "The effects of cue exposure on reaction time in male alcoholics," *Journal of Studies in Alcoholism,* 55(5), 629–633 (September 1994).

ALCOHOLISM AND ALCOHOL ABUSE

1. Newman, J.C., Holden, R.J., "The 'cerebral diabetes' paradigm for unipolar depression," *Medical Hypotheses,* 41(5), 391–408 (November 1993).

2. Opie, L.H., "Role of carnitine in fatty acid metabolism of normal and ischemic myocardium," *American Heart Journal,* 97, 375–388 (1979).

3. Rossi, C.S., Siliprandi, N., "Effects of carnitine on serum HDL-cholesterol: report of two cases," *Johns Hopkins Medical Journal,* 150, 51–54 (1982).

4. Jermain, D.M., Crismon, M.L., Nisbet, R.B., "Controversies over the use of magnesium sulfate in delirium tremens," *Annals of Pharmacotherapy,* 26, 650–652 (1992).

5. Abbott, L., Nadler, J., Rude, R.K., "Magnesium deficiency in alcoholism," *Alcoholism in Clinical and Experimental Research,* 18, 1076–1082 (1994).

6. Suematsu, T., Matsumura, T., Sato, N., et al., "Lipid peroxidation in alcoholic liver disease in humans," *Alcoholism in Clinical and Experimental Research,* 5, 427–430 (1981).

7. Porea, T.J., Belmont, J.W., Mahoney, D.H., Jr., "Zinc-induced anemia and neutropenia in an adolescent," *Journal of Pediatrics,* 136(5), 688–690 (1980).

8. McMartin, K.E., Collins, T.D., Bairnsfather, L., "Cumulative excess urinary excretion of folate in rats after repeated ethanol treatment," *Journal of Nutrition,* 116, 1316–1325 (1986).

9. Murray, M., Pizzorno, J., *Encyclopedia of Nutrition* (London: Churchill-Livingstone, 1999), p. 1962.

ALLERGIES

1. Evans, R., III., "Epidemiology and natural history of asthma, allergic rhinitis, and atopic dermatitis." In: Middleton, E. Jr., Reed, C.E., Ellis, E.F., Adkinson, N.F., Yunginger, J.W., Busse, W.W., eds. *Allergy Principles and Practice,* Fourth Edition. (St. Louis, Missouri: Mosby, 1993) pp. 1109–1136.

2. Marshall, P.S., "Effects of allergy season on mood and cognitive function," *Annals of Allergy,* 71, 251–258 (1993).

3. Meltzer, E.O., Nathan, R.A., Seiner, J.C., Storms, W., "Quality of life and rhinitic symptoms: results of a nationwide survey with the SF-36 and RQLQ questionnaires," *Journal of Allergy and Clinical Immunology,* 99, 815–819 (1997).

4. Milgrom, H., Bender, B., "Adverse effects of medications for rhinitis," *Annals of Allergy, Asthma, and Immunology,* 78, 439–444 (1997).

5. Rimoldi, R., Ginesu, F., Giura, R., "The use of bromelain in pneumological therapy," *Drugs in Experimental Clinical Research,* 4, 55–66 (1978).

6. Ako, H., Cheung, A., Matsura, P., "Isolation of a fibrinolysis enzyme activator from commercial bromelain," *Archives of International Pharmacodynamics,* 254, 157–167 (1981).

7. Sheffner, A., "The reduction in vitro in viscosity of mucoprotein solution by a new mucolytic agent, n-acetyl-l-cysteine," *Annals of the New York Academy of Sciences,* 106, 298–310 (1963).

8. Jansen, D.F., Schouten, J.P., Vonk, J.M., Rijcken, B., Timens, W., Weiss, S.T., Postma, D.S., "Smoking and airway hyperresponsiveness especially in the presence of blood eosinophilia increase the risk to develop respiratory symptoms: a 25-year follow-up study in the general adult population," *American Journal of Respiratory Critical Care,* 160(1), 259–264 (July 1999).

9. Otsuka, H., Inaba, M., Fujikura, T., Kunitomo, M., "Histochemical and functional characteristics of metachromic cells in the nasal epithelium in allergic rhinitis: studies of nasal scrapings and their dispersed cells," *Journal of Allergy and Clinical Immunology,* 96, 528–536 (1995).

10. Taussig, S., "The mechanism of the physiological action of bromelain," *Medical Hypotheses,* 6, 99–104 (1980).

11. Murray, M.T., "A comprehensive review of vitamin C, *American Journal of Natural Medicine,* 3, 0–21 (1996).

12. Clemetson, C.A., "Histamine and ascorbic acid in human blood," *Journal of Nutrition,* 110, 662–668 (1980).

13. Podoshin, L., Gertner, R., Fradis, M., "Treatment of perennial allergic rhinitis with ascorbic acid solution," *Ear, Nose, and Throat Journal,* 70, 54–55 (1991).

14. Melmon, K.L., Rocklin, R.E., Rosenkranz, R.P., "Autocoids as modulators of the inflammatory and immune response," *American Journal of Medicine,* 71, 100–106 (1981).

15. Horton, B.T., "The clinical use of histamine," *Postgraduate Medicine,* 9, 1–11 (1951).

16. Mittman, P., "Randomized, double-blind study of freeze dried *Urtica dioica* in the treatment of allergic rhinitis," *Planta Medica,* 56, 44–47 (1990).

17. Zhou, R.L., Zhang, J.C., "An analysis of combined desensitizing acupoints therapy in 419 cases of allergic rhinitis accompanying asthma [MedLine abstract]", *Zhongguo Zhong Xi Yi Jie He Za Zhi,* 17(10), 587–589 (October 1997).

ALOPECIA AREATA

1. Shimizu, T., Mizue, Y., Abe, R., Watanabe, H., Shimizu, H., "Increased macrophage migration inhibitory factor (MIF) in sera of patients with extensive alopecia areata," *Journal of Investigational Dermatology,* 118(3), 555–557 (March 2002).

2. Hay, I.C., Jamieson, M., Ormerod, A.D., "Randomized trial of aromatherapy. Successful treatment for alopecia areata," *Archives of Dermatology,* 134(11), 1349–1352 (November 1998).

3. Tritrungtasna, O., Jerasutus, S., Suvanprakorn, P., "Treatment of alopecia areata with khellin and UVA (letter)," *International Journal of Dermatology* 32(9), 690 (1993).

4. Chen, M.F., Shimada, F., Kato, H., Yano, S., Kanaoka, M., "Effect of glycyrrhizin on the pharmacokinetics of prednisolone following low dosage of prednisolone hemisuccinate," *Endocronologica Japonica,* 37, 331–341 (1990).

5. Wiseman, M.C., Shapiro, J., MacDonald, N., Lui, H., "Predictive model for immunotherapy of alopecia areata with diphencyprone," *Archives of Dermatology,* 137, 1063–1068 (August 2001).

6. Garcia-Bravo, B., Rodriguez-Pichardo, A., Sanchez-Pedreno, P., "Nickel sulphate in the treatment of alopecia areata," *Contact Dermatitis.* 20, 228–229 (1989).

7. Rhodes, E.L., Dolman, W., Kennedy, C., Taylor, R.R., "Alopecia areata regrowth induced by *Primula obconica*," *British Journal of Dermatology,* 104, 339–340 (1981).

8. Neve, H.J., Bhatti, W.A., Soulsby, C., Kincey, J., Taylor, T.V., "Reversal of hair loss following vertical gastroplasty when treated with zinc sulfate," *Obesity Surgery,* 6(1), 63–65 (February 1996).

ALTITUDE SICKNESS

1. Lawless, N.P., Dillard, T.A., Torrington, K.G., Davis, H.Q., Kamimori, G., "Improvement in hypoxemia at 4600 meters of simulated mountain with carbohydrate ingestion," *Aviation, Space, and Environmental Medicine,* 70, 874–878 (1999).

2. Swenson, E.R., MacDonald, A., Vatheuer, M., Maks, C., Treadwell, A., Allen, R., Schoene, R.B., "Acute altitude sickness is not altered by a high carbohydrate diet nor associated with elevated circulating cytokines," *Aviation, Space, and Environmental Medicine,* 68, 499–503 (1997).

3. Gray, D., Milne, D., "Effect of dietary supplements on acute altitude sickness," *Perceptual and Motor Skills,* 63, 873–874 (1986).

4. Bailey, D.M., Davies, B., "Acute altitude sickness; prophylactic benefits of antioxidant vitamin supplementation at high mountain," *High Mountain Medicine and Biology,* 2, 21–29 (2001).

5. Roncin, J.P., Schwartz, F., D'Arbigny, P., "EGb 761 in control of acute altitude sickness and vascular reactivity to cold exposure," *Aviation, Space, and Environmental Medicine,* 67, 445–452 (1996).

6. Jefferson, J.A., Escudero, E., Hurtado, M.E., Pando, J., Tapia, R., Swenson, E.R., Prchal, J., Schreniner, G.F., Schoene, R.B., Hurtado, A., Johnson, R.J., "Excessive erythrocytosis, chronic altitude sickness, and serum cobalt levels," *Lancet,* 359(9304), 407–408 (2 Feburary 2002).

7. Kaur, C., Srinivisan, K.N., Singh, J., Peng, C.M., Ling, E.A., "Plasma melatonin, pinealocyte morphology, and surface receptors/antigen expression on macrophages/microglia in the pineal gland following a high-mountain exposure," *Journal of Neuroscience Research,* 67(4), 533–543 (15 February 2002).

8. Honigman, B., Noordewier, E., Kleinman, D., Yaron, M., "High altitude retinal hemorrhages in a Colorado skier," *High Mountain Medicine and Biology,* 2(4), 539–544 (Winter 2001).

ALZHEIMER'S DISEASE

1. Braunwald, E., Fauci, A.S., Kasper, D.L., Hauser, S.L., Longo, D.L., Jameson, J.L., editors. *Harrison's Principles of Internal Medicine,* Fifteenth Edition (New York: McGraw-Hill, 2001), p. 2391.

2. in t' Veld, B.A., Ruitenberg, A., Hofman, A., Launer, L.J., van Duijn, C.M., Stijnen, T., Bretler, M.M., Stricker, B.H., "Nonsteroidal anti-inflammatory drugs and the risk of Alzheimer's disease," *New England Journal of Medicine,* 345 (21), 1515–1521 (22 November 2001).

3. Shin, R.W., "Interaction of aluminum with paired helical filament tau is involved in neurofibrillary pathology in Alzheimer's disease," *Gerontology,* 43 (Suppl 1), 16–23 (1997).

4. Zapatero, M.D., Garcia de Jalon, A., Pascual, F., Calvo, M.L., Escanero, J., Marro, A., "Serum aluminum levels in Alzheimer's disease and other senile dementias," *Biological Trace Element Research,* 47, 235–240 (1995).

5. Frolich, L., Riederer, P., "Free radical mechanisms in dementia of the Alzheimer's type and the potential for antioxidative treatment," *Drug Research,* 45 443–446 (1995).

6. Matthews, K.A., Kuller, L.H., Wing, R.R., Meilahn, E.N., Plantinga, P., "Prior to use of estrogen replacement therapy, are users healthier than nonusers?" *American Journal of Epidemiology,* 143, 971–978 (1996).

7. Rieder, C.R., Fricke, D., "Vitamin B(12) and folate in relation to the development of Alzheimer's disease," *Neurology,* 57(9), 1742–1743 (13 November 2001).

8. Martin, D.C., Francis, J., Protetch, J., Huff, F.J., "Time dependency of cognitive recovery with cobalamin replacement: a report of a pilot study," *Journal of the American Geriatric Society,* 40, 168–172 (1992).

9. Ho, P.I., Collins, S.C., Dhitavat, S., Ortiz, D., Ashline, D., Rogers, E., Shea, T.B., "Homocysteine potentiates beta-amyloid neurotoxicity: role of oxidative stress," *Journal of Neurochemistry,* 78(2), 249–253 (July 2001).

10. Sano, M., Ernesto, C., Thomas, R.G., Lauber, M.R., Schafer, K., Grundman, M., Woodbury, P., Growdon, J., Cotman, C.W., Pfeiffer, E., Schneider, L.S., Thal, L.J., "A controlled trial of selegiline, alpha-tocopherol, or both as treatment for Alzheimer's disease: the alzheimer's disease cooperative study," *New England Journal of Medicine,* 3336(17), 1216–1222 (24 April 1997).

11. Tabet, N., Birks, J., Grimley Evans, J., "Vitamin E for Alzheimer's disease," *Cochrane Database Systems Review,* 2000(4):CD002854.

12. Brooks, J.O., III, Yesavage, J.A., Carta, A., Bravi, D., "Acetyl-l-carnitine slows decline in younger patients with Alzheimer's disease: a reanalysis of a

double-blind, placebo-controlled study using the trilinear approach," *International Psychogeriatrics,* 10, 193–203 (1998).

13. Geula, C., Mesulam, M., "Cortical cholinergic fibers in aging and Alzheimer's: a morphometric study," *Neuroscience,* 33, 469–481 (1989).

14. West, M.J., Coleman, P.D., Flood, D.G., Troncoso, J.C., "Differences in the pattern of hippocampal neuronal loss in normal aging and Alzheimer's disease," *Lancet,* 344, 769–772 (1994).

15. Nunzi, M.G., Milan, F., Guidolin, D., Toffano, G., "Dendritic spine loss in hippocampus of aged rats. Effect of brain phosphatidylserine administration," *Neurobiology of Aging,* 8, 501–510 (1987).

16. Crook, T.H., Tinklenberg, J., Yesavage, J., Petrie, W., Nunzi, M.G., Massari, D.C., "Effects of phosphatidylserine in age-associated memory impairment," *Neurology,* 41, 644–649 (1991).

17. Nerozzi, D., Magnani, A., Sforza, V., et al., "Early cortisol escape phenomenon reversed by phosphatidylserine in elderly normal subjects," *Clinical Trials Journal,* 26, 33–38 (1989).

18. Kidd, P.M., "A review of nutrients and botanicals in the integrative management of cognitive dysfunction," *Alternative Medicine Review,* 4(3), 144–161 (June 1999).

19. Le Bars, P.L., Katz, M.M., Berman, N., et al., "A placebo-controlled, double-blind, randomized trial of an extract of *Ginkgo biloba* for dementia. North American EGb study group," *Journal of the American Medical Association,* 278, 1327–1332 (1997).

20. Le Bars, P.L., Velasco, F.M., Ferguson, J.M., Dessain, E.C., Kieser, M., Hoerr, R., "Influence of the severity of cognitive impairment on the effect of the *Ginkgo biloba* extract EGb 761 in Alzheimer's disease," Neuropsychobiology, 45(1), 19–26 (2002).

21. Rister, R., "Kampo Medicine," *Let's Live* (February 2001).

22. Snowdon, D.A., Greiner, L.H., Mortimer, J.A., Riley, K.P., Greiner, P.A., Markesbery, W.R., "Brain infarction and the clinical expression of Alzheimer disease: the nun study," *Journal of the American Medical Association,* 277, 813–817 (1997).

23. Small, G.W., "The pathogenesis of Alzheimer's disease," *Journal of Clinical Psychiatry,* 59, 7–14 (1998).

AMBLYOPIA IN CHILDHOOD

1. The Pediatric Eye Disease Investigator Group, "The clinical profile of moderate amblyopia in children younger than 7 years," *Archives of Ophthalmology,* 120(3), 281–287 (March 2002).

2. The Pediatric Eye Disease Investigator Group, "A randomized trial of atropine vs. patching for treatment of moderate amblyopia in children," *Archives of Ophthalmology,* 120(3), 268–278 (March 2002).

3. Campos, E.C., Bolzani, R., Schiavi, C., Baldi, A., Porciatti, V., "Cytidine-5-diphosphocholine enhances the effect of part-time occlusion in amblyopia," *Documenti di Ophthalmologia,* 93(3), 247–263 (1996–1997).

AMENORRHEA

1. Miller, K.K., Parulekar, M.S., Schoenfeld, E., et al., "Decreased leptin levels in normal weight women with hypothalamic amenorrhea: the effects of body composition and nutritional intake," *Journal of Clinical Endocrinology and Metabolism,* 83, 2309–2312 (1998).

2. Snow, R.C., Schneider, J.L., Barbieri, R.L., "High dietary fiber and low saturated fat intake among oligomenorrheic undergraduates," *Fertility and Sterility,* 54, 632–637 (1990).

3. Laughlin, G.A., Dominguez, C.E., Yen, S.S., "Nutritional and endocrine-metabolic aberrations in women with functional hypothalamic amenorrhea," *Journal of Clinical Endocrinology and Metabolism,* 83, 25–35 (1998).

4. Benson, J.E., Engelbert-Fenton, K.A., Eisenman, P.A., "Nutritional aspects of amenorrhea in the female athlete triad," *International Journal of Sports Nutrition,* 6, 134–145 (1996).

5. Frederick, L., Hawkins, S.T., "A comparison of nutrition knowledge and attitudes, dietary practices, and bone densities of postmenopausal women, female college athletes, and nonathletic college women," *Journal of the American Dietetic Association,* 92, 299–305 (1992).

6. Hirschberg, A.L., Hagenfeldt, K., "Athletic amenorrhea and its consequences. Hard physical training at an early age can cause serious bone damage, *Lakartidningen,* 95, 5765–5770 (1998).

7. Kleiner, S.M., Bazzarre, T.L., Ainsworth, B.E., "Nutritional status of nationally ranked elite bodybuilders," *International Journal of Sports Nutrition,* 4, 54–69 (1994).

8. Kalkwarf, H.J., Specker, B.L., Ho, M., "Effects of calcium supplementation on calcium homeostasis and bone turnover in lactating women," *Journal of Clinical Endocrinology and Metabolism,* 84, 464–470 (1999).

9. Couzinet, B., Young, J., Brailly, S., et al., "Functional hypothalamic amenorrhoea, a partial and reversible gonadotrophin deficiency of nutritional origin," *Clinical Endocrinology* (Oxford), 50, 229–235 (1999).

10. Kemmann, E., Pasquale, S.A., Skaf, R., "Amenorrhea associated with carotenemia," *Journal of the American Medical Association,* 249, 926–929 (1983).

11. Martin-Du Pan, R.C., Hermann, W., Chardon, F., "Hypercarotenemia, amenorrhea and a vegetarian diet," *Journal de gynecologie, obstetrique et biologie de la reproduction* (Paris), 19(3), 290–294 (1990).

12. Mühlenstedt, D., Bohnet, H.G., Hanker, J.P., Schneider, H.P., "Short luteal phase and prolactin," *International Journal of Fertility,* 23(3), 213–218 (1978).

13. Loch, E.G., Katzorke, T., "Diagnosis and treatment of dyshormonal menstrual periods in general practice," *Gynäkologische Praxis,* 14, 489–495 (1990).

14. Gerhard, I., Postneek, F., "Possibilities of therapy by ear acupuncture in female sterility," *Geburtshilfe Frauenheilkunde,* 48, 165–171 (1988).

15. Kubista, E., Boschitsch, E., Spona, J., "Effect of ear-acupuncture on the LH-concentration in serum in patients with secondary amenorrhea," *Wiener Medizinische Wochenschrift,* 131, 123–126 (1981).

AMYOTROPHIC LATERAL SCLEROSIS (ALS)

1. Plaitakis, A., Caroscio, J.T., "Abnormal glutamate metabolism in amyotrophic lateral sclerosis," *Annals of Neurology,* 22, 575–579 (1987).

2. Blackstone, C.D., Huganir, R.L., "Molecular structure of glutamate receptor channels" In Stone, T.W., editor, *Neurotransmitters and Neuromodulators* (Boca Raton, Florida: CRC Press, 1995), 53–67.

3. Olney, J.W., "Excitotoxic food additives: functional teratological aspects," *Progress in Brain Research,* 18, 283–294 (1988).

4. Desnuelle, C., Dib, M., Garrei, C., Favier, A., "A double-blind, placebo-controlled randomized clinical trial of alpha-tocopherol (vitamin E) in the treatment of amyotrophic lateral sclerosis. ALS riluzole-tocopherol Study Group," *Amyotrophic Lateral Sclerosis and Other Motor Neuron Disorders,* 2(1), 9–18 (March 2001).

5. Plaitakis, A., Smith, J., Mandeli, J., Yahr, M.D., "Pilot trial of branched-chain amino acids in amyotrophic lateral sclerosis," *Lancet,* 1(8593), 1015–1018 (7 May 1988).

6. Tandan, R., Bromberg, M.B., Forshew, D., Fries, T.J., Badger, G.J., Carpenter, J., Krusinski, P.B., Betts, E.F., Arciero, K., Nau, K., "A controlled trial of amino acid therapy in amyotrophic lateral sclerosis: I. Clinical, functional, and maximum isometric torque data," *Neurology,* 47(5), 1220–1226 (November 1996).

ANAL FISSURES

1. Wehrli, H., "Etiology, pathogenesis and classification of anal fissure," *Swiss Surgeon,* 1, 14–17 (1996).

2. Oh, C., Divino, C.M., Steinhagen, R.M., "Anal fissure, 20-year experience," *Diseases of the Colon and Rectum,* 38(4), 378–382 (April 1995).

3. Nelson, R., "Operative procedures for fissure in ano," *Cochrane Database Systems Review,* 1: CD0–02199 (2002).

4. Meier zu Eissen, J., "Chronic anal fissure therapy," *Kongressblatt der Deutsche Gesellschaft für Churgerie,* 118, 654–656 (2001).

5. McCallion, K., Gardiner, K.R., "Progress in the understanding and treatment of chronic anal fissure," *Postgraduate Medicine,* 77(914), 753–758 (December 2001).

6. Brisinda, G., Maria, G., Sganga, G., Bentivoglio, A.R., Albanese, A., Castagneto, M., "Effectiveness of higher doses of botulinum toxin to induce healing in patients with chronic anal fissures," *Surgery*, 131(2), 179–184 (February 2002).

7. McCallion, K., Gardiner, K.R., ibid.

8. Tankova, L., Yoncheva, K., Muhtarov, M., Kadyan, H., Draganov, V., "Topical mononitratetreatment in patients with anal fissure," *Alimentary Pharmacology and Therapy*, 16(1), 101–103 (January 2002).

9. Metcalf, A., "Anorectal disorders. Five common causes of pain, itching, and bleeding," *Postgraduate Medicine*, 98(5), 81–84, 87–89 (November 1995).

10. Iacono, G., Cavataio, F., Montalto, G., Florena, A., Tumminello, M., Soresi, M., Notarbartolo, A., Carroccio, A., "Intolerance of cow's milk and chronic constipation in children," *New England Journal of Medicine*, 339(16), 1100–1104 (15 October 1998).

11. Cheney, G., "Anti-peptic ulcer dietary factor," *Journal of the American Dietetic Association*, 26, 668–672 (1950).

12. Hughes, Gerson, C.D., Fabry, E.M., "Ascorbic acid deficiency and fistula formation in regional enteritis," *Gastroenterology*, 467, 428–433 (1974).

13. Accatino, L., Pizarro, M., Solis, N., Koenig, C.S., "Effects of diosgenin, a plant-derived steroid, on bile secretion and hepatocellular cholestasis induced by estrogens in the rat," *Hepatology*, 28(1), 129–140 (July 1998).

14. Yamada, T., Hoshino, M., Hayakawa, T., Ohhara, H., Yamada, H., Nakazawa, T., Inagaki, T., Lida, M., Ogasawara, T., Uchida, A., Hasegawa, C., Maurasaki, C., Miyaji, M., Hirata, A., Takeuchi, T., "Dietary diosgenin attenuates subacute intestinal inflammation associated with indomethacin in rats," *American Journal of Physiology*, 273(2 Part 1), G355–364 (August 1997).

15. Beveridge, R.J., Stoddard, J.F., Szarek, W.A., Jones, J.K.N., "Some structural features of the mucilage from the bark of *Ulmus fulva* (slippery elm mucilage)," *Carbohydrate Research*, 9, 429–439 (1969).

16. Mehanna, D., Platell, C., "Investigating chronic, bright red, rectal bleeding," *Australia New Zealand Journal of Surgery*, 71(12), 720–722 (December 2001).

ANAL ITCH

1. Pfenninger, J.L., Zainea, G.G., "Common anorectal conditions: Part I. symptoms and complaints," *American Family Physician*, 63(12), 2391–2398 (15 June 2001).

2. Accatino, L., Pizarro, M., Solis, N., Koenig, C.S., "Effects of diosgenin, a plant-derived steroid, on bile secretion and hepatocellular cholestasis induced by estrogens in the rat," *Hepatology*, 28(1), 129–140 (July 1998).

3. Beveridge, R.J., Stoddard, J.F., Szarek, W.A., Jones, J.K.N., "Some structural features of the mucilage from the bark of *Ulmus fulva* (slippery elm mucilage)," *Carbohydrate Research*, 9, 429–439 (1969).

4. Wiedemann, B., "Gluteal pruritis: not necessarily a mycotic etiology and especially don't recommend chamomile bath," *MMW: Münchener Medizinische Wochenschrift*, 143(37), 6–8 (13 September 2001).

ANAPHYLAXIS, PREVENTING RECURRENCES

1. Chen, M.F., et al., "Effect of glycyrrhizin on the pharmacokinetics of prednisolone following low dosage of prednisolone hemisuccinate," *Endocronologica Japonica*, 37, 331–341 (1990).

2. Shiozaki, T., Sugiyama, K., Nakazato, K., Takeo, T., "Effect of tea extracts, catechin and caffeine against type-I allergic reaction," *Yakugaku Zasshi*, 117(7), 448–454 (July 1997).

3. Murray, M.T., "A comprehensive review of vitamin C, *American Journal of Natural Medicine*, 3, 8–21 (1996).

4. Clemetson, C.A., "Histamine and ascorbic acid in human blood," *Journal of Nutrition*, 110, 662–668 (1980).

5. Feigen, G.A., Smith, B.H., Dix, C.E., Flynn, C.J., Peterson, N.S., Rosenberg,L.T., Pavlovic, S., Leibovitz, B., "Enhancement of antibody production and protection against systemic anaphylaxis by large doses of vitamin C," *Research Communications in Chemical Pathology and Pharmacology*, 38(2), 313–333 (November 1982).

6. Dalal, I., Binson, I., Reifen, R., Amitai, Z., Shohat, T., Rahmani, S., Levine,

A., Ballin, A., Somekh, E., "Food allergy is a matter of geography after all: sesame as a major cause of severe IgE-mediated food allergic reactions among infants and young children in Israel," *Allergy*, 57(4), 362–365 (April 2002).

7. Pastorello, E.A., Vieths, S., Pravettoni, V., Farioli, L., Trambaioli, C., Fortunato, D., Luttkopf, D., Calamari, M., Ansaloni, R., Scibilia, J., Ballmer-Weber, B.K., Poulsen, L.K., Wutrich, B., Hansen, K.S., Robino, A.M., Ortolani, C., Conti, A., "Identification of hazelnut major allergens in sensitive patients with positive double-blind, placebo-controlled food challenge results," *Journal of Allergy and Clinical Immunology*, 109(3), 563–570 (March 2002).

8. Hosey, R.G., Carek, P.J., Goo, A., "Exercise-induced anaphylaxis and urticaria," *American Family Physician*, 64(8), 1367–1372 (15 October 2001).

9. Rueff, F., Wenderoth, A., Przybilla, B., "Patients still reacting to a sting challenge while receiving conventional *Hymenoptera* venom immunotherapy are protected by increased venom doses," *Journal of Allergy and Clinical Immunology*, 108(6), 1027–1032 (December 2001).

ANEMIA, IRON-DEFICIENCY

1. For example, Mejia, L.A., Chew, F., "Hematological effect of supplementing anemic children with vitamin A alone and in combination with iron," *American Journal of Clinical Nutrition*, 48, 595–600 (1988).

2. Hunt, J.R., Gallagher, S.K., Johnson, L.K., "Effect of acorbic acid on apparent iron absorption by women with low iron stores," *American Journal of Clinical Nutrition*, 59, 1381–1385 (1991).

3. Sandoval, C., Berger, E., Ozkaynak, M.F., Tugal, O., Jayabose, S., "Severe iron deficiency anemia in 42 pediatric patients," *Pediatric Hematology and Oncology*, 19(3), 157–161 (March–April 2002).

4. Braunwald, E., Fauci, A.S., Kasper, D.L., Hauser, S.L., Longo, D.L., Jameson, J.L., editors, *Harrison's Principles of Internal Medicine*, Fifteenth Edition (New York: McGraw-Hill, 2001), p. 662.

5. Morck, T.A., Lynch, S.R., Cook, J.D., "Inhibition of food iron absorption by coffee," *American Journal of Clinical Nutrition*, 37, 416–420 (1983).

6. Mehta, S.W., Pritchard, M.E., Stegman, C., "Contribution of coffee and tea to anemia among NHANES II participants," *Nutrition Research*, 12, 209–222 (1992).

7. Kaltwasser, J.P., Werner, E., Schalk, K., et al., "Clinical trial on the effect of regular tea drinking or ion accumulation in genetic haemochromatosis," *Gut*, 43, 699–704 (1998).

ANEMIA, PERNICIOUS AND MEGALOBLASTIC

1. Fafouti, M., Paparrigopoulos, T., Liappas, J., Mantouvalos, V., Typaldou, R., Christodoulou, G., "Mood disorder with mixed features due to vitamin B_{12} and folate deficiency," *General Hospital Psychiatry*, 24(2), 106–109 (March–April 2002).

2. Braunwald, E., Fauci, A.S., Kasper, D.L., Hauser, S.L., Longo, D.L., Jameson, J.L., editors, *Harrison's Principles of Internal Medicine*, Fifteenth Edition (New York: McGraw-Hill, 2001), pp. 674–680.

3. Pittock, S.J., Payne, T.A., Harper, C.M., "Reversible myelopathy in a 34-year-old man with vitamin B_{12} deficiency," *Mayo Clinic Proceedings*, 77(3), 291–294 (March 2002).

4. Miyamoto, M., Takahashi, H., Sakata, I., Adachi, Y., "Hepatitis-associated aplastic anemia and transfusion-transmitted virus infection," *Internal Medicine*, 39(12), 1068–1070 (December 2000).

5. Dagnelie, P.C., van Staveren, W.A., van den Berg, H., "Vitamin B_{12} from algae appears not to be bioavailable," *American Journal of Cinical Nutrition*, 53, 695–697 (1991).

ANEURYSM

1. Heller, L.J., Mohrman, D.E., Prohaska, J.R., "Decreased passive stiffness of cardiac myocytes and cardiac tissue from copper-deficient rat hearts," *American Journal of Physiology Heart and Circulatory Physiology*, 278(6), H1840–H1847 (June 2000).

2. Iskra, M., Patelski, J., Majewski, W., "Relationship of calcium, magnesium, zinc and copper concentrations in the arterial wall and serum in atherosclerosis obliterans and aneurysm," *Journal of Trace Elements in Medicine and Biology*, 11(4), 248–252 (December 1997).

3. Tornwall, M.E., Virtamo, J., Haukka, J.K., Albanes, D., Huttunen J.K., "Alpha-tocopherol (vitamin E) and beta-carotene supplementation does not affect the risk for large abdominal aortic aneurysm in a controlled trial," *Atherosclerosis*, 157(1) 167–73 (July, 2001)

4. Wijnen, M.H., Roumen, R.M., Vader, H.L., Goris, R.J., "A multiantioxidant supplementation reduces damage from ischaemia reperfusion in patients after lower torso ischaemia. A randomized trial," *European Journal of Vascular and Endovascular Surgery*, 23(6), 486–490 (June 2002).

ANGINA

1. Folkers, K., Yamamura. Y., editors. *Biomedical and clinical aspects of conezyme* Q$_{10}$. Volumes *1–4* (Amsterdam: Elsevier, 1977, 1980, 1982, 1984).

2. Kamikawa, T., Kobayashi, A., Yamashita, T., Hayashi, H., Yamazaki, N., "Effects of coenzyme Q$_{10}$ on exercise tolerance in chronic stable angina pectoris," *American Journal of Cardiology*, 56, 247 (1985).

3. Tran, M.T., Mitchell, T.M., Kennedy, D.T., Giles, J.T., "Role of coenzyme Q$_{10}$ in chronic heart failure, angina, and hypertension," *Pharmacotherapy*, 21(7), 797–806 (July 2001).

4. Nagao, B., Kobayashi, A., Yamazaki, N., "Effects of L-carnitine on phospholipids in the ischemic myocardium," *Japanese Heart Journal*, 28(2), 243–251 (March 1987).

5. Cherchi, A., Lai, C., Angelino, F., Trucco, G., Caponnetto, S., Mereto, P.E., Rosolen, G., Manzoli, U., Schiavoni, G., Reale, A., et al., "Effects of L-carnitine on exercise tolerance in chronic stable angina: a multicenter, double-blind, randomized, placebo controlled crossover study," *International Journal of Clinical Pharmacology and Therapeutic Toxicology*, 23(10), 579–582 (October 1985).

6. Donati, C., Bertieri, R.S., Barbi, G., "Pantethine, diabetes mellitus and atherosclerosis. Clinical study of 1045 patients," *La Clinica Terapeutica*, 128, 411–422 (1989).

7. Turlapaty, P.D.M.V., Altura, B.M., "Magnesium deficiency produce spasms of coronary arteries. Relationship to etiology of sudden death ischemic heart disease," *Science*, 208, 199–200 (1980).

8. Murray, M., Pizzorno, J., *Encyclopedia of Natural Medicine* (London: Churchill-Livingstone, 1999), p. 1081.

9. Schüssler, M., Hölzl, J., Fricke, U., "Myocardial effects of flavonoids from *Crataegus* species," *Arzneimittel Forschung*, 45, 842–845 (1995).

10. Ceriana, P., "Effect of myocardial ischaemia-reperfusion on granulocyte elastase release," *Anaesthia and Intensive Care*, 20, 187–190 (1992).

11. Rajendran, S., Deepalakshmi, P.D., Parasakthy, K., Devaraj, H., Devaraj, S.N., "Effect of tincture of *Crataegus* on the LDL-receptor activity of hepatic plasma membrane of rats fed an atherogenic diet," *Atherosclerosis*, 123, 235–241 (1996).

12. Schüssler ,M., Hölzl, J., Rump, A.F., Fricke, U., "Functional and antiischaemic effects of monoacetyl-vitexinrhamnoside in different in vitro models," *General Pharmacology*, 26, 1565–1570 (1995).

13. Nasa, Y., Hashizume, H., Hoque, A.N., Abiko, Y., "Protective effect of *Crataegus* extract on the cardiac mechanical dysfunction in isolated perfused working rat heart," *Arzneimittel Forschung*, 43, 945–949 (1993).

14. Dwivedi, S., Agarwal. M.P., "Anti-anginal and cardioprotective effects of *Terminalia arjuna*, an indigenous drug, in coronary artery disease," *Journal of the Association of Physicians of India*, 42, 287–289 (1994).

15. Tripathi, S.N., Upadhyaya, B.N., Gupka, V.K., "Beneficial effect of *Inula racemosa* (Pushkarmoola) in Angina pectoris: a preliminary report," *Indian Journal of Physiology and Pharmacology*, 28, 73–75 (1984).

16. Singh, R.P., Singh, R., Ram, P., Batliwala, P.G., "Use of Pushkar-Guggul, an indigenous antiischemic combination, in the management of ischemic heart disease," *International Journal of Pharmacognosy*, 31, 147–160 (1993).

17. Parker, J.O., Parker, J.D., Caldwell, R.W., Farrell, B., Kaesemeyer, W.H., "The effect of supplemental L-arginine on tolerance development during continuous transdermal nitroglycerin therapy," *Journal of the American College of Cardiology*, 39(7), 1199–1203 (3 April 2002).

18. Cabiedes, J., Cabral, A.R., Lopez-Mendoza, A.T., Cordero-Esperon, H.A., Huerta, M.T., Alarcon-Segovia, D., "Characterization of anti-phosphatidylcholine polyreactive natural autoantibodies from normal human subjects," *Journal of Autoimmunity*, 18(2), 181–190 (March 2002).

ANIMAL BITES

1. Chakrabarty, K.H., Heaton, M., Dalley. A.J., Dawson, R.A., Freedlander, E., Khaw, P.T., Mac Neil, S., "Keratinocyte-driven contraction of reconstructed human skin," *Wound Repair and Regeneration*, 9(2), 95–110 (March–April 2001).

2. Silverstein, R.J., Landsman, A.S., "The effects of a moderate and high dose of vitamin C on wound healing in a controlled guinea pig model," *Journal of Foot and Ankle Surgery*, 38(5), 333–338 (September–October 1998).

3. Fulton, J.E., Jr., "The stimulation of postdermabrasion wound healing with stabilized aloe vera gel-polyethylene oxide dressing," *Journal of Dermatologic Surgery* and *Oncology*, 16(5), 460–467 (May 1990).

4. Kohyama, T., Ertl, R.F., Valenti, V., Spurzem, J., Kawamoto, M., Nakamura, Y., Veys, T., Allegra, L., Romberger, D., Rennard, S.I., "Prostaglandin E(2) inhibits fibroblast chemotaxis," *American Journal of Physiology Lung Cell Molecular Physiology*, 281(5), L1257–1263 (November 2001).

5. Bosse, J.P., Papillon, J., Frenette, G., Dansereau, J., Cadotte, M., Le Lorier, J., "Clinical study of a new antikeloid agent," *Annals of Plastic Surgery*, 3(1), 13–21 (July 1979).

6. Meijia, K., Reng, R., *Plantas medicinales de uso popular en la Amazonia Peruviana* (Lima, Peru: AECI and IIAP, 1995), p. 75.

7. Cooper, W.E., Perez-Mellado, V., Vitt, L.J., "Lingual and biting responses to selected lipids by the lizard *Podarcis lilfordi*," *Physiology and Behavior*, 75(1–2), 237–241 (1 February 2002).

8. Rothe, M., Rudy, T., Stankovic, P., "Treatment of bites to the hand and wrist—is the primary antibiotic prophylaxis necessary," *Handchirurgie · Mikrochirurgie · Plastische Chirurgie*, 34(1), 22–29 (January 2002).

ANOREXIA

1. Hewitt, P.L., Coren, S., Steel, G.D., "Death from anorexia nervosa: age span and sex differences," *Aging and Mental Health*, 5(1), 41–46 (February 2001).

2. Hullye, A.J., Hill, A.J., "Eating disorders and health in elite women distance runners," *International Journal of Eating Disorders*, 30(3), 312–317 (November 2001).

3. Farrow, J.A., "The adolescent male with an eating disorder," *Pediatric Annals*, 21(11), 769–774 (November 1992).

4. Hirata, Y., Sawada, M., Minami, M., Arai, H., Iizuka, R., Nagatsu, T., "Tryosine hydroxylase, tryptophan hydroxylase, biopterin, and neopterin in the brain of anorexia nervosa," *Journal Neural Transmission* (*Genetics Section*), 80(2), 145–150 (1990).

5. Avraham, Y., Hao, S., Mendelson, S., Berry, E.M., "Tyrosine improves appetite, cognition, and exercise tolerance in activity anorexia," *Medical Science in Sports and Exercise*, 33(12), 2104–2110 (December 2001).

6. Russell, J.D, Mira, M., Allen, B.J., Stewart, P.M., Vizzard, J., Arthur, B., Beumont, P.J., "Protein repletion and treatment in anorexia nervosa," *American Journal of Clinical Nutrition*, 59(1), 98–102 (January 1994).

7. Hadigan, C.M., Anderson, E.J., Miller, K.K., Hubbard, J.L, Herzog, D.B., Klibanski, A., Grinspoon, S.K., "Assessment of macronutrient and micronutrient intake in women with anorexia nervosa," *International Journal of Eating Disorders*, 28(3), 284–292 (November 2000).

8. Gilliland, K., Bullick, W., "Caffeine: a potential drug of abuse," *Advances in Alcohol and Substance Abuse*, 3, 53–73 (1984).

9. Neil, J.F., Himmelhoch, J.M., Mallinger, A.C., Mallinger J., Hanin I., "Caffeinism complicating hypersomnic depressive disorders," *Comprehensive Psychiatry*, 19, 377–385 (July–August 1978).

10. Greden, J., Fontaine, P., Lubetsky, M., Chamberlain, K., "Anxiety and depression associated with caffeinism among psychiatric patients," *American Journal of Psychiatry*, 135(8), 963–966 (August 1978).

11. Bolton, S., Null, G., "Caffeine, psychological effects, use and abuse," *Journal of Orthomolecular Psychiatry*, 10, 202–211 (1981).

12. Charney, D., Henninger, G., Jatlow, P., "Increased anxiogenic effects of caffeine in panic disorders," *Archives of General Psychiatry*, 42, 233–243 (1984).

13. Avraham, Y., Hao, S., Mendelson, S., Berry, E.M., ibid.

14. van Praag, H.M., "In search of the mode of action of antidepressants. 5-HTP/tyrosine mixtures in depression." *Advances in Biochemical Pscychopharmacology*, 39, 301–314 (1984).

15. Coppen, A., Bailey, J., "Enhancement of the antidepressant action of fluoxetine by folic acid: a randomized, placebo controlled trial," *Journal of Affective Disorders*, 60, 121–130 (2000).

16. Barbenel, D.M., Yusufi, B., O'Shea, D., Bench, C.J., "Mania in a patient receiving testosterone replacement postorchidectomy taking St John's wort and sertraline," *Journal of Psychopharmacology*, 14, 84–86 (2000).

17. Poldinger, W., Calanchini, B., Schwarz, W. A., "Functional-dimensional approach to depression: serotonin deficiency as a target syndrome in a comparison of 5-hydroxytryptophan and fluvoxamine," *Psychopathology*, 24, 53–81 (1991).

18. Sternberg, E.M., Van Woert, M.H., Young, S.N., Magnussen, I., Baker, H., Gauthier, S., Osterland, C.K., "Development of a scleroderma-like illness during therapy with L 5 hydroxytryptophan and carbidopa," *New England Journal of Medicine*, 303, 782–787 (1980).

19. Joly, P., Lampert, A., Thomine, E., Lauret, P., "Development of pseudobullous morphea and scleroderma-like illness during therapy with L-5-hydroxytryptophan and carbidopa," *Journal of the American Academy of Dermatology*, 25(2 Pt 1), 332–333 (1991).

20. Vorbach, E.U., Hübner, W.D., Arnold, K.H., "Effectiveness and tolerance of the hypericum extract LI 160 in comparison with imipramine: randomized double-blind study with 135 outpatients," *Journal of Geriatric Psychiatry and Neurology*, 7 Suppl 1, S19–S23 (October 1994).

21. Woelk, H., "Comparison of St. John's wort and imipramine for treating depression: randomized controlled trial," *British Medical Journal*, 321, 536–539 (2 September 2000).

22. Schrader, E., "Equivalence of St. John's wort extract (Ze 117) and fluoxetine: a randomized, controlled study in mild-moderate depression," *International Clinical Psychopharmacology*, 15(2), 61–68 (March 2000).

23. Brenner, R., Azbel, V., Madhusoodanan, S., Pawlowska, M., "Comparison of an extract of hypericum (LI 160) and sertraline in the treatment of depression: a double-blind, randomized pilot study," *Clinical Therapies*, 22(4), 411–419 (April 2000).

24. Butterweck, V., Winterhoff, H., Herkenham, M., "St John's wort, hypericin, and imipramine: a comparative analysis of mRNA levels in brain areas involved in HPA axis control following short-term and long-term administration in normal and stressed rats," *Molecular Psychiatry*, 6(5), 547–564 (September 2001).

25. Shelton, R.C., Keller, M.B., Gelenberg, A., Dunner, D.L., Hirschfeld, R., Thase, M.E., Russell, J., Lydiard, R.B., Crits-Cristoph, P., Gallop, R., Todd, L., Hellerstein, D., Goodnick, P., Keitner, G., Stahl, S.M., Halbreich, U., "Effectiveness of St John's wort in major depression: a randomized controlled trial," *Journal of the American Medical Association*, 285(15), 1978–1986 (18 April 2001).

26. Barbenel, D.M., Yusufi, B., O'Shea, D., Bench, C.J., "Mania in a patient receiving testosterone replacement postorchidectomy taking St John's wort and sertraline," *Journal of Psychopharmacology*, 14, 84–86 (2000).

27. Peebles, K.A., Baker, R.K., Kurz, E.U., Schneider, B.J., Kroll, D.J., "Catalytic inhibition of human DNA topoisomerase II alpha by hypericin, a naphthodianthrone from St. John's wort (*Hypericum perforatum*)," *Biochemical Pharmacology*, 62(8), 1059–1070 (15 October 2001).

28. Ruschitzka, F., Meier, P.J., Turina, M., Luscher, T.F., Noll, G., "Acute heart transplant rejection due to Saint John's wort." *Lancet*, 355, 547 (12 February 2000).

29. Johne, A., Brockmoller, J., Bauer, S., Maurer, A., Langheinrich, M., Roots, I., "Pharmacokinetic interaction of digoxin with an herbal extract from St. John's wort (*Hypericum perforatum*)," *Clinical Pharmacology and Therapeutics*, 66, 338–345 (October 1999).

30. Piscitelli, S.C., Burstein, A.H., Chaitt, D., Alfaro, R.M., Falloon, J., "Indinavir concentrations and St. John's wort [letter]," *Lancet*, 355,548 (12 February 2000).

31. Nebel, A., Schneider, B.J., Baker, R.K., Kroll, D.J., "Potential metabolic interaction between St. John's wort and theophylline," *Annals of Pharmacotherapy*, 33, 502 (1999).

32. Maurer, A., "Interaction of St. John's wort extract with phenprocoumon," *European Journal of Clinical Pharmacology*, 55, A22, Abstract 79 (1999).

33. Birmingham, C.L., Goldner, E.M., Bakan, R., "Controlled trial of zinc supplementation in anorexia nervosa," *International Journal of Eating Disorders*, 3, 251–255 (15 April 1994).

34. Hill, K., Bucuvalas, J., McClain, C., Kryscio, R., Martini, R.T., Alfaro, M.P., Maloney, M., "Pilot study of growth hormone administration during the refeeding of malnourished anorexia nervosa patients," *Journal of Child and Adolescent Psychopharmacology*, 10(1), 3–8 (Spring 2000).

35. Gross, H., et al., "A double-blind trial of alpha-9-tetrahydrocannabinol in the treatment of anorexia nervosa," Psychopharmocology, 3, 165–171 (1983).

ANTHRAX, CUTANEOUS

1. Hanna, P.C., Acosta, D., Collier, R.J., "On the role of macrophages in anthrax," *Proceedings of the National Academy of Sciences of the USA*, 90(21), 10198–101201 (1 November 1993).

2. Shin, S., Hur, G.H., Kim, Y.B., Yeon, G.B., Park, K.J., Park, Y.M., Lee, W.S., "Dehydroepiandrosterone and melatonin prevent *Bacillus anthracis* lethal toxin-induced TNF production in macrophages," *Cell Biology and Toxicology*, 16(3), 165–174 (2000).

3. Ide, N., Lau, B.H., "Garlic compounds minimize intracellular oxidative stress and inhibit nuclear factor-kappa b activation," *Journal of Nutrition*, 131(3s),1020S-1026S (March 2001).

ANXIETY (GENERALIZED ANXIETY DISORDER)

1. Freud, S., "The justification from neurasthenia of a particular syndrome: The anxiety neurosis," In *Collected Papers*, Volume 1 (New York: Basic Books, 1959), 76–106.

2. Wittchen, H.U., Zhao, S., Kessler, R.C., Eaton, W.W., "DSM-III-R generalized disorder in the National Comorbidity Survey," *Archives of General Psychiatry*, 51, 355–364 (1994).

3. Noyes, R., Jr., "Revision of the DSM III classification of anxiety disorders." In Noyes, R., Jr., Roth, M., Burrows, G.D., Eds., *Handbook of Anxiety* (Amsterdam: Elsevier Science Publishers, 1988), 81–107.

4. Eaton, W.W., Dryman, A., Weissman, M.M., "Panic and phobia." In Robins, L.N., Regier, D.A., editors, *Psychiatric Disorders in America: the ECA study* (New York: The Free Press, 1991), pp. 155–179.

5. Morgane, P.J., Jacobs, M.S., "Raphe projections to the locus coeruleus in the rat," *Brain Research Bulletin*, 4(4), 519–534 (1979).

6. Aston-Jones, G., Ennis, M., Pieribone, V.A., Nickell, W.T., Shipley, M.T., "The brain nucleus locus coeruleus: restricted afferent control of a broad efferent network," *Science*, 234, 734–737 (1986).

7. Charney, D., Henninger, C., Jatlow, P., "Increased anxiogenic effects of caffeine in panic disorders," *Archives of General Psychiatry*, 42, 233–243 (1984).

8. Chou, T., "Wake up and smell the coffee. Caffeine, coffee, and the medical consequences," *Western Medical Journal*, 157, 544–553 (1992).

9. Pizzorno, Jr., J.E., Murray, M.T. *Textbook of Natural Medicine*, Volume 2, Second Edition (Edinburgh: Churchill-Livingstone, 1999), p. 1044.

10. Altar, C., Bennett, B., Wallace, R., Yuwiler, A., "Glucocorticoid induction of tryptophan oxygenase," *Biochemical Pharmacology*, 32, 979–984 (1983).

11. File, S.E., Fluck, E., Leahy, A., "Nicotine has calming effects on stress-induced mood changes in females, but enhances aggressive mood in males," *International Journal of Neuropsychopharmacology*, 4(4), 371–376 (December 2001).

12. Dursun, S.M., Kutcher, S., "Smoking, nicotine and psychiatric disorders: evidence for therapeutic role, controversies and implications for future research," *Medical Hypotheses*, 52(2), 101–109 (February 1999).

13. Kahn, R.S., Asnis, G.M., Wetzler, S., Van Praag, H.M., "Neuroendocrine evidence of serotonin receptor hypersensitivity in panic disorder," *Psychopharmacology*, 96(3), 360–364 (1988).

14. Carroll, D., Ring, C., Suter, M., Willemsem, C., "The effects of an oral multivitamin combination with calcium, magnesium, and zinc on psychological well-being in healthy young male volunteers: a double-blind placebo-controlled trial," *Psychopharmacology* (*Berlin*), 150, 220–225 (2000).

15. Steiner, G.G., "The correlation between cancer incidence and kava consumption," *Hawaii Medical Journal*, 59(11), 420–422 (November 2000).

16. Dinh, L.D., Simmen, U., Bueter, K.B., Bueter, B., Lundstrom, K., Schaffner, W., "Interaction of various Piper methysticum cultivars with CNS receptors in vitro," *Planta Medica*, 67(4), 306–311 (June 2001).

17. Seitz, U., Schule, A., Gleitz, J., "[3H]-monoamine uptake inhibition properties of kava pyrones," *Planta Medica*, 63, 548–549 (1997).

18. Kretzschmar, R., Meyer, H.J., "Comparative studies on the anticonvulsant activity of the pyrone compounds of *Piper methysticum* Forst." *Archives of International Pharmacodynamics*, 177, 261–267 (1969).

19. Woelk, H., Kapoula, O., Lehrl, S., et al., "The treatment of patients with anxiety. A double-blind study: kava extract WS 1490 versus benzodiazepine," *Zeitschrift für Allgemeiner Medizin*, 69, 271–277 (1993).

20. Warnecke, G., "Psychosomatic dysfunctions in the female climacteric. Clinical effectiveness and tolerance of Kava Extract WS 1490," *Fortshritte für Medizin*, 109(4), 119–122 (10 February 1991).

21. Volz, H.P., Lieser, M., "Kava-kava extract WS 1490 versus placebo in anxiety disorders: a randomized placebo-controlled 25-week outpatient trial," *Pharmacopsychiatry*, 30(1), 1–5 (January 1997).

22. Watkins L.L., Connor K.M., Davidson, J.R., "Effect of kava extract on vagal cardiac control in generalized anxiety disorder: preliminary findings J, "*Psychopharmacol* 15(4), 283–286 (December 2001)

23. Watkins, L.L., Grossman, P., Krishnan, R., Sherwood, A., "Anxiety and vagal control of heart rate," *Psychosomatic Medicine*, 60(4), 498–502 (July–August 1998).

24. Blumenthal, M., "Kava safety questioned due to case reports of liver toxicity: expert analyses of case reports say insufficient evidence to make causal connection," *Herbalgram*, 55, 26–30 (2002).

25. Schmidt, M., Narstadt, A., "Is kava hepatotoxic?" Deutsche Apotheker Zeitung, 142(9), 58–63 (2002).

26. National Institutes of Health, National Institute of Mental Health, Anxiety Disorders Association of America, News Advisory, 15 December 1998.

27. Bradwejn, J., Zhou, Y., Koxzycki, D., Shlike, J., "A double-blind, placebo-controlled study on the effects of Gotu Kola (*Centella asiatica*) on acoustic startle response in healthy subjects," *Journal of Clinical Psychopharmacology*, 20(6), 680–684 (December 2000).

28. Eich, H., Agelink, M.W., Lehmann, E., Lemmer, W., Klieser, E., "Acupuncture in patients with minor depressive episodes and generalized anxiety. Results of an experimental study," *Fortschritte für Neurologie und Psychiatrie*, 68(3), 137–144 (March 2000).

29. Harvey, B.H., Brink, C.B., Seedat, S., Stein, D.J., "Defining the neuromolecular action of myo-inositol: application to obsessive-compulsive disorder," *Progress in Neuropsychopharmacology and Biological Psychiatry*, 26(1), 21–32 (January 2002).

30. Gelber, D., Levine, J., Belmaker, R.H., "Effect of inositol on bulimia nervosa and binge eating," *International Journal of Eating Disorders*, 29(3), 345–348 (January 2001).

31. Palatnik, A., Frolov, K., Fux, M., Benjamin, J., "Double-blind, controlled, crossover trial of inositol versus fluvoxamine for the treatment of panic disorder," *Journal of Clinical Psychopharmacology*, 21(3), 335–9 (June 2001).

32. Grimaldi, B.L., "The central role of magnesium deficiency in Tourette's syndrome: causal relationships between magnesium deficiency, altered biochemical pathways and symptoms relating to Tourette's syndrome and several reported comorbid conditions," *Medical Hypotheses*, 58(1), 47–60 (January 2002).

33. Kara, H., Sahin, N., Ulusan, V., Aydogdu, T., "Magnesium infusion reduces perioperative pain," *European Journal of Anaesthesiology*, 19(1), 52–56 (January 2002).

34. Lerner, V., Miodownik, C., Kaptsan, A., Cohen, H., Loewenthal, U., Kotler, M., "Vitamin B$_6$ as add-on treatment in chronic schizophrenic and schizoaffective patients: a double-blind, placebo-controlled study," *Journal of Clinical Psychiatry*, 63(1), 54–58 (January 2002).

35. Walach, H., Rilling, C., Engelke, U., "Efficacy of Bach-flower remedies in test anxiety: a double-blind, placebo-controlled, randomized trial with partial crossover," *Journal of Anxiety Disorders*, 15(4), 359–366 (July-August 2001).

36. Krall, E.A., Garvey, A.J., Garcia, R.I, "Smoking relapse after 2 years of abstinence: findings from the VA Normative Aging Study," *Nicotine and Tobacco Research*, 4(1), 95–100 (February 2002).

ARSENIC EXPOSURE

1. Gibson, R., Gage, L., "Changes in hair arsenic levels in breast and bottle fed infants during the first year of infancy," *The Science of the Total Environment*, 26, 33–40 (1982).

2. Chen, C.J., Chiiou, H.Y., Chiang, M.H., et al., "Arsenic levels in human blood, urine, and hair in response to exposure via drinking water," *Environmental Research*, 20, 24–32 (1979).

3. Hopenhayn-Rich, C., Biggs, M.I., Fuchs, A., et al, "Bladder cancer mortality associated with arsenic in drinking in Argentina," *Epidemiology*, 7, 117–124 (1996).

4. Liu, S.X., Athar, M., Lippai, I., Waldren, C., Hei, T.K., "Induction of oxyradicals by arsenic: Implication for mechanism of genotoxicity," *Proceedings of the National Academy of Sciences of the USA*, 98(4), 1643–1648 (13 February 2001).

5. Nakadaira, H., Endoh, K., Katagiri, M., Yamamoto, M., "Elevated mortality from lung cancer associated with arsenic exposure for a limited duration," *Journal of Occupational and Environmental Medicine*, 44(3), 291–299 (March 2002).

6. Liu, S.X., Athar, M., Lippai, I, Waldren, C., Hei, T.K., ibid.

7. Shaffrali, F.C., McDonagh, A.J., Messenger, A.G., "Hair darkening in porphyria cutanea tarda," *British Journal of Dermatology*, 146(2), 325–329 (February 2002).

8. Liu, S.X., Athar, M., Lippai, I., Waldren, C., Hei, T.K., ibid.

ASTHMA

1. Lang, D.M., Polansky, M., "Patterns of asthma mortality in Philadelphia from 1969 to 1991," *New England Journal of Medicine*, 331, 1542–1546 (1994).

2. Mannino, D.M., "Environmental tobacco smoke and childhood asthma: when is exposure most important? Program and abstracts of the 96th International Conference of the American Thoracic Society; May 5–10, 2000; Toronto, Ontario, Canada. Educational Tracks Session ALA24: Childhood Asthma: Is Change in Lifestyle the Key?" accessed from organizer website 21 February 2002.

3. Stein, R.T., Sherrill, D., Morgan, W.T., et al., "Respiratory syncytial virus in early life and the subsequent risk of wheezing and allergic sensitization: a longitudinal analysis," *Lancet*, 354, 541–545 (1999).

4. Platts-Mills, T.A. "Indoor environment and lifestyle: What are their roles in the etiology of childhood asthma? Program and abstracts of the 96th International Conference of the American Thoracic Society; May 5–10, 2000; Toronto, Ontario, Canada. Educational Tracks Session ALA24: Childhood Asthma: Is Change in Lifestyle the Key?" accessed from organized website 22 February 2002.

5. For example, Anderson, S.D., "Is there a unifying hypothesis for exercise-induced asthma?" *Journal of Allergy and Clinical Immunology*, 73, 660–665 (1984).

6. Miller, A.L., "The Etiologies, Pathophysiology, and Alternative/Complementary Treatment of Asthma," *Alternative Medicine Review*, 6(1), 20–47 (February 2001).

7. Peat, J.K., Saolme, C.M., Woolcock, A.J., "Factors associated with bronchial hyperresponsiveness in Australian adults and children," *European Respiratory Journal*, 5, 921–929 (1992).

8. Hodge, L., Solme, C.M., Peat, J.K., et al., "Consumption of oily fish and childhood asthma risk," *Medical Journal of Australia*, 164, 137–140 (1996).

9. Takemura, Y., Sakurai, Y., Honjo, S., Tokimatsu, A., Gibo, M., Hara, T., Kusakari, A., Kugai, N., "The relationship between fish intake and the prevalence of asthma: the Tokorozawa childhood asthma and pollinosis study," *Preventive Medicine*, 34(2), 221–225 (February 2002).

10. Broughton, K.S., Johnson, C.S., Pace, B.K., Liebman, M., Kleppinger, K.M., "Reduced asthma symptoms with n-3 fatty acid ingestion are related to

5-series leukotriene production," *American Journal of Clinical Nutrition,* 65, 1011–1017 (1995).

11. Harari, M., Barzillai, R., Shani, J., "Magnesium in the management of asthma: critical review of acute and chronic treatments, and Deutsches Medizinisches Zentrum's (DMZ's) clinical experience at the Dead Sea," *Journal of Asthma,* 35, 525–536 (1998).

12. Britton, J., Pavord, I., Richards, K., et al., "Dietary magnesium, lung function, wheezing, and airway hyperreactivity in a random adult population sample," *Lancet,* 344, 357–362 (1994).

13. Hill, J., Micklewright, A., Lewis, S., Britton, J., "Investigation of the effect of short-term change in dietary magnesium intake in asthma," *European Respiratory Journal,* 110, 2225–2229 (1997).

14. Feillet-Coudray, C., Coudray, C., Tressol, J.C., Pépin, D., Mazur, A., Abrams, S.A., Rayssiguier, Y., "Exchangeable magnesium pool masses in healthy women: effects of magnesium supplementation," *American Journal of Clinical Nutrition,* 75(1), 72–78 (January 2002).

15. Collipp, P.J., Goldzier, S., Weiss, N., et al., "Pyridoxine treatment of childhood bronchial asthma," *Annals of Allergy,* 35, 93–97 (1975).

16. Sur, S., Camara, M., Buchmeier, A., et al., "Double-blind trial of pyridoxine (vitamin B$_6$) in the treatment of steroid-dependent asthma," *Annals of Allergy,* 70, 147–152 (1993).

17. Reynolds, R.D., Natta, C.L., "Depressed plasma pyridoxal phosphate concentrations in adult asthmatics," *American Journal of Clinical Nutrition,* 41, 684–688 (1985).

18. Schwartz, J., Weiss, S.T., "Relationship between dietary vitamin C intake and pulmonary function in the first national health and nutrition examination survey (NHANES 1)," *American Journal of Clinical Nutrition,* 59, 110–114 (1994).

19. Ammon, H.P., Safayhi, H., Mack, T., Sabieraj, J., "Mechanism of anti-inflammatory actions of curcumin and boswellic acids," *Journal of Ethnopharmacology,* 38, 113–119 (1993).

20. Sharma, M.L., Khajuria, A., Kaul, A., et al., "Effect of salia guggal ex-*Boswellia serrata* on cellular and humoral immune responses and leucocyte migration," *Agents and Actions,* 24, 161–164 (1988).

21. Gupta, I., Gupta, V., Parihar, A., et al., "Effects of *Boswellia serrata* gum resin in patients with bronchial asthma: results of a double-blind, placebo-controlled, 6-week clinical study," *European Journal of Medical Research,* 3, 511–514. (1988).

22. Udupa, A.L., Udupa, S.L., Guruswamy, M.N., "The possible site of anti-asthmatic action of *Tylophora asthmatica* on pituitary-adrenal axis in albino rats," *Planta Medica* 57, 409–413 (1991).

23. Shivpuri, D.N., Menon, M.P.S., Prakash, D., "A crossover double-blind study on *Tylophora indica* in the treatment of asthma and allergic rhinitis," *Journal of Allergy,* 43, 145–150 (1969).

24. Nagarathna, R., Nagendra, H.R., "Yoga for bronchial asthma: a controlled study", *British Medical Journal,* 291, 1077–1079 (1985).

25. Lai, X., Li, Y., Fan, Z., Zhang, J., Liu, B., "An analysis of therapeutic effect of drug acupoint application in 209 cases of allergic asthma," *Journal of Traditional Chinese Medicine,* 21(2), 122–126 (June 2001).

26. Field, T., Henteleff, T., Hernandez-Reif, M., et al., "Children with asthma have improved pulmonary functions after massage therapy," *Journal of Pediatrics,* 132, 854–858 (1998).

27. Kern-Buell, C.L., McGrady, A.V., Conran, P.B., Nelson, L.A., "Asthma severity, psychophysiological indicators of arousal, and immune function in asthma patients undergoing biofeedback-assisted relaxation," *Applied Psychophysiology and Biofeedback,* 25, 79–91 (2000).

28. Denson, K., W., "Passive smoking in infants, children and adolescents. The effects of diet and socioeconomic factors," *International Archives of Environmental and Occupational Health,* 74(3), 527–535 (October 2001).

ATHEROSCLEROSIS

1. Rajaratnam, R.A., Gylling, H., Miettinen. T.A., "Cholesterol absorption, synthesis, and fecal output in postmenopausal women with and without coronary artery disease," *Arteriosclerosis and Thrombosis: A Journal of Vascular Biology* (American Heart Association), 21(10), 1650–1655 (October 2001).

2. Navab, M., Berliner, J.A., Subbanagounder, G., Hama, S., Lusis, A.J., Castellani, L.W., Reddy, S., Shih, D., Shi, W., Watson, A.D., Van Lenten, B.J., Vora, D., Fogelman, A.M., "HDL and the inflammatory response induced by LDL-derived oxidized phospholipids," *Arteriosclerosis, Thrombosis, and Vascular Biology,* 21(4), 481–488 (April 2001).

3. Navab, M., Hama, S.Y., Anantharamaiah, G.M., Hassan, K., Hough, G.P., Watson, A.D., Reddy, S.T., Sevanian, A., Fonarow, G.C., Fogelman, A.M., "Normal high density lipoprotein inhibits three steps in the formation of mildly oxidized low density lipoprotein: steps 2 and 3," *Journal of Lipid Research,* 41(9), 1495–1508 (September 2000).

4. Spieker, L.E., Sudano, I., Hurlimann, D., Lerch, P.G., Lang, M.G., Binggeli, C., Corti, R., Ruschitzka, F., Luscher, T.F., Noll, G., "High-density lipoprotein restores endothelial function in hypercholesterolemic men," *Circulation,* 105(12), 1399–1402 (26 March 2002).

5. Turpeinen, O., "Effect of cholesterol-lowering diet on mortality from coronary heart disease and other causes," *Circulation,* 59, 1–7 (1979).

6. Han, S.N., Leka, L.S., Lichtenstein, A.H., Ausman, L.M., Schaefer, E.J., Meydani, S.N., "Effect of hydrogenated and saturated, relative to polyunsaturated, fat on immune and inflammatory responses of adults with moderate hypercholesterolemia," *Journal of Lipid Research,* 43(3), 445–452 (March 2002).

7. Doherty, T.M., Uzui, H., Fitzpatrick, L.A., Tripathi, P.V., Dunstan, C.R., Asotra, K., Rajavashisth, T.B., "Rationale for the role of osteoclast-like cells in arterial calcification," *Federation of the American Societies for Experimental Biology* (FASEB) *Journal,* 16(6), 577–582 (April 2002).

8. Braunwald, E., "Shattuck lecture cardiovascular medicine at the turn of the millennium: triumphs, concerns, and opportunities," *New England Journal of Medicine,* 337(19), 1360–1369 (1997).

9. Gruberg, L., Weissman, N.J., Waksman, R., Fuchs, S., Deible, R., Pinnow, E.E., Ahmed, L.M., Kent, K.M., Pichard, A.D., Suddath, W.O., Satler, L.F., Lindsay, J. Jr., "The impact of obesity on the short-term and long-term outcomes after percutaneous coronary intervention: the obesity paradox," *Journal of the American College of Cardiology,* 39(4), 578–584 (20 February 2002).

10. Wilson, T., Porcari, J.P., Harbin, D., "Cranberry extract inhibits low density lipoprotein oxidation," *Life Sciences,* 62(24), PL381–PL3866 (1998).

11. Osakabe, N., Natsume, M., Adachi, T., Yamagishi, M., Hirano, R., Takizawa, T., Itakura, H., Kondo, K., "Effects of cacao liquor polyphenols on the susceptibility of low-density lipoprotein to oxidation in hypercholesterolemic rabbits," *Journal of Atherosclerosis and Thrombosis,* 7(3), 164–168 (2000).

12. Wakabayashi, Y., "Effect of germanium-132 on low-density lipoprotein oxidation and atherosclerosis in Kurosawa and Kusanagi hypercholesterolemic rabbits," *Bioscience, Biotechnology, and Biochemistry,* 65(8), 1893–1896 (August 2001).

13. Lee, M.J., Chou, F.P., Tseng, T.H., Hsieh, M.H., Lin, M.C., Wang, C.J., "Hibiscus protocatechuic acid or esculetin can inhibit oxidative LDL induced by either copper ion or nitric oxide donor," *Journal of Agricultural Food Chemistry,* 50(7), 2130–2136 (27 March 2002).

14. McQuillan, B.M., Hung, J., Beilby, J.P., Nidorf, M., Thompson, P.L., "Antioxidant vitamins and the risk of carotid atherosclerosis. The perth carotid ultrasound disease assessment study (CUDAS)," *Journal of the American College of Cardiology,* 38(7), 1788–1794 (December 2001).

15. Kelly, M.R., Loo, G., "Melatonin inhibits oxidative modification of human low-density lipoprotein," *Journal of Pineal Research,* 22(4), 203–209 (May 1997).

16. Makino, T., Ono, T., Muso, E., Honda, G., "Effect of *Perilla frutescens* on nitric oxide production and DNA synthesis in cultured murine vascular smooth muscle cells," *Phytotherapy Research,* 16 Suppl 1, 19–23 (March 2002).

17. Vahouny, G.V., Connor, W.E., Roy, T., Lin, D.S., Gallo, L.L., "Lymphatic absorption of shellfish sterols and their effects on cholesterol absorption," *American Journal of Clinical Nutrition,* 34, 507–513 (1981).

18. Patrick, L., Uzick, M., "Cardiovascular disease: C-reactive protein and the inflammatory disease paradigm: HMG-CoA reductase inhibitors, alpha-tocopherol, red yeast rice, and olive oil polyphenols. A review of the literature," *Alternative Medicine Review,* 6(3), 248–271 (June 2001).

19. de Lorgeril, M., Salen, P., Martin, J.L., Monjaud, I., Delaye, J., Mamelle,

N., "Mediterranean diet, traditional risk factors, and the rate of cardiovascular complications after myocardial infarction: final report of the Lyon Diet Heart Study," *Circulation*, 99(6), 779–785 (16 February 1999).

20. Leaf, A., "Dietary prevention of coronary heart disease: The Lyon Diet Heart Study," *Circulation*, 99, 733–735 (16 February 1999).

21. Tomeo, A.C., Geller, M., Watkins, T.R., Gapor, A., Bierenbaum, M.L., "Antioxidant effects of tocotrienols in patients with hyperlipidemia and carotid stenosis," *Lipids*, 30(12), 1179–1183 (December 1995).

22. Terentis, A.C., Thomas, S.R., Burr, J.A., Liebler, D.C., Stocker, R., "Vitamin E oxidation in human atherosclerotic lesions," *Circulatory Research*, 90(3), 333–339 (22 February 2002).

23. Wang, J., Lu, Z., Chi, J., et al., "Multicenter clinical trial of the serum lipid-lowering effects of a *Monascus purpureus* (red yeast) rice preparation from traditional Chinese medicine," Current Therapies in Research, 58, 964–978 (1997).

24. Heber, D., Yip, I., Ashley, J.M., Elashoff, D.A., Elashoff, R.M., Liang, V., Go, W., "Cholesterol-lowering effects of a proprietary Chinese red-yeast-rice dietary supplement," *American Journal of Clinical Nutrition*, 69(2), 231–236 (February 1999).

25. Yang, W.S., Lee, W.J., Funahashi, T., Tanaka, S., Matsuzawa, Y., Chao, C.L., Chen, C.L., Tai, T.Y., Chuang, L.M., "Weight reduction increases plasma levels of an adipose-derived anti-inflammatory protein, adiponectin," *Journal of Clinical Endocrinology and Metabolism*, 86(8), 3815–3819 (August 2001).

26. Brattström, L, Wilcken, D.E.L, "Homocysteine and cardiovascular disease: cause or effect," *American Journal of Clinical Nutrition*, 72(2), 315–322 (August 2000).

27. Borstelmann, S., "Mit Allium sativum das kardiale risiko verringern," *Gesundes Leben*, 75, 63–65 (1998).

28. Linde, K., ter Riet, G., Hondras, M., Vickers, A., Saller, R., Melchart, D., "Systematic reviews of complementary therapies - an annotated bibliography. Part 2: Herbal medicine," *BMC Complementary and Alternative Medicine*, 1(1), 5 (2001).

29. Lau, B.H., "Suppression of LDL oxidation by garlic," *Journal of Nutrition*, 131(3s), 985S-988S (March 2001).

30. Lee, M.J., Chou, F.P., Tseng, T.H., Hsieh, M.H., Lin, M.C., Wang, C.J., "Hibiscus protocatechuic acid or esculetin can inhibit oxidative LDL induced by either copper ion or nitric oxide donor," *Journal of Agricultural Food Chemistry*, 50(7), 2130–2136 (27 March 2002).

31. Dietrich, M., Block, G., Hudes, M., Morrow, J.D., Norkus, E.P., Traber, M.G., Cross, C.E., Packer, L., "Antioxidant supplementation decreases lipid peroxidation biomarker F(2)-isoprostanes in plasma of smokers," *Cancer Epidemiology, Biomarkers, and Prevention*, 11(1), 7–13 (January 2002).

32. Kaikkonen, J., Porkkala-Sarataho, E., Morrow, J.D., Roberts, L.J., 2nd, Nyyssonen, K., Salonen, R., Tuomainen, T.P., Ristonmaa, U., Poulsen, H.E., Salonen, J.T., "Supplementation with vitamin E but not with vitamin C lowers lipid peroxidation in vivo in mildly hypercholesterolemic men," *Free Radical Research*, 35(6), 967–978 (December 2001).

33. King, M.S., Carr, T., D'Cruz, C., "Transcendental meditation, hypertension and heart disease," *Australian Family Physician*, 31(2), 164–168 (February 2002).

34. Beck, J.D., Elter, J.R., Heiss, G., Couper, D., Mauriello, S.M., Offenbacher, S., "Relationship of periodontal disease to carotid artery intima-media wall thickness: the atherosclerosis risk in communities (ARIC) study," *Arteriosclerosis and Thrombosis: A Journal of Vascular Biology* (American Heart Association), 21(11), 1816–1822 (November 2001).

35. Suwa, T., Hogg, J.C., Quinlan, K.B., Ohgami, A., Vincent, R., van Eeden, S.F., "Particulate air pollution induces progression of atherosclerosis," *Journal of the American College of Cardiology*, 39(6), 935–942 (20 March 2002).

36. Gaenzer, H., Neumayr, G., Marschang, P., Sturm, W., Lechleitner, M., Foger, B., Kirchmair, R., Patsch, J., "Effect of insulin therapy on endothelium-dependent dilation in type 2 diabetes mellitus," *American Journal of Cardiology*, 89(4), 431–434 (15 February 2002).

ATHLETE'S FOOT

1. Greenberg, H.L., Shwayder, T.A., Bieszk, N., Fivenson, D.P., "Clotrima-

zole/Betamethasone dipropironate: a review of costs and complications in the treatment of common cutaneous fungal infections," *Pediatric Dermatology*, 19(1), 78–81 (January–February 2002).

2. Klein, P.A., Clark, R.A., Nicol, N.H., "Acute infection with *Trichophyton rubrum* associated with flares of atopic dermatitis," *Cutis*, 63(3), 171–172 (March 1999).

3. Ninomiya, J., Ide, M., Ito, Y., Takiuchi, I., "Experimental penetration of *Trichophyton mentagrophytes* into human stratum corneum," *Mycopathologia*, 141(3), 153–157 (1998).

4. Tong, M.M., Altman, P.M., Barnetson, R.S., "Tea tree oil in the treatment of tinea pedis," *Australian Journal of Dermatology*, 33, 145–149 (1992).

5. Eaton, S.A., Allen, D., Eades, S.C., Schneider, D.A., "Digital Starling forces and hemodynamics during early laminitis induced by an aqueous extract of black walnut (*Juglans nigra*) in horses," *American Journal of Veterinary Research*, 56(10), 1338–1344 (October 1995).

6. Pattnaik, S., Subramanyam, V.R., Kole, C., "Antibacterial and antifungal activity of ten essential oils in vitro," *Microbios*, 86(349), 237–246 (1996).

AUTISM

1. Tsai, L.Y., "Psychopharmacology in autism," *Psychosomatic Medicine*, 61, 651–665 (1999).

2. Van der Does, A.J., "The effects of trytophan depletion on mood and psychiatric disorders," *Journal of Affective Disorders*, 64(2–3), 107–19 (May 2001).

3. Reichelt, K.L., Ekrem, J., Scott, H., "Gluten, milk products and autism: Dietary intervention effects on behavior and peptide excretion," *Journal of Applied Nutrition*, 42, 2–10 (1990).

4. Martineau, J., Barthelemy, C., Garreau, B., Lelord, G., "Vitamin B$_6$, magnesium, and combined B$_6$-Mg: therapeutic effects in childhood autism," *Biological Psychiatry*, 20(5), 467–478 (May 1985).

5. Lelord, G., Callaway, E., Muh, J.P., "Clinical and biological effects of high doses of vitamin B$_6$ and magnesium on autistic children." *Acta Vitaminologica et Enzymologica*, 4(1–2), 27–44 (1982).

6. McGuire, J.K., Kulkarni, M.S., Baden, H.P., "Fatal hypermagnesemia in a child treated with megavitamin/megamineral therapy," *Pediatrics*, 105, E18 (2000).

7. Kulman, G., Lissoni, P., Rovelli, F., Roselli, M.G., Brivio, F., Sequeri, P., "Evidence of pineal endocrine hypofunction in autistic children," *Neuroendocrinology Letters*, 21(1), 31–34 (2000).

8. Ishizaki, A., Sugama, M., Takeuchi, N., "Usefulness of melatonin for developmental sleep and emotional/behavior disorders—studies of melatonin trial on 50 patients with developmental disorders," *No To Hattatsu*, 31(5), 428–437 (October 1999).

9. Hayashi, E., "Effect of melatonin on sleep-wake rhythm: the sleep diary of an autistic male," *Psychiatry and Clinical Neuroscience*, 54(3), 383–384 (June 2000).

10. Latif, A., Heinz, P., Cook, R., "Iron deficiency in autism and Asperger syndrome," *Autism*, 6(1), 103–114 (March 2002).

11. Charlton, C.G., "Secretin modulation of behavioral and physiological functions in the rat," *Peptides*, 4(5), 739–742 (1983).

12. Barbarcyz, E., Szabo, G., Telegdy, G., "Effects of secretin on acute and chronic effects of morphine," *Pharmacology, Biochemistry & Behavior*, 51, 469–472 (1995).

13. Horvath, K., Stefanatos, K. G., Sokolski, K.N., Wachtel, R., Nabors, L., Toldon, J.T., "Improved social and language skills after secretin administration in patients with autistic spectrum disorders," *Journal of the Association for Academic Minority Physicians*, 9, 9–15 (1998).

14. Lightdale, J.R., Thayer, C., Duer, A., Lind-White, C., Jenkins, S., Siegel, B., Elliott, G.R., Heyman, M.B., "Effects of intravenous secretin on language and behavior of children with autism and gastrointestinal symptoms: a single-blinded, open-label study," *Pediatrics*, 108(5), 90 (November 2001).

BACK PAIN

1. Cassidy, J.D., Carroll, L.J, Cote, P., "The Saskatchewan health and back pain

survey. The prevalence of low back pain and related disability in Saskatchewan adults," *Spine,* 23(17), 1860–1867 (1 September 1998).

2. Kelsey, J.L., Githens, P.B., O'Conner, T., Weil, U., Calogero, J.A., Holford, T.R., White, A.A., 3rd, Walter, S.D., Ostfeld, A.M., Southwick, W.O., "Acute prolapsed lumbar intervertebral disc. An epidemiologic study with special reference to driving automobiles and cigarette smoking," *Spine,* 9(6), 608–13 (September 1984).

3. Thomas, E., Silman, A.J., Croft, P.R., Papageorgiou, A.C., Jayson, M.I., Macfarlane, G.J., "Predicting who develops chronic low back pain in primary care: a prospective study," *British Medical Journal,* 318(7199), 1662–1667 (19 June 1999).

4. Carrasco, S., Codoceo, R., Prieto, G., et al., "Effect of taurine supplements on growth, fat absorption and bile acid on cystic fibrosis," *Acta Universitatis Carolinae,* 36, 152–156 (1990).

5. Booth, S.L., Tucker, K.L., Chen, H., et al., "Dietary vitamin K intakes are associated with hip fracture but not with bone mineral density in elderly men and women," *American Journal of Clinical Nutrition,* 71, 1201–1208 (2000).

6. Green, M.R., Buchanan, E., Weaver, L.T., "Nutritional management of the infant with cystic fibrosis," *Archives of Diseases in Childhood,* 72, 452–456 (1995).

7. Kuhlwein, A., Meyer, H.J., Koehler, C.O., "Reduced diclofenac administration by B vitamins: results of a randomized double-blind study with reduced daily doses of diclofenac (75 mg diclofenac versus 75 mg diclofenac plus B vitamins) in acute lumbar vertebral syndromes," *Klinische Wochenschrift,* 68(2), 107–115 (19 January 1990).

8. Vetter, G., Bruggemann, G., Lettko, M., Schwieger, G., Asbach, H., Biermann, W., Blasius, K., Brinkmann, R., Bruns, H., Dorn, E., et al., "Shortening diclofenac therapy by B vitamins. Results of a randomized double-blind study, diclofenac 50 mg versus diclofenac 50 mg plus B vitamins, in painful spinal diseases with degenerative changes," *Zeitschrift für Rheumatologie,* 47(5), 351–362 (September-October 1988).

9. Schnitzer, T.J., "Non-NSAID pharmacologic treatment options for the management of chronic pain," *American Journal of Medicine,* 105(1B), 45S-52S (27 July 1998).

10. Lisi, A.J., "The centralization phenomenon in chiropractic spinal manipulation of discogenic low back pain and sciatica," *Journal of Manipulative Physiology and Therapy,* 24(9), 596–602 (November–December 2001).

11. Nyiendo, J., Haas, M., Goldberg, B., Lloyd, C., "A descriptive study of medical and chiropractic patients with chronic low back pain and sciatica: management by physicians (practice activities) and patients (self-management)," *Journal of Manipulative Physiology and Therapy,* 24(9), 543–551 (November–December 2001).

12. Waddell, G., Feder, G., Lewis, M., "Systematic reviews of bed rest and advice to stay active for acute low back pain," *British Journal of General Practice,* 47(423), 647–652 (October 1997).

13. Allen, C., Glasziou, P., Del Mar, C., "Bed rest: a potentially harmful treatment needing more careful evaluation," *Lancet,* 354(9186), 1229–1233 (9 October 1999).

14. Hansen, F.R., Bendix, T., Skov, P., Jensen, C.V., Kristensen, J.H., Krohn, L., Schioeler, H., "Intensive, dynamic back-muscle exercises, conventional physiotherapy, or placebo-control treatment of low-back pain. A randomized, observer-blind trial," *Spine,* 18(1), 98–108 (January 1993).

15. Cherkin, D.C., Eisenberg, D., Sherman, K.J., Barlow, W., Kaptchuk, T.J., Street, J., Deyo, R.A., "Randomized trial comparing traditional Chinese medical acupuncture, therapeutic massage, and self-care education for chronic low back pain," *Archives of Internal Medicine,* 161(8), 1081–1088 (April 2001).

16. Ehrenpreis, S., "Analgesic properties of enkephalinase inhibitors: animal and human studies," *Progress in Clinical and Biological Research,* 192, 363–370 (1985).

BALANITIS AND BALANOPOSTHITIS

1. Albertini, J.G., Holck, D.E., Farley, M.F., "Zoon's balanitis treated with Erbium: YAG laser ablation," *Lasers in Surgery and Medicine,* 30(2), 123–126 (2002).

2. Mitscher, L., Park, Y., Clark, D., "Antimicrobial agents from higher plants, "Glycyrrhiza glabra L. var. typica," *Journal of Natural Products,* 43, 259–269 (1980).

BARBER'S ITCH

1. Klein, P.A., Clark, R.A., Nicol, N.H., "Acute infection with *Trichophyton rubrum* associated with flares of atopic dermatitis," *Cutis,* 63(3), 171–172 (March 1999).

2. Ninomiya, J., Ide, M., Ito, Y., Takiuchi, I., "Experimental penetration of *Trichophyton mentagrophytes* into human stratum corneum," *Mycopathologia,* 141(3), 153–157 (1998).

3. Tong, M.M., Altman, P.M., Barnetson, R.S., "Tea tree oil in the treatment of tinea pedis," *Australian Journal of Dermatology,* 33, 145–149 (1992).

4. Eaton, S.A., Allen, D., Eades, S.C., Schneider, D.A., "Digital Starling forces and hemodynamics during early laminitis induced by an aqueous extract of black walnut (*Juglans nigra*) in horses," *American Journal of Veterinary Research,* 56(10), 1338–1344 (October 1995).

5. Pattnaik, S., Subramanyam, V.R., Kole, C., "Antibacterial and antifungal activity of ten essential oils in vitro," *Microbios,* 86(349), 237–246 (1996).

BAROTITIS MEDIA

1. Stangerup, S.E., Tjernstrom, O., Harcourt, J., Klokker, M., Stokholm, J., "Brotitis in children after aviation: prevalence and treatment with Otovent," *Journal of Laryngology and Otolaryngology,* 110(7), 625–628 (July 1996).

2. Kuhn, O., untitled article, *Arzneimittel-Forschung,* 3, 194–200 (1953).

3. Facino, R.M., Carini, M., Aldini, G., Marinello, C., Arlandini, E., Franzoi, L., Colombo, M., Pietta, P., Mauri, P., "Direct characterization of caffeoyl esters with antihyaluronidase activity in crude extracts from *Echinacea angustifolia* roots by fast atom bombardment tandem mass spectrometry," *Farmaco,* 48(10), 1447–1461 (October 1993).

4. Budzinski, J.W., Foster, B.C., Vandenhoek, S., Arnason, J.T., "An in vitro evaluation of human cytochrome P405 3A4 inhibition by selected commercial herbal extracts and tinctures," *Phytomedicine,* 7(4), 273–282 (July 2000).

5. Luettig, B., Steinmuller, C., Gifford, G.E., Wagner, H., Lohmann-Matthes, M.L., "Macrophage activation by the polysaccharide arabinogalactan isolated from plant cell cultures of *Echinacea purpurea,*" *Journal of the National Cancer Institute,* 81(9), 669–675 (3 May 1989).

6. Blumenthal, M., Goldberg, A., Brinckmann, J., *Herbal Medicine: Expanded Commission E Monographs* (Boston, Integrative Medicine, 2000), p. 88.

7. Drew, S., Davies, E., "Effectiveness of *Ginkgo biloba* in treating tinnitus: double blind, placebo controlled trial," *British Medical Journal,* 322(7278), 73 (13 January 2001).

8. Weiss, M.H., Frost, J.O., "May children with otitis media with effusion safely fly?" *Clinical Pediatrics* (Philadelphia), 26(11), 567–568 (November 1987).

BASAL CELL CARCINOMA

1. Miller, J.H., "Mutagenic specificity of ultraviolet light," *Journal of Molecular Biology,* 182, 45–68 (1985).

2. Michalovitz, D. Halvey, O., Oren, M., "Conditional inhibition of transformation and of cell proliferation by a temperature-sensitive mutant of p53," *Cell,* 62, 671–680 (1990).

3. Stewart, M.S., Cameron, G.S., Pence, B.C., "Antioxidant nutrients protect against UVB-induced oxidative damage to DNA of mouse keratinocytes in culture," *Journal of Investigational Dermatology,* 106, 1086–1089 (1996).

4. Miyachi, Horio, T., Imamura, S., "Sunburn cell formation is prevented by scavenging oxygen intermediates," *Clinical and Experimental Dermatology,* 8, 305–310 (1983).

5. Hanada, K., Gange, R.W., Connor, M.J., "Effect of glutathione depletion on sunburn cell formation in the hairless mouse," *Journal of Investigational Dermatology,* 96, 838–840 (1991).

6. Sansone, G., Reisner, R., "Differential rates of conversion of testosterone to dihydrotestosterone in acne and normal human skin—a possible pathogenic factor in acne," *Journal of Investigational Dermatology,* 56, 366–372 (1971).

7. Jansen, D.F., Schouten, J.P., Vonk, J.M., Rijcken, B., Timens, W., Weiss, S.T., Postma, D.S., "Smoking and airway hyperresponsiveness especially in the

presence of blood eosinophilia Increase the risk to develop respiratory symptoms: a 25-year follow-up study in the general adult population," *American Journal of Respiratory Critical Care,* 160(1), 259–264 (July 1999).

BASHFUL BLADDER SYNDROME

1. Kaplan, S.A., Santarosa, R.P., D'Alisera, P.M., Fay, B.J., Ikeguchi, E.F., Hendricks, J., Klein, L., Te, A.E., "Pseudodyssynergia (contraction of the external sphincter during voiding) misdiagnosed as chronic nonbacterial prostatitis and the role of biofeedback as a therapeutic option," *Journal of Urology,* 157(6), 2234–2237 (June 1997).

2. Rosario, D.J., Chapple, C.R., Tophill, P.R., Woo, H.H., "Urodynamic assessment of the bashful bladder," *Journal of Urology,* 163(1), 215–220 (January 2000).

BECHTEREW'S DISEASE

1. Hüber, R., Herdrich, A., Rostock, M., Vogel, T., "Clinical remission of an HLA B27-positive sacroiliitis on vegan diet ," *Forschrift für Komplementarmedizin und Klassiche Naturheilkunde,* 8(4), 228–231 (August 2001).

BED SORES

1. van Marum, R.J., Meijer, J.H., Ooms, M.E., Kostense, P.J., van Eijk, J.T., Ribbe, M.W., "Relationship between internal risk factors for development of decubitus ulcers and the blood flow response following pressure load," *Angiology,* 52(6), 409–416 (June 2001).

2. Thomas, D.R., "Improving outcome of pressure ulcers with nutritional interventions: a review of the evidence," *Nutrition,* 17(2), 121–125 (February 2001).

3. Aquilani, R., Boschi, F., Contardi, A., Pistarini, C., Achilli, M.P., Fizzotti, G., Moroni, S., Catapano, M., Verri, M., Pastoris, O., "Energy expenditure and nutritional adequacy of rehabilitation paraplegics with asymptomatic *bacteriuria* and pressure sores," *Spinal Cord,* 39(8), 437–441 (August 2001).

4. Chakrabarty, K.H., Heaton, M., Dalley. A.J., Dawson, R.A, Freedlander, E., Khaw, P.T., Mac Neil, S., "Keratinocyte-driven contraction of reconstructed human skin," *Wound Repair and Regeneration,* 9(2), 95–110 (March–April 2001).

5. Silverstein, R.J., Landsman, A.S., "The effects of a moderate and high dose of vitamin C on wound healing in a controlled guinea pig model," *Journal of Foot and Ankle Surgery,* 38(5), 333–338 (Septembe–October 1998).

6. Fulton, J.E., Jr., "The stimulation of postdermabrasion wound healing with stabilized aloe vera gel-polyethylene oxide dressing," *Journal of Dermatologic Surgery* and *Oncology,* 16(5), 460–467 (May 1990).

BEDWETTING

1. Rushton, H.G., Belman, A.B., Zaontz, M., Skoog, S.J., Sihelnik, S., "Response to desmopressin as a function of urine osmolality in the treatment of monosymptomatic nocturnal enuresis: A double-blind prospective study," *Journal of Urology,* 154, 2(2), 749–753 (August 1995).

2. Ghosh, P.M., Mikhailova, M., Bedolla, R., Kreisberg, J.I., "Arginine vasopressin stimulates mesangial cell proliferation by activating the epidermal growth factor receptor," *American Journal of Physiology—Renal Physiology,* 280(6), F972–F979 (June 2001).

3. Eiberg, H., "Total genome scan analysis in a single extended family for primary nocturnal enuresis: evidence for a new locus (ENUR3) for primary nocturnal enuresis on chromosome 22q1," *European Urologist,* 33(Suppl 3), 34–36 (1998).

4. Hansen, A., Hansen, B., Dahm, T.L., "Urinary tract infection, day wetting and other voiding symptoms in seven- to eight-year-old Danish children," *Acta Paediatrica,* 86(12), 1345–1349 (December 1997).

5. Hunsballe, J.M., "Increased delta component in computerized sleep electroencephalographic analysis suggests abnormally deep sleep in primary monosymptomatic nocturnal enuresis," *Scandinavian Journal of Urology and Nephrology,* 34(5), 294–302 (October 2000).

6. Friman, P.C., Handwerk, M.L., Swearer, S.M., Mcginnis, J.C., Warzak, W.J., "Do children with primary nocturnal enuresis have clinically significant behavior problems?" *Archives of Pediatrics* & *Adolescent Medicine,* 152(6), 537–539 (June 1998).

7. Kruse, S., Hellstrom, A.L., Hjalmas, K., "Daytime bladder dysfunction in therapy-resistant nocturnal enuresis. A pilot study in urotherapy," *Scandinavian Journal of Urology and Nephrology,* 33(1), 49–52 (February 1999).

8. Braff, D.L., Geyer, M.A., Swerdlow, N.R., "Human studies of prepulse inhibition of startle: normal subjects, patient groups, and pharmacological studies," *Psychopharmacology* (Berlin), 156(2–3), 234–258 (July 2001).

9. van Londen, A., van Londen-Barentsen, M., van Son, M., Mulder, G., "Arousal training for children suffering from nocturnal enuresis: a 2–1/2 year follow up," *Behavioral Research and Therapy,* 31, 613–615 (1993).

10. Hussein Mohamed, E.E., "The role of pelvic traction in the management of primary monosymptomatic nocturnal enuresis," *BJU International,* 89(4), 416–419 (March 2002).

11. Butler, R.J., "Combination Therapy for Nocturnal Enuresis," *Scandinavian Journal of Urology and Nephrology,* 35, 364–369 (October 2001).

12. Hunsballe, J.M., Hansen, T.K., Rittig, S., Pedersen, E.B., Djurhuus, J.C., "The efficacy of DDAVP is related to the circadian rhythm of urine output in patients with persisting nocturnal enuresis," *Clinical Endocrinology* (Oxford), 49(6), 793–801 (December 1998).

13. Caione, P., Arena, F., Biraghi, M., Cigna, R., Chendi, D., Chiozza, M., et al., "Nocturnal enuresis and daytime wetting: a multicentric trial with oxybutynin and desmopressin," *European Urologist,* 31, 459–463 (1997).

14. Hammer, F., "Therapie der Enuresis Nocturna mit Spezial-Präparat Noxenur," *MMW Münchener Medizinische Wochenschrift,* 116(10), 525–526 (8 March 1974).

15. Rona, R.J., Li, L., Chinn, S., "Determinants of nocturnal enuresis in England and Scotland in the 90's," *Development and Medical Child Neurology,* 39(10), 677–681 (October 1997).

16. Balch, P.A., *Prescription for Herbal Healing* (New York: Avery Press, 2002), 201–202.

17. Wieting, J.M., Dykstra, D.D., Ruggiero, M.P., Robbins, G.B., Galusha, K., "Central nervous system ischemia after varicella infection and desmopressin therapy for enuresis," *Journal of the American Osteopathic Association,* 97(5), 293–295 (May 1997).

18. Hunsballe, J.M., Rittig, S., Pedersen, E.B., Djuhuus, J.C., "Smokeless nicotinergic stimulation of vasopressin secretion in patients with persisting nocturnal enuresis and controls," *Scandinavian Journal of Urology and Nephrology,* 35(2), 117–121 (April 2001).

BEE AND WASP STINGS

1. Teelucksingh, S., Mackie, A.D., Burt, D., McIntyre, M.A., Brett, L., Edwards, C.R., "Potentiation of hydrocortisone activity in skin by glycyrrhetinic acid," *Lancet,* 335(8697), 1060–1063 (5 May 1990).

2. Chen, M.F., Shimada, F., Kato, H., Yano, S., Kanaoka, M., "Effect of glycyrrhizin on the pharmacokinetics of prednisolone following low dosage of prednisolone hemisuccinate," *Endocronologica Japonica,* 37, 331–341 (1990).

3. Shiozaki, T., Sugiyama, K., Nakazato, K., Takeo, T., "Effect of tea extracts, catechin and caffeine against type-I allergic reaction," *Yakugaku Zasshi,* 117(7), 448–454 (July 1997).

4. Murray, M.T., "A comprehensive review of vitamin C," *American Journal of Natural Medicine,* 3, 8–21 (1996).

5. Clemetson, C.A., "Histamine and ascorbic acid in human blood," *Journal of Nutrition,* 110, 662–668 (1980).

6. Feigen, G.A., Smith, B.H., Dix, C.E., Flynn, C.J., Peterson, N.S., Rosenberg,L.T., Pavlovic, S., Leibovitz, B., "Enhancement of antibody production and protection against systemic anaphylaxis by large doses of vitamin C," *Research Communications in Chemical Pathology and Pharmacology,* 38(2), 313–333 (November 1982).

7. Rueff, F., Wenderoth, A., Przybilla, B., "Patients still reacting to a sting challenge while receiving conventional *Hymenoptera* venom immunotherapy are protected by increased venom doses," *Journal of Allergy and Clinical Immunology,* 108(6), 1027–1032 (December 2001).

8. Visscher, P.K., Vetter, R.S., Camazine, S., "Removing bee stings," *Lancet*, 348 (9023), 301–302 (3 August 1996).

BELCHING AND BURPING

1. Kahrilas, P.J., Dodds, W.J., Dent, J.B., Wyman, J.B., Hogan, W.J., Arndorfer, R.C., "Upper esophageal sphincter function during belching," *Gastroenterology*, 91, 133–140 (1986).

2. Wilmshurst, P.T., "Tachyarrhythmias triggered by swallowing and belching," *Heart*, 81(3), 313–315 (March 1999).

3. Pimentel, M., Bonorris, G.G., Chow, E.J., Lin, H.C., "Peppermint oil improves the manometric findings in diffuse esophageal spasm," *Journal of Clinical Gastroenterology*, 33(1), 8–10 (July 2001).

BELL'S PALSY

1. Dowriero, R.R., Fidler, V.J., "Atmospheric pressure and idiopathic facial paralysis (Bell's palsy)," *Aviation, Space, and Environmental Medicine*, 48, 672–673 (1977).

2. Herbert, I., Nolte, E., Eicchorn, T., "Wetterlage und Häufigkeit von idiopathischen Fazialisparesen, Vestibularisausfällen, Ménière-Anfällen und Hörstürzen," *Laryngologie, Rhinologie, und Otolaryngologie*, 66, 249–250 (1987).

3. Danielides, V., Patrikako, G., Nousia, C.S., Bartzoka, A., Haralampos, J.M., Lolis, C. Skevas, A., "Weather conditions and Bell's palsy: five-year study and review of the literature," *BMC Neurology*, 1(7), 1471–1477 (5 December 2001).

4. Jalaludin, M.A., "Methylcobalamin treatment of Bell's palsy," *Methods and Findings in Clinical and Experimental Pharmacology*, 17(8), 539–544 (October 1995).

5. Sheridan, J., Kern, E., Martin, A., Booth, A., "Evaluation of antioxidant healing formulations in topical therapy of experimental cutaneous and genital herpes simplex virus infections," *Antiviral Research*, 36(30), 157–166 (December 1997).

6. Xing, W., Yang, S., Guo, X., "Treating old facial nerve paralysis of 260 cases with the acupuncture treatment skill of pause and regress in six parts," *Chen Tzu Yen Chiu*, 19(2), 8–10 (1994). Read in abstract on MedLine.

BENIGN PROSTATIC HYPERPLASIA (BPH)

1. Oesterling, J.E., "Benign prostatic hyperplasia: a review of its histogenesis and natural history," *Prostate*, 6, 67–73 (1996).

2. Xia, S.J., Xu, C.X., Tang, X.D., Wang, W.Z., Du, D.L., "Apoptosis and hormonal milieu in ductal system of normal prostate and benign prostatic hyperplasia," *Asian Journal of Andrology*, 3(2), 131–134 (June 2001).

3. Kramer, G., Steiner, G.E., Handisurya, A., Stix, U., Haitel, A., Knerer, B., Gessl, A., Lee, C., Marberger, M., "Increased expression of lymphocyte-derived cytokines in benign hyperplastic prostate tissue, identification of the producing cell types, and effect of differentially expressed cytokines on stromal cell proliferation," *Prostate*, 52(1), 43–58 (15 June 2002).

4. Suzuki, S., Platz, E.A., Kawachi, I., Willett, W.C., Giovannucci, E., "Intakes of energy and macronutrients and the risk of benign prostatic hyperplasia," *American Journal of Clinical Nutrition*, 75(4), 689–697 (April 2002).

5. Hart, J.P., Cooper, W.L., *Vitamin F in the treatment of prostatic hyperplasia. Report Number 1.* (Milwaukee, Wisconsin: Lee Foundation for Nutritional Research), 1941.

6. Weber, K.S., Setchell, K.D., Stocco, D.M., Lephart, E.D., "Dietary soy-phytoestrogens decrease testosterone levels and prostate weight without altering LH, prostate 5alpha-reductase or testicular steroidogenic acute regulatory peptide levels in adult male Sprague-Dawley rats," *Journal of Endocrinology*, 170(3), 591–599 (September 2001).

7. Adlercreutz, H., "Epidemiology of phytoestrogens," *Baillieres' Best Practice and Research: Clinical Endocrinology and Metabolism*, 12(4), 605–623 (December 1998).

8. Buck, A.C., "Phytotherapy for the prostate," *British Journal of Urology*, 78, 325–336 (1996).

9. Sokeland, J., "Combined sabal and urtica extract compared with finasteride in men with benign prostatic hyperplasia: analysis of prostate volume and therapeutic outcome," *BJU International*, 86(4), 439–442 (September 2000).

10. Vacherot, F., Azzouz, M., Gil-Diez-De-Medina, S., Colombel, M., De La Taille, A., Lefrere Belda, M.A., Abbou, C.C., Raynaud, J.P., Chopin, D.K., "Induction of apoptosis and inhibition of cell proliferation by the lipido-sterolic extract of *Serenoa repens* (LSESr, Permixon) in benign prostatic hyperplasia," *Prostate*, 45(3), 259–266 (1 November 2000).

11. Debruyne, F., Koch, G., Boyle, P., Da Silva, F.C., Gillenwater, J.G., Hamdy, F.C., Perrin, P., Teillac, P., Vela-Navarrete, R., Raynaud, J.P., "Comparison of a phytotherapeutic agent (Permixon) with an alpha-blocker (Tamsulosin) in the treatment of benign prostatic hyperplasia: a 1-year randomized international study," *European Urology*, 41(5), 497–507 (May 2002).

12. Buck, A.C., Cox, R., Rees, R.W., Ebeling, L., John, A., "Treatment of outflow tract obstruction due to benign prostatic hyperplasia with the pollen extract, Cernilton. A double-blind, placebo-controlled study," *British Journal of Urology*, 66, 398–404 (1990).

13. Andro, M.C., Riffaud, J.P., "Pygeum africanum extract for the treatment of patients with benign prostatic hyperplasia: a review of 25 years of published experience," *Current Therapeutic Research*, 56, 796–817 (1995).

14. Chyou, P.H., Nomura, A.M., Stemmermann, G.N., Hankin, J.H., "A prospective study of alcohol, diet, and other lifestyle factors in relation to obstructive uropathy," *Prostate*, 22(3), 253–264 (1993).

BIPOLAR DISORDER (MANIC DEPRESSION)

1. Kessler, R.C., McGonagle, K.A., Zhao, S., et al: "Lifetime and 12-month prevalence of DSM-III-R psychiatric disorders in the United States," *Archives of General Psychiatry*, 51, 8–19 (1994).

2. Naylor, G., Smith, A., Bryce-Smith, D., Ward, N., "Tissue vanadium levels in manic-depressive psychosis," *Psychological Medicine*, 14, 767–772 (1984).

3. Naylor, G., "Vanadium and affective disorders," *Biological Psychiatry*, 18, 103–112 (1983).

4. Myron, D., Givand, S., Nielsen, F., "Vanadium content of selected foods as determined by flameless atomic absorption spectroscopy," *Journal of Agricultural and Food Chemistry*, 25, 297–300 (1977).

5. Stoll, A.L., Locke, C.A., Marangell, L.B., Rueter, S., Zboyan, H.A., Diamond, E., Cress, K.K., "Omega-3 fatty acids and bipolar disorder: a review," *Prostaglandins, Leukotrienes, and Essential Fatty Acids*, 60, 329–337 (1999).

6. Barton, P.G., Gunstone, F.D., "Hydrocarbon chain packing and molecular motion in phospholipid bilayers formed from unsaturated lecithins. Synthesis and properties of sixteen positional isomers of 1,2-dioctadecenolyl-sn-glycero-3-phosphorylcholine," *Journal of Biological Chemistry*, 250(12), 4470–4476 (1975).

7. Stoll, A.L., Severus, W.E., "Mood stabilizers: shared mechanisms of action at postsynaptic signal-transduction and kindling processes," *Harvard Review of Psychiatry*, 4(2), 77–89 (1996).

8. Carney, M.W., Chary, T.K., Bottiglieri, T., et al., "Switch and S-adenosylmethionine," *Alabama Journal of Medical Science*, 25, 316–319 (1988).

9. Mebane, A.H., "L-Glutamine and mania [letter]," *American Journal of Psychiatry*, 141, 1302–1303 (1984).

10. Kampo formulas are discussed in much greater depth in Rister, R., *Medicine of the Five Rings* (M. Evans & Company, 2002).

11. Nierenberg, A.A., Burt, T., Matthews, J., Weiss, A.P., "Mania associated with St. John's wort," *Biological Psychiatry*, 46(12), 1707–1708 (1999).

12. Krauthammer, C., Klerman, G.L., "Secondary mania: Manic syndromes associated with antecedent physical illness of drugs," *Archives of General Psychiatry*, 35, 1333–1379 (1978).

BLADDER CANCER

1. Weyer, P.J., Cerhan, J.R., Kross, B.C., Hallberg, G.R., Kantamneni, J., Breuer, G., Jones, M.P., Zheng, W., Lynch, C.F., "Municipal drinking water nitrate level and cancer risk in older women: the Iowa Women's Health Study," *Epidemiology*, 12(3), 327–338 (May 2001).

2. Vinh, P.Q., Sugie, S., Tanaka, T., Hara, A., Yamada, Y., Katayama, M., Deguchi, T., Mori, H., "Chemopreventive effects of a flavonoid antioxidant silymarin on N-butyl-N-(4-hydroxybutyl)nitrosamine-induced urinary bladder carcinogenesis in

male ICR mice," *Japanese Journal of Cancer Research*, 93(1), 42–49 (January 2002).

3. Miller, B.A., Kolonel, L.N., Bernstein, L., Young, J.L., Jr., Swanson, G.M., West, D., Key, C.R., Liff, J.M., Glover, C.S., Alexander, G.A., et al. (eds). Racial/Ethnic Patterns of Cancer in the United States 1988–1992, NIH Pub. No. 96–4104. (Bethesda, Maryland: National Cancer Institute, 1996).

4. Michaud, D.S., Spiegelman, D., Clinton, S.K., Rimm, E.B., Willett, W.C., Giovannucci, E.L., "Fruit and vegetable intake and incidence of bladder cancer in a male prospective cohort," *Journal of the National Cancer Institute*, 90, 1072–1079, 1028–1029 (1998).

5. Steinmaus, C.M., Nunez, S., Smith, A.H., "Diet and bladder cancer: a meta-analysis of six dietary variables," *American Journal of Epidemiology*, 151(7), 693–702 (1 April 2000).

6. Augustsson, K., Skog, K., Jagerstad, M., Dickman, P.W., Steineck, G., "Dietary heterocyclic amines and cancer of the colon, rectum, bladder, and kidney: a population-based study," *Lancet*, 353(9154), 703–707 (27 February 1999).

BLEPHARITIS

1. Proctor, M., Wilkenson, D., Orenberg, E., Farber, E.M., "Lowered cutaneous and urinary levels of polyamines with clinical improvement in treated psoriasis," *Archives of Dermatology*, 115, 945–949 (1979).

2. Kalman, J., Gecse, A., Farkas, T., Joo, F., Telegdy, G., Lajtha, A., "Dietary manipulation with high marine fish oil intake of fatty acid composition and arachidonic acid metabolism in rat cerebral microvessels," *Neurochemical Research*, 17(2), 167–172 (February 1992).

3. Nisenson, A., "Treatment of seborrheic dermatitis with biotin and vitamin B complex," *Journal of Pediatrics*, 81, 630–631 (1972).

4. Roe, D.A., *Drug-Induced Nutritional Deficiencies* (Westport, CT: AVI Publications, 1976), 168–177.

5. Schreiner, A., Rockewell, E., Vilter, R., "A local defect in the metabolism of pyridoxine in the skin of persons with seborrheic dermatitis of the 'sicca' type," *Journal of Investigational Dermatology*, 19, 95–96 (1952).

6. Al-Waili, N.S., "Therapeutic and prophylactic effects of crude honey on chronic seborrheic dermatitis and dandruff," *European Journal of Medical Research*, 30, 6(7), 306–308 (July 2001).

7. Schreiner, A., Slinger, W., Hawkins, V., et al., ibid.

BLOATING

1. Brunetton, J. *Pharmacognosy, Phytochemistry, Medicinal Plants* (Paris: Lavoisier Publishing, 1995), p. 444.

2. Safayhi, H., Sabieraj, J., Sailer, E.R., Ammon, H.P., "Chamazulene: an antioxidant-type inhibitor of leukotriene B4 formation," *Planta Medica*, 60(5), 410–413 (October 1994).

3. Miller, T., Wittstock, U., Lindequist, U., Teuscher, E., "Effects of some components of the essential oil of chamomile, *Chamomilla recutita*, on histamine release from rat mast cells," *Planta Medica*, 62(1), 60–61 (1 February 1996).

4. Kawakishi, S., Morimitsu, Y., Osawa, T., "Chemistry of ginger components and inhibitory factors of the arachidonic acid cascade," in Ho, C.T., Osawa, T., Huang, M.T., Rosen, R. (eds). *Food Phytochemicals for Cancer Prevention II: Teas, Spices, and Herbs* (Washington: American Chemical Society, 1994), pp. 244–249.

5. Bisset, N.G., Editor. *Herbal Drugs and Phytopharmaceuticals: A Handbook for Practice on a Scientific Basis* (Stuttgart, Germany: Medpharm Scientific Publishers, 1994), 538.

6. Bracken, J., "Ginger as an antiemetic: possible side effect due to its thromboxane synthetase activity," *Anaesthesia*, 46, 705–706 (1991).

7. Buchbauer, G., Jirovetz, L., Jager, W., Dietrich, H., Plank, C., "Aromatherapy: evidence for sedative effects of the essential oil of lavender after inhalation," *Zeitschrift für Naturforschung*, 46(11–12), 1067–1072 (November–December 1991).

8. Dew, M.J., Evans, B.K., Rhodes, J., "Peppermint oil for the irritable bowel syndrome: a multicentre trial," *British Journal of Clinical Practice*, 38, 394–398 (1984).

9. Suarez, F.L., Furne, J., Springfield, J., Levitt, M.D., "Failure of activated charcoal to reduce the release of gases produced by colonic flora," *American Journal of Gastroenterology*, 94(1), 208–212 (January 1999).

10. Suarez, F.L., Springfield, J., Levitt, M.D., "Identification of gases responsible for the odour of human flatus and evaluation of a device purported to reduce this odour," *Gut*, 43(1), 100–104 (July 1998).

BOILS AND CARBUNCLES

1. Payne, M.C., Wood, H.F., Karakawa, W., Gluck, L., "A prospective study of staphylococcal colonization and infections in newborns and their families," *American Journal of Epidemiology*, 82, 305–316 (1966).

2. Wadlvogel, F.A. *Staphylococcus aureus* (including staphylococcal toxic shock). In: Mandell, G.L., Bennett, J.E., Dolin, R., editors. *Principles and Practice of Infectious Diseases*, Fifth Edition (Philadelphia: Churchill Livingstone, 2000), pp. 2072–2073.

3. Ross, S., Rodriguez, W., Controni, G., Khan, W., "Staphylococcal susceptibility to penicillin G: the changing pattern among community isolates," *Journal of the American Medical Association*, 2229, 1075–1077 (1974).

4. Sanford, M.D., Widmer, A.F, Bale, M.J., Jones, R.N., Wenzel, R.P., "Efficient detection and long-term persistence of the carriage of methicillin-resistant *Staphylococcus aureus*," *Clinical Infectious Disease*, 19, 1123–1128 (1994).

5. Havsteen, B., "Flavonoids, a class of natural products of high pharmacological potency," *Biochemical Pharmacology*, 32, 1141–1148 (1983).

6. Rimoldi, R., Ginesu, F., Giura, R., "The use of bromelain in pneumological therapy," *Drugs in Experimental Clinical Research*, 4, 55–66 (1978).

7. Ako, H., Cheung, A., Matsura, P., "Isolation of a fibrinolysis enzyme activator from commercial bromelain," *Archives of International Pharmacodynamics*, 254, 157–167 (1981).

8. Bliznakov, E., Casey, A., Kishi, T., "Coenzyme Q deficiency in mice following infection with Friend leukemia virus," *International Journal of Vitamin and Nutrition Research*, 45, 388–395 (1975).

9. Cazzola, P., Mazzanti, P., Bossi, G., "In vivo modulating effect of a calf thymus acid lysate on human T lymphocyte subsets and CD4+/CD8+ ratio in the course of difference diseases," *Current Therapies Research*, 42, 1011–1017 (1987).

10. Seifter, E., Rettura, G., Seiter, J., "Thymotrophic action of vitamin A," *Federal Proceedings*, 32, 947 (1973).

11. Semba, R.D., "Vitamin A, immunity, and infection," *Clinical Infectious Disease*, 19, 489–499 (1994).

12. Ginter, E., "Optimum intake of vitamin C for the human organisms," *Nutrition and Health*, 1, 66–77 (1982).

13. Gabor, M., "Pharmacologic effects of flavonoids on blood vessels," *Angiologica*, 9, 355–374 (1972).

14. Prasad, A., "Clinical, biochemical and nutritional spectrum of zinc deficiency in human subjects. An update," *Nutrition Review*, 41, 197–208 (1983).

15. Porea, T.J., Belmont, J.W., Mahoney, D.H., Jr., "Zinc induced anemia and neutropenia in an adolescent," *Journal of Pediatrics*, 136(5), 688–690.

16. Klein, A.D., Penneys, N.S., "*Aloe vera*," *Journal of the American Academy of Dermatology*, 18, 714–719 (1988).

17. Chu, D.T., Wong, W.L., Mavlight, G.M., "Immunotherapy with Chinese medicinal herbs," *Journal of Clinical and Laboratory Immunology*, 25, 119–129 (1988).

18. Zhao, K.S., Mancini, C., Doria, G., "Enhancement of the immune response in mice by *Astragalus membranaceus*," *Immunopharmacology*, 20, 225–233 (1990).

19. Wildfeuer, A., Mayerhofer, D., "The effects of plant preparations on cellular functions in body defense," *Arzneimittel-Forschung*, 44(3), 361–366 (March 1994).

20. Tragni, E., Tubaro, A., Melis, S., Galli, C.L., "Evidence from two classic irritation tests for an anti-inflammatory action of a natural extract, Echinacina B," *Food Chemistry and Toxicology*, 23, 317–319 (1985).

21. Facino, R.M., Carini, M., Aldini, G., Marinello, C., Arlandini, E., Franzoi, L., Colombo, M., Pietta, P., Mauri, P., "Direct characterization of caffeoyl esters

with antihyaluronidase activity in crude extracts from *Echinacea angustifolia* roots by fast atom bombardment tandem mass spectrometry," *Farmaco,* 48(10), 1447–1461 (October 1993).

22. Murray, M., Pizzorno, J., *Encyclopedia of Natural Medicine* (Rocklin, California: 1998), p. 223.

BREAST CANCER

1. Summarizing figures published by the National Cancer Institute and the Ministries of Health of Australia, Canada, Japan, and the United Kingdom.

2. Lynch, J., Pattekar, R., Barnes, D.M., Hanby, A.M., Camplejohn, R.S., Ryder, K., Gillett, C.E., "Mitotic counts provide additional prognostic information in grade II mammary carcinoma," *Journal of Pathology,* 196(3), 275–9 (March 2002).

3. Selim, A.G., El-Ayat, G., Wells, C.A., "Androgen receptor expression in ductal carcinoma in situ of the breast: relation to oestrogen and progesterone receptors," *Journal of Clinical Pathology,* 55(1), 14–16 (January 2002).

4. Wang-Gohrke, S., Becher, H., Kreienberg, R., Runnebaum, I.B., Chang-Claude, J., "Intron 3 16 bp duplication polymorphism of p53 is associated with an increased risk for breast cancer by the age of 50 years," *Pharmacogenetics,* 12(3), 269–272 (April 2002).

5. Conway, K., Edmiston, S.N., Cui, L., Drouin, S.S., Pang, J., He, M., Tse, C.K., Geradts, J., Dressler, L., Liu, E.T., Millikan, R., Newman, B., "Prevalence and spectrum of p53 mutations associated with smoking in breast cancer," *Cancer Research,* 62(7), 1987–1995 (1 April 2002).

6. Hoyer, A.P., Gerdes, A.M., Jorgensen, T., Rank, F., Hartvig, H.B., "Organochlorines, p53 mutations in relation to breast cancer risk and survival. A Danish cohort-nested case-controls study," *Breast Cancer Research and Treatment,* 71(1), 59–65 (January 2002).

7. Grant, W.B., "An ecologic study of dietary and solar ultraviolet-B links to breast carcinoma mortality rates," *Cancer,* 194(1), 272–281 (January 2002).

8. Colston, K.W., Mork Hansen, C., "Mechanisms implicated in the growth regulatory effects of vitamin D in breast cancer," *Endocrine-Related Cancer,* 9(1), 45–59 (March 2002).

9. Hecht, S.S., "Tobacco smoke carcinogens and breast cancer," *Environmental and Molecular Mutagenesis,* 39(2–3), 119–126 (2002).

10. Byrne, C., Rockett, H., Holmes, M.D., "Dietary fat, fat subtypes, and breast cancer risk: lack of an association among postmenopausal women with no history of benign breast disease," *Cancer Epidemiology, Biomarkers, and Prevention,* 11(3), 261–265 (March 2002).

11. Terry, P., Suzuki, R., Hu, F.B., Wolk, A., "A prospective study of major dietary patterns and the risk of breast cancer," *Cancer Epidemiology, Biomarkers, and Prevention,* 10(12), 1281–1285 (December 2001).

12. Rock, C.L., Thomson, C., Caan, B.J., Flatt, S.W., Newman, V., Ritenbaugh, C., Marshall, J.R., Hollenbach, K.A., Stefanick, M.L., Pierce, J.P., "Reduction in fat intake is not associated with weight loss in most women after breast cancer diagnosis: evidence from a randomized controlled trial," *Cancer,* 91(1), 25–34 (1 January 2001).

13. van den Brandt, P.A., Spiegelman, D., Yaun, S.S., Adami, H.O., Beeson, L., Folsom, A.R., Fraser, G., Goldbohm, R.A., Graham, S., Kushi, L., Marshall, J.R., Miller, A.B., Rohan, T., Smith-Warner, S.A., Speizer, F.E., Willett, W.C., Wolk, A., Hunter, D.J., "Pooled analysis of prospective cohort studies on height, weight, and breast cancer risk," *American Journal of Epidemiology,* 152(6), 514–527 (15 September 2000).

14. Ching, S., Ingram, D., Hahnel, R., Beilby, J., Rossi, E., "Serum levels of micronutrients, antioxidants and total antioxidant status predict risk of breast cancer in a case control study", *Journal of Nutrition,* 132, 303–306 (2002).

15. Shao, Z.M., Shen, Z.Z., Liu, C.H., Sartippour, M.R., Go, V.L., Heber, D., Nguyen, M., "Curcumin exerts multiple suppressive effects on human breast carcinoma cells," *International Journal of Cancer,* 98(2), 234–240 (10 March 2002).

16. Khafif, A., Schantz, S.P., Chou, T.C., Edelstein, D., Sacks, P.G., "Quantitation of chemopreventive synergism between (-)epigalocatechin 3-gallate and curcumin in normal, premalignant, and malignant human oral epithelial cells," *Carcinogenesis,* 19(3), 419–424 (March 1998).

17. Rahman, K.M., Sarkar, F.H., "Steroid hormone mimics: molecular mechanisms of cell growth and apoptosis in normal and malignant mammary epithelial cells," *Journal of Steroid Biochemistry and Molecular Biology,* 80(2), 191–201 (February 2002).

18. Eichholzer, M., Luthy, J., Moser, U., Fowler, B., "Folate and the risk of colorectal, breast and cervix cancer: the epidemiological evidence," *Swiss Medical Weekly,* 131(37–38), 539–549 (22 September 2001).

19 Lockwood, K., Moesgaard, S., Hanioka, T., Folkers, K., "Apparent partial remission of breast cancer in 'high risk' patients supplemented with nutritional antioxidants, essential fatty acids and coenzyme Q_{10}," *Molecular Aspects of Medicine,* 15 Suppl, S231–S240 (1994).

20 Morabia, A., Bernstein, M., Heritier, S., Khatchatrian, N., "Relation of breast cancer with passive and active exposure to tobacco smoke," *American Journal of Epidemiology,* 143(9), 918–928 (1 May 1996).

21 Zheng, W., Xie, D., Cerhan, J.R., Sellers, T.A., Wen, W., Folsom, A.R., "Sulfotransferase 1A1 polymorphism, endogenous estrogen exposure, well-done meat intake and breast cancer risk," *Cancer Epidemiology, Biomarkers and Prevention,* 10(2), 89–94 (February 2001).

22. Missmer, S.A., Smith-Warner, S.A., Spiegelman, D., Yaun, S.S., Adami, H.O., Beeson, W.L., van Den Brandt, P.A., Fraser, G.E., Freudenheim, J.L., Goldbohm, R.A., Graham, S., Kushi, L.H., Miller, A.B., Potter, J.D., Rohan, T.E., Speizer, F.E., Toniolo, P., Willett, W.C., Wolk, A., Zeleniuch-Jacquotte, A., Hunter, D.J., "Meat and dairy food consumption and breast cancer: a pooled analysis of cohort studies," *International Journal of Epidemiology,* 31(1), 78–85 (February 2002).

23. Lamartiniere, C.A., "Protection against breast cancer with genistein: a component of soy," *American Journal of Clinical Nutrition,* 71(6), 1705S-1707S (June 2000).

24. Messina, M.J., Loprinzi, C.L., "Soy for breast cancer survivors: a critical review of the literature," *Journal of Nutrition,* 131(11 Suppl), 3095S-3108S (November 2001).

25. Hargreaves, D.F., Potten, C.S., Harding, C., Shaw, L.E., Morton, M.S., Roberts, S.A., Howell, A., Bundred, N.J., "Two-week dietary soy supplementation has an estrogenic effect on normal premenopausal breast," *Journal of Clinical Endocrinology and Metabolism,* 84(11), 4017–4024 (November 1999).

26 Funahashi, H., Imai, T., Mase, T., Sekiya, M., Yokoi, K., Hayashi, H., Shibata, A., Hayashi, T., Nishikawa, M., Suda, N., Hibi, Y., Mizuno, Y., Tsukamura, K., Hayakawa, A., Tanuma, S., "Seaweed prevents breast cancer," *Japanese Journal of Cancer Research,* 92(5), 483–487 (May 2001).

27. Hebert, J.R., Hurley, T.G., Ma, Y., "The effect of dietary exposures on recurrence and mortality in early stage breast cancer," *Breast Cancer Research and Treatment,* 51(1), 17–28 (September 1998).

28. Fleischauer, A.T., Arab, L., "Garlic and cancer: a critical review of the epidemiologic literature," *Journal of Nutrition,* 131(3s), 1032S–1040S (March 2001).

29. Goodwin, P.J., Ennis, M., Pritchard, K.I., Trudeau, M.E., Koo, J., Madarnas, Y., Hartwick, W., Hoffman, B., Hood, N., "Fasting insulin and outcome in early-stage breast cancer: results of a prospective cohort study," *Journal of Clinical Oncology,* 20(1), 42–51 (1 January 2002).

30. Davis, S., Mirick, D.K., Stevens, R.G., "Night shift work, light at night, and risk of breast cancer," *Journal of the National Cancer Institute,* 17, 93(20), 1557–1562 (October 2001).

31. Haus, E., Dumitriu, L., Nicolau, G.Y., Bologa, S., Sackett-Lundeen, L., "Circadian rhythms of basic fibroblast growth factor (bFGF), epidermal growth factor (EGF), insulin-like growth factor-1 (IGF-1), insulin-like growth factor binding protein-3 (IGFBP-3), cortisol, and melatonin in women with breast cancer," *Chronobiology International,* 18(4), 709–727 (June–July 2001).

32. Collaborative Group on Hormonal Factors in Breast Cancer, "Breast cancer and hormonal contraceptives: collaborative reanalysis of individual data on 53,297 women with breast cancer and 100,239 women without breast cancer from 54 epidemiological studies," *Lancet,* 347, 1713 (1996).

33. Spigel, J.J., Evans, W.P., Grant, M.D., Langer, T.G., Krakos, P.A., Wise, D.K., "Male inflammatory breast cancer," *Clinical Breast Cancer,* 2(2), 153–155 (July 2001).

34. Koc, M., Polat, P., "Epidemiology and aetiological factors of male breast cancer: a ten years retrospective study in eastern Turkey," *European Journal of Cancer Prevention,* 10(6), 531–534 (December 2001).

BRITTLE NAILS

1. Lubach, D., Cohrs, W., Wurzinger, R., "Incidence of brittle nails," *Dermatologica*, 172(3), 144–147 (1986).

2. Colombo, V.E., Gerber, F., Bronhofer, M., Florsheim, G.L., "Treatment of brittle fingernails and onychoschizia with biotin: scanning electron microscopy," *Journal of the American Academy of Dermatology*, 23, 1128–1132 (1990).

3. Hochman, L.G., Scher, R.K., Meyerson, M.S., "Brittle nails: response to daily biotin supplementation," *Cutis*, 51(4), 303–305 (April 1993).

BRONCHITIS, CHRONIC

1. Rautalahti, M., Virtamo, J., Haukka, J., Heinonen, O.P., Sundvall, J., Albanes, D., Huttunen, J.K., "The effect of alpha-tocopherol and beta-carotene supplementation on COPD symptoms," *American Journal of Respiratory Critical Care Medicine*, 156(5), 1447–1452 (November 1997).

2. Frankfort, J.D., Fischer, C.E., Stansbury, D.W., et al., "Effects of high- and low-carbohydrate meals on maximum exercise performance in chronic airflow obstruction," *Chest*, 100, 792–795 (1991).

3. Fujimoto, S., Kurihara, N., Hirata, K., et al., "Effects of coenzyme-Q_{10} administration on pulmonary function and exercise performance in patients with chronic lung diseases," *Clinical Investigations*, 71, S162–S166 (1993).

4. Koichiro, M., Aizawa, H., Inoue, H., Shigyo, M., Takata, S., Hara, N., "Thromboxane causes airway hyperresponsiveness after cigarette smoke-induced neurogenic inflammation," *Journal of Applied Physiology*, 81(6), 2358–2364 (December 1996).

5. Sharp, D.S., Rodriguez, B.L., Shahar, E., Hwang, L.J., Burchfiel, C.M., "Fish consumption may limit the damage of smoking on the lung," *American Journal of Respiratory Critical Care*, 150(4), 983–984 (October 1994).

6. Shahar, E., Folsom, A.R., Melnick, S.L., Tockman, M.S., Comstock, G.W., Gennaro, V., Higgins, M.W., Sorlie, P.D., Ko, W.J., Szklo, M., "Dietary n-3 polyunsaturated fatty acids and smoking-related chronic obstructive pulmonary disease. Atherosclerosis risk in communities study investigators," *New England Journal of Medicine*, 331(4), 228–233 (July 1994).

7. Rimoldi, R., Ginesu, F., Giura, R., "The use of bromelain in pneumological therapy," *Drugs in Experimental Clinical Research*, 4, 55–66 (1978).

8. Stagnaro, R., Pierri, I., Piovano, P., et al., "Thio containing antioxidant drugs and the human immune system," *Bulletin Europeen de Physiopathologie Respiratoire*, 23, 303–307 (1987).

9. Grandjean, E.M., Berthet, P., Ruffmann, R., Leuenberger, P., "Efficacy of oral long-term N-acetyl cysteine in chronic bronchopulmonary disease: a meta-analysis of published double-blind, placebo-controlled clinical trials," *Clinical Therapeutics*, 22(2), 209–221 (February 2001).

10. Jansen, D.F., Schouten, J.P., Vonk, J.M., Rijcken, B., Timens, W., Weiss, S.T., Postma, D.S., "Smoking and airway hyperresponsiveness especially in the presence of blood eosinophilia increase the risk to develop respiratory symptoms: A 25-year follow-up study in the general adult population," *American Journal of Respiratory Critical Care*, 160(1), 259–264 (July 1999).

11. Rautalahti, M., Virtamo, J., Haukka, J., Heinonen, O.P., Sundvall, J., Albanes, D., Huttunen, J.K., ibid.

12. Miedema, I., Feskens, E.J.M., Heederiks, D., Kromhout, D., "Dietarydeterminants of long-term incidence of chronic nonspecific lung disease," *American Journal of Epidemiology*, 138, 37–45 (1993).

13. De, M., De, A.K., Sen, P., Banerjee, A.B., "Antimicrobial properties of star anise (*Illicium verum* Hook f)," *Phytotherapy Research*, 16(1), 94–95 (February 2002).

14. Elgayyar, M., Draughon, F.A., Golden, D.A., Mount, J.R., "Antimicrobial activity of essential oils from plants against selected pathogenic and saprophytic microorganisms," *Journal of Food Protection*, 64(7), 1019–1024 (July 2001).

15. Gay-Crosier, F., Schreiber, G., Hauser, C., "Anaphylaxis from inulin in vegetables and processed food," *New England Journal of Medicine*, 342, 1372 (4 May 2000).

16. Chandra, R., Barron, J.L., "Anaphylactic reaction to intravenous sinistrin (Inutest)," *Annals of Clinical Biochemistry*, 39(Pt 1), 76 (January 2002).

17. El Bardai, S., Lyoussi, B., Wibo, M., Morel, N., "Pharmacological evidence of hypotensive activity of *Marrubium vulgare* and *Foeniculum vulgare* in spontaneously hypertensive rat," *Clinical Experiments in Hypertension*, 23(4), 329–343 (May 2001).

18. De Jesus, R.A., Cechinel-Filho, V., Oliveira, A.E., Schlemper, V., "Analysis of the antinociceptive properties of marrubiin isolated from *Marrubium vulgare*," *Phytomedicine*, 7(2), 111–115 (April 2000).

19. Trute, A., Gross, J., Mutschler, E., Nahrstedt, A., "In vitro antispasmodic compounds of the dry extract obtained from *Hedera helix*," *Planta Medica*, 63(2), 125–129 (April 1997).

20. Dwoskin, L.P., Crooks, P.A., "A novel mechanism of action and potential use for lobeline as a treatment for psychostimulant abuse," *Biochemical Pharmacology*, 3(2), 89–98 (15 January 2002).

21. Deep, V., Singh, M., Ravi, K., "Role of vagal afferents in the reflex effects of capsaicin and lobeline in monkeys," *Respiratory Physiology*, 125(3), 155–168 (April 2001).

22. Miller, D.K., Crooks, P.A., Teng, L., Witkin, J.M., Munzar, P., Goldberg, S.R., Acri, J.B., Dwoskin, L.P., "Lobeline inhibits the neurochemical and behavioral effects of amphetamine," *Journal of Pharmacology and Experimental Therapy*, 296(3), 1023–1034 (March 2001).

23. Bergner, P., "Is lobelia toxic," *Medical Herbalism*, 10(1), 15–32 (1998).

24. Blumenthal M., Busse, W.R., Goldberg, A., Gruenwald, W., Hall, T., Klein S., Riggins, C., Rister, R., (eds), *The Complete Commission E Monographs: Therapeutic Guide to Herbal Medicines* (Boston, Massachusetts: Integrative Medicine Communications, 1998) 166–167.

25. Nosal'ova, G., Strapkova, A., Kardosova, A., Capek, P., Zathurecky, L., Bukovska, E., "Antitussive action of extracts and polysaccharides of marsh mallow (*Althea officinalis* L., var. *robusta*)," *Pharmazie*, 47(3), 224–226 (March 1992).

26. Sarrell, E.M., Mandelberg, A., Cohen, H.A., "Efficacy of naturopathic extracts in the management of ear pain associated with acute otitis media," *Archives of Pediatric and Adolescent Medicine*, 155(7), 796–799 (July 2001).

27. Serkedjieva, J., "Combined antiinfluenza virus activity of Flos verbasci infusion and amantadine derivatives," *Phytotherapy Research*, 14(7), 571–574 (November 2000).

28. Kim, D.H., Kim, B.R., Kim, J.Y., Jeong, Y.C., "Mechanism of covalent adduct formation of aucubin to proteins," *Toxicology Letters*, 114(1–3), 181–188 (3 April 2000).

29. Michaelsen, T.E., Gilje, A., Samuelsen, A.B., Hogasen, K., Paulsen, B.S., "Interaction between human complement and a pectin type polysaccharide fraction, PMII, from the leaves of *Plantago major* L.," *Scandinavian Journal of Immunology*, 52(5), 483–490 (November 2000).

30. Schinella, G.R., Tournier, H.A., Prieto, J.M., Mordujovich, D., Rios, J.L., "Antioxidant activity of anti-inflammatory plant extracts," *Life Sciences*, 70(9), 1023–1033 (18 January 2002).

31. Ma, S.C., Du, J., But, P.P., Deng, X.L., Zhang, Y.W., Ooi, V.E., Xu, H.X., Lee, S.H., Lee, S.F., "Antiviral Chinese medicinal herbs against respiratory syncytial virus," *Journal of Ethnopharmacology*, 79(2), 205–211 (February 2002).

32. Kohlert, C., *Systemische Verfügbarkeit und Pharmakokinetik von Thymol nach oraler Applikation einer thymianhaltigen Zubereitung im Menschen* (Würzburg, University of Würzburg, 2000). Doctoral disseration.

33. Meister, R., Wittig, T., Beuscher, N., et al., "Efficacy and tolerability of Myrtol standardized in long-term treatment of chronic bronchitis. A double-blind, placebo-controlled study. Study Group Investigators," *Arzneimittel Forschung*, 49, 351–358 (1999).

34. Linder, J.A., Sim, I., "Antibiotic treatment of acute bronchitis in smokers: a systematic review," *Journal of General Internal Medicine*, 17(3), 230–234 (March 2002).

BRUISES

1. Galley, P., Thiollet, M., "A double-blind, placebo-controlled trial of a new veno-active flavonoid fraction (S 5682) in the treatment of symptomatic capillary fragility," *International Angiology*, 12, 69–72 (1993).

2. Miller, M.J., "Injuries to athletes. Evaluation of ascorbic acid and water soluble citrus bioflavonoids in the prophylaxis of injuries in athletes," *Medical Times*, 88, 313–316 (1960).

3. Schorah, C.J., Tormey, W.P., Brooks, G.H., et al., "The effect of vitamin C supplements on body weight, serum proteins, and general health of an elderly population," *American Journal of Clinical Nutrition,* 34, 871–8746 (1981).

4. Maffei Facino, R., Carini, M., Aldini, G., et al., "Free radicals scavenging action and anti-enzyme activities of procyanidines from *Vitis vinifera:* a mechanism for their capillary protective action," *Arzneimittel Forschung,* 44, 592–601 (1994).

5. Amella, M., Bronner, C., Briancon, F., et al.," Inhibition of mast cell histamine release by flavonoids and bioflavonoids," *Planta Medica,* 51, 16–20 (1985).

6. Bionstein, J.L., "Control of swelling in boxing injuries," *Practitioner,* 203, 206 (1969).

7. Masson, M., "Bromelain in blunt injuries of the locomotor system. A study of observed applications in general practice," *Fortschrift für Medizin,* 113(19), 303–306 (10 July 1995).

8. Calabrese, C., Preston, P., "Report of the results of a double-blind, randomized, single-dose trial of a topical 2% escin gel versus placebo in the acute treatment of experimentally-induced hematoma in volunteers," *Planta Medica,* 59(5), 394–397 (October 1993).

9. Stamenova, P.K., Marchetti, T., Simeonov, I., "Efficacy and safety of topical hirudin (Hirudex): a double-blind, placebo-controlled study," *European Review of Medicine and Pharmacological Science,* 5(2), 37–42 (March-April 2001).

BRUXISM

1. Braunwald, E., Fauci, A.S., Kasper, D.L., Hauser, S.L., Longo, D.L., Jameson, J.L., editors, *Harrison's Principles of Internal Medicine,* Fifteenth Edition (New York: McGraw-Hill, 2001), p. 162.

2. Ohayon, M.M., Li, K.K., Guilleminault, C., "Risk factors for sleep bruxism in the general population," *Chest,* 119(1), 53–61 (January 2001).

3. Lobbezoo, F., Naeije, M., "Etiology of bruxism: morphological, pathophysiological and psychological factors," *Nederlandische Tijdschrift vor Tandheelkunde,* 107(7), 275–280 (July 2000).

4. Brown, E.S., Hong, S.C., "Antidepressant-induced bruxism successfully treated with gabapentin," *Journal of the American Dental Association,* 130(10), 1467–1469 (October 1999).

5. Nakazawa, M., Tadataka, M., Takeda, H., "High-dose vitamin B_6 therapy for infantile spasms—the effect and adverse reactions," *Brain Development,* 5, 193–197 (1983).

6. Boonen, G., Haberlein H., "Influence of genuine kavapyrone enantiomers on the GABAA binding site," *Planta Medica,* 64, 504–506 (1998).

7. Jussofie, A., Schmiz, A., Hiemke, C., "Kavapyrone enriched extract from *Piper methysticum* as modulator of the GABA binding site in different regions of rat brain," *Psychopharmacology* (Berlin), 116, 469–474(1994).

8. Woelk, H., Kapoula, O., Lehrl, S., et al., "The treatment of patients with anxiety. A double blind study: kava extract WS 1490 versus benzodiazepines," *Zeitschrift für Allgemeiner Medizin,* 69, 271–277 (1993).

9. Blumenthal, M., "Kava safety questioned due to case reports of liver toxicity: expert analyses of case reports say insufficient evidence to make causal connection," *Herbalgram,* 55, 26–30 (2002).

10. Schmidt, M., Narstadt. A., "Is kava hepatotoxic?" *Deutsche Apotheker Zeitung,* 142(9), 58–63 (2002).

11. Leathwood, P.D., Chauffard, F., "Aqueous extract of valerian reduces latency to fall asleep in man," *Planta Medica,* 50, 144–148 (1984).

12. Mennini, T., Bernasconi, P., Bombardelli, E., et al., "In vitro study on the interaction of extracts and pure compounds from *Valeriana officinalis* roots with GABA, benzodiazepine, and barbiturate receptors in rat brain," *Fitoterapia,* 64, 291–300 (1993).

13. Leathwood, P.D., Chauffard, F., ibid.

BULIMIA

1. Harvey, B.H., Brink, C.B., Seedat, S., Stein, D.J., "Defining the neuromolecular action of myo-inositol: application to obsessive-compulsive disorder," *Progress in Neuropsychopharmacology and Biological Psychiatry,* 26(1), 21–32 (January 2002).

2. Gelber, D., Levine, J., Belmaker, R.H., "Effect of inositol on bulimia nervosa and binge eating," *International Journal of Eating Disorders,* 29(3), 345–348 (January 2001).

3. Rohr, U.D., Herold, J., 'Melatonin deficiencies in women," *Maturitas,* 41 Suppl 1, 85–104 (15 April 2002).

4. Ohanian, V., "Imagery rescripting within cognitive behavior therapy for bulimia nervosa: an illustrative case report," *International Journal of Eating Disorders,* 31(3), 352–357 (April 2002).

BUNIONS

1. Simoncini, L., Giuriati, L., Giannini, S., "Clinical evaluation of the effective use of magnetic fields in podology," *La Chirurgia Degli Organi Di Movimento,* 86(3), 243–247 (July–September 2001).

BURNS

1. Chakrabarty, K.H., Heaton, M., Dalley, A.J., Dawson, R.A., Freedlander, E., Khaw, P.T., MacNeil, S., "Keratinocyte-driven contraction of reconstructed human skin," *Wound Repairand Regeneration,* 9(2), 95–106 (March–April 2001).

2. Silverstein, R.J., Landsman, A.S., "The effects of a moderate and high dose of vitamin C on wound healing in a controlled guinea pig model," *J Foot and Ankle Surgery,* 38(5), 333–338 (September–October 1999).

3. Visuthikosol, V., Chowchuen, B., Sukwanarat, Y., Sriurairatana, S., Boonpucknavig, V., "Effect of aloe vera gel to healing of burn wound: a clinical and histologic study," *Journal of the Medical Association of Thailand,* 78(8), 403–409 (August 1995).

4. Fulton, J.E., Jr., "The stimulation of postdermabrasion wound healing with stabilized aloe vera gel-polyethylene oxide dressing," *Journal of Dermatologic Surgery & Oncology,* 16(5), 460–467 (May 1990).

5. Kohyama, T., Ertl, R.F., Valenti, V., Spurzem, J., Kawamoto, M., Nakamura, Y., Veys, T., Allegra, L., Romberger, D., Rennard, S.I,. "Prostaglandin E(2) inhibits fibroblast chemotaxis," *American Journal of Physiology Lung Cell Molecular Physiology,* 281(5), L1257–1263 (November 2001).

6. Bosse, J.P., Papillon, J., Frenette, G., Dansereau, J., Cadotte, M., Le Lorier, J., "Clinical study of a new antikeloid agent," *Annals of Plastic Surgery,* 3(1), 13–21 (July 1979).

7. Lis-Balchin, M., Hart, S., "Studies on the mode of action of the essential oil of lavender (*Lavandula angustifolia* P. Miller)." *Phytotherapy Research,* 13(6), 540–542 (September 1999).

8. Meijia, K., Reng, R., *Plantas medicinales de uso popular en la Amazonia Peruviana* (Lima, Peru: AECI and IIAP, 1995), 75.

BURSITIS

1. Kannus, P., "Etiology and pathophysiology of chronic tendon disorders in sports," *Scandinavian Journal of Medicine and Science of Sport,* 7(2), 78–85 (April 1997).

2. Klemes, I.S., "Vitamin B_{12} in acute subdeltoid bursitis," *Industrial Medicine and Surgery,* 26, 290–292 (1957).

3. Chadwick, V.S., Schlup, M.M., Ferry, D.M., Chang, A.R., Butt, T.J., "Measurements of unsaturated vitamin B_{12}-binding capacity and methylperoxidase as indices of severity of acute inflammation in serial colonoscopy biopsy specimens from patients with inflammatory bowel disease," *Scandinavian Journal of Gastroenterology,* 25(12), 1196–1204 (December 1990).

4. Klein, G., Küllich, W., "Reducing pain by oral enzyme therapy in rheumatic diseases," *Wienerischer Medizinische Wochenschrift,* 149(21–22), 577–580 (1999).

5. Chen, M.F., Shimada, F., Kato, H., Yano, S., Kanaoka, M., "Effect of glycyrrhizin on the pharmacokinetics of prednisolone following low dosage of prednisolone hemisuccinate," *Endocronologica Japonica,* 37, 331–341 (1990).

6. MacGregor, R.R., Safford, M., Shalit, M., "Effect of ethanol on functions required for the delivery of neutrophils to sites of inflammation," *Journal of Infectious Disease,* 157(4), 682–689 (April 1988).

7. de Jesús Banderas Vargas, T., "Eficacia de la auriculoterapia y combinación de ariculoterapia y tuina en la bursitis de hombro," *Revista Cubana de Enfermedad,* 17(1), 14–19 (2001).

CANKER SORES

1. Ship, I.I., Merritt, A.D., Stanley, H.R., "Recurrent aphthous ulcers," *American Journal of Medicine,* 32, 32–43 (1962).

2. Ferguson, R., Bashu, M.K., Asquith, P., Cooke, W.T., "Jejunal mucosal abnormalities in patients with recurrent aphthous ulcerations," *British Medical Journal* 1, 11–13 (1975).

3. Nolan, A., McIntosh, W.B., Allam, B.F., Lamey, P.J., "Recurrent aphthous ulceration. Vitamin B_1, B_2, and B_6 status and response to replacement therapy," *Journal of Oral Pathology and Medicine,* 20, 389–391 (1991).

4. Wray, D., Ferguson, M.M., Mason, D.K., Hutcheon, A.W., Dagg, J.H., "Recurrent aphthae: treatment with vitamin B_{12}, folic acid, and iron," *British Medical Journal,* 2, 490–493 (1975).

5. O'Farrelly, C., O'Mahony, C., Graeme-Cook, F., Feighery, C., McCartan, B.E., Weir, D.G., "Gliadin antibodies identify gluten-sensitive oral ulceration in the absence of villous atrophy," *Oral Surgery, Oral Medicine, Oral Pathology,* 57, 504–507 (1984).

6. Nolan, A., McIntosh, W.B., Allan, B.F., Larne, P.J., "Recurrent aphthous ulceration, Vitamin B_1, B_2, and B_6 status and response to replacement therapy," *Journal of Oral Pathology and Medicine,* 20, 389–391 (1991).

7. Merchant, H.L., Gangers, L.J., Glassman, I.B., Sobel, R.E., "Zinc sulfate supplementation for treatment of recurring oral ulcers," *Southern Medical Journal,* 70, 559–561 (1977).

8. No authors listed, "Oral ulcers remedy gets FDA clearance," *Journal of the American Dental Association,* 125(10), 1308, 1310 (October 1994).

9. Safayhi, H., Sabieraj, J., Sailer, E.R., Ammon, H.P., "Chamazulene: an antioxidant-type inhibitor of leukotriene B4 formation," *Planta Medica,* 60(5), 410–413 (October 1994).

10. Miller, T., Wittstock, U., Lindequist, U., Teuscher, E., "Effects of some components of the essential oil of chamomile, *Chamomilla recutita,* on histamine release from rat mast cells," *Planta Medica,* 62(1), 60–61 (1 February 1996).

11. Das, S.K., Gulati, A.K., Singh, V.P., "Deglycyrrhizinated licorice in apthous ulcers," *Journal of the Association of Physicians of India,* 37, 647 (1989).

12. Herlofson, B.B., Barkvoll, P., "The effect of two toothpaste detergents on the frequency of recurrent aphthous ulcers," *Acta Odontologica Scandinavica,* 54(3), 150–153 (June 1996).

13. Healy, C.M., Paterson, M., Joyston-Bechal, S., Williams, D.M., Thornhill, M.H., "The effect of a sodium lauryl sulfate-free dentifrice on patients with recurrent oral ulceration," *Oral Disease,* 5(1), 39–43 (January 1999).

14. Fakhry-Smith, S., Din, C., Nathoo, S.A., Gaffar, A., "Clearance of sodium lauryl sulphate from the oral cavity," *Journal of Clinical Periodontology,* 24(5), 313–317 (May 1997).

15. Srinivasan, U., Weir, D.G., Feighery, C., O'Farrelly, C., "Lesson of the week: emergence of classic enteropathy after longstanding gluten sensitive oral ulceration," BMJ, 316, 3076–207 (17 January 1999).

CARDIOMYOPATHY

1. Sodi-Pallares, personal conversation, 23 January 2001.

2. Folkers, K., Yamamura, Y., editors, *Biomedical and Clinical Aspects of Conezyme* Q_{10}. Volumes 1–4 (Amsterdam: Elsevier, 1977, 1980, 1982, 1984).

3. Crestanello, J.A., Doliba, N.M., Babsky, A.M., Niborii, K., Osbakken, M.D., Whitman, G.J., "Effect of coenzyme Q_{10} supplementation on mitochondrial function after myocardial ischemia reperfusion," *Journal of Surgical Research,* 102(2), 221–228 (February 2002).

4. Kamikawa, T., Kobayashi, A., Yamashita, T., Hayashi, H., Yamazaki, N., "Effects of coenzyme Q_{10} on exercise tolerance in chronic stable angina pectoris," *American Journal of Cardiology,* 56, 247 (1985).

5. Munkholm, H., Hansen, H.H., Rasmussen, K., "Conezyme Q_{10} treatment in serious heart failure," *Biofactors,* 9(2–4), 285–289 (1999).

6. Langsjoen, P.H., Langsjoen, A., Willis, R., Folkers, K., "Treatment of hypertrophic cardiomyopathy with coenzyme Q_{10}," *Molecular Aspects of Medicine,* 18 Suppl, S145–S151 (1997).

7. Rebuzzi, A.G., Schiavoni, G., Amico, C.M., et al., "Beneficial effects of L-carnitine in the reduction of the necrotic area in acute myocardial infarction," *Drugs in Experimental Clinical Research,* 18, 355–365 (1984).

8. Cherchi, A., Lai, C., Angelino, F., Trucco, G., Caponnetto, S., Mereto, P.E., Rosolen, G., Manzoli, U., Schiavoni, G., Reale, A., et al., "Effects of L-carnitine on exercise tolerance in chronic stable angina: a multicenter, double-blind, randomized, placebo controlled crossover study," *International Journal of Clinical Pharmacology and Therapeutic Toxicology,* 23(10), 579–582 (October 1985).

9. Donati, C., Bertieri, R.S., Barbi, G., "Pantethine, diabetes mellitus and atherosclerosis. Clinical study of 1045 patients," *La Clinica Terapeutica,* 128, 411–422 (1989).

10. Schüssler, M., Hölzl, J., Fricke, U., "Myocardial effects of flavonoids from *Crataegus* species," *Arzneimittel Forschung,* 45, 842–845 (1995).

11. Ceriana, P., "Effect of myocardial ischaemia-reperfusion on granulocyte elastase release," *Anaesthia and Intensive Care,* 20, 187–190 (1992).

12. Rajendran, S., Deepalakshmi, P.D., Parasakthy, K., Devaraj, H., Devaraj, S.N., "Effect of tincture of *Crataegus* on the LDL-receptor activity of hepatic plasma membrane of rats fed an atherogenic diet," *Atherosclerosis,* 123, 235–241 (1996).

13. Schüssler ,M., Hölzl, J., Rump, A.F., Fricke, U.," Functional and antiischaemic effects of monoacetyl-vitexinrhamnoside in different in vitro models," *General Pharmacology,* 26, 1565–1570 (1995).

14. Nasa, Y., Hashizume, H., Hoque, A.N., Abiko, Y., "Protective effect of *Crataegus* extract on the cardiac mechanical dysfunction in isolated perfused working rat heart," *Arzneimittel Forschung,* 43, 945–949 (1993).

15. Dwivedi, S., Agarwal. M.P.. "Anti-anginal and cardioprotective effects of *Terminalia arjuna,* an indigenous drug, in coronary artery disease," *Journal of the Association of Physicians of India,* 42, 287–289 (1994).

16. Dwivedi, S., Jauhari, R., "Beneficial effects of Terminalia arjuna in coronary artery disease," *Indian Heart Journal,* 49(5), 507–510 (September–October 1997).

17. Tripathi, S.N., Upadhyaya, B.N., Gupka, V.K., "Beneficial effect of *Inula racemosa* (Pushkarmoola) in Angina pectoris: a preliminary report," *Indian Journal of Physiology and Pharmacology,* 28, 73–75 (1984).

18. Singh, R.P., Singh, R., Ram, P., Batliwala, P.G., "Use of Pushkar-Guggul, an indigenous antiischemic combination, in the management of ischemic heart disease," *International Journal of Pharmacognosy,* 31, 147–160 (1993).

19. Johne, A., Brockmoller, J., Bauer, S., Maurer, A., Langheinrich, M., Roots, I., "Pharmacokinetic interaction of digoxin with an herbal extract from St. John's wort (*Hypericum perforatum*)," *Clinical Pharmacology and Therapeutics,* 66, 338–345 (October 1999).

20. Liu, Y., Chiba, M., Inaba, Y., Kondo, M., "Keshan disease—a review from the aspect of history and etiology," *Nippon Eiseigaku Zasshi,* 56(4), 641–648 (January 2002).

21. Burke, M.P., Opeskin, K., "Fulminant heart failure due to selenium deficiency cardiomyopathy (Keshan disease)," *Medicine, Science, and the Law,* 42(1), 10–13 (January 2002).

CARPAL TUNNEL SYNDROME

1. Singer, G., Ashworth, C.R., "Anatomic variations and carpal tunnel syndrome: 10-year clinical experience," *Clinical Orthopedics,* 392, 330–340 (November 2001).

2. Allampallam, K., Chakraborty, J., Robinson, J., "Effect of ascorbic acid and growth factors on collagen metabolism of flexor retinaculum cells from individuals with and without carpal tunnel syndrome," *Journal of Occupational and Environmental Medicine,* 42(3), 251–259 (March 2000).

3. Villareal, D.T., Morley, J.E., "Trophic factors in aging. Should older people receive hormonal replacement therapy?" *Drugs and Aging,* 4(6), 492–509 (June 1994).

4. Brenstein, A.L., Dinesen, J.S., "Brief communication: effect of pharmacologic doses of vitamin B_6 on carpal tunnel syndrome, electroencephalograph-

ic results, and pain," *Journal of the American College of Nutrition,* 12(1), 73–76 (February 1993).

5. Keniston, R.C., Nathan, P.A., Leklem, J.E., Lockwood, R.S., "Vitamin B$_6$, vitamin C, and carpal tunnel syndrome. A cross-sectional study of 441 adults," *Journal of Occupational and Environmental Medicine,* 39(10), 949–959 (October 1997).

6. Klein, G., Küllich, W., "Reducing pain by oral enzyme therapy in rheumatic diseases," *Wienerischer Medizinische Wochenschrift,* 149(21–22), 577–580 (1999).

7. Chen, M.F., Shimada, F., Kato, H., Yano, S., Kanaoka, M., "Effect of glycyrrhizin on the pharmacokinetics of prednisolone following low dosage of prednisolone hemisuccinate," *Endocronologica Japonica,* 37, 331–341 (1990).

8. Carter, C., Hall, T., Aspy, C.B., "The effectiveness of magnet therapy for treatment of wrist pain attributed to carpal tunnel syndrome," *Journal of Family Practice,* 51(1), 38–40 (January 2002).

9. Davis, P.T., Hulbert, J.R., Kassak, K.M., Meyer, J.J., "Comparative efficacy of conservative and chiropractic treatment for carpal tunnel syndrome: a randomized clinical trial," *Journal of Manipulative Physiology andl Therapy,* 21, 317–326 (1998).

CAT SCRATH FEVER

1. Bosch, X., "Hypercalcemia due to endogenous overproduction of active vitamin D in identical twins with cat-scratch disease," *Journal of the American Medical Association,* 279(7), 532–534 (18 February 1998).

CATARACTS

1. Braunwald, E., Fauci, A.S., Kasper, D.L., Hauser, S.L., Longo, D.L., Jameson, J.L., editors, *Harrison's Principles of Internal Medicine,* Fifteenth Edition (New York: McGraw-Hill, 2001), p. 172.

2. Young, R.W., "The family of sunlight-related eye diseases," *Optometry and Vision Science,* 71, 125–144 (1994).

3. Christen, W.G., Glynn, R.J., Ajani, U.A., Schaumberg, D.A., Buring, J.E., Hennekens, C.H., Manson, J.E., "Smoking cessation and risk of age-related cataract in men," *Journal of the American Medical Association,* 284(6), 713–716 (August 2000).

4. Taylor, H.R., "Epidemiology of age-related cataract," *Eye,* 13, 445–448 (1999).

5. Schaumberg, D.A., Glynn, R.J., Christen, W.G., Hankinson, S.E., Hennekens, C.H., "Relations of body fat distribution and height with cataract in men," *American Journal of Clinical Nutrition,* 72, 1495–1502 (2000).

6. Cekic, O., Bardak, Y., Totan, Y., Kavakli, S., Akyol, O., Ozdemir, O., Karel, F., "Nickel, chromium, manganese, iron and aluminum levels in human cataractous and normal lenses," *Ophthalmological Research,* 31, 332–336 (1999).

7. Cekic, O., "Effect of cigarette smoking on copper, lead, and cadmium accumulation in human lens," *British Journal of Ophthalmology,* 82, 186–188 (1998).

8. Braunwald, E., Fauci, A.S., Kasper, D.L., Hauser, S.L., Longo, D.L., Jameson, J.L., editors, *Harrison's Principles of Internal Medicine,* Fifteenth Edition (New York: McGraw-Hill, 2001), p. 172.

9. Harding, J.J., "Cataract: sanitation or sunglasses," *Lancet,* 1(8262), 39 (1982).

10. Sasaki, H., Kojima, M., Sasaki, H., Jonasson, F., Ono, M., Nagata, M., Sasaki, K., "UV-light exposure and pure cortical cataract: a population bases case-control study in Iceland," cited by Trevithick, J.R., Mitton, K.P., 'Antioxidants and Diseases of the Eye' in Papas, A.M., editor, *Antioxidant Status, Diet, Nutrition, and Health* (Boca Raton, Florida: CRC Press, 1999), p. 561.

11. Hayes, R.P., Fisher, R.F., "Influence of a prolonged period of low dosage x-rays on the optic and ultrastructural appearance of cataract of the human lens," *British Journal Ophthalmology,* 63, 457–464 (1979).

12. Rao, G.N., Sadasivudu, B., Cotlier, E., "Studies of glutathione s-transferase, glutathione peroxidase and glutathione reductase in human normal and cataractous lenses," *Ophthalmic Research,* 15, 173–179 (1983).

13. Reddy, V.N., Giblin, F.J., "Metabolism and function of glutathione in the lens. Human Cataract Formation," *Ciba Foundation Symposium,* 106, 65–87 (1984).

14. Robertson, J., Donner, A.P., Trevithick, J.R., "A possible role for vitamin C and E in cataract prevention," *Annals of the New York Academy of Sciences,* 40, 372–382 (1989).

15. Robertson, J., Donner, A.P., Trevithick, J.R., "A possible role for vitamins C and E in cataract prevention," *American Journal of Clinical Nutrition,* 53, 3465–34515 (1991).

16. Leske, M.C., Chylack, L.T., Jr., He, Q., Wu, S.Y., Schoenfeld, E., Friend, J., Wolfe, J., "Antioxidant vitamins and nuclear opacies: the longitudinal study of cataract," *Ophthalmology,* 105, 831–836 (1998).

17. Jacques, P.F., Taylor, A., Hankinson, S.E., Willett, W.C., Mahnken, B., Lee, Y., Vaid, K., Lahav, M., "Long-term vitamin C supplement use and prevalence of early age-related opacities," *American Journal of Clinical Nutrition,* 66, 911–916 (1997).

10. Nudulin, G., Rubman, L.D., McCarty, C.A., Nudulin, G., Rubman, L.D., McCarty, C.A., Garrett, S.K., McNeil, J.J., Taylor, H.R., "The role of past intake of vitamin E in early cataract changes," *Ophthalmic Epidemiology,* 6, 105–112 (1999).

19. Karakucuk, S., Ertugrul Mirza, G., Faruk Ekinciler, O., Saraymen, R., Karakucuk, I., Ustdal, M., "Selenium concentrations in serum, lens and aqueous humour of patients with senile cataract," *Acta Ophthalmologica Scandinavica,* 73, 329–332 (1995).

20. Tavani, A., Negri, E., La Vecchia, C., "Food and nutrient intake and risk of cataract," *Annals of Epidemiology,* 6, 41–46 (1966).

21. Chasan-Taber, L., Willet, W.C., Seddon, J.M., Stampfer, M.J., Rosner, B., Colditz, G.A., Speizer, F.E., Hankinson, S.E., "A prospective study of carotenoid and vitamin A intakes and risk of cataract extraction in U.S. women," *American Journal of Clinical Nutrition,* 70, 509–516 (1999).

22. Brown, L., Rimm, E.B., Seddon, J.M., Giovannucci, E.L., Chasan-Taber, L., Spiegelman, D., Willett, W.C., Hankinson, S.E., "A prospective study of carotenoid intake and risk of cataract extraction in U.S. men," *American Journal of Clinical Nutrition,* 70, 517–524 (1999).

23. Moeller, S.M., Jacques, P.F., Blumberg, J.B., "The potential role of dietary xanthophylls in cataract and age-related macular degeneration," *Journal of the American College of Nutrition,* 19, 522S–527S (2000).

24. Brown, L., Rimm, E.B., Seddon, J.M., Giovannucci, E.L., Chasan-Taber, L., Spiegelman, D., Willett, W.C., Hankinson, S.E., ibid.

25. Chasan-Taber, L., Willet, W.C., Seddon, J.M., Stampfer, M.J., Rosner, B., Colditz, G.A., Speizer, F.E., Hankinson, S.E., ibid.

26. Sperduto, R.D., Hu, T.S., Milton, R.C., Zhao, J.L., Everett, D.F., Cheng, Q.F., Blot, W.J., Bing, L., Taylor, P.R., Li, J.Y., et al., "The Linxian cataract studies. Two nutrition intervention trials," *Archives of Ophthalmology,* 111, 1246–1253 (1993).

27. Bravetti, G., "Preventive medical treatment of senile cataract with vitamin E and anthocyanosides: clinical evaluation," *Annali di ottalmologia e clinica oculistica,* 115, 109 (1989).

28. Sasaki, H., Kojima, M., Sasaki, H., Jonasson, F., Ono, M., Nagata, M., Sasaki, K., ibid.

29. Linetsky, M., James, H.L., Ortwerth, B.J., "The generation of superoxide anion by the UVA irradiation of human lens proteins," *Experimental Eye Research,* 63, 67–74 (1996).

30. Sperduto, R.D., Hu, T.S., Milton, R.C., Zhao, J.L., Everett, D.F., Cheng, Q.F., Blot, W.J., Bing, L., Taylor, P.R., Li, J.Y., et al., "The Linxian cataract studies," *Archives of Ophthalmology,* 111, 1246–53 (1993).

CELIAC DISEASE

1. Dickey, W., "Low serum vitamin B$_{12}$ is common in coeliac disease and is not due to autoimmune gastritis,," *European Journal of Gastroenterology,* 14(4), 425–427 (April 2002).

2. Jublin, L., Edqvist, L.E., Ekman, L.G., Ljunghall K., Olsson, M., "Blood glutathione-peroxidase levels in skin diseases: effect of selenium and vitamin E treatment," *Acta Dermatologica et Venereologica,* 62, 211–214 (1982).

3. Kalita, B., Nowak, P., Slimok, M., Sikora, A., Szkilnik, R., Obuchowicz, A., Sulej, J., Sabat, D., "Selenium plasma concentrations in children with celiac

disease in different stages of diagnosis," *Polski Merkuriusz Lekarski: Organ Polskiego Towarzystwa Lekarskiego,* 12(67), 32–34 (January 2002).

4. Srinivasan, U., Weir, D.G., Feighery, C., O'Farrelly, C., "Lesson of the week: emergence of classic enteropathy after longstanding gluten sensitive oral ulceration," *BMJ,* 316, 3076–207 (17 January 1999).

5. Sanders, D.S., "Management of infertility–don't forget coeliac disease," *BMJ,* 325, 28 (24 July 2002).

6. Hozyasz, K.K., "Is low male sex ratio in offspring of celiacs an advantage?" *American Journal of Gastroenterology,* 97(6), 1574 (June 2002).

7. Annibale, B., Severi, C., Chistolini, A., Antonelli, G., Lahner, E., Marcheggiano, A., Iannoni, C., Monarca, B., Delle Fave, G., "Efficacy of gluten-free diet alone on recovery from iron deficiency anemia in adult celiac patients," *American Journal of Gastroenterology,* 96(1), 132–137 (January 2001).

CELLULITE

1. Nurnberger F., Muller, G., "So-called cellulite: an invented disease," *Journal of Dermatological Surgery and Oncology,* 4(3), 221–229 (March 1978).

2. Lotti, T., Ghersetich, I., Grappone, C., Dini, G., "Proteoglycans in so-called cellulite," *International Journal of Dermatology,* 29(4), 272–274 (May 1990).

3. Pierard, G.E., Nizet, J.L., Pierard-Franchimont, C., "Cellulite: from standing fat herniation to hypodermal stretch marks," *American Journal of Dermatopathology,* 22(1), 34–37 (February 2000).

4. Hexsel, D.M., Mazzuco, R., "Subcision: a treatment for cellulite," *International Journal of Dermatology,* 39 (7), 539–544 (July 2000).

5. Bertin, C., Zunino, H., Pittet, J.C., Beau, P., Pineau, P., Massonneau, M., Robert, C., Hopkins, J., "A double-blind evaluation of the activity of an anticellulite product containing retinol, caffeine, and ruscogenine by a combination of several non-invasive methods," *Journal of Cosmetic Science,* 52(4), 199–210 (July–August 2001).

6. Goodpaster, B.H., Thaete, F.L., Kelley, D.E., "Thigh adipose tissue distribution is associated with insulin resistance in obesity and in type 2 diabetes mellitus," *American Journal of Clinical Nutrition,* 71, 885–892 (2000).

7. Ryan, A.S., Nicklas, B.J., Berman, D.M., Bennis, K.E., "Dietary restriction and walking reduce fat deposition in the midthigh in obese older women," *American Journal of Clinical Nutrition,* 72, 708–713 (2000).

8. Auteri, A., Pasqui, A.L., Bruni, F., Di Renzo, M., Bova, G., Chiarion, C., Delchambre, J., "Pharmacodynamics and pharmacokinetics of Veliten (rutine, alpha-tocopherol and ascorbic acid) in patients with chronic venous insufficiency," *International Journal of Clinical Pharmacology Research,* 14(3), 95–100 (1994).

9. Bertin, C., Zunino, H., Pittet, J.C., Beau, P., Pineau, P., Massonneau, M., Robert, C., Hopkins, J., ibid.

10. Aichinger, F., Giss, G., Vogel, G., "New findings regarding the phamacodyanmics of bioflavonoids and the horse chestnut saponin aescin as the basis for their use in therapy," *Arzneimittel Forschung,* 14, 892 (1964).

11. Bisler, H., Pfeifer, R., Kluken, N., Pauschinger, P., "Wirkung von Roßkastaniensamenextrakt auf die transkapillare filtration bei chronischer venöser insuffizienz," *Deutsche Medizinischer Wochenschrift,* 111, 1321–1328 (1986).

12. Incandela, L, Cesarone, M.R., Cacchio, M., De Sanctis, M.T., Santavenere, C., D'Auro, M.G., Bucci, M., Belcaro, G., "Total triterpenic fraction of Centella asiatica in chronic venous insufficiency and in high-perfusion microangiopathy," *Angiology* 52 Suppl 2, S9–S13 (October 2001).

13. Incandela, L., Belcaro, G., De Sanctis, M.T., Cesarone, M.R., Griffin, M., Ippolito, E., Bucci, M., Cacchio, M., "Total triterpenic fraction of Centella asiatica in the treatment of venous hypertension: a clinical, prospective, randomized trial using a combined microcirculatory model," *Angiology* 52 Suppl 2, S61–S67 (October 2001).

14. Grimaldi, R., De Ponti, F., D'Angelo, L., Caravaggi, M., Guidi, G., Lecchini, S., Frigo, G.M., Crema, A., "Pharmacokinetics of the total triterpenic fraction of Centella asiatica after single and multiple administrations to healthy volunteers. A new assay for asiatic acid," *Journal of Ethnopharmacology,* 28(2), 235–241 (February 1990).

15. Draelos, Z.D., Marenus, K.D., "Cellulite. Etiology and purported treatment." *Dermatological Surgery,* 23(12), 1177–1181 (December 1997).

16. Collis, N., Elliot, L.A., Sharpe, C., Sharpe, D.T., "Cellulite treatment: a

myth or reality: a prospective randomized, controlled trial of two therapies, endermologie and aminophylline cream." *Plastic and Reconstructive Surgery,* 104(4), 1110–1114, discussion 1115–1117 (September 1999).

17. Adcock, D., Paulsen, S., Jabour, K., Davis, S., Nanney, L.B., Shack, R.B., "Analysis of the effects of deep mechanical massage in the porcine model." *Plastic and Reconstructive Surgery,* 108(1), 233–240 (July 2001).

CELLULITIS

1. Cervin, A., "The anti-inflammatory effect of erythromycin and its derivatives, with special reference to nasal polyposis and chronic cellulitis," *Acta Otolaryngolica,* 121(1), 183–192 (January 2001).

2. Cazzola, P., Mazzanti, P., Bossi, G., "In vivo modulating effect of a calf thymus acid lysate on human T lymphocyte subsets and CD4+/CD8+ ratio in the course of difference diseases," *Current Therapies Research,* 42, 1011–1017 (1987).

3. Seifter, E., Rettura, G., Seiter, J., "Thymotrophic action of vitamin A," *Federal Proceedings,* 32, 947 (1973).

4. Semba, R.D., "Vitamin A, immunity, and infection," *Clinical Infectious Disease,* 19, 489–499 (1994).

5. Ginter, E., "Optimum intake of vitamin C for the human organisms," *Nutrition and Health,* 1, 66–77 (1982).

6. Gabor, M., "Pharmacologic effects of flavonoids on blood vessels," *Angiologica,* 9, 355–374 (1972).

7. Prasad, A., "Clinical, biochemical and nutritional spectrum of zinc deficiency in human subjects. An update," *Nutrition Review,* 41, 197–208 (1983).

8. Erhard, M., "Effect of echinacea, aconitum, lachesis, and apis extracts, and their combinations of phagocytosis of human granulocytes," *Phytotherapy Research,* 8, 14–77 (1994).

9. Stoll, A., Renz, J., Brack, A., "Antibacterial substances II. Isolation and constitution of echnacoside, a glycoside from the roots of *Echinacea angustifolia,*" *Helvetica Chimica Acta,* 33, 1877–1893 (1950).

10. Zhang, L., Yang, L.W., Yang, L.J., "Relation between *Helicobacter pylori* and pathogenesis of chronic atrophic gastritis and the research of its prevention and treatment," *Chung-Kuo Chung Hsi I Chieh Ho Tsa Chih-Chinese Journal of Modern Developments in Traditional Medicine,* 12(9), 515–516 (September 1992).

11. Latino, H., "Pylori implicated in allergies," *Medical Tribune,* March 24, 1994, p. 1.

CEREBRAL PALSY

1. Perlman, J.M., "Intrapartum hypoxic-ischemic cerebral injury and subsequent cerebral palsy: medicolegal issues," *Pediatrics,* 99, 851–859 (1997).

2. Maclennan, A., "For the international cerebral palsy task force. A template for defining a causal relation between acute intrapartum events and cerebral palsy: International Consensus Statement," *British Medical Journal,* 319, 1054–1059 (1999).

3. Azcue, M.P., Zello, G.A., Levy, L.D., Pencharz, P.B., "Energy expenditure and body composition in children with spastic quadriplegic cerebral palsy," *Journal of Pediatrics,* 129(6), 870–876 (December 1996).

4. Newnham, R.E., "Essentiality of boron for healthy bones and joints," *Environmental Health Perspectives,* 102 (Suppl 7), 83–85 (1994).

5. Penland, J.G., "The importance of boron nutrition for brain and psychological function," *Biological Trace Element Research,* 66, 299–317 (1998).

6. Mittendorf, R., Pryde, P.G., "An overview of the possible relationship between antenatal pharmacologic magnesium and cerebral palsy," *Journal of Perinatal Medicine,* 28(4), 286–293 (2000).

7. Prabhala, A., Garg, R., Dandona, P., "Severe myopathy associated with vitamin D deficiency in Western New York," *Archives of Internal Medicine,* 160, 1199–1203 (2000).

8. McGibbon, N.H., Andrade, C.K., Widener, G., Cintas, H.L., "Effect of an equine-movement therapy program on gait, energy expenditure, and motor function in children with spastic cerebral palsy: a pilot study," *Developmental Medicine and Child Neurology,* 40(11), 754–762 (November 1998).

9. Montgomery, D., Goldberg, J., Amar, M., Lacroix, V., Lecomte, J., Lambert,

J., Vanasse, M., Marois, P., "Effects of hyperbaric oxygen therapy on children with spastic diplegic cerebral palsy: a pilot project," *Undersea and Hyperbaric Medicine*, 26(4), 235–242 (Winter 1999).

10. Collet, J.P., Vanasse, M., Marois, P., Amar, M., Goldberg, J., Lambert, J., Lassonde, M., Hardy, P., Fortin, J., Tremblay, S.D., Montgomery, D., Lacroix, J., Robinson, A., Majnemer, A., "Hyperbaric oxygen for children with cerebral palsy: a randomised multicentre trial. HBO-CP Research Group," *Lancet*, 357(9256), 582–586 (24 February 2001).

CHAGAS DISEASE

1. Fraker, P.J., Caruso, R., Kierszenbaum, F., "Alteration of the immune and nutritional status of mice by synergy between zinc deficiency and infection with *Trypanosoma cruzi*," *Journal of Nutrition*, 112(6), 1224–1229 (June 1982).

2. Porea, T.J., Belmont, J.W., Mahoney, D.H., Jr., "Zinc induced anemia and neutropenia in an adolescent," *Journal of Pediatrics*, 176(5), 688–690.

3. Gao, W., Pereira, M.A., "Interleukin-6 is required for parasite specific response and host resistance to *Trypanosoma cruzi*," *International Journal of Parasitology*, 32(2), 167–170 (February 2002).

4. Lemaire, I., Assinewe, V., Cano, P., Awang, D.V., Arnason, J.T., "Stimulation of interleukin-1 and -6 production in alveolar macrophages by the neotropical liana, *Uncaria tomentosa* (uña de gato)," *Journal of Ethnopharmacology*, 64(2), 109–115 (February 1999).

5. Pinto, C.N., Dantas, A.P., de Moura, K.C., Emery, F.S., Polequevitch, P.F., Pinto, M.C., de Castro, S.L, Pinto, A.V., "Chemical reactivity studies with naphthoquinones from *Tabeuia* with anti-trypanosomal efficacy," *Arzneimittel-Forschung*, 50(12), 1120–1128 (December 2000).

6. Oliveira, M.M., Einicker-Lamaa, M., "Inositol metabolism in Trypanosoma cruzi: potential target for chemotherapy against Chagas' disease," *Anais da Academia Brasiliera de Ciências*, 72(3), 413–419 (September 2000).

7. Oliveira, E., Ribeiro, A.L., Assis Silva, F., Torres, R.M., Rocha, M.O., "The Valsalva maneuver in Chagas disease patients without cardiopathy," *International Journal of Cardiology*, 82(1), 49–54 (January 2002).

8. López, A., Crocco, L., Morales, G., Catalá, S., "Feeding frequency and nutritional status of peridomestic populations of *Triatoma infestans* from Argentina," *Acta Tropica*, 73(3), 275–281 (15 October 1999).

CHICKEN POX

1. Pollard, A.J., Isaacs, A., Lyall, E.G.H., Curtis, N., Lee, K., Walters, S., Levin, M., "Lesson of the week: potentially lethal bacterial infection associated with varicella zoster virus," *British Medical Journal*, 313, 283–285 (3 August 1996)

2. Guess, H.A., Broughton, D.D., Melton, L.J., Kurland, L.T., "Chickenpox hospitalizations among residents of Olmsted County, Minnesota, 1962 through 1981. A population based study," *American Journal of Disease of Childhood*, 138, 1055–1057 (1984).

3. Billigmann P., "Enzyme therapy—an alternative in treatment of herpes zoster. A controlled study of 192 patients," *Fortschrift für Medizin*, 113(4), 43–48 (10 February 1995).

4. Kleine, M.W., Stauder, G.M., Beese, E.W., "The intestinal absorption of orally administered hydrolytic enzymes and their effects in the treatment of acute herpes zoster as compared with those of oral acyclovir therapy," *Phytomedicine*, 2, 7–15 (1995).

5. Powell, C.J., "Pancreatic enzymes and fibrosing colonopathy," *Lancet*, 354, 251 (1999).

6. Heyblon, R., "Vitamin B$_{12}$ in herpes zoster," *Journal of the American Medical Association*, 149, 1338 (1950).

7. Cochrane, T., "Post-herpes zoster neuralgia: response to vitamin E therapy," *Archives of Dermatology*, 111, 296 (1975).

CHLAMYDIA

1. Westrom, L., "Genital chlamydial infections in the female," *Archives of Gynecology*, 238, 811–818 (1985).

2. Matyszak, M.K., Young, J.L., Gaston, J.S., "Uptake and processing of chlamydia trachomatis by human dendritic cells," *European Journal of Immunology*, 32(3), 742–751 (March 2002).

3. Stamm, W.E., Hicks, C.B., Martin, D.H., et al., "Azithromycin for empirical treatment of the nongonococcal urethritis syndrome in men: a randomized double-blind study," *Journal of the American Medical Association*, 274, 545–549 (1995).

4. Hillier, S.L., et al., "The relationship of hydrogen peroxide-producing *Lactobacilli* to bacterial vaginosis in genital microflora in pregnant women," *Obstetrics and Gynecology*, 79, 369–373 (1992).

5. Cazzola, P., Mazzanti, P., Bossi, G., "In vivo modulating effect of a calf thymus acid lysate on human T lymphocyte subsets and CD4+/CD8+ ratio in the course of difference diseases," *Current Therapies Research*, 42, 1011–1017 (1987).

6. Seifter, E., Rettura, G., Seiter, J., "Thymotrophic action of vitamin A," *Federal Proceedings*, 32, 947 (1973).

7. Semba, R.D., "Vitamin A, immunity, and infection," *Clinical Infectious Disease*, 19, 489–499 (1994).

8. Scholer, J., Ollinger, K., Kvarnstrom, M., Soderlund, G., Kohlstrom, E., "*Chlamydia trachomatis*-induced apoptosis occurs in uninfected McCoy cells late in the developmental cycle and is regulated by the intracellular redox state," *Microbiology and Pathology*, 31(4), 173–184 (October 2001).

9. Prasad, A., "Clinical, biochemical and nutritional spectrum of zinc deficiency in human subjects. An update," *Nutrition Review*, 41, 197–208 (1983).

10. Erhard, M., "Effect of echinacea, aconitum, lachesis, and apis extracts, and their combinations of phagocytosis of human granulocytes," *Phytotherapy Research*, 8, 14–77 (1994).

11. Facino, R.M., Carini, M., Aldini, G., Marinello, C., Arlandini, E., Franzoi, L., Colombo, M., Pietta, P., Mauri, P., "Direct characterization of caffeoyl esters with antihyaluronidase activity in crude extracts from *Echinacea angustifolia* roots by fast atom bombardment tandem mass spectrometry," *Farmaco*, 48(10), 1447–1461 (October 1993).

12. Budzinski, J.W., Foster, B.C., Vandenhoek, S., Arnason, J.T., "An in vitro evaluation of human cytochrome P405 3A4 inhibition by selected commercial herbal extracts and tinctures," *Phytomedicine*, 7(4), 273–282 (July 2000).

13. Luettig, B., Steinmuller, C., Gifford, G.E., Wagner, H., Lohmann-Matthes, M.L., "Macrophage activation by the polysaccharide arabinogalactan isolated from plant cell cultures of *Echinacea purpurea*," *Journal of the National Cancer Institute*, 81(9), 669–675 (3 May 1989).

14. Blumenthal, M., Goldberg, A., Brinckmann, J. *Herbal Medicine: Expanded Commission E Monographs* (Boston, Integrative Medicine, 2000), p. 88.

15. Rehman, J., Dillow, J.M., Carter, S.M., Chou, J., Le, B., Maisel, A.S., "Increased production of antigen-specific immunoglobulins G and M following in vivo treatment with the medical plants *Echinacea angustifolia* and *Hydrastis canadensis*," *Immunology Letters*, 68(2–3), 391–395 (1 June 1999).

16. Wang, S.K., Patton, D.L., Kuo, C.C., "Effects of ascorbic acid on *Chlamydia trachomatis* infection and on erythromycin treatment in primary cultures of human amniotic cells," *Journal of Clinical Microbiology*, 30(10), 2551–2554 (October 1992).

17. Reeve, P., "The inactivation of chlamydia trachomatis by Providone-iodine," *Journal of Antimicrobial Chemotherapy*, 2, 77–80 (1976).

CHRONIC FATIGUE SYNDROME

1. Jason, L.A., Richman, J.A., Rademaker, A.W., Jordan, K.M., Plioplys, A.V., Taylor, R.R., McCready, W., Huang, C.F., Plioplys, S., "A community-based study of chronic fatigue syndrome," *Archives of Internal Medicine*, 159, 2129–2137 (1999).

2. Ichise, M., Salit, I.E., Abbey, S.E., Chung, D.G., Gray, B., Kirsh, J.C., Freedman, M., "Assessment of regional cerebral perfusion by 99Tcm-HMPAO SPECT in chronic fatigue syndrome," *Nuclear Medicine Communications*, 13, 767–772 (1992).

3. Natelson, B.H., Cohen, J.M., Brassloff, I., Lee, H.J., "A controlled study of brain magnetic resonance imaging in patients with the chronic fatigue syndrome," *Journal of Neurological Science*, 120, 213–217 (1993).

4. Furman, J.M., "Testing of vestibular function: an adjunct in the assessment of chronic fatigue syndrome," *Review of Infectious Diseases*, 13, S109–S111 (1991).

5. Saggini, R., Pizzigallo, E., Vecchiet, J., Macellari, V., Giacomozzi, C., "Alter-

ation of spatial-temporal parameters of gait in chronic fatigue syndrome patients," *Journal of Neurological Science,* 154, 18–25 (1998).

6. Bennett, A.L., Chao, C.C., Hu, S., et al., "Elevation of bioactive transforming growth factor-beta in serum from patients with chronic fatigue syndrome," *Journal of Clinical Immunology,* 17, 160–166 (1997).

7. Chao, C.C., Janoff, E.N., Hu, S.X., Thomas, K., Gallagher, M., Tsang, M., Peterson, P.K., "Altered cytokine release in peripheral blood mononuclear cell cultures from patients with chronic fatigue syndrome," *Cytokine,* 3, 292–298 (1991).

8. Patarca, R., Klimas, N.G., Lugtendorf, S., Antoni, M., Fletcher, M.A., "Dis-regulated expression of tumor necrosis factor in chronic fatigue syndrome: interrelations with cellular sources and patterns of soluble immune mediator expression," *Clinical Infectious Disease,* 18, S147–S153 (1994).

9. Pall, M.L., "Elevated, sustained peroxynitrite levels as the cause of chronic fatigue syndrome," *Medical Hypotheses,* 54, 115–125 (2000).

10. Komaroff, A.L., Fagioli, L.R., Geiger, A.M., Doolittle, T.H., Lee, J., Kornish, R.J., Gleit, M.A., Guerriero, R.T., "An examination of the working case definition of chronic fatigue syndrome," *American Journal of Medicine,* 100, 56–64 (1996).

11. Miller, C.S., Prihoda, T.J., "A controlled comparison of symptoms and chemical intolerances reported by Gulf War veterans, implant recipients and persons with multiple chemical sensitivity," *Toxicology and Industrial Health,* 15, 386–397 (1999).

12. Dunstan, R.H., Donohoe, M., Taylor, W., Roberts, T.K., Murdoch, R.N., Watkins, J.A., McGregor, N.R., "A preliminary investigation of chlorinated hydrocarbons and chronic fatigue syndrome," *Medical Journal of Australia,* 163, 294–297 (1995).

13. Miller, C.S., Prihoda, T.J., ibid.

14. Reported in Logan, A.C., Wong, C., "Chronic fatigue syndrome: oxidative stress and dietary modifications," *Alternative Medicine Review,* 6(5), 450–459 (2001).

15. Han, D., Tritschler, H.J., Packer, L., "Alpha-lipoic acid increases intracellular glutathione in a human T-lymphocyte Jurkat cell line," *Biochemistry and Biophysics Research Communications,* 207, 258–264 (1995).

16. Packer, L., Tritschler, H.J., Wessel. K., "Neuroprotection by the metabolic antioxidant alpha-lipoic acid," *Free Radicals in Biology and Medicine,* 22, 359–378 (1997).

17. Bridges, R.J., Koh, J.Y., Hatalski, C.G., Cotman, C.W., "Increased excito-toxic vulnerability of cortical cultures with reduced levels of glutathione," *European Journal of Pharmacology,* 192, 199–200 (1991).

18. Matthews, R.T., Yang, L., Browne, S., Baik, M., Beal, M.F., "Coenzyme Q_{10} administration increases brain mitochondrial concentrations and exerts neuroprotective effects," *Proceedings of the National Academy of Sciences of the USA,* 95, 8892–889 (1998).

19. Manuel y Keenoy, B., Moorkens, G., Vertommen, J., De Leeuw, I., "Magnesium status and parameters of the oxidant-antioxidant balance in patients with chronic fatigue: effects of supplementation with magnesium," *Journal of the American College of Nutrition,* 19, 374–382 (2000).

20. Jansen, D.F., Schouten, J.P., Vonk, J.M., Rijcken, B., Timens, W., Weiss, S.T., Postma, D.S., "Smoking and airway hyperresponsiveness especially in the presence of blood eosinophilia increase the risk to develop respiratory symptoms: a 25-year follow-up study in the general adult population," *American Journal of Respiratory Critical Care,* 160(1), 259–264 (July 1999).

21. Baschetti, R., "Chronic fatigue syndrome and liquorice (letter)," *New Zealand Medical Journal,* 108, 156–157 (1995).

22. Bohn, B., Nebe, C.T., Birr, C., "Flow-cytometeric studies with *Eleuthercoccus senticosus* extract as an immunomodulatory agent," *Arzneimittel Forschung,* 37, 1193–1196 (1987).

CIRRHOSIS OF THE LIVER

1. Lieber C.S., "Liver diseases by alcohol and hepatitis C: early detection and new insights in pathogenesis lead to improved treatment," *American Journal of Addiction,* 10 (Suppl), 29–50 (2001).

2. Lieber, C.S., de Carl, L.M., Mak, K.M., Kim, C.I., Leo, M.A., "Attenuation of alcohol-induced hepatic fibrosis by polyunsaturated lecithin," *Hepatology,* 12, 1390–1398 (1990).

3. Mato, J.M., Camara, J., Fernandez de Paz, J., Caballeria. L., Coll, S., Caballero, A., Garcia-Buey, L., Beltran, J., Benita, V., Caballeria, J., Sola, R., Moreno-Otero, R., Barrao, F., Martin-Duce, A., Correa, J.A., Pares, A., Barrao, E., Garcia-Magaz, I., Puerta, J.L., Moreno, J., Boissard, G., Ortiz, P., Rodes, J., "S-adnosylmethionine in alcoholic liver cirrhosis: a randomized, placebo-controlled, double-blind, multicenter clinical trial," *Journal of Hepatology,* 30, 1081–1089 (1999).

4. Miglio, F., Stefanini, G.F., Corazza, G.R., D'Ambro, A., Gasbarrini, G., "Double-blind studies of the therapeutic action of s-adenosylmethionine in oral administration in liver cirrhosis and other chronic hepatitides," *Minerva Medica,* 66, 1595–1599 (1975).

5. Lieber, C.S., "Alcohol: Its metabolism and interaction with nutrients," *Annual Review* of *Nutrition,* 20, 395–430 (2000).

6. Deulofeu, R., Pares, A., Rubio, M., Gasso, M., Roman, J., Gimenez, A., Varela-Moreiras, G., Caballeria, J., Ballesta, A.M., Mato, J.M., Rodes, J., "S-adenosylmethionine prevents hepatic tocopherol depletion in carbon tetrachloride-injured rats," *Clinical Science* (London), 99(4), 315–320 (October 2000).

7. Naveau, S., Abella, A., Raynard, B., Balian, A., Giraud, V., Montembault, S., Mathurin, P., Keros, L.G., Portier, A., Capron, F., Emilie, D., Galanaud, P., Chaput, J.C., "Tumor necrosis factor soluble receptor p55 and lipid peroxidation in patients with acute alcoholic hepatitis," *American Journal of Gastroenterology,* 96(12), 3361–3367 (December 2001).

8. Buzzelli, G., Moscarella, S., Giusti, A., Duchini, A., Marena, C., Lampertico, M., "A pilot study on the liver protective effect of silybin-phosphatidylcholine complex (IdB1016) in chronic active hepatitis," *International Journal of Clinical Pharmacology and Therapeutics,* 31(9), 456–460 (September 1993).

9. Ferenci, P., Dragosics, B., Dittrich, H., Frank, H., Benda, L., Lochs, H., Meryn, S., Base, W., Schneider, B., "Randomized controlled trial of silymarin treatment in patients with cirrhosis of the liver," *Journal of Hepatology,* 9, 105–113 (1989).

10. Farghali, H., Kamenikova, L., Hynie, S., Kmonickova E., "Silymarin effects of intracellular calcium and cytotoxicity: a study in perfused rat hepatocytes after oxidative stress injury," *Pharmacological Research,* 41, 231–237 (2000).

11. Sonnenbichler, J., Zetl, I., "Biochemical effects of the flavonolignane silibinin on RNA, protein and DNA synthesis in rat livers." In Cody, V., Middleton, E., Harborne, J.B., editors, *Plant Flavonoids in Biology and Medicine: Biochemical, Pharmacological and Structure-Activity Relations.* (New York: Liss, 1986), 319–331.

12. Frenci, P., Dragosics, B., Dittrich, H., et al., "Randomized controlled trial of silymarin treatment in patients with cirrhosis of the liver," *Journal of Hepatology,* 9, 105–113 (1989).

13. Yamamoto, S., Ohmoto, K., Ideguchi, S., Yamamoto, R., Mitsui, Y., Shimabara, M., Iguchi, Y., Ohumi, T., Takatori, K., "Painful muscle cramps in liver cirrhosis and effects of oral taurine administration," *Nippon Shokakibyo Gakkai Zasshi,* 91(7), 1205–1209 (July 1994).

14. Ferenci ,P., Wewalka, F., "Parenteral feeding of patients with liver cirrhosis with hepatic encephalopathy," *Infusionstherapie und Klinische Ernährung,* 7(2), 72–78 (1980).

15. Marchesini, G., Bianchi, G., Rossi, B., Brizi, M., Melchionda, N., "Nutritional treatment with branched-chain amino acids in advanced liver cirrhosis," *Journal of Gastroenterology,* 35(Suppl), 7–12 (2000).

16. Watson, J.P., Jones, D.E., James, O.F., Cann, P.A., Bramble, M.G., "Case report: oral antioxidant therapy for the treatment of primary biliary cirrhosis: a pilot study," *Journal of Gastroenterology and Hepatology,* 14(10), 1034–1040 (October 1999).

CLEFT LIP AND CLEFT PALATE

1. Faron, G., Drouin, R., Pedneault, L., Poulin, L.D., Laframboise, R., Garrido-Russo, M., Fraser, W.D., "Recurrent cleft lip and palate in siblings of a patient with malabsorption syndrome, probably caused by hypovitaminosis a associated with folic acid and vitamin B(2) deficiencies," *Tetralogy,* 63(3), 61–63 (March 2001).

CLUSTER HEADACHES

1. Mendizabal, J., "Cluster Headache," *eMedicine,* 2(12) (21 November 2001).

2. Pringsheim, T., "Cluster headache: evidence for a disorder of circadian rhythm and hypothalamic function," *Canadian Journal of Neurological Science,* 29(1), 33–40 (February 2002).

3. Peres, M.F., Rozen, T.D., "Melatonin in the preventive treatment of chronic cluster headache," *Cephalgia,* 10 993–995 (December 2001).

4. Kudrow, L., "Response of cluster headache attacks to oxygen inhalation," *Headache,* 21, 1–4 (1981).

5. Barclay, L., "Intranasal civamide helps prevent episodic cluster headache," *Archives of Neurology,* 59, 990–994 (2002).

COLD SORES

1. Fleming, D.T., McQuillan, G.M., Johnson, R.E., Nahmias, A.J., Aral, S.O., Lee, F.K., St. Louis, M.E., "Herpes simplex virus type 2 in the United States, 1976 to 1994," *New England Journal of Medicine,* 337, 1105–1111 (1997).

2. Wonnacott, K.M., Bonneau, R.H., "The effects of stress on memory cytotoxic T lymphocyte-mediated protection against herpes simplex virus infection at mucosal sites," *Brain, Behavior, and Immunology,* 16(2), 104–117 (April 2002).

3. Field, H.J., "Herpes simplex virus antiviral drug resistance—current trends and future prospects," *Journal of Clinical Virology,* 21(3), 261–269 (June 2001).

4. Naesens, L., De Clercq, E., "Recent developments in herpesvirus therapy," *Herpes,* 8(1), 12–16 (March 2001).

5. Griffith, R., DeLong, D., Nelson, J., "Relation of arginine-lysine antagonism to herpes simplex growth in tissue culture," *Chemotherapy,* 27, 209–213 (1981).

6. DiGiovanna, J., Blank, H., "Failure of lysine in frequently recurrent herpes simplex infection," *Archives of Dermatology,* 120, 48–51 (1984).

7. Weber, P.C., Spatz, S.J., Nordby, E.C., "Stable ubiquitination of the ICP0R protein of herpes simplex virus type 1 during productive infection," *Virology,* 20, 253(2), 288–298 (January 1999).

8. Fitzherbert, J., "Genital herpes and zinc," *Medical Journal of Australia,* 1, 399 (1979).

9. Godfrey, H.R., Godfrey, N.J., Godfrey, J.C., Riley, D., "A randomized clinical trial on the treatment of oral herpes with topical zinc oxide/glycine," *Alternative Therapies in Health and Medicine,* 7(3), 49–56 (May–June 2001).

10. Basile, A.C., Sertie, J.A., Freitas, P.C., Zanini, A.C., "Anti-inflammatory activity of oleoresin from Brazilian *Copaifera,*" *Journal of Ethnopharmacology,* 22(1), 101–109 (January 1988).

11. Williams, M., "Immuno-protection against herpes simplex type II infection by eleutherococcus root extract," *International Journal of Alternative and Complementary Medicine,* 13, 9–12 (1995).

12. Nagasaka, K., Kurokawa, M., Imakita, M., Terasawa, K., Shiraki, K., "Efficacy of *kakkon-to,* a traditional herbal medicine, in herpes simplex virus type 1 infection in mice," *Journal of Medical Virology,* 46(1), 28–34 (May 1995).

13. Utsunomiya, T., Kobayashi, M., Herndon, D.N., Pollard, R.B., Suzuki, F., "Glycyrrhizin (20 beta-carboxy-11-oxo-30-norolean-12-en-3 beta-yl-2-O-beta-D-glucopyranuronosyl-alpha-D-glucopyranosiduronic acid) improves the resistance of thermally injured mice to opportunistic infection of herpes simplex virus type 1," *Immunology Letters,* 44(1), 59–66 (January 1995).

14. Robe, P.A., Princen, F., Martin, D., Malgrange, B., Stevenaert, A., Moonen, G., Gielen, J., Merville, M., Bours, V., "Pharmacological modulation of the bystander effect in the herpes simplex virus thymidine kinase/ganciclovir gene therapy system: effects of dibutyryl adenosine 3',5'-cyclic monophosphate, alpha-glycyrrhetinic acid, and cytosine arabinoside," *Biochemical Pharmacology,* 60(2), 241–249 (15 July 2000).

15. Koytchev, R., Alken, R.G., Dundarov, S., "Balm mint extract (Lo-701) for topical treatment of recurring herpes labialis," *Phytomedicine,* 6(4), 225–230 (October 1999).

16. Carson, C.F., Ashton, L., Dry, L., Smith, D.W., Riley, T.V., "*Melaleuca al-*

ternifolia (tea tree) oil gel (6%) for the treatment of recurrent herpes labialis," *Journal of Antimicrobial Chemotherapy,* 48(3), 450–451 (September 2001).

17. Saller, R., Buechi, S., Meyrat, R., Schmidhauser, C., "Combined herbal preparation for topical treatment of Herpes labialis," *Forschende Komplementarmedizin und Klassische Naturheilkunde,* 8(6), 373–382 (December 2001).

COLDS

1. Braunwald, E., Fauci, A.S., Kasper, D.L., Hauser, S.L., Longo, D.L., Jameson, J.L., editors, *Harrison's Principles of Internal Medicine,* Fifteenth Edition (New York: McGraw-Hill, 2001), p. 1121.

2. Hayden, F.G., Diamond, L., Wood, P.B., Korts, D.C., Wecker, M.T., "Effectiveness and safety of intranasal ipratropium bromide in common colds: a randomized, double-blind, placebo-controlled trial," *Annals of Internal Medicine,* 125, 89–97 (1996).

3. Cohen, S., Tyrrell, D.A.J., Smith, A.P. "Negative life events, received stress, negative affect, and susceptibility to the common cold," *Journal of Personality and Social Psychology,* 64, 131–140 (1993).

4. Cohen, S., Doyle, W.J., Skoner, D.P., Fireman, P., Gwaltney, J.M., Jr., Newsom, J.T., "State and trait negative affect as predictors of objective and subjective symptoms of respiratory viral infections," *Journal of Personality and Social Psychology,* 68, 159–169 (1995).

5. Cohen, S., Tyrrell, D.A., Russell, M.A., Jarvis, M.J., Smith, A.P., "Smoking, alcohol consumption, and susceptibility to the common cold," *American Journal of Public Health,* 83, 1277–1283 (1993).

6. Cohen, S., Doyle, W.J., Skoner, D.P., Rabin, B.S., Gwaltney, J.M., Jr., "Social ties and susceptibility to the common cold," *Journal of the American Medical Association,* 277, 1940–1944, 1997.

7. McMillan, J.A., Weiner, L.B., Higgins, A.M., Macknight, K., "Rhinovirus infection associated with serious illness among pediatric patients," *Pediatric Infectious Disease Journal,* 12, 321–325 (1993).

8. Schmidt, H.J., Fink, R.J., "Rhinovirus as a lower respiratory pathogen in infants," *Pediatric Infectious Disease Journal,* 10, 700–702 (1991).

9. Nicholson, K.G., Kent, J., Hammersley, V., Cancio, E., "Risk factors for lower respiratory complications of rhinovirus infections in elderly people living in the community: Prospective cohort study," *British Medical Journal,* 313, 1119–1123 (1996).

10. Whimbey, E., Champlin, R.E., Couch, R.B., Cancio, E., "Community respiratory virus infections among hospitalized adult bone marrow transplant recipients," *Clinical Infectious Disease,* 22, 778–782 (1996).

11. Wald, T.G., Shult, P., Krause, P., Miller, B.A., Drinka, P., Gravenstein, S., "A rhinovirus outbreak among residents of a long-term care facility," *Annals of Internal Medicine,* 123, 588–593 (1995).

12. Elkhatieb, A., Hipskind, G., Woerner, D., Hayden, F.G., Middle ear abnormalities during natural rhinovirus colds in adults," *Journal of Infectious Disease,* 168, 618–621 (1993).

13. Pitkäranta, A., Arruda, E., Malmberg, H., Hayden, F.G., "Detection of rhinovirus in sinus brushings of patients with acute community-acquired sinusitis by reverse transcription-PCR," *Journal of Clinical Microbiology,* 35(7), 1791–1793 (1997).

14. Nicholson, K.G., Kent, J., Ireland, D.C., "Respiratory viruses and exacerbations of asthma in adults," *British Medical Journal,* 307, 982–986 (1993).

15. Smyth, A.R., Smyth, R.L., Tong, C.Y., Hart, C.A., Heaf, D.P., "Effect of respiratory virus infections including rhinovirus on clinical status in cystic fibrosis," *Archives of Diseases of Childhood,* 73, 117–120 (1995).

16. Sheretz, R.J., Reagan, D.R., Hampton, K.D., Robertson, K.L., Streed, S.A., Hoen, H.M., Thomas, R., Gwaltney, J.M., Jr., "A cloud adult: The *Staphylococcus aureus*- virus interaction revisited," *Annals of Internal Medicine,* 124, 539–547 (1996).

17. Diehl, H.S., "Medicinal treatment of the common cold," *Journal of the American Medical Association,* 101, 2042–2049 (1933).

18. Mainous, A.G., Hueston, W.J., Clark, J.R., "Antibiotics and upper respiratory infection: do some folks think there is a cure for the common cold?" *Journal of Family Practice,* 42, 357–361 (1996).

19. Åberg, N., Åberg, B., Alestig, K., "The effect of inhaled and intranasal

sodium chromoglycate on symptoms of upper respiratory tract infections," *Clinical Experience in Allergy* 26, 1045–1050 (1996).

20. Gwaltney, J.M., Jr., Park, J., Paul, R.A., Edelman, D.A., O'Connor, R.R., Turner, R.B., "Randomized controlled trial of clemastine fumarate for treatment of experimental rhinovirus colds," *Clinical Infectious Disease, 22*, 656–662 (1996).

21. Turner, R.B., Sperber, S.J., Sorrentino, J.V., O'Connor, R.R., Rogers, J., Batouli, A.R., Gwaltney, J.M., Jr., "Effectiveness of clemastine fumarate for treatment of rhinorrhea and sneezing associated with the common cold," *Clinical Infectious Disease, 25*, 824–830 (1997).

22. Hirt, M., Nobel, S., Barron, E., "Zinc nasal gel for the treatment of common cold symptoms: a double-blind, placebo-controlled trial," *Ear, Nose, and Throat Journal, 79*, 778–781 (2000).

23. Belongia, E.A., Berg, R., Liu, K., "A randomized trial of zinc nasal spray for the treatment of upper respiratory illness in adults," *American Journal of Medicine, 111*, 103–108 (2001).

24. Mossad, S.B., Macknin, M.L., Medendorp, S.V., Mason, P., "Zinc gluconate lozenges for treating the common cold: a randomized, double-blind, placebo-controlled study," *Annals of Internal Medicine, 125*, 81–88 (1996).

25. Prasad, A.S., Fitzgerald, J.T., Bao, B., Beck, F.W., Chandrasekar, P.H., "Duration of symptoms and plasma cytokine levels in patients with the common cold treated with zinc acetate. A randomized, double-blind, placebo-controlled trial," *Annals of Internal Medicine, 133*, 245–252 (2000).

26. Hoheisel, O., Sandberg, M., Bertram, S., et al., "Echinagard treatment shortens the course of the common cold: a double-blind, placebo-controlled clinical trial," *European Journal of Clinical Research, 9*, 261–268 (1997).

27. Grimm, W., Müller, H.H., "A randomized controlled trial of the effect of fluid extract of Echinacea purpurea on the incidence and severity of colds and respiratory infections," *American Journal of Medicine, 106*(2), 138–143 (1999).

28. Facino, R.M., Carini, M., Aldini, G., Marinello, C., Arlandini, E., Franzoi, L., Colombo, M., Pietta, P., Mauri, P., "Direct characterization of caffeoyl esters with antihyaluronidase activity in crude extracts from *Echinacea angustifolia* roots by fast atom bombardment tandem mass spectrometry," *Farmaco, 48*(10), 1447–1461 (October 1993).

29. Budzinski, J.W., Foster, B.C., Vandenhoek, S., Arnason, J.T., "An in vitro evaluation of human cytochrome P405 3A4 inhibition by selected commercial herbal extracts and tinctures," *Phytomedicine, 7*(4), 273–282 (July 2000).

30. Luettig, B., Steinmuller, C., Gifford, G.E., Wagner, H., Lohmann-Matthes, M.L., "Macrophage activation by the polysaccharide arabinogalactan isolated from plant cell cultures of *Echinacea purpurea,*" *Journal of the National Cancer Institute, 81*(9), 669–675 (3 May 1989).

31. Blumenthal, M., Goldberg, A., Brinckmann, J. *Herbal Medicine: Expanded Commission E Monographs* (Boston, Integrative Medicine, 2000), p. 88.

32. Hemila, H., "Does vitamin C alleviate the symptoms of the common cold?—A review of current evidence," *Scandinavian Journal of Infectious Disease, 26*, 1–6 (1994).

33. Hemila, H., "Vitamin C supplementation and common cold symptoms: factors affecting the magnitude of the benefit," *Medical Hypotheses, 52*, 171–178 (1999).

34. Podoshin, L., Gertner, R., Fradis, M., "Treatment of perennial allergic rhinitis with ascorbic acid solution," *Ear, Nose, and Throat Journal, 70*, 54–55 (1991).

35. De, M., De, A.K., Sen, P., Banerjee, A.B., "Antimicrobial properties of star anise (*Illicium verum* Hook f)," *Phytotherapy Research, 16*(1), 94–95 (February 2002).

36. Elgayyar, M., Draughon, F.A., Golden, D.A., Mount, J.R., "Antimicrobial activity of essential oils from plants against selected pathogenic and saprophytic microorganisms," *Journal of Food Protection, 64*(7), 1019–1024 (July 2001).

37. Gay-Crosier, F., Schreiber, G., Hauser, C., "Anaphylaxis from inulin in vegetables and processed food," *New England Journal of Medicine, 342*, 1372 (4 May 2000).

38. Chandra, R., Barron, J.L., "Anaphylactic reaction to intravenous sinistrin (Inutest)," *Annals of Clinical Biochemisty, 39*(Pt 1), 76 (January 2002).

39. El Bardai, S., Lyoussi, B., Wibo, M., Morel, N., "Pharmacological evidence of hypotensive activity of *Marrubium vulgare* and *Foeniculum vulgare* in spontaneously hypertensive rat," *Clinical Experiments in Hypertension, 23*(4), 329–343 (May 2001).

40. De Jesus, R.A., Cechinel-Filho, V., Oliveira, A.E., Schlemper, V., "Analysis of the antinociceptive properties of marrubiin isolated from *Marrubium vulgare,*" *Phytomedicine, 7*(2), 111–115 (April 2000).

41. Trute, A., Gross, J., Mutschler, E., Nahrstedt, A., "In vitro antispasmodic compounds of the dry extract obtained from *Hedera helix,*" *Planta Medica, 63*(2), 125–129 (April 1997).

42. Dwoskin, L.P., Crooks, P.A., "A novel mechanism of action and potential use for lobeline as a treatment for psychostimulant abuse," *Biochemical Pharmacology, 3*(2):89–98 (15 January 2002).

43. Deep, V., Singh, M., Ravi, K., "Role of vagal afferents in the reflex effects of capsaicin and lobeline in monkeys," *Respiratory Physiology, 125*(3), 155–168 (April 2001).

44. Miller, D.K., Crooks, P.A., Teng, L., Witkin, J.M., Munzar, P., Goldberg, S.R., Acri, J.B., Dwoskin, L.P., "Lobeline inhibits the neurochemical and behavioral effects of amphetamine," *Journal of Pharmacology and Experimental Therapy, 296*(3), 1023–1034 (March 2001).

45. Bergner, P., "Is lobelia toxic?," *Medical Herbalism, 10*(1), 15–32 (1998).

46. Blumenthal, M., Busse, W.R., Goldberg, A., Gruenwald, W., Hall, T., Klein, S., Riggins, C., Rister, R. (eds). *The Complete Commission E Monographs: Therapeutic Guide to Herbal Medicines* (Boston, Massachusetts: Integrative Medicine Communications, 1998), p. 166–167.

47. Nosal'ova, G., Strapkova, A., Kardosova, A., Capek, P., Zathurecky, L., Bukovska, E., "Antitussive action of extracts and polysaccharides of marsh mallow (*Althea officinalis* L., var. *robusta*)," *Pharmazie, 47*(3), 224–226 (March 1992).

48. Sarrell, E.M., Mandelberg, A., Cohen, H.A., "Efficacy of naturopathic extracts in the management of ear pain associated with acute otitis media," *Archives of Pediatric and Adolescent Medicine, 155*(7), 796–799 (July 2001).

49. Serkedjieva, J., "Combined antiinfluenza virus activity of Flos verbasci infusion and amantadine derivatives," *Phytotherapy Research, 14*(7), 571–574 (November 2000).

50. Kim, D.H., Kim, B.R., Kim, J.Y., Jeong, Y.C., "Mechanism of covalent adduct formation of aucubin to proteins," *Toxicology Letters, 114*(1–3), 181–188 (3 April 2000).

51. Michaelsen, T.E., Gilje, A., Samuelsen, A.B., Hogasen, K., Paulsen, B.S., "Interaction between human complement and a pectin type polysaccharide fraction, PMII, from the leaves of *Plantago major* L.," *Scandinavian Journal of Immunology, 52*(5), 483–490 (November 2000).

52. Schinella, G.R., Tournier, H.A., Prieto, J.M., Mordujovich, D., Rios, J.L., "Antioxidant activity of anti-inflammatory plant extracts," *Life Sciences, 70*(9), 1023–1033 (18 January 2002).

53. Ma, S.C., Du, J., But, P.P., Deng, X.L., Zhang, Y.W., Ooi, V.E., Xu, H.X., Lee, S.H., Lee, S.F., "Antiviral Chinese medicinal herbs against respiratory syncytial virus," *Journal of Ethnopharmacology, 79*(2), 205–211 (February 2002).

54. Kohlert, C., *Systemische Verfügbarkeit und Pharmakokinetik von Thymol nach oraler Applikation einer thymianhaltigen Zubereitung im Menschen* (Würzburg, University of Würzburg, 2000). Doctoral disseration.

55. Meister, R., Wittig, T., Beuscher, N., et al., "Efficacy and tolerability of Myrtol standardized in long-term treatment of chronic bronchitis. A double-blind, placebo-controlled study. Study group investigators," *Arzneimittel Forschung, 49*, 351–358 (1999).

56. Barenboim, G.M., Koslova, N.B., "Eleutherococcus extract as an agent increasing the biological resistance of man exposed to unfavorable factors," in *Eleutherococcus: Strategy of the Use and New Fundamental Data* (Moscow: MedExport, not dated).

57. Wagner, H., Proksch, A., Riess-Maurer, I., Vollmar, A., Odenthal, S., Stuppner, H., Jurcic, K., Le Turdu, M., Fang, J.N., "Immunostimulatory effects of polysaccharides (heteroglycans) of higher plants," *Arzneimittel-Forschung, 35*(7), 1069–1075 (1985).

58. Murray, M., *Healing Power of Herbs* (Rocklin, California: Prima Publishing, 1991), p. 56.

59. Sosnova, T., "The effect of E. spinosus on the color distinction function of the optic analyzer in persons with normal trichromatic vision," *Vestnik Oftalmologii,* 82(5), 59–61 (1969).

60. Melchior, J., Palm, S., Wikman, G., "Controlled clinical study of standardized *Andrographis paniculata* extract in common cold–a pilot trial," *Phytomedicine,* 3, 315–318 (1996/1997).

61. Cáceres, D.D., Hancke, J.L., Burgos, R.A., Sandberg, F., Wikman, G.K., "Use of visual analogue scale measurements (VAS) to assess the effectiveness of standardizing *Andrographis paniculata* extract SHA-10 in reducing the symptoms of common cold. A randomized double blind-placebo study," *Phytomedicine,* 6(4), 217–223 (1999).

62. Caceres, D.D., Hancke, J.L., Burgos, R.A., et al., "Use of visual analogue scale measurements (VAS) to assess the effectiveness of standardized *Andrographis paniculata* extract SHA-10 in reducing the symptoms of common cold. A randomized double blind-placebo study," *Phytomedicine,* 6, 217–223 (1999).

63. Burgos, R.A., Caballero, E.E., Sanchez, N.S., Sandberg, F., Wikman, G.K., "Testicular toxicity assessment of *Andrographis paniculata* dried extract in rats," *Journal of Ethnopharmacology,* 58, 219–224 (1997).

64. Peters, E.M., Goetzsche, J.M., Grobbelaar, B., Noakes, T.D., "Vitamin C supplementation reduces the incidence of postrace symptoms of upper-respiratory-tract infection in ultramarathon runners," *American Journal of Clinical Nutrition,* 57, 170–174 (1993).

COLIC

1. Wade, S., Kilgour, T., "Colic in Infants," *British Medical Journal,* 323, 437–440 (25 August 2001).

2. Lucas, A., St James-Roberts, I., "Crying, fussing and colic behaviour in breast and bottle-fed infants," *Early Human Development,* 53, 9–19 (1998).

3. Crowcroft, N.S., Strachan, D.P., "The social origins of infantile colic; questionnaire study covering 76,747 infants," *British Medical Journal,* 314, 1325–1328 (1997).

4. Parkin, P.C., Schwartz, C.J., Manuel, B.A., "Randomized controlled trial of three interventions in the management of persistent crying of infancy," *Pediatrics,* 92, 197–201 (1993).

5. Taubman, B., "Parental counselling compared with elimination of cow's milk or soy milk protein for the treatment of infant colic syndrome: a randomized trial," *Pediatrics,* 81, 756–761 (1988).

6. Barr, R.G., McMullen, S.J., Spiess, H., Leduc, D.G., Yaremko, J., Barfield, R., et al., "Carrying as a colic 'therapy': a randomized controlled trial," *Pediatrics,* 87, 623–630 (1991).

7. Metcalf, T.J., Irons, T.G., Sher, L.D., Young, P.C., "Simethicone in the treatment of infantile colic: a randomized, placebo-controlled, multicenter trial," *Pediatrics,* 94, 29–34 (1994).

8. Garrison, M.M., Christakis, D.A., "A systematic review of treatments for infant colic. *Pediatrics,* 106, 184–190 (2000).

9. Lucassen, P.L.B.J., Assendelf, W.J.J., Gubbels, J.W., van Eijk, J.T.M., Douwes, A.C., "Infantile colic: crying time reduction with a whey hydrolysate: a double-blind, randomized, placebo-controlled trial," *Pediatrics,* 106(6), 1349–1354 (6 December 2000).

10. Weizman, Z., Alkrinawi, S., Goldfarb, D., Bitran, C., "Efficacy of herbal tea preparation in infantile colic," *Journal of Pediatrics,* 122, 650–652 (1993).

11. Wiberg, J.M., Nordsteen, J., Nilsson, N., "The short term effect of spinal manipulation in the treatment of infantile colic: a randomized controlled clinical trial with a blinded observer," *Journal of Manipulative Physioliogical Therapy,* 22, 517–522 (1999).

12. Sondergaard, C., Henriksen, T.B., Obel, C., Wisborg, K., "Smoking during pregnancy and infantile colic," *Pediatrics,* 108(2), 342–346 (August 2001).

COLORECTAL CANCER

1. Jarvis, J.K., Miller, G.D., "Overcoming the barrier of lactose intolerance to reduce health disparities," *Journal of the National Medical Association,* 94(2), 55–66 (February 2002).

2. Boutron-Ruault, M.C., Senesse, P., Meance, S., Belghiti, C., Faivre, J., "Energy intake, body mass index, physical activity, and the colorectal adenoma-carcinoma sequence," *Nutrition and Cancer,* 39(1), 50–57 (2001).

3. Nakaji, S., Shimoyama, T., Umeda, T., Sakamoto, J., Katsura, S., Sugawara, K., Baxter, D., "Dietary fiber showed no preventive effect against colon and rectal cancers in Japanese with low fat intake: an analysis from the results of nutrition surveys from 23 Japanese prefectures," *BMC Cancer,* 1(1), 14 (2001).

4. Nilsen, T.I., Vatten, L.J., "Prospective study of colorectal cancer risk and physical activity, diabetes, blood glucose and BMI: exploring the hyperinsulinaemia hypothesis," *British Journal of Cancer,* 84(3), 417–422 (2 February 2001).

5. Slattery, M.L., Anderson, K., Curtin, K., Ma, K., Schaffer, D., Edwards, S., Samowitz, W., "Lifestyle factors and Ki-ras mutations in colon cancer tumors," *Mutation Research,* 483(1–2), 73–81 (1 November 2001).

6. Wu, K., Willett, W.C., Fuchs, C.S., Colditz, G.A., Giovannucci, E.L., "Calcium intake and risk of colon cancer in women and men," *Journal of the National Cancer Institute,* 94(6), 437–446 (20 March 2002).

7. Sesink, A.L., Termont, D.S., Kleibeuker, J.H., Van Der Meer, R., "Red meat and colon cancer: dietary haem, but not fat, has cytotoxic and hyperproliferative effects on rat colonic epithelium," *Carcinogenesis,* 21(10), 1909–1915 (October 2000).

8. Sesink, A.L., Termont, D.S., Kleibeuker, J.H., Van der Meer, R., "Red meat and colon cancer: dietary haem-induced colonic cytotoxicity and epithelial hyperproliferation are inhibited by calcium," *Carcinogenesis,* 22(10), 1653–1659 (October 2001).

9. Darmoul, D., Marie, J.C., Devaud, H., Gratio, V., Laburthe, M., "Initiation of human colon cancer cell proliferation by trypsin acting at protease-activated receptor-2," *British Journal of Cancer,* 85(5), 772–779 (1 September 2001).

10. Jarvinen, R., Knekt, P., Hakulinen, T., Aromaa, A., "Prospective study on milk products, calcium and cancers of the colon and rectum," *European Journal of Clinical Nutrition,* 55(11), 1000–1007 (November 2001).

11. Bolognani, F., Rumney, C.J., Pool-Zobel, B.L., Rowland, I.R., "Effect of lactobacilli, bifidobacteria and inulin on the formation of aberrant crypt foci in rats," *European Journal of Nutrition,* 40(6), 293–300 (December 2001).

12. Holt, P.R., Arber, N., Halmos, B., Forde, K., Kissileff, H., McGlynn, K.A., Moss, S.F., Fan, K., Yang, K., Lipkin, M., "Colonic epithelial cell proliferation decreases with increasing levels of serum 25-hydroxy vitamin D," *Cancer Epidemiology, Biomarkers, and Prevention,* 11(1), 113–119 (January 2002).

13. Tangpricha, V., Flanagan, J.N., Whitlatch, L.W., Tseng, C.C., Chen, T.C., Holt, P.R., Lipkin, M.S., Holick, M.F., "25-hydroxyvitamin D-1alpha-hydroxylase in normal and malignant colon tissue, *Lancet,* 26, 357(9269), 1673–1674 (May 2001).

14. Tang, R., Wang, J.Y., Lo, S.K., Hsieh, L.L., "Physical activity, water intake and risk of colorectal cancer in Taiwan: a hospital-based case-control study," *International Journal of Cancer,* 82(4), 484–489 (12 August 1999).

15. Hong, J., Smith, T.J., Ho, C.T., August, D.A., Yang, C.S., "Effects of purified green and black tea polyphenols on cyclooxygenase- and lipoxygenase-dependent metabolism of arachidonic acid in human colon mucosa and colon tumor tissues," *Biochemical Pharmacology,* 62(9), 1175–1183 (1 November 2001).

16. Finley, J.W., Davis, C.D., "Selenium (Se) from high-selenium broccoli is utilized differently than selenite, selenate and selenomethionine, but is more effective in inhibiting colon carcinogenesis," *Biofactors,* 14(1–4), 191–196 (2001).

17. Fuchs, C.S., Willett, W.C., Colditz, G.A., Hunter, D.J., Stampfer, M.J., Speizer, F.E., Giovannucci, E.L., "The influence of folate and multivitamin use on the familial risk of colon cancer in women," *Cancer Epidemiology, Biomarkers, and Prevention,* 11(3), 227–234 (March 2002).

18. Iizaka, M., Furukawa, Y., Tsunoda, T., Akashi, H., Ogawa, M., Nakamura, Y., "Expression profile analysis of colon cancer cells in response to sulindac or aspirin," *Biochemistry and Biophysics Research Communications,* 292(2), 498–512 (29 March 2002).

19. Lin, S.Y., Liu, J.D., Chang, H.C., Yeh, S.D., Lin, C.H., Lee, W.S., "Magnolol suppresses proliferation of cultured human colon and liver cancer cells by inhibiting DNA synthesis and activating apoptosis," *Journal of Cellular Biochemistry,* 84(3), 532–544 (2002).

CONGESTIVE HEART FAILURE

1. Folkers, K., Yamamura. Y., editors, *Biomedical and Cinical Aspects of Conezyme* Q$_{10}$. Volumes 1–4 (Amsterdam: Elsevier, 1977, 1980, 1982, 1984).

2. Crestanello, J.A., Doliba, N.M., Babsky, A.M., Niborii, K., Osbakken, M.D., Whitman, G.J., "Effect of coenzyme Q$_{10}$ supplementation on mitochondrial function after myocardial ischemia reperfusion," *Journal of Surgical Research,* 102(2), 221–228 (February 2002).

3. Kamikawa, T., Kobayashi, A., Yamashita, T., Hayashi, H., Yamazaki, N., "Effects of coenzyme Q$_{10}$ on exercise tolerance in chronic stable angina pectoris," *American Journal of Cardiology,* 56, 247 (1985).

4. Munkholm, H., Hansen, H.H., Rasmussen, K., "Conezyme Q$_{10}$ treatment in serious heart failure," *Biofactors,* 9(2–4), 285–289 (1999).

5. Langsjoen, P.H., Langsjoen, A., Willis, R., Folkers, K., "Treatment of hypertrophic cardiomyopathy with coenzyme Q$_{10}$," *Molecular Aspects of Medicine,* 18 Suppl, S145–S151 (1997).

6. Rebuzzi, A.G., Schiavoni, G., Amico, C.M., et al., "Beneficial effects of L-carnitine in the reduction of the necrotic area in acute myocardial infarction," *Drugs in Experimental Clinical Research,* 18, 355–365 (1984).

7. Cherchi, A., Lai, C., Angelino, F., Trucco, G., Caponnetto, S., Mereto, P.E., Rosolen, G., Manzoli, U., Schiavoni, G., Reale, A., et al., "Effects of L-carnitine on exercise tolerance in chronic stable angina: a multicenter, double-blind, randomized, placebo controlled crossover study," *International Journal of Clinical Pharmacology and Therapeutic Toxicology,* 23(10), 579–582 (October 1985).

8. Cohen, N., Alon, I., Almoznino-Sarafian, D., Zaidenstein, R., Weissgarten, J., Gorelik, O., Berman, S., Modai, D., Golik, A., "Metabolic and clinical effects of oral magnesium supplementation in furosemide-treated patients with severe congestive heart failure," *Clinical Cardiology,* 23(6), 433–6 (June 2002).

9. Oladapo, O.O., Falase, A.O., "Congestive heart failure and ventricular arrhythmias in relation to serum magnesium," *African Journal of Medicine and Medical Sciences,* 29(3–4), 265–268 (January 2000).

10. Tauchert, M., "Efficacy and safety of crataegus extract WS 1442 in comparison with placebo in patients with chronic stable New York Heart Association class-III heart failure," *American Heart Journal,* 143(5), 910–915 (May 2002).

11. Schüssler, M., Hölzl, J., Fricke, U., "Myocardial effects of flavonoids from *Crataegus* species," *Arzneimittel Forschung,* 45, 842–845 (1995).

12. Ceriana, P., "Effect of myocardial ischaemia-reperfusion on granulocyte elastase release," *Anaesthia and Intensive Care,* 20, 187–190 (1992).

13. Rajendran, S., Deepalakshmi, P.D., Parasakthy, K., Devaraj, H., Devaraj, S.N., "Effect of tincture of *Crataegus* on the LDL-receptor activity of hepatic plasma membrane of rats fed an atherogenic diet," *Atherosclerosis,* 123, 235–241 (1996).

14. Schüssler ,M., Hölzl, J., Rump, A.F., Fricke, U.," Functional and antiischaemic effects of monoacetyl-vitexinrhamnoside in different in vitro models," *General Pharmacology,* 26, 1565–1570 (1995).

15. Nasa, Y., Hashizume, H., Hoque, A.N., Abiko, Y., "Protective effect of *Crataegus* extract on the cardiac mechanical dysfunction in isolated perfused working rat heart," *Arzneimittel Forschung,* 43, 945–949 (1993).

16. Dwivedi, S., Agarwal. M.P., "Anti-anginal and cardioprotective effects of *Terminalia arjuna,* an indigenous drug, in coronary artery disease," *Journal of the Association of Physicians of India,* 42, 287–289 (1994).

17. Dwivedi, S., Jauhari, R., "Beneficial effects of Terminalia arjuna in coronary artery disease," *Indian Heart Journal,* 49(5), 507–510 (September–October 1997).

18. Tripathi, S.N., Upadhyaya, B.N., Gupka, V.K., "Beneficial effect of *Inula racemosa* (Pushkarmoola) in Angina pectoris: a preliminary report," *Indian Journal of Physiology and Pharmacology,* 28, 73–75 (1984).

19. Singh, R.P., Singh, R., Ram, P., Batliwala, P.G., "Use of Pushkar-Guggul, an indigenous antiischemic combination, in the management of ischemic heart disease," *International Journal of Pharmacognosy,* 31, 147–160 (1993).

20. Johne, A., Brockmoller, J., Bauer, S., Maurer, A., Langheinrich, M., Roots, I., "Pharmacokinetic interaction of digoxin with an herbal extract from St. John's wort (*Hypericum perforatum*)," *Clinical Pharmacology and Therapeutics,* 66, 338–345 (October 1999).

CONJUNCTIVITIS

1. Boniface, R., Robert, A.M., "Effect of anthocyanins on human connective tissue metabolism in humans," *Klinische Monatsblätter für Augenheilkunde,* 209, 368–372 (1996).

2. Detre, Z., Jellinek, H., Miskulin, M., Robert, A.M., "Studies on vascular permeability in hypertension: action of anthocyanosides," *Clinical Physiology and Biochemistry,* 4, 143–149 (1986).

3. Cazzola, P., Mazzanti, P., Bossi, G., "In vivo modulating effect of a calf thymus acid lysate on human T lymphocyte subsets and CD4+/CD8+ ratio in the course of difference diseases," *Current Therapies Research,* 42, 1011–1017 (1987).

4. Rankov, B.G., "Vitamin A and carotene concentrations in serum in patients with chronic conjunctivitis and pterygium," *Internationale Zeitschrift fur Vitamin- und Ernährungsforschung,* 46, 454–457 (1976).

5. Seifter, E., Rettura, G., Seiter, J., "Thymotrophic action of vitamin A," *Federal Proceedings,* 32, 947 (1973).

6. Semba, R.D., "Vitamin A, immunity, and infection," *Clinical Infectious Disease,* 19, 489–499 (1994).

7. Ringsdorf, W., Cheraskin, E., "Vitamin C and human wound healing," *Oral Surgery,* 53(3), 231–236 (March 1982).

8. Gabor, M., "Pharmacologic effects of flavonoids on blood vessels," *Angiologica,* 9, 355–374 (1972).

9. Prasad, A., "Clinical, biochemical and nutritional spectrum of zinc deficiency in human subjects. An update," *Nutrition Review,* 41, 197–208 (1983).

10. Kuhn, O., untitled article, *Arzneimittel-Forschung,* 3, 194–200 (1953).

11. Erhard, M., "Effect of echinacea, aconitum, lachesis, and apis extracts, and their combinations of phagocytosis of human granulocytes," *Phytotherapy Research,* 8, 14–77 (1994).

12. Facino, R.M., Carini, M., Aldini, G., Marinello, C., Arlandini, E., Franzoi, L., Colombo, M., Pietta, P., Mauri, P., "Direct characterization of caffeoyl esters with antihyaluronidase activity in crude extracts from *Echinacea angustifolia* roots by fast atom bombardment tandem mass spectrometry," *Farmaco,* 48(10), 1447–1461 (October 1993).

13. Rehman, J., Dillow, J.M., Carter, S.M., Chou, J., Le, B., Maisel, A.S., "Increased production of antigen-specific immunoglobulins G and M following in vivo treatment with the medical plants, *Echinacea angustifolia* and *Hydrastis canadensis,*" *Immunology Letters,* 68(2–3), 391–395 (1 June 1999).

CONSTIPATION

1. Petticrew, M., Watt, I., Sheldon, T., "Systematic review of the effectiveness of laxatives in the elderly," *United Kingdom Health Technology Assessment Program Report,* 1, 13 (1997).

2. Jacobs, E.J., White, E., "Constipation, laxative use, and colon cancer among middle-aged adults," *Epidemiology,* 9, 371–372, 385–391 (July 1998).

3. Cann, P.A., Read, N.W., Holdsworth, C.D., "What is the benefit of coarse wheat bran in patients with irritable bowel syndrome?" *Gut,* 25(2), 168–173 (February 1984).

4. McIntyre, A., Vincent, R.M., Perkings, A.C., Spiller, R.C., "Effect of bran, isphagula, and inert plastic particles on gastric emptying and small bowel transit in humans: the role of physical factors," *Gut,* 40(2), 223–227 (February 1997).

5. Vincent, R., Roberts, A., Frier, M., Perkins, A.C., MacDonald, I.A., Spiller, R.C., "Effect of bran particle size on gastric emptying and small bowel transit in humans: a scintigraphic study," *Gut,* 37(2), 216–219 (August 1995).

6. Hebden, J.M., Blackshaw, P.E., Perkins, A.C., d'Amato, M., Spiller, R.C., "Small bowel transit of a bran meal residue in humans: sieving of solids from liquids and response to feeding," *Gut,* 42(5), 685–689 (May 1998).

7. Stacewicz-Sapuntzakis, M., Bowen, P.E., Hussain, E.A., Damayanti-Wood, B.I., Farnsworth, N.R., "Chemical composition and potential health effects of prunes: a functional food" *Critical Reviews in Food Science and Nutrition,* 41(4), 251–286 (May 2001).

8. Russo, A., Fraser, R., Horowitz, M., "The effect of cute hyperglycemia on small intestinal motility in normal subjects," *Diabetologia,* 39, 984–989 (1989).

9. Pizzorno, J.E., Jr., Murray, M.T., *Textbook of Natural Medicine* (London: Churchill Livingstone, 1999), 1360–1361.

10. Brown, W.J., Mishra, G., Lee, C., Bauman, A., "Leisure time physical activity in Australian women: relationship well being and symptoms," *Research Questions in Exercise and Sport,* 71(3), 206–216 (September 2000).

11. Meshkinpour, H., Selod, S., Movahedi, H., Nami, N., James, N., Wilson, A., "Effects of regular exercise in management of chronic idiopathic constipation," *Digestive Diseases and Sciences,* 43, 2379–2383 (1998).

12. Yagi, T., Yamauchi, K., Kuwano, S., "The synergistic purgative action of aloe-emodin anthrone and rhein anthrone in mice, synergism in large intestinal propulsion and water secretion," *Journal of Pharmacy* & *Pharmacology,* 49(1), 22–25 (January 1997).

13. Taubman, B., Buzby, M., "Overflow encopresis and stool toileting refusal during toilet training: a prospective study on the effect of therapeutic efficacy," *Pediatrics,* 99, 54–58 (November 1997).

COUGH, SMOKER'S

1. Lee, L.Y., Widdicombe, J.G., "Modulation of airway sensitivity to inhaled irritants: role of inflammatory mediators," *Environmental Health Perspectives,* 109 Suppl 4, 585–589 (August 2001).

2. Xu, X., B. Rijcken, J. P., Schouten, Weiss, S.T., "Airways responsiveness and development and remission of chronic respiratory symptoms in adults," *Lancet,* 350, 1431–1434 (1997).

3. Sherman, C.B., Xu, X., Speizer, F.E., Ferris, B.G., Jr., Weiss, S.T., Dockery, D.W., "Longitudinal lung function decline in subjects with respiratory symptoms," *American Review of Respiratory Diseases,* 146, 855–859 (1992).

4. Jansen, D.F., Schouten, J.P., Vonk, J.M., Rijcken, B., Timens, W., Weiss, S.T., Postma, D.S., "Smoking and airway hyperresponsiveness especially in the presence of blood eosinophilia increase the risk to develop respiratory symptoms: a 25-year follow-up study in the general adult population," *American Journal of Respiratory Critical Care,* 160(1), 259–264 (July 1999).

5. Frankfort, J.D., Fischer, C.E., Stansbury, D.W., et al., "Effects of high- and low-carbohydrate meals on maximum exercise performance in chronic airflow obstruction," *Chest,* 100, 792–795 (1991).

6. Fujimoto, S., Kurihara, N., Hirata, K., et al., "Effects of coenzymeQ$_{10}$ administration on pulmonary function and exercise performance in patients with chronic lung diseases," *Clinical Investigations,* 71, S162–S166 (1993).

7. Koichiro, M., Aizawa, H., Inoue, H., Shigyo, M., Takata, S., Hara, N., "Thromboxane causes airway hyperresponsiveness after cigarette smoke-induced neurogenic inflammation," *Journal of Applied Physiology,* 81(6), 2358–2364 (December 1996).

8. Sharp, D.S., Rodriguez, B.L., Shahar, E., Hwang, L.J., Burchfiel, C.M., "Fish consumption may limit the damage of smoking on the lung," *American Journal of Respiratory Critical Care,* 150(4), 983–984 (October 1994).

9. Shahar, E., Folsom, A.R., Melnick, S.L., Tockman, M.S., Comstock, G.W., Gennaro, V., Higgins, M.W., Sorlie, P.D., Ko, W.J., Szklo, M., "Dietary n-3 polyunsaturated fatty acids and smoking-related chronic obstructive pulmonary disease. Atherosclerosis risk in communities study investigators," *New England Journal of Medicine,* 331(4), 228–233 (July 1994).

10. Meister, R., Wittig, T., Beuscher, N., et al., "Efficacy and tolerability of Myrtol standardized in long-term treatment of chronic bronchitis. A double-blind, placebo-controlled study. Study group investigators," *Arzneimittel Forschung,* 49, 351–358 (1999).

CUTS AND SCRAPES

1. Chakrabarty, K.H., Heaton, M., Dalley. A.J., Dawson, R.A, Freedlander, E., Khaw, P.T., Mac Neil, S., "Keratinocyte-driven contraction of reconstructed human skin," *Wound Repair and Regeneration,* 9(2), 95–110 (March–April 2001).

2. Silverstein, R.J., Landsman, A.S., "The effects of a moderate and high dose of vitamin C on wound healing in a controlled guinea pig model," *Journal of Foot and Ankle Surgery,* 38(5), 333–338 (September–October 1998).

3. Fulton, J.E., Jr., "The stimulation of postdermabrasion wound healing with stabilized aloe vera gel-polyethylene oxide dressing," *Journal of Dermatologic Surgery* & *Oncology,* 16(5), 460–467 (May 1990).

4. Kohyama, T., Ertl, R.F., Valenti, V., Spurzem, J., Kawamoto, M., Nakamura, Y., Veys, T., Allegra, L., Romberger, D., Rennard, S.I., "Prostaglandin E(2) inhibits fibroblast chemotaxis," *American Journal of Physiology Lung Cell Molecular Physiology,* 281(5), L1257–1263 (November 2001).

5. Bosse, J.P., Papillon, J., Frenette, G., Dansereau, J., Cadotte, M., Le Lorier, J., "Clinical study of a new antikeloid agent," *Annals of Plastic Surgery,* 3(1), 13–21 (July 1979).

6. Meijia, K., Reng, R., *Plantas Medicinales de Uso Popular en la Amazonia Peruviana* (Lima, Peru: AECI and IIAP, 1995), p. 75.

7. Rothe, M., Rudy, T., Stankovic, P., "Treatment of bites to the hand and wrist—is the primary antibiotic prophylaxis necessary?" *Handchirurgie · Mikrochirurgie · Plastische Chirurgie,* 34(1), 22–29 (January 2002).

CYSTIC FIBROSIS

1. Zielenski, J., Tsui, L-C., "Cystic fibrosis: genotypic and phenotypic variations," *Annual Review of Genetics,* 29, 777–807 (1995).

2. Sereth, H., Shoshani, T., Bashan, N., Kerem, B.S., "Extended haplotype analysis of cystic fibrosis mutations and its implications for the selective advantage hypothesis," *Human Genetics,* 92, 289–295 (1993).

3. Meindl, R.S., "Hypothesis: a selective advantage for cystic fibrosis heterozygotes," *American Journal of Physical Anthropology,* 74, 39–45 (1987).

4. Tomezsko, J.L., Stallings, V.A., Kawchak, D.A., et al., Energy expenditure and genotype of children with cystic fibrosis," *Pediatric Research,* 35, 451–460 (1994).

5. Konstan, M.W., Bryard, P.J., Hoppel, C.L., "Effect of high dose ibuprofen in patients with cystic fibrosis," *New England Journal of Medicine,* 332, 848–854 (1995).

6. Govan, J.W.R., Nelson, J.W.," Microbiology of lung infection in cystic fibrosis," *British Medical Bulletin,* 48, 912–930 (1992).

7. Rosenfeld, M., Ramsey, B., "Evolution of airway microbiology in the infant with cystic fibrosis: role of nonpseudomonal and pseudomonal pathogens," *Seminars in Respiratory Infection,* 7, 158–167 (1992).

8. Steinkamp, G., Demmelmair, H., Ruhl-Bagheri, I., von der Hardt, H., Koletzko, B., "Energy supplements rich in Linoleic acid improve body weight and essential fatty acid status of cystic fibrosis patients," *Journal of Pediatric Gastroenterology and Nutrition,* 31(4), 418–423 (October 2000).

9. Winklhofer-Roob, B.M., van't Hof, M.A., Shmerling, D.H., "Response to oral beta-carotene supplementation in patients with cystic fibrosis: a 16-month follow-up study," *Acta Paediatrica,* 84, 1132–1136 (1995).

10. Mayer, P., Hamberger, H., Drews, J., "Differential effects of ubiquinone Q7 and ubiquinone analogs on macrophage activation and experimental infections in granulocytopenic mice," *Infection,* 8, 256–261 (1980).

11. Krumdieck, C., Butterworth, C.E., "Ascorbate-cholesterol-lecithin interactions: Factors of potential importance in the pathogenesis of atherosclerosis," *American Journal of Clinical Nutrition,* 27, 866–876 (1974).

12. Ulane, M.M., Butler, J.D., Peri, A., Miele, L., Ulane, R.E., Hubbard, V.S., "Cystic fibrosis and phosphatidylcholine biosynthesis," *Clinica Chimica Acta,* 239(2), 109–116 (31 October 1994).

13. Stagnaro, R., Pierri, I., Piovano, P., et al., "Thio containing antioxidant drugs and the human immune system," *Bulletin Europeen de Physiopathologie Respiratoire,* 23, 303–307 (1987).

14. Smith, U., Lacaille, F., Lepage, G., et al., "Taurine decreases fecal fatty acid and sterol excretion in cystic fibrosis. A randomized double-blind study," *American Journal of Diseases in Childhood,* 145, 1401–1404 (1995).

15. Carrasco, S., Codoceo, R., Prieto, G., et al., "Effect of taurine supplements on growth, fat absorption and bile acid on cystic fibrosis," *Acta Universitatis Carolinae,* 36, 152–156 (1990).

16. Winklhofer-Roob, B.M., Puhl, H., Khoschsorur, G., et al., "Enhanced resistance to oxidation of low density lipoproteins and decreased lipid peroxide formation during beta-carotene supplementation in cystic fibrosis," *Free Radicals in Biology and Medicine,* 18, 849–859 (1995).

17. Green, M.R., Buchanan, E., Weaver, L.T., "Nutritional management of the infant with cystic fibrosis," *Archives of Diseases in Childhood,* 72, 452–456 (1995).

18. Ramsey, B.W., Dorkin, H.L., Eisenberg, J.P., et al., "Efficacy of aerosolized tobramycin in patients with cystic fibrosis," *New England Journal of Medicine,* 328, 1740–1746 (1993).

19. Hutler, M., Schnabel, D., Staab, D., Tacke, A., Wahn, U., Boning, D., Beneke, R., "Effect of growth hormone on exercise tolerance in children with cystic fibrosis," *Medical Science in Sports and Exercise,* 34(4), 567–572 (April 2002).

20. Blau, H., Mussaffi-Georgy, H., Fink, G., Kaye, C., Szeinberg, A., Spitzer, S.A., Yahav, J., "Effects of an intensive 4-week summer cAMP on cystic fibrosis(*) : pulmonary function, exercise tolerance, and nutrition," *Chest,* 121(4), 1117–1122 (April 2002).

CYSTITIS

1. Manges, A.R., Johnson, J.R., Foxman, B., O'Bryan, T.T., Fullerton, K.E., Riley, L.W., "Widespread distribution of urinary tract infections caused by a multidrug-resistant *Escherichia coli* clonal group," *New England Journal of Medicine;* 345, 1007–1013 (2001).

2. Murray, M., Pizzorno, J., *Encyclopedia of Natural Medicine* (Philadelphia: Churchill-Livingstone, 1999), p. 1184.

3. Sanchez, A., Reeser, J.L., Lau, H.S., et al., "Role of sugars in human neutrophilic phagocytosis," *American Journal of Clinical Nutrition,* 26, 1180–1184 (1973).

4. Manges, A.R., Johnson, J.R., Foxman, B., O'Bryan, T.T., Fullerton, K.E., Riley, L.W., ibid.

5. Howell, A.B., Foxman, B., "Cranberry Juice and Adhesion of antibiotic-resistant uropathogens," *Journal of the American Medical Association,* 287(23), 3082–3083 (19 June 2002).

6. Garcia-Calatayud, S., Larreina Cordoba, J.J., Lozano De La Torre, M.J., "Intoxicación grave por zumo de arándanos," *Añales Españoles de Pediátrica,* 56(1), 72–74 (1 March 2002).

7. Erhard, M., "Effect of echinacea, aconitum, lachesis, and apis extracts, and their combinations of phagocytosis of human granulocytes," *Phytotherapy Research,* 8, 14–77 (1994).

8. Murray, M., Pizzorno, J., p. 1184.

9. Rehman, J., Dillow, J.M., Carter, S.M., Chou, J., Le, B., Maisel, A.S., "Increased production of antigen-specific immunoglobulins G and M following in vivo treatment with the medical plants *Echinacea angustifolia* and *Hydrastis canadensis,*" *Immunology Letters,* 68(2–3), 391–395 (1 June 1999).

10. Facino, R.M., Carini, M., Aldini, G., Marinello, C., Arlandini, E., Franzoi, L., Colombo, M., Pietta, P., Mauri, P., "Direct characterization of caffeoyl esters with antihyaluronidase activity in crude extracts from *Echinacea angustifolia* roots by fast atom bombardment tandem mass spectrometry," *Farmaco,* 48(10), 1447–1461 (October 1993).

11. Budzinski, J.W., Foster, B.C., Vandenhoek, S., Arnason, J.T., "An in vitro evaluation of human cytochrome P405 3A4 inhibition by selected commercial herbal extracts and tinctures," *Phytomedicine,* 7(4), 273–282 (July 2000).

12. Luettig, B., Steinmuller, C., Gifford, G.E., Wagner, H., Lohmann-Matthes, M.L., "Macrophage activation by the polysaccharide arabinogalactan isolated from plant cell cultures of *Echinacea purpurea,*" *Journal of the National Cancer Institute,* 81(9), 669–675 (3 May 1989).

13. Eenham, I., "Pelvic inflammatory disease," *Australian Family Physician,* 15, 254–256 (1986).

14. Cromer, B., Heald, F., "Pelvic inflammatory disease associated with *Neisseria gonorrhoeae* and *Chlamydia trachomatis.* Clinical correlates," *Sexually Transmitted Diseases,* 14, 125–129 (1987).

15. Mori, S., Ojima, Y., Hirose, T., et al., "The clinical effect of proteolytic enzyme containing bromelain and trypsin on urinary tract infection evaluated by double blind method," *Acta Obstetrica et Gynaecologica Japonica,* 19, 147–153. (1972).

16. Cornelissenm C.N., Kelley, M., Hobbs, M.M., Anderson, J.E., Cannon, J.G., Cohen, M.S., Sparling, P.F., "The transferrin receptor expressed by gonococcal strain FA1090 is required for the experimental infection of human male volunteers," *Molecular Microbiology,* 27(3), 611–616 (February 1998).

17. Payne, S.M., Finkelstein, R.A., "Pathogenesis and immunology of experimental gonococcal infection: role of iron in virulence," *Infection and Immunology,* 12(6), 1313–1318 (1975).

DANDRUFF

1. Garbe, C., Husak, R., Orfanos, C.E., "HIV-associated dermatoses and their prevalence in 456 HIV-infected patients. Relation to immune status and its importance as a diagnostic marker," *Hautarzt,* 45(9), 623–629 (September 1994).

2. Andrews, G., Post, C., Domonkos, A., "Seborrheic dermatitis supplementation treatment with vitamin B$_{12}$," *New York State Journal of Medicine,* 50, 1921–1925 (1950).

3. Proctor, M., Wilkenson, D., Orenberg, E., Farber, E.M., "Lowered cutaneous and urinary levels of polyamines with clinical improvement in treated psoriasis," *Archives of Dermatology,* 115, 945–949 (1979).

4. Kalman, J., Gecse, A., Farkas, T., Joo, F., Telegdy, G., Lajtha, A., "Dietary manipulation with high marine fish oil intake of fatty acid composition and arachidonic acid metabolism in rat cerebral microvessels," *Neurochemical Research,* 17(2), 167–172 (February 1992).

5. Nisenson, A., "Treatment of seborrheic dermatitis with biotin and vitamin B complex," *Journal of Pediatrics,* 81, 630–631 (1972).

6. Roe, D.A., *Drug-Induced Nutritional Deficiencies* (Westport, CT: AVI Publications, 1976), 168–177.

7. Schreiner, A., Rockewell, E., Vilter, R., "A local defect in the metabolism of pyridoxine in the skin of persons with seborrheic dermatitis of the 'sicca' type," *Journal of Investigational Dermatology,* 19, 95–96 (1952).

8. Vardy, D.A., Cohen, A.D., Tchetov, T., Medvedovsky, E., Biton, A., "A double-blind, placebo-controlled trial of an Aloe vera (*A. barbadensis*) emulsion in the treatment of seborrheic dermatitis," *Journal of Dermatological Treatment,* 10, 7–11 (October 1999),

9. Al-Waili, N.S., "Therapeutic and prophylactic effects of crude honey on chronic seborrheic dermatitis and dandruff," *European Journal of Medical Research,* 30, 6(7), 306–308 (July 2001).

10. Scheriner, A., Slinger, W., Hawkins, V., et al., "Seborrheic dermatitis. A local metabolic defect involving pyridoxine," *Journal of Laboratory and Clinical Medicine,* 40, 121–130 (1952).

DENGUE FEVER

1. Sanchez, I., Gomez-Garibay, F., Taboada, J., Ruiz, B.H., "Antiviral effect of flavonoids on the dengue virus," *Phytotherapy Research,* 14(2), 89–92 (March 2000).

DEPRESSION

1. Robins, L.N., Regier, D.A., *Psychiatric disorders in America: the epidemiologic catchment area study.* (New York, NY: The Free Press; 1991).

2. Weissman, M.M., Bland, R.C., Canino, G.J., Faravelli, C., Greenwald, S., Hwu, H.G., Joyce, P.R., Karam, E.G., Lee, C.K., Lellouch, J., Lepine, J.P., Newman, S.C., Rubio-Stipec, M., Wells, J.E., Wickramaratne, P.J., Wittchen, H., Yeh, E.K., "Cross-national epidemiology of major depression and bipolar disorder," *Journal of the American Medical Association,* 276, 293–299 (1996).

3. Akiskal, H.S., "Mood disorders: introduction and overview." In: Kaplan, H.I., Sadock, B.J., eds., *Comprehensive Textbook of Psychiatry,* Sixth Edition (Baltimore: Lippincott, Williams & Wilkins; 1995) 1067–1079.

4. Ladd, C.O., Huot, R.L., Thrivikraman, K.V., Nemeroff, C.B., Meaney, M.J., Plotsky, P.M., "Long-term behavioral and neuroendocrine adaptations to adverse early experience," *Progress in Brain Research,* 122, 81–103 (2000).

5. Duman, R.S., Malberg, J., Thome, J., "Neural plasticity to stress and antidepressant treatment," *Social and Biological Psychiatry,* 46, 1181–1191 (1999).

6. Holsboer, F., Barden, N., "Antidepressants and hypothalamic-pituitary-adrenocortical regulation," *Endocrinology Review,* 17, 187–205 (1996).

7. Gilliand, K., Bullick, W., "Caffeine: a potential drug of abuse," *Advances in Alcohol and Substance Abuse,* 3, 53–73 (1984).

8. Neil, J.F., Himmelhoch, J.M., Mallinger, A.C., Mallinger J., Hanin I., "Caffeinism complicating hypersomnic depressive disorders," *Comprehensive Psychiatry,* 19, 377–385 (July–August 1978).

9. Greden, J., Fontaine, P., Lubetsky, M., Chamberlain, K., "Anxiety and depression associated with caffeinism among psychiatric patients," *American Journal of Psychiatry,* 135(8), 963–966 (August 1978).

10. Bolton, S., Null, G., "Caffeine, psychological effects, use and abuse," *Journal of Orthomolecular Psychiatry,* 10, 202–211 (1981).

11. Charney, D., Henninger, G., Jatlow, P., "Increased anxiogenic effects of caffeine in panic disorders," *Archives of General Psychiatry,* 42, 233–243 (1984).

12. Christensen, L., "Psychological distress and diet—effects of sucrose and caffeine," *Journal of Applied Nutrition,* 40, 44–50 (1988).

13. Kreitsch, K., "Prevalence, presenting symptoms, and psychological characteristics of individuals experiencing a diet-related mood disturbance," *Behavioral Therapies,* 19, 593–594 (1985).

14. Poldinger, W., Calanchini, B., Schwarz, W. A., "Functional-dimensional approach to depression: Serotonin deficiency as a target syndrome in a comparison of 5-hydroxytryptophan and fluvoxamine," *Psychopathology,* 24, 53–81 (1991).

15. Sternberg, E.M., Van Woert, M.H., Young, S.N., Magnussen, I., Baker, H., Gauthier, S., Osterland, C.K., "Development of a scleroderma-like illness during therapy with L-5-hydroxytryptophan and carbidopa," *New England Journal of Medicine,* 303, 782–787 (1980).

16. Joly, P., Lampert, A., Thomine, E., Lauret, P., "Development of pseudobullous morphea and scleroderma-like illness during therapy with L-5-hydroxytryptophan and carbidopa," *Journal of the American Academy of Dermatology,* 25(2 Pt 1), 332–333 (1991).

17. Mischoulon, D., Fava, M., "Docosahexanoic acid and omega-3 fatty acids in depression," *The Psychiatric Clinics of North America,* 23(4), 785–794 (December 2000).

18. Coppen, A., Bailey, J., "Enhancement of the antidepressant action of fluoxetine by folic acid: a randomized, placebo controlled trial," *Journal of Affective Disorders,* 60, 121–130 (2000).

19. Delle Chiaie, R., Pancheri, P., "Combined analysis of two controlled, multicentric, double blind studies to assess efficacy and safety of Sulfo-Adenosyl-Methionine (SAMe) vs. placebo (MC1) and SAMe vs. clomipramine (MC2) in the treatment of major depression [in Italian; English abstract]," *Gioornale Italiano di Psicopatologia,* 5, 1–16 (1999).

20. Iruela, L.M., Minguez, L., Merino, J., Monedero, G., "Toxic interaction of S-adenosylmethionine and clomipramine [letter]," *American Journal of Psychiatry,* 150, 522 (1993).

21. Vorbach, E.U., Hübner, W.D., Arnold, K.H., "Effectiveness and tolerance of the hypericum extract LI 160 in comparison with imipramine: randomized double-blind study with 135 outpatients," *Journal of Geriatric Psychiatry and Neurology,* 7 Suppl 1, S19–S23 (October 1994).

22. Woelk, H., "Comparison of St. John's wort and imipramine for treating depression: randomized controlled trial," *British Medical Journal,* 321, 536–539 (2 September 2000).

23. Schrader, E., "Equivalence of St. John's wort extract (Ze 117) and fluoxetine: a randomized, controlled study in mild-moderate depression," *International Clinical Psychopharmacology,* 15(2), 61–68 (March 2000).

24. Brenner, R., Azbel, V., Madhusoodanan, S., Pawlowska, M., "Comparison of an extract of hypericum (LI 160) and sertraline in the treatment of depression: a double-blind, randomized pilot study," *Clinical Therapies,* 22(4), 411–419 (April 2000).

25. Butterweck, V., Winterhoff, H., Herkenham, M., "St John's wort, hypericin, and imipramine: a comparative analysis of mRNA levels in brain areas involved in HPA axis control following short-term and long-term administration in normal and stressed rats," *Molecular Psychiatry,* 6(5), 547–564 (September 2001).

26. Shelton, R.C., Keller, M.B., Gelenberg, A., Dunner, D.L., Hirschfeld, R., Thase, M.E., Russell, J., Lydiard, R.B., Crits-Cristoph, P., Gallop, R., Todd, L., Hellerstein, D., Goodnick, P., Keitner, G., Stahl, S.M., Halbreich, U., "Effectiveness of St John's wort in major depression: a randomized controlled trial," *Journal of the American Medical Association,* 285(15), 1978–1986 (18 April 2001).

27. Barbenel, D.M., Yusufi, B., O'Shea, D., Bench, C.J., "Mania in a patient receiving testosterone replacement postorchidectomy taking St John's wort and sertraline," *Journal of Psychopharmacology,* 14, 84–86 (2000).

28. Peebles, K.A., Baker, R.K., Kurz, E.U., Schneider, B.J., Kroll, D.J., "Catalytic inhibition of human DNA topoisomerase IIalpha by hypericin, a naphthodianthrone from St. John's wort (*Hypericum perforatum*)," *Biochemical Pharmacology,* 62(8), 1059–1070 (15 October 2001).

29. Ruschitzka, F., Meier, P.J., Turina, M., Luscher, T.F., Noll, G., "Acute heart transplant rejection due to Saint John's wort." *Lancet,* 355, 547 (12 February 2000).

30. Johne, A., Brockmoller, J., Bauer, S., Maurer, A., Langheinrich, M., Roots, I., "Pharmacokinetic interaction of digoxin with an herbal extract from St. John's wort (*Hypericum perforatum*)," *Clinical Pharmacology and Therapeutics,* 66, 338–345 (October 1999).

31. Piscitelli, S.C., Burstein, A.H., Chaitt, D., Alfaro, R.M., Falloon, J., "Indinavir concentrations and St. John's wort [letter]," *Lancet,* 355,548 (12 February 2000).

32. Nebel, A., Schneider, B.J., Baker, R.K., Kroll, D.J., "Potential metabolic interaction between St. John's wort and theophylline," *Annals of Pharmacotherapy,* 33, 502 (1999).

33. Maurer, A., "Interaction of St. John's wort extract with phenprocoumon," *European Journal of Clinical Pharmacology,* 55, A22, Abstract 79 (1999).

34. Huguet, F., Drieu, K., Piriou, A., "Decreased cerebral 5-HT$_{1A}$ receptors during aging: reversal by *Ginkgo biloba* extract (EGv 761)," *Journal of Pharmacy and Pharmacology,* 46, 316–318 (1994).

35. Schubert, H., Halama, P., "Depressive episode primarily unresponsive to therapy in elderly patients: efficacy of *Ginkgo biloba* extract EGb 761 in combination with antidepressants [translated from German]," *Geriatrische Forschung,* 3, 45–53 (1993).

36. Lane, A.M., Lovejoy, D.J., "The effects of exercise on mood changes: the moderating effect of depressed mood," *Journal of Sports Medicine and Physical Fitness,* 41(4), 539–545 (December 2001).

37. Brown, M.A., Goldstein-Shirley, J., Robinson, J., Casey, S., "The effects of a multi-modal intervention trial of light, exercise, and vitamins on women's mood," *Women's Health,* 34(3), 93–112 (2001).

DERMATITIS HERPETIFORMIS

1. Garioch, J.J., Lewis, H.M., Sargent, S.A., Leonard, J.N., Fry, L., "25 years' experience of a gluten-free diet in the treatment of dermatitis herpetiformis," *British Journal of Dermatology,* 131(4), 541–545 (October 1994).

2. Lewis, H.M., Renaula, T.J., Garioch, J.J., "Protective effect of gluten-free diet against development of lymphomas in dermatitis herpetiformis," *British Journal of Dermatology,* 1335, 363–367 (1996).

3. Barnes, R.M.R., Lewis-Jones, M.S., "Isotype distribution and serial levels of antibodies reactive with dietary protein antigens in dermatitis herpetiformis," *Journal of Clinical and Laboratory Immunology,* 30, 87–01 (1989).

4. Kadunce, D.P., Mcmurry, M.P., Avots-Avotins, A., "The effect of an elemental diet with and without gluten on disease activity in dermatitis herpetiformis," *Journal of Investigational Dermatology,* 97, 175–182 (1991).

5. Zarafonctis, C.J., Johnwick, E.B., Kirkman, L.W., Curtis, A.C., "para-aminobenzoic acid in dermatitis herpetiformis," *Archives of Dermatology and Syphilis,* 63, 115–132 (1951).

6. Jublin, L., Edqvist, L.E., Ekman, L.G., Ljunghall, K., Olsson M., "Blood glutathione-peroxidase levels in skin diseases: effect of selenium and vitamin E treatment," *Acta Dermatologica et Venereologica,* 62. 211–214 (1982).

7. Ljunbhall, K., Jublin, L., Edqvist, L.E., Plantin, L.O., "Selenium, glutathione-peroxidase and dermatitis herpetiformis," *Acta Dermatologica et Venereologica,* 64, 546–547 (1984).

DIABETES

1. Couper, J.J., "Environmental triggers of type 1 diabetes," *Journal of Paediatrics and Child Health,* 37(3), 218–220 (June 2001).

2. Paronen, J., Knip, M., Savilahti, E., Virtanen, S.M., Ilonen, J., Akerblom, H.K., Vaarala, O., "Effect of cow's milk exposure and maternal type 1 diabetes on cellular and humoral immunization to dietary insulin in infants at genetic risk for type 1 diabetes. Finnish trial to reduce IDDM in the genetically at risk study group," *Diabetes,* 49(10), 1657–1665 (October 2000).

3. Lewis, G.F., Carpentier, A., Adeli, K., Giacca, A., "Disordered fat storage and mobilization in the pathogenesis of insulin resistance and type 2 diabetes," *Endocrinology Review,* 23(2), 201–229 (April 2002).

4. Steppan, C.M., Lazar, M.A., "Resistin and obesity-associated insulin resistance," *Trends in Endocrinology and Metabolism,* 13(1), 18–23 (January–February 2002).

5. Evans, J.L., Heymann, C.J., Goldfine, I.D., Gavin, L.A., "Pharmacokinetics, tolerability, and fructosamine-lowering effect of a novel, controlled-release formulation of alpha-lipoic acid," *Endocrine Practice,* 8(1), 29–35 (January–February 2002).

6. Greene, E.L., Nelson, B.A., Robinson, K.A., Buse, M.G., "Alpha-Lipoic acid prevents the development of glucose-induced insulin resistance in 3T3–L1 adipocytes and accelerates the decline in immunoreactive insulin during cell incubation," *Metabolism,* 50(9), 1063–1069 (September 2001).

7. El Midaoui, A., de Champlain, J., "Prevention of hypertension, insulin resistance, and oxidative stress by alpha-lipoic acid," *Hypertension,* 39(2), 303–307 (February 2002).

8. Eason, R.C., Archer, H.E., Akhtar, S., Bailey, C.J., "Lipoic acid increases glucose uptake by skeletal muscles of obese-diabetic ob/ob mice," *Diabetes, Obesity, Metabolism,* 4(1), 29–35 (January 2002).

9. Saengsirisuwan, V., Perez, F.R., Kinnick, T.R., Henriksen, E.J., "Effects of exercise training and antioxidant R-ALA on glucose transport in insulin-sensitive rat skeletal muscle," *Journal of Applied Physiology,* 92(1), 50–58 (January 2002).

10. Thampy, G.K., Haas, M.J., Mooradian, A.D., "Troglitazone stimulates acetyl-CoA carboxylase activity through a post-translational mechanism," *Life Sciences,* 68(6), 699–708 (29 December 2000).

11. Yoshikawa, H., Tajiri, Y., Sako, Y., Hashimoto, T., Umeda, F., Nawata, H., "Effects of biotin on glucotoxicity or lipotoxicity in rat pancreatic islets," *Metabolism,* 51(2), 163–168 (February 2002).

12. McCarty, M.F., "Hepatothermic therapy of obesity: rationale and an inventory of resources," *Medical Hypotheses,* 57(3), 324–336 (September 2001).

13. Bender, D.A., "Optimum nutrition: thiamin, biotin and pantothenate," *Proceedings of the Nutrition Society,* 58(2), 427–433 (May 1999).

14. Alcolado, J.C., Laji, K., Gill-Randall, R., "Maternal transmission of diabetes," *Diabetes in Medicine,* 19(2), 89–98 (February 2002).

15. Morris, B.W., MacNeil, S., Hardisty, C.A., et al., "Chromium homeostasis in patients with type II (NIDDM) diabetes," *Journal of Trace Elements in Medicine and Biology,* 13, 57–61 (1999).

16. Kim, D.S., Kim, T.W., Park, I.K., Kang, J.S., Om, A.S., "Effects of chromium picolinate supplementation on insulin sensitivity, serum lipids, and body weight in dexamethasone-treated rats," *Metabolism,* 51(5), 589–594 (May 2002).

17. Bahijiri, S.M., Mira, S.A., Mufti, A.M., Ajabnoor, M.A., "The effects of inorganic chromium and brewer's yeast supplementation on glucose tolerance, serum lipids and drug dosage in individuals with type 2 diabetes," *Saudi Medical Journal,* 21(9), 831–837 (September 2000).

18. Bahijiri, S.M., Mufti, A.M., "Beneficial effects of chromium in people with type 2 diabetes, and urinary chromium response to glucose load as a possible indicator of status," *Biological Trace Element Research,* 85(2), 97–109 (February 2002).

19. Urberg, M., Zemel, M.B., "Evidence for synergism between chromium and nicotinic acid in the control of glucose tolerance in elderly humans," *Metabolism,* 36(9), 896–899 (September 1987).

20. Evans, W.J., "Vitamin E, vitamin C, and exercise," *American Journal of Clinical Nutrition,* 72(2), 647S–652S (August 2000).

21. Baydas, G., Canatan, H., Turkoglu, A., "Comparative analysis of the protective effects of melatonin and vitamin E on streptozocin-induced diabetes mellitus," *Journal of Pineal Research,* 32(4), 225–230 (May 2002).

22. Lefebvre, P.J., Paolisso, G., Scheen, A.J., "Magnesium and glucose metabolism," *Therapie,* 49, 1–7. (1994).

23. Halberstam, M., Cohen, N., Shlimovich, P., et al., "Oral vanadyl sulfate improves insulin sensitivity in NIDDM but not in obese nondiabetic subjects," *Diabetes,* 45, 659–666 (1996).

24. Meloni, C., Morosetti, M., Suraci, C., Pennafina, M.G., Tozzo, C., Taccone-Gallucci, M., Casciani, C.U., "Severe dietary protein restriction in overt diabetic nephropathy: Benefits or risks," *Journal of Renal Nutrition,* 12(2), 96–101 (April 2002).

DIAPER RASH

1. Ward, B.H., Flesicher, A.B., Jr., Feldman, S.R., Krowchuk, D.P., "Characterization of diaper dermatitis in the United States," *Archives of Pediatric and Adolescent Medicine,* 154(9), 943–946 (September 2000).

2. Berg, R.W., Milligan, M.C., Sarbaugy, F.C., "Association of skin wetness and pH with diaper dermatitis," *Pediatric Dermatology,* 11(1), 18–20 (March 1994).

3. Brook, L., "The effects of amoxicillin therapy on skin flora in infants," *Pediatric Dermatology,* 17(5), 360–363 (September–October 2000).

4. Ward, B.H., Flesicher, A.B., Jr., Feldman, S.R., Krowchuk, D.P., ibid.

5. Penna, R.P., Coprrigan, L.L., Walsh, J., *Handbook of Nonprescription Drugs,* Sixth Edition (Washington, DC: American Pharmaceutical Association, 1979), p. 424.

6. Akin, F., Spraker, M., Aly, R., Leyden, J., Raynor, W., Landin. W., "Effects of breathable disposable diapers: reduced prevalence of *Candida* and common diaper dermatitis," *Pediatric Dermatology,* 18(4), 282–290 (July–August 2001).

7. Draelos, Z.C., "Hydrogel barrier/repair creams and contact dermatitis," *American Journal of Contact Dermatology,* 11(4), 222–225 (December 2000).

8. Cant, A.J., Bailes, J.A., Marsden, R.A., Hewitt, D., "Effect of maternal dietary exclusion on breast-fed infants with eczema," *British Medical Journal,* 293, 231–233 (1986).

9. Casimir, G.J., Cuchaateau, J., Gosssart, B., Cuvelier, P., Vandaele, F., Vis, H.L., "Atopic dermatitis: role of food and house dust mite allergens," *Pediatrics,* 92(2), 252–256, (August 1993).

10. Teelucksingh, S., Mackie, A.D., Burt, D., McIntyre, M.A., Brett, L., Edwards, C.R., "Potentiation of hydrocortisone activity in skin by glycyrrhetinic acid," *Lancet,* 335(8697), 1060–1063 (5 May 1990).

DIARRHEA

1. Loeb, H., Vandenplas, Y., Wursch, P., Guesry, P., "Tannin-rich pod for treatment of acute-onset diarrhea," *Journal of Pediatric Gastroenterology and Nutrition;* 8, 480–485 (1989).

2. Pothoulakis, C., Kelly, C.P., Joshi, M.A., Gao, N., O'Keane, C.J., Castagliuolo, I., Lamont, J.T., "*Saccharomyces boulardii* inhibits *Clostridium difficile* toxin A binding and enterotoxicity in rat ileum," *Gastroenterology* 104, 1108–1115 (1993).

3. Bleichner, G., Blehaut, H., Mentec, H., Moyse, D., "*Saccharomyces boulardii* prevents diarrhea in critically ill tube-fed patients. A muticenter, randomized, double-blind placebo-controlled trial," *Intensive Care Medicine,* 23, 517–523 (1997).

4. Surzwicz, C.M., Elmer, G.W., Speelman, P., et al., "Prevention of antibiotic-associated diarrhea by *Saccharomyces boulardii:* a prospective study," *Gastroenterology,* 96, 981–988 (1989).

5. Plein, K., Hotz, J., "Therapeutic effects of *Saccharomyces* on mild residual symptoms in a stable phase of Crohn's disease with special respect to chronic diarrhea—a pilot study," *Zeitschrift für Gastroenterologie,* 31, 129–134 (1993).

6. Saavedra, J., "Probiotics and infectious diarrhea," *American Journal of Gastroenterology,* 95, S16–S18 (2000).

7. No authors given, "Monograph: Berberine," Alternative Medicine Review, 5(2), 175–177 (April 2000).

8. Williams, J.E., "Review of antiviral and immunomodulating properties of

plants of the peruvian rainforest with a particular emphasis on uña de gato and sangre de grado," *Alternative Medicine Review,* 6(6), 567–579 (December 2001).

9. Blumenthal, M., Busse, W.R., Goldberg, A., Gruenwald, W., Hall, T., Klein, S., Riggins, C., Rister, R. (eds). *The Complete Commission E Monographs: Therapeutic Guide to Herbal Medicines* (Boston, Massachusetts: Integrative Medicine Communications, 1998) p. 91.

10. Blumenthal, M., Busse, W.R., Goldberg, A., Gruenwald, W., Hall, T., Klein, S., Riggins, C., Rister, R., (eds)., ibid., p. 175–176.

11. Blumenthal M., Busse, W.R., Goldberg, A., Gruenwald, W., Hall, T., Klein, S., Riggins, C., Rister, R., (eds)., ibid., p. 376

12. Blumenthal M., Busse, W.R., Goldberg, A., Gruenwald, W., Hall, T., Klein, S., Riggins, C., Rister, R., (eds)., ibid, p. 107.

13. Beveridge, R.J., Stoddard, J.F., Szarek, W.A., Jones, J.K.N., "Some structural features of the mucilage from the bark of *Ulmus fulva* (slippery elm mucilage)," *Carbohydrate Research,* 9, 429–439 (1969).

14. Lin, Y., Zhou, Z., Shen, W., Shen, J., Hu, M., Zhang, F., Hu, P., Xu, M., Huang, S., Zheng, Y., "Clinical and experimental studies on shallow needling technique for treating childhood diarrhea," *Journal of Traditional Chinese Medicine,* 13, 107–114 (1993).

15. Okhuysen, P.C., Chappell, C.L., Crabb, J., Valdez, L.M., Douglass, E.T., DuPont, H.L., "Prophylactic effect of bovine anti-Cryptosporidium hyperimmune colostrum immunoglobulin in healthy volunteers challenged with Cryptosporidium parvum," *Clinical Infectious Disease,* 26, 1324–1329 (1998).

16. Saavedra, J.M., Bauman, N.A., Oung, I., Perman, J.A., Yolken, R.H., "Feeding of Bifidobacterium bifidum and Streptococcus thermophilus to infants in hospital for prevention of diarrhea and shedding of rotavirus," *Lancet,* 344, 1046–1049 (1994).

17. Van Niel, C.W., Feudtner, C., Garrison, M.M., Christakis, D.A., "Lactobacillus therapy for acute infectious diarrhea in children: a meta-analysis", *Pediatrics* 109(4) 678–84 (April 2002).

DIPHTHERIA

1. Ramos, A.C., Barrucand, L., Elias, P.R., Pimentel, A.M., Pires, V.R., "Carnitine supplementation in diphtheria," *Indian Pediatrics,* 29(12), 1501–1505 (December 1992).

2. Rahman, M.M., Mahalanabis, D., Hossain, S., Wahed, M.A., Alvarez, J.O., Siber, G.R., Thompson, C., Santosham, M., Fuchs, G.J., "Simultaneous vitamin A administration at routine immunization contact enhances antibody response to diphtheria vaccine in infants younger than six months," *Journal of Nutrition,* 129(12), 2192–2195 (December 1999).

3. Jonas, W.B., Lin, Y., Tortella, F., "Neuroprotection from glutamate toxicity with ultra-low dose glutamate," *Neurology Reports,* 12, 335–339 (2001).

4. Hoover, T., "Homoepathic prophylaxis," *Journal of the American Institute of Homeopathy,* 3, 168–175 (2001).

DIVERTICULITIS AND DIVERTICULOSIS

1. Aldoori, W.H., Giovannucci, E.L., Rockett, H.R., Sampson, L., Rimm, E.B., Willett, W.C., "A prospective study of dietary fiber types and symptomatic diverticular disease in men," *Journal of Nutrition,* 128(4), 714–719 (April 1998).

2. Papi, C., Ciaco, A., Koch, M., Capurso, L., "Efficacy of rifaximin in the treatment of symptomatic diverticular disease of the colon. A multicentre double-blind placebo-controlled trial," *Alimentary Pharmacology and Therapy,* 9(1), 33–39 (February 1995).

3. Marzio, L., Del Bianco, R., Donne, M.D., Pieramico, O., Cuccurullo, F., "Mouth-to-cecum transit time in patients affected by chronic constipation: effect of glucomannan," *American Journal of Gastroenterology,* 84(8), 888–891 (August 1989).

4. Matsuura, Y., "Degradation of konjac glucomannan by enzymes in human feces and formation of short-chain fatty acids by intestinal anaerobic bacteria," *Journal of Nutrition Science and Vitaminology* (Tokyo), 44(3), 423–436 (June 1998).

5. Petrakis, I., Sakellaris, G., Kogerakis, N., Zacharioudakis, G., Kourtis, D.,

Xynos, E., Chalkiadakis, G., "New perspectives in the management of sigmoid diverticulitis," *Panminerva Medica,* 43(4), 289–293 (December 2001).

6. Lin, O.S., Soon, M.S., Wu, S.S., Chen, Y.Y., Hwang, K.L., Triadafilopoulos, G., "Dietary habits and right-sided colonic diverticulosis," *Diseases of the Colon and Rectum,* 43(10), 1412–1418 (October 2000).

DOWN SYNDROME

1. Seven, M., Cengiz, M., Tuzgen, S., Iscan, M.Y., "Plasma carnitine levels in children with Down syndrome," *American Journal of Human Biology,* 13(6), 721–725 (November–December 2001).

2. De Falco, F.A., D'Angelo, E., Grimaldi, G., Scafuro, F., Sachez, F., Caruso, G., "Effect of the chronic treatment with L-acetylcarnitine in Down's syndrome," *Clinica Terapeutica,* 144(2), 123–127 (February 1994).

DUCHENNE MUSCULAR DYSTROPHY

1. Passaquin, A.C., Renard, M., Kay, L., Challet, C., Mokhtarian, A., Wallimann, T., Ruegg, U.T., "Creatine supplementation reduces skeletal muscle degeneration and enhances mitochondrial function in mdx mice," *Neuromuscular Disorders,* 12(2), 174–182 (February 2002).

2. Hankard, R., Mauras, N., Hammond, D., Haymond, M., Darmaun, D., "Is glutamine a 'conditionally essential' amino acid in Duchenne muscular dystrophy?" *Clinical Nutrition,* 18(6), 365–369 (December 1999).

3. Camina, F., Novo-Rodriguez, M.I., Rodriguez-Segade, S., Castro-Gago, M., "Purine and carnitine metabolism in muscle of patients with Duchenne muscular dystrophy," *Clinica Chimica Acta,* 243(2), 151–164 (29 December 1995).

DUPUYTREN'S CONTRACTURE

1. Ross, D.C., "Epidemiology of Dupuytren's disease," *Hand Clinician,* 15(1), 53–62, vi (February 1999).

2. Tomasek, J.J., Vaughan, M.B., Haaksma, C.J., "Cellular structure and biology of Dupuytren's disease," *Hand Clinician,* 15(1), 21–34 (February 1999).

3. Kirk, J.E., Chieffli, M., "Tocopherol administration in patients with Dupuytren's contracture: effect on plasma tocopherol levels and degree of contracture," *Proceedings of the Society for Experimental Biology and Medicine,* 80, 565–568 (1952).

4. Richards, H.J., "Dupuytren's contracture treated with vitamin E," *British Medical Journal,* 1328 (1952).

5. Kaneko, M., Kawakita, T., Kumazawa, Y., Takimoto, H., Nomoto, K., Yoshikawa, T., "Accelerated recovery from cyclphosphamide-induced leucopenia in mice administered a Japanese ethical herbal drug hochu-ekki-to," *Immunopharmacology,* 44(3), 223–231 (November 1999).

DYSLEXIA

1. Stordy, B.J., "Dark adaptation, motor skills, docosahexaenoic acid, and dyslexia," *American Journal of Clinical Nutrition,* 71(suppl), 323S–326S (2000).

2. Stein, J., "The magnocellular theory of developmental dyslexia," *Dyslexia,* 7(1), 12–36 (January–March 2001).

3. Taylor, K.E., Higgins, C.J., Calvin, C.M., Hall, J.A., Easton, T., McDaid, A.M., Richardson, A.J., "Dyslexia in adults is associated with clinical signs of fatty acid deficiency," *Prostaglandins, Leukotrienes, and Essential Fatty Acids,* 63(1–2), 75–78 (July–August 2000).

4. Taylor, K.E., Richardson, A.J., "Visual function, fatty acids and dyslexia," *Prostaglandins, Leukotrienes, and Essential Fatty Acids,* 63(1–2), 89–93 (July–August 2000).

5. Stevens, L.J., Zentall, S.S., Abate, M.L., Watkins, B.A., Kuczek, T., Burgess, J.R., "Omega-3 fatty acids in boys with behavior, learning, and health problems," *Physiology of Behavior,* 59, 915–920 (1996).

6. Stordy, B.J., "Dark adaptation, motor skills, docosahexaenoic acid, and dyslexia," *American Journal of Clinical Nutrition,* 71(Suppl), 323S–326S (2000).

7. Stordy, B.J., "Benefit of docosahexaenoic acid supplements to dark adaptation in dyslexics," *Lancet,* 346, 385 (1995).

DYSMENORRHEA

1. Clark, A.D., "Dysmenorrhea," *eMedicine Journal,* 3(3), 11 March 2002.

2. Granot, M., Yarnitsky, D., Itskovitz-Eldor, J., Granovsky, Y., Peer, E., Zimmer, E.Z., "Pain perception in women with dysmenorrhea," *Obstetrics and Gynecology,* 98(3), 407–411 (September 2001).

3. Thys-Jacobs, S., Starkey, P., Bernstein, D., Tian, J., "Calcium carbonate and the premenstrual syndrome: effects on premenstrual and menstrual symptoms. Premenstrual syndrome study group," *American Journal of Obstetrics and Gynecology,* 179(2), 444–452 (August 1998).

4. Alvir, J.M., Thys-Jacobs, S., "Premenstrual and menstrual symptom clusters and response to calcium treatment," *Psychopharmacology Bulletin,* 27(2), 145–148 (1991).

5. Ostad, S.N., Soodi, M., Shariffzadeh, M., Khorshidi, N., Marzban, H., "The effect of fennel essential oil on uterine contraction as a model for dysmenorrhea, pharmacology and toxicology study," *Journal of Ethnopharmacology,* 76(3), 299–304 (August 2001).

6. Ziaei, S., Faghihzadeh, S., Sohrabvand, F., Lamyian, M., Emamgholy, T., "A randomized placebo-controlled trial to determine the effect of vitamin E in treatment of primary dysmenorrhoea," *BJOG: An International Journal of Obstetrics and Gynecology,* 108(11), 1181–1183 (November 2001).

7. Chen, C., Cho, S.I., Damokosh, A.I., Chen, D., Li, G., Wang, X., Xu, X., "Prospective study of exposure to environmental tobacco smoke and dysmenorrhea," *Environmental Health Perspectives,* 108(11), 1019–1022 (November 2000).

8. Proctor, M.L., Hing, W., Johnson, T.C., Murphy, P.A., "Spinal manipulation for primary and secondary dysmenorrhoea," *Cochrane Database Systems Review,* 4, CD002119 (2001).

9. Alonso, C., Coe, C.L., "Disruptions of social relationships accentuate the association between emotional distress and menstrual pain in young women," *Health and Psychology,* 20(6), 411–416 (November 2001).

10. Yuqin, Z., "A report of 49 cases of dysmenorrhea treated by acupuncture," *Journal of Traditional Chinese Medicine,* 4, 101–102. (1984).

E. COLI INFECTION

1. Lievin-Le Moal, V., Amsellem, R., Servin, A.L., Coconnier, M.H., "*Lactobacillus acidophilus* (strain LB) from the resident adult human gastrointestinal microflora exerts activity against brush border damage promoted by a diarrhoeagenic *Escherichia coli* in human enterocyte-like cells," *Gut,* 50(6), 803–811 (June 2002).

EAR INFECTIONS

1. Thrasher, R., "Middle Ear: Otitis Media with Effusion," *eMedicine,* 3(2) (15 February 2002).

2. Thrasher, R., ibid.

3. Lieu, J.E., Feinstein, A.R., "Effect of gestational and passive smoke exposure on ear infections in children," *Archives of Pediatric and Adolescent Medicine,* 156(2), 147–154 (February 2002).

4. Ryding, M., Konradsson, K., Kalm, O., Prellner, K., "Auditory consequences of recurrent acute purulent otitis media," *Annals of Otology, Rhinology, and Laryngology,* 111(3 Pt 1), 261–266 (March 2002).

5. Linday, L.A., Dolitsky, J.N., Shindledecker, R.D., Pippenger, C.E., "Lemon-flavored cod liver oil and a multivitamin-mineral supplement for the secondary prevention of otitis media in young children: pilot research," *Annals of Otology, Rhinology, and Laryngology,* 111(7 Pt 1), 642–652 (July 2002).

6. Qiu, J., Hendrixson, D.R., Baker, E.N., Murphy, T.F., St Geme, J.W., 3rd, Plaut, A.G., "Human milk lactoferrin inactivates two putative colonization factors expressed by *Haemophilus influenzae,*" *Proceedings of the National Academy of Sciences of the USA,* 95(21), 12641–12646 (13 October 1998).

7. Tully, S.B., Bar-Haim,Y., Bradley, R.L., "Abnormal tympanography after supine bottle feeding," *Journal of Pediatrics,* 126(6), S105–111 (June 1995).

8. Uhari, M., Kontiokari, T., Niemelä, M., "A novel use of xylitol sugar in preventing acute otitis media," *Pediatrics,* 102(4), 879–884 (4 October 1998).

9. Tapiainen, T., Luotonen, L., Kontiokari, T., Renko, M., Uhari, M., "Xylitol

administered only during respiratory infections failed to prevent acute otitis media," *Pediatrics,* 109(2), E19 (February 2002).

10. Frei, H., Thurneysen, A., "Homeopathy in acute otitis media in children: treatment effect or spontaneous resolution," *British Journal of Homeopathy,* 90(4), 178–179 (October 2001).

11. Jacobs, J., Springer, D.A., Crothers, D., "Homeopathic treatment of acute otitis media in children: a preliminary randomized placebo-controlled trial," *Pediatric Infectious Disease,* 20(2), 178–183(February 2001).

ECZEMA

1. Casimir, G.J., Cuchaateau, J., Gosssart, B., Cuvelier, P., Vandaele, F., Vis, H.L., "Atopic dermatitis: role of food and house dust mite allergens," *Pediatrics,* 92(2), 252–256, (August 1993).

2. Hansen, A.E., "A study of iodine number of serum fatty acids in infantile eczema," *Proceedings of the Society for Experimental Biology and Medicine,* 30, 1198–1199 (1933).

3. Galli, E., Picardo, M., Chini, L, "Analysis of polyunsaturated fatty acids in newborn sera: a screening tool for atopic disease," *British Journal of Dermatology,* 130, 752–756 (1994).

4. Burr, G.O, Murr, M.M.," A new deficiency disease produced by the rigid exclusion of fat from the diet," *Journal of Biological Chemistry,* 82, 5345–5367 (1929).

5. Horrobin, D.F., "Essential fatty acid metabolism and its modification in atopic eczema," *American Journal of Clinical Nutrition,* 71 (Suppl), 367S–372S (2000).

6. Pettit, J.H.S., "The use of unsaturated fatty acids in eczemas of childhood," *British Medical Journal,* 1, 79–81 (1954).

7. Lowe, N.J., DeQuoy, P.R., "Linoleic acid effects on epidermal DNA synthesis and cutaneous prostaglandin levels in essential fatty acids deficiency," *Journal of Investigational Dermatology,* 70, 200–203 (1978).

8. Prottey, C., "Investigation of functions of essential fatty acids in the skin," *British Journal of Dermatology,* 9, 29–38 (1977).

9. Ziboh, V.A., "Biochemical abnormalities in essential fatty acid deficiency," *Models in Dermatology,* 3, 106–111 (1987).

10. Lee, T.H., Arm, J.P., Horton, C.E., Crea, A.E., Mencai-Huerta, J.M., Spurt, B.W., "Effects of dietary fish oil lipids on allergic and inflammatory diseases," *Allergy Proceedings,* 12(5), 299–303 (September–October 1991).

11. Saarinen, U.M., Kajosaari, M., "Breastfeeding as prophylaxis against atopic disease. Prospective follow-up study until 17 years old," *Lancet,* 346, 1065–1069 (1995).

12. Cant, A.J., Bailes, J.A., Marsden, R.A., Hewitt, D., "Effect of maternal dietary exclusion on breast-fed infants with eczema," *British Medical Journal,* 293, 231–233 (1986).

13. Casimir, G.J, Cuchaateau, J., Gosssart, B., Cuvelier, P., Vandaele, F., Vis, H.L., "Atopic dermatitis: role of food and house dust mite allergens," *Pediatrics,* 92(2), 252–256, (August 1993).

14. Werfel, T., Ahlers, G., Schmidt, P., Boeker, M., Kapp, A., Neumann, C., "Milk-responsive atopic dermatitis is associated with a casein-specific lymphocyte response in adolescent and adult patients," *Journal of Allergy and Clinical Immunology,* 22 (1 Pt 1), 124–133 (January 1997).

15. Fiocchi, A., Restani, P., Riva, E., "Beef allergy in children," *Nutrition,* 16(6), 454–457 (June 2000).

16. Wefel, S.J., Cooke, S.K., Sampson, H.A., "Clinical reactivity to beef in children allergic to cow's milk," *Journal of Allergy and Clinical Immunology,* 99(1), 293–300 (March 1997).

17. Isolauri, E., Arvola, T., Sutas, Y., Moilanen, E., Salminen, S., "Probiotics in the management of atopic eczema," *Clinical Experience in Allergy,* 30(11), 1604–1610 (November 2000).

18. Pessi, T., Sutas, Y., Hurme, M., Isolauri, E., "Interleukin-10 generation in atopic children following oral *Lactobacillus rhamnosus* GG," *Clinical Experience in Allergy,* 30(12), 1804–1808 (December 2000).

19. Kalliomaki, M., Salminen, S., Arviolommi, H., Kero, P., Koskinen, P., Isolauir, E., "Probiotics in primary prevention of atopic disease: a randomized placebo-controlled trial," *Lancet,* 357(9262), 1976–1979 (April 2001).

20. Manku, M.S., Horrobin, D.F., Morse, N., Kyte, V., Jenkins, K., Wright, S., Burton, J.L., "Reduced levels of prostaglandin precursors in the blood of atopic patients: defective delta-6-desaturase function as a biochemical basis for atopy," *Prostaglandins and Leukotrienes in Medicine,* 9(6), 615–628 (December 1982).

21. Shimasaki, H., "PUFA content and effect of dietary intake of gamma-linolenic acid-rich oil on profiles of n-6, n-3 metabolites in plasma of children with atopic eczema," *Journal of Clinical Biochemistry and Nutrition,* 19, 183–192 (1995).

22. Courage, B., Nissen, H.P., Wehrmann, W., Biltz, H., "Influence of polyunsaturated fatty acids on the plasma catecholamines of patients with atopic eczema," *Zeitschrift für Hautkrankheit,* 66, 509–510 (1991).

23. Nissen, H.P., Wehrmann, W., Kroll, U., Kreyse, H.W., "Influence of polyunsaturated fatty acids on the plasma phospholipids of atopic patients," *Fat Science and Technology,* 90, 268–271 (1988).

24. Anstey, A., Quigley, M., Wilkinson, J.D., "Topical evening primrose oil as treatment for atopic eczema," *Journal of Dermatological Treatment,* 1, 199–201 (1991).

25. Guenther, L., Wexler, D., "Efamol in the treatment of atopic dermatitis," *Journal of the American Academy of Dermatology,* 17(5 Pt 1), 860 (November 1987).

26. Humphreys, F., Symons, J.A., Brown, H.K., Duff, G.N., Hunter, J.A., "The effects of gamma-linolenic acid on adult atopic eczema and premenstrual exacerbation of eczema," *European Journal of Dermatology,* 4, 598–603. (1994).

27. Horrobin, D.F., Stewart, C., "Evening primrose oil in atopic eczema," *Lancet* 335, 864–865 (1990).

28. Horrobin, D.F., Stewart, C., "Evening primrose oil and atopic eczema," *Lancet,* 336, 50 (1990).

29. Horrobin, D.F., Stewart, C., "Evening primrose oil and atopic eczema," *Lancet,* 345, 260–261 (1995).

30. Middleton, E., Drzewiecki, G., "Naturally occurring flavonoids and human basophil histamine release," *International Archives of Allergy and Applied Immunology,* 77, 155–157 (1985).

31. Yoshimoto, T., Furukawa, M., Yamamoto, S., Horie, T., Watanabe-Kohno, S., "Flavonoids: potent inhibitors of arachidonate 5-lipoxygenase," *Biochemistry and Biophysics Research Communications,* 116(2), 612–618 (31 October 1983).

32. Worm, M., Herz, U., Krab, J.M., Renz, H., Henz, B.M., "Effects of retinoids on in vitro and in vivo IgE production," *International Archives of Allergy and Immunology,* 124(1–3), 233–236 (January–March 2001).

33. Tobe, M., Isobe, Y., Goto, Y., Obara, F., Tsuchiya, M., Matsui, J., Hirota, K., Hayashi, H., "Synthesis and biological evaluation of CX-659S and its related compounds for their inhibitory effects on the delayed-type hypersensitivity reaction," *Bioorganic Medicinal Chemistry,* 8(8), 2037–2047 (August 2000).

34. Fairris, G.M., Perkins, P.J., Lloyd, B., Hinks, L., Clayton, E.B., "The effect on atopic dermatitis of supplementation with selenium and vitamin E.," *Acta Dermatologica et Venereologica,* 69(4), 359–362 (1989).

35. Del Toro, R., Baldo, Capotorti, G., Ginalanella, G., Miraglia del Giudice, M., Moro, R., Perrone, L., "Zinc and copper status in allergic children," *Acta Paediatrica Scandinavica,* 76(4), 612–617 (July 1987).

36. el-Kholy, M.S., Gas Allah, M.A., el-Shimi, S., el-Baz, F., el-Tayeh, H., Abdel-Hamid M.S., "Zinc and copper status in children with bronchial asthma and atopic dermatitis," *Egyptian Public Health Association Newsletter,* 65(5–6), 657–668 (1990).

37. Kreft, B., Wohlrab, J., Fischer, M., Uhlig, H., Skölziger, R., Marsch, W.C., "Analysis of serum zinc level in patients with atopic dermatitis, psoriasis vulgaris and in probands with healthy skin," *Hautarzt,* 51(120) 931–934 (December 2000).

38. Solomons, N.W., "Mild human zinc deficiency produces an imbalance between cell-mediated and humoral immunity," *Nutrition Review,* 26, 27–28 (1998).

39. Cooper, P.D., Carter, M., "Anti-complementary action of polymorphic 'solubility forms' of particulate inulin," *Molecular Immunology,* 23, 895–901 (1985).

40. Pizzorno, J.E., Jr., Murray, M.T., *Textbook of Natural Medicine* (London: Churchill Livngstone, 1999), p. 1128.

41. Schichijo, M., Shimizu, Y., Hiramatsu, K., Inagaki, N., Tagaki, K., Nagai, H., "Cyclic AMP-elevating agents inhibit mite-antigen-induced IL-4 and IL-13 release from basophil-enriched leukocyte preparation," *International Archives of Allergy and Immunology,* 114(4), 348–353 (December 1997).

42. Teelucksingh, S., Mackie, A.D., Burt, D., McIntyre, M.A,, Brett, L., Edwards, C.R,. "Potentiation of hydrocortisone activity in skin by glycyrrhetinic acid," *Lancet,* 335(8697), 1060–1063 (5 May 1990).

43. Evans, F.A., The rational use of glycyrrhetinic acid in dermatology," *British Journal of Clinical Practice,* 12, 269–279 (1958).

44. Rekka, E.A., Kourounakis, A.P., Kourounakis, P.N., "Investigation of the effect of chamazulene on lipid peroxidation and free radical processes," *Research Communications in Molecular Pathology* & *Pharmacology,* 92(3), 361–364 (June 1996).

45. Safayhi, H., Sabieraj, J., Sailer, E.R., Ammon, H.P., "Chamazulene: an antioxidant-type inhibitor of leukotriene B4 formation," *Planta Medica,* 60(5), 410–413 (October 1994).

46. Miller, T., Wittstock, U., Lindequist, U., Teuscher, E., "Effects of some components of the essential oil of chamomile, *Chamomilla recutita,* on histamine release from rat mast cells," *Planta Medica,* 62(1), 60–61 (1 February 1996).

47. Korting, H.C., Schafer-Koring, M., Hart, H., Laux, P., Schmid, M., "Anti-inflammatory activity of hamamelis distillate applied topically to the skin. Influence of vehicle and dose," *European Journal of Clinical Pharmacology,* 44(4), 315–318 (1993).

48. Gloor, M., Haus, C., Fluhr, J., Gehring, W., "Do shake lotions, zinc oil and polyethylene glycol gels produce dehydration or moisturization?" *Skin Pharmacology and Applied Skin Physiology,* 14(10), 34–43 (January–February 2001).

Emphysema

1. Rautalahti, M., Virtamo, J., Haukka, J., Heinonen, O.P., Sundvall, J., Albanes, D., Huttunen, J.K., "The effect of alpha-tocopherol and beta-carotene supplementation on COPD symptoms," *American Journal of Respiratory Critical Care Medicine,* 156(5), 1447–1452 (November 1997).

2. Frankfort, J.D., Fischer, C.E., Stansbury, D.W., et al., "Effects of high- and low-carbohydrate meals on maximum exercise performance in chronic airflow obstruction," *Chest,* 100, 792–795 (1991).

3. Fujimoto, S., Kurihara, N., Hirata, K., et al., "Effects of coenzymeQ10 administration on pulmonary function and exercise performance in patients with chronic lung diseases," *Clinical Investigations,* 71, S162–S166 (1993).

4. Koichiro, M., Aizawa, H., Inoue, H., Shigyo, M., Takata, S., Hara, N., "Thromboxane causes airway hyperresponsiveness after cigarette smoke-induced neurogenic inflammation," *Journal of Applied Physiology,* 81(6), 2358–2364 (December 1996).

5. Sharp, D.S., Rodriguez, B.L., Shahar, E., Hwang, L.J., Burchfiel, C.M., "Fish consumption may limit the damage of smoking on the lung," *American Journal of Respiratory Critical Care,* 150(4), 983–984 (October 1994).

6. Shahar, E., Folsom, A.R., Melnick, S.L., Tockman, M.S., Comstock, G.W., Gennaro, V., Higgins, M.W., Sorlie, P.D., Ko, W.J., Szklo, M., "Dietary n-3 polyunsaturated fatty acids and smoking-related chronic obstructive pulmonary disease. Atherosclerosis risk in communities study investigators," *New England Journal of Medicine,* 331(4), 228–233 (July 1994).

7. Stagnaro, R., Pierri, I., Piovano, P., et al., "Thio containing antioxidant drugs and the human immune system," *Bulletin Europeen de Physiopathologie Respiratoire,* 23, 303–307 (1987).

8. Grandjean, E.M., Berthet, P., Ruffmann, R., Leuenberger, P., "Efficacy of oral long-term N-acetylcysteine in chronic bronchopulmonary disease: a meta-analysis of published double-blind, placebo-controlled clinical trials," Clinical Therapeutics, 22(2), 209–221 (February 2001).

9. Jansen, D.F., Schouten, J.P., Vonk, J.M., Rijcken, B., Timens, W., Weiss, S.T., Postma, D.S., "Smoking and airway hyperresponsiveness especially in the presence of blood eosinophilia increase the risk to develop respiratory symptoms: A 25-year follow-up study in the general adult population," *American Journal of Respiratory Critical Care,* 160(1), 259–264 (July 1999).

10. Meister, R., Wittig, T., Beuscher, N., et al., "Efficacy and tolerability of Myrtol standardized in long-term treatment of chronic bronchitis. A double-blind, placebo-controlled study. Study group investigators," *Arzneimittel Forschung,* 49, 351–358 (1999)..

11. Rautalahti, M., Virtamo, J., Haukka, J., Heinonen, O.P., Sundvall, J., Albanes, D., Huttunen, J.K., ibid.

12. Miedema, I., Feskens, E.J.M., Heederiks, D., Kromhout, D., "Dietarydeterminants of long-term incidence of chronic nonspecific lung disease," *American Journal of Epidemiology,* 138, 37–45 (1993).

ENDOMETRIOSIS

1. Schenken, R.S., "Pathogenesis of endometriosis," *Journal of the SGI,* 9, 9 (20 March 2002).

2. Cooke, P., "Estrogen and progesterone action in endometrium," *Journal of the SGI,* 9, 9 (20 March 2002).

3. Chwalisz, K., Elger, W., McCrary, K., Beckman, P.M., Larsen, L., "Reversible suppression of menstruation in normal women irrespective of the effect on ovulation with the novel selective progesterone receptor modulator (SPRM) J867," *Journal of the SGI,* 9, 82A. Abstract 49 (20 March 2002).

4. Harel, Z., Biro, F.M., Kottenhahn, R.K., Rosenthal, S.L., "Supplementation with omega-3 polyunsaturated fatty acids in the management of dysmenorrhea in adolescents," *American Journal of Obstetrics and Gynecology,* 174, 1335–1338. (1996).

5. Grodstein, F., Goldman, M.B., Ryan, L., Cramer, D.W., "Relation of female infertility to consumption of caffeinated beverages," *American Journal of Epidemiology,* 137(12), 1353–1360 (15 June 1993).

6. Carpenter, S.E., Tjaden, B., Rock, J.A., Kimball, A., "The effect of regular exercise on women receiving danazol for treatment of endometriosis," *International Journal of Gynaecology and Obstetrics,* 49(3), 299–304 (June 1995).

7. Mai, A., Horibe, S., Fuseya, S., Iida, K., Takagi, H., Tamaya, T., "Possible evidence that the herbal medicine *shakuyaku-kanzo-to* decreases prostaglandin levels through suppressing arachidonate turnover in endometrium," *Journal of Medicine,* 26(3–4), 163–174 (1995).

EPIDIDYMITIS

1. Koff, S.A., "Altered bladder function and non-specific epidiymitis," *Journal of Urology,* 116, 589–592 (1976).

2. Berger, B., Alexander, R.E., Monda, G., "*Chlamydia trachomatis* as a cause of acute 'idiopathic' epididymitis," *New England Journal of Medicine,* 298, 301–304 (February 1978).

3. Berger, R., Kessle, D., Holmes, K., "Etiology and manifestations of epidiymitis in young men. Correlations with sexual orientation," *Journal of Infectious Disease,* 155, 1341–1343 (1987).

4. Cazzola, P., Mazzanti, P., Bossi, G., "In vivo modulating effect of a calf thymus acid lysate on human T lymphocyte subsets and CD4+/CD8+ ratio in the course of difference diseases," *Current Therapies Research,* 42, 1011–1017 (1987).

5. Seifter, E., Rettura, G., Seiter, J., "Thymotrophic action of vitamin A," *Federal Proceedings,* 32, 947 (1973).

6. Semba, R.D., "Vitamin A, immunity, and infection," *Clinical Infectious Disease,* 19, 489–499 (1994).

7. Ginter, E., "Optimum intake of vitamin C for the human organisms," *Nutrition and Health,* 1, 66–77 (1982).

8. Gabor, M., "Pharmacologic effects of flavonoids on blood vessels," *Angiologica,* 9, 355–374 (1972).

9. Prasad, A., "Clinical, biochemical and nutritional spectrum of zinc deficiency in human subjects. An update," *Nutrition Review,* 41, 197–208 (1983).

10. Neubauer, R., "A plant protease and possible replacement of antibiotics," *Experimental Medicine and Surgery,* 19, 1430–169 (1961).

11. Kuhn, O., untitled article, *Arzneimittel-Forschung,* 3, 194–200 (1953).

12. Erhard, M., "Effect of echinacea, aconitum, lachesis, and apis extracts, and their combinations of phagocytosis of human granulocytes," *Phytotherapy Research,* 8, 14–77 (1994).

13. Facino, R.M., Carini, M., Aldini, G., Marinello, C., Arlandini, E., Franzoi, L.,

Colombo, M., Pietta, P., Mauri, P., "Direct characterization of caffeoyl esters with antihyaluronidase activity in crude extracts from *Echinacea angustifolia* roots by fast atom bombardment tandem mass spectrometry," *Farmaco,* 48(10), 1447–1461 (October 1993).

14. Budzinski, J.W., Foster, B.C., Vandenhoek, S., Arnason, J.T., "An in vitro evaluation of human cytochrome P405 3A4 inhibition by selected commercial herbal extracts and tinctures," *Phytomedicine,* 7(4), 273–282 (July 2000).

15. Luettig, B., Steinmuller, C., Gifford, G.E., Wagner, H., Lohmann-Matthes, M.L., "Macrophage activation by the polysaccharide arabinogalactan isolated from plant cell cultures of *Echinacea purpurea,*" *Journal of the National Cancer Institute,* 81(9), 669–675 (3 May 1989).

16. Rehman, J., Dillow, J.M., Carter, S.M., Chou, J., Le, B., Maisel, A.S., "Increased production of antigen-specific immunoglobulins G and M following in vivo treatment with the medical plants *Echinacea angustifolia* and *Hydrastis canadensis,*" *Immunology Letters,* 68(2–3), 391–395 (1 June 1999).

17. Iinuma, M., Tanaka, T., Sakakibara, N., Mizuno, M., Matsuda, H., Shiomoto, H., Kubo, M., "Phagocytic activity of leaves of Epimedium species on mouse reticuloendothelial system," *Yakugaku Zasshi,* 110(3), 179–185 (March 1990).

EPILEPSY

1. Coppola, G., Veggiotti, P., Cusmai, R., Bertoli, S., Cardinali, S., Dionisi-Vici, C., Elia, M., Lispi, M.L., Sarnelli, C., Tagliabue, A., Toraldo, C., Pascotto, A., "The ketogenic diet in children, adolescents and young adults with refractory epilepsy: an Italian multicentric experience," *Epilepsy Research,* 48(3),221–227 (February 2002).

2. Ogunmekan, A.O., Hwang, P.A., "A randomized, double-blind, placebo-controlled, clinical trial of D-alpha-tocopheryl acetate (vitamin E), as add-on therapy, for epilepsy in children," *Epilepsia,* 30, 84–89 (1989).

ERECTILE DYSFUNCTION

1. de Tejada, I.S., Kim, N.N., Goldstein, I.I., Traish, A.M., "Regulation of pre-synaptic alpha adrenergic activity in the corpus cavernosum," *International Journal of Impotence Research,* 12(S1), S20–S25 (March 2000).

2. Kunelius, P., Hakkinen, J., Lukkarinen, O., "Is high-dose yohimbine hydrochloride effective in the treatment of mixed-type impotence? A prospective, randomized, controlled double-blind crossover study," *Urology,* 49(3), 441–444 (March 1997).

3. Vogt, H.J., Brandl, P., Kockott, G., Schmitz, J.R., Wiegand, M.H., Schadrack, J., Gierend, M., "Double-blind, placebo-controlled safety and efficacy trial with yohimbine hydrochloride in the treatment of nonorganic erectile dysfunction," *International Journal of Impotence Research,* 9(3), 155–161 (September 1997).

4. Betz, J.M., White, K.D., der Marderosian, A.H., "Gas chromatographic determination of yohimbine in commercial yohimbe products," *Journal of the AOAC International,* 78(5), 1189–1194 (September–October 1995).

5. Honing, M.L.H., Morrison, P.J., Banga, J.D., Stroes, E.S.K., Rabelink, T.J., "Nitric oxide availability in diabetes mellitus," *Diabetes and Metabolism Review,* 14, 241–49 (1998).

6. Ziegler, D., Gries, F.A., "Alpha-lipoic acid in the treatment of diabetic peripheral and cardiac autonomic neuropathy," *Diabetes,* 46 Suppl 2, S62–S66 (September 1997).

7. Zorgniotti, A.W., Lizza, E.F., "Effect of large doses of the nitric oxide precursor, L-arginine, on erectile dysfunction," *International Journal of Impotence Research,* 6, 33–36 (1994).

8. Chen, J., Wollman, Y., Chernichovsky, T., et al., "Effect of oral administration of high-dose nitric oxide donor L-arginine in men with organic erectile dysfunction: results of a double-blind, randomized study," *BJU International,* 83, 269–273 (1999).

FEMALE INFERTILITY

1. Jensen, T.K., Hjollund, N.H.I., Henriksen, T.B., Scheike, T., Kolstad, H., Giwercman, A., Ernst, E., Bonde, J.P., Skakkebæk, N.E., Olsen, J., "Does moderate alcohol consumption affect fertility? Follow up study among couples planning first pregnancy," *BMJ,* 317, 505–510 (17 August 1999).

2. Clausson, B., Granath, F., Ekbom, A., Lundgren, S., Nordmark, A., Signorello, L.B., Cnattingius, S., "Effect of caffeine exposure during pregnancy on birth weight and gestational age," *American Journal of Epidemiology*, 155(5), 429–436 (1 March 2002).

3. Gocze, P.M., Szabo, I., Freeman, D.A., "Influence of nicotine, cotinine, anabasine and cigarette smoke extract on human granulosa cell progesterone and estradiol synthesis," *Gynecology and Endocrinology*, 13(4), 266–272 (August 1999).

4. Czeizel, A.E., Metneki, J., Dudas, I., "The effect of preconceptional multivitamin supplementation on fertility," *International Journal of Vitaminology and Nutrition* Research, 66(1), 55–58 (1996).

5. Bergmann, J., Luft, B., Boehmann, S., Runnebaum, B., Gerhard, I., "The efficacy of the complex medication Phyto-Hypophyson L in female, hormone-related sterility. A randomized, placebo-controlled clinical double-blind study," *Forschrift für Komplementarmedizin und Klassische Naturheilkunde*, 7(4), 190–199 (August 2000).

6. Schultz,W.W., van Andel, P., Sabelis, I., Mooyaart, E., "Magnetic resonance imaging of male and female genitals during coitus and female sexual arousal," *BMJ*, 319, 1596–1600 (18 December 1999).

FETAL ALCOHOL SYNDROME

1. Zachman, R.D., Grummer, M.A., "The interaction of ethanol and vitamin A as a potential mechanism for the pathogenesis of fetal alcohol syndrome," *Alcoholism in Clinical and Experimental Research*, 22(7), 1544–1556 (October 1998).

2. Keppen, L.D., Moore, D.J., Cannon, D.J., "Zinc nutrition in fetal alcohol syndrome," *Neurotoxicology*, 11(2), 375–380 (Summer 1990).

FIBROCYSTIC BREAST DISEASE

1. Roubidoux, M.A., "Breast fibroadenoma," *eMedicine*, 3(6) (21 June 2002).

2. Petrakis, N.L., King, E.B., "Cytological abnormalities in nipple aspirates of breast fluid from women with severe constipation," *Lancet*, 2, 1203–1205 (1981).

3. Ernster, V.L., Mason, L., Goodson, W.H., et al., "Effects of caffeine-free diet on benign breast disease. A random trial," *Surgery*, 91, 263–267 (1982).

4. Ferrini, R.L., Barrett-Connor, E., "Caffeine intake and endogenous sex steroid levels in postmenopausal women. The rancho bernardo study," *American Journal of Epidemiology*, 144(7), 642–644 (1 October 1996).

5. Rammer, E., Friedrich, F., "Enzyme therapy in treatment of mastopathy. A randomized double-blind clinical study," *Wiener Klinischer Wochenschrift*, 108(6), 103–108 (1996).

6. Band, P.R., Deschamps, M., Falardeau, M., et al., "Treatment of benign breast disease with vitamin A," *Preventive Medicine*, 13, 549–554 (1984).

FIBROIDS

1. Faerstein, E., Szklo, M., Rosenshein, N.B., "Risk factors for uterine leiomyoma, a practice-based case-control study, II Atherogenic risk factors and potential sources of uterine irritation," *American Journal of Epidemiology*, 153(1), 11–19 (1 January 2001).

2. Chiaffarino, F., Parazzini, F., La Vecchia, C., Chatenoud, L., Di Cintio, E., Marsico, S., "Diet and uterine myomas," *Obstetrics and Gynecology*, 94(3), 395–398 (September 1999).

3. Zierau, O., Bodinet, C., Kolba, S., Wulf, M., Vollmer, G., "Antiestrogenic activities of *Cimicifuga racemosa* extracts," *Journal of Steroid Biochemistry and Molecular Biology*, 80(1), 125–130 (January 2002).

4. Freudenstein, J., Dasenbrock, C., Nisslein, T., "Lack of promotion of estrogen-dependent mammary gland tumors in vivo by an isopropanolic *Cimicifuga racemosa* extract," *Cancer Research*, 62(12), 3448–3452 (15 June 2002).

5. Düker, E.M., Kopanski, L., Jarry, H., Wuttke, W., "Effects of extracts from *Cimicifuga racemosa* on gonadotropin release in menopausal women and ovariectomized rats," *Planta Medica*, 57(5), 420–424 (October 1991).

6. Somekawa, Y., Chiguchi, M., Ishibashi, T., Wakana, K., Aso, T., "Efficacy of ipriflavone in preventing adverse effects of leuprolide," *Journal of Clinical Endocrinolgoy and Metabolism*, 86(7), 3202–3206 (July 2001).

FLATULENCE

1. Brunetton, J., *Pharmacognosy, Phytochemistry, Medicinal Plants* (Paris: Lavoisier Publishing, 1995), p. 444.

2. Safayhi, H., Sabieraj, J., Sailer, E.R., Ammon, H.P., "Chamazulene: an antioxidant-type inhibitor of leukotriene B4 formation," *Planta Medica*, 60(5), 410–413 (October 1994).

3. Miller, T., Wittstock, U., Lindequist, U., Teuscher, E., "Effects of some components of the essential oil of chamomile, *Chamomilla recutita*, on histamine release from rat mast cells," *Planta Medica*, 62(1), 60–61 (1 February 1996).

4. Kawakishi, S., Morimitsu, Y., Osawa, T., "Chemistry of ginger components and inhibitory factors of the arachidonic acid cascade," in Ho, C.T., Osawa, T., Huang, M.T., Rosen, R. (eds), *Food Phytochemicals for Cancer Prevention II: Teas, Spices, and Herbs* (Washington: American Chemical Society, 1994), pp. 244–249.

5. Bisset, N.G., Editor, *Herbal Drugs and Phytopharmaceuticals. A Handbook for Practice on a Scientific Basis* (Stuttgart, Germany: Medpharm Scientific Publishers, 1994), p. 538.

6. Bracken, J., "Ginger as an antiemetic: possible side effect due to its thromboxane synthetase activity," *Anaesthesia*, 46, 705–706 (1991).

7. Buchbauer, G., Jirovetz, L., Jager, W., Dietrich, H., Plank, C., "Aromatherapy: evidence for sedative effects of the essential oil of lavender after inhalation," *Zeitschrift für Naturforschung*, 46(11–12), 1067–1072 (November–December 1991).

8. Dew, M.J., "Peppermint oil for the irritable bowel syndrome: a multicentre trial," *British Journal of Clinical Practice*, 38, 394–398 (1984).

9. Suarez, F.L., Springfield, J., Levitt, M.D., "Identification of gases responsible for the odour of human flatus and evaluation of a device purported to reduce this odour," *Gut*, 43(1), 100–104 (July 1998).

10. Suarez, F.L., Furne, J., Springfield, J., Levitt, M.D., "Failure of activated charcoal to reduce the release of gases produced by colonic flora," *American Journal of Gastroenterology*, 94(1), 208–212 (January 1999).

FLU

1. Hawkes, W.C., Kelley, D.S., Taylor, P.C., "The effects of dietary selenium on the immune system in healthy men," *Biological Trace Elements Research*, 81(3), 189–213 (September 2001).

2. Rayman, M.P., Rayman, M.P., "The argument for increasing selenium intake," *Proceedings of the Nutrition Society*, 61(2), 203–215 (May 2002).

3. Visseren, F.L., Verkerk, M.S., van der Bruggen, T., Marx, J.J., van Asbeck, B.S., Diepersloot, R.J., "Iron chelation and hydroxyl radical scavenging reduce the inflammatory response of endothelial cells after infection with *Chlamydia pneumoniae* or influenza A," *European Journal of Clinical Investigation*, 32 Suppl 1, 84–90 (March 2002).

4. Gorton, H.C., Jarvis K., "The effectiveness of vitamin C in preventing and relieving the symptoms of virus-induced respiratory infections," *Journal of Manipulative Physiology and Therapy*, 22(8), 530–533 (October 1999).

5. Mileva, M., Bakalov, R., Tancheva, L., Galabov, A., Ribarov, S., "Effect of vitamin E supplementation on lipid peroxidation in blood and lung of influenza virus infected mice," *Comparative Immunology, Microbiology, and Infectious Disease*, 25(1), 1–11 (January 2002).

6. Hoheisel, O., Sandberg, M., Bertram, S., et al., "Echinagard treatment shortens the course of the common cold: a double-blind, placebo-controlled clinical trial," *European Journal of Clinical Research*, 9, 261–268 (1997).

7. Grimm, W., Müller, H.H., "A randomized controlled trial of the effect of fluid extract of *Echinacea purpurea* on the incidence and severity of colds and respiratory infections," *American Journal of Medicine*, 106(2), 138–143 (1999).

8. Facino, R.M., Carini, M., Aldini, G., Marinello, C., Arlandini, E., Franzoi, L., Colombo, M., Pietta, P., Mauri, P., "Direct characterization of caffeoyl esters with antihyaluronidase activity in crude extracts from *Echinacea angustifolia* roots by fast atom bombardment tandem mass spectrometry," *Farmaco*, 48(10), 1447–1461 (October 1993).

9. Budzinski, J.W., Foster, B.C., Vandenhoek, S., Arnason, J.T., "An in vitro evaluation of human cytochrome P405 3A4 inhibition by selected commercial herbal extracts and tinctures," *Phytomedicine*, 7(4), 273–282 (July 2000).

10. Luettig, B., Steinmuller, C., Gifford, G.E., Wagner, H., Lohmann-Matthes, M.L., "Macrophage activation by the polysaccharide arabinogalactan isolated from plant cell cultures of *Echinacea purpurea*," *Journal of the National Cancer Institute*, 81(9), 669–675 (3 May 1989).

11. Blumenthal, M., Goldberg, A., Brinckmann, J. *Herbal Medicine: Expanded Commission E Monographs* (Boston, Integrative Medicine, 2000), p. 88.

12. Barak, V., Halperin, T., Kalickman, I., "The effect of Sambucol, a black elderberry-based, natural product, on the production of human cytokines: I. Inflammatory cytokines," *European Cytokine Network*, 12(2), 290–296 (April–June 2001).

13. Zakay-Rones, Z., Varsano, N., Zlotnik, M., Manor, O., Regev, L., Schlesinger, M., Mumcuoglu, M., "Inhibition of several strains of influenza virus in vitro and reduction of symptoms by an elderberry extract (*Sambucus nigra* L.) during an outbreak of influenza B Panama, *Journal of Alternative and Complementary Medicine*, 1(4), 361–369 (Winter 1995).

14. Sarrell, E.M., Mandelberg, A., Cohen, H.A., "Efficacy of naturopathic extracts in the management of ear pain associated with acute otitis media," *Archives of Pediatric and Adolescent Medicine*, 155(7), 796–799 (July 2001).

15. Serkedjieva, J., "Combined antiinfluenza virus activity of Flos verbasci infusion and amantadine derivatives," *Phytotherapy Research*, 14(7), 571–574 (November 2000).

FOOT ODOR

1. Spielman, A.I., Sunavala, G., Harmony, J.A., Stuart, W.D., Leyden, J.J., Turner, G., Vowels, B.R., Lam, W.C., Yang, S., Preti, G., "Identification and immunohistochemical localization of protein precursors to human axillary odors in apocrine glands and secretions," *Archives of Dermatology*, 134(7), 813–818 (July 1998).

2. Carson, C.F., Riley, T.V., "The antimicrobial activity of tea tree oil," *Medical Journal of Australia*, 160, 236 (1994).

FOOT ULCERS (DIABETIC COMPLICATION)

1. Rodriguez-Moran, M., Guerrero-Romero, F., "Low serum magnesium levels and foot ulcers in subjects with type 2 diabetes," *Archives of Medical Research*, 32(4), 300–303 (July–August 2001).

2. Mudge, B.P., Harris, C., Gilmont, R.R., Adamson, B.S., Rees, R.S., "Role of glutathione redox dysfunction in diabetic wounds," *Wound Repair and Regeneration*, 10(1), 52–58 (January 2002).

FROSTBITE

1. Mechem, C.C., "Frostbite," *eMedicine*, 2(4) (26 April 2001).

2. Roncin, J.P., Schwartz, F., D'Arbigny, P., "EGb 761 in control of acute altitude sickness and vascular reactivity to cold exposure," *Aviation, Space, and Environmental Medicine*, 67, 445–452 (1996).

GALACTORRHEA

1. Küpper, C., Loch, E.G., "Prämenstruelles Syndrom," *Deutsche Apotheker Zeitung*, 136, 23–29 (1996).

2. Hobbs, C., "The chaste tree: vitex agnus castus," *Pharmacological History*, 23, 19–24 (1991).

3. Brugisser, R., Burkard, W., Simmen, U., Schaffner, W., "Untersuchungen an Opiod-Rezeptoren mit Vitrex agnus-castus L." In Agni-casti-fructus—Neue Erkenntnisse zur Qualität under Wirksamkeit," *Zeitschrift für Phytotherapie*, 20, 140–158 (1999).

4. Schellenberg, R., "Treatment for the premenstrual syndrome with agnus castus fruit extract: prospective, randomized, placebo controlled study," *British Medical Journal*, 322, 134–137 (20 January 2001).

5. Cahill, D.J., Fox, R., Wardel, P.G., Harlow, C.R., "Multiple follicular development associated with herbal medicine," *Human Reproduction*, 9(8), 1469–1470 (August 1994).

6. Bhargava, S.K., "Antiandrogenic effects of a flavonoid-rich fraction of *Vitex negundo* seeds: a histological and biochemical study in dogs," *Journal of Ethnopharmacology*, 27(3), 327–339 (December 1989).

GALLSTONES

1. Tierney, L.M., McPhee, S.J., Papadakis, M.A., *Current medical diagnosis and treatment*. (Appleton, Wisconsin: Lange. 1997) pp. 630–632.

2. Martinez de Pancorbo, C., Carballo, F., Horcajo, P., Aldeguer, M., de la Villa, I., Nieto, E., Gaspar, M.J., de la Morena, J., "Prevalence and associated factors for gallstone disease: results of a population survey in Spain," *Journal of Clinical Epidemiology*, 50(12),1347–1355 (December 1997).

3. Tomlinson, B., Chan, P., Lan, W., "How well tolerated are lipid-lowering drugs?" *Drugs and Aging*, 18(9), 665–683 (2001).

4. Misciagna, G., Guerra, V., Di Leo, A., Correale, M., Trevisan, M., "Insulin and gallstones: a population case control study in southern Italy," *Gut*, 47(1), 144–147 (July 2000).

5. Pakula, R., Konikoff, F.M., Moser, A.M., Greif, F., Tietz, A., Gilat, T., Rubin, M., "The effects of short term lipid infusion on plasma and hepatic bile lipids in humans," *Gut*, 45(3), 453–438 (September 1999).

6. Mendez-Sanchez, N., Gonzalez, V., Aguayo, P., Sanchez, J.M., Tanimoto, M.A., Elizondo, J., Uribe, M., "Fish oil (n-3) polyunsaturated fatty acids beneficially affect biliary cholesterol nucleation time in obese women losing weight," *Journal of Nutrition*, 131(9), 2300–2303 (September 2001).

7. Watts, J.M., Jablonski, P., Toouli, J., "The effect of added bran to the diet on the saturation of bile in people without gallstones," *American Journal of Surgery*, 135, 321–324 (1978).

8. McDougall, R.M., Kakymyshyn, L., Walker, K., Thurston, O.G., "Effect of wheat bran on serum lipoproteins and biliary lipids," *Canadian Journal of Surgery*, 21, 433–435 (1978).

9. Simon, J.A., Hunninghake, D.B., Agarwal, S.K., Lin, F., Cauley, J.A., Ireland, C.C., Pickar, J.H., "Effect of estrogen plus progestin on risk for biliary tract surgery in postmenopausal women with coronary artery disease. The heart and estrogen/progestin replacement study," *Annals of Internal Medicine*, 135(7), 493–501 (2 October 2001).

10. Pavel, S., "Sunbathing and gallstones," *Lancet*, 339, 241 (1992).

11. Leitzmann, M.F., Giovannucci, E.L., Rimm, E.B., Stampfer, M.J., Spiegelman, D., Wing, A.L., Willett, W.C., "The relation of physical activity to risk for symptomatic gallstone disease in men," *Annals of Internal Medicine*, 128(6), 417–425 (15 March 1998).

12. Leitzmann, M.F., Rimm, E.B., Willett, W.C., Spiegelman, D., Grodstein, F., Stampfer, M.J., Colditz, G.A., Giovannucci, E., "Recreational physical activity and the risk of cholecystectomy in women," *New England Journal of Medicine*, 341(11), 777–784 (9 September 1999).

13. Gustafsson, U., Wang, F.-H., Axelson, M., et al., "The effect of vitamin C in high doses on plasma and biliary lipid composition in patients with cholesterol gallstones: prolongation of the nucleation time," *European Journal of Clinical Investigation*, 27, 387–391 (1997).

14. Kratzer, W., Kachele, V., Mason, R.A., Muche, R., Hay, B., Wiesneth, M., Hill, V., Beckh, K., Adler, G., "Gallstone prevalence in relation to smoking, alcohol, coffee consumption, and nutrition. The Ulm Gallstone Study," *Scandinavian Journal of Gastroenterology*, 32(9), 953–958 (September 1997).

15. Leitzmann, M.F., Willett, W.C., Rimm, E.B., Stampfer, M.J., Spiegelman, D., Colditz, G.A., Giovannucci, E., "A prospective study of coffee consumption and the risk of symptomatic gallstone disease in men," *Journal of the American Medical Association*, 281(22), 2106–2112 (9 June 1999).

16. Dukas, L., Leitzmann, M.F., Willett, W.C., Colditz, G.A., Giovannucci, E.L., "Association of bowel movement frequency and use of laxatives with the occurrence of symptomatic gallstone disease in a prospective study of women," *American Journal of Gastroenterology*, 96(3), 715–721 (March 2001).

17. Leitzmann, M.F., Giovannucci, E.L., Stampfer, M.J., Spiegelman, D., Colditz, G.A., Willett, W.C., Rimm, E.B., "Prospective study of alcohol consumption patterns in relation to symptomatic gallstone disease in men," *Alcoholism in Clinical and Experimental Research*, 23(5), 835–841 (May 1999).

GASTRITIS

1. Beil, W., Birkholz, C., Sewing, K.F., "Effects of flavonoids on parietal cell acid secretion, gastric mucosal prostaglandin production and *Helicobacter pylori* growth," *Arzneimittel Forschung*, 45(6), 697–700 (1995).

2. Spirichev, V.B., Levachev, M.M., Rymarenko, T.V., et al., "The effect of administration of beta-carotene in an oil solution on its blood serum level and antioxidant status of patients with duodenal ulcer and erosive gastritis," *Voprosii Medizineho Khimii,* 38(6), 44–47 (1992).

3. Best, R., Lewis, D.A., Nasser, N., "The anti-ulcerogenic activity of the unripe plantain banana (*Musa* species)," *British Journal of Pharmacology,* 82, 107–116 (1984).

4. Sanyal, A.K., Gupa, K.K., Chowdhury, N.K., "Banana and experimental peptic ulcer," *Journal of Pharmacy and Pharmacology,* 15, 283–284 (1963).

5. Cicero, A.F., Gaddi, A., "Rice bran oil and gamma-oryzanol in the treatment of hyperlipoproteinaemias and other conditions," *Phytotherapy Research,* 15(4), 277–289 (June 2001).

6. Takemoto, T., Miyoshi, H., Nagashima, H., "Clinical trial of Hi-Z fine granules (gamma-oryzanol) on gastrointestinal symptoms at 375 hospitals (Japan)," *Shinyaku To Rinsho,* 25, 124 (1977)

7. Armuzzi, A., Cremonini, F., Ojetti, V., Bartolozzi, F., Canducci, F., Candelli, M., Santarelli, L., Cammarota, G., De Lorenzo, A., Pola, P., Gasbarrini, G., Gasbarrini, A., "Effect of *Lactobacillus* GG supplementation on antibiotic-associated gastrointestinal side effects during *Helicobacter pylori* eradication therapy: a pilot study," *Digestion,* 63, 1–7 (2001).

8. Sakamoto, I., Igarashi, M., Kimura, K., Takagi, A., Miwa, T., Koga, Y., "Suppressive effect of *Lactobacillus gasseri* OLL 2716 (LG21) on *Helicobacter pylori* infection in humans," *Journal of Antimicrobial Chemotherapy,* 47(5), 709–710 (May 2001).

9. Jarosz, M., Dzieniszewski, J., Dabrowska-Ufinarz, E., et al, "Effects of high dose vitamin C treatment on *Helicobacter pylori* infection and total vitamin C concentration in gastric juice," *European Journal of Cancer Prevention,* 7, 449–454 (1998).

10. Farinati, F., Della Libera, G., Cardin, R., Molari, A., Plebani, M., Rugge, M., Di Mario, F., Naccarato, R., "Gastric antioxidant, nitrites, and mucosal lipoperoxidation in chronic gastritis and *Helicobacter pylori* infection," Journal of Clinical Gastroenterology, 22(4), 275–281 (June 1996).

11. Sobala, G.M., Schorah, C.J., Shjires, S., et al., "Effect of eradication of *Helicobacter pylori* on gastric juice ascorbic acid concentrations," *Gut* 34, 1038–1041 (1993).

12. Schorah, C.J., Sobala, G.M., Sanderson, M., et al, "Gastric juice and ascorbic acid: effects of disease and implications for gastric carcinogenesis," *American Journal of Clinical Nutrition,* 53, 287–293S (1991).

GASTROPARESIS (DIABETIC COMPLICATION)

1. De Block, C.E., De Leeuw, I.H., Pelckmans, P.A., Callens, D., Maday, E., Van Gaal, L.F., "Delayed gastric emptying and gastric autoimmunity in type 1 diabetes," *Diabetes Care,* 25(5), 912–917 (May 2002).

2. Gutfreund, A.E., Taussig, S.J., Morris, A.K., "Effect of oral bromelain on blood pressure and heart rate of hypertensive patients," *Hawaii Medical Journal,* 37, 143–146 (1978).

3. Suarez, F., Levitt, M.D., Adshead, J., Barkin, J.S., "Pancreatic supplements reduce symptomatic response of healthy subjects to a high fat meal," *Digestive Diseases and Sciences,* 44, 1317–1321 (1999).

4. Andersen, T., Fogh, J., "Weight loss and delayed gastric emptying following a South American herbal preparation in overweight patients," *Journal of Human Nutrition and Dietetics,* 14(3), 243–250 (June 2001).

5. Chang, C.S., Ko, C.W., Wu, C.Y., Chen, G.H., "Effect of electrical stimulation on acupuncture points in diabetic patients with gastric dysrhythmia: a pilot study," *Digestion,* 64(3), 184–190 (2001).

GENITAL WARTS

1. Carson, S., "Human papillomatous virus infection update: impact on women's health. *The Nurse Practitioner,* 22, 24–35 (1997).

2. Kiviat, N.B., Koutsky, L.A., Paavonen, J.A., Galloway, D.A., Critchlow, C.W., Beckmann, A.M, McDougall, J.K., Peterson, M.L., Stevens, C.E., Lipinski ,C.M., et al, "Prevalence of genital papillomavirus infection among women attending a college student health clinic or a sexually transmitted disease clinic," *Journal of Infectious Disease,* 159(2), 293–302 (February 1989).

3. Romney, S.I., Palan, B.R., Basu, J., Mikhail, M., "Nutrient antioxidants in the pathogenesis and prevention of cervical dysplasias and cancer," *Journal of Cellular Biochemistry,* 23 (Suppl), 96–103 (1995).

4. Bendich, A., "Beta-carotene and the immune response," *Proceedings of the Nutrition Society,* 50, 263–274 (1991).

5. Underwood, B., "Vitamin A in animal and human nutrition." In *The Retinoids,* Volume I (Orlando, Florida, Academic Press, 1984), pp. 282–392.

6. Harper, J.M., Levine, A.J., Rosenthal, D.L., "Erythrocyte folate levels, oral contraceptive use, and abnormal cervical cytology," *Acta Cytologica,* 38, 324–330 (1994).

7. Beisel, W., Edelman, R., Nauss, K., Suskind, R., "Single-nutrient effects on immunologic functions," *Journal of the American Medical Association,* 245, 53–538 (1981)

8. Yeo, A.S., Schiff M.A., Montoya G., Masuk, M., van Asselt-King, L., Becker, T.M., "Serum micronutrients and cervical dysplasia in Southwestern American Indian women," *Nutrition and Cancer,* 38(2), 141–150 (2000).

9. Dowd, P., Heatley, R., "The influence of undernutrition on immunity," *Clinical Science,* 66, 241–418 (1984).

10. Ramaswamy, P., Natarajan, R., "Vitamin B status in patients with cancer of the uterine cervix," *Nutrition and Cancer,* 6, 176–180 (1984).

11. Dawson, E., Nosovitch, J., Harrigan, E., "Serum vitamin and selenium changes in cervical dysplasia," *Federation Proceedings,* 43, 612 (1984).

12. Mason, B., Ghanee, N., Haigh, W.G., Lee, S.P., Oda, D., "Effect of vitamins A, C and E on normal and HPV-immortalized human oral epithelial cells in culture," *Anticancer Research,* 19(6B), 5469–5474 (November–December 1999).

13. Hamilton, I.M., Gilmore, W.S., Benzie, I.F., Mulholland, C.W., Strain, J.J., "Interactions between vitamins C and E in human subjects," *British Journal of Nutrition,* 84(3), 261–267 (September 2000).

14. Kubena, K.S., McMurray, D.N., "Nutrition and the immune system: a review of nutrient-nutrient interactions," *Journal of the American Dietetic Association,* 96(11), 1156–1164 (November 1996).

15. Wassertheil-Smoller, S., Romney, S.L., Wylie-Rosett, J., Slagle, S., Miller, G., Lucido, D., Duttagupta, C., Palan, P.R., "Dietary vitamin C and uterine cervical dysplasia," *American Journal of Epidemiology,* 114, 714–724 (1981).

16. Mann, G., Newton, P., "The membrane transport of ascorbic acid," *Annals of the New York Academy of Sciences,* 258, 243–251 (1975).

17. Kellhere, J., "Vitamin E and the immune response," *Proceedings of the Nutrition Society,* 50, 245–249 (1991).

18. Liu, T., Soong, S.J., Alvarez, R.D., Butterworth, C.E., "A longitudinal analysis of human papillomavirus 16 infection, nutritional status, and cervical dysplasia progression," *Cancer Epidemiology, Biomarkers, and Prevention,* 4, 373–380 (1995).

19. Moore, T.O., Moore, A.Y., Carrasco, D., Vander Straten, M., Arany, I., Au, W., Tyring, S.K., "Human papillomavirus, smoking, and cancer," *Journal of Cutaneous Medicine and Surgery,* 5(4), 323–328 (July–August 2001).

GIARDIASIS

1. Pennardt, A., "Giardiasis," *eMedicine,* 2(4) (19 April 2001).

2. Choudhry, V.P., Sabir, M., Bhide, V.N., "Berberine in giardiasis," *Indian Pediatriacian,* 9, 143–146 (1972).

3. Moya-Camarena, S.Y., Sotelo, N., Valencia, M.E., "Effects of asymptomatic *Giardia intestinalis* infection on carbohydrate absorption in well-nourished Mexican children," *American Journal of Tropical Medicine and Hygiene,* 66(3), 255–259 (March 2002).

4. Ertan, P., Yereli, K., Kurt, O., Balcioglu, I.C., Onag, A., "Serological levels of zinc, copper and iron elements among *Giardia lamblia* infected children in Turkey," *Pediatrics International,* 44(3), 286–288 (June 2002).

GILBERT'S SYNDROME

1. Bombardieri, G., "Effects of S-adenosyl-methionine (SAMe) in the treatment of Gilbert's syndrome," *Current Therapeutic Research,* 37, 580–585 (1985).

GINGIVITIS

1. Murray, M., Pizzorno, J., *Encyclopedia of Natural Medicine* (London: Churchill-Livingstone, 1999), p. 1486.

2. Page, R., Schroeder, H., "Current status of the host response in chronic marginal periodontitis," *Journal of Periodontal Dentistry,* 52, 477–491 (1981).

3. Otake, S., Makimura, M., Kuroki, T., Nishihara, Y., Hirasawa, M., "Anti-caries effects of polyphenolic compounds from Japanese green tea," *Caries Research* (Switzerland), 25(6), 438–443 (1991).

4. Murray, M., Pizzorno, J., p. 1488.

5. Addya, S., Chakravarti, K., Basu, A., et al., ibid.

6. Prasad, A., "Clinical, biochemical and nutritional spectrum of zinc deficiency in human subjects: an update," *Nutrition Review,* 41, 197–308 (1983).

7. Freeland, J., Cousins, R., Schwartz, R., "Relationship of mineral status and intake to periodontal disease," *American Journal of Clinical Nutrition,* 29, 745–749 (1976).

8. Addya, S., Chakravarti, K., Basu, A., et al., "Effects of mercuric chloride on several scavenging enzymes in rat kidney and influence of vitamin E supplementation," *Acta Vitaminologica et Enzymologica,* 6, 103–107 (1984).

9. Godkowsky, K.C.," Antimicrobial action of sanguinarine," *Journal of Clinical Dentistry,* 1, 96–101 (1989).

GLAUCOMA, CHRONIC

1. Braunwald, E., Fauci, A.S., Kasper, D.L., Hauser, S.L., Longo, D.L., Jameson, J.L., editors. *Harrison's Principles of Internal Medicine,* Fifteenth Edition (New York: McGraw-Hill, 2001), pp. 172–173.

2. Bhuyan, K.C., Bhuyan, D.K., "Molecular mechanism of cataractogenesis: III. Toxic metabolites of oxygen as initiators of lipid peroxidation and cataract," *Current Eye Research,* 3, 67–81 (1984).

3. Knepper, P.A., Goossens, W., Palmberg, P.F., "Glycosaminoglycan stratification of the juxtacanalicular tissue in normal and primary open-angle glaucoma," *Investigational Ophthalmology,* 37, 2414–2425 (1996).

4. Knepper, P.A., McLone, D.G., "Glycosaminoglycans and outflow pathways of the eye and brain," *Pediatric Neuroscience,* 12, 240–251 (1985).

5. Bunin, A.I., Filina, A.A., Erichev, V.P.," Glutathione deficiency in open-angle glaucoma and the approaches to its correction," *Vestnik Optamologii,* 108(4–6), 13–15 (July–December 1992).

6. Kurysheva, N.I., Vinetskaia, M.I., Erichev, V.P., Demchuk, M.L., Kuryshev, S.I., "Contribution of free-radical reactions of chamber humor to the development of primary open-angle glaucoma *Vestnik Optamologii,* 112(4), 3–5 (September–October 1996).

7. Beers, M.H., Berkow, R., eds., *Merck Manual,* Centennial Edition (Whitehouse Station, NJ: Merck Research Laboratories; 1999).

8. Filina, A.A., Davydova, N.G., Kolomoitseva, E.M., "The effect of lipoic acid on the components of the glutathione system in the lacrimal fluid of patients with open-angle glaucoma," *Vestnik Oftalmologii,* 109, 5–7 (1993).

9. Bunin, A.I., Filina, A.A., Erichev, V.P., "A glutathione deficiency in open-angle glaucoma and the approaches to its correction," *Vestnik Oftalmologii,* 108, 13–15 (1992).

10. Filina, A.A., Davydova, N.G., Endrikhovskii, S.N., Shamshinova, A.M., "Lipoic acid as a means of metabolic therapy of open-angle glaucoma," *Vestnik Oftalmologii,* 111 (4), 16–18 (October 1995).

11. Caselli, L., "Clinical and electroretinographic study on activity of anthocyanosides," *Archivio di Medicina Interna,* 37, 29–35 (1985).

12. Bindoli, A., Valente, M., Cavallini, L., "Inhibitory action of quercetin on xanthine oxidase and xanthine dehydrogenase activity," *Pharmacology Research Communications,* 17, 831–839 (1985).

13. Gaspar, A.Z., Gasser, P., Flammer, J., "The influence of magnesium on visual field and peripheral vasospasm in glaucoma," *Ophthalmologica,* 209(1), 11–13 (1995).

14. Samples, J.R., Krause, G., Lewy, A.J., "Effect of melatonin on intraocular pressure," *Current Eye Research,* 7, 649–653. (1998).

15. Asregadoo, E.R., "Blood levels of thiamine and ascorbic acid in chronic open-angle glaucoma," *Annals of Ophthalmology,* 11, 1095–1100 (1979).

16. Sakai, T., "Effect of long-term treatment of glaucoma with vitamin B_{12}," *Glaucoma,* 14, 167–170 (1992).

17. Virno, M., Bucci, M., Pecori-Giraldi, J., Missiroli, A., "Oral treatment of glaucoma with vitamin C," *Eye Ear Nose Throat Monthly,* 46, 1502–1508 (1967),

18. Schachtschabel, D.O., Binninber, E., "Stimulatory effects of ascorbic acid in hyaluronic acid synthesis of in vitro cultured normal and glaucomatous trabecular meshwork cells of the human eye," *Zeitschrift für Gerontologie,* 26, 243–246 (1993).

19. Takahashi, N., Iwasaka, T., Sugiura, T., Onoyama, H., Kurihara, S., Inada, M., Miki, H., Uyama, M., "Effect of coenzyme Q_{10} on hemodynamic response to ocular timolol," *Journal of Cardiovascular Pharmacology,* 14(3), 264–468 (September 1989).

20. Tengroth, B., Ammitzboll, T., "Changes in the content and composition of collagen in the glaucomatous eye—basis for a new hypothesis for the genesis of chronic open-angle glaucoma," *Acta Ophthalmologica,* 62, 999–1008 (1984).

GONORRHEA

1. Dodson, P.S., "The polymicrobial etiology of acute pelvic inflammatory disease and treatment regimens," *Review of Infectious Disease,* 7, S6996–S7002 (1985).

2. Stoner, B.P., Douglas, J.M., Jr., Martin, D.H., Hook, E.W., 3rd, Leone, P., McCormack, W.M., Mroczkowski, T.F., Jones, R., Yang, J., Baumgartner, T., "Single-dose gatifloxacin compared with Ofloxacin for the treatment of uncomplicated gonorrhea: a randomized, double-blind, multicentre trial," *Sexually Transmitted Diseases,* 28(3), 136–142 (March 2001).

3. Brunham, R.C., "Therapy for acute pelvic inflammatory disease: a critique of recent treatment trials," *American Journal of Obstetrics and Gynecology,* 148, 235–240 (1985).

4. Cazzola, P., Mazzanti, P., Bossi, G., "In vivo modulating effect of a calf thymus acid lysate on human T lymphocyte subsets and CD4+/CD8+ ratio in the course of difference diseases," *Current Therapies Research,* 42, 1011–1017 (1987).

5. Seifter, E., Rettura, G., Seiter, J., "Thymotrophic action of vitamin A," *Federal Proceedings,* 32, 947 (1973).

6. Semba, R.D., "Vitamin A, immunity, and infection," *Clinical Infectious Disease,* 19, 489–499 (1994).

7. Roberts, N. "Pelvic Inflammatory Disease." In Pizzorno, Jr., J.E., Murray, M.T., *Textbook of Natural Medicine* (London: Churchill Livingstone, 1999), p. 1474.

8. Ringsdorf, W., Cheraskin, E., "Vitamin C and human wound healing," *Oral Surgery,* 53(3), 231–236 (March 1982).

9. Gabor, M., "Pharmacologic effects of flavonoids on blood vessels," *Angiologica,* 9, 355–374 (1972).

10. Prasad, A., "Clinical, biochemical and nutritional spectrum of zinc deficiency in human subjects. An update," *Nutrition Review,* 41, 197–208 (1983).

11. Neubauer, R., "A plant protease and possible replacement of antibiotics," *Experimental Medicine and Surgery,* 19, 1430–169 (1961).

12. Shipochliev, T., Dimitrov, A., Aleksandrova, E., "Anti-inflammatory action of a group of plant extracts," *Veterinarskii i Medinitzskii Nauki,* 18(6), 87–94 (1981).

13. Kuhn, O., untitled article, *Arzneimittel-Forschung,* 3, 194–200 (1953).

14. Erhard, M., "Effect of echinacea, aconitum, lachesis, and apis extracts, and their combinations of phagocytosis of human granulocytes," *Phytotherapy Research,* 8, 14–77 (1994).

15. Facino, R.M., Carini, M., Aldini, G., Marinello, C., Arlandini, E., Franzoi, L., Colombo, M., Pietta, P., Mauri, P., "Direct characterization of caffeoyl esters with antihyaluronidase activity in crude extracts from *Echinacea angustifolia* roots by fast atom bombardment tandem mass spectrometry," *Farmaco,* 48(10), 1447–1461 (October 1993).

16. Budzinski, J.W., Foster, B.C., Vandenhoek, S. Arnason, J.T., "An in vitro evaluation of human cytochrome P405 3A4 inhibition by selected commercial herbal extracts and tinctures," *Phytomedicine*, 7(4), 273–282 (July 2000).

17. Luettig, B., Steinmuller, C., Gifford, G.E., Wagner, H., Lohmann-Matthes, M.L., "Macrophage activation by the polysaccharide arabinogalactan isolated from plant cell cultures of *Echinacea purpurea*," *Journal of the National Cancer Institute*, 81(9), 669–675 (3 May 1989).

18. Rehman, J., Dillow, J.M., Carter, S.M., Chou, J., Le, B., Maisel, A.S., "Increased production of antigen-specific immunoglobulins G and M following in vivo treatment with the medical plants *Echinacea angustifolia* and *Hydrastis canadensis*," *Immunology Letters*, 68(2–3), 391–395 (1 June 1999).

19. Iinuma, M., Tanaka, T., Sakakibara, N., Mizuno, M., Matsuda, H., Shiomoto, H., Kubo, M., "Phagocytic activity of leaves of Epimedium species on mouse reticuloendotherial system," *Yakugaku Zasshi*, 110(3),179–185 (March 1990).

20. Cornelissen, C.N., Kelley, M., Hobbs, M.M., Anderson, J.L., Cannon, J.G., Cohen, M.S., Sparling, P.F., "The transferrin receptor expressed by gonococcal strain FA1090 is required for the experimental infection of human male volunteers," *Molecular Microbiology*, 27(3), 611–616 (February 1998).

21. Payne, S.M., Finkelstein, R.A., "Pathogenesis and immunology of experimental gonococcal infection: role of iron in virulence," *Infection and Immunology*, 12(6), 1313–1318 (1975).

22. Mertz, K.J., Finelli, L., Levine, W.C., Mognoni, R.C., Berman, S.M., Fishbein, M., Garnett, G., St. Louis, M.E., "Gonorrhea in male adolescents and young adults in Newark, New Jersey: implications of risk factors and patient preferences for prevention strategies," *Sexually Transmitted Diseases*, 27(4), 201–207 (April 2000).

23. Diseker, R.A., 3rd, Peterman, T.A., Kamb, M.L., Kent, C., Zenilman, J.M., Douglas, J.M., Jr., Rhodes, F., Iatesta, M., "Circumcision and STD in the United States: cross sectional and cohort analyses," *Sexually Transmitted Diseases*, 76(6), 474–479 (December 2000).

24. Marchbanks, P., Lee, N.C., Peterson, H.B., "Cigarette smoking as a risk factor for pelvic inflammatory disease," *American Journal of Obstetrics and Gynecology*, 162, 639–644 (1990).

25. Scholes, D., "Current cigarette smoking and risk of acute pelvic inflammatory disease," *American Journal of Public Health*, 82, 1352–1355 (1992).

26. Tucker, M.E., "Douching raises pelvic inflammatory disease risk," *Family Practice News*, (15 August 1996).

27. Ndimbie, O.K., Kingsley, L.A., Nedjar, S., Rinaldo, C.R., "Hepatitis C virus infection in a male homosexual cohort: risk factor analysis," *Genitourinary Medicine*, 72(30), 213–216 (June 1996).

28. Keith, L., Berger, G., Edelman, D., Newton, W., Fullan, N., Bailey, R., Friberg, J., "On the causation of pelvic disease," *American Journal of Obstetrics and Gynecology*, 149, 215–224 (1984).

29. Eenham, I., "Pelivc inflammatory disease," *Australian Family Physician*, 15, 254–256 (1986).

30. Cromer, B., Heald, F., "Pelvic inflammatory disease associated with *Neisseria gonorrhoeae* and *Chlamydia trachomatis*. Clinical correlates," *Sexually Transmitted Diseases*, 14, 125–129 (1987).

GOUT

1. Braunwald, E., Fauci, A.S., Kasper, D.L., Hauser, S.L., Longo, D.L., Jameson, J.L., editors, *Harrison's Principles of Internal Medicine*, Fifteenth Edition (New York: McGraw-Hill, 2001), p. 1994.

2. Barceloux, D.G., "Molybdenum," *Journal of Toxicology and Clinical Toxicology*, 37(2), 231–237 (1999).

3. Struthers, A.D., Donnan, P.T., Lindsay, P., McNaughton, D., Broomhall, J., MacDonald, T.M., "Effect of allopurinol on mortality and hospitalisations in chronic heart failure: a retrospective cohort study," *Heart*, 87(3), 229–234 (March 2002).

4. Hisatome, I., Kitamura, H., Saito, M., Kinugawa, T., Miyakoda, H., Kotake, H., Mashiba, H., Azumi, T., Ohno, K., Takeda, A,, et al., "Excess release of hypoxanthine from exercising muscle in two gout patients with partial HG-PRTase deficiency: lack of ammonium release," *American Journal of Medicine*, 90(4), 533–535 (April 1991).

5. Dessein, P.H., Shipton, E.A., Stanwix, A.E., Joffe, B.I., Ramokgadi, J., "Beneficial effects of weight loss associated with moderate calorie/carbohydrate restriction, and increased proportional intake of protein and unsaturated fat on serum urate and lipoprotein levels in gout: a pilot study," *Annals of Rheumatic Disease*, 59(7), 539–543 (July 2000).

6. Havsteen, B., "Flavonoids, a class of natural products of high pharmacological potency," *Biochemical Pharmacology*, 32, 1141–1148 (1983).

7. Caspi, D., Lubart, E., Graff, E., Habot, B., Yaron, M., Segal, R., "The effect of mini-dose aspirin on renal function and uric acid handling in elderly patients," *Arthritis and Rheumatology*, 43(1), 103–108 (January 2000).

8. Kiefer, G., "Twenty-year-old patient with pseudogout," *Schweizer Rundschau für Medizin Praxis*, 90(51–52), 2295–2297 (20 December 2001).

9. Petty, H.R., Fernando, M., Kindzelskii, A.L., Zarewych, B.N., Ksebati, M.B., Hryhorczuk, L.M., Mobashery, S., "Identification of colchicine in placental blood from patients using herbal medicines," *Chemical Research and Toxicology*, 14(9), 1254–1258 (September 2001).

HAIR LOSS, MALE-PATTERN

1. Prager, K., Bickett, N., French, N., Marcovici, G., "A randomized, double-blind, placebo controlled to determine the effectiveness of biologically derived inhibitors of 5–reductase in the treatment of androgenetic alopecia," *Journal of Alternative and Complementary Medicine*, 2(8), 143–152 April 2002).

HALITOSIS

1. Page, R., Schroeder, H., "Current status of the host response in chronic marginal periodontitis," *Journal of Periodontal Dentistry*, 52, 477–491 (1981).

2. Otake, S., Makimura, M., Kuroki, T., Nishihara, Y., Hirasawa, M., "Anticaries effects of polyphenolic compounds from Japanese green tea," *Caries Research* (Switzerland), 25(6), 438–443 (1991).

3. Murray, M., Pizzorno, J., *Textbook of Natural Medicine* (London: Churchill-Livingstone, 1999), p. 1488.

4. Addya, S., Chakravarti, K., Basu, A., et al., "Effects of mercuric chloride on several scavenging enzymes in rat kidney and influence of vitamin E supplementation," *Acta Vitaminologica et Enzymologica*, 6, 103–107 (1984).

5. Prasad, A., "Clinical, biochemical and nutritional spectrum of zinc deficiency in human subjects: an update," *Nutrition Review*, 41, 197–308 (1983).

6. Freeland, J., Cousins, R., Schwartz, R., "Relationship of mineral status and intake to periodontal disease," *American Journal of Clinical Nutrition*, 29, 745–749 (1976).

7. Addya, S., Chakravarti, K., Basu, A., et al., "Effects of mercuric chloride on several scavenging enzymes in rat kidney and influence of vitamin E supplementation," *Acta Vitaminologica et Enzymologica*, 6, 103–107 (1984).

8. Godkowsky, K.C., "Antimicrobial action of sanguinarine," *Journal of Clinical Dentistry*, 1, 96–101 (1989).

HEARTBURN

1. Rodriguez-Stanley, S., Collings, K.L., Robinson, M., Owen, W., Miner, P.B., Jr., "The effects of capsaicin on reflux, gastric emptying and dyspepsia," *Alimentary Pharmcology and Therapy*, 14(1), 129–134 (January 2000).

2. Terry, P., Lagergren, J., Wolk, A., Nyren, O., "Reflux inducing dietary factors and risk of adenocarcinoma of the esophagus and gastric cardia," *Nutrition and Cancer*, 28(2), 186–191 (2000).

3. Colombo, P., Mangano, M., Bianchi, P.A., Penagini, R., "Effect of calories and fat on postprandial gastro-oesophageal reflux," *Scandinavian Journal of Gastroenterology*, 37(1), 3–5 (January 2002).

4. Morgan, A.G., Pacsoo, C., McAdam, W.A.F., "Maintenance therapy: a two-year comparison between Caved-S and cimetidine treatment in the prevention of symptomatic gastric ulcer recurrence," *Gut*, 26, 599–602 (1985).

5. Kassir, Z.A., "Endoscopic controlled trial of four drug regimens in the treatment of chronic duodenal ulceration," *Irish Medical Journal*, 78, 153–156 (1985).

HEAVY PERIODS (MENORRHAGIA)

1. Hallberg, L., Hogdahl, A., Nilsson, L., Rybo, G., "Menstrual blood loss—a population study," *Acta Obstetrica et Gynaecologica Scandinavica,* 45, 320–351 (1966).

2. Lusher, J.M., "Systemic causes of excessive uterine bleeding," *Seminars in Hematology,* 36(3 Suppl 4), 10–20 (July 1999).

3. Lithgow, D.M., Politzer, W.M., "Vitamin A in the treatment of menorrhagia," *South African Medical Journal,* 51(7), 191–193 (February 1977).

4. Tielens, J.A., "Vitamin C for paroxetine- and fluvoxamine-associated bleeding," *American Journal of Psychiatry,* 154(6), 883–884 (June 1997).

5. Dasgupta, P.R., Dutta, S., Banerjee, P., Majumdar, S., "Vitamin E (alpha tocopherol) in the management of menorrhagia associated with the use of intrauterine contraceptive devices (IUCD)," *International Journal of Fertility,* 28(1), 55–56 (1983).

6. Taymor, M.L., Sturgis, S.H., Yahia, C., "The etiological role of chronic iron deficiency in production of menorrhagia," *Journal of the American Medical Association,* 187, 323–327 (1964).

7. Jensen, J.T., Speroff, L., "Health benefits of oral contraceptives," *Obstetrics and Gynecology Clinics of North America,* 27(4), 705–721 (December 2000).

8. Hope, S., "10-minute consultation: menorrhagia," *British Medical Journal,* 321, 935 (14 October 2000).

HEMORRHOIDS

1. Pizzorno, J.E., Jr., Murray, M.T., *Textbook of Natural Medicine* (London: Churchill Livingstone, 1999), 1262.

2. Gopal, D.V., "Diseases of the rectum and anus: a clinical approach to common disorders," *Clinical Cornerstones,* 4(4), 34–48 (2002).

3. Delco, F., Sonnenberg, A., "Associations between hemorrhoids and other diagnoses," *Diseases of the Colon and Rectum,* 41(12), 1534–1541, discussion 1541–1542 (December 1998).

4. Johanson, J.F., "Association of hemorrhoidal disease with diarrheal disorders: potential pathogenic relationship," *Diseases of the Colon and Rectum,* 40(2), 215–219, discussion 219–221 (February 1997).

5. Godeberg, P., "Daflon 500 mg in the treatment of hemorrhoidal disease: a demonstrated efficacy in comparison with placebo," *Angiology,* 45(6 Pt. 2), 574–578 (June 1994).

6. Cospite, M., "Double-blind, placebo-controlled evaluation of clinical activity and safety of Daflon 500 mg in the treatment of acute hemorrhoids," *Angiology,* 45(6 Pt. 2), 566–573 (June 1994).

7. Misra, M.C., Parshad, R., "Randomized clinical trial of micronized flavonoids in the early control of bleeding from acute internal haemorrhoids," *British Journal of Surgery,* 87(7), 868–872 (2000).

8. Russo, A., Fraser, R., Horowitz, M., "The effect of cute hyperglycemia on small intestinal motility in normal subjects," *Diabetologia,* 39, 984–989 (1989).

9. Pizzorno, J.E., Jr., Murray, M.T., *Textbook of Natural Medicine* (London: Churchill Livingstone, 1999), 1360–1361.

HEPATITIS A

1. Gilroy, R., "Hepatitis A," *eMedicine,* 3(2) (11February 2002).

HEPATITIS B

1. Lee, D.H., Kim, J.H., Nam, J.J., Kim, H.R., Shin, H.R., "Epidemiological findings of hepatitis B infection based on 1998 national health and nutrition survey in Korea," *Journal of Korean Medical Science,* 17(4), 457–462 (August 2002).

2. Kessler, A.T., "Hepatitis B," *eMedicine,* 3 (1) (4 January 2002).

3. Andreone, Fiorino, S., Cursaro, C., Gramenzi, A., Margotti, M., Di Giammarino, L., Biselli, M., Miniero, R., Gasbarrini, G., Bernardi, M., "Vitamin E as treatment for chronic hepatitis B: results of a randomized controlled pilot trial," *Antiviral Research,* 49(2), 75–81 (February 2001).

4. Kakumu, S., Yoshioka, K., Wakita, T., Ishikawa, T., "Effects of TJ-9 Sho-saiko-

to (kampo medicine) on interferon gamma and antibody production specific for hepatitis B virus antigen in patients with type B chronic hepatitis," *International Journal of Pharmacology,* 13(2–3), 141–146 (1991).

5. Barbieri, B., Lund, B., Lundstrom, B., Scaglione, F., "Coenzyme Q$_{10}$ administration increases antibody titer in hepatitis B vaccinated volunteers—a single blind placebo-controlled and randomized clinical study," *Biofactors,* 9(2–4), 351–357 (1999).

6. Meydani, S.N., Meydani, M., Blumberg, J.B., Leka, L.S., Siber, G., Loszewski, R., Thompson, C., Pedrosa, M.C., Diamond, R.D., Stollar, B.D., "Vitamin E supplementation and in vivo immune response in healthy elderly subjects. A randomized controlled trial," *Journal of the American Medical Association,* 277(17), 1380–1386 (7 May 1997).

7. Andreone, Fiorino, S., Cursaro, C., Gramenzi, A., Margotti, M., Di Giammarino, L., Biselli, M., Miniero, R., Gasbarrini, G., Bernardi, M., ibid.

HEPATITIS C

1. Dhawan, V.K, "Hepatitis C," *eMedicine,* 3(4) (5 April 2002).

2. Hickman, I.J., Clouston, A.D., Macdonald, G.A., Purdie, D.M., Prins, J.B., Ash, S., Jansson, J.R., Powell, E.E., "Effect of weight reduction on liver histology and biochemistry in patients with chronic hepatitis C," *Gut,* 51, 89–94 (July 2002).

3. Naveau, S., Abella, A., Raynard, B., Balian, A., Giraud, V., Montembault, S., Mathurin, P., Keros, L.G., Portier, A., Capron, F., Emilie, D., Galanaud, P., Chaput, J.C., "Tumor necrosis factor soluble receptor p55 and lipid peroxidation in patients with acute alcoholic hepatitis," *American Journal of Gastroenterology,* 96(12), 3361–3367 (December 2001).

4. Buzzelli, G., Moscarella, S., Giusti, A., Duchini, A., Marena, C., Lampertico, M., "A pilot study on the liver protective effect of silybin-phosphatidylcholine complex (IdB1016) in chronic active hepatitis," *International Journal of Clinical Pharmacology and Therapeutics,* 31(9), 456–460 (September 1993).

5. Ferenci, P., Dragosics, B., Dittrich, H., Frank, H., Benda, L., Lochs, H., Meryn, S., Base, W., Schneider, B., "Randomized controlled trial of silymarin treatment in patients with cirrhosis of the liver," *Journal of Hepatology,* 9, 105–113 (1989).

6. Farghali, H., Kamenikova, L., Hynie, S., Kmonickova, E., "Silymarin effects of intracellular calcium and cytotoxicity: a study in perfused rat hepatocytes after oxidative stress injury," *Pharmacological Research,* 41, 231–237 (2000).

7. Sonnenbichler, J., Zetl, I., "Biochemical effects of the flavonolignane silibinin on RNA, protein and DNA synthesis in rat livers." In Cody, V., Middleton, E., Harborne, J.B., editors, *Plant Flavonoids in Biology and Medicine: Biochemical, Pharmacological and Structure-Activity Relations.* (New York: Liss, 1986), 319–331.

8. Frenci, P., Dragosics, B., Dittrich, H., et al., "Randomized controlled trial of silymarin treatment in patients with cirrhosis of the liver," *Journal of Hepatology,* 9, 105–113 (1989).

9. Yamamoto, S., Ohmoto, K., Ideguchi, S., Yamamoto, R., Mitsui, Y., Shimabara, M., Iguchi, Y., Ohumi, T., Takatori, K., "Painful muscle cramps in liver cirrhosis and effects of oral taurine administration," *Nippon Shokakibyo Gakkai Zasshi,* 91(7), 1205–1209 (July 1994).

10. Ferenci ,P., Wewalka, F., "Parenteral feeding of patients with liver cirrhosis with hepatic encephalopathy," *Infusionstherapie und Klinische Ernährung,* 7(2), 72–78 (1980).

11. Marchesini, G., Bianchi, G., Rossi, B., Brizi, M., Melchionda, N., "Nutritional treatment with branched-chain amino acids in advanced liver cirrhosis," *Journal of Gastroenterology,* 35(Suppl), 7–12 (2000).

HERPES

1. Fleming, D.T., McQuillan, G.M., Johnson, R.E., Nahmias, A.J., Aral, S.O., Lee, F.K., St. Louis, M.E.. "Herpes simplex virus type 2 in the United States, 1976 to 1994," *New England Journal of Medicine,* 337, 1105–1111 (1997).

2. Corey, I., Wald. A., "New developments in the biology of genital herpes," In Sacks, S.I., Straus, S.F., Whitley, R.J., Griffiths, P.D., eds., *Clinical Management of Herpes Viruses* (Washington, DC: IOS Press, 1995), 45–53.

3. Lovie, S.R., Kaplowitz, L.G., "Management of genital herpes infection," *Seminars in Dermatology,* 13, 248–255 (1994).

4. Sacks, S.I., "Genital herpes simplex virus infection and treatment," In Sacks, S.I., Straus, S.F., Whitley, R.J., Griffiths, P.D., eds., *Clinical Management of Herpes Viruses* (Washington, D.C.: IOS Press, 1995), pp. 55–67.

5. Griffith, R., DeLong, D., Nelson, J., "Relation of arginine-lysine antagonism to herpes simplex growth in tissue culture," *Chemotherapy,* 27, 209–213 (1981).

6. DiGiovanna, J., Blank, H., "Failure of lysine in frequently recurrent herpes simplex infection," *Archives of Dermatology,* 120, 48–51 (1984).

7. Weber, P.C., Spatz, S.J., Nordby, E.C.,. "Stable ubiquitination of the ICP0R protein of herpes simplex virus type 1 during productive infection," *Virology,* 20, 253(2), 288–298 (January 1999).

8. McCune, M.A., Perry, H.O., Muller, S.A., "Treatment of recurrent herpes simplex infections with L-lysine monohydrochloride," *Cutis,* 175, 183–190 (1987).

9. DiGiovanna, J., Blank, H., "Failure of lysine in frequently recurrent herpes simplex infection," *Archives of Dermatology,* 120, 48–51 (1984).

10. Terezhalmy, G.T., Bottomley, W.K., Pelleu, G.B., "The use of water-soluble bioflavonoid-ascorbic acid complex in the treatment of recurrent herpes labialis," *Oral Surgery, Oral Medicine, Oral Pathology,* 45(1), 56–62 (January 1978).

11. Vynograd, N., Vynograd, I., Sosnowski, Z., "A comparative multi-centre study of the efficacy of propolis, acyclovir and placebo in the treatment of genital herpes (HSV)," *Phytomedicine,* 7(1), 1–6 (March 2000).

12. Amoros, M., Lurton, E., Boustie, J., Girre, L., Sauvager, F., Cormier, M., "Comparison of the anti-herpes simplex virus activities of propolis and 3-methyl-but-2-enyl caffeate," *Journal of Natural Products,* 57(5), 644–647 (May 1994).

13. Amoros, M., Simoes, C.M., Girre, L., Sauvager, F., Cormier, M., "Synergistic effect of flavones and flavonols against herpes simplex virus type 1 in cell culture: comparison with the antiviral activity of propolis," *Journal of Natural Products,* 55(12), 1732–1740 (December 1992).

14. Aiuti, F., Sirianni, M.C., Paganelli, R., Stella, A., Turbessi, G., Fiorilli, M., "A placebo-controlled trial of thymic hormone treatment of recurrent herpes simplex labialis infection in immunodeficient hosts," *International Journal of Clinical Pharmacology and Therapeutic Toxicology,* 21(2), 81–86 (February 1986).

15. Mostad, S.B., Kreiss, J.K., Ryncarz, A.J., Mandaliya, K., Chohan, B., Ndinya-Achola, J., Bwayo, J.J., Corey, L., "Cervical shedding of herpes simplex virus in human immunodeficiency virus-infected women: effects of hormonal contraception, pregnancy, and vitamin A deficiency," *Journal of Infectious Disease,* 181(1), 58–63 (January 2000).

16. Fitzherbert, J., "Genital herpes and zinc," *Medical Journal of Australia,* I, 399 (1979).

17. Godfrey, H.R., Godfrey, N.J., Godfrey, J.C., Riley, D., "A randomized clinical trial on the treatment of oral herpes with topical zinc oxide/glycine," *Alternative Therapies in Health and Medicine,* 7(3), 49–56 (May–June 2001).

18. Basile, A.C., Sertie, J.A., Freitas, P.C., Zanini, A.C., "Anti-inflammatory activity of oleoresin from Brazilian *Copaifera,*" *Journal of Ethnopharmacology,* 22(1), 101–109 (January 1988).

19. Williams, M., "Immuno-protection against herpes simplex type II infection by eleutherococcus root extract," *International Journal of Alternative and Complementary Medicine,* 13, 9–12 (1995).

20. Nagasaka, K., Kurokawa, M., Imakita, M., Terasawa, K., Shiraki, K., "Efficacy of *kakkon-to,* a traditional herbal medicine, in herpes simplex virus type 1 infection in mice," *Journal of Medical Virology,* 46(1), 28–34 (May 1995).

21. Utsunomiya, T., Kobayashi, M., Herndon, D.N., Pollard, R.B., Suzuki, F., "Glycyrrhizin (20 beta-carboxy-11-oxo-30-norolean-12-en-3 beta-yl-2-O-beta-D-glucopyranuronosyl-alpha-D-glucopyranosiduronic acid) improves the resistance of thermally injured mice to opportunistic infection of herpes simplex virus type 1," *Immunology Letters,* 44(1), 59–66 (January 1995).

22. Robe, P.A., Princen, F., Martin, D., Malgrange, B., Stevenaert, A., Moonen, G., Gielen, J., Merville, M., Bours, V., "Pharmacological modulation of the bystander effect in the herpes simplex virus thymidine kinase/ganciclovir gene therapy system: effects of dibutyryl adenosine 3',5'-cyclic monophosphate, alpha-glycyrrhetinic acid, and cytosine arabinoside," *Biochemical Pharmacology,* 60(2), 241–249 (15 July 2000).

23. Koytchev, R., Alken, R.G., Dundarov, S., "Balm mint extract (Lo-701) for topical treatment of recurring herpes labialis," *Phytomedicine,* 6(4), 225–230 (October 1999).

HICCUPS

1. Dodds, W.J., Dent, J., Hogan, Walter, J., et al., "Mechanisms of gastroesophageal reflux in patients with reflux esophagitis," *New England Journal of Medicine,* 307, 1547–1552 (1983).

2. Shay, S.D.S., Myers, R.L., Johnson, L.F., "Hiccups associated with reflux esophagitis," *Gastroenterology,* 87, 204–207 (1984).

3. Stacher, G., Schmeierer, G., Landgraf, M., "Tertiary esophageal contractions evoked by acoustical stimuli," *Gastroenterology,* 77, 49–54 (1979).

4. Boyle, J.T., Altschuler, S.M., Patterson, B.L., et al., "Reflex inhibition of the lower esophageal sphincter following stimulation of pulmonary afferent receptors," *Gastroenterology,* 90, 1353 (1986).

HIGH CHOLESTEROL

1. Navab, M., Berliner, J.A., Subbanagounder, G., Hama, S., Lusis, A.J., Castellani, L.W., Reddy, S., Shih, D., Shi, W., Watson, A.D., Van Lenten, B.J., Vora, D., Fogelman, A.M., "HDL and the inflammatory response induced by LDL-derived oxidized phospholipids," *Arteriosclerosis, Thrombosis, and Vascular Biology,* 21(4), 481–488 (April 2001).

2. Navab, M., Hama, S.Y., Anantharamaiah, G.M., Hassan, K., Hough, G.P., Watson, A.D., Reddy, S.T., Sevanian, A., Fonarow, G.C., Fogelman, A.M., "Normal high density lipoprotein inhibits three steps in the formation of mildly oxidized low density lipoprotein: steps 2 and 3," *Journal of Lipid Research,* 41(9), 1495–1508 (September 2000).

3. Gotto, A.M., Whitney, E., Stein, E.A., Shapiro, D.R., Clearfield, M., Weis, S., Jou, J.Y., Langendörfer, A., Beere, P.A., Watson, D.J., Downs, J.R., de Cani, J.S., "Relation between baseline and on-treatment lipid parameters and first acute major coronary events in the air force/texas coronary atherosclerosis prevention study (AFCAPS/TexCAPS)," *Circulation,* 101(5), 477–484 (8 February 2000).

4. Santos, M.J., Lopez-Jurado, M., Llopis, J., et al., "Influence of dietary supplementation with fish on plasma total cholesterol and lipoprotein cholesterol fractions in patients with coronary heart disease," *Journal of Nutritional Medicine,* 3, 107–115 (1992).

5. Arjmandi, B.H., Khan, D.A., Juma, S., et al., "Whole flaxseed consumption lowers serum LDL-cholesterol and lipoprotein(a) concentrations in postmenopausal women," *Nutrition Research,* 18, 1203–1214 (1998).

6. Warshafsky, S., Kamer, R.S., Sivak, S.L., "Effect of garlic on total serum cholesterol—a meta-analysis," *Annals of Internal Medicine,* 119, 599–605 (1993).

7. Durak, I., Köksal, I., Kaçmaz, M., et al., "Hazelnut supplementation enhances plasma antioxidant potential and lowers plasma cholesterol levels," *Clinica Chimica Acta,* 284, 113–115 (1999).

8. Curb, J.D., Wergowski, G., Abbott, R.D., et al., "High mono-unsaturated fat macadamia nut diets: effects on serum lipids and lipoproteins," *FASEB Journal,* 12, A506 (1998).

9. Edwards, K., Kwaw, I., Matud, J., Kurtz, I., "Effect of pistachio nuts on serum lipid levels in patients with moderate hypercholesterolemia," *Journal of the American College of Nutrition,* 18, 229–32 (1999).

10. Ripsin, C.M., Keenan, J.M., Jacobs, D.R., et al., "Oat products and lipid lowering—a meta-analysis," *Journal of the American Medical Association,* 267, 3317–3325 (1992).

11. Anderson, J.W., Allgood, L.D., Lawrence, A., et al., "Cholesterol-lowering effects of psyllium intake adjunctive to diet therapy in men and women with hypercholesterolemia: meta-analysis of 8 controlled trials," *American Journal of Clinical Nutrition,* 71, 472–479 (2000).

12. Baum, J.A., Teng, H., Erdman, J.W., Jr., et al., "Long-term intake of soy protein improves blood lipid profiles and increases mononuclear cell low-density-lipoprotein receptor messenger RNA in hypercholesterolemic, postmenopausal women," *American Journal of Clinical Nutrition,* 68, 545–551 (1998).

13. Hallikainen, M.A., Sarkkinen, E.S., Uusitupa, M.I., "Plant stanol esters af-

fect serum cholesterol concentrations of hypercholesterolemic men and women in a dose-dependent manner," *Journal of Nutrition,* 130, 767–776 (2000).

14. Anderson, J.W., Gilliland, S.E., "Effect of fermented milk (yogurt) containing *Lactobacillus acidophilus* L1 on serum cholesterol in hypercholesterolemic humans," *Journal of the American College of Nutrition,* 18, 43–50 (1999).

15. Wilson, T., Porcari, J.P., Harbin, D., "Cranberry extract inhibits low density lipoprotein oxidation," *Life Sciences,* 62(24), PL381–PL3866 (1998).

16. Osakabe, N., Natsume, M., Adachi, T., Yamagishi, M., Hirano, R., Takizawa, T., Itakura, H., Kondo, K., "Effects of cacao liquor polyphenols on the susceptibility of low-density lipoprotein to oxidation in hypercholesterolemic rabbits," *Journal of Atherosclerosis and Thrombosis,* 7(3), 164–168 (2000).

17. Wakabayashi, Y., "Effect of germanium-132 on low-density lipoprotein oxidation and atherosclerosis in Kurosawa and Kusanagi hypercholesterolemic rabbits," *Bioscience, Biotechnology, and Biochemistry,* 65(8), 1893–1896 (August 2001).

18. Lee, M.J., Chou, F.P., Tseng, T.H., Hsieh, M.H., Lin, M.C., Wang, C.J., "Hibiscus protocatechuic acid or esculetin can inhibit oxidative LDL induced by either copper ion or nitric oxide donor," *Journal of Agricultural Food Chemistry,* 50(7), 2130–2136 (27 March 2002).

19. McQuillan, B.M., Hung, J., Beilby, J.P., Nidorf, M., Thompson, P.L., "Antioxidant vitamins and the risk of carotid atherosclerosis. The perth carotid ultrasound disease assessment study (CUDAS)," *Journal of the American College of Cardiology,* 38(7), 1788–1794 (December 2001).

20. Kelly, M.R., Loo, G., "Melatonin inhibits oxidative modification of human low-density lipoprotein," *Journal of Pineal Research,* 22(4), 203–209 (May 1997).

21. Makino,T., Ono,T., Muso, E., Honda, G., "Effect of *Perilla frutescens* on nitric oxide production and DNA synthesis in cultured murine vascular smooth muscle cells," *Phytotherapy Research,* 16 Suppl 1, 19–23 (March 2002).

22. Vahouny, G.V., Connor, W.E., Roy, T., Lin, D.S., Gallo, L.L., "Lymphatic absorption of shellfish sterols and their effects on cholesterol absorption," *American Journal of Clinical Nutrition,* 34, 507–513 (1981).

23. Wang, J., Lu, Z., Chi, J., et al., "Multicenter clinical trial of the serum lipid-lowering effects of a *Monascus purpureus* (red yeast) rice preparation from traditional Chinese medicine," *Current Therapies in Research,* 58, 964–978 (1997).

24. Heber, D., Yip, I., Ashley, J.M., Elashoff, D.A., Elashoff, R.M., Liang, V., Go, W., "Cholesterol-lowering effects of a proprietary Chinese red-yeast-rice dietary supplement," *American Journal of Clinical Nutrition,* 69(2), 231–236 (February 1999).

25. de Lorgeril, M., Salen, P., Martin, J.L., Monjaud, I., Delaye, J., Mamelle, N., "Mediterranean diet, traditional risk factors, and the rate of cardiovascular complications after myocardial infarction: final report of the Lyon Diet Heart Study," *Circulation,* 99(6), 779–785 (16 February 1999).

26. Leaf, A., "Dietary prevention of coronary heart disease: The Lyon Diet Heart Study," *Circulation,* 99, 733–735 (16 February 1999).

27. Tomeo, A.C., Geller, M., Watkins, T.R., Gapor, A., Bierenbaum, M.L., "Antioxidant effects of tocotrienols in patients with hyperlipidemia and carotid stenosis," *Lipids,* 30(12), 1179–1183 (December 1995).

28. Terentis, A.C., Thomas, S.R., Burr, J.A., Liebler, D.C., Stocker, R., "Vitamin E oxidation in human atherosclerotic lesions," *Circulatory Research,* 90(3), 333–339 (22 February 2002).

29. Yang, W.S., Lee, W.J., Funahashi, T., Tanaka, S., Matsuzawa, Y., Chao, C.L., Chen, C.L., Tai, T.Y., Chuang, L.M., "Weight reduction increases plasma levels of an adipose-derived anti-inflammatory protein, adiponectin," *Journal of Clinical Endocrinology and Metabolism,* 86(8), 3815–3819 (August 2001).

30. Volek, J.S., Gomez, A.L., Love, D.M., Weyers, A.M., Hesslink, R., Jr., Wise, J.A., Kraemer, W.J., "Effects of an 8-week weight-loss program on cardiovascular disease risk factors and regional body composition," *European Journal of Clinical Nutrition,* 56(7), 585–592 (July 2002).

31. Hooper, L., Summerbell, C.D., Higgins, J.P., Thompson, R.L., Clements, G., Capps, N., Davey, S., Riemersma, R.A., Ebrahim, S., "Reduced or modified dietary fat for preventing cardiovascular disease," *Cochrane Database System Review,* 3, CD002137 (2001).

32. Borstelmann, S., "Mit Allium sativum das kardiale risiko verringern," *Gesundes Leben,* 75, 63–65 (1998).

33. Linde, K., ter Riet, G., Hondras, M., Vickers, A., Saller, R., Melchart, D., "Systematic reviews of complementary therapies–an annotated bibliography. Part 2: Herbal medicine," *BMC Complementary and Alternative Medicine,* 1(1), 5 (2001).

34. Lau, B.H., "Suppression of LDL oxidation by garlic," *Journal of Nutrition,* 131(3s), 985S-988S (March 2001).

35. Lee, M.J., Chou, F.P., Tseng, T.H., Hsieh, M.H., Lin, M.C., Wang, C.J., "Hibiscus protocatechuic acid or esculetin can inhibit oxidative LDL induced by either copper Ion or nitric oxide donor," *Journal of Agricultural Food Chemistry,* 50(7), 2130–2136 (27 March 2002).

36. Dietrich, M., Block, G., Hudes, M., Morrow, J.D., Norkus, E.P., Traber, M.G., Cross, C.E., Packer, L., "Antioxidant supplementation decreases lipid peroxidation biomarker F(2)-isoprostanes in plasma of smokers," *Cancer Epidemiology, Biomarkers, and Prevention,* 11(1), 7–13 (January 2002).

37. Kaikkonen, J., Porkkala-Sarataho, E., Morrow, J.D., Roberts, L.J., 2nd, Nyyssonen, K., Salonen, R., Tuomainen, T.P., Ristonmaa, U., Poulsen, H.E., Salonen, J.T., "Supplementation with vitamin E but not with vitamin C lowers lipid peroxidation in vivo in mildly hypercholesterolemic men," *Free Radical Research,* 35(6), 967–978 (December 2001).

38. King, M.S., Carr, T., D'Cruz, C., "Transcendental meditation, hypertension and heart disease," *Australian Family Physician,* 31(2), 164–168 (February 2002).

39. Beck, J.D., Elter, J.R., Heiss, G., Couper, D., Mauriello, S.M., Offenbacher, S., "Relationship of periodontal disease to carotid artery intima-media wall thickness: the atherosclerosis risk in communities (ARIC) study," *Arteriosclerosis and Thrombosis: A Journal of Vascular Biology* (American Heart Association), 21(11), 1816–1822 (November 2001).

40. Gaenzer, H., Neumayr, G., Marschang, P., Sturm, W., Lechleitner, M., Foger, B., Kirchmair, R., Patsch, J., "Effect of insulin therapy on endothelium-dependent dilation in type 2 diabetes mellitus," *American Journal of Cardiology,* 89(4), 431–434 (15 February 2002).

41. Sodi-Pallares, D., personal communication (21 January 2001).

42. Matvienko, O.A., Lewis, D.S., Swanson, M., Arndt, B., Rainwater, D.L., Stewart, J., Alekel, D.L., "A single daily dose of soybean phytosterols in ground beef decreases serum total cholesterol and LDL cholesterol in young, mildly hypercholesterolemic men," *American Journal of Clinical Nutrition,* 76(1), 57–64 (July 2002).

HIGH HOMOCYSTEINE

1. Marchesini, G., Manini, R., Bianchi, G., Sassi, S., Natale, S., Chierici, S., Visani, F., Baraldi, L., Forlani, G., Melchionda, N., "Homocysteine and psychological traits: a study in obesity," *Nutrition,* 18(5), 403–407 (May 2002).

2. Volek, J.S., Gomez, A.L., Love, D.M., Weyers, A.M., Hesslink, R., Jr., Wise, J.A., Kraemer, W.J., "Effects of an 8-week weight-loss program on cardiovascular disease risk factors and regional body composition," *European Journal of Clinical Nutrition,* 56(7), 585–592 (July 2002).

HIGH TRIGLYCERIDES

1. Lee, I.K., Kim, H.S., Bae, J.H., "Endothelial dysfunction: its relationship with acute hyperglycaemia and hyperlipidemia," *International Journal of Clinical Practice,* 129, 59–64 (July 2002).

2. Lemieux, I., Almras, N., Maurige, P., Blanchet, C., Dewailly, E., Bergeron, J., Despres, J.P., "Prevalence of 'hypertriglyceridemic waist' in men who participated in the Quebec health survey: association with atherogenic and diabetogenic metabolic risk factors," *Canadian Journal of Cardiology,* 18(7), 725–732, (June 2002).

3. Couillard, C., Bergeron, N., Pascot, A., Almeras, N., Bergeron, J., Tremblay, A., Prud'homme, D., Despres, J.P., "Evidence for impaired lipolysis in abdominally obese men: postprandial study of apolipoprotein B-48– and B-100-containing lipoproteins," *American Journal of Clinical Nutrition,* 76(2), 311–318 (August 2002).

4. Lee, I.K., Kim, H.S., Bae, J.H., ibid.

5. Soria, A., Chicco, A., Eugenia D'Alessandro, M., Rossi, A., Lombardo, Y.B.,

"Dietary fish oil reverse epididymal tissue adiposity, cell hypertrophy and insulin resistance in dyslipemic sucrose fed rat model small star, filled," *Journal of Nutritional Biochemistry,* 13(4), 209–218 (April 2002).

6. Citkowitz, E., "Hypertriglyceridemia," *eMedicine,* 2(10) (21 October 2001).

HIV AND AIDS

1. Selik, R.M., Byers, R.H., Jr., Dworkin, M.S., "Trends in diseases reported on U.S. death certificates that mentioned HIV infection, 1987–1999," *Journal of Acquired Immune Deficiency Syndrome,* 29(4), 378–387 (1 April 2002).

2. Kilter, D.B., Tierney, A.A., Culpepper-Morgan, J.A., Pierson, R.N., "Effect of home total parental nutrition on body composition in patients with acquired immunodeficiency syndrome," *Journal of Parenteral and Enteral Nutrition,* 14, 454–458 (1990).

3. Garter, R., Seefried, M., Vorlberding, P., "Dronabinol effects on weight in patients with HIV infections," *AIDS,* 6, 127 (1992).

4. Kaiser, F.E., Silver, A.J., Morley, J.E., "The effect of recombinant growth human growth hormone on malnourished older individuals," *Journal of the American Geriatric Society,* 39, 235–240 (1991).

5. Swanson, B., Keithley, J.K., Zeller, J.M., Sha, B.E., "A pilot study of the safety and efficacy of supplemental arginine to enhance immune function in persons with HIV/AIDS," *Nutrition,* 18(7–8), 688–690 (July–August 2002).

6. Clark, R.H., Feleke, G., Din, M., Yasmin, T., Singh, G., Khan, F.A., Rathmacher, J.A., "Nutritional treatment for acquired immunodeficiency virus-associated wasting using beta-hydroxy beta-methylbutyrate, glutamine, and arginine: a randomized, double-blind, placebo-controlled study," *Journal of Parenteral and Enteral Nutrition,* 24(3), 133–139 (May–June 2000).

7. Austgen, T.R., Chen, M.K., Dudrick, P.S., Dudrick, P.S., Copeland, E.M., Souba, W.W., "Cytokine regulation of intestinal glutamine utilization," *American Journal of Surgery,* 163, 174–179 (1992).

8. Weglicki, W.B., Phillips, T.M., Mak, I.T., et al., "Cytokines, neuropeptides, and reperfusion injury during magnesium deficiency," *Annals of the New York Academy of Sciences,* 723, 246–257 (1994).

9. Lissoni, P., Paolorossi, F., Tancini, G., Barni, S., Ardizzoia, A., Brivio, F., Zubelewicz, B., Chatikhine, V., "Is there a role for melatonin in the treatment of neoplastic cachexia?" *European Journal of Cancer,* 32A(8), 1340–1343 (July 1996).

10. Lissoni, P., Rovelli, F., Malugani, F., Bucovec, R., Conti, A., Maestroni, G.J., "Anti-angiogenic activity of melatonin in advanced cancer patients," *Neuroendocrinology Letters,* 22(1), 45–47 (2001).

11. Sandoval, M., Charbonnet, R.M., Okuhama, N.N., Roberts, J., Krenova, Z., Trentacosti, A.M., Miller, M.J., "Cat's claw inhibits TNFalpha production and scavenges free radicals: role in cytoprotection," *Free Radicals in Biology and Medicine,* 29(1), 71–78 (1 July 2000).

12. Brocker, P., Vellas, B., Albarede, J., Poynard, T. "A two centre, randomized, double-blind trial of ornithine oxoglutarate in 194 elderly, ambulatory, convalescent subjects," *Age and Aging,* 23, 303–306 (1994).

13. Pi-Sunyer, F.X., "Overnutrition and undernutrition as modifiers of metabolic processes in disease states," *American Journal of Clinical Nutrition,* 72(2), 533S–537S (August 2000).

14. Luettig, B., Steinmuller, C., Gifford, G.E., Wagner, H., Lohmann-Matthes, M.L., "Macrophage activation by the polysaccharide arabinogalactan isolated from plant cell cultures of *Echinacea purpurea,*" *Journal of the National Cancer Institute,* 81(9), 669–675 (3 May 1989).

15. Blumenthal, M., Goldberg, A., Brinckmann, J. *Herbal Medicine: Expanded Commission E Monographs* (Boston, Integrative Medicine, 2000), p. 88.

HIVES

1. Pizzorno, J.E., Jr., Murray, M.T. *Textbook of Natural Medicine* (Churchill-Livingstone: Edinburgh, 1999), p. 1561.

2. Supramaniam, G., Warner, J.O, "Artificial food additive intolerance in patients with angio-oedema and urticaria," *Lancet,* 88, 907–909 (1986)

3. Asad, S.I., Youlten, L.J.F., Lessof, M.H., "Specific desensitization in aspirin sensitive urticaria," *Clinical Allergy,* 13, 459–466 (1983).

4. Sanchez Borges, M., Capriles-Hulett, A., Caballero-Fonseca, F., Perez, C.R., "Tolerability to new COX-2 inhibitors in NSAID-sensitive patients with cutaneous reactions," *Annals of Allergy, Asthma, and Immunology,* 87(3), 201–204 (September 2001).

5. Allison, J.R., "The relation of hydrochloric acid and vitamin B complex deficiency in certain skin diseases," *Southern Medical Journal,* 38, 235–241 (1945).

6. Davies, D., James, T.G., "An investigation into the gastric secretion of a hundred normal persons over the age of sixty," *British Journal of Medicine,* I, 1–14 (1930).

7. Kowalski, M.L., Grzelewiski-Ryzmowski, I., Roznieki, J., Szmidt, M., "Aspirin-induced tolerance in aspirin sensitive asthmatics," *Allergy,* 39, 171–178 (1984).

8. Collins-Williams, C., "Clinical spectrum of adverse reactions to tartrazine," *Journal of Asthma,* 22, 139–143 (1985).

9. Swain, A.R., Dutton, S.P., Truswell, A.S., "Salicylates in foods," *Journal of the American Dietetic Association,* 85, 950–960 (1985).

10. Kulcycki, A., "Aspartame-induced urticaria," *Annals of Internal Medicine,* 104, 207–208 (1984).

11. Winkelmann, R.K., "Food sensitivity and urticaria or vasculitis," in Brostoff, J., Challacombe, S.J., eds., *Food Allergy and Intolerance* (Philadelphia: W.B. Saunders, 1987), pp. 602–617.

12. Juhlin, L., "Recurrent urticaria: clinical investigation of 330 patients," *British Journal of Dermatology,* 104, 369–381 (1981).

13. Michaelsson, G., Juhlin, L., "Urticaria induced by preservatives and dye additives to food and drugs," *British Journal of Dermatology,* 88, 525–534 (1973).

14. Czarnetzki, B.M., *Urticaria* (New York, New York: Springer-Verlag, 1986).

15. Schwartz, H.J., Sher, T.H., "Anaphylaxis to penicillin in a frozen dinner," *Annals of Allergy,* 5, 342–343 (1984).

16. Ormerod, A.D., Reid, T.M.S., Main, R.A., "Penicillin in milk—its importance in urticaria," *Clinical Allergy,* 17, 229–234 (1987).

17. Wicher, K., Reisman, R.E., "Anaphylactic reaction to penicillin in a soft drink," *Journal of Allergy and Clinical Immunology,* 66, 155–157 (1980).

18. Boonk, W.J., Van Ketel, W.G., "The role of penicillin in the pathogenesis of chronic urticaria," *British Journal of Dermatology,* 106, 183–190 (1982).

19. Middleton, E., Drzewiecki, G., "Naturally occurring flavonoids and human basophil histamine release," *International Archives of Allergy and Applied Immunology,* 77, 155–157 (1985).

20. Yoshimoto, T., Furukawa, M., Yamamoto, S., Horie T., Watanabe-Kohno, S., "Flavonoids: potent inhibitors of arachidonate 5-lipoxygenase," *Biochemistry and Biophysics Research Communications,* 116(2), 612–618 (31 October 1983).

21. Jacobson, D.W., Simon, R.A., Singh, M., "Sulfite oxidase deficiency and cobalamin protection in sulfite sensitive asthmatics," *Journal of Allergy and Clinical Immunology,* 73 (Suppl), 135 (1984).

22. Rekka, E.A., Kourounakis, A.P., Kourounakis, P.N., "Investigation of the effect of chamazulene on lipid peroxidation and free radical processes," *Research Communications in Molecular Pathology & Pharmacology,* 92(3), 361–364 (June 1996).

23. Safayhi, H., Sabieraj, J., Sailer, E.R., Ammon, H.P., "Chamazulene: an antioxidant-type inhibitor of leukotriene B4 formation," *Planta Medica,* 60(5), 410–413 (October 1994).

24. Miller, T., Wittstock, U., Lindequist, U., Teuscher, E., "Effects of some components of the essential oil of chamomile, *Chamomilla recutita,* on histamine release from rat mast cells," *Planta Medica,* 62(1), 60–61 (1 February 1996).

25. Teelucksingh, S., Mackie, A.D., Burt, D., McIntyre, M.A., Brett, L., Edwards, C.R., "Potentiation of hydrocortisone activity in skin by glycyrrhetinic acid," *Lancet,* 335(8697), 1060–1063 (5 May 1990).

HOT FLASHES

1. Grisso, J.A., Richardson, M.C., "Racial differences in menopause informa-

tion and the experience of hot flashes," *Journal of General Internal Medicine,* 14, 98–103 (February 1999).

2. Hlatky, M.A., Boothroyd, D., Vittinghoff, E., Sharp, P., Whooley, M.A., Heary, T., Estrogen/Progestin Replacement Study Research Group, "Quality-of-life and depressive symptoms in postmenopausal women after receiving hormone therapy: results from the heart and estrogen/progestin replacement study trial," *Journal of the American Medical Association,* 287, 591–596 (2002).

3. Writing Group for the Women's Health Initiative Investigators, "Risks and benefits of estrogen plus progestin in healthy postmenopausal women: principal results from the women's health initiative randomized controlled trial," *Journal of the American Medical Association,* 288, 321–333 (17 July 2002).

4. Rodriguez, C., Patle, A.V., Calle, E.E., Jacob, E.J., Thun, M.J., "Estrogen Replacement therapy and ovarian cancer mortality in a large prospective study of U.S. women," *Journal of the American Medical Association,* 285, 1460–1465 (2001).

5. Han, K.K., Soares, J.M., Jr., Haidar, M.A., de Lima, G.R., Baracat, E.C., "Benefits of soy isoflavone therapeutic regimen on menopausal symptoms," *Obstetrics and Gynecology,* 99(3), 389–394 (March 2002).

6. Knight, D.C., Howes, J.B., Eden, J.A., "The effect of Promensil, an isoflavone extract, on menopausal symptoms," *Climacteric,* 2(2), 79–84 (June 1999).

7. Upmalis, D.H., Lobo, R., Bradley, L., Warren, M., Cone, F.L., Lamia, C.A., "Vasomotor symptom relief by soy isoflavone extract tablets in postmenopausal women: a multicenter, double-blind, randomized, placebo-controlled study," *Menopause,* 7(4), 236–242 (July–August 2000).

8. Scambia, G., Mango, D., Signorile, P.G., Anselmi Angeli, R.A., Palena, C., Gallo, D., Bombardelli, E., Morazzoni, P., Riva, A., Mancuso, S., "Clinical effects of a standardized soy extract in postmenopausal women: a pilot study," *Menopause,* 7(2),105–111 (March–April 2000).

9. Stoll, W., "A phythotherapeutic agent affects atrophic vaginal epithelium. Double-blind study: Cimicifuga vs. an estrogen preparation," *Therapeutikon,* 1, 23–31 (1987).

10. Makkonen, M., Simpanen, A.L., Saarikoski, S., Uusitupa, M., Penttila, I., Silvasti, M., Korhonen, P., "Endocrine and metabolic effects of guar gum in menopausal women," *Gynecology and Endocrinology,* 7(2), 135–141 (June 1993).

11. Jacobson, J.S., Troxel, A.B., Evans, J., Klaus, L., Vahdat, L., Kinne, D., Lo, K.M., Moore, A., Rosenman, P.J., Kaufman, E.L., Neugut, A.I., Grann, V.R., "Randomized trial of black cohosh for the treatment of hot flashes among women with a history of breast cancer," *Journal of Clinical Oncology,* 19(10), 2739–2745 (15 May 2001).

12. Van Patten, C.L., Olivotto, I.A., Chambers, G.K., Gelmon, K.A., Hislop, T.G., Templeton, E., Wattie, A., Prior, J.C., "Effect of soy phytoestrogens on hot flashes in postmenopausal women with breast cancer: a randomized, controlled clinical trial," *Journal of Clinical Oncology,* 20(6),1449–1455 (15 March 2002).

13. Tanaka, T., "Effects of herbal medicines on menopausal symptoms induced by gonadtropin-releasing hormone agonist therapy," *Clinical and Experimental Obstetrics and Gynecology,* 28(1), 20–23 (2001).

14. Wang, C.C., Chen, L.G., Yang, L.L., "Inducible nitric oxide synthase inhibitor of the Chinese herb I. *Saposhnikovia divaricata* (Turcz.) Schischk.," *Cancer Letters,* 145(1–2), 151–157 (18 October 1999).

15. Hirata, J.D., Swiersz, L.M., Zell, B., Small, R., Ettinger, B., "Does dong quai have estrogenic effects in postmenopausal women? A double-blind, placebo-controlled trial," *Fertility and Sterility,* 68(6), 981–986 (December 1997).

16. Carpenter, J.S., Wells, N., Lambert, B., Watson, P., Slayton, T., Chak, B., Hepworth, J.T., Worthington, W.B., "A pilot study of magnetic therapy for hot flashes after breast cancer," *Cancer Nursing,* 25(2), 104–109 (April 2002).

17. Kam, I.W., Dennehy, C.E., Tsourounis, C., "Dietary supplement use among menopausal women attending a San Francisco health conference," *Menopause,* 9(1), 72–78 (January–February 2002).

HUMAN BITES

1. Chakrabarty, K.H., Heaton, M., Dalley. A.J., Dawson, R.A., Freedlander, E., Khaw, P.T., Mac Neil, S., "Keratinocyte-driven contraction of reconstructed

human skin," *Wound Repair and Regeneration,* 9(2), 95–110 (March–April 2001).

2. Silverstein, R.J., Landsman, A.S., "The effects of a moderate and high dose of vitamin C on wound healing in a controlled guinea pig model," *Journal of Foot and Ankle Surgery,* 38(5), 333–338 (September–October 1998).

3. Fulton, J.E., Jr., "The stimulation of postdermabrasion wound healing with stabilized aloe vera gel-polyethylene oxide dressing," *Journal of Dermatologic Surgery & Oncology,* 16(5), 460–467 (May 1990).

4. Kohyama, T., Ertl, R.F., Valenti, V., Spurzem, J., Kawamoto, M., Nakamura, Y., Veys, T., Allegra, L., Romberger, D., Rennard, S.I., "Prostaglandin E(2) inhibits fibroblast chemotaxis," *American Journal of Physiology Lung Cell Molecular Physiology,* 281(5), L1257–1263 (November 2001).

5. Bosse, J.P., Papillon, J., Frenette, G., Dansereau, J., Cadotte, M., Le Lorier, J., "Clinical study of a new antikeloid agent," *Annals of Plastic Surgery,* 3(1), 13–21 (July 1979).

6. Meijia, K, Reng, R. *Plantas medicinales de uso popular en la Amazonia Peruviana* (Lima, Peru: AECI and IIAP, 1995), p. 75.

HUNTINGTON'S DISEASE

1. Scherzinger, E., Lurz, R., Turmaine, M., Mangiarini, L., Hollenbach, B., Hasenbank, R., Bates, G.P., Davies, S.W., Lehrach, H., Wanker, E.E., "Huntington-encoded polyglutamine expansion forms amyloid-like protein aggregates in vitro and in vivo," *Cell,* 90, 549–558 (1997).

2. Olney, J.W., "Excitotoxic food additives: functional teratological aspects," *Progress in Brain Research,* 18, 283–294 (1988).

3. Koroshetz, W.J., Jenkins, B.G., Rosen, B.R., Beal, M.F., "Energy metabolism defects in Huntington's disease and effects of coenzyme Q_{10}," *Annals of Neurology,* 41(2), 160–165 (February 1997).

4. Reiter, R.J., Cabrera, J., Sainz, R.M., Mayo, J.C., Manchester, L.C., Tan, D.X., "Melatonin as a pharmacological agent against neuronal loss in experimental models of Huntington's disease, Alzheimer's disease and parkinsonism," *Annals of the New York Academy of Sciences,* 890, 471–485 (1999).

5. Scherzinger, E., Sittler, A., Schweiger, K., Heiser, V., Lurz, R., Hasenbank, R., Bates, G.P., Lehrach, H., Wanker, E.E., "Self-assembly of polyglutamine-containing huntingtin fragments into amyloid-like fibrils: implications for Huntington's disease pathology," *Proceedings of the National Academy of Sciences of the USA,* 13;96(8), 4604–4609 (April 1999).

6. Peyser, C.E., Folstein, M., Chase, G.A., Starkstein, S., Brandt, J., Cockrell, J.R., Bylsma, F., Coyle, J.T., McHugh, P.R., Folstein, S.E., "Trial of d-alpha-tocopherol in Huntington's disease," *American Journal of Psychiatry,* 152(12), 1771–1775 (December 1995).

HYPERTENSION

1. Vasan, R.S., Beiser, Z., Seshadri, S., Larson, M.G., Kannel, W.B., D'Agostino, R.A., Levy, D., "Residual lifetime risk for developing hypertension in middle-aged women and men: the framingham heart study, *Journal of the American Medical Association,* 287(8), (27 February 2002).

2. Chatrattanakunchai, S., Fraser, T., Stobart, K., "Sesamin inhibits lysophosphatidylcholine acyltransferase in *Mortierella alpine,*" *Biochemical Society Transactions,* 28(6), 718–721 (December 2000).

3. Prisco, D., Paniccia, R., Bandinelli, B., Filippini, M., Francalanci, I., Giusti, B., Giurlani, L., Gensini, G.F., Abbate, R., Neri Serneri, G.G., "Effect of medium-term supplementation with a moderate dose of n-3 polyunsaturated fatty acids on blood pressure in mild hypertensive patients," *Thrombosis Research,* 91(3), 105–112 (1 August 1998).

4. Abe, Y., El-Masri, B., Kimball, K.T., et al., "Soluble cell adhesion molecules in hypetriglyceridemia and potential significance on monocytes adhesion," *Arteriosclerosis, Thrombosis, and Vascular Biology,* 18, 723–731 (1998).

5. Arnesen, H., "n-3 fatty acids and revascularization procedures," *Lipids,* 36 Suppl, S103–S106 (2001).

6. Devaraj, S., Li, D., Jialal, I., "The effects of alpha tocopherol supplementation on monocyte function. Decreased lipid oxidation, interleukin 1beta, and monocyte adhesion to endothelium," *Journal of Clinical Investigation,* 98, 756–763 (1996).

7. Weber, C., Erl, W., Weber, K., Weber, P.C., "Increased adhesiveness of iso-

lated monocytes to endothelium is prevented by vitamin C intake in smokers," *Circulation,* 93, 1488–1492 (1996).

8. Davi, G., Romano, M., Mezzetti, A., et al., "Increased levels of soluble P-selectin in hypercholesterolemic patients," Circulation, 97, 953–957. (1998).

9. Block, G., "Ascorbic acid, blood pressure, and the American diet," *Annals of the New York Academy of Sciences,* 959, 180–187 (April 2002).

10. HOPE Investigators, "Vitamin E supplementation and cardiovascular events in high-risk patients," *New England Journal of Medicine,* 342, 154–160 (2000).

11. Raitakari, O.T., Adams, M.R., McCredie, R.J., Griffiths, K.A., Stocker, R., Celermajer, D.S., "Oral vitamin C and endothelial function in smokers: short-term improvement, but no sustained beneficial effect," *Journal of the American College of Cardiology,* 35, 1616–1621 (2000).

12. Hamilton, I.M., Gilmore, W.S., Benzie, I.F., Mulholland, C.W., Strain, J.J., "Interactions between vitamins C and E in human subjects," *British Journal of Nutrition,* 84(3), 261–267 (September 2000).

13. Wilmink, H.W., Stroes, E.S., Erkelens, W.D., et al., "Influence of folic acid on postprandial endothelial dysfunction," *Arteriosclerosis, Thrombosis, and Vascular Biology,* 20, 185–188. (2000).

14. Verhaar, M.C., Wever, R.M., Kastelein, J.J., et al., "Effects of oral folic acid supplementation on endothelial function in familial hypercholesterolemia. A randomized placebo-controlled trial," *Circulation,* 100, 335–338 (1999).

15. Hu, F.B., Stampfer, M.J., Manson, J.E., et al., "Dietary protein and risk of ischemic heart disease in women," *American Journal of Clinical Nutrition,* 70, 221–227 (1999).

16. Clarkson, P., Adams, M.R., Powe, A.J., et al., "Oral L-arginine improves endothelium-dependent dilation in hypercholesterolemic young adults," *Journal of Clinical Investigation,* 97, 1989–1994 (1996).

17. Adams, M.R., McCredie, R., Jessup, W., Robinson, J., Sullivan, D., Celermajer, D.S., "Oral L-arginine improves endothelium-dependent dilatation and reduces monocyte adhesion to endothelial cells in young men with coronary artery disease," *Atherosclerosis,* 129, 261–269 (1997).

18. Lennan, A., Burnett, J.C., Jr., Higano, S.T., McKinley, L.J., Holmes, D.R., "Long-term L-Arginine supplementation improves small-vessel coronary endothelial function in humans, *Circulation,* 97, 2123–2128 (1998).

19. Burke, B.E., Neuenschwander, R., Olson, R.D., "Randomized, double-blind, placebo-controlled trial of coenzyme Q10 in isolated systolic hypertension," *Southern Medical Journal,* 94(11), 1112–1117 (November 2001).

20. Klag, M.J., Wang, N.Y., Meoni, L.A., Brancati, F.L., Cooper, L.A., Liang, K.Y., Young, J.H., Ford, D.E., "Coffee intake and risk of hypertension: the Johns Hopkins precursors study," *Archives of Internal Medicine,* 162(6), 657–662 (25 March 2002).

21. Rakic, V., Burke, V., Beilin, L.J., "Effects of coffee on ambulatory blood pressure in older men and women: a randomized controlled trial," *Hypertension,* 33(3), 869–873 (March 1999).

22. Hsu, Y.H., Liu, J.C., Kao, P.F., Lee, C.N., Chen, Y.J., Hsieh, M.H., Chan, P., "Antihypertensive effect of stevioside in different strains of hypertensive rats," *Zhonghua Yi Xue Za Zhi* (Taipei), 65, 1–6 (January 2002).

23. Appel, L.J., Moore, T.J., Obarzanek, E., Vollmer, W.M.N., Svetkey, L.P., Sacks, F.M., Bray, G.A., Vogt, T.M., Cutler, J.A., Windhauser, M.M., Pao-Hwa, L., Kranja, N., for the DASH Collaborative Research Group, "A clinical trial of the effects of dietary patterns on blood pressure," *New England Journal of Medicine,* 336, 1117–1124 (1997).

24. Pizzorno, J.E., Jr., Murray, M.T., *Textbook of Natural Medicine* (London: Churchill Livingstone, 1999), p. 1305.

25. Andrianova, I.V., Fomchenkov, I.V., Orekhov, A.N., "Hypotensive effect of long-acting garlic tablets allicor (a double-blind placebo-controlled trial)," *Terapiicheskii Arkhiv,* 74(3), 76–78 (2002).

HYPOCHLORHYDRIA

1. Rood, J.C., Ruiz, B., Fonthma, E.T., Malcom, G.T., Hunger, F.M., Sobhan, M., Johnson, W.D., Correa, P., "*Helicobacter pylori* associated gastritis and the ascorbic acid concentration in gastric juice," *Nutrition and Cancer,* 22(1), 65–72 (1994).

2. Phull, P.S., Price, A.B., Thorniley, M.S., et al., "Vitamin E concentrations in

the human stomach and duodenum—correlation with *Helicobacter pylori* infection," *Gut,* 39, 31–35 (1996).

3. Baik, S.C., Youn, H.S., Chung, M.H., Lee. W.K., Cho, M.J., Ko, G.H., Park, C.K., Kasai, H., Rhee, K.H., "Increased oxidative DNA damage in *Helicobacter pylori*-infected human gastric mucosa," *Cancer Research,* 56, 1279–1282 (1996).

4. Johnson, B., McIssac, R., "Effect of some anti-ulcer agents on mucosal blood flow," *British Journal of Pharmacology,* 1, 308 (1981).

5. Kang, J.Y., Tay, H.H., Wee, A., Guan, R., Math, M.V., Yap, I., "Effect of colloidal bismuth subcitrate on symptoms and gastric histology in non-ulcer dyspepsia. A double blind placebo controlled study," *Gut,* 31(4), 476–480 (April 1990).

HYPOGLYCEMIA

1. Kim, D.S., Kim, T.W., Park, I.K., Kang, J.S., Om, A.S., "Effects of chromium picolinate supplementation on insulin sensitivity, serum lipids, and body weight in dexamethasone-treated rats," *Metabolism,* 51(5), 589–594 (May 2002).

2. Lefebvre, P.J., Paolisso, G., Scheen, A.J., "Magnesium and glucose metabolism," *Therapie,* 49, 1–7. (1994).

HYPOTHYROIDISM

1. Cruz, M.W., Tendrich, M., Vaisman, M., Novis, S.A., "Electroneuromyography and neuromuscular findings in 16 primary hypothyroidism patients," *Arquivos de Neuropsiquiatria,* 54, 12–18 (1996).

2. Perros, P., Singh, R.K., Ludlam, C.A., Frier, B.M., "Prevalence of pernicious anaemia in patients with Type 1 diabetes mellitus and autoimmune thyroid disease," *Diabetic Medicine: A Journal of the British Diabetic Association,* 17(10), 749–751 (October 2000).

3. Vanderpas, J.B., Contempre, B., Duale, N.L., Deckx, H., Bebe, N., Longombe, A.O., Thilly, C.H., Diplock, A.T., Dumont, J.E., "Selenium deficiency mitigates hypothyroxinemia in iodine-deficient subjects," *American Journal of Clinical Nutrition,* 47, 271S-275S (1993).

4. O'Brien, T., Silverberg, J.D., Nguyen, T.T., "Nicotinic acid-induced toxicity associated with cytopenia and decreased levels of thyroxine-binding globulin," *Mayo Clinic Proceedings,* 67, 465–468. (1992).

5. Luboshitzky, R., Aviv, A., Herer, P., Lavie, L., "Risk factors for cardiovascular disease in women with subclinical hypothyroidism," *Thyroid,* 12(5), 421–425 (May 2002).

6. Zha, L.L., "Relation of hypothyroidism and deficiency of kidney yang," *Chung Kuo Chung Hsi I Chieh Ho Tsa Chih,* 13, 202–204 (1993).

7. Konno, N., Makita, H., Yuri, K., Iizuka, N., Kawasaki, K., "Association between dietary iodine intake and prevalence of subclinical hypothyroidism in the coastal regions of Japan," *Journal of Clinical Endocrinology and Metabolism,* 78(2), 393–397 (February 1994).

8. Nagata, K., Takasu, N., Akamine, H., Ohshiro, C., Komiya, I., Murakami, K., Suzawa, A., Nomura, T., "Urinary iodine and thyroid antibodies in Okinawa, Yamagata, Hyogo, and Nagano, Japan: the differences in iodine intake do not affect thyroid antibody positivity," *Endocrinology Journal,* 45(6), 797–803 (December 1998).

9. Bunevicius, R., Prange, A.J. Jr., "Mental improvement after replacement therapy with thyroxine plus triiodothyronine: relationship to cause of hypothyroidism," *International Journal of Neuropsychopharmacology,* 3(2), 167–174 (June 2000).

INFLAMMATORY BOWEL DISEASE

1. Raouf, A.H., Hildrey, V., Daniel, J., et al., "Enteral feeding as sole treatment for Crohn's disease: controlled trial of whole protein v amino acid based feed and a case study of dietary challenge," *Gut,* 32, 702–707 (1991).

2. Rigaud, D., Cosnes, J., Le Quintrec, Y., et al., "Controlled trial comparing two types of enteral nutrition in treatment of active Crohn's disease: elemental versus polymeric diet, *Gut,* 32, 1492–1497 (1991).

3. Alic, M., "Baker's yeast in Crohn's disease—can it kill you?" *American Journal of Gastroenterology,* 94, 1711 (1999).

4. Sturniolo, G.C., Mestriner, C., Lecis, P.E., D'Odorico, A., Venturi, C., Irato, P., Cecchetto, A., Tropea, A., Longo, G., D'Inca, R., "Altered plasma and mucosal concentrations of trace elements and antioxidants in active ulcerative colitis," *Scandinavian Journal of Gastroenterology*, 33(6), 644–649 (June 1998).

5. Dibble, J.B., Sheridan, P., Losowsky, M.S., "A survey of vitamin D deficiency in gastrointestinal and liver disorders," *Quarterly Journal of Medicine*, 53(209), 119–134 (Winter 1984).

6. Gionchetti, P., Rizzello, F., Venturi, A., Brigidi, P., Matteuzzi, D., Bazzocchi, G., Poggioli, G., Miglioli, M., Campieri, M., "Oral bacteriotherapy as maintenance treatment in patients with chronic pouchitis: a double-blind, placebo-controlled trial," *Gastroenterology*, 119(2), 584–587 (August 2000).

7. Loeschke, K., Ueberschaer, B., Pietsch, A., Gruber, E., Ewe, K., Wiebecke, B., Heldwein, W., Lorenz, R., "n-3 fatty acids only delay early relapse of ulcerative colitis in remission," *Digestive Disease Science*, 41(10), 2098–2094 (August 1996).

8. Krasinski, S.D., Russell, R.M., Furie, B.C., Kruger, S.F., Jacques, P.F., Furie, B.., "The prevalence of vitamin K deficiency in chronic gastrointestinal disorders," *American Journal of Clinical Nutrition*, 41(3), 639–643 (March 1985).

9. Ainley, C.C., Cason, J., Carlsson, L.K., Slavin, B.M., Thompson, R.P.," Zinc status in inflammatory bowel disease," *Clinical Science*, 75(3), 277–283 (September 1988).

INSECT, SPIDER, AND TICK BITES

1. Fradin, M.S., Day, J.F., "Comparative efficacy of insect repellents against mosquito bites," *New England Journal of Medicine*, 347(1), 13–18 (4 July 2002).

2. Teelucksingh, S., Mackie, A.D., Burt, D., McIntyre, M.A., Brett, L., Edwards, C.R., "Potentiation of hydrocortisone activity in skin by glycyrrhetinic acid," *Lancet*, 335(8697), 1060–1063 (5 May 1990).

INSOMNIA

1. Balter, M.B., Uhlenhuth, E.H., "New epidemiologic findings about insomnia and its treatment," *Journal of Clinical Psychiatry*, 53(Suppl 12), 34–39 (1992).

2. Mellinger, G.D., Balter, M.B., Uhlenhuth, E.H., "Insomnia and its treatment: prevalence and correlates," *Archives of General Psychiatry*, 42, 225–232. (1985).

3. Ford, D.E., Kamerow, D.B., "Epidemiologic study of sleep disturbances and psychiatric disorders," *Journal of the American Medical Association*, 262, 1479–1484. (1989).

4. Foley, D.J., Monjan, A.A., Brown, L., Simnsick, E.M., Wallace, R.B., Blazer, D.B., "Sleep complaints among elderly persons: an epidemiologic study of three communities," *Sleep*, 18, 425–432 (1995).

5. Roth, T., Ancoli-Israel, S., "Daytime consequences and correlates of insomnia in the United States: results of the 1991 National Sleep Foundation Survey II" *Sleep*, 22(Suppl 2), S354–S358 (1999).

6. Zammit, G.K., Weiner, J., Damato, N., Sillup, G.P., McMillan, C.A., "Quality of life in people with insomnia," *Sleep*, 22 (Suppl 2), S379–S385 (1999).

7. Roth, T., Ancoli-Israel, S., ibid.

8. Zammit, G.K., Weiner, J., Damato, N., Sillup, G.P., McMillan, C.A., ibid.

9. Shochat, T., Umphress, J., Israel, A.G., Ancoli-Israel, S., "Insomnia in primary care patients," *Sleep*, 22(Suppl 2), S359–S365 (1999).

10. Wheatley, D., "Kava and valerian in the treatment of stress-induced insomnia," *Phytotherapy Research*, 15(6), 549–551 (September 2001).

11. Attele, A.S., Xie, J.T., Yuan, C.S., "Treatment of insomnia: an alternative approach," *Alternative Medicine Review*, 5(3), 249–259 (2000).

12. Rechshaffen, A., Kales, A., "A manual of standardized terminology, techniques, and scoring system for sleep stages of human subjects," *NIH Report No. 204* (Bethesda, Maryland: National Institutes of Health, 1968).

13. Irwin, M., Smith, T.L., Gilling, J.C., "Electroencephalographic sleep and natural killer activity in depressed patients and control subjects," *Psychosomatic Medicine*, 54, 107–126 (1992).

14. Vgontzas, A.N., Papanicolaou, D.A., Bixler, E.O., et al, "Circadian interleukin-6 secretion and quantity and depth of sleep," *Journal of Clinical Endocrinology and Metabolism*," 84, 2603–2607 (1999).

15. Vgontzas, A.N., Papanicolaou, D.A., Bixler, E.O., Kales, A., Tyson, K., Chrousos, G.P., "Elevation of plasma cytokines in disorders of excessive daytime sleepiness: role of sleep disturbance and obesity," *Journal of Clinical Endocrinology and Metabolism*, 82, 1313–1316 (1997).

16. Everson, C.A., "Sustained sleep deprivation impairs host defense," *American Journal of Physiology*, 34, R1148–R1154 (1993).

17. Vitaliano, P.P., Scanlan, J.M., Moe, K., Siegler, I.C., Prinz, P.N., Ocsh, H.D., "Stress, sleep problems, and immune function in persons with cancer histories," *Cancer Research, Therapeutics, and Control*, 00, 1–16 (1999).

18. Crofford, L.J., Kalogeras, K.T., Mastorakos, G., et al., "Circadian relationships between interleukin (IL)-6 and hypothalamic-pituitary-adrenal axis hormones: failure of IL-6 to cause sustained hypercortisolism in patients with early untreated rheumatoid arthritis," *Journal of Clinical Endocrinology and Metabolism*, 82, 1279–1283 (1997).

19. Spiegel, K., Leproult, R., Van Cauter, E., ibid.

20. Redwine, L., Hauger, R.L., Gillin, J.C., Irwin, M., "Effects of sleep and sleep deprivation on interleukin-6, growth hormone, cortisol, and melatonin levels in humans," *Journal of Clinical Endocrinology and Metabolism*, 85, 10, 3597–3603 (2000).

21. George, C.F., Millar, T.W., Hanly, P.J., Kryger, M.H., "The effect of L-tryptophan on daytime sleep latency in normals: correlation with blood levels," *Sleep*, 12(4), 345–353 (August 1989).

22. Birdsall, T.C., "5–Hydroxytryptophan: a clinically-effective serotonin precursor," *Alternative Medicine Review*, 3(4), 271–280 (1998).

23. Martin, T.G., "Serotonin syndrome," *Annals of Emergency Medicine*, 28, 520–526 (1996).

24. Van Praag, H.M., Lemus, C., "Monoamine precursors in the treatment of psychiatric disorders." In Wurtman, R.J., Wurtman, J.J., eds., *Nutrition and the Brain* (New York, Raven Press, 1986), 89–139.

25. Wyatt, R.J., Zarcone, V., Engelman, K., et al, "Effect of 5-hydroxytryptophan on the sleep of normal human subjects," *Electroencephalography and Clinical Neurophysiology*, 34, 177–184 (1973).

26. Zhdanova, I.V., Wurtman, R.J., Regan, M.M., Taylor, J.A., Shi, J.P., Leclair, O.U., "Melatonin treatment for age-related insomnia," *Journal of Clinical Endocrinology and Metabolism*, 86(10), 4727–4730 (October 2001).

27. Smits, M.G., Nagtegaal, E.E., van der Heijden, J., Coenen, A.M., Kerkhof, G.A., "Melatonin for chronic sleep onset insomnia in children: a randomized placebo-controlled trial," *Journal of Child Neurology*, 16(2), 86–92 (February 2001).

28. Speroni, E., Minghetti, A., "A neuropharmacological activity of extracts from *Passiflora incarnate*," *Planta Medica*, 54, 488–491 (1988).

29. Paladini, A.C., Marder, M., Viola, H., Wolfman, C., Wasowski, C., Medina, J.H., "Flavonoids and the central nervous system: from forgotten factors to potent anxiolytic compounds," *Journal of Pharmacy and Pharmacology*, 51(5), 519–526 (May 1999).

30. Foster, S., Tyler, V.E., "Valerian," in *Tyler's Honest Herbal* (New York: Haworth Press, 1999), 377–378.

31. Santos, M.S., Ferreira, F., Faro, C., et al., "The amount of GABA present in aqueous extracts of valerian is sufficient to account for [3H]GABA release in synaptosomes," *Planta Medica*, 60, 2475–2476 (1994).

32. Leathwood, P.D., Chauffard, F., "Aqueous extract of valerian reduces latency to fall asleep in man," *Planta Medica*, 50, 144–148 (1984).

33. Schulz, H., Solz, C., Muller, J., "The effect of valerian extract on sleep polygraphy in poor sleepers: a pilot study," *Pharmacopsychiatry*, 27, 147–151 (1994).

34. Fussel, A., Wolf, A., Brattstrom, A., "Effect of a fixed valerian-hop extract combination (Ze91019) on sleep polygraphy in patients with non-organic insomnia: a pilot study," *European Journal of Medical Research*, 3(9), 385–390 (18 September 2000).

35. Tode, T., Kikuchi, Y., Hirata, J., Kita, T., Nakata, H., Nagata, I., "Effect of Korean red ginseng on psychological functions in patients with severe climacteric syndromes," *International Journal of Gynaecology and Obstetrics*, 67(3), 169–174 (December 1999).

36. Rim, B.M., "Ultrastructural studies on the effects of Korean *Panax ginseng* on the theca interna of rat ovary," *American Journal of Chinese Medicine,* 7(4), 333–344 (Winter 1979).

37. Leproult, R., Colecchia, E.F., L'Hermite-Baleriaux, M., Van Cauter, E., "Transition from dim to bright light in the morning induces an immediate elevation of cortisol levels," *Journal of Clinical Endocrinology and Metabolism,* 86(1), 151–157 (January 2001).

38. Buxton, O.M., L'Hermite-Baleriaux, M., Turke, F.W., Van Cauter, E., "Daytime naps in darkness phase shift the human circadian rhythms of melatonin and thyrotropin secretion," *American Journal of Physiological Regulation and Integrated Comprehensive Physiology,* 278(2), R373–382 (February 2000).

39. Spiegel, K., Leproult, R., Van Cauter, E., "Impact of sleep debt on metabolic and endocrine function," *Lancet,* 354 (9188), 1435–1439 (23 October 1999).

40. Mishima, K., Okawa, M., Shimizu, T., Hishikawa, Y., "Diminished melatonin secretion in the elderly caused by insufficient environmental illumination," *Journal of Clinical Endocrinology and Metabolism,* 86(1), 129–134 (January 2001).

41. Lin, Y., "Acupuncture treatment for insomnia and acupuncture analgesia," *Psychiatry and Clinical Neuroscience,* 409, 119–120 (1995).

42. Ruiz-Vega, G., Perez-Ordaz, L., Proa-Flores, P., Aguilar-Diaz, Y., "An evaluation of Coffea cruda effect on rats," *British Journal of Homeopathy,* 89(3), 122–126 (July 2000).

IRREGULAR HEARTBEAT

1. Tsuji, H., Venditti, F.J., Jr., Manders, E.S., Evans, J.C., Larson, M.G., Feldman, C.L., Levy, D., "Reduced heart rate variability and mortality risk in an elderly cohort: the Framingham Heart Study," *Circulation,* 90, 878–883 (1994).

2. Tsuji, H., Venditti, F.J., Evans, J.C., Larson, M.G., Levy, D., "The associations of levels of serum potassium and magnesium with ventricular premature complexes (the Framingham Heart Study)," *American Journal of Cardiology,* 74, 232–235 (1994).

3. Bashir, Y., Sneddon, J.F., Staunton, H.A., Haywood, G.A., Simpson, J.A., McKenna, W.J., Camm, A.J., "Effects of long-term oral magnesium chloride replacement in congestive heart failure secondary to coronary artery disease," *American Journal of Cardiology,* 72(15), 1156–1162 (November 1993).

4. Klevay, L.M., Milne, D.B., "Low dietary magnesium increases supraventricular ectopy," *American Journal of Clinical Nutrition,* 75(3), 550–554 (March 2002).

5. Jing, X.K., Leaf, A., "Prevention of fatal cardiac arrhythmias by polyunsaturated fatty acids," *American Journal of Clinical Nutrition,* 71(1), 202–207 (January 2000).

6. Lumme, J.A., Jounela, A.J., "The effect of potassium and potassium plus magnesium supplementation in ventricular exstrasystoles in mild hypertensives treated with hydrochlorothiazide," *International Journal of Cardiology,* 25, 93–98 (1989).

7. Dobmeyer, D.J., Stine, R.A., Leier, C.V., Greenberg, R, Schaal, S.F., "The arrhythmogenic effects of caffeine in human beings," *New England Journal of Medicine,* 308, 614–616 (7 April 1983).

IRRITABLE BOWEL SYNDROME

1. Pizzorno, J.E., Jr., Murray, M.T., *Textbook of Natural Medicine* (London: Churchill Livingstone, 1999), p. 1361.

2. Tanum, L., Malt, U.F., "Personality traits predict treatment outcome with an antidepressant in patients with functional gastrointestinal disorder," *Scandinavian Journal of Gastroenterology,* 35(9), 935–941 (September 2000).

3. Engel, C.C., Jr., Walker, E.A., Katon, W.J., "Factors related to dissociation among patients with gastrointestinal complaints," *Journal of Psychosomatic Research,* 40(6), 643–653 (June 1996).

4. Masand, P.S., Kaplan, D.S., Gupta, S., Bhandary, A.N., "Irritable bowel syndrome and dysthymia. Is there a relationship?" Psychosomatics, 38(1), 63–69 (January–February 1997).

5. Mendall, M.A., Kumar, D., "Antibiotic use, childhood affluence and irritable bowel syndrome (IBS)," *European Journal of Gastroenterology and Hepatology,* 10(1), 59–62 (January 1998).

6. Fowlie, S., Eastwood, M.A., Ford, M.J., "Irritable bowel syndrome: the influence of psychological factors on the symptom complex," *Journal of Psychosomatic Research,* 36(2), 169–173 (February 1992).

7. Freidman, G., "Nutritional therapy of irritable bowel syndrome," *Gastroenterology Clinician North America,* 18(3), 513–524 (September 1989).

8. Lucey, M.R., Clark, M.L., Lowndes, J., Dawson, A.M., "Is bran efficacious in irritable bowel syndrome? A double blind placebo controlled crossover study," *Gut,* 28(2), 221–225 (February 1987).

9. Cann, P.A., Read, N.W., Holdsworth, C.D., "What is the benefit of coarse wheat bran in patients with irritable bowel syndrome?" *Gut,* 25(2), 168–173 (February 1984).

10. Russo, A., Fraser, R., Horowitz, M., "The effect of cute hyperglycemia on small intestinal motility in normal subjects," *Diabetologia,* 39, 984–989 (1989).

11. Pizzorno, J.E., Jr., Murray, M.T., *Textbook of Natural Medicine* (London: Churchill Livingstone, 1999), 1360–1361.

12. King, T.S., Elia, M., Hunter, J.O., "Abnormal colonic fermentation in irritable bowel syndrome," *Lancet,* 352(9135), 1187–1189 (10 October 1998).

13. Jones, V., McLaughlin, P., Shorthouse, "Food intolerance. A major factor in the pathogenesis of irritable bowel syndrome," *Lancet,* II, 1115–1118 (1982).

14. Nanda, R., James, R., Smith, H., "Food intolerance and the irritable bowel syndrome," *Gut,* 30, 1099–1104 (1989).

15. Nobaek, S., Johansson, M.L., Molin, G., Ahrne, S., Jeppsson, B., "Alteration of intestinal microflora is associated with reduction in abdominal bloating and pain in patients with irritable bowel syndrome," *American Journal of Gastroenterology,* 95(5), 1231–1238 (May 2000).

16. Middleton, E., Drzewiecki, G., "Naturally occurring flavonoids and human basophil histamine release," *International Archives of Allergy and Applied Immunology,* 77, 155–157 (1985).

17. Yoshimoto, T., Furukawa, M., Yamamoto, S., Horie T., Watanabe-Kohno, S., "Flavonoids: potent inhibitors of arachidonate 5-lipoxygenase," *Biochemistry and Biophysics Research Communications,* 116(2), 612–618 (31 October 1983).

18. Asao, T., Mochiki, E., Suzuki, H., Nakamura, J., Hirayama, I., Morinaga, N., Shoji, H., Shitara, Y., Kuwano, H., "An easy method for the intraluminal administration of peppermint oil before colonoscopy and its effectiveness in reducing colonic spasm," *Gastrointestinal Endoscopy,* 53(2), 172–177 (February 2001).

19. Beesley, A., Hardcastle, J., Hardcastle, P.T., Taylor, C.J., "Influence of peppermint oil on absorptive and secretory processes in rat small intestine," *Gut,* 39(2), 214–219 (August 1996).

20. Kline, R.M., Kline, J.J., Di Palma, J., Barbero, G.J., "Enteric-coated, pH-dependent peppermint oil capsules for the treatment of irritable bowel syndrome in children," *Journal of Pediatrics,* 138(1), 125–128 (January 2001).

21. Bivol, G.K., "Gastric secretory function in peptic ulcer in youth and the effect on it of diet therapy," *Voprosii Pitanskii,* 4, 57–63 (July–August 1977).

22. Wichtl, M., ed., Grainger Bisset, N., trans. *Herbal Drugs and Phytopharmaceuticals: A Handbook for Practice on a Scientific Basis* (Boca Raton, Florida: CRC Press, 1994), p. 66.

23. Zhang, L., Yang, L.W., Yang, L.J., "Relation between *Helicobacter pylori* and pathogenesis of chronic atrophic gastritis and the research of its prevention and treatment," *Chung-Kuo Chung Hsi I Chieh Ho Tsa Chih-Chinese Journal of Modern Developments in Traditional Medicine,* 12(9), 515–516 (September 1992).

JELLYFISH STINGS

1. Bellezo, J.M., "Jellyfish stings," *eMedicine,* 2(4), (29 April 2001).

2. Lee, N.S., Wu, M.L., Tsai, W.J., Deng, J.F., "A case of jellyfish sting," *Veterinary and Human Toxicology,* 43(4), 203–205 (August 2001).

JET LAG

1. Arendt, J., Aldhous, M., Marks, V., "Alleviation of jet-lag by melatonin: Preliminary results of controlled double-blind trial," *British Medical Journal,* 292, 1170 (1986).

2. Comperatore, C.A., Lieberman, H.R., Kirby, A.W., Adams, B., Crowley, J.S., "Melatonin efficacy in aviation missions requiring rapid deployment and night operations," *Aviation, Space, and Environmental Medicine,* 67(6), 520–524 (1996).

3. Lieberman, H.R., Waldhauser, F., Garfield, G., et al., "Effects of melatonin on human mood and performance," *Brain Research* (Netherlands), 323(2), 201–207 (1984).

4. Suhner, A., Schlagenhauf, P., Hofer, I., Johnson, R., Tschopp, A., Steffen, R., "Effectiveness and tolerability of melatonin and zolpidem for the alleviation of jet lag," *Aviation, Space, and Environmental Medicine,* 72(7), 638–646 (July 2001).

KIDNEY STONES

1. Bihl, G., Meyers, A., "Recurrent renal stone disease advances in pathogenesis and clinical management," *Lancet,* 358(9282), 651–656 (25 August 2001).

2. Hall, W.D., Pettinger, M., Oberman, A., Watts, N.B., Johnson, K.C., Paskett, E.D., Limacher, M.C., Hays, J., "Risk factors for kidney stones in older women in the southern United States," *American Journal of Medical Science,* 322(1), 12–18 (July 2001).

3. Kinder, J.M., Clark, C.D., Coe, B.J., Asplin, J.R., Parks, J.H., Coe, F.L., "Urinary stone risk factors in the siblings of patients with calcium renal stones," *Journal of Urology,* 167(5), 1965–1967 (May 2002).

4. Terris, M.K., Issa, M.M., Tacker, J.R., "Dietary supplementation with cranberry concentrate tablets may increase the risk of nephrolithiasis," *Urology,* 57(1), 26–9 (January 2001).

5. Borghi, L., Meschi, T., Guerra, A., Briganti, A., Schianchi, T., Allegri, F., Novarini, A., "Essential arterial hypertension and stone disease," *Kidney International,* 55(6), 2397–2406 (June 1999).

6. Kinder, J.M., Clark, C.D., Coe, B.J., Asplin, J.R., Parks, J.H., Coe, F.L., ibid.

7. Furth, S.L., Casey, J.C., Pyzik, P.L., Neu, A.M., Docimo, S.G., Vining, E.P., Freeman, J.M., Fivush, B.A., "Risk factors for urolithiasis in children on the ketogenic diet," *Pediatric Nephrology,* 15(1–2), 125–128 (November 2000).

8. Curhan, G.C., Willett, W.C., Rimm, E.B., Spiegelman, D., Stampfer, M.J., "Prospective study of beverage use and the risk of kidney stones," *American Journal of Epidemiology,* 143(3), 240–7 (1 February 1996).

9. Borghi, L., Schianchi, T., Meschi, T., Guerra, A., Allegri, F., Maggiore, U., Novarini, A., "Comparison of two diets for the prevention of recurrent stones in idiopathic hypercalciuria," *New England Journal of Medicine,* 346(2), 77–84 (10 January 2002).

10. Levine, B.S., Rodman, J.S., Wienerman, S., Bockman, R.S., Lane, J.M., Chapman, D.S., "Effect of calcium citrate supplementation on urinary calcium oxalate saturation in female stone formers: Implications for prevention of osteoporosis," *American Journal of Clinical Nutrition,* 60(4), 592–596 (October 1994).

11. Nguyen, Q.V., Kalin. A., Drouve, U., Casez, J.P., Jaeger, P., "Sensitivity to meat protein intake and hyperoxaluria in idiopathic calcium stone formers," *Kidney International,* 59(6), 2273–2281 (June 2001).

12. Ettinger, B., Pak, C.Y., Citron, J.T., et al., "Potassium-magnesium citrate is an effective prophylaxis against recurrent calcium oxalate nephrolithiasis," *Journal of Urology,* 158, 2069–2073 (1997).

13. Grases, F., Simonet, B.M., Vucenik, I., Perello, J., Prieto, R.M., Shamsuddin, A.M., "Effects of exogenous inositol hexakisphosphate (InsP(6)) on the levels of InsP(6) and of inositol trisphosphate (InsP(3)) in malignant cells, tissues and biological fluids," *Life Sciences,* 71(13), 1535–1546 (16 August 2002).

14. Curhan, G.C., Willett, W.C., Speizer, F.E., Stampfher, M.J., "Intake of vitamins B_6 and C and the risk of kidney stones in women," *Journal of the American Society for Nephrology,* 10, 840–845 (1999).

15. Curhan, G.C., Willett, W.C., Rimm, E.B., Stampfer, M.J., "A prospective study of the intake of vitamins C and B_6, and the risk of kidney stones in men," *Journal of Urology,* 155, 1847–1851 (1996).

16. Kessler, T., Hesse, A., "Cross-over study of the influence of bicarbonate-rich mineral water on urinary composition in comparison with sodium potassium citrate in healthy male subjects," *British Journal of Nutrition,* 84(6), 865–871 (December 2000).

17. Martini, L.A., Cuppari, L., Colugnati, F.A., Sigulem, D.M., Szejnfeld, V.L., Schor, N., Heilberg, I.P., "High sodium chloride intake is associated with low bone density in calcium stone-forming patients," *Clinical Nephrology,* 54(2), 85–93 (August 2000).

18. Simon, J.A., Hudes, E.S., "Relation of serum ascorbic acid to serum vitamin B_{12}, serum ferritin, and kidney stones in U.S. adults," *Archives of Internal Medicine,* 159, 619–624 (1999).

19. Auer, B.L., Auer, D., Rodgers, A.L., "Relative hyperoxaluria, crystalluria and haematuria after megadose ingestion of vitamin C," *European Journal of Clinical Investigation,* 28, 695–700 (August 1998).

KNEE PAIN

1. Messier, S.P., Glasser, J.L., Ettinger, W.H., Jr., Craven, T.E., Miller, M.E., "Declines in strength and balance in older adults with chronic knee pain: a 30-month longitudinal, observational study," *Arthritis and Rheumatism,* 47(2), 141–148 (15 April 2002).

2. Fitzgerald, G.K., Childs, J.D., Ridge, T.M., Irrgang, J.J., "Agility and perturbation training for a physically active individual with knee osteoarthritis," *Physical Therapy,* 82(4), 1–10 (April 2002).

3. Pienimaki, T., "Cold exposure and musculoskeletal disorders and diseases. A review," *International Journal of Circumpolar Health,* 61(2), 173–182 (May 2002).

4. Hinman, M.R., Ford, J., Heyl, H., "Effects of static magnets on chronic knee pain and physical function: a double-blind study," *Alternative Therapies in Health and Medicine,* 8(4), 50–55 (July–August 2002).

5. Berger, R., Nowak, H., "A new medical approach to the treatment of osteoarthritis. Report of an open phase IV study with ademetionine (Gumbaral)," *American Journal of Medicine,* 83, 84–88 (1987).

6. Konig, B., "A long term (two years) clinical trial with S-adenosylmethionine for the treatment of osteoarthritis," *American Journal of Medicine,* 83, 89–94 (1987).

7. Singh, B.G., Atal, C.K., "Pharmacology of an extract of Sali guggal ex-*Boswellia serrata,* a new non-steroidal anti-inflammatory agent," *Agents and Actions,* 18, 407–412 (1986).

8. Beg, M., Singhal, K.C., Afzaal, S., "A study of effect of guggulsterone of hyperlipidemia of secondary glomerulopathy," *Indian Journal of Physiology and Pharmacology,* 40(3), 237–240 (July 1996).

9. Schnitzer, T.J., "Non-NSAID pharmacologic treatment options for the management of chronic pain," *American Journal of Medicine,* 105(1B), 45S-52S (27 July 1998).

10. McCleane, G., "The analgesic efficacy of topical capsaicin is enhanced by glyceryl trinitrate in painful osteoarthritis: a randomized, double blind, placebo controlled study," *European Journal of Pain,* 4(4), 355–360 (2000).

11. Murray, M., Pizzorno, J., *Encyclopedia of Natural Medicine* (London: Churchill-Livingstone, 1999), p. 1448.

12. Agafonov, A., personal correspondence, 22 July 2002.

KWASHIORKOR

1. Mahalanabis, D., Bhan, M.K., "Micronutrients as adjunct therapy of acute illness in children: impact on the episode outcome and policy implications of current findings," *British Journal of Nutrition,* 85 Suppl 2, S151–S158 (May 2001).

2. Carvalho, N.F., Kenney, R.D., Carrington, P.H., Hall, D.E., "Severe nutritional deficiencies in toddlers resulting from health food milk alternatives," *Pediatrics,* 107(4), E46 (April 2001).

LACTATION, INSUFFICIENT

1. Hartmann, P., Cregan, M., "Lactogenesis and the effects of insulin-dependent diabetes mellitus and prematurity, *Journal of Nutrition,* 131(11), 3016S-3020S (November 2001).

2. Rasmussen, K.M., Hilson, J.A., Kjolhede, C.L., "Obesity may impair lactogenesis II," *Journal of Nutrition,* 131(11), 3009S-3011S (November 2001).

3. Dewey, K.G., Nommsen-Rivers, L.A., "Differences in morbidity between

breast-fed and formula-fed infants," *Journal of Pediatrics,* 126, 696–702 (1995).

4. Wright, A.L., Bauer, M., Naylor, A., Sutcliffe, E., Clark, L., "Increasing breastfeeding rates to reduce infant illness at the community level," *Pediatrics,* 101(5), 837–844 (1998).

5. Mayer, E.J., Hamman, R.F., Gay, E.C., Lezotte, D.C., Savitz, D.A., Klingensmith, G.J., "Reduced risk of IDDM among breast-fed children: The Colorado IDDM Registry," *Diabetes,* 37, 1625–1632 (1988).

6. Koletzo, S., Sherman, P., Corey, M., Griffiths A., Smith C., "Role of infant feeding practices in development of Crohn's disease in childhood," *British Medical Journal,* 298, 1617–1618 (1989).

7. Davis, M., Savitz, D., Graubard, B.I., "Infant feeding and childhood cancer," *Lancet,* 1992, 365–368 (August 1988).

8. Dewey, K.G., Nommsen-Rivers, L.A., ibid.

9. Nylander, G., "Unsupplemented breastfeeding in the maternity ward. Positive long-term effects," *Acta Obstetrica et Gynaecologica Scandinavica,* 70(3), 205–209 (1991).

10. Menella, J.A., Beauchamp., G.K.," The effects of repeated exposure to garlic-flavored milk on the nursling's behavior," *Pediatric Research,* 36(6), 805–808 (1993).

LARYNGITIS

1. Brodnitz, F.S., "Hormones and the human voice," *Bulletin of the New York Academy of Medicine,* 47(2), 183–191 (February 1971).

2. DelGaudio, J.M., "Steroid inhaler laryngitis: dysphonia caused by inhaled fluticasone therapy," *Archives of Otolaryngological and Head and Neck Surgery,* 128(6), 677–81 (June 2002).

3. De, M., De, A.K., Sen, P., Banerjee, A.B., "Antimicrobial properties of star anise (*Illicium verum* Hook f)," *Phytotherapy Research,* 16(1), 94–95 (February 2002).

4. Elgayyar, M., Draughon, F.A., Golden, D.A., Mount, J.R., "Antimicrobial activity of essential oils from plants against selected pathogenic and saprophytic microorganisms," *Journal of Food Protection,* 64(7), 1019–1024 (July 2001).

5. Gay-Crosier, F., Schreiber, G., Hauser, C., "Anaphylaxis from inulin in vegetables and processed food," *New England Journal of Medicine,* 342, 1372 (4 May 2000).

6. Chandra, R., Barron, J.L., "Anaphylactic reaction to intravenous sinistrin (Inutest)," *Annals of Clinical Biochemisty,* 39(Pt 1), 76 (January 2002).

7. Trute, A., Gross, J., Mutschler, E., Nahrstedt, A., "In vitro antispasmodic compounds of the dry extract obtained from *Hedera helix,*" *Planta Medica,* 63(2), 125–129 (April 1997).

8. Dwoskin, L.P., Crooks, P.A., "A novel mechanism of action and potential use for lobeline as a treatment for psychostimulant abuse," *Biochemical Pharmacology,* 3(2), 89–98 (15 January 2002).

9. Deep, V., Singh, M., Ravi, K., "Role of vagal afferents in the reflex effects of capsaicin and lobeline in monkeys," *Respiratory Physiology,* 125(3), 155–168 (April 2001).

10. Miller, D.K., Crooks, P.A., Teng, L., Witkin, J.M., Munzar, P., Goldberg, S.R., Acri, J.B., Dwoskin, L.P., "Lobeline inhibits the neurochemical and behavioral effects of amphetamine," *Journal of Pharmacology and Experimental Therapy,* 296(3), 1023–1034 (March 2001).

11. Bergner, P., "Is lobelia toxic?," *Medical Herbalism,* 10(1), 15–32 (1998).

12. Blumenthal, M., Busse, W.R., Goldberg, A., Gruenwald, W., Hall, T., Klein S., Riggins, C., Rister, R. (eds), *The Complete Commission E Monographs: Therapeutic Guide to Herbal Medicines* (Boston, Massachusetts: Integrative Medicine Communications, 1998) 166–167.

13. Nosal'ova, G., Strapkova, A., Kardosova, A., Capek, P., Zathurecky, L., Bukovska, E., "Antitussive action of extracts and polysaccharides of marsh mallow (*Althea officinalis* L., var. *robusta*)," *Pharmazie,* 47(3), 224–226 (March 1992).

14. Sarrell, E.M., Mandelberg, A., Cohen, H.A., "Efficacy of naturopathic extracts in the management of ear pain associated with acute otitis media," *Archives of Pediatric and Adolescent Medicine,* 155(7), 796–799 (July 2001).

15. Serkedjieva, J., "Combined antiinfluenza virus activity of Flos verbasci infusion and amantadine derivatives," *Phytotherapy Research,* 14(7), 571–574 (November 2000).

16. Kim, D.H., Kim, B.R., Kim, J.Y., Jeong, Y.C., "Mechanism of covalent adduct formation of aucubin to proteins," *Toxicology Letters,* 114(1–3), 181–188 (3 April 2000).

17. Michaelsen, T.E., Gilje, A., Samuelsen, A.B., Hogasen, K., Paulsen, B.S., "Interaction between human complement and a pectin type polysaccharide fraction, PMII, from the leaves of *Plantago major* L.," *Scandinavian Journal of Immunology,* 52(5), 483–490 (November 2000).

18. Schinella, G.R., Tournier, H.A., Prieto, J.M., Mordujovich, D., Rios, J.L., "Antioxidant activity of anti-inflammatory plant extracts," *Life Sciences,* 70(9), 1023–1033 (18 January 2002).

19. Ma, S.C., Du, J., But, P.P., Deng, X.L., Zhang, Y.W., Ooi, V.E., Xu, H.X., Lee, S.H., Lee, S.F., "Antiviral Chinese medicinal herbs against respiratory syncytial virus," *Journal of Ethnopharmacology,* 79(2), 205–211 (February 2002).

20. Kohlert, C. *Systemische Verfügbarkeit und Pharmakokinetik von Thymol nach oraler Applikation einer thymianhaltigen Zubereitung im Menschen* (Würzburg, University of Würzburg, 2000). Doctoral disseration.

21. Meister, R., Wittig, T., Beuscher, N., et al., "Efficacy and tolerability of Myrtol standardized in long-term treatment of chronic bronchitis. A double-blind, placebo-controlled study. Study Group Investigators," *Arzneimittel Forschung,* 49, 351–358 (1999).

LEAD EXPOSURE

1. Conners, G.P., "Lead toxicity," *eMedicine,* 3(7), 17 July 2002.

2. Rodrigo, M.J., Moskovitz, J., Salamini, F., Bartels, D., "Reverse genetic approaches in plants and yeast suggest a role for novel, evolutionarily conserved, selenoprotein-related genes in oxidative stress defense," *Molecular Genetics and Genomics,* 267(5), 613–612 (July 2002).

3. Zeng, H., "Selenite and selenomethionine promote HL-60 cell cycle progression," *Journal of Nutrition,* 132(4), 674–679 (April 2002).

4. Courtney, J.G., Ash, S., Kilpatrick, N., Buchanan, S., Meyer, P., Kim, D., Brown, L., "Childhood lead poisoning associated with tamarind candy and folk remedies–California, 1999–2000," *CDC Reporter,* 51(31), 684–686 (8 August 2002).

LENNOX-GASTAUT SYNDROME

1. Ohtsuka, Y., Matsuda, M., Ogino, T., Kobayashi, K., Ohtahara, S., "Treatment of the west syndrome with high-dose pyridoxal phosphate," *Brain Development,* 9(4), 418–421 (1987).

LEUKOPLAKIA

1. Bartsch, H., Nair, U., Risch, A., Rojas, M., Wikman, H., Alexandrov, K., "Genetic polymorphism of CYP genes, alone or in combination, as a risk modifier of tobacco-related cancers," *Cancer Epidemiology, Biomarkers, and Prevention,* 91(1), 3–28 (January 2000).

2. Bouquot, J.E., Gnepp, D.R., "Laryngeal precancer—a review of the literature and comparison with oral leukoplakia," *Head and Neck,* 13, 488–497 (1991).

3. Mihail, R.C., "Oral leukoplakia caused by cinnamon food allergy," *Journal of Otolaryngology,* 21(5), 366–367 (October 1992).

4. Gupta, P.C., Hebert, J.R., Bhonsie, R.B., Murti, P.R., Mehta, H., Mehta, F.S., "Influence of dietary factors or oral precancerous lesions in a population-based case-control study in Kerala, India," *Cancer,* 85(9), 1885–1893 (1 May 1999).

5. Lippman, S.M., Batsakis, J.G., Toth, B.B., Weber, R.S., Lee, J.J., Martin, J.W., Hays, G.L., Goepfe, H., Hong, W., "Comparison of low-dose isotretinoin with beta carotene to prevent oral carcinogenesis," *New England Journal of Medicine,* 328(1), 15–20 (7 January 1993).

6. Epstein, J.B., Gorsky, M., "Topical application of vitamin A to oral leukoplakia: a clinical case series," *Cancer,* 86(6), 921–927 (15 September 1999).

7. Stich, H.F., Rosin, M.P., Vallejera, M.O., "Reduction with vitamin A and

beta-carotene administration of proportion of micronucleated buccal mucosal cells in Asian betel nut and tobacco chewers," *Lancet,* 1(8388), 1204–1206 (2 June 1984).

8. Stich, H.F., Rosin, M.P., Hornby, A.P., et al., "Remission of oral leukoplakias and micronuclei in tobacco/betel quid chewers treated with beta-carotene and with beta-carotene plus vitamin A," *International Journal of Cancer,* 42, 195–199 (1995).

9. Kaugars, G.E., Silverman S., Jr., Lovas, J.G., Brandt, R.B., Riley, W.T., Dao, Q., Singh, V.N., Gall, J., "A clinical trial of antioxidant supplements in the treatment of oral leukoplakia," *Oral Surgery Oral Medicine Oral Pathology,* 78(4), 462–468 (October 1994).

10. Benner, S.E., Wargovich, M.J., Lippman, S.M., Fisher, R., Velasco, M., Winn, R.J., Hong, W.K., "Reduction in oral mucosa micronuclei frequency following alpha-tocopherol treatment of oral leukoplakia," *Cancer Epidemiology, Biomarkers, and Prevention,* 3(1), 73–76 (January–February 1994).

11. Benner, S.E., Winn, R.J., Lippman, S.M., Poland, J., Hansen, K.S., Luna, M.A., Hong, W.K., "Regression of oral leukoplakia with alpha-tocopherol: a community clinical oncology program chemoprevention study," *Journal of the National Cancer Institute,* 85(1), 44–47 (6 January 1993).

12. Nagao, T., Ikeda, N., Warnakulasuriya, S., Fukano, H., Yuasa, H., Yano, M., Miyazaki, H., Ito, P., "Serum antioxidant micronutrients and the risk of oral leukoplakia among Japanese," *Oral Oncology,* 36(5), 466–470 (September 2000).

13. Garewal, H.S., Katz, R.V., Meyskens, F., Pitcock, J., Morse, D., Friedman, S., Peng, Y., Pendrys, D.G., Mayne, S., Alberts, D., Kiersch, T., Graver, E., "Beta-carotene produces sustained remissions in patients with oral leukoplakia: results of a multicenter prospective trial," *Archives of Otolaryngological and Head and Neck Surgery,* 125(12), 1305–1310 (December 1999).

14. Fettig, A., Pogrel, M.A., Silverman S., Jr., Bramanti, T.E., da Costa, M., Regezi, J.A., "Proliferative verrucous leukoplakia of the gingiva," *Oral Surgery, Oral Medicine, Oral Pathology, Oral Radiology, and Endodontics,* 90(6), 723–730 (December 2000).

15. Lippman, S.M., Shin, D.M., Lee, J.J., Batsakis, J.G., Lotan, R., Tainsky, M.A., Hittelman, W.N., Hong, W.K., "p53 and retinoid chemoprevention of oral carcinogenesis," *Cancer Research,* 55(1), 16–19 (1 January 1995).

16. Shin, D.M., Xu, X.C., Lippman, S.M., Lee, J.J., Lee, J.S., Batsakis, J.G., Ro, J.Y., Martin, J.W., Hittelman, W.N., Lotan, R., Hong, W.K., "Accumulation of p53 protein and retinoic acid receptor beta in retinoid chemoprevention," *Clinical Cancer Research,* 3(6), 875–880 (June 1997).

17. Khafif, A., Schantz, S.P., Chou, T.C., Edelstein, D., Sacks, P.G., "Quantitation of chemopreventive synergism between (-)epigalocatechin 3-gallate and curcumin in normal, premalignant, and malignant human oral epithelial cells," *Carcinogenesis,* 19(3), 419–424 (March 1998).

18. Li, N., Sun, Z., Liu, Z., Han, C., "Study on the preventive effect of tea on DNA damage of the buccal mucosa of cells in oral leukoplakias induced by cigarette smoking," *Wei Sheng Yan Jiu,* 27(3), 173–174 (May 1998).

LIPOSUCTION, HEALING AFTER

1. Foulds, I.S., Barker, A.T., "Human skin battery potentials and their role in wound healing," *British Journal of Dermatology,* 109, 515 (1983).

2. Markov, M.S., "Electric current and electromagnetic field effects on soft tissue: implication for wound healing," *Wounds,* 7, 94 (1995).

3. Man, D., Man, B., Plosker, H., "The influence of permanent magnetic field therapy on wound healing in suction lipectomy patients: a double-blind study," *Plastic and Reconstructive Surgery,* 104(7), 2261–2268 (December 1999).

LIVER CANCER

1. Kuper, H., Tzonou, A., Kaklamani, E., Hsieh, C.C., Lagiou, P., Adami, H.O., Trichopoulos, D., Stuver, S.O., "Tobacco smoking, alcohol consumption and their interaction in the causation of hepatocellular carcinoma," *International Journal of Cancer,* 85(4), 498–502 (15 February 2002).

2. Yu, M.W., Chiu, Y.H., Chiang, Y.C., Chen, C.H., Lee, T.H., Santella, R.M., Chern, H.D., Liaw, Y.F., Chen, C.J., "Plasma carotenoids, glutathione S-transferase M1 and T1 genetic polymorphisms, and risk of hepatocellular carcinoma: independent and interactive effects," *American Journal of Epidemiology,* 149(7), 621–629 (1 April 1999).

3. Yu, M.W., Horng, I.S., Hsu, K.H., Chiang, Y.C., Liaw, Y.F., Chen, C.J., "Plasma selenium levels and risk of hepatocellular carcinoma among men with chronic hepatitis virus infection," *American Journal of Epidemiology,* 150(4), 367–374 (15 August 1999).

4. Mandishona, E., MacPhail, A.P., Gordeuk, V.R., Kedda, M.A., Paterson, A.C., Rouault, T.A., Kew, M.C., "Dietary iron overload as a risk factor for hepatocellular carcinoma in Black Africans," 27(6), 1563–1566 (June 1998).

5. Yamamoto, Y., Yamashita, S., Fujisawa, A., Kokura, S., Yoshikawa, T., "Oxidative stress in patients with hepatitis, cirrhosis, and hepatoma evaluated by plasma antioxidants," *Biochemistry and Biophysics Research Communications,* 247(1), 166–170 (9 June 1998).

6. Kang, J.H., Shi, Y.M., Zheng, R.L., "Effects of ascorbic acid and DL-alpha-tocopherol on human hepatoma cell proliferation and redifferentiation," *Acta Pharmacologica Sinica,* 21(4), 348–352 (April 2000).

7. Igarashi, M., Miyazawa, T., "The growth inhibitory effect of conjugated linoleic acid on a human hepatoma cell line, HepG2, is induced by a change in fatty acid metabolism, but not the facilitation of lipid peroxidation in the cells," *Biochimica et Biophysica Acta,* 1530(2–3), 162–71 (26 February 2001).

8. Kodama, N., Komuta, K., Nanba, H., "Can maitake-D fraciton aid cancer patients?" *Alternative Medicine Review,* 7(3), 236–239 (July 2002).

9. Kakumu, S., Yoshioka, K., Wakita, T., Ishikawa, T., "Effects of TJ-9 Sho-saiko-to (kampo medicine) on interferon gamma and antibody production specific for hepatitis B virus antigen in patients with type B chronic hepatitis," *International Journal of Pharmacology,* 13(2–3), 141–146 (1991).

10. Grossmann, M., Hoermann, R., Weiss, M., Jauch, K.W., Oertel, H., Staebler, A., Mann, K., Engelhardt, D., "Spontaneous regression of hepatocellular carcinoma," *American Journal of Gastroenterology,* 90(9), 1500–1503 (September 1995).

11. Duthie, S.J., Johnson, W., Dobson, V.L., "The effect of dietary flavonoids on DNA damage (strand breaks and oxidised pyrimdines) and growth in human cells," *Mutation Research,* 390(1–2), 141–151 (24 April 1997).

12. Balkau, B., Kahn, H.S., Courbon, D., Eschwege, E., Ducimetiere, P., "Paris prospective study. Hyperinsulinemia predicts fatal liver cancer but is inversely associated with fatal cancer at some other sites," *Diabetes Care,* 24(5), 843–849 (May 2001).

LOSS OF SEXUAL DESIRE IN MEN

1. Lund, B.C., Bever-Stille, K.A., Perry, P.J., "Testosterone and andropause: the feasibility of testosterone replacement therapy in elderly men," *Pharmacotherapy,* 19(8), 951–956 (August 1999).

2. Luboshitzky, R., Aviv, A., Hefetz, A., Herer, P., Shen-Orr, Z., Lavie, L., Lavie, P., "Decreased pituitary-gonadal secretion in men with obstructive sleep apnea," *Journal of Endocrinology and Metabolism,* 87(7), 3394–3398 (July 2002).

3. King, D.S., Sharp, R.L., Vukovich, M.D., et al., 'Effect of oral androstenedione on serum testosterone and adaptations in resistance training in young men. A randomized controlled trial," *Journal of the American Medical Association* 282, 2020–2028 (1999).

LOSS OF SEXUAL DESIRE IN WOMEN

1. DeCherney, A.H., "Hormone receptors and sexuality in the human female," *Journal of Women's Health and Gender Base Medicine,* 9 (Supl 1), S9–S13 (2000).

2. Shoupe, D., "Androgens and bone: clinical implications for menopausal women," *American Journal of Obstetrics and Gynecology,* 180 (3 Pt 2), 329–333 (March 1999).

3. Bachmann, G.A., "Androgen therapy in menopause: evolving benefits and challenges," *American Journal of Obstetrics and Gynecology,* 180 (3 Pt 2), 308–311 (March 1999).

4. Sherwin, B.B., Gelfand, M.M., "Differential symptom response to parenteral estrogen and/or androgen administration in the surgical menopause," *American Journal of Obstetrics and Gynecology,* 151, 153–160 (1995).

5. Hoeger, K., Guzick, D.S., "The use of androgens in menopause, *Clinical Obstetrics and Gynecology,* 42(4), 883–894 (December 1999).

6. Redmond, G.P., "Hormones and sexual function," *International Journal of Women's Medicine,* 44(4), 193–197 (June–August 1999).

7. Morales, A.J., Nolan, J.J., Nelson, J.C., Yen, S.S., "Effects of replacement dose of dehydroepiandrosterone in men and women of advancing age," *Journal of Clinical Endocrinology and Metabolism,* 78(6), 130–1367 (June 1994).

8. Cohen, A.J., Bartlik, B., "Ginkgo biloba for antidepressant-induced sexual dysfunction," *Journal of Sex and Marital Therapy,* 24(2), 139–143 (April–June 1998).

9. Ito, T.Y., Trant, A.S., Polan, M.L., "A double-blind placebo-controlled study of Arginmax, a nutritional supplement for enhancement of female sexual function," *Journal of Sex and Marital Therapy,* 27(5), 541–549 (October–December 2001).

LUNG CANCER

1. Kuper, H., Adami, H.O., Boffetta, P., "Tobacco use, cancer causation and public health impact," *Journal of Internal Medicine,* 251(6), 455–466 (June 2002).

2. Tapei, H.S., Roberfroid, M.B., "Inulin/oligofructose and anticancer therapy," *British Journal of Nutrition,* 87(S2), S283–S286 (2002).

3. The Canadian Cancer Registries Epidemiology Research Group, "Risk factors for lung cancer among Canadian women who have never smoked," *Cancer Detection and Prevention,* 26(2), 129–138 (2002).

4. Lissoni, P., Rovelli, F., Malugani, F., Bucovec, R., Conti, A., Maestroni, G.J. "Anti-angiogenic activity of melatonin in advanced cancer patients," *Neuroendocrinology Letters,* 22(1), 45–47 (2001).

5. Ohlmann, C.H., Jung, C., Jaques, G., "Is growth inhibition and induction of apoptosis in lung cancer cell lines by fenretinide [N-(4-hydroxyphenyl)retinamide] sufficient for cancer therapy?," *Interantional Journal of Cancer Therapy,* 100(5), 520–526 (10 August 2002).

6. Tsubaki, K., Horiuchi, A., Kitani, T., et al., "Investigation of the preventive effect of CoQ_{10} against the side-effects of anthracycline antineoplastic agents," *Gan To Kagaku Ryoho,* 11, 1420–1427 (1984).

7. Unverferth, D.V., Jagadeesh, J.M., Unverferth, B.J., et al., "Attempt to prevent doxorubicin induced acute human myocardial morphologic damage with acetylcysteine," *Journal of the National Cancer Institute,* 71, 917–920 (1983).

8. Olson, R.D., Stroo, W.E., Boerth, R.C., "Influence of N-acetylcysteine on the antitumor activity of doxorubicin," *Seminars in Oncology,* 10, S29–S34 (1983).

9. Schmitt-Graff, A., Scheulen, M.E., "Prevention of Adriamycin cardiotoxicity by niacin, isocitrate, or N-acetylcysteine in mice,' *Pathology in Research and Practice,* 181, 168–174 (1986).

10. Scambia, G., Ranelletti, F.O., Panici, P.B., et al., "Quercetin potentiates the effect of Adriamycin in a multidrug-resistant MCF-7 human breast cancer cell line: P-glycoprotein as a possible target," *Cancer Chemotherapy and Pharmacology,* 34, 459–464 (1994).

11. Critchfield, J.W., Welsh, C.J., Phang, J.M., Yeh, G.C., "Modulation of Adriamycin accumulation and efflux by flavonoids in HCT-15 colon cells," *Biochemical Pharmacology,* 48, 1437–1445 (1994).

12. Doyle, L.A., Giangiulo, D., Hussain, A., "Differentiation of human variant small cell lung cancer cell lines to a classic morphology by retinoic acid," *Cancer Research,* 49, 6745–6751 (1989).

13. Shimpo, K., Nagatsu, T., Yamada, K., et al., "Ascorbic acid and Adriamycin toxicity," *American Journal of Clinical Nutrition,* 54, 1298S-1301S (1991).

14. Myers, C.E., McGuire, W.P., Liss, R.H., et al., "Adriamycin: the role of lipid peroxidation in cardiac toxicity and tumor response," *Science,* 197, 165–167 (1977).

15. Sonneveld, P., "Effect of alpha-tocopherol on the cardiotoxicity of Adriamycin in the rat," *Cancer Treatment Reports,* 62, 1033–1036 (1978).

LUPUS

1. GL601 Study Group, "Effects of prasterone on corticosteroid requirements of women with systemic lupus erythematosus: a double-blind, randomized, placebo-controlled trial," *Arthritis and Rheumatism,* 46(7), 1280–1829 (June 2002).

2. Walton, A.J.E., Snaith, M.L., Locniskar, M., et al., "Dietary fish oil and the severity of symptoms in patients with systemic lupus erythematosus," *Annals of Rheumatological Disease,* 50, 463–466 (1991).

LYME DISEASE

1. Edlow, J.A., "Lyme disease and related tick-borne illnesses," *Annals of Emergency Medicine,* 33(6), 680–693 (1999).

2. Sellati, T.J., Bouis, D.A., Kitchens, R.L., Darveau, R.P., Pugin, J., Ulevitch, R.J., Gaugloff, S.C., Goyert, S.M., Norgard, M.V., Radolf, J.D., "*Treponema pallidum* and *borrelia burgdorferi* lipoproteins and synthetic lipopeptides activate monocytic cells via a CD14–dependent path distinct from that used by lipopolysaccharide," *Journal of Immunology,* 160, 5455–5464 (1998).

3. Sigal, L.H., Williams, S., "A monoclonal antibody to *borrelia burgdorferi* flagellin modifies neuroblastoma cell neuritogenesis in vitro: a possible role for autoimmunity in the neuropathy of lyme disease," *Infection and Immunity,* 65(3), 1722–1728 (May 1997).

4. Seifter, E., Rettura, G., Seiter, J., "Thymotrophic action of vitamin A," *Federal Proceedings,* 32, 947 (1973).

5. Semba, R.D., "Vitamin A, immunity, and infection," *Clinical Infectious Disease,* 19, 489–499 (1994).

6. Prasad, A., "Clinical, biochemical and nutritional spectrum of zinc deficiency in human subjects. An update," *Nutrition Review,* 41, 197–208 (1983).

7. Seamon, K.B., Daly, J.W., "Forskolin: A unique diterpene activator of cAMP-generating systems," *Journal of Cyclic Nucleotide Research,* 7, 201–224 (1981).

8. Jie, Y.H., Cammisuli, S., Baggiolini, M., "Immunomodulatory effects of *Panax ginseng* C.A., Meyer in the mouse," *Agents and Actions,* 15, 386–391 (1984).

9. Kick, H.P., Basher, J., Toffler, E., "Silymarin. Potent inhibitor of cyclic AMP phosphodiesterase," *Methods and Findings in Experimental and Clinical Pharmacy,* 7, 409–413 (1985).

LYMPHEDEMA

1. Lee, Y.M., Mak, S.S., Tse, S.M., Chan, S.J., "Lymphoedema care of breast cancer patients in a breast care clinic: a survey of knowledge and health practice," *Supportive Care for Cancer,* 9(8), 634–641 (November 2001).

2. Johansson, K., Ohlsson, K., Ingvar, C., Albertsson, M., Ekdahl, C., "Factors associated with the development of arm lymphedema following breast cancer treatment: a match pair case-control study," *Lymphology,* 35(2), 59–71 (June 2002).

3. Korpan, M.I., Fialka, V., "Wobenzym and diuretic therapy in lymphedema after breast surgery," *Wiener Medizinischer Wochenschrift,* 146(4), 67–72, 74 (1996).

4. Loprinzi, C.L., Kugler, J.W., Soan, J.A., Rooke, T.W., Quella, S.K., Novotny, P., Mowat, R.B., Michalak, J.C., Stella, P.J., Levitt, R., Tschetter, L.K., Windschitl, H., "Lack of effect of coumarin in women with lymphedema after treatment for breast cancer," *New England Journal of Medicine,* 340(5), 346–350 (4 February 1999).

5. Soria, P., Cuesta, A., Romero, H., Martinez, F.J., Sastre, A., "Dietary treatment of lymphedema by restriction of long-chain triglycerides," *Angiology,* 45(8), 703–707 (August 1994).

6. Friis, H., Kaestel, P., Nielsen, N., Simonsen, P.E., "Serum ferritin, alpha-tocopherol, beta-carotene and retinol levels in lymphatic filariasis," *Transactions of the Royal Society for Tropical Medicine and Hygiene,* 96(2), 151–156 (March–April 2002).

7. Ohkuma, M., "Treatment of peripheral lymphedema by concomitant application of magnetic fields, vibration and hyperthermia: a preliminary report," *Lymphology,* 35(2), 87–90 (June 2002).

8. de Godoy, J.M., Batigalia, F., de Godoy, F., "Preliminary evaluation of a new, more simplified physiotherapy technique for lymphatic drainage," *Lymphology,* 35(2),91–93 (June 2002).

9. Ruocco, V., Schwartz, R.A., Ruocco, E., "Lymphedema: an immunologically vulnerable site for development of neoplasms," *Journal of the American Academy of Dermatology,* 47(1), 124–127 (July 2002).

MACULAR DEGENERATION

1. Goldberg, J., Flowerdew, G., Smith, E., et al., "Factors associated with age-related macular degeneration," *American Journal of Epidemiology,* 128, 700–710 (1988).

2. Seddon, J.M., Ajani, U.A., Sperduto, R.D., et al., "Dietary carotenoids, vitamins A, C, and E, and advanced age-related macular degeneration," *Journal of the American Medical Association,* 272, 1413–1420 (1994).

3. VandenLangenberg, G.M., Mares-Perlman, J.A., Klein, R., et al., "Associations between antioxidant and zinc intake and the 5-year incidence of early age-related maculopathy in the Beaver Dam Eye Study," *American Journal of Epidemiology,* 148, 204–214 (1998).

4. Eye Disease Case-Control Study Group, "Antioxidant status and neovascular age-related macular degeneration," *Archives of Ophthalmology,* 111, 104–109 (1994).

5. Organisciak, D.T., Wang, H.M., Kou, A.L., "Ascorbate and glutathione levels in the developing normal and dystrophic rat retina: effect of intense light exposure," *Current Eye Research,* 3, 257–267 (1984).

6. West, S., Vitale, S., Hallfrisch, J., et al., "Are antioxidants or supplements protective for age-related macular degeneration?" *Archives of Ophthalmology,* 112, 222–227 (1994).

7. Christen, W.G., "Antioxidant vitamins and age-related eye disease," *Proceedings of the Association of American Physicians,* 3, 16–21 (1999).

8. Stoyanovsky, D.A., Goldman, R., Darrow, R.M., et al., "Endogenous ascorbate regenerates vitamin E in the retinal directly and in combination with exogenous dihydrolipoic acid," *Current Eye Research,* 14, 181–189 (1995).

9. Newsome, D.A., Swartz, M., Leone, N.C., "Oral zinc in macular degeneration," Archives of Ophthalmology, 106, 192–198 (1988).

10. Stur, M., Tittle, M., Reitner, A., "Oral zinc and the second eye in age-related macular degeneration," *Investigational Ophthalmology and Visual Science,* 37, 1225–1235 (1996).

11. Scharrer, A., Ober, N.M., "Anthocyanosides in the treatment of retinopathies," *Klinische Monatsblätter der Augenheilkunde,* 178, 386–389 (1981).

12. Murray, M., Pizzorno, J., *Encyclopedia of Natural Medicine* (London: Churchill-Livingstone, 1999), p. 1375.

13. Hammond, B.R, Jr., Wooten, B.R., Snoderlt, D.M., "Cigarette smoking and retinal carotenoids: implications for age-related macular degeneration," *Vision Research,* 36, 3003–3009 (1996).

14. Hammond, B.R., Jr., Curran-Celentano, J., Judd, S., et al., "Sex differences in macular pigment optical density: relation to plasma carotenoid concentrations and dietary patterns," *Vision Research,* 36, 2001–2012 (1996).

MALE INFERTILITY

1. Purvis, K., Christiansen, E., "Male infertility: current concepts," *Annals of Medicine,* 24, 258–272 (1992).

2. Purvis, K., Christiansen, E., "Infection in the male reproductive tract. Impact, diagnosis and treatment in relation to male infertility," *International Journal of Andrology,* 16, 1–13 (1993).

3. Wong, W.Y., Merkus, H.M., Thomas, C.M., Menkveld, R., Zielhuis, G.A., Steegers-Theunissen, R.P., "Effects of folic acid and zinc sulfate on male factor subfertility: a double-blind, randomized, placebo-controlled trial," *Fertility and Sterility,* 77(3), 491–498 (March 2002).

4. Costa, M., Canale, D., Filicori, M., et al., "L-carnitine in idiopathic asthenozoospermia: a multicenter study. Italian Study Group on Carnitine and Male Infertility," *Andrologia,* 26, 155–159. (1994).

5. Vitali, G., Parente, R., Melotti, C., "Carnitine supplementation in human idiopathic asthenospermia: clinical results," *Drugs in Experimental and Clinical Research,* 21, 157–159. (1995).

6. Purvis, K., Christiansen, E., (1993), ibid.

7. Dawson, E.B., Harris, W.A., Teter, M.C., Powell, L.C., "Effect of ascorbic acid supplementation on the sperm quality of smokers," *Fertility and Sterility,* 58, 1034–1039. (1992).

8. Sudo, K., Honda, K., Taki, M., Kanitani, M., Fujii, Y., Aburada, M., Hosoya, E., Kimura, M., Orikasa, S., "Effects of TJ-41 (Tsumura *Hochu-ekki-to*) on spermatogenic disorders in mice under current treatment with adriamycin," *Nippon Yakurigaku Zasshi - Folia Pharmacologica Japonica,* 92(4), 251–61 (October 1988).

MASTITIS

1. Payne, M.C., Wood, H.F., Karakawa, W., Gluck, L., "A prospective study of staphylococcal colonization and infections in newborns and their families," *American Journal of Epidemiology,* 82, 305–316 (1966).

2. Waldvogel, F.A. "*Staphylococcus aureus* (including staphylococcal toxic shock)," In: Mandell, G.L., Bennett, J.E., Dolin, R., editors, *Principles and Practice of Infectious Diseases,* Fifth Edition (Philadelphia: Churchill Livingstone, 2000), pp. 2072–2073.

3. Ross, S., Rodriguez, W., Controni, G., Khan, W., "Staphylococcal susceptibility to penicillin G: The changing pattern among community isolates," *Journal of the American Medical Association,* 2229, 1075–1077 (1974).

4. Sanford, M.D., Widmer, A.F., Bale, M.J., Jones, R.N., Wenzel, R.P., "Efficient detection and long-term persistence of the carriage of methicillin-resistant *Staphylococcus aureus,*" *Clinical Infectious Disease,* 19, 1123–1128 (1994).

5. Havsteen, B., "Flavonoids, a class of natural products of high pharmacological potency," *Biochemical Pharmacology,* 32, 1141–1148 (1983).

6. Bliznakov, E., Casey, A., Kishi, T., "Coenzyme Q deficiency in mice following infection with Friend leukemia virus," *International Journal of Vitamin and Nutrition Research,* 45, 388–395 (1975).

7. Cazzola, P., Mazzanti, P., Bossi, G., "In vivo modulating effect of a calf thymus acid lysate on human T lymphocyte subsets and CD4+/CD8+ ratio in the course of difference diseases," *Current Therapies Research,* 42, 1011–1017 (1987).

8. Seifter, E., Rettura, G., Seiter, J., "Thymotrophic action of vitamin A," *Federal Proceedings,* 32, 947 (1973).

9. Semba, R.D., "Vitamin A, immunity, and infection," *Clinical Infectious Disease,* 19, 489–499 (1994).

10. Ginter, E., "Optimum intake of vitamin C for the human organisms," *Nutrition and Health,* 1, 66–77 (1982).

11. Gabor, M., "Pharmacologic effects of flavonoids on blood vessels," *Angiologica,* 9, 355–374 (1972).

12. Prasad, A., "Clinical, biochemical and nutritional spectrum of zinc deficiency in human subjects: An update," *Nutrition Review,* 41, 197–308 (1983).

13. Porea, T.J., Belmont, J.W., Mahoney, D.H., Jr., "Zinc induced anemia and neutropenia in an adolescent," *Journal of Pediatrics,* 136(5), 688–690.

14. Klein, A.D., Penneys, N.S., "*Aloe vera,*" *Journal of the American Academy of Dermatology,* 18, 714–719 (1988).

15. Chu, D.T., Wong, W.L., Mavlight, G.M., "Immunotherapy with Chinese medicinal herbs," *Journal of Clinical and Laboratory Immunology,* 25, 119–129 (1988).

16. Zhao, K.S., Mancini, C., Doria, G., "Enhancement of the immune response in mice by *Astragalus membranaceus,*" *Immunopharmacology,* 20, 225–233 (1990).

17. Erhard, M., "Effect of echinacea, aconitum, lachesis, and apis extracts, and their combinations of phagocytosis of human granulocytes," *Phytotherapy Research,* 8, 14–77 (1994).

18. Stoll, A., Renz, J., Brack, A., "Antibacterial substances II. Isolation and constitution of echnacoside, a glycoside from the roots of *Echinacea angustifolia,*" *Helvetica Chimica Acta,* 33, 1877–1893 (1950).

19. Murray, M., Pizzorno, J., *Encyclopedia of Natural Medicine* (Rocklin, California: 1998), p. 223.

20. Andiman, W.A., "Transmission of HIV-1 from mother to infant," *Current Opinion in Pediatrics,* 14(1), 78–85 (February 2002).

MEASLES

1. D'Souza, R.M., D'Souza, R., "Vitamin A for treating measles in children," Cochrane Database Syst Review, *(1):CD001479 (2002).*

MEMORY LOSS

1. Brooks, J.O., 3rd, Yesavage, J.A., Carta, A., Bravi, D., "Acetyl-l-carnitine slows decline in younger patients with Alzheimer's disease: a reanalysis of a double-blind, placebo-controlled study using the trilinear approach," *International Psychogeriatrics,* 10, 193–203 (1998).

2. Geula, C., Mesulam, M., "Cortical cholinergic fibers in aging and Alzheimer's: a morphometric study," *Neuroscience,* 33, 469–481 (1989).

3. West, M.J., Coleman, P.D., Flood, D.G., Troncoso, J.C., "Differences in the pattern of hippocampal neuronal loss in normal aging and Alzheimer's disease," *Lancet,* 344, 769–772 (1994).

4. Nunzi, M.G., Milan, F., Guidolin, D., Toffano, G., "Dendritic spine loss in hippocampus of aged rats. Effect of brain phosphatidylserine administration," *Neurobiology of Aging,* 8, 501–510 (1987).

5. Crook, T.H., Tinklenberg, J., Yesavage, J., Petrie, W., Nunzi, M.G., Massari, D.C., "Effects of phosphatidylserine in age associated memory impairment," *Neurology,* 41, 644–649 (1991).

6. Nerozzi, D., Magnani, A., Sforza, V., et al., "Early cortisol escape phenomenon reversed by phosphatidylserine in elderly normal subjects," *Clinical Trials Journal,* 26, 33–38 (1989).

7. Solomon, P.R., Adams, F., Silver, A., Zimmer, J., DeVeaux, R., "Ginkgo for memory enhancement: A randomized controlled trial," *Journal of the American Medical Association,* 288(7), 835–840 (20 August 2002).

8. Mix, J.A., Crews, W.D., "A double-blind, placebo-controlled, randomized trial of *Ginkgo biloba* extract EGb 761 in a sample of cognitively intact older adults: neuropsychological findings," *Human Psychopharmacology in Clinical Experience,* 17, 267–277 (2002).

9. Snowdon, D.A., Greiner, L.H., Mortimer, J.A., Riley, K.P., Greiner, P.A., Markesbery, W.R., "Brain infarction and the clinical expression of Alzheimer disease: The Nun Study," *Journal of the American Medical Association,* 277, 813–817 (1997).

10. Small, G.W., "The pathogenesis of Alzheimer's disease," *Journal of Clinical Psychiatry,* 59, 7–14 (1998).

MÉNIÈRE'S DISEASE

1. Moser, M., Ranacher, G., Wilmot, T.J., Golden, G.J., "A double-blind clinical trial of hydroxyethylrutosides in Meniere's disease," *Journal of Laryngoogy and Otology,* 98, 265–272 (1984).

2. Kraft, J.R., "Hyperinsulinemia: A merging history with idiopathic tinnitus, vertigo, and hearing loss," *International Tinnitus Journal,* 4(2), 127–130 (1998).

3. Simpson, J.J., Donaldson, I., Davies, W.E., "Use of homeopathy in the treatment of tinnitus," *British Journal of Audiology,* 32(4), 227–233 (August 1998).

MENKE'S DISEASE

1. Lott, I.T., Dipaolo, R., Raghavan, S.S., Clopath, P., Milunsky, A., Robertson, W.C., Jr., Kanfer, J.N., "Abnormal copper metabolism in Menke's steely-hair syndrome," *Pediatric Research,* 13(7), 845–850 (July 1979).

MIGRAINE

1. Malapira, A., "Migraine Headache," *eMedicine,* 3(7) (16 July 2002).

2. Lipton, R.B., Stewart, W.F., "Migraine in the United States: A review of epidemiology and healthcare use," *Neurology,* 43, S6–S10 (1993).

3. Trauninger, A., Pfund, Z., Koszegi, T., Czopf, J., "Oral magnesium load test in patients with migraine," *Headache,* 42(2), 114–119 (February 2002).

4. Mauskop, A., Altura, B.T., Altura, B.M., "Serum ionized magnesium levels and serum ionized calcium/ionized magnesium ratios in women with menstrual migraine," *Headache,* 42(4), 242–248 (April 2002).

5. Bigal, M.E., Bordini, C.A., Tepper, S.J., Speciali, J.G., "Intravenous magnesium sulphate in the acute treatment of migraine without aura and migraine with aura. A randomized, double-blind, placebo-controlled study," *Cephalalgia,* *22(5),* 345–353 *(June 2002).*

6. Peikert, A., Wilimzig, C., Kohne-Volland, R., "Prophylaxis of migraine with oral magnesium: results from a prospective, multi-center, placebo-controlled and double-blind randomized study," *Cephalalgia,* 16, 257–263 (1996).

7. Gagnier, J.D., "The therapeutic potential of melatonin in migraines and other headache types," *Alternative Medicine Review,* 6(5), 488–494 (2001).

8. Schoenen, J., Jacquy, J., Lenaerts, M., "Effectiveness of high-dose riboflavin in migraine prophylaxis. A randomized controlled trial," *Neurology,* 50, 466–470 (1998).

MITRAL VALVE PROLAPSE

1. Lichodziejewska. B., Klos, J., Rezler, J., Grudzka, K., Dluzniewska, M., Budaj, A., Ceremuzynski, L., "Clinical symptoms of mitral valve prolapse are related to hypomagnesemia and attenuated by magnesium supplementation," *American Journal of Cardiology,* 79(6), 768–772 (15 March 1997).

2. Oda, T., "Effect of coenzyme Q_{10} on stress-induced cardiac dysfunction in paediatric patients with mitral valve prolapse: a study by stress echocardiography," *Drugs in Experimental and Clinical Research,* 11(8), 557–576 (1985).

MORNING SICKNESS

1. Michelini, G.A., "Hyperemesis Gravidarum," *eMedicine,* 3(7) (12 July 2002).

2. Niebyl, J.R., Goodwin, T.M., "Overview of nausea and vomiting of pregnancy with an emphasis on vitamins and ginger," *American Journal of Obstetrics and Gynecology,* 186, S253–S255 (2002).

3. Vutyavanich, T., Wongtra-ngan, S., Ruangsri, R., "Pyridoxine for nausea and vomiting of pregnancy: a randomized, double-blind, placebo-controlled trial," *American Journal of Obstetrics and Gynecology,* 173, 881–884 (1995).

4. Fischer-Rasmussen, W., Kjaer, S.K., Dahl, C., et al., "Ginger treatment of hyperemesis gravidarum," *European Journal of Obstetrics, Gynecology, and Reproductive Biology,* 38, 19–24 (1991).

MOTION SICKNESS

1. Triesman, M., "Motion sickness: an evolutionary hypothesis," *Science,* 197, 493–495 (1977).

2. Lindseth, G., Lindseth, P.D., "The relationship of diet to airsickness," *Aviation, Space, and Environmental Medicine,* 66(6), 537–541 (June 1995).

3. Bagshaw, M., Stott, J.R.R., "The desensitization of chronically motion sick aircrew in the Royal Air Force," *Aviation, Space, and Environmental Medicine,* 56, 1144–1151 (1985).

4. Skoromnyi, N.A., "The effect of pyridoxine on cerebral hemodynamics in vestibular disorders," *Farmakologii i Toksikologii,* 52(6), 43–46 (November 1989).

5. Wood, C.D., Manno, J.E., Wood, M.J., Manno, B.R., Mims, M.E., "Comparison of efficacy of ginger with various antimotion sickness drugs," *Clinical Research and Practice in Drug Regulatory Affairs,* 6(2), 129–136 (1988).

6. Stewart, J.J., Wood, M.J., Wood, C.D., Mims, M.E., "Effects of ginger on motion sickness susceptibility and gastric function," *Pharmacology,* 42(2), 111–120 (1991).

7. European Scientific Cooperative on Phytotherapy. *Zingiberis rhizoma* (*ginger*). Exeter, UK: ESCOP; 1996–1997. Monographs on the Medicinal Uses of Plant Drugs, Fascicule 1.

8. Grontved, A., Brask, T., Kambskard, J., et al. "Ginger root against seasickness. A controlled trial on the open sea." *Acta Otolaryngol,* 105, 45–49 (1998).

9. Grontved, A., Hentzer, E., "Vertigo-reducing effect of ginger root. A controlled clinical study," *ORL J Otorhinolaryngol Relat Spec.,* 48, 282–286 (1986).

10. Qian, D.S., Liu, Z.S., "Pharmacologic studies on antimotion sickness actions of ginger," *Zhongguo Zhong Xi Yi Jie He Za Zhi,* 12(2), 95–98, 70 (February 1992).

MSG SENSITIVITY

1. Folkers, K., Shizukuishi, S., Scudder, S.L., Willis, R., Takemura, K., Longenecker, J.B.., "Biochemical evidence for a deficiency of vitamin B_6 in subjects reacting

to monosodium-L-glutamate by the Chinese restaurant syndrome," *Biochemistry and Biophysics Research Communications,* 100, 972–977 (1981).

2. Folkers, K., Shizukuishi, S., Willis, R., Scudder, S.L., Takemura, K., Longenecker, J.B., "The biochemistry of vitamin B_6 is basic to the cause of the Chinese restaurant syndrome," *Hoppe Seylers Zeitschrift für Physiologie und Chemie,* 365(3), 405–414 (March 1984).

MULTIPLE SCLEROSIS (MS)

1. Anderson, D.W., Ellenberg, J.H., Leventhal, C.M., et al., "Revised estimate of the prevalence of multiple sclerosis in the United States," *Annals of Neurology,* 31, 333–336 (1992).

2. Kidd, P.M., "Multiple sclerosis, an autoimmune inflammatory disease: prospects for its integrative management," *Alternative Medicine Review,* 6(6), 540–566 (December 2001).

3. Pizzorno, J.E., Jr., Murray, M.T., *Textbook of Natural Medicine* (London: Churchill Livingstone, 1999), p. 1416.

4. Landtblom, A.M., Flodin, U., Karlsson, M., et al., "Multiple sclerosis and exposure to solvents, ionizing radiation, and animals," *Scandinavian Journal of Work and Environmental Health,* 19, 399–404 (1993).

5. Swank, R.L., Dugan, B.B., "Effect of low saturated fat diet in early and late cases of multiple sclerosis," *Lancet,* 336, 37–39 (1990).

6. Nordvik, I., Myhr, K.M., Nyland, H., Bjerve, K.S., "Effect of dietary advice and n-3 supplementation in newly diagnosed MS patients," *Acta Neurologica Scandinavica,* 102(3), 143–149 (September 2000).

7. McCarty, M.F., "Upregulation of lymphocyte apoptosis as A strategy for preventing and treating autoimmune disorders: a role for whole-food vegan diets, fish oil and dopamine agonists," *Medical Hypotheses,* 57(2), 258–275. (August 2001).

8. Korwin-Piotrowska, T., Nocon, D., Stankowska-Chomicz, A., Starkiewicz, A., Wojcicki, J., Samochowiec, L., "Experience of Padma 28 in multiple sclerosis," *Phytotherapy Research,* 6, 133–136. (1992).

9. Winter, A., "New treatment for multiple sclerosis," *Neurol Orthop J Med Surg.,* 5, 39–43 (1984).

10. Hauser, S.L., Doolittle, T.H., Lopez-Bresnahan, M., et al., "An antispasticity effect of threonine in multiple sclerosis," *Archives of Neurology,* 49, 923–926 (1992).

11. Lee, A., Patterson, V., "A double-blind study of L-threonine in patients with spinal spasticity," *Acta Neurologica Scandinavica,* 88, 334–338 (1993).

12. Huggins, H.A., Levy, T.E., "Cerebrospinal fluid protein changes in multiple sclerosis after dental amalgam removal," *Alternative Medicine Review,* 3(4), 295–300 (August 1998).

13. Gilson, G., Wright, J.V., DeLack, E., Ballasiotes, G., "Transdermal histamine in multiple sclerosis: Part one–clinical experience," *Alternative Medicine Review,* 4(6), 424–428 (December 1999).

14. Rodriguez, F.J., Lluch, M., Dot, J., et al., "Histamine modulation of glutamate release from hippocampal synaptosomes," *European Journal of Pharmacology,* 323, 283–286 (1997).

15. van der Pouw Kraan, T.C., Snijders, A., Boeije, L.C., et al., "Histamine inhibits the production of interleukin-12 through interaction with H_2 receptors," *Journal of Clinical Investigation,* 102, 1866–1873. (1998).

MULTISYSTEM VASCULITIS

1. Terasawa, K., Bacowsky, H., Gerz, A., *Kampo, Japanese-Oriental Medicine: Insights from Clinical Cases* (Tokyo: K.K. Standard McIntyre, 1993), pp. 26–27.

MYASTHENIA GRAVIS

1. Lewis, S.J., Smith, P.E., "Osteoporosis prevention in myasthenia gravis: a reminder," *Acta Neurologica Scandinavica,* 103(5), 320–322 (May 2001).

NAIL INFECTIONS

1. Buck, D.S., Nidorf, D.M., Addino, J.G., "Comparison of two topical preparations for the treatment of onychomycosis: *Melaleuca alternifolia* (tea tree) oil and clotrimazole," *Journal of Family Practice,* 38(6), 601–605 (June 1994).

2. Dumenil, G., Chemli, R., Balansard, C., Guiraud, H., Lallemand, M., "Evaluation of antibacterial properties of marigold flowers (*Calendula officinalis* L.) and other homeopathic tinctures of *C. officinalis* L. and *C. arvensis* L.," *Ann. Pharm. Franç,* 38, 493 (1980).

NEUROPATHY (DIABETIC COMPLICATION)

1. Hounsom, L., Corder, R., Patel, J., Tomlinson, D.R., "Oxidative stress participates in the breakdown of neuronal phenotype in experimental diabetic neuropathy," *Diabetologia,* 44(4), 424–428 (April 2001).

2. Vincent, A.M., Brownlee, M., Russell, J.W., "Oxidative stress and programmed cell death in diabetic neuropathy," *Annals of the New York State Academy of Sciences,* 959, 369–383 (2002).

3. Gomez Viera, N., Soto Lavastida, A., Rosello Silva, H., Gomez e Molina Iglesias, M., "Risk factors involved in symmetrical distal diabetic neuropathy," *Revista de Neurología,* 32(9), 806–812 (16 May 2001).

4. Ziegler, D., Reljanovic, M., Mehnert, H., Gries, F.A., "Alpha-lipoic acid in the treatment of diabetic polyneuropathy in Germany: current evidence from clinical trials," *Experimental and Clinical Endocrinology and Diabetes,* 107(7), 421–430 (1999).

5. Ziegler, D., Gries, F.A., "Alpha-lipoic acid in the treatment of diabetic peripheral and cardiac autonomic neuropathy," *Diabetes,* 46 Suppl 2, S62–S66 (September 1997).

6. Goodnick, P.J., Breakstone, K., Wen, X.L., "Acupuncture and Neuropathy (letter)," *American Psychiatric Journal,* 157, 1342–1343 (August 2000).

NIGHT TERRORS IN CHILDREN

1. Paroli, E., "Opioid peptides from food (the exorphins)," *World Review of Nutrition and Dietetics,* 55, 58–97 (1988).

NIGHT VISION, IMPAIRED

1. Muth, E.R., Laurent, J.M., Jasper, P., "The effect of bilberry nutritional supplementation on night visual acuity and contrast sensitivity," *Alternative Medicine Review,* 5, 164–173 (2000).

2. Zadok, D., Levy, Y., Glovinsky, Y., et al., "The effect of anthocyanosides on night vision tests," *Investigations in Ophthalmology and Visual Science,* 38 (Suppl), 633 (1997).

3. Christian, P., West, K.P., Jr., Khatry, S.K., Katz, J., LeClerq, S., Pradhan, E.K., Shrestha, S.R., "Vitamin A or carotene supplementation reduces but does not eliminate maternal night blindness in Nepal," *The Journal of Nutrition,* 128(9), 1458–1463 (9 September 1998).

4. McCaleb, R. "Bilberry: health from head to toe," *Better Nutrition for Today's Living,* 29–31 (June 1991).

5. Jayle, G.E., Aubert, L., "Action des glucosides d'anthocyanes sur la vision scotopique et mesopique du sujet normal," *Therapie,* 19, 171–185 (1964).

6. Belleoud, L., Leluan, D., Boyer, Y.," Study on the effects of anthocyanin glycosides on the nocturnal vision of air traffic controllers," *Revue de Medicine Aeronautique et Spatiale,* 2, 18 (1966).

NOSEBLEEDS

1. Galley, P., Thiollet, M., "A double-blind, placebo-controlled trial of a new veno-active flavonoid fraction (S 5682) in the treatment of symptomatic capillary fragility," *International Angiology,* 12, 69–72 (1993).

2. Maffei Facino, R., Carini, M., Aldini, G., et al., "Free radicals scavenging action and anti-enzyme activities of procyanidines from *Vitis vinifera:* a mechanism for their capillary protective action," *Arzneimittel Forschung,* 44, 592–601 (1994).

3. Amella, M., Bronner, C., Briancon, F., et al.," Inhibition of mast cell histamine release by flavonoids and bioflavonoids," *Planta Medica,* 51, 16–20 (1985).

OBSESSIVE-COMPULSIVE DISORDER (OCD)

1. Pizzorno, J.E., Jr., Murray, M.T., *Textbook of Natural Medicine,* Volume 2, Second Edition (Edinburgh: Churchill-Livingstone, 1999), p. 787.

2. Poldinger, W., Calachini, B., Schwarz, W., "A functional-dimensional approach to depression. Serotonin deficiency as a target syndrome in comparison of 5-hydroxytryptophan and fluvoxamine," *Psychopathology*, 24, 53–81 (1991).

OSGOOD-SCHLATTER DISEASE

1. Chang, A.K., "Osgood-schlatter disease," *eMedicine Journal*, 2(5), (21 May 2001).

2. Hirano, A., Fukubayashi, T., Ishii, T., Ochiai, N., "Magnetic resonance imaging of Osgood-Schlatter disease: the course of the disease," *Skeletal Radiology*, 31(6), 334–342 (June 2002).

3. Nordstrom, P., Nordstrom, G., Thorsen, K., Lorentzon, R., "Local bone mineral density, muscle strength, and exercise in adolescent boys: a comparative study of two groups with different muscle strength and exercise levels," *Calciferous Tissue International*, 58(6), 402–408 (June 1996).

OSTEOARTHRITIS

1. Murray, M., Pizzorno, J. *Textbook of Natural Medicine* (London: Churchill-Livingstone, 1999), pp. 1441–1442.

2. Flugsrud, G.B., Nordsletten, L., Espehaug, B., Havelin, L.I., Meyer, H.E., "Risk factors for total hip replacement due to primary osteoarthritis: A cohort study in 50,034 persons," *Arthritis and Rheumatism*, 46(3), 675–682 (March 2002).

3. Bland, J.H., Cooper, S.M., "Osteoarthritis: a review of the cell biology involved and evidence for reversibility. Management rationally related to known genesis and pathophysiology," *Seminars in Arthritis and Rheumatology*, 14, 106–133 (1984).

4. Perry, G.H., Smith, M.J.G., Whiteside, C.G., "Spontaneous recovery of the hip joint space in degenerative hip disease," *Annals of Rheumatic Disease*, 31, 440–448 (1972).

5. Dingle, J.T., "The effects of NSAIDs on the matrix of human articular cartilages," *Zeitschrift für Rheumatologie*, 58(3), 125–129 (June 1999).

6. Hogue, J.H., Mersfelder, T.L., "Pathophysiology and first-line treatment of osteoarthritis," *Annals of Pharmacotheapy*, 36(4), 679–686 (April 2002).

7. Travers, R.L., Rennie, G.C., Newnham, R.E., "Boron and arthritis: the results of a double-blind pilot study," *Journal of Nutritional Medicine*, 1, 127–132 (1990).

8. Schachtschabel, D.O., Binninber, E., "Stimulatory effects of ascorbic acid in hyaluronic acid synthesis of in vitro cultured normal and glaucomatous trabecular meshwork cells of the human eye," *Zeitschrift für Gerontologie*, 26, 243–246 (1993).

9. Vaz, A.L., "Double-blind clinical evaluation of the relative efficacy of ibuprofen and glucosamine sulfate in the management of osteoarthrosis of the knee in out-patients," *Current Medical Research Opinions*, 8, 145–149 (1982).

10. Müller-Fassbiner, H., et al, "Glucosamine sulfate compared to ibuprofen in osteoarthritis of the knee," *Osteoarthritis and Cartilage*, 2, 61–69 (1994).

11. Reichelt, A., Forster, K.K., Fischer, M., et al., "Efficacy and safety of intramuscular glucosamine sulfate in osteoarthritis of the knees. A randomized, placebo-controlled, double-blind study," *Arzneimittel Forschung*, 44, 75–80 (1994).

12. Reichelt, A., Forster, K.K., Fischer, M., et al., ibid.

13. Tapadinhas, M.J., Revera, I.C., Bignamni, A.A., et al., "Oral glucosamine sulfate in the management of arthrosis. Report on a multi-centre open investigation in Portugal," *Pharmacotherapeutica*, 3, 157–168 (1982).

14. Bucsi, L, Poor, G., "Efficacy and tolerability of oral chondroitin sulfate as a symptomatic low-acting drug for osteoarthritis (SYSADOA) in the treatment of knee arthritis," *Osteoarthritis and Cartilage*, 6 (Suppl A), 31–36 (1998).

15. Berger, R., Nowak, H., "A new medical approach to the treatment of osteoarthritis. Report of an open phase IV study with ademetionine (Gumbaral)," *American Journal of Medicine*, 83, 84–88 (1987).

16. Konig, B., "A long term (two years) clinical trial with S-adenosylmethionine for the treatment of osteoarthritis," *American Journal of Medicine*, 83, 89–94 (1987).

17. Singh, B.G., Atal, C.K., "Pharmacology of an extract of Sali guggal ex-

Boswellia serrata, a new non-steroidal anti-inflammatory agent," *Agents and Actions*, 18, 407–412 (1986).

18. Beg, M., Singhal, K.C., Afzaal, S., "A study of effect of guggulsterone of hyperlipidemia of secondary glomerulopathy," *Indian Journal of Physiology and Pharmacology*, 40(3), 237–240 (July 1996).

19. Schnitzer, T.J., "Non-NSAID pharmacologic treatment options for the management of chronic pain," *American Journal of Medicine*, 105(1B), 45S–52S (27 July 1998).

20. McCleane, G., "The analgesic efficacy of topical capsaicin is enhanced by glyceryl trinitrate in painful osteoarthritis: a randomized, double blind, placebo controlled study," *European Journal of Pain*, 4(4), 355–360 (2000).

21. Murray, M., Pizzorno, J., *Encyclopedia of Natural Medicine* (London: Churchill-Livingstone, 1999), p. 1448.

22. Lequesne, M., Maheu, E., Cadet, C., Dreiser, R.L., "Structural effect of avocado/soybean unsaponifiables on joint space loss in osteoarthritis of the hip," *Arthritis and Rheumatism*, 17(1), 50–58 (February 2002).

23. Tillu, A., Tillu, S., Vowler, S., "Effect of acupuncture on knee function in advanced osteoarthritis of the knee: a prospective, non-randomized controlled study," *Acupuncture Medicine*, 20(1), 19–21 (March 2002).

24. Creamer, P., Singh, B.B., Hochberg, M.C., Berman, B.M., "Are psychosocial factors related to response to acupuncture among patients with knee osteoarthritis?" *Alternative Therapies in Health and Medicine*, 5(4), 72–76 (July 1999).

25. Kwon, Y.B., Kim, J.H., Yoon, J.H., Lee, J.D., Han, H.J., Mar, W.C., Beitz, A.J., Lee, J.H., "The analgesic efficacy of bee venom acupuncture for knee osteoarthritis: a comparative study with needle acupuncture," *American Journal of Chinese Medicine*, 29(2), 187–199 (2001).

26. Krampla, W., Mayrhofer, R., Malcher, J., Kristen, K.H., Urban, M., Hruby, W., "MR imaging of the knee in marathon runners before and after competition," *Skeletal Radiology*, 30(2), 72–76 (February 2001).

27. Parcell, S., "Sulfur in human nutrition and its applications in medicine," *Alternative Medicine Review*, 7(1), 22–44 (February 2002).

OSTEOMALACIA

1. Smith, U., Lacaille, F., Lepage, G., et al., "Taurine decreases fecal fatty acid and sterol excretion in cystic fibrosis. A randomized double-blind study," *American Journal of Diseases in Childhood*, 145, 1401–1404 (1995).

2. Carrasco, S., Codoceo, R., Prieto, G., et al., "Effect of taurine supplements on growth, fat absorption and bile acid on cystic fibrosis," *Acta Universitatis Carolinae*, 36, 152–156 (1990).

3. Booth, S.L., Tucker, K.L, Chen, H., et al., "Dietary vitamin K intakes are associated with hip fracture but not with bone mineral density in elderly men and women," *American Journal of Clinical Nutrition*, 71, 1201–1208 (2000).

4. Green, M.R., Buchanan, E., Weaver, L.T., "Nutritional management of the infant with cystic fibrosis," *Archives of Diseases in Childhood*, 72, 452–456 (1995).

OSTEOPOROSIS

1. Slipman, C.W., Whyte, W., Lenrow, D., "Osteoporosis," *eMedicine*, 3(6) (17 June 2002).

2. New, S.A., New, S.A., "The role of the skeleton in acid-base homeostasis," *Proceedings of the Nutrition Society*, 61(2), 151–164 (May 2002).

3. Kerstetter, J.E., Looker, A.C., Insogna, K.L., "Low dietary protein and low bone density," *Calcified Tissue International*, 66, 313 (2000).

4. Wortsman, J., Matsuoka, L.Y., Chen, T.C., Lu, Z., Holick, M.F., "Decreased bioavailability of vitamin D in obesity," *American Journal of Clinical Nutrition*, 72, 690–693 (2000).

5. Cleghorn, D.B., O'Loughlin, P.D., Schroeder, B.J., Nordin, B.E., "An open, crossover trial of calcium-fortified milk in prevention of early postmenopausal bone loss," *Medical Journal of Australia*, 175(5), 242–245 (3 September 2001).

6. Nieves, J.W., Komar, L., Cosman, F., Lindsay, R., "Calcium potentiates the effect of estrogen and calcitonin on bone mass: review and analysis," *American Journal of Clinical Nutrition*, 67, 18–24 (1998).

7. Brot, C., Jorgensen, N., Madsen, O.R., et al., "Relationships between bone mineral density, serum vitamin D metabolites and calcium: phosphorus intake in healthy perimenopausal women," *Journal of Internal Medicine*, 245, 509–516 (1999).

8. Hidaka, T., Hasegawa, T., Fujimura, M., Sakai, M., Saito, S., "Treatment for patients with postmenopausal osteoporosis who have been placed on HRT and show a decrease in bone mineral density: effects of concomitant administration of vitamin K(2)," *Journal of Bone Mineral Metabolism*, 20(4), 235–239 (2002).

9. Shiomi, S., Nishiguchi, S., Kubo, S., Tamori, A., Habu, D., Takeda, T., Ochi, H., "Vitamin K2 (menatetrenone) for bone loss in patients with cirrhosis of the liver," *American Journal of Gastroenterology*, 97(4), 978–981 (April 2002).

10. Elmståhl, S., Gullberg, B., Janzon, L., et al., "Increased incidence of fractures in middle-aged and elderly men with low intakes of phosphorus and zinc," *Osteoporos Inernational*, 8, 333–340 (1988).

11. Garrett, I.R., Gutierrez, G., Mundy, G.R., "Statins and bone formation," *Current Pharmacy*, 7(8), 715–736 (May 2001).

12. Iwasaki, T., Mukai, M., Tsujimura, T., Tatsuta, M., Nakamura, H., Terada, N., Akedo, H., "Ipriflavone inhibits osteolytic bone metastasis of human breast cancer cells in a nude mouse model," *International Journal of Cancer*, 100(4), 381–387 (1 August 2002).

OVARIAN CANCER

1. Kushi, L.H., Mink, P.J., Folsom, A.R., Anderson, K.E., Zheng, W., Lazovich, D., Sellers, T.A., "Prospective study of diet and ovarian cancer," *American Journal of Epidemiology*, 149(1), 21–31 (1 January 1999).

2. Pinto, V., Marinaccio, M., Garofalo, S., Vittoria Larocca, A.M., Geusa, S., Lanzilotti, G., Orsini, G., "Preoperative evaluation of ferritinemia in primary epithelial ovarian cancer," *Tumori*, 83(6), 927–929 (November–December 1997).

3. Cramer, D.W., Kuper, H., Harlow, B.L., Titus-Ernstoff, L., "Carotenoids, antioxidants and ovarian cancer risk in pre- and postmenopausal women," *International Journal of Cancer*, 94(1), 128–134 (1 October 2001).

4. Fleischauer, A.T., Olson, S.H., Mignone, L., et al., "Dietary antioxidants, supplements, and risk of epithelial ovarian cancer," *Nutrition and Cancer*, 4, 92–98 (2002)

5. Dickerson, R.N., White, K.G., Curcillo, P.G., 2nd, King, S.A., Mullen, J.L., "Resting energy expenditure of patients with gynecologic malignancies," *Journal of the American College of Nutrition*, 14(5), 448–454 (October 1995).

6. Shen, F., Weber, G., "Synergistic action of quercetin and genistein in human ovarian carcinoma cells," *Oncology Research*, 9(11–12), 597–602 (1997).

7. Rodriguez, C., Patle, A.V., Calle, E.E., Jacob, E.J., Thun, M.J., "Estrogen replacement therapy and ovarian cancer mortality in a large prospective study of U.S. women," *Journal of the American Medical Association*, 285, 1460–1465 (2001).

8. Smyth, J.F., Bowman, A., Parren, T., et al., "Glutathione reduces the toxicity and improves quality of life of women diagnosed with ovarian cancer treated with cisplatin: Results of a double-blind, randomized trial," *Annals of Oncology*, 8, 569–573 (1997).

9. Cascinu, S., Cordella, L., Del Ferro, E., et al., "Neuroprotective effect of reduced glutathione on cisplatin-based chemotherapy in advanced gastric cancer: a randomized double-blind placebo-controlled trial," *Journal of Clinical Oncology*, 13, 26–32 (1995).

10. Di Re, F., Bohm, S., Oriana, S., et al., "High-dose cisplatin and cyclophosphamide with glutathione in the treatment of advanced ovarian cancer," *Annals of Oncology*, 4, 55–61 (1993).

PAGET'S DISEASE

1. Agnusdei, D., Camporeale, A., Gonnelli, S., Gennari, C., Baroni, M.C., Passeri, M., "Short-term treatment of Paget's disease of bone with ipriflavone," *Bone Minerals*, 19 Suppl 1, S35–S42 (October 1992).

2. Bisbocci, D., Gallo, V., Damiano, P., Cantoni, R., Suriano, A., Chiandussi, L.,

"Paget's disease: prospects with ipriflavone," *Recenti Progressi in Medicina*, 83(12), 701–706 (December 1992).

3. Naiken, V.S., "Did Beethoven have Paget's disease of the bone?" *Annals of Internal Medicine*, 74, 995–999 (1971).

PANCREATITIS

1. Meskar, A., Plee-Gautier, E., Amet, Y., Berthou, F., Lucas, D., "Alcohol-xenobiotic interactions. Role of cytochrome P450 2E1," *Pathologie-Biologie* (Paris), 49(9), 696–702 (November 2001).

2. Bansi, D.S., Price, A., Russell, C., Sarner, M., "Fibrosing colonopathy in an adult owing to over use of pancreatic enzyme supplements," *Gut*, 46, 283–285 (2000).

3. Bagchi, D., Bagchi, M., Stohs, S., Ray, S.D., Sen, C.K., Preuss, H.G., "Cellular protection with proanthocyanidins derived from grape seeds," *Annals of the New York Academy of Sciences*, 957, 260–270 (May 2002).

4. Uden, S., Bilton, D., Nathan, L., Hunt, L.P., Main, C., Braganza, J.M., "Antioxidant therapy for recurrent pancreatitis: placebo-controlled trial," *Alimentary Pharmacological Therapy*, 4(4), 357–371 (August 1990).

PARASITES, INTESTINAL

1. Huh, S., "Pinworms," eMedicine, 2(9) (6 September 2001).

2. Joubert, J.R., van Schalwyk, D.J., Turner, K.J. "*Ascaris lumbricoides* and the human immunogenic response: enhanced IgE-mediated reactivity to common inhaled allergens," *South African Medical Journal*, 57, 409–412 (1980).

3. Aderel, W.I., Odenwole, O., "*Ascaris* and bronchial asthma in children," *African Journal of Medical Sciences*, 11, 161–166 (1982).

4. Jeliffe, E.F., Jellife, D.B., "Ascariasis and malnutrition: a worm's eye view," *American Journal of Clinical Nutrition*, 34, 1976–1977 (1982).

5. Krause, S., Moraleda, L., Leon, G., et al., "Intestinal absorption of Vitamin A and D-xylose in asymptomatic *Ascaris lumbriocides* infected school children," *Boletina Chilena de Parasitologia*, 41, 62–67 (1982).

6. Kaleysa, R.R., "Screening of indigenous plants for anthelmintic action against *Ascaris lumbricoides*. Part 1," *Indian Journal of Physiology and Pharmacology*, 19, 47–49 (1975).

7. Leung, A.Y., *Encyclopedia of Common Natural Ingredients Used in Food*, (New York: John Wiley, 1980), 162–163.

PARKINSON'S DISEASE

1. Franco-Maside, A., Coamano, J., Gomez, M.J., Cacabelos, R., "Brain mapping activity and mental performance after treatment with CDP-choline in Alzheimer's disease," *Methods and Findings in Experimental and Clinical Pharmacology*, 16, 597–607 (1994).

2. Dizdar, N., Kagdeal, B., Lindvall, B., "Treatment of Parkinson's disease with NADH," *Acta Neurologica Scandinavica*, 49, 345–347 (1994).

PELVIC ADHESIONS

1. Diamond, M.P., "Surgical aspects of infertility." In Sciarra, J.J., editor, *Gynecology and Obstetrics* (Philadelphia: Harper & Row, 1995), 1–26.

2. di Zerega, G.S., "Contemporary adhesion prevention," *Fertility and Sterility*, 61, 219–235 (1994).

3. Diamond, M.P., Hershlag, A., "Adhesion formation/reformation." In di Zerega, G.D., et al, editors, *Treatment of Postsurgical Adhesions* (New York: Alan R. Liss, 1990).

4. Eddy, C.A., Asch, R.H., Balmaceda, J.P., "Pelvic adhesion following microsurgical and macrosurgical wedge resection of the ovaries," *Fertility and Sterility*, 33, 557 (1980).

5. Canopoulos, A.N., et al., "Inhibition of leukocyte migration by progesterone in vivo and in vitro," *Society for Gynecological Investigation*, 8, 110 (1977).

6. Nakagawa, H., et al., "Anti-inflammatory action of progesterone on carrageenin-induced inflammation in rats," *Japanese Journal of Pharmacology*, 29, 509 (1970).

7. Evans, D.M., McAree, K., Guyton, D.P., Hawkins, N., Stakleff, K., "Dose de-

pendency and wound healing aspects of the use of tissue plasminogen activator in the prevention of intra-abdominal adhesions," *American Journal of Surgery,* 165, 229 (1993).

8. Ako, H., Cheung, A., Matsura, P., "Isolation of a fibrinolysis enzyme activator from commercial bromelain," *Archives of International Pharmacodynamics,* 254, 157–167 (1981).

9. Zatuchni, G.I., Colombi, D.J., "Bromelains therapy for the prevention of episiotomy pain," *Obstetrics and Gynecology,* 29, 275–278 (1967).

10. Howat, R.C., Lewis, G.D., "The effect of bromelain therapy on episiotomy wounds—a double-blind controlled clinical trial," *Journal of Obstetrics and Gynaecology of the British Commonwealth,* 79, 951–953 (1972).

11. Burns, J.W., Burgess, L, Shinner, K., Rose, R., Celt, M.J., Diamond, M.P., "A hyaluronate-based gel for the prevention of postsurgical adhesion: evaluation in two animal species," *Fertility and Sterility,* 66, 814 (1996).

12. Urnan, B., Gomel, V., Jetha, N., "Effect of hyaluronic acid on postoperative intraperitoneal adhesion formation in the rat model," *Fertility and Sterility,* 56, 563 (1991).

13. Taussig, S., "The mechanism of the physiological action of bromelain," *Medical Hypotheses,* 6, 99–104 (1980).

14. Murray, M.T., "A comprehensive review of vitamin C," *American Journal of Natural Medicine,* 3, 8–21 (1996).

15. Clemetson, C.A., "Histamine and ascorbic acid in human blood," *Journal of Nutrition,* 110, 662–668 (1980).

16. Harmon, D., Gardiner, J., Harrison, R., Kelly, A., "Acupressure and the prevention of nausea and vomiting after laparoscopy," *British Journal of Anaethesiology,* 82(3), 387–390 (March 1999).

17. Harmon, D., Gardiner, J., Harrison, R., Kelly, A., "Acupressure and prevention of nausea and vomiting during and after spinal anaesthesia for caesarean section," *British Journal of Anaesthesiology,* 84(4), 463–467 (April 2000).

18. Ho, C.M., Hseu. S.S., Tsai. S.K., Lee, T.Y., "Effect of P-6 acupressure on prevention of nausea and vomiting after epidural morphine for post-cesarean section pain relief," *Acta Anaethesiologica Scandinavica,* 40(3), 372–375 (March 1996).

19. Brown, C.S., Parker, N., Ling, F., et al.," Effect of magnets on chronic pelvic pain," *Obstetrics and Gynecology,* 95, S29 (2000).

PELVIC INFLAMMATORY DISEASE

1. Washington, A.E., Arno, P., Brooks, A., "The economic cost of pelvic inflammatory disease," *Journal of the American Medical Association,* 255, 1735–1738 (1986).

2. Dodson, P.S., "The polymicrobial etiology of acute pelvic inflammatory disease and treatment regimens," *Review of Infectious Disease,* 7, S6996–S7002 (1985).

3. Roberts, N. "Pelvic inflammatory disease." In Pizzorno, J.E., Jr., Murray, M.T., *Textbook of Natural Medicine* (London: Churchill Livingstone, 1999), p. 1470.

4. Ward, M., Watt, P., Robertson, J., "The human fallopian tubes: a laboratory model for gonococcal infection," *Journal of Infectious Disease,* 129, 650–659 (1974).

5. Kinghorn, G.R., Waugh, M.A., "Oral contraceptive use and prevalence of infection with *Chlamydia trachomatis* in women," *British Journal of Venereal Disease,* 57, 187–190 (1981).

6. Friberg, J., "Chlamydia attached to spermatozoa," *Journal of Infectious Disease,* 152, 854 (1985).

7. Kinghorn, G.R., Waugh, M.A., ibid.

8. Thompson, S., Washington, E., "Epidemiology of sexually transmitted *Chlamydia trachomatis* infections," *Epidemiology Review,* 5, 96–123 (1983).

9. Gudeian, A.M., Trobough, G., "Residues of pelvic inflammatory disease in intrauterine device users. A result of intrauterine devices or *Chlamydia trachomatis* infection," *American Journal of Obstetrics and Gynecology,* 154, 497–503 (1986).

10. Kinghorn, G.R., Waugh, M.A., ibid.

11. Shafer, M., Irwin, C., Sweet, R., "Acute salpingitis in the adolescent female," *Journal of Pediatrics,* 100, 339–350 (1982).

12. Cromer, B., Heald, F., "Pelvic inflammatory disease associated with *Neisseria gonorrhoeae* and *Chlamydia trachomatis.* Clinical correlates," *Sexually Transmitted Diseases,* 14, 125–129 (1987).

13. Cornelissenm, C.N., Kelley, M., Hobbs, M.M., Anderson, J.E., Cannon, J.G., Cohen, M.S., Sparling, P.F., "The transferrin receptor expressed by gonococcal strain FA1090 is required for the experimental infection of human male volunteers," *Molecular Microbiology,* 27(3), 611–616 (February 1998).

14. Payne, S.M., Finkelstein, R.A., "Pathogenesis and immunology of experimental gonococcal infection: role of iron in virulence," *Infection and Immunology,* 12(6), 1313–1318 (1975).

15. Mertz, K.J., Finelli, L., Levine, W.C., Mognoni, R.C., Berman, S.M., Fishbein, M., Garnett, G., St. Louis, M.E., "Gonorrhea in male adolescents and young adults in Newark, New Jersey: implications of risk factors and patient preferences for prevention strategies," *Sexually Transmitted Diseases,* 27(4), 201–207 (April 2000).

16. Handsfield, H., Lipman, T., Harnisch, J., Tronca, F., Holmes, K.K., "Asymptomatic gonorrhea in men: diagnosis, natural course, prevalence and significance," *New England Journal of Medicine,* 290, 117–123 (1974).

17. Diseker, R.A., 3rd, Peterman, T.A., Kamb, M.L., Kent, C., Zenilman, J.M., Douglas, J.M., Jr., Rhodes, F., Iatesta, M., "Circumcision and STD in the United States: cross sectional and cohort analyses," *Sexually Transmitted Diseases,* 76(6), 474–479 (December 2000).

18. Marchbanks, P., Lee, N.C., Peterson, H.B., "Cigarette smoking as a risk factor for pelvic inflammatory disease," *American Journal of Obstetrics and Gynecology,* 162, 639–644 (1990).

19. Scholes, D., "Current cigarette smoking and risk of acute pelvic inflammatory disease," *American Journal of Public Health,* 82, 1352–1355 (1992).

20. Tucker, M.E., "Douching raises pelvic inflammatory disease risk," *Family Practice News* (15 August 1996).

21. Keith, L., Berger, G., Edelman, D., Newton, W., Fullan, N., Bailey, R., Friberg, J., "On the causation of pelvic disease," *American Journal of Obstetrics and Gynecology,* 149, 215–224 (1984).

22. Eenham, I., "Pelvic inflammatory disease," *Australian Family Physician,* 15, 254–256 (1986).

23. Cromer, B., Heald, F., "Pelvic inflammatory disease associated with *Neisseria gonorrhoeae* and *Chlamydia trachomatis.* Clinical correlates," *Sexually Transmitted Diseases,* 14, 125–129 (1987).

24. Cazzola, P., Mazzanti, P., Bossi, G., "In vivo modulating effect of a calf thymus acid lysate on human T lymphocyte subsets and CD4+/CD8+ ratio in the course of difference diseases," *Current Therapies Research,* 42, 1011–1017 (1987).

25. Seifter, E., Rettura, G., Seiter, J., "Thymotrophic action of vitamin A," *Federal Proceedings,* 32, 947 (1973).

26. Semba, R.D., "Vitamin A, immunity, and infection," *Clinical Infectious Disease,* 19, 489–499 (1994).

27. Roberts, N., "Pelvic inflammatory disease." In Pizzorno, J.E., Jr., Murray, M.T. *Textbook of Natural Medicine* (London: Churchill Livingstone, 1999), p. 1474.

28. Ringsdorf, W., Cheraskin, E., "Vitamin C and human wound healing," *Oral Surgery,* 53(3), 231–236 (March 1982).

29. Gabor, M., "Pharmacologic effects of flavonoids on blood vessels," *Angiologica,* 9, 355–374 (1972).

30. Prasad, A., "Clinical, biochemical and nutritional spectrum of zinc deficiency in human subjects. An update," *Nutrition Review,* 41, 197–208 (1983).

31. Neubauer, R., "A plant protease and possible replacement of antibiotics," *Experimental Medicine and Surgery,* 19, 1430–169 (1961).

32. Shipochliev, T., Dimitrov, A., Aleksandrova, E., "Anti-inflammatory action of a group of plant extracts," *Veterinarskii i Medinitzskii Nauki,* 18(6), 87–94 (1981).

33. Kuhn, O., untitled article, *Arzneimittel-Forschung,* 3, 194–200 (1953).

34. Erhard, M., "Effect of echinacea, aconitum, lachesis, and apis extracts, and their combinations of phagocytosis of human granulocytes," *Phytotherapy Research,* 8, 14–77 (1994).

35. Facino, R.M., Carini, M., Aldini, G., Marinello, C., Arlandini, E., Franzoi, L., Colombo, M., Pietta, P., Mauri, P., "Direct characterization of caffeoyl esters with antihyaluronidase activity in crude extracts from *Echinacea angustifolia* roots by fast atom bombardment tandem mass spectrometry," *Farmaco,* 48(10), 1447–1461 (October 1993).

36. Budzinski, J.W., Foster, B.C., Vandenhoek, S. Arnason, J.T., "An in vitro evaluation of human cytochrome P405 3A4 inhibition by selected commercial herbal extracts and tinctures," *Phytomedicine,* 7(4), 273–282 (July 2000).

37. Luettig, B., Steinmuller, C., Gifford, G.E., Wagner, H., Lohmann-Matthes, M.L., "Macrophage activation by the polysaccharide arabinogalactan isolated from plant cell cultures of *Echinacea purpurea,*" *Journal of the National Cancer Institute,* 81(9), 669–675 (3 May 1989).

38. Rehman, J., Dillow, J.M., Carter, S.M., Chou, J., Le, B., Maisel, A.S., "Increased production of antigen-specific immunoglobulins G and M following in vivo treatment with the medical plants *Echinacea angustifolia* and *Hydrastis canadensis,*" *Immunology Letters,* 68(2–3), 391–395 (1 June 1999).

39. Iinuma, M., Tanaka, T., Sakakibara, N., Mizuno, M., Matsuda, H., Shiomoto, H., Kubo, M., "Phagocytic activity of leaves of Epimedium species on mouse reticuloendotherial system," *Yakugaku Zasshi,* 110(3), 179–185 (March 1990).

PEPTIC ULCER DISEASE

1. Braunwald, E., Fauci, A.S., Kasper, D.L., Hauser, S.L., Longo, D.L., Jameson, J.L., editors, *Harrison's Principles of Internal Medicine,* Fifteenth Edition (New York: McGraw-Hill, 2001), p. 1651.

2. Treiber, G., Lambert, J.R., "The impact of Helicobacter *pylori* eradication on peptic ulcer healing," *American Journal of Gastroenterology,* 93, 1080–1084 (1993).

3. Cutler, A.F., "Eradicating *Helicobacter pylori* infection," *Patient Care,* 91–100 (15 April 2000).

4. Soll, A.H., "Consensus conference. Medical treatment of peptic ulcer disease. Practice guidelines. Practice Parameters Committee of the American College of Gastroenterology," *Journal of the American Medical Association,* 275, 622–629 (1996).

5. Hawkey, C.J., Tulassay, Z., Szcaepanski, L., van Rensburg, C.J., Flipowicz-Sosnowska, A., Lanas, A., Wason, C.M., Peacock, R.A., Gillon, K.R., "Randomized controlled trial of *Helicobacter pylori* eradication in patients on non-steroidal anti-inflammatory drugs: HELP NSAIDs study. *Helicobacter* eradication for lesion prevention," *Lancet,* 352 (9133), 1016–1021 (26 September 1998).

6. Graham, D.Y., Anderson, S.Y., Lang, T., "Garlic or jalapeno peppers for treatment of *Helicobacter pylori* infection," *American Journal of Gastroenterology,* 94(5), 1200–1202 (May 2000).

7. Ernst, E., "Is garlic an effective treatment of *Helicobacter pylori* infection? (letter)," *Archives of Internal Medicine,* 159(20), (8 November 1999).

8. McNulty, C.A.M., Wilson, M.P., Havinga, W., Johnston, B., Maslin, D.T., "A pilot study to determine the effectiveness of garlic oil capsules in the treatment of dyspeptic patients with *Helicobacter pylori,*" *Report to the South West R & D Directorate,* 2001.

9. Holzer, P., Pabst, M.A., Lippe, I.T., "Intragastric capsaicin protects against aspirin-induced lesion formation and bleeding in the rat gastric mucosa," *Gastroenterology,* 96(6), 1425–1433 (June 1989).

10. Yeoh, K.G., Kang, J.Y., Yap, I., Guan, R., Tan, C.C., Wee, A., Teng, C.H., "Chili protects against aspirin-induced gastroduodenal mucosal injury in humans," *Digestive Diseases and Sciences,* 40(3), 580–583 (March 1995).

11. Best, R., Lewis, D.A., Nasser, N., "The anti-ulcerogenic activity of the unripe plantain banana (*Musa* species)," *British Journal of Pharmacology,* 82, 107–116 (1984).

12. Sanyal, A.K., Gupa, K.K., Chowdhury, N.K., "Banana and experimental peptic ulcer," *Journal of Pharmacy and Pharmacology,* 15, 283–284 (1963).

13. Beil, W., Birkholz, C., Sewing, K.F., "Effects of flavonoids on parietal cell acid secretion, gastric mucosal prostaglandin production and *Helicobacter pylori* growth," *Arzneimittel Forschung,* 45(6), 697–700 (1995).

14. Armuzzi, A., Cremonini, F., Ojetti, V., Bartolozzi, F., Canducci, F., Candelli, M., Santarelli, L., Cammarota, G., De Lorenzo, A., Pola, P., Gasbarrini, G.,

Gasbarrini, A., "Effect of *Lactobacillus* GG supplementation on antibiotic-associated gastrointestinal side effects during *Helicobacter pylori* eradication therapy: a pilot study," *Digestion,* 63, 1–7 (2001).

15. Sakamoto, I., Igarashi, M., Kimura, K., Takagi, A., Miwa, T., Koga, Y., "Suppressive effect of *Lactobacillus gasseri* OLL 2716 (LG21) on *Helicobacter pylori* infection in humans," *Journal of Antimicrobial Chemotherapy,* 47(5), 709–710 (May 2001).

16. Schumpelik, V.V., Farthmann, E., "Investigation into the protective efficacy of vitamin A against the development of stress ulcers in the rat," *Arzneimittel Forschung,* 26, 386 (1976).

17. Harris, P.I., "Dietary production of gastric ulcers in rats and prevention by tocopherol administration," *Proceedings for the Society for Experimental Biology in Medicine,* 4, 273–277 (1947), cited by Pizzorno, J.E., Jr., Murray, M.T., *Textbook of Natural Medicine* (London: Churchill Livingstone, 1999), p. 1483.

18. Carmel, R., Aruangzeb, I., Qian, D., "Associations of food-cobalamin malabsorption with ethnic origin, age, *Helicobacter pylori* infection, and serum markers of gastritis," *American Journal of Gastroenterology,* 96, 63–70 (1996).

19. Kaptan, K., Beyan, C., Ural, A.U., et al., "*Helicobacter pylori:* is it a novel causative agent in vitamin B_{12} deficiency?" *Archives of Internal Medicine,* 160, 1349–1353 (2000).

20. Jarosz, M., Dzieniszewski, J., Dabrowska-Ufinarz, E., et al, "Effects of high dose vitamin C treatment on *Helicobacter pylori* infection and total vitamin C concentration in gastric juice," *European Journal of Cancer Prevention,* 7, 449–454 (1998).

21. Farinati, F., Della Libera, G., Cardin, R., Molari, A., Plebani, M., Rugge, M., Di Mario, F., Naccarato, R., "Gastric antioxidant, nitrites, and mucosal lipoperoxidation in chronic gastritis and *Helicobacter pylori* infection," *Journal of Clinical Gastroenterology,* 22(4), 275–281 (June 1996).

22. Sobala, G.M., Schorah, C.J., Shjires, S., et al., "Effect of eradication of *Helicobacter pylori* on gastric juice ascorbic acid concentrations," *Gut* 34, 1038–1041 (1993).

23. Schorah, C.J., Sobala, G.M., Sanderson, M., et al, "Gastric juice and ascorbic acid: effects of disease and implications for gastric carcinogenesis," *American Journal of Clinical Nutrition,* 53, 287–293S (1991).

24. Rodrigues, L.E., Paes, I.B., Jacobnia, H., "Role of lysosomes on human ulcerogenic gastropathies. Effect of zinc ion on lysosomal stability," *Arquivos Gastroenterologias,* 35(4), 247–251 (October–December 1998).

25. Agafonov, A., letter, (7 January 2002).

26. Morgan, A.G., Pacsoo, C., McAdam, W.A.F., "Maintenance therapy: a two-year comparison between Caved-S and cimetidine treatment in the prevention of symptomatic gastric ulcer recurrence," *Gut,* 26, 599–602 (1985).

27. Kassir, Z.A., "Endoscopic controlled trial of four drug regimens in the treatment of chronic duodenal ulceration," *Irish Medical Journal,* 78, 153–156 (1985).

28. Huwez, F.U., Al-Habbal, M.J., "Mastic in treatment of benign gastric ulcers," *Gastroenterology Japan,* 21, 273–274 (1986).

29. Al-Habbal, M.J., Al-Habbal, Z., Huwez, F.U., "A double-blind controlled clinical trial of mastic and placebo in the treatment of duodenal ulcer," *Clinical and Experimental Pharmacology and Physiology,* 11, 541–544 (1984).

PERIPHERAL VASCULAR DISEASE

1. Drabaek, H., Mehlsen, J., Himmelstrup, H., Winther, K., "A botanical compound, Padma 28, increases walking distance in stable intermittent claudication," *Angiology,* 44(11), 863–867 (1993).

PEYRONIE'S DISEASE

1. Lauman, A., "Peyronie Disease," *eMedicine,* 3(4) (1 April 2002).

2. Carson, C.C., "Potassium para-aminobenzoate for treatment of Peyronie's disease: is it effective?" *Techniques of Urology,* 3, 135–139 (1997).

PHENYLKETONURIA (PKU)

1. Ercal, N., Aykin-Burns, N., Guerer-Ohan, H., McDonald, J.D., "Oxidative

stress in a phenylketonuria animal model.," *Free Radicals in Biology and Medicine,* 32(9), 906–911 (May 2002).

2. Koch, R., Moseley, K., Ning, J., et al., "Long-term beneficial effects of the phenylalanine-restricted diet in late-diagnosed individuals with phenylketonuria," *Molecular Genetics and Metabolism,* 67, 148–155 (1999).

3. Walter, J.H., White, F.J., Hall, S.K., MacDonald, A., Rylance, G., Boneh, A., Francis, D.E., Shortland, G.J., Schmidt, M., Vail, A., "How practical are recommendations for dietary control in phenylketonuria?" *Lancet,* 360(9326), 55–57 (6 July 2002).

4. Berry, H.K., Brunner, R.L., Hunt, M.M., et al., "Valine, isoleucine, and leucine. A new treatment for phenylketonuria," *American Journal of the Diseases of Childhood,* 144, 539–543 (1990).

5. Agostoni, C., Riva, E., Biasucci, G., et al., "The effects of n-3 and n-6 polyunsaturated fatty acids on plasma lipids and fatty acids of treated phenylketonuric children," *Prostaglandins Leukotrienes, and Essential Fatty Acids,* 53, 401–404 (1995).

6. Jochum, F., Terwolbeck, K., Meinhold, H., et al., "Effects of a low selenium state in patients with phenylketonuria," *Acta Paediatrica,* 86, 775–777 (1997).

7. Mackey, S.A., Berlin, C.M., Jr., "Effect of dietary aspartame on plasma concentrations of phenylalanine and tyrosine in normal and homozygous phenylketonuric patients," *Clinical Pediatrics* (Philadelphia), 31(7), 394–399 (July 1992).

8. Sievers, E., Arpe, T., Schleyerbach, U., Schaub, J., "Molybdenum supplementation in phenylketonuria diets: adequate in early infancy?" *Journal of Pediatric Gastroenterology and Nutrition,* 31, 57–62 (2000).

PHLEBITIS

1. Maurer, H.R., "Bromelain: biochemistry, pharmacology, and medical use," *Cellular and Molecular Life Sciences,* 58(9), 1234–1245 (August 2001).

2. Neubauer, R., "A plant protease for the potentiation of a possible replacement of antibiotics," *Experimental Medicine and Surgery,* 19, 143–160 (1961).

3. Felton, G., "Does kinin released by pineapple stem bromelain stimulate production of prostaglandin E_1-like compounds?" *Hawaii Medical Journal,* 36, 39–47 (1977).

4. Taussig, S., Nieper, H., "Bromelain: its use in prevention and treatment of cardiovascular disease. Present status," *Journal of the International Association for Preventative Medicine,* 6, 139–151 (1979).

5. Seligman, B., "Oral bromelains as adjuncts in the treatment of acute thrombophlebitis," *Angiology,* 20, 22–26 (1969).

PLUMMER-VINSON SYNDROME

1. For example, Mejia, L.A., Chew, F., "Hematological effect of supplementing anemic children with vitamin A alone and in combination with iron," *American Journal of Clinical Nutrition,* 48, 595–600 (1988).

2. Hunt, J.R., Gallagher, S.K., Johnson, L.K., "Effect of acorbic acid on apparent iron absorption by women with low iron stores," *American Journal of Clinical Nutrition,* 59, 1381–1385 (1991).

PNEUMONIA

1. Marston, B.J., Plouffe, J.F., File, T.M. Jr., et al., "Incidence of community-acquired pneumonia requiring hospitalization. Results of a population-based active surveillance study in Ohio. The community-based pneumonia incidence study group," *Archives of Internal Medicine,* 157(15), 1709–1718 (1997).

2. Wichtl, M., Grainger Bisset, N., eds. *Herbal Drugs and Phytopharmaceuticals: A Handbook for Practice on a Scientific Basis.* (Stuttgart, Germany: MedPharm, 1994), p. 474

3. Rimoldi, R., Ginesu, F., Giura, R., "The use of bromelain in pneumological therapy," *Drugs in Experimental Clinical Research,* 4, 55–66 (1978).

4. Hunt, C., Chakravorty, N.K., Anna, G., Habibzadeh, N., Schorah, C.J., "The clinical effects of vitamin C supplementation in elderly hospitalized patients with acute respiratory infections," *International Journal of Vitaminology and Nutrition Research,* 64(3), 212–219 (1994).

5. Nagibina, M.V., Neifakh, E.A., Krylov, V.F., Braginskii, D.M., Kulagina., M.G., "The treatment of pneumonias in influenza using antioxidants," *Terpevticheskii Arkhiv,* 68(11), 33–35 (1996).

6. Wildfeuer, A., Mayerhofer, D., "The effects of plant preparations on cellular functions in body defense," *Arzneimittel-Forschung,* 44(3), 361–366 (March 1994).

7. Kuhn, O., untitled article, *Arzneimittel-Forschung,* 3, 194–200 (1953).

8. Budzinski, J.W., Foster, B.C., Vandenhoek, S., Arnason, J.T., "An in vitro evaluation of human cytochrome P405 3A4 inhibition by selected commercial herbal extracts and tinctures," *Phytomedicine,* 7(4), 273–282 (July 2000).

POISON IVY, POISON OAK, AND POISON SUMAC

1. Teelucksingh, S., Mackie, A.D., Burt, D., McIntyre, M.A., Brett, L., Edwards, C.R., "Potentiation of hydrocortisone activity in skin by glycyrrhetinic acid," *Lancet,* 335(8697), 1060–1063 (5 May 1990).

2. Manku, M.S., Horrobin, D.F., Morse, N., Kyte, V., Jenkins, K., Wright, S., Burton, J.L., "Reduced levels of prostaglandin precursors in the blood of atopic patients: defective delta-6-desaturase function as a biochemical basis for atopy," *Prostaglandins and Leukotrienes in Medicine,* 9(6), 615–628 (December 1982).

3. Courage, B., Nissen, H.P., Wehrmann, W., Biltz, H., "Influence of polyunsaturated fatty acids on the plasma catecholamines of patients with atopic eczema," *Zeitschrift für Hautkrankheit,* 66, 509–510 (1991).

4. Nissen, H.P., Wehrmann, W., Kroll, U., Kreyse, H.W., "Influence of polyunsaturated fatty acids on the plasma phospholipids of atopic patients," *Fat Science and Technology,* 90, 268–271 (1988).

5. Middleton, E., Drzewiecki, G., "Naturally occurring flavonoids and human basophil histamine release," *International Archives of Allergy and Applied Immunology,* 77, 155–157 (1985).

6. Yoshimoto, T., Furukawa, M., Yamamoto, S., Horie, T., Watanabe-Kohno, S., "Flavonoids: potent inhibitors of arachidonate 5-lipoxygenase," *Biochemistry and Biophysics Research Communications,* 116(2), 612–618 (31 October 1983).

7. Worm, M., Herz, U., Krab, J.M., Renz, H, Henz, B.M., "Effects of retinoids on in vitro and in vivo IgE production," International *Archives of Allergy and Immunology,* 124(1–3), 233–236 (January-March 2001).

8. Tobe, M., Isobe, Y., Goto, Y., Obara, F., Tsuchiya, M., Matsui, J., Hirota, K., Hayashi, H., "Synthesis and biological evaluation of CX-659S and its related compounds for their inhibitory effects on the delayed-type hypersensitivity reaction," *Bioorganic Medicinal Chemistry,* 8(8), 2037–2047 (August 2000).

9. Del Toro, R., Baldo, Capotorti G., Ginalanella, G., Miraglia del Giudice, M., Moro, R., Perrone, L., "Zinc and copper status in allergic children," *Acta Paediatrica Scandinavica,* 76(4), 612–617 (July 1987).

10. el-Kholy, M.S., Gas Allah, M.A., el-Shimi, S., el-Baz, F., el-Tayeh, H., Abdel-Hamid M.S., "Zinc and copper status in children with bronchial asthma and atopic dermatitis," *Egyptian Public Health Association Newsletter,* 65(5–6), 657–668 (1990).

11. Cooper, P.D., Carter, M., "Anti-complementary action of polymorphic 'solubility forms' of particulate inulin," *Molecular Immunology,* 23, 895–901 (1985).

12. Schichijo, M., Shimizu, Y., Hiramatsu, K., Inagaki, N., Tagaki, K., Nagai, H., "Cyclic AMP-elevating agents inhibit mite-antigen-induced IL-4 and IL-13 release from basophil-enriched leukocyte preparation," *International Archives of Allergy and Immunology,* 114(4), 348–353 (December 1997).

13. Teelucksingh, S., Mackie, A.D., Burt, D., McIntyre, M.A., Brett, L., Edwards, C.R., ibid.

PREECLAMPSIA AND ECLAMPSIA

1. Hubel, C.A., Kozlov, A.V., Kagan, V.E., Evans, R.W., Advidge, S.T., McLaughlin, M.K., Roberts, J.M., "Decreased transferrin and increased transferrin saturation in sera of women with preeclampsia: implications for oxidative stress," *American Journal of Obstetrics and Gynecology,* 175 (3 Pt 1), 692–700 (September 1996).

2. Hubel, C.A., Kagan, V.E., Kisin, E.R., McLaughlin, M.K., Roberts, J.M., "Increased ascorbate radical formation and ascorbate depletion in plasma from

women with preeclampsia: implications for oxidative stress," *Free Radicals in Biology and Medicine,* 23(4), 597–609 (1997).

3. Tyurin, V.A., Liu, S.Z., Tyurina, Y.Y., Sussman, N.B., Hubel, C.A., Roberts, J.M., Taylor, R.N., Kagan, V.E., "Elevated levels of S-nitrosoalbumin in preeclampsia plasma," *Circulatory Research,* 88(11), 1210–1215 (8 June 2001).

4. Atallah, A.N., Hofmeyr, G.J., Duley, L., "Calcium supplementation during pregnancy for preventing hypertensive disorders and related problems," *Cochrane Database System Review,* CD0001059 (2000).

5. Levine, R.J., Hauth, J.C., Curet, L.B., Sibai, B.M., Catalano, P.M., Morris, C.D., DerSimonian, R., Esterlitz, J.R., Raymond, E.G., Bild, D.E., Clemens, J.D., Cutler, J.A., "Trial of calcium to prevent preeclampsia," *New England Journal of Medicine,* 337(2), 69–76 (10 July 1997).

6. Hertz-Picciotto, I., Schramm, M., Watt-Morse, M., Chantala, K., Anderson, J., Osterloh, J., "Patterns and determinants of blood lead during pregnancy," *American Journal of Epidemiology,* 152(9), 829–827 (1 November 2000).

7. Sibai, B.M., Villar, M.A., Bray, E., "Magnesium supplementation during pregnancy: a double-blind randomized controlled clinical trial," *American Journal of Obstetrics and Gynecology,* 163(1 Pt 1), 240–241 (July 1990).

8. Spatling, L., Spatling, G., "Magnesium supplementation in pregnancy. A double-blind study," *British Journal of Obstetrics and Gynaecology,* 95(2), 120–125 (February 1988).

9. Rudnicki, M., Frolich, A., Rasmussen, W.F., McNair, P., "The effect of magnesium on maternal blood pressure in pregnancy-induced hypertension. A randomized double-blind placebo-controlled trial," *Acta Obstretrica et Gynaecologica Scandinavica,* 70(6), 445–450 (1991).

10. Laurence, K.M., James, N., Miller, M.H., Tennant, G.B., Campbell, H., "Double-blind randomized controlled trial of folate treatment before conception to prevent recurrence of neural-tube defects,:" *British Medical Journal (Clinical Research and Education),* 282(6275), 1509–1511 (9 May 1981).

11. Velie, E.M., Block, G., Shaw, G.M., Samuels, S.J., Schaffer, D.M., Kulldorff, M., "Maternal supplemental and dietary zinc intake and the occurrence of neural tube defects in California," *American Journal of Epidemiology,* 150(6), 605–616 (15 September 1999).

12. Chappell, L.C., Seed, P.T., Briley, A.L., Kelly, F.J., Lee, R., Hunt, B.J., Parmar, K., Bewley, S.J., Shennan, A.H., Steer, P.J., Poston, L., "Effect of antioxidants on the occurrence of pre-eclampsia in women at increased risk: a randomized trial," *Lancet,* 357(9267), 1534 (12 May 2001).

13. Hubel, C.A., Kozlov, A.V., Kagan, V.E., Evans, R.W., Advidge, S.T., McLaughlin, M.K., Roberts, J.M., ibid.

PREMENSTRUAL SYNDROME (PMS)

1. Christensen, M., Tybring, G., Mihara, K., Yasui-Furokori, N., Carrillo, J.A., Ramos, S.I., Andersson, K., Dahl, M.L., Bertilsson, L., "Low daily 10-mg and 20-mg doses of fluvoxamine inhibit the metabolism of both caffeine (cytochrome P4501A2) and omeprazole (cytochrome P4502C19)," *Clinical Pharmacology and Therapy,* 71(3), 141–152 (March 2002).

2. Wyatt, K.M., Dimmock, P.W., Frischer, M., Jones, P.W., O'Brien, S.P., "Prescribing patterns in premenstrual syndrome," *BMC Women's Health,* 2(1), 4 (19 June 2002).

3. Thys-Jacobs, S., Starkey, P., Bernstein, D., Tian, J., "Calcium carbonate and the premenstrual syndrome: effects on premenstrual and menstrual symptoms," *American Journal of Obstetrics and Gynecology,* 179, 444–452 (1998).

4. De Souza, M.C., Walker, A.F., Robinson, P.A., Bolland, K., "A synergistic effect of a daily supplement for 1 month of 200 mg magnesium plus 50 mg vitamin B$_6$ for the relief of anxiety-related premenstrual symptoms: a randomized, double-blind, crossover study," *Journal of Women's Health and Gender Based Medicine,* 9(2), 131–139 (March 2002).

5. Schellenberg, R., "Treatment for the premenstrual syndrome with agnus castus fruit extract: prospective, randomized, placebo controlled study," *BMJ,* 322, 134–137 (20 January 2001).

PROSTATE CANCER

1. Hughes-Fulford, M., Chen, Y., Tjandrawinata, R.R., "Fatty acid regulates

gene expression and growth of human prostate cancer PC-3 cells," *Carcinogenesis,* 22, 701–707 (2001).

2. Attiga, F.A., Fernandez, P.M., Weeraratna, A.T., et al. "Inhibitors of prostaglandin synthesis inhibit human prostate tumor cell invasiveness and reduce the release of matrix metalloproteinases," *Cancer Research,* 60, 4629–4637 (2000).

3. Kristal, A.R., Cohen, J.H., Qu, P., Stanford, J.L., "Associations of energy, fat, calcium, and vitamin D with prostate cancer risk," *Cancer Epidemiology, Biomarkers, and Prevention,* 11(8), 719–725 (August 2002).

4. Clark, L.C., Combs, G.G., Turnbull, B.W., et al., "Effects of selenium supplementation for cancer prevention in patients with carcinoma of the skin. A randomized controlled trial. Nutritional Prevention of Cancer Study Group," *Journal of the American Medical Association,* 276, 1957–1963 (1996).

5. Giovannucci, E., "Tomatoes, tomato-based products, lycopene and cancer. Review of the epidemiologic literature," *Journal of the National Cancer Institute,* 91, 317–331 (1999).

6. Cohen, L.A., "Nutrition and Prostate Cancer," *Annals of the New York Academy of Sciences,* 963, 148–155 (August 2002).

7. Stahl, W., Junghams, A., De Boer, B., et al., "Carotenoid mixtures protect multilamellar liposomes against oxidative damage: synergistic effects of lycopene and lutein," *FEBS Letters,* 427, 305–308 (1998).

8. Cacciola, S.A., Cohen, L.A., Kashfi, K., "Lycopene inhibits proliferation and regulates cyclooxygenase-2 gene expression in neoplastic rat mammary epithelial cells," *FASEB Journal,* 13, Abstract 441–2 (1999).

9. Stahl, W., Von Laar, J., Martin, H.D. et al., Stimulation of gap junctional communication: comparison of acyclo-retinoic acid and lycopene," *Archives of Biochemistry and Biophysics,* 323, 271–274 (2000).

10. Van Veldhuizen, P.J., Taylor, S.A., Williamson, S., Drees, B.M., "Treatment of vitamin D deficiency in patients with metastatic prostate cancer may improve bone pain and muscle strength," *Journal of Urology,* 163, 187–190 (2000).

11. Hsieh, T.C., Xiong, W., Traganos, F., Darzynkiewicz, Z., Wu, J.M., "Effects of PC-SPES on proliferation and expression of AR/PSA in androgen-responsive LNCaP cells are independent of estrodiol," *Anticancer Research,* 22(4), 2051–2060 (July–August 2002).

PROSTATITIS

1. Yavascaoglu, I., Oktay, B., Simsek, U., Ozyurt, M., "Role of ejaculation in the treatment of chronic non-bacterial prostatitis," *International Journal of Urology,* 6, 130–134 (1999).

2. Buck, A.C., Rees, R.W., Ebeling, L., "Treatment of chronic prostatitis and prostadynia with pollen extract," *British Journal of Urology,* 64, 496–499 (1989).

PSORIASIS

1. Strom, T.B., Carpenter, C.B., "Cyclic nucleotides in immunosuppression—neuroendocrine pharmacologic manipulation and in vivo immunoregulation of immunity acting via second messenger systems," *Transplant Procedures,* 12(2), 304–310 (June 1980).

2. Ferreira, G.G., Brascher, H.K., Javierre, M.Q., Sassine, W.A., Lima, A.O., "Rosette formation by human T and B lymphocytes in the presence of adrenergic and cholinergic drugs," *Experientia,* 32(12), 1594–1596 (15 December 1976).

3. Gallin, J.I., Sandler, J.A., Clyman, R.I., Manganiello, V.C., Vaughan, M., "Agents that increase cyclic AMP inhibit accumulation of cGMP and depress human monocyte locomotion," *Journal of Immunology,* 120(2), 492–496 (February 1978).

4. Nagpal, S., Chandraratna, R.A., "Vitamin A and regulation of gene expression," *Current Opinion in Clinical Nutrition and Metabolic Care,* 1(4), 341–346 (July 1998).

5. Saurat,. J.H., "Retinoids and psoriasis: novel issues in retinoid pharmacology and implications for psoriasis treatment," *Journal of the American Academy of Dermatology,* 41(3 Pt 2), S2–S6 (September 1999).

6. Serwin, A.B., Chodynicka, B., Wasowicz W., Gromadzinska, J., "Selenium nutritional status and the course of psoriasis [abstract on MedLine]," *Pol*

Merkuriusz Lek, 6(35), 263–265 (May 1999).

7. Frank, S., Munz, B., Werner, S., "The human homologue of a bovine non-selenium glutathione peroxidase is a novel keratinocyte growth factor-regulated gene," *Oncogene,* 27, 14(8), 915–921 (February 1997).

8. Fairris, G.M., Lloyd, B., Hinks, L., Perkins, P.J., Clayton, B.E., "The effect of supplementation with selenium and vitamin E in psoriasis," *Annals of Clinical Biochemistry,* 26(Pt 1), 83–88 (January 1989).

9. Azzini, M., Girelli, D., Olivieri, O., Guarini, P., Stanzial, A.M., Frigo, A., Milanino, R., Bambara, L.M., Corrocher, R., "Fatty acids and antioxidant micronutrients in psoriatic arthritis," *Journal of Rheumatology,* 22(1), 103–108 (January 1995).

10. Syed, T.A., Ahmad, S.A, Holt, A.H., Ahmad S.A., Ahmad, S.H., Afzal, M., "Management of psoriasis with Aloe vera extract in a hydrophilic cream: a placebo-controlled, double-blind study," *Tropical Medicine and International Health,* 1(4), 505–509 (August 1996).

11. Stucker, M., Memmel, U., Hoffmann, M., Hartung, J., Altmeyer, P., "Vitamin b(12) cream containing avocado oil in the therapy of plaque psoriasis," *Dermatology,* 203(2), 141–147 (2001).

12. Reimann, S., Luger, T., Metze, D., "Topische anwendung von capsaicin in der dermatologie zur therapie von juckreiz und schmerz," *Hautarzt,* 51(3), 164–172 (March 2000).

13. Rekka, E.A., Kourounakis, A.P., Kourounakis, P.N., "Investigation of the effect of chamazulene on lipid peroxidation and free radical processes," *Research Communications in Molecular Pathology & Pharmacology,* 92(3), 361–364 (June 1996).

14. Safayhi, H., Sabieraj, J., Sailer, E.R., Ammon, H.P., "Chamazulene, an antioxidant-type inhibitor of leukotriene B4 formation," *Planta Medica,* 60(5), 410–413 (October 1994).

15. Miller, T., Wittstock, U., Lindequist, U., Teuscher, E., "Effects of some components of the essential oil of chamomile, *Chamomilla recutita,* on histamine release from rat mast cells," *Planta Medica,* 62(1), 60–61 (1 February 1996).

16. Yamada, K., Miura, T., Mimaki, Y., Sashida, Y., "Effect of inhalation of chamomile oil vapour on plasma ACTH level in ovariectomized-rat under restriction stress," *Biological & Pharmaceutical Bulletin,* 19(9), 1244–1246 (September 1996).

17. Teelucksingh, S., Mackie A.D., Burt, D., McIntyre, M.A., Brett, L., Edwards, C.R., "Potentiation of hydrocortisone activity in skin by glycyrrhetinic acid," *Lancet,* 335(8697), 1060–1063 (5 May 1990).

18. Editorial, "Polyamines in psoriasis," *Journal of Investigational Dermatology,* 81, 385–387 (1983).

19. Proctor, M.S., Wilkinson, D.I., Orenberg, E.K., Farber, E.M., "Lowered cutaneous and urinary levels of polyamines with clinical improvement in treated psoriasis," *Archives of Dermatology,* 115(8), 945–9 (August 1979).

20. Rosenberg, E., Belew, P., "Microbial factors in psoriasis," *Archives of Dermatology,* 118, 1434–1444 (1982).

21. Skottova, N., Krecman, V., Walterova, D., Ulrichova, J., Kosina, P., Smianek, V., "Effect of silymarin on serum cholesterol levels in rats," *Acta Universitatis Palackianae Olomucensis Facultatis Medicae,* 141, 87–89 (1998).

22. Thurmon, F.M., "The treatment of psoriasis with sarsaparilla compound," *New England Journal of Medicine,* 227, 128–133 (1942).

23. Seidl, H., Kreimer-Erlache, H., Back, B., Soyer, H.P., Hofler, G., Kerl, H., Wolf, P., "Ultraviolet exposure as the main initiator of p53 mutations in basal cell carcinomas from psoralen and ultraviolet A-treated patients with psoriasis," *Journal of Investigational Dermatology,* 117(2), 365–370 (August 2001).

24. Boer, J., Hermans, J., Schothorst, A., Suurmond, D., "Comparison of phototherapy (UV-B) and photochemotherapy (PUVA) for clearing and maintenance therapy of psoriasis," *Archives of Dermatology,* 120, 52–57 (1984).

25. Seidl, H., Kreimer-Erlacher, H., Back, B., Soyer, H.P., Hofler, G., Kerl, H., Wolf, P., ibid.

26. Ishizaki, C., Oguro, T., Yoshida, T., Wen, C.Q., Sueki, H., Iijima, M., "Enhancing effect of ultraviolet A on ornithine decarboxylase induction and dermatitis evoked by 12-o-tetradecanoylphorbol-13-acetate and its inhibition by curcumin in mouse skin," *Dermatology,* 193(4), 311–317 (1996).

27. Urabe, H., Nishitani, K., Kohda, H., "Hyperthermia in the treatment of psoriasis," *Archives of Dermatology,* 117, 770–774 (1981).

28. Orenberg, E., Deneau, D., Farber, E., "Response of chronic psoriatic plaques to localized heating induced by ultrasound," *Archives of Dermatology,* 116, 893–897 (1980).

RADON EXPOSURE

1. Neuberger, J.S., "Residential radon exposure and lung cancer: an overview of published studies," *Cancer Detection and Prevention,* 15(6), 435–441 (1991).

2. Sullivan, M., Reummler, P., "Absorption of U, Np, NP, Am, and Cm from the gastrointestinal tracts of rats fed on iron deficient diet," *Health Physics,* 54, 311–316 (1988).

3. Murray, M., Pizzorno, J., *Encyclopedia of Natural Medicine* (London: Churchill-Livingstone, 1999), p. 169.

RAYNAUD'S PHENOMENON

1. Lau, C.S., Khan, F., Brown, R., McCallum, P., Belch, J.J., "Digital blood flow response to body warming, cooling, and rewarming in patients with Raynaud's phenomenon," *Angiology,* 46(1), 1–10 (January 1995).

2. Lau, C.S., O'Dowd, A., Belch, J.J., "White blood cell activation in Raynaud's phenomenon of system sclerosis and vibration induced white finger syndrome," *Annals of Rheumatic Disease,* 51(2), 249–252 (February 1992).

3. Braunwald, E., Fauci, A.S., Kasper, D.L., Hauser, S.L., Longo, D.L., Jameson, J.L., editors, *Harrison's Principles of Internal Medicine,* Fifteenth Edition (New York: McGraw-Hill, 2001), pp. 1438–1439.

4. Watson, H.R., Robb, R., Belcher, G., Belch, J.J., "Seasonal variation of Raynaud's phenomenon secondary to systemic sclerosis," *Journal of Rheumatology,* 26(8), 1734–1737 (August 1999).

5. Belch, J.J., Shaw, B., O'Dowd, A., Saniabadi, A., Leiberman, P., Sturrock, R.D., Frobes, C.D., "Evening primrose oil (Efamol) in the treatment of Raynaud's phenomenon: a double blind study," *Thrombosis and Haemostasis,* 54(2), 490–494 (August 1985).

6. DiGiacomo, R.A., Kremer, J.M., Shah, D.M., "Fish-oil supplementation in patients with Raynaud's phenomenon: a double-blind, controlled, prospective study," *American Journal of Medicine,* 86(2), 158–164 (February 1989).

7. Belch, J.J., Land, D., Park, R.H., McKillop, J.H., MacKenzie, J.F., "Decreased oesophageal blood flow in patients with Raynaud's phenomenon," *British Journal of Rheumatology,* 27(6), 426–240 (December 1988).

RESTLESS LEGS SYNDROME

1. Chabli, A., Michaud, M., Montplaisir, J., "Periodic arm movements in patients with the restless legs syndrome," *European Neurologist,* 44(3), 133–138 (2000).

2. Bassetti, C.L., Mauerhofer, D., Gugger, M., Mathis, J., Hess, C.W., "Restless legs syndrome: a clinical study of 55 patients," *European Neurologist,* 45(2), 67–74 (2001).

3. Walters, A.S., Hickey, K., Maltzman, J., Verrico, T., Joseph, D., Hening, W., Wilson, V., Chokroverty, S., "A questionnaire study of 138 patients with restless legs syndrome: the 'Night-Walkers' survey," *Neurology,* 1996, 46(1), 92–95 (1996).

4. Polydefkis, M., Allen, R.P., Hauer, P., Earley, C.J., Griffin, J.W., McArthur, J.C., "Subclinical sensory neuropathy in late-onset restless legs syndrome," *Neurology,* 55(8), 1115–1121 (2000).

5. Turjanski, N., Lees, A.J., Brooks, D.J., "Striatal dopaminergic function in restless legs syndrome: 18F-dopa and 11C-raclopride PET studies," *Neurology,* 52(5), 932–937 (1999).

6. Montplaisir, J., Godbout, R., Poirier, G., Bedard, M.A., "Restless legs syndrome and periodic movements in sleep: physiopathology and treatment with L-dopa," *Clinical Neuropharmacology,* 9(5), 456–463 (1986).

7. Sun, E.R., Chen, C.A., Ho, G., Earley, C.J., Allen, R.P., "Iron and the restless legs syndrome," *Sleep,* 21(4), 371–377 (1998).

8. Allen, R.P., Barker, P.B., Wehrl, F., Song, H.K., Earley, C.J., "MRI measure-

ment of brain iron in patients with restless legs syndrome," *Neurology,* 56(2), 263–265 (2001).

9. Kanter, A.H., "The effect of sclerotherapy on restless legs syndrome," *Dermatological Surgery,* 21(4), 328–332 (1995).

10. Botez, M.I., Fontaine, F., Botez, T., Bachevalier, J., "Folate-responsive neurological and mental disorders: report of 16 cases. Neuropsychological correlates of computerized transaxial tomography and radionuclide cisternography in folic acid deficiencies," *European Neurologist,* 16(1–6), 230–246 (1977).

11. Popoviciu, L., Asgian, B., Delast-Popoviciu, D., Alexandrescu, A., Petrutiu, S., Bagathal, I., "Clinical, EEG, electromyographic and polysomnographic studies in restless legs syndrome caused by magnesium deficiency," *Romanian Journal of Neurology and Psychiatry,* 31(1), 55–61 (1993),

12. Hornyak M., Voderholzer, U., Hohagen, F., Berger, M., Riemann, D., "Magnesium therapy for periodic leg movements-related insomnia and restless legs syndrome: an open pilot study," *Sleep,* 21(5), 501–505 (1998).

13. Hornyak M., Voderholzer, U., Hohagen, F., Berger, M., Riemann, D., ibid.

14. Barton, J.C., Wooten, V.D., Acton, R.T., "Hemochromatosis and iron therapy of restless legs syndrome," *Sleep Medicine,* 3(2), 249–251 (2001).

RETINITIS PIGMENTOSA

1. Lodi, R., Iotti, S., Scorolli, L., Scorolli, L., Bargossi, A.M., Sprovieri, C., Zaniol, P., Meduri, R., Barbiroli, B., "The use of phosphorus magnetic resonance spectroscopy to study in vivo the effect of coenzyme Q_{10} treatment in retinitis pigmentosa," *Molecular Aspects of Medicine,* 15, S221–S230 (1994).

2. Banas, I., Buntner, B., Niebroj, T., Ostrowska, Z., "Levels of melatonin in serum of patients with retinitis pigmentosa," *Kliniczka Oczna,* 97, 321–323 (1995).

3. Schmidt, S.Y., Berson, E.L., Hayes, K.C., "Retinal degeneration in cats fed casein. I: Taurine deficiency," *Investigations in Ophthalmology,* 15, 47–52 (1976).

4. Airaksinen, E.M., Sihvola, P., Airaksinen, M.M., Sihvola, M., Tuovinen, E., "Uptake of taurine by platelets in retinitis pigmentosa," *Lancet,* 1(8114), 474–475 (3 March 1979).

5. Berson, E.L., Rosner, B., Sandberg, M.A., Hayes, K.C., Nicholson. B.W., Weigel-DiFranco, C., Willett, W., "A randomized trial of vitamin A and vitamin E supplementation for retinitis pigmentosa," *Archives of Ophthalmology,* 111, 761–772 (1993).

RETINOPATHY, DIABETIC

1. Kohner, E.M., Stratton, I.M., Aldington, S.J., Holman, R.R., Matthews, D.R., UK Prospective Diabetes Study (IKPDS) Group, "Relationship between the severity of retinopathy and progression to photocoagulation in patients with Type 2 diabetes mellitus in the UKPDS (UKPDS 52)," *Diabetes Medicine,* 18(3), 178–184 (March 2001).

2. Hsieh, P.S., Huang, W.C., "Neonatal chemical sympathectomy attenuates fructose-induced hypertriglyceridemia and hypertension in rats," *Chinese Journal of Physiology,* 44(1), 25–31 (31 March 2001).

3. McNair, P., Christiansen, C., Madsbad, S., et al., "Hypomagnesemia, a risk factor in diabetic retinopathy," *Diabetes,* 27, 1075–1078 (1978).

4. Erasmus, R.T., Olukoga, A.O., Alanamu, R.A., et al., "Plasma magnesium and retinopathy in black African diabetics," *Trop Geogr Med,* 41, 234–237 (1989).

5. Cunningham, J., "Reduced mononuclear leukocyte ascorbic acid content in adults with insulin-dependent diabetes mellitus consuming adequate dietary vitamin C," *Metabolism,* 40, 146–149 (1991).

6. Cunningham, J.J., Mearkle, P.L., Brown, R.G.," Vitamin C. An aldose reductase inhibitor that normalizes erythrocyte sorbitol in insulin-dependent diabetes mellitus," *Journal of the American College of Nutrition,* 4, 344–350 (1994).

7. Bursell, S.E., Schlossman, D.K., Clermont, A.C., Aiello, L.P., Aiello, L.M., Feener, E.P., Laffel, L., King, G.L., "High-dose vitamin E supplementation normalizes retinal blood flow and creatinine clearance in patients with type 1 diabetes," *Diabetes Care,* 22, 1245–1251 (1999).

8. Maffei Facino, R., Carini, M., Aldini, G., et al., "Free radicals scavenging ac-

tion and anti-enzyme activities of procyanidines from *Vitis vinifera:* a mechanism for their capillary protective action," *Arzneimittel Forschung,* 44, 592–601 (1994).

9. Amella, M., Bronner, C., Briancon, F., et al.," Inhibition of mast cell histamine release by flavonoids and bioflavonoids," *Planta Medica,* 51, 16–20 (1985).

10. Perossini M, et al., "Diabetic and hypertensive retinopathy therapy with *Vaccinium myrtillus* anthocyanosides (Tegens(r)): double-blind placebo controlled clinical trial.," *Annale Ottalmologica et Clinica Ocula,* 113, 1173 (1987)

11. Lanthony, P., Cosson, J.P., "The course of color vision in early diabetic retinopathy treated with Ginkgo biloba extract. A preliminary double-blind versus placebo study," *Journal Francaise d' Ophtalmologie,* 11, 671–474 (1988).

RETINOPATHY OF PREMATURITY (RETROLENTAL FIBROPLASIA)

1. Braunwald, E., Fauci, A.S., Kasper, D.L., Hauser, S.L., Longo, D.L., Jameson, J.L., editors, *Harrison's Principles of Internal Medicine,* Fifteenth Edition (New York: McGraw-Hill, 2001), pp. 527.

2. Finer, N.N., Schindler, R.F., Grant, G., Hill, G.B., Peters, K., "Effect of intramuscular vitamin E on frequency and severity of retrolental fibroplasia: a controlled trial," *Lancet,* 15, 1087–1091 (1982).

3. Hittner, H.M., Rudolph, A.J., Kretzer, F.L., "Suppression of severe retinopathy of prematurity with vitamin E supplementation. Ultrastructural mechanism of clinical efficacy," *Ophthalmology,* 91, 1512–1523 (1984).

4. Hittner, H.M., Kretzer, F.L., "Vitamin E and retrolental fibroplasia: ultrastructural mechanism of clinical efficacy," *Ciba Foundation Symposia,* 101, 165–185. (1983).

RHEUMATOID ARTHRITIS

1. Scherak, O., Kolaz, G., "Vitamin E and rheumatoid arthritis," *Arthritis and Rheumatology,* 34, 1205 (1991).

2. Honkanen, V., Kontinnen, Y.T., Mussalo-Rauhamaa, M.H., "Vitamin A, E, zinc, and retinol binding protein in rheumatoid arthritis," *Clinical Experience in Rheumatology,* 7, 465 (1989).

3. Maurice, M.M., Nakamura, H., van derVoort, E.A.M., et al., "Evidence for the role of an altered redox state in hyporesponsiveness of synovial T cells in rheumatoid arthritis," *Journal of Immunology,* 158, 1458 (1997).

4. Fairburn, K., Grootveld, M., Ward, R.J., et al., "Alpha-tocopherol, lipids and lipoproteins in knee-joint synovial fluid and serum from patients with inflammatory joint disease" *Clinical Science,* 83, 657 (1992).

5. Hicklin, J.A., McEwen, L.M., Morgan. J.E., "The effect of diet in rheumatoid arthritis," *Clinical Allergy,* 10, 463 (1980).

6. Kjeldsen-Kragh, J., Haugen, M., Borchgrevink, C.F., Forre, O., "Vegetarian diet for patients with rheumatoid arthritis - status: two years after introduction of the diet," *Clinical Rheumatology,* 13, 475–482 (1994).

7. Nesher, G., Mates, M., "Palindromic rheumatism: effect of dietary manipulation," *Clinical Experience in Rheumatology,* 18(3), 375–378 (May–June 2000).

8. Hanninen, O., Kaartinen, K., Rauma, A.L., Nenonen, M., Torronen, R., Hakkinen, A.S., Adlercreutz, H., Laakso, J., "Antioxidants in vegan diet and rheumatic disorders," *Toxicology,* 155(1–3), 45–53 (30 November 2000).

9. Darlington, L.G., Ramsey, N.W., "Diets for rheumatoid arthritis," *Lancet,* 338, 1209 (1991).

10. Following Darlington, L.G., "Dietary therapy for arthritis," *Rheumatological Disease Clinicians of North America,* 17, 273–285 (1991).

11. Agafonov, A., personal communication, 26 February 2002.

12. Lee, H.A., Hughes, D.A., "Alpha-lipoic acid modulates NF-kappaB activity in human monocytic cells by direct interaction with DNA," *Experimental Gerontology,* 37(2–3), 401–410 (3 January 2002).

13. Helmy, M., Shohayeb, M., Helmy, M.H., el-Bassiouni, E.A., "Antioxidants as adjuvant therapy in rheumatoid disease. A preliminary study," *Arzneimittel-Forschung,* 51(4), 293–298 (2001).

14. Bandt, M.D., Grossin, M., Driss, F., Pincemail, J., Babin-Chevaye, C., Pasquier, C., "Vitamin E uncouples joint destruction and clinical inflammation in a transgenic mouse model of rheumatoid arthritis," *Arthritis and Rheumatism,* 46(2), 522–532 (February 2002).

15. Knekt, P., Heliovaara, M., Aho, K., Alfthan, G., Marniemi, J., Aromaa, A., "Serum selenium, serum alpha-tocopherol, and the risk of rheumatoid arthritis," *Epidemiology,* 11(4), 402–405 (July 2000).

16. Romas, E., Gillespie, M.T., Martin, T.J., "Involvement of receptor activator of NF[kappa]B ligand and tumor necrosis factor-[alpha] in bone destruction in rheumatoid arthritis," *Bone,* 30(2), 340–346 (February 2002).

17. McCarty, M.F., Russell, A.L., "Niacinamide therapy for osteoarthritis—does it inhibit nitric oxide xynthase induction by interleukin 1 in chondrocytes," *Medical Hypotheses,* 53(4), 350–360 (October 1999).

18. Vaz, A.L., "Double-blind clinical evaluation of the relative efficacy of ibuprofen and glucosamine sulfate in the management of osteoarthrosis of the knee in out-patients," *Current Medical Research Opinions,* 8, 145–149 (1982).

19. Müller-Fassbiner, H., et al, "Glucosamine sulfate compared to ibuprofen in osteoarthritis of the knee," *Osteoarthritis and Cartilage,* 2, 61–69 (1994).

20. Reichelt, A., Forster, K.K., Fischer, M., et al., "Efficacy and safety of intramuscular glucosamine sulfate in osteoarthritis of the knees. A randomized, placebo-controlled, double-blind study," *Arzneimittel Forschung,* 44, 75–80 (1994).

21. Tapadinhas, M.J., Revera, I.C., Bignamni, A.A., et al., "Oral glucosamine sulfate in the management of arthrosis. Report on a multi-centre open investigation in Portugal," *Pharmacotherapeutica,* 3, 157–168 (1982).

22. Bucsi, L., Poor, G., "Efficacy and tolerability of oral chondroitin sulfate as a symptomatic low-acting drug for osteoarthritis (SYSADOA) in the treatment of knee arthritis," *Osteoarthritis and Cartilage,* 6 (Suppl A), 31–36 (1998).

23. Berger, R., Nowak, H., "A new medical approach to the treatment of osteoarthritis. Report of an open phase IV study with ademetionine (Gumbaral)," *American Journal of Medicine,* 83, 84–88 (1987).

24. Konig, B., "A long term (two years) clinical trial with S-adenosylmethionine for the treatment of osteoarthritis," *American Journal of Medicine,* 83, 89–94 (1987).

25. Walker, W.R., Keats, D.M., "An investigation of the therapeutic value of the 'copper bracelet:' dermal assimilation of copper in arthritic/rheumatoid conditions," *Agents and Actions,* 6, 454–459 (1976).

26. Mazzetti, I., Grigolo, B., Pulsatelli, L., Dolzani, P., Silvestri, T., Roseti, L., Meliconi, R., Facchini, A., "Differential roles of nitric oxide and oxygen radicals in chondrocytes affected by osteoarthritis and rheumatoid arthritis," *Clinical Science* (London), 101(6), 593–599 (December 2001).

27. Leventhal, L.J., Boyce, E.G., Zurier, R.B., "Treatment of rheumatoid arthritis with gammalinolenic acid," *Annals of Internal Medicine,* 119, 867–873 (1993).

28. Ergas, D., Eilat, E., Mendlovic, S., Sthoeger, Z.M., "n-3 fatty acids and the immune system in autoimmunity," *Israeli Medical Association Journal,* 4(1), 34–38 (January 2002).

29. Schnitzer, T.J., "Non-NSAID pharmacologic treatment options for the management of chronic pain," *American Journal of Medicine,* 105(1B), 45S–52S (27 July 1998).

30. McCleane, G., "The analgesic efficacy of topical capsaicin is enhanced by glyceryl trinitrate in painful osteoarthritis: a randomized, double blind, placebo controlled study," *European Journal of Pain,* 4(4), 355–360 (2000).

31. Parcell, S., "Sulfur in human nutrition and its applications in medicine," *Alternative Medicine Review,* 7(1), 22–44 (February 2002).

32. Ishiguro, N., Ito, T., Oguchi, T., Kojima, T., Iwata, H., Ionescu, M., Poole, A.R., "Relationships of matrix metalloproteinases and their inhibitors to cartilage proteoglycan and collagen turnover and inflammation as revealed by analyses of synovial fluids from patients with rheumatoid arthritis," *Arthritis and Rheumatism,* 44(11), 2503–2511 (November 2001).

RICKETS

1. Centers for Disease Control and Prevention, "From the Centers for Disease Control and Prevention. Severe malnutrition among young children—Geor-

gia, January 1997–June 1999," *Journal of the American Medical Association,* 285(20), 2573–2474 (23–30 May 2001).

2. Pugliese, M.T., Blumberg, D.L., Hludzinski, J., Kay, S., "Nutritional rickets in suburbia," *Journal of the American College of Nutrition,* 17(6), 637–641 (December 1998).

3. Grover, S.R., Morley, R., "Vitamin D deficiency in veiled or dark-skinned pregnant women," *Medical Journal of Australia,* 175(5), 251–252 (3 September 2001).

4. Booth, S.L., Tucker, K.L., Chen, H., et al., "Dietary vitamin K intakes are associated with hip fracture but not with bone mineral density in elderly men and women," *American Journal of Clinical Nutrition,* 71, 1201–1208 (2000).

5. Green, M.R., Buchanan, E., Weaver, L.T., "Nutritional management of the infant with cystic fibrosis," *Archive of Diseases in Childhood,* 72, 452–456 (1995).

RINGWORM

1. Bronson, D.M., Desai, D.R., Barsky, S., Foley, S.M., "An epidemic of infection with Trichophyton tonsurans revealed in a 20-year survey of fungal infections in Chicago," *Journal of the American Academy of Dermatology,* 8, 322–330 (1983).

2. Tong, M.M., Altman, P.M., Barnetson, R.S., "Tea tree oil in the treatment of tinea pedis," *Australian Journal of Dermatology,* 33, 145–149.

ROSACEA

1. Marks, R., "Concepts in the pathogenesis of rosacea," *British Journal of Dermatology,* 80, 170 (1968).

2. Rosen, T., Stone, M.S., "Acne rosacea in blacks," *Journal of the American Academy of Dermatology,* 17, 70–73 (1987).

3. Shiotani, A., Okada, K., Yanaoka, K., Itoh, H., Nishioka, S., Sakurane, M., Matsunaka, M., "Beneficial effect of *Helicobacter pylori* eradication in dermatologic disease," *Helicobacter,* 6, 60–65 (September 2001).

4. Marks, R., Harcourt-Webster, J.N., "Histopathology of rosacea," *Archives of Dermatology,* 100, 682 (1969).

5. Rufli, T., Buchner, S.A., "T-cell subsets in acne rosacea lesions and the possible role of *Demodex folliculorum,*" *Dermatologica,* 169, 1 (1984).

6. Tulipan, L., "Acne rosacea: a vitamin B complex deficiency," *New York State Journal of Medicine,* 29, 1063–1064 (1929).

7. Starr, P.A.H., McDonald, A., "Oculocutaneous aspects of rosacea," *Proceedings of the Royal Society for Medicine,* 62, 9 (1969).

8. Marks, R., Harcourt-Webster, J.N., ibid.

9. Mondino, B.J., "Inflammatory diseases of the peripheral cornea," *Ophthalmology,* 95, 463–472 (1988).

10. Toyoda, M., Morohashi, M., "Pathogenesis of acne," *Medical Electron Microscopy,* 34(1), 29–40 (March 2001).

11. Abdel, K.M., El Mofty, A., Ismail, A., Bassili, F., "Glucose tolerance in blood and skin of patients with acne vulgaris I.," *Journal of Investigational Dermatology,* 40, 259–261 (1963).

12. Starr, P.A.H., McDonald, A., ibid.

13. Kuhnau, J., "The flavonoids. A class of semi-essential food components: their role in human nutrition," *World Review of Nutrition and Dietetics,* 24, 117–191 (1976).

14. Gabor, M., "Pharmacologic effects of flavonoids on blood vessels," *Angiologica,* 9, 355–374 (1972).

15. Beil, W., Birkholz, C., Sewing, K.F., "Effects of flavonoids on parietal cell acid secretion, gastric mucosal prostaglandin production and *Helicobacter pylori* growth," *Arzneimittel Forschung,* 45, 697–400 (1995).

16. Ihme, N., Kieswetter, H., Jung, F., Hoffman, K.H., Birk, A., Müller, A., Grützner, K.I., "Leg edema protection from buckwheat herb tea in patients with chronic venous insufficiency: a single-center randomized, double-blind, placebo-controlled clinical trial," *European Journal of Clinical Pharmacology,* 50, 443–447 (1995).

17. Tulipan, L., ibid.

18. Beil, W., Birkholz, C., Sewing, K.F., "Effects of flavonoids on parietal cell

acid secretion, gastric mucosal prostaglandin production and *Helicobacter pylori* growth," *Arzneimittel Forschung,* 45, 697–400 (1995).

19. Rendi, M., Mayer, C., Weniger, W., Tschachler, E., "Topically applied lactic acid increases spontaneous secretion of vascular endothelial growth factor by human reconstructed epidermis," *British Journal of Dermatology,* 145(1), 3–9 (July 2001).

20. Ryle, J., Barber, H., "Gastric analysis in acne rosacea," *Lancet,* 11, 1195–1196 (1920).

21. Barba, A., Rosa, B., Angelini, G., Sapuppo, A., Brocco, G., Scuro, L.A., Cavallini, G., "Pancreatic exocrine function in rosacea," *Dermatologica,* 165, 601–606 (1982).

ROTATOR CUFF TENDONITIS

1. Khan, K.M., Cook, J.L., Kannus, P., Maffulli, N., Bonar, S.F., "Time to abandon the 'tendinitis' myth," *British Medical Journal,* 324, 626–627 (16 March 2002).

2. Khan, K.M., Cook, J.L., Bonar, F., Harcourt, P., Astrom, M., "Histopathology of common overuse tendon conditions: update and implications for clinical management," *Sports Medicine,* 27, 393–408 (1999).

3. Klein, G., Küllich, W., "Reducing pain by oral enzyme therapy in rheumatic diseases," *Wienerischer Medizinische Wochenschrift,* 149(21–22), 577–580 (1999).

4. Schnitzer, T.J., "Non-NSAID pharmacologic treatment options for the management of chronic pain," *American Journal of Medicine,* 105(1B), 45S-52S (27 July 1998).

5. McCleane, G., "The analgesic efficacy of topical capsaicin is enhanced by glyceryl trinitrate in painful osteoarthritis: a randomized, double blind, placebo controlled study," *European Journal of Pain,* 4(4), 355–360 (2000).

6. Brenstein, A.L., Dinesen, J.S., "Brief communication: effect of pharmacologic doses of vitamin B_6 on carpal tunnel syndrome, electroencephalographic results, and pain," *Journal of the American College of Nutrition,* 12(1), 73–76 (February 1993).

7. Keniston, R.C., Nathan, P.A., Leklem, J.E., Lockwood, R.S., "Vitamin B_6, vitamin C, and carpal tunnel syndrome. A cross-sectional study of 441 adults," *Journal of Occupational and Environmental Medicine,* 39(10), 949–959 (October 1997).

8. Bito, T., Roy, S., Sen, C.K., Packer, L., "Pine bark extract pycnogenol downregualtes IFN-gamma-induced adhesion of T cells to human keratinocytes by inhibiting inducible ICAM-1 expression," *Free Radicals in Biology and Medicine,* 28, 219–227 (2000).

9. Chen, M.F., Shimada, F., Kato, H., Yano, S., Kanaoka, M., "Effect of glycyrrhizin on the pharmacokinetics of prednisolone following low dosage of prednisolone hemisuccinate," *Endocronologica Japonica,* 37, 331–341 (1990).

10. Kuhlwein, A., Meyer, H.J., Koehler, C.O., "Reduced diclofenac administration by B vitamins: results of a randomized double-blind study with reduced daily doses of diclofenac (75 mg diclofenac versus 75 mg diclofenac plus B vitamins) in acute lumbar vertebral syndromes," *Klinisches Wochenschrift,* 68(2), 107–115 (19 January 1990).

11. Vetter, G., Bruggemann, G., Lettko, M., Schwieger, G., Asbach, H., Biermann, W., Blasius, K., Brinkmann, R., Bruns, H., Dorn, E., et al., "Shortening diclofenac therapy by B vitamins. Results of a randomized double-blind study, diclofenac 50 mg versus diclofenac 50 mg plus B vitamins, in painful spinal diseases with degenerative changes," *Zeitschrift für Rheumatologie,* 47(5), 351–362 (September–October 1988).

12. Ehrenpreis, S., "Analgesic properties of enkephalinase inhibitors: animal and human studies," *Progress in Clinical and Biological Research,* 192, 363–370 (1985).

13. Parcell, S., "Sulfur in human nutrition and its applications in medicine," *Alternative Medicine Review,* 7(1), 22–44 (February 2002).

14. Ishiguro, N., Ito, T., Oguchi, T., Kojima, T., Iwata, H., Ionescu, M., Poole, A.R., "Relationships of matrix metalloproteinases and their inhibitors to cartilage proteoglycan and collagen turnover and inflammation as revealed by analysis of synovial fluids from patients with rheumatoid arthritis," *Arthritis and Rheumatism,* 44(11), 2503–2511 (November 2001).

SARCOIDOSIS

1. Caserio, R.J., Eaglstein, W.H., Allen,C.J., "Treatment of granuloma annulare with potassium iodide," *Journal of the American Academy of Dermatology,* 10, 294 (1984).

SCHIZOPHRENIA

1. Vaughan, K., McConaghy, N., "Megavitamin and dietary treatment in schizophrenia: a randomized, controlled trial," *Australia-New Zealand Journal of Psychiatry,* 33(1), 84–88 (February 1999).

2. Reichelt, K.L., Seim, A.R., Reichelt, W.H., "Could schizophrenia be reasonably explained by Dohan's hypothesis on genetic interaction with a dietary peptide overload?" *Progress in Neuropsychopharmacology and Biological Psychiatry,* 20(7), 1083–1114 (October 1996).

3. De Santis, A., Addolorato, G., Romito, A., Caputo, S., Giordano, A., Gambassi, G., Taranto, C., Manna, R., Gasbarrini, G., "Schizophrenic symptoms and SPECT abnormalities in a coeliac patient: regression after a gluten-free diet," *Journal of Internal Medicine,* 242(5), 241–243 (1997).

4. Peet, M., Horrobin, D.F., E-E Multicentre Study Group, "A dose-ranging exploratory study of the effects of ethyl-eicosapentaenoate in patients with persistent schizophrenic symptoms," *Journal of Psychiatric Research,* 36(1), 7–18 (January-February 2002).

5. Fenton, W.S., Dickerson, F., Boronow, J., Hibbeln, J.R., Knable, M., "A placebo-controlled trial of omega-3 fatty acid (ethyl eicosapentaenoic acid) supplementation for residual symptoms and cognitive impairment in schizophrenia," *American Journal of Psychiatry,* 158(12), 2071–2074 (December 2001).

6. Joy, C.B., Mumby-Croft, R., Joy, L.A., "Polyunsaturated fatty acid (fish or evening primrose oil) for schizophrenia," *Cochrane Database System Review,* (2):CD001257 (2000).

SCLERODERMA

1. Zarafonetis, C.J., Dabich, L., Skovronshki, J.J., et al., "Retrospective studies in scleroderma: skin responses to potassium para-aminobenzoate therapy," *Clinical Experience in Rheumatology,* 6, 261–268 (1998).

SEASONAL AFFECTIVE DISORDER (SAD)

1. Palinkas, L.A., Reed, H.L., Reedy, K.R., Do, N.V., Case, H.S., Finney, N.S., "Circannual pattern of hypothalamic-pituitary-thyroid (HPT) function and mood during extended Antarctic residence," *Psychoneuroimmunology,* 26(4), 421–431 (May 2001).

2. Sher, L., "The role of brain thyroid hormones in the mechanisms of seasonal changes in mood and behavior," *Medical Hypotheses,* 55(1), 55–59 (July 2000).

3. Gaist, P.A., Obarzanek, E., Skwerer, R.G., Duncan, C.C., Shultz, P.M., Rosenthal, N.E., "Effects of bright light on resting metabolic rate in patients with seasonal affective disorder and control subjects," *Biological Psychiatry,* 28(11), 989–996 (1 December 1990).

4. Neumeister, A., Praschak-Rieder, N., Hesselmann, B., Vitouch, O., Rauh, M., Barocka, A., Kasper, S., "Rapid tryptophan depletion in drug-free depressed patients with seasonal affective disorder," *American Journal of Psychiatry,* 154(8), 1153–1155 (August 1997).

5. Partonen, T., "Possible pathophysiological mechanisms regulating food intake in seasonal affective disorder," *Medical Hypotheses,* 47(3), 215–216 (August 1996).

6. Pinchasov, B.B., Shurgaja, A.M., Grischin, O.V., Putilov, A.A., "Mood and energy regulation in seasonal and non-seasonal depression before and after midday treatment with physical exercise or bright light," *Psychiatry Research,* 94(1), 29–42 (24 April 2000).

7. Kräuchi, K., Wirz-Justice, A., Graw, P., "High intake of sweets late in the day predicts a rapid and persistent response to light therapy in winter depression," *Psychiatry Research,* 46(2), 107–117 (February 1993).

8. Wirz-Justice, A., Graw, P., Kräuchi, K., Sarrafzadeh, A., English, J., Arendt, J., Sand, L., "'Natural light treatment of seasonal affective disorder," *Journal of Affective Disorders,* 37, 109–120 (1996).

9. Partonen, T., ibid.

10. Kolvisto, V.A., Yuki-Harvinen, H., "Fructose and insulin sensitivity in patients with type 2 diabetes," *Journal of Internal Medicine*, 233, 145–153 (1993).

11. Levine, R., Streeten, D., Doisy, R., "Effect of oral chromium supplementation on the glucose tolerance of elderly human subjects," *Metabolism*, 17, 114–125 (1968).

12. Ibid.

13. Honma, K., Kohsaka, M., Fukuda, N., Morita, N., Honma, S., "Effects of vitamin B$_{12}$ on plasma melatonin rhythm in humans. Increased light sensitivity phase-advances the circadian clock," *Experientia*, 48, 716–720 (1992).

14. Zhdanova, I.V., Wuirtman, R.J., Lynch, H.J., Ives, J.R., Dollins, A.B., Morabito, C., Matheson, J.K., Schomer, D.L., "Sleep-inducing effects of low doses of melatonin ingested in the evening," *Clinical Pharmacology and Therapeutics*, 57, 552–558 (1995).

15. Kripke, D., Risch, S., Jonowsky, D., "Bright white light alleviates depression," *Psychiatric Research* 10, 105–112 (1983).

16. Gordon, J.B., "SSRIs and St. John's wort: Possible toxicity," *American Family Physician*, 57, 950, 953 (1998).

17. DeMott, K., "St. John's wort tied to serotonin syndrome." *Clinical Psychiatry News*, 26, 28 (1998).

18. Lane-Brown, M.M., "Photosensitivity associated with herbal preparations of St John's wort (*Hypericum perforatum*) [letter]," *Medical Journal of Australia*, 172, 302 (2000).

19. Rosenthal, N.E., Sack, D.A., Gillin, J.C., et al., "Seasonal affective disorder. A description of the syndrome and preliminary findings with light therapy," *Archives of General Psychiatry*, 41, 72–79 (1984).

20. Waldhauser, F., Ehrhart, B., Forster, E., "Clinical aspects of the melatonin action," *Experientia*, 49, 671–681 (1993).

21. Wilson, B.W., Wright, C.W., Morris, J.E., Buschborn, R.L., Brown, D.P., Miller, D.L., et al., "Effect of an artificial magnetic field on serotonin N-acetyltransferase activity and melatonin content of the rat pineal gland," *Experimental Brain Research*, 50, 426–432 (1983).

SEBORRHEIC DERMATITIS

1. Garbe, C., Husak, R., Orfanos, C.E., "HIV-associated dermatoses and their prevalence in 456 HIV-infected patients. Relation to immune status and its importance as a diagnostic marker," *Hautarzt*, 45(9), 623–629 (September 1994).

2. Andrews, G., Post, C., Domonkos, A., "Seborrheic dermatitis supplementation treatment with vitamin B$_{12}$," *New York State Journal of Medicine*, 50, 1921–1925 (1950).

3. Proctor, M., Wilkenson, D., Orenberg, E., Farber, E.M., "Lowered cutaneous and urinary levels of polyamines with clinical improvement in treated psoriasis," *Archives of Dermatology*, 115, 945–949 (1979).

4. Kalman, J., Gecse, A., Farkas, T., Joo, F., Telegdy, G., Lajtha, A., "Dietary manipulation with high marine fish oil intake of fatty acid composition and arachidonic acid metabolism in rat cerebral microvessels," *Neurochemical Research*, 17(2), 167–172 (February 1992).

5. Nisenson, A., "Treatment of seborrheic dermatitis with biotin and vitamin B complex," *Journal of Pediatrics*, 81, 630–631 (1972).

6. Roe, D.A., *Drug-Induced Nutritional Deficiencies* (Westport, CT: AVI Publications, 1976), 168–177.

7. Schreiner, A., Rockewell, E., Vilter, R., "A local defect in the metabolism of pyridoxine in the skin of persons with seborrheic dermatitis of the 'sicca' type," *Journal of Investigational Dermatology*, 19, 95–96 (1952).

8. Vardy, D.A., Cohen, A.D., Tchetov, T., Medvedovsky, E., Biton, A. "A double-blind, placebo-controlled trial of an *Aloe vera* (*A. barbadensis*) emulsion in the treatment of seborrheic dermatitis," *Journal of Dermatological Treatment*, 10, 7–11 (October 1999),

9. Al-Waili, N.S., "Therapeutic and prophylactic effects of crude honey on chronic seborrheic dermatitis and dandruff," *European Journal of Medical Research*, 30, 6(7), 306–308 (July 2001).

10. Scheriner, A., Slinger, W., Hawkins, V., et al., "Seborrheic dermatitis. A lo-

cal metabolic defect involving pyridoxine," *Journal of Laboratory and Clinical Medicine*, 40, 121–130 (1952).

SHINGLES

1. Guess, H.A., Broughton, D.D., Melton, I.J., III, Kurland, L.T., "Epidemiology of herpes zoster in children and adolescents: a population-based study," *Pediatrics*, 76 512–517 (1985).

2. Horne, K., Cirelli, H., Lee, P., Tyring, S.K., "Antiviral therapy of acute herpes zoster in older patients," *Drugs and Aging*, 8, 97–112 (1996).

3. Helgason, S., Petursson, G., Gudmondsson, S., Sigurdsson J.A., "Prevalence of postherpetc neuralgia after a first episode of herpes zoster: prospective study with long term follow up," *British Medical Journal*, 321, 794 (30 September 2000).

4. Nikkela, A.F., Pierard, G.F., "Recognition and treatment of shingles," *Drugs*, 48, 528–548 (1994).

5. Nikkela, A.F., Pierard, G.F., ibid.

6. Billigmann P., "Enzyme therapy—an alternative in treatment of herpes zoster. A controlled study of 192 patients," *Fortschrift für Medizin*, 113(4), 43–48 (10 February 1995).

7. Kleine, M.W., Stauder, G.M., Beese, E.W., "The intestinal absorption of orally administered hydrolytic enzymes and their effects in the treatment of acute herpes zoster as compared with those of oral acyclovir therapy," *Phytomedicine*, 2, 7–15 (1995).

8. Powell, C.J., "Pancreatic enzymes and fibrosing colonopathy," *Lancet*, 354, 251 (1999).

9. Heyblon, R., "Vitamin B$_{12}$ in Herpes zoster," *Journal of the American Medical Association*, 149, 1338 (1950).

10. Ayres, S., Jr., Mihan, R., "Post-herpes zoster neuralgia: response to vitamin E therapy," *Archives of Dermatology*, 108, 855–858 (1973).

11. Cochrane, T., "Post-herpes zoster neuralgia: response to vitamin E therapy," *Archives of Dermatology*, 111, 296 (1975).

12. Sheridan, J., Kern, E., Martin, A., Booth, A., "Evaluation of antioxidant healing formulations in topical therapy of experimental cutaneous and genital herpes simplex virus infections," *Antiviral Research*, 36(30), 157–166 (December 1997).

13. Ibid.

14. Peikert, A., Heinrich, M., Ochs, G., "Topical 0.025% capsaicin in chronic post-herpetic neuralgia: efficacy, predictors of response and long-term course," *Journal of Neurology*, 238(8), 452–456 (December 1991).

15. Westerman, R.A., Roberts, R.G., Kotzmann, R.R., Westerman, D.A., Delaney, C., Widdop, R.E., Carter, B.E., "Effects of topical capsaicin on normal skin and affected dermatomes in herpes zoster," *Clinical and Experimental Neurology*, 25, 71–84 (1988).

SICKLE CELL ANEMIA

1. Singhal, A., Parker, S., Linsell, L., Serjeant, G., "Energy intake and resting metabolic rate in preschool Jamaican children with homozygous sickle cell disease," *American Journal of Clinical Nutrition*, 75(6), 1093–1097 (June 2002).

2. Fung, E.B., Malinauskas, B.M., Kawchak, D.A., Koh, B.Y., Zemel, B.S., Gropper, S.S., Ohene-Frempong, K., Stallings, V.A., "Energy expenditure and intake in children with sickle cell disease during acute illness," *Clinical Nutrition*, 20(2), 131–138 (April 2001).

3. Fung, E.B., Barden, E.M., Kawchak, D.A., Zemel, B.S., Ohene-Frempong, K., Stallings, V.A., "Effect of hydroxyurea therapy on resting energy expenditure in children with sickle cell disease," *Journal of Pediatric Hematology and Oncology*, 23(9), 604–608 (December 2001).

4. Shankar, A.H., Prasad, A.S., "Zinc and immune function: the biological basis of altered resistance to infection," American Journal of Clinical Nutrition, 68, 447S–463S (1998).

5. Zemel, B.S., Kawchak, D.A., Fung, E.B., Ohene-Frempong, K., Stallings, V.A., "Effect of zinc supplementation on growth and body composition in children with sickle cell disease," *American Journal of Clinical Nutrition*, 75(2), 300–307 (February 2002).

6. Tangney, C.C., Phillips, G., Bell, R.A., Fernandes, P., Hopkins, R., Wu, S.M., "Selected indices of micronutrient status in adult patients with sickle cell anemia (SCA)," *American Journal of Hematology*, 32(3), 161–166 (November 1989).

7. Buchowski, M.S., Townsend, K.M., Williams, R., Chen, K.Y., "Patterns and energy expenditure of free-living physical activity in adolescents with sickle cell anemia," *Journal of Pediatrics*, 140(1), 86–92 (January 2002).

8. Barbeau, P., Woods, K.F., Ramsey, L.T., Litaker, M.S., Pollock, D.M., Pollock, J.S., Callahan, L.A., Kutlar, A., Mensah, G.A., Gutin, B., "Exercise in sickle cell anemia: effect on inflammatory and vasoactive mediators," *Endothelium*, 8(2), 147–155 (2001).

9. Wirthwein, D.P., Spotswood, S.D., Barnard, J.J., Prahlow, J.A., "Death due to microvascular occlusion in sickle-cell trait following physical exertion," *Journal of Forensic Science*, 46(2), 399–401 (March 2001).

10. Laurencem B., Reid, B.C., Katz, R.V., "Sickle cell anemia and dental caries: a literature review and pilot study," *Special Care Dentistry*, 22(2), 70–74 (March–April 2002).

SIDS, LOWERING RISK OF

1. Rinaldo, P., Stanley, C.A., Hsu, B.Y., Sanchez, L.A., Stern, H.J., "Sudden neonatal death in carnitine transporter deficiency," *Journal of Pediatrics*, 131(2), 304–305 (August 1997).

2. Caddell, J.L., "The apparent impact of gestational magnesium (Mg) deficiency on the sudden infant death syndrome (SIDS)," *Magnesium Research*, 14(4), 291–303 (December 2001).

3. Reid, G.M., Tervit, H., "Sudden infant death syndrome and placental disorders: the thyroid-selenium link," *Medical Hypotheses*, 48(4), 317–324 (April 1997).

SINUSITIS

1. Braunwald, E., Fauci, A.S., Kasper, D.L., Hauser, S.L., Longo, D.L., Jameson, J.L., editors, *Harrison's Principles of Internal Medicine*, Fifteenth Edition (New York: McGraw-Hill, 2001), pp. 188–189.

2. Stone, S., Gonzales, R., Maselli, J., Lowenstein, S.R., "Antibiotic prescribing for patients with colds, upper respiratory tract infections, and bronchitis: a national study of hospital-based emergency departments," *Annals of Emergency Medicine*, 36(4), 320–327 (October 2000).

3. Cervin, A., "The anti-inflammatory effect of erythromycin and its derivatives, with special reference to nasal polyposis and chronic sinusitis," *Acta Otolaryngolica*, 121(1), 183–192 (January 2001).

4. Cazzola, P., Mazzanti, P., Bossi, G., "In vivo modulating effect of a calf thymus acid lysate on human T lymphocyte subsets and CD4+/CD8+ ratio in the course of difference diseases," *Current Therapies Research*, 42, 1011–1017 (1987).

5. Seifter, E., Rettura, G., Seiter, J., "Thymotrophic action of vitamin A," *Federal Proceedings*, 32, 947 (1973).

6. Semba, R.D., "Vitamin A, immunity, and infection," *Clinical Infectious Disease*, 19, 489–499 (1994).

7. Ginter, E., "Optimum intake of vitamin C for the human organisms," *Nutrition and Health*, 1, 66–77 (1982).

8. Gabor, M., "Pharmacologic effects of flavonoids on blood vessels," *Angiologica*, 9, 355–374 (1972).

9. Prasad, A., "Clinical, biochemical and nutritional spectrum of zinc deficiency in human subjects. An update," *Nutrition Review*, 41, 197–208 (1983).

10. Erhard, M., "Effect of echinacea, aconitum, lachesis, and apis extracts, and their combinations of phagocytosis of human granulocytes," *Phytotherapy Research*, 8, 14–77 (1994).

11. Stoll, A., Renz, J., Brack, A., "Antibacterial substances II. isolation and constitution of echnacoside, a glycoside from the roots of *Echinacea angustifolia*," *Helvetica Chimica Acta*, 33, 1877–1893 (1950).

12. Zhang, L., Yang, L.W., Yang, L.J., "Relation between *Helicobacter pylori* and pathogenesis of chronic atrophic gastritis and the research of its prevention and treatment," *Chung-Kuo Chung Hsi I Chieh Ho Tsa Chih-Chinese Journal of Modern Developments in Traditional Medicine*, 12(9), 515–516 (September 1992).

13. Latino, "H. pylori implicated in allergies," *Medical Tribune*, March 24, 1994, p. 1

SJÖGREN'S SYNDROME

1. Francis, M.L., "Sjögren Syndrome," *eMedicine*, 3(4) (24 April 2002).

2. Manthorpe, R., Hagen Petersen, S., Prause, J.U., "Primary Sjögren's syndrome treated with Efamol/Efavit. A double-blind cross-over investigation," *Rheumatology Internation*, 4(4), 165–167 (1984).

3. Theander, E., Horrobin, D.F., Jacobsson, L.T., Manthorpe, R., "Gammalinolenic acid treatment of fatigue associated with primary Sjögren's syndrome," *Scandinavian Journal of Rheumatology*, 31(2), 72–79 (2002).

SKIN TAGS

1. Terlikowska, A., Patterson, W.M., Schwartz, R.A., "Acrochordons," *eMedicine Journal*, 26 November 2001.

2. Agarwal, J.K., Nigam, P.K., "Acrochordon: a cutaneous sign of carbohydrate intolerance," *Australasian Journal of Dermatology*, 28(3), 132–133 (December 1987).

3. Evans, J.L., Heymann, C.J., Goldfine, I.D., Gavin, L.A., "Pharmacokinetics, tolerability, and fructosamine-lowering effect of a novel, controlled-release formulation of alpha-lipoic acid," *Endocrine Practice*, 8(1), 29–35 (January–February 2002).

4. Greene, E.L., Nelson, B.A., Robinson, K.A., Buse, M.G., "Alpha-lipoic acid prevents the development of glucose induced insulin resistance in 3T3–L1 adipocytes and accelerates the decline in immunoreactive insulin during cell incubation," *Metabolism*, 50(9), 1063–1069 (September 2001).

5. El Midaoui, A., de Champlain, J., "Prevention of hypertension, insulin resistance, and oxidative stress by alpha-lipoic acid," *Hypertension*, 39(2), 303–307 (February 2002).

6. Eason, R.C., Archer, H.E., Akhtar, S., Bailey, C.J., "Lipoic acid increases glucose uptake by skeletal muscles of obese-diabetic ob/ob mice," *Diabetes, Obesity, and Metabolism*, 4(1), 29–35 (January 2002).

7. Saengsirisuwan, V., Perez, F.R., Kinnick, T.R., Henriksen, E.J., "Effects of exercise training and antioxidant R-ALA on glucose transport in insulin-sensitive rat skeletal muscle," *Journal of Applied Physiology*, 92(1), 50–58 (January 2002).

8. Morris, B.W., MacNeil, S., Hardisty, C.A., et al., "Chromium homeostasis in patients with type II (NIDDM) diabetes," *Journal of Trace Elements in Medicine and Biology*, 13, 57–61 (1999).

9. Kim, D.S., Kim, T.W., Park, I.K., Kang, J.S., Om, A.S., "Effects of chromium picolinate supplementation on insulin sensitivity, serum lipids, and body weight in dexamethasone-treated rats," *Metabolism*, 51(5), 589–594 (May 2002).

10. Bahijiri, S.M., Mira, S.A., Mufti, A.M., Ajabnoor, M.A., "The effects of inorganic chromium and brewer's yeast supplementation on glucose tolerance, serum lipids and drug dosage in individuals with type 2 diabetes," *Saudi Medical Journal*, 21(9), 831–837 (September 2000).

11. Urberg, M., Zemel, M.B., "Evidence for synergism between chromium and nicotinic acid in the control of glucose tolerance in elderly humans," *Metabolism*, 36(9), 896–899 (September 1987).

SPINA BIFIDA, PREVENTION OF

1. Honein, M.A., Paulozzi, L.J., Mathews, T.J., Erickson, J.D., Wong, L-Y. C., "Impact of folic acid fortification of the U.S. food supply on the occurrence of neural tube defects," *Journal of the American Medical Association*, 285, 2891 (20 June 2001).

STREP THROAT

1. Pizzorno, J.E., Jr., Murray, M.T., *Textbook of Natural Medicine* (London: Churchill Livingstone, 1999), p. 1553.

2. Budzinski, J.W., Foster, B.C., Vandenhoek, S., Arnason, J.T., "An in vitro evaluation of human cytochrome P405 3A4 inhibition by selected commercial herbal extracts and tinctures," *Phytomedicine*, 7(4), 273–282 (July 2000).

3. Luettig, B., Steinmuller, C., Gifford, G.E., Wagner, H., Lohmann-Matthes,

M.L., "Macrophage activation by the polysaccharide arabinogalactan isolated from plant cell cultures of *Echinacea purpurea*," *Journal of the National Cancer Institute*, 81(9), 669–675 (3 May 1989).

4. Blumenthal, M., Goldberg, A., Brinckmann, J., *Herbal Medicine: Expanded Commission E Monographs* (Boston, Integrative Medicine, 2000), p. 88.

STRETCH MARKS

1. Watson, R.E., Parry, E.J., Humphries, J.D., Jones, C.J., Polson, D.W., Kielty, C.M., Griffiths, C.E., "Fibrillin microfibrils are reduced in skin exhibiting striae distensae," *British Journal of Dermatology*, 138(6), 931–937 (June 1998).

2. Rangel, O., Arias, I., Garcia, E., Lopez-Padilla, S., "Topical tretinoin 0.1% for pregnancy-related abdominal striae: an open-label, multicentre, prospective study," *Advances in Therapeutics*, 18(4), 181–186 (July–August 2001).

3. Ash, K., Lord J., Zukowski, M., McDaniel, D.H., "Comparison of topical therapy for striae alba (20% glycolic acid/0.05% tretinoin versus 20% glycolic acid/10% L-ascorbic acid)," *Dermatological Surgery*, 24(8), 849–838 (August 1998).

4. Young, G.L., Jewell, D., "Creams for preventing stretch marks in pregnancy," *Cochrane Database System Review*, 2000, (2): CD 000066.

STROKE

1. Bazzano, L.A., He, J., Ogden, L.G., Loria, C., Vupputuri, S., Myers, L., Whelton, P.K., "Dietary intake of folate and risk of stroke in U.S. men and women: NHANES I epidemiologic follow-up study. National health and nutrition examination survey," *Stroke*, 33(5), 1183–1189 (May 2002).

2. Bazzano, L.A., He, J., Ogden, L.G., Loria, C., Vupputuri, S., Myers, L., Whelton, P.K., "Dietary potassium intake and risk of stroke in U.S. men and women: National health and nutrition examination survey I epidemiologic follow-up study," *Stroke*, 32(7), 1473–1480 (July 2001). Discussion in *Stroke*, 33(5), 1178–1179 (May 2002).

3. Bazzano, L.A., He, J., Ogden, L.G., Loria, C., Vupputuri, S., Myers, L., Whelton, P.K., "Fruit and vegetable intake and risk of cardiovascular disease in U.S. adults: The first national health and nutrition examination survey epidemiologic follow-up study," *American Journal of Clinical Nutrition*, 76(1), 93–99 (July 2002).

4. Bazzano, L.A., He, J., Ogden, L.G., Loria, C., Vupputuri, S., Myers, L., Whelton, P.K., "Legume consumption and risk of coronary heart disease in U.S. men and women: NHANES I epidemiologic follow-up study," *Archives of Internal Medicine*, 161(21), 2573–2578 (26 November 2001).

5. He, J., Ogden, L.G., Vupputuri, S., Bazzano, L.A., Loria, C., Whelton, P.K., "Dietary sodium intake and subsequent risk of cardiovascular disease in overweight adults," *Journal of the American Medical Association*, 282(21), 2027–2034 (1 December 1999).

6. Liu, S., Buring, J.E., Sesso, H.D., Rimm, E.B., Willett, W.C., Manson, J.E., "A prospective study of dietary fiber intake and risk of cardiovascular disease among women," *Journal of the American College of Cardiology*, 39(1), 49–56 (2 January 2002).

7. Liu, S., Manson, J.E., Stampfer, M.J., Rexrode, K.M., Hu, F.B., Rimm, E.B., Willett, W.C., "Whole grain consumption and risk of ischemic stroke in women: a prospective study," *Journal of the American Medical Association*, 284(12), 1534–1540 (27 September 2000).

8. Gillman, M.W., Cupples, L.A., Millen, B.E., Ellison, R.C., Wolf, P.A., "Inverse association of dietary fat with development of ischemic stroke in men," *Journal of the American Medical Association*, 278(24), 2145–2150 (24–31 December 1997).

9. Gillum, R.F., Mussolino, M.E., Madans, J.H., "The relationship between fish consumption and stroke incidence. The NHANES I epidemiologic follow-up study (national health and nutrition examination survey)," *Archives of Internal Medicine*, 156(5), 537–542 (11 March 1996).

10. McCulloch, J., Dewar, D., "A radical approach to stroke therapy," *Proceedings of the National Academy of Sciences of the U.S.A.*, 98(20), 10989–10991 (25 September 2001).

11. Mori, M., Hojo, E., Takano, K., "Action of *oren-gedoku-to* on platelet aggregation in vitro," *American Journal of Chinese Medicine*, 19(2), 131–143 (1991).

12. Fushitani, S., Minakuchi, K., Tsuchiya, K., Takasugi, M., Murakami, K., "Studies on attenuation of post-ischemic brain injury by kampo medicines-inhibitory effects of free radical production," *Yakugaku Zasshi*, 115(8), 611–617 (August 1995).

13. van Es, R.F., Jonker, J.J., Verheugt, F.W., Deckers, J.W., Grobbee, D.E., "Antithrombotics in the secondary prevention of events in coronary thrombosis-2 (ASPECT-2) research group. Aspirin and coumadin after acute coronary syndromes (the ASPECT-2 study): a randomized controlled trial," *Lancet*, 360(9327), 109–113 (13 July 2002).

STUFFY NOSE

1. Niven, R.M., Fletcher, A.M., Pickering,C.A., Faragher, E.B., Potter, I.N., Booth, W.B., Jones, T.J., Potter, P.D., "Building sickness syndrome in healthy and unhealthy buildings: an epidemiological and environmental assessment with cluster analysis," *Occupational and Environmental Medicine*, 57(9), 627–634 (September 2000).

2. Loehrl, T.A., Smith, T.L., Darling, R.J., Torrico, L., Prieto, T.E., Shaker, R., Toohill, R.J., Jaradeh, S.S., "Autonomic dysfunction, vasomotor rhinitis, and extraesophageal manifestations of gastroesophageal reflux," *Otolaryngological, Head, and Neck Surgery*, 126(4), 382–387 (April 2002).

3. De, M., De, A.K., Sen, P., Banerjee, A.B., "Antimicrobial properties of star anise (*Illicium verum* Hook f)," *Phytotherapy Research*, 16(1), 94–95 (February 2002).

4. Elgayyar, M., Draughon, F.A., Golden, D.A., Mount, J.R., "Antimicrobial activity of essential oils from plants against selected pathogenic and saprophytic microorganisms," *Journal of Food Protection*, 64(7), 1019–1024 (July 2001).

5. El Bardai, S., Lyoussi, B., Wibo, M., Morel, N., "Pharmacological evidence of hypotensive activity of *Marrubium vulgare* and *Foeniculum vulgare* in spontaneously hypertensive rat," *Clinical Experiments in Hypertension*, 23(4), 329–343 (May 2001).

6. De Jesus, R.A., Cechinel-Filho, V., Oliveira, A.E., Schlemper, V., "Analysis of the antinociceptive properties of marrubiin isolated from *Marrubium vulgare*," *Phytomedicine*, 7(2), 111–115 (April 2000).

7. Baudoin, T., Kalogjera, L., Hat, J., "Capsaicin significantly reduces sinonasal polyps," *Acta Otolaryngologica*, 120(2), 307–311 (March 2000).

8. Sarrell, E.M., Mandelberg, A., Cohen, H.A., "Efficacy of naturopathic extracts in the management of ear pain associated with acute otitis media," *Archives of Pediatric and Adolescent Medicine*, 155(7), 796–799 (July 2001).

9. Serkedjieva, J., "Combined antiinfluenza virus activity of Flos verbasci infusion and amantadine derivatives," *Phytotherapy Research*, 14(7), 571–574 (November 2000).

10. Meister, R., Wittig, T., Beuscher, N., et al., "Efficacy and tolerability of Myrtol standardized in long-term treatment of chronic bronchitis. A double-blind, placebo-controlled study. Study group investigators," *Arzneimittel Forschung*, 49, 351–358 (1999).

11. Aoyagi, M., Watanabe, H., Sekine, K., Nishimuta, T., Konno, A., Shimojo, N., Kohno, Y., "Circadian variation in nasal reactivity in children with allergic rhinitis: correlation with the activity of eosinophils and basophilic cells," *International Archives of Allergy and Immunology*, 120 Suppl 1, 95–99 (1999).

SUNBURN

1. Mathews-Roth, M.M., Pathak, M.A., Parrish J., Fitzpatrick, T.B., Kass, E.H., Toda, K., Clemens, W., "A clinical trial of the effects of oral beta-carotene on the responses of human skin to solar radiation.," *Journal of Investigational Dermatology*, 59(4), 349–353 (October 1972).

2. Clausen, W.W., "Carotenemia and resistance to infection," *Transactions of the American Pediatric Society*, 43, 27–30 (1931).

3. Carughim, A., Hooper, P. G., "Plasma carotenoid concentrations before and after supplementation with a carotenoid mixture," *American Journal of Clinical Nutrition*, 59, 896–899 (1994).

4. Ben-Amotz, A., Mokadya, S., Edelstein, S., Avron, M., "Bioavailability of a natural isomer mixture as compared with synthetic all-trans-beta-carotene in rats and chicks," *Journal of Nutrition*, 119(7), 1013–1019 (July 1989).

5. Stampfer, M.J., Willett, W., Hennekens, C.H., "Carotene, carrots, and neutropenia," *Lancet,* II, 615 (1982).

6. Kemmann, E., Pasquale, S.A., Skaf, R., "Amenorrhea associated with carotenemia," *Journal of the American Medical Association,* 249, 926–929 (1983).

7. Gollnick, H.P.M., Hopfenmuller, W., Hemmes, C., et al., "Systemic beta carotene plus topical UV sunscreen are an optimal protection against harmful effects of natural UV-sunlight: results of the Berlin-Eilath study," *European Journal of Dermatology,* 6, 200–205 (1996).

8. Lee, J., Jiang, S., Levine, N., et al., "Carotenoid supplementation reduces erythema in human skin after simulated solar radiation exposure," *Proceedings of the Society for Experimental Biology and Medicine,* 223, 170–174 (2000).

9. Stahl, W., Heinrich, U., Jungmann, H., et al., "Carotenoids and carotenoids plus vitamin E protect against ultraviolet light-induced erythema in humans," *American Journal of Clinical Nutrition,* 71, 795–798 (2000).

10. Garmyn, M., Ribaya-Mercardo, J.D., Russel, R.M., et al., "Effect of beta-carotene supplementation on the human sunburn reaction," *Experimental Dermatology,* 4, 104–111 (1995).

11. Wolf, C., Steiner, A., Honigsmann, H., et al., "Do oral carotenoids protect human skin against UV erythema, psoralen phototoxicity, and UV-induced DNA damage?" *Journal of Investigational Dermatology,* 90, 55–57 (1988).

12. Darr, D., Dunston, S., Faust, H., et al., "Effectiveness of antioxidants (vitamin C and E) with and without sunscreens as topical photoprotectants," *Acta Dermatologica et Venereologica,* 76, 264–268 (1996).

13. Ibid.

14. Alpha-Tocopherol, Beta-Carotene Cancer Prevention Study Group, "The effect of vitamin E and beta-carotene on the incidence of lung cancer and other cancers in male smokers," *New England Journal of Medicine,* 330, 1029–1035 (1994).

15. Omenn, G.S., Goodman, G.E., Thornquist, M.D., et al., "Effects of a combination of beta carotene and vitamin A on lung cancer and cardiovascular disease," *New England Journal of Medicine,* 334, 1150–1155 (1996).

16. Krinsky, N.J., "The biological properties of carotenoids," *Pure and Applied Chemistry,* 66, 1003–1010 (1994).

17. Krinsky, N.J., "Antioxidant functions of carotenoids," *Free Radicals in Biology and Medicine,* 7, 617–635 (1989).

18. Widyarini, S., Spinks, N., Husband, A.J., Reeve, V.E., "Isoflavonoid compounds from red clover (*Trifolium pratense*) protect from inflammation and immune suppression induced by UV radiation," *Photochemistry and Photobiology,* 74(3), 465–470 (September 2001).

19. Crowell, J., Penneys, N., "The effects of aloe vera on cutaneous erythema and blood flow following ultraviolet B (UVB) exposure," *Clinical Research,* 35, 676A (1987).

20. Katiyar, S.K., Elmets, C.A., Agarwal, R., Mukhtar, H., "Protection against ultraviolet-B radiation-induced local and systemic suppression of contact hypersensitivity and edema responses in C3H/HeN mice by green tea polyphenols," *Photochemistry and Photobiology,* 62, 855–861 (1995).

21. Katiyar, S.K., Matsui, M.S., Elmets, C.A., Katiyar, S.K., Matsui, M.S., Elmets, C.A., "Polyphenolic antioxidant (–)-epigallocatechin-3-gallate from green tea reduces UVB-induced inflammatory responses and infiltration of leukocytes in human skin," *Photochemistry and Photobiology,* 69, 148–153 (1999).

22. Katiyar, S.K., Matsui, M.S., Elmets, C.A., Mukhtar, H., "Polyphenolic antioxidant(–)-epigallocatechin-3-gallate from green tea reduces UVB-induced inflammatory responses and infiltration of leukocytes in human skin," *Photochemistry and Photobiology,* 69, 148–153 (1999).

23. Elmets, C.A., Singh, D., Tubesing, K., Matsui, M., Katiyar, S., Mukhtar, H., "Cutaneous photoprotection from ultraviolet injury by green tea polyphenols," *Journal of the American Academy of Dermatology,* 44, 425–432 (2001).

SYPHILIS

1. Cardin de Stefani, E., Costa, C., "Tryptophan metabolism in syphilis infections," *Bolletina de la Societa Italiana de la Biologia Sperimentale,* 60(8), 1541–1547 (31 August 1984).

2. Montero, J.Q., Zaulyanov, L.L., Houston, S.H., Sinnott, J.T., "Chancroid: An update," *Infections in Medicine,* 19(4), 174–178 (2002).

TARDIVE DYSKINESIA

1. Rotrosen, J., Adler, L., Lohr, J., Edson, R., Lavori, P.,"Antioxidant treatment of tardive dyskinesia," *Prostaglandins, Leukotrienes, and Essential Fatty Acids,* 55, 77–81 (1996).

2. Richardson, M.A., Bevans, M.L., Weber, J.B., Gonzalez, J.J., Flynn, C.J., Amira, L., Read, L.L., Suckow, R.F., Maher, T.J., "Branched chain amino acids decrease tardive dyskinesia symptoms," *Psychopharmacology* (Berlin), 143(4), 358–364 (April 1999).

3. Adler, L.A., Edson, R., Lavori, P., Peselow, E., Duncan, E., Rosenthal, M., Rotrosen, J., "Long-term treatment effects of vitamin E for tardive dyskinesia," *Biological Psychiatry,* 43(12), 868–872 (15 June 1998).

4. Tkacz, C., "A preventive measure for tardive dyskinesia," *Journal of the International Academy of Preventive Medicine,* 8(5), 5–8 (1984).

TENNIS ELBOW

1. Khan, K.M., Cook, J.L., Kannus, P., Maffulli, N., Bonar, S.F., "Time to abandon the 'tendinitis' myth," *British Medical Journal,* 324, 626–627 (16 March 2002).

2. Khan, K.M., Cook, J.L., Bonar, F., Harcourt, P., Astrom, M., "Histopathology of common overuse tendon conditions: update and implications for clinical management," *Sports Medicine,* 27, 393–408 (1999).

3. Klein, G., Küllich, W., "Reducing pain by oral enzyme therapy in rheumatic diseases," *Wienerischer Medizinische Wochenschrift,* 149(21–22), 577–580 (1999).

4. Schnitzer, T.J., "Non-NSAID pharmacologic treatment options for the management of chronic pain," *American Journal of Medicine,* 105(1B), 45S-52S (27 July 1998).

5. McCleane, G., "The analgesic efficacy of topical capsaicin is enhanced by glyceryl trinitrate in painful osteoarthritis: a randomized, double-blind, placebo controlled study," *European Journal of Pain,* 4(4), 355–360 (2000).

6. Brenstein, A.L., Dinesen, J.S., "Brief communication: effect of pharmacologic doses of vitamin B$_6$ on carpal tunnel syndrome, electroencephalographic results, and pain," *Journal of the American College of Nutrition,* 12(1), 73–76 (February 1993).

7. Keniston, R.C., Nathan, P.A., Leklem, J.E., Lockwood, R.S., "Vitamin B$_6$, vitamin C, and carpal tunnel syndrome. A cross-sectional study of 441 adults," *Journal of Occupational and Environmental Medicine,* 39(10), 949–959 (October 1997).

8. Bito, T., Roy, S., Sen, C.K., Packer, L., "Pine bark extract pycnogenol downregaltes IFN-gamma-induced adhesion of T cells to human keratinocytes by inhibiting inducible ICAM-1 expression," *Free Radicals in Biology and Medicine,* 28, 219–227 (2000).

9. Chen, M.F., Shimada, F., Kato, H., Yano, S., Kanaoka, M., "Effect of glycyrrhizin on the pharmacokinetics of prednisolone following low dosage of prednisolone hemisuccinate," *Endocronologica Japonica,* 37, 331–341 (1990).

10. Kuhlwein, A., Meyer, H.J., Koehler, C.O., "Reduced diclofenac administration by B vitamins: results of a randomized double-blind study with reduced daily doses of diclofenac (75 mg diclofenac versus 75 mg diclofenac plus B vitamins) in acute lumbar vertebral syndromes," *Klinische Wochenschrift,* 68(2), 107–115 (19 January 1990).

11. Vetter, G., Bruggemann, G., Lettko, M., Schwieger, G., Asbach, H., Biermann, W., Blasius, K., Brinkmann, R., Bruns, H., Dorn, E., et al., "Shortening diclofenac therapy by B vitamins. Results of a randomized double-blind study, diclofenac 50 mg versus diclofenac 50 mg plus B vitamins, in painful spinal diseases with degenerative changes," *Zeitschrift für Rheumatologie,* 47(5), 351–362 (September–October 1988).

12. Ehrenpreis, S., "Analgesic properties of enkephalinase inhibitors: animal and human studies," *Progress in Clinical Biological Research,* 192, 363–370 (1985).

13. Parcell, S., "Sulfur in human nutrition and its applications in medicine," *Alternative Medicine Review,* 7(1), 22–44 (February 2002).

14. Ishiguro, N., Ito, T., Oguchi, T., Kojima, T., Iwata, H., Ionescu, M., Poole, A.R., "Relationships of matrix metalloproteinases and their inhibitors to cartilage proteoglycan and collagen turnover and inflammation as revealed by analyses of synovial fluids from patients with rheumatoid arthritis," *Arthritis and Rheumatism,* 44(11), 2503–2511 (November 2001).

TENSION HEADACHES

1. Diamond, S., "Tension-type headache," *Clinical Cornerstones,* 1(6), 33–44 (1999).

2. De Giorgis, G., Miletto, R., Iannuccelli, M., Camuffo, M., Scerni, S., "Headache in association with sleep disorders in children: a psychodiagnostic evaluation and controlled clinical study—L-5-HTP versus placebo," *Drugs in Experimental and Clinical Research,* 13(7):425–433 (1987).

3. Gobel, H., Fresenius, J., Heinze, A., Dworschak, M., Soyka, D., "Effectiveness of Oleum menthae piperitae and paracetamol in therapy of headache of the tension type," *Nervenarzt,* 67(8), 672–681 (August 1996).

4. Nilsson, N., Christensen, H.W., Hartvigsen, J., "The effect of spinal manipulation in the treatment of cervicogenic headache," *Journal of Manipulative Physiology and Therapy,* 20, 326–330 (1997).

TINNITUS

1. Rüedi, L., "Vitamin A und schwerhörigkeit," *Wissenschäftlicher Dienst Roche,* 1952.

2. Shemesh, Z., Attias, J., Ornan, M., Shapira, N., Shahar, A., "Vitamin B_{12} deficiency in patients with chronic-tinnitus and noise-induced hearing loss," *American Journal of Otolaryngology,* 14(2), 94–99 (March–April 1993).

3. Lamm, K., Arnold, W., "The effect of blood flow promoting drugs on cochlear blood flow, perilymphatic pO(2) and auditory function in the normal and noise-damaged hypoxic and ischemic guinea pig inner ear," *Hearing Research,* 141(1–2), 199–219 (March 2000).

4. Stange, G., Benning, C.D., "The influence on sound damages by an extract of *Ginkgo biloba,*" *Archiv der Otorhinolaryngolie,* 209(3), 203–215 (8 July 1975).

5. Vavrina, J., Müller, W., "Therapeutic effect of hyperbaric oxygenation in acute acoustic trauma. physiological mechanisms of HBO responsible for the clinical success in AAT," *Revue de Laryngologie-Otologie-Rhinologie* (Bordeaux),116(5), 377–380 (1995).

6. Drew, S., Davies, E., 'Effectiveness of *Ginkgo biloba* in treating tinnitus: double blind, placebo controlled trial," *British Medical Journal,* 322(7278), 73 (13 January 2001).

7. Morgenstern, C., Biermann, E., "The efficacy of ginkgo extract EGb 761 in patients with tinnitus," *International Journal of Pharmacological Therapy,* 40(5), 188–107 (May 2002).

8. Dineen, R., Doyle, J., Bench, J., Perry, A., "The influence of training on tinnitus perception: an evaluation 12 months after tinnitus management training," *British Journal of Audiology,* 29–51 (February 1999).

9. Bayazit, Y.A., Gursoyt, S., Oxzer, E., Karakurum, G., Madenci, E., "Neurotologic manifestations of the fibromyalgia syndrome," *Journal of Neurological Sciences,* 196(1–2), 77–80 (15 April 2002).

10. Simpson, J.J., Donaldson, I., Davies, W.E., "Use of homeopathy in the treatment of tinnitus," *British Journal of Audiology,* 32(4), 227–233 (August 1998).

TOURETTE'S SYNDROME

1. Grimaldi, B.L., "The central role of magnesium deficiency in Tourette's syndrome: causal relationships between magnesium deficiency, altered biochemical pathways and symptoms relating to Tourette's syndrome and several reported comorbid conditions," *Medical Hypotheses,* 58(1), 47–60 (January 2002).

TRACHOMA

1. Boniface, R., Robert, A.M., "Effect of anthocyanins on human connective tissue metabolism in humans," *Klinische Monatsblätter für Augenheilkunde,* 209, 368–372 (1996).

2. Detre, Z., Jellinek, H., Miskulin, M., Robert, A.M., "Studies on vascular permeability in hypertension: action of anthocyanosides," *Clinical Physiology and Biochemistry,* 4, 143–149 (1986).

3. Cazzola, P., Mazzanti, P., Bossi, G., "In vivo modulating effect of a calf thymus acid lysate on human T lymphocyte subsets and CD4+/CD8+ ratio in the course of difference diseases," *Current Therapies Research,* 42, 1011–1017 (1987).

4. Seifter, E., Rettura, G., Seiter, J., "Thymotrophic action of vitamin A," *Federal Proceedings,* 32, 947 (1973).

5. Semba, R.D., "Vitamin A, immunity, and infection," *Clinical Infectious Disease,* 19, 489–499 (1994).

6. Ringsdorf, W., Cheraskin, E., "Vitamin C and human wound healing," *Oral Surgery,* 53(3), 231–236 (March 1982).

7. Gabor, M., "Pharmacologic effects of flavonoids on blood vessels," *Angiologica,* 9, 355–374 (1972).

8. Prasad, A., "Clinical, biochemical and nutritional spectrum of zinc deficiency in human subjects. An update," *Nutrition Review,* 41, 197–208 (1983).

9. Kuhn, O., untitled article, *Arzneimittel-Forschung,* 3, 194–200 (1953).

10. Erhard, M., "Effect of echinacea, aconitum, lachesis, and apis extracts, and their combinations of phagocytosis of human granulocytes," *Phytotherapy Research,* 8, 14–77 (1994).

11. Facino, R.M., Carini, M., Aldini, G., Marinello, C., Arlandini, E., Franzoi, L., Colombo, M., Pietta, P., Mauri, P., "Direct characterization of caffeoyl esters with antihyaluronidase activity in crude extracts from *Echinacea angustifolia* roots by fast atom bombardment tandem mass spectrometry," *Farmaco,* 48(10), 1447–1461 (October 1993).

12. Budzinski, J.W., Foster, B.C., Vandenhoek, S., Arnason, J.T., "An in vitro evaluation of human cytochrome P405 3A4 inhibition by selected commercial herbal extracts and tinctures," *Phytomedicine,* 7(4), 273–282 (July 2000).

13. Luettig, B., Steinmuller, C., Gifford, G.E., Wagner, H., Lohmann-Matthes, M.L., "Macrophage activation by the polysaccharide arabinogalactan isolated from plant cell cultures of *Echinacea purpurea,*" *Journal of the National Cancer Institute,* 81(9), 669–675 (3 May 1989).

14. Rehman, J., Dillow, J.M., Carter, S.M., Chou, J., Le, B., Maisel, A.S., "Increased production of antigen-specific immunoglobulins G and M following in vivo treatment with the medical plants *Echinacea angustifolia* and *Hydrastis canadensis,*" *Immunology Letters,* 68(2–3), 391–395 (1 June 1999).

TRENCH MOUTH

1. Addya, S., Chakravarti, K., Basu, A., et al., "Effects of mercuric chloride on several scavenging enzymes in rat kidney and influence of vitamin E supplementation," *Acta Vitaminologica et Enzymologica,* 6, 103–107 (1984).

2. Godkowsky, K.C.," Antimicrobial action of sanguinarine," *Journal of Clinical Dentistry,* 1, 96–101 (1989).

3. Page, R., Schroeder, H., "Current status of the host response in chronic marginal periodontitis," *Journal of Periodontal Dentistry,* 52, 477–491 (1981).

4. Otake, S., Makimura, M., Kuroki, T., Nishihara, Y., Hirasawa, M., "Anticaries effects of polyphenolic compounds from Japanese green tea," *Caries Research* (Switzerland), 25(6), 438–443 (1991).

5. Murray, M., Pizzorno, J., p. 1488.

6. Addya, S., Chakravarti, K., Basu, A., et al., ibid.

7. Prasad, A., "Clinical, biochemical and nutritional spectrum of zinc deficiency in human subjects: an update," *Nutrition Review,* 41, 197–308 (1983).

8. Freeland, J., Cousins, R., Schwartz, R., "Relationship of mineral status and intake to periodontal disease," *American Journal of Clinical Nutrition,* 29, 745–749 (1976).

TUBERCULOSIS

1. Lauzardo, M., Ashkin, D., "Phthisiology at the dawn of the new century," *Chest,* 117, 1455–1473 (2000).

2. Karyadi, E., West, C.E., Schultink, W., Nelwan, R.H., Gross, R., Amin, Z., Dolmans, W.M., Schlebusch, H., van der Meer, J.W., "A double-blind, place-

bo-controlled study of vitamin A and zinc supplementation in persons with tuberculosis in Indonesia: effects on clinical response and nutritional status," *American Journal of Clinical Nutrition*, 75(4), 720–727 (April 2002).

UNCOMBABLE HAIR SYNDROME

1. de Luna, M.M., Rubinson, R., de Kohan, Z.B., "Pili trianguli canaliculi: uncombable hair syndrome in a family with apparent autosomal dominant inheritance," *Pediatric Dermatology*, 2(4), 324–327 (July 1985).

2. Shelley, W.B., Shelley, E.D., "Uncombable hair syndrome: observations on response to biotin and occurrence in sibling with ectodermal dysplasia," *Journal of the American Academy of Dermatology*, 13(1), 97–102 (July 1985).

VAGINAL DRYNESS

1. Cauci, S., Driussi, S., De Santo, D., Penacchioni, P., Iannicelli, T., Lanzafame, P., De Seta, F., Quadrifoglio, F., de Aloysio, D., Guaschino, S., "Prevalence of bacterial vaginosis and vaginal flora changes in peri- and postmenopausal women," *Journal of Clinical Microbiology*, 40(6), 2147–2152 (June 2002).

2. Williams, A., Yu, C., Tashima, K., et al., "Weekly treatment for prophylaxis of Candida vaginitis. Presentation. 7th Conference on Retroviruses and Opportunistic infections," *Foundation for Retrovirology and Human Health in collaboration with the (U.S.) National Institute of Allergy and Infectious Diseases and the Centers for Disease Control and Prevention.* January 30–February 2, 2000.

3. Holzman, C., Leventhal, J.M., Qiu, H., Jones, N.M., Wang, J. (BV Study Group), "Factors linked to bacterial vaginosis in nonpregnant women," *American Journal of Public Health*, 91(10), 1664–1670 (October 2001).

4. Moodley, P., Connolly, C., Sturm, A.W., "Interrelationships among human immunodeficiency virus type 1 infection, bacterial vaginosis, trichomoniasis, and the presence of yeasts," *Journal of Infectious Disease*, 185(1), 69–73 (1 January 2002).

5. Sorvillo, F., Smith, L., Kerndt, P., Ash, L., "Trichomonas vaginalis, HIV, and African-Americans," *Emerging Infectious Diseases*, 7(6), 927–932 (November–December 2001).

VAGINOSIS

1. Moodley, P., Connolly, C., Sturm, A.W., "Interrelationships among human immunodeficiency virus type 1 infection, bacterial vaginosis, trichomoniasis, and the presence of yeasts," *Journal of Infectious Disease*, 185(1), 69–73 (1 January 2002).

2. Sorvillo, F., Smith, L., Kerndt, P., Ash, L., "Trichomonas vaginalis, HIV, and African-Americans," *Emerging Infectious Diseases*, 7(6), 927–932 (November–December 2001).

3. Holzman, C., Leventhal, J.M., Qiu, H., Jones, N.M., Wang, J., (BV Study Group), "Factors linked to bacterial vaginosis in nonpregnant women," *American Journal of Public Health*, 91(10), 1664–1670 (October 2001).

4. Williams, A., Yu, C., Tashima, K., et al., "Weekly treatment for prophylaxis of Candida vaginitis. Presentation. 7th Conference on Retroviruses and Opportunistic infections". *Foundation for Retrovirology and Human Health in collaboration with the (U.S.) National Institute of Allergy and Infectious Diseases and the Centers for Disease Control and Prevention.* January 30–February 2, 2000.

VARICOSE VEINS

1. Tuchsen, B.F., Krause, N., Hannerz, H., et al., "Standing at work and varicose veins," *Scandinavian Journal of Work and Environmental Health*, 26, 414–420 (2000).

2. Evans, C.J., Fowkes, F.G., Ruckley, C.V., Lee, A.J., "Prevalence of varicose veins and chronic venous insufficiency in men and women of the general population: Edinburgh Vein Study," *Journal of Epidemiology and Community Health*, 53, 149–153 (1999).

3. Ducimetiere, P., Richard, J.L., Pequignot, G., Warnet, J.M., "Varicose veins: a risk for atherosclerotic disease in middle-aged men," *International Journal of Epidemiology*, 10(4), 329–335 (December 1981).

4. Diehm, C., et al., "Comparison of leg compression stocking and oral horse-chestnut seed extract therapy in patients with chronic venous insufficiency," *Lancet*, 347, 292–294 (1996).

5. Arpaia, M.R., Ferrone, R., Amitrano, M., et al., "Effects of *Centella asiatica* extract on mucopolysaccharide metabolism in subjects with varicose veins," *International Journal of Clinical Pharmacological Research*, 4, 229–233 (1990).

6. Incandela, L., Belcaro, G., De Sanctis, M.T., Cesarone, M.R., Griffin, M., Ippolito, E., Bucci, M., Cacchio, M., "Total triterpenic fraction of Centella asiatica in the treatment of venous hypertension: a clinical, prospective, randomized trial using a combined microcirculatory model," *Angiology* 52 Suppl 2, S61–S67 (October 2001).

7. Belcaro, G.V., Rulo, A., Grimaldi, R., "Capillary filtration and ankle edema in patients with venous hypertension treated with TTFCA," Angiology, 41, 12–18. (1990).

8. Pointel, J.P., Boccalon, H., Cloarec, M., et al., "Titrated extract of *Centella asiatica* (TECA) in the treatment of venous insufficiency of the lower limbs," *Angiology*, 38, 46–50. (1987).

9. Thebaut, J.F., Thebaut, P., Vin ,F., "Study of endotelon(r) in functional manifestations of peripheral venous insufficiency," *Gazette Medicale de France*, 92, 96–100 (1985).

10. Arcangeli, P., "Pycnogenol in chronic venous insufficiency," *Fitoterapia*, 71, 236–244 (2000).

11. Kiesewetter, H., Koscielny, J., Kalus, U., Vix, J.M., Peil, H., Petrini, O., van Toor, B.S., de Mey, C., "Efficacy of orally administered extract of red vine leaf AS 195 (*folia vitis viniferae*) in chronic venous insufficiency (stages I–II)," *Arzneimittelforschung*, 50, 109–117 (2000).

12. Lohr, E., Garanin, G., Jesau, P., et al., "Anti-edemic therapy in chronic venous insufficiency with tendency to formation of edema," *Münchener Medizinischer Wochenschrift*, 128, 579–581 (1986).

13. Ihme, N., Kiesewetter, H., Jung, F., Hoffmann, K.H., Birk, A., Muller, A., Grutzner, K.I., "Leg edema protection from a buckwheat herb tea in patients with chronic venous insufficiency: a single-centre, randomized, double-blind, placebo-controlled clinical trial," *European Journal of Clinical Pharmacology*, 50(6), 443–447 (1996).

VITILIGO

1. D'Amelio, R. Frati, C., Fattorossi, A., Aiuti, F., "Peripheral T-cell subset imbalance in patients with vitiligo and in their apparently healthy first-degree relatives," *Annals of Allergy*, 65, 143–145 (1990).

2. Ogg, G.S., Rod Dunbar, P., Romero, P., Chen, J.L., Cerundolo, V., "High frequency of skin-homing melanocyte-specific cytotoxic T lymphocytes in autoimmune vitiligo," *Journal of Experimental Medicine*, 188, 1203–1208 (1998).

3. Moretti, S., Spallanzani, A., Amato, L., Hautmann, G., Gallerani, I., Fabiani, M., Fabbri, P., "New insights into the pathogenesis of vitiligo: imbalance of epidermal cytokines at sites of lesions," *Pigment Cell Research*, 15(2), 87–92 (April 2002).

4. Pedersen, Ls. L.O., Vetter, C.S., Mingari, M.C., Andersen, M.H., thor Straten, P., Brocker, E.B., Becker, J.C., "Differential expression of inhibitory or activating CD94/NKG2 subtypes on MART-1–reactive T cells in vitiligo versus melanoma: a case report," *Journal of Investigational Dermatology*, 118(4), 595–599 (April 2002).

5. Ajjan, R.A., Kemp, E.H., Waterman, E.A., Watson, P.F., Endo, T., Onaya, T., Weetman, A.P., "Detection of binding and blocking autoantibodies to the human sodium-iodide symporter in patients with autoimmune thyroid disease," *Journal of Clinical Endocrinology and Metabolism*, 85(5), 2020–2027 (May 2000).

6. Macaron, C., Winter, R.J., Traisman, H.S., Kahan, B.D., Lasser, A.E., Green, O.C., "Vitiligo and juvenile diabetes mellitus," *Archives of Dermatology*, 113, 1515–1517 (1977).

7. Sharma, V.K., Dawn, G., Kumar, B., "Profile of alopecia areata in Northern India," *International Journal of Dermatology*, 35, 22–27 (1996).

8. Mandry, R.C., Ortiz, L.J., Lugo-Somolinos, A., Sanchez, J.L., "Organ-specific autoantibodies in vitiligo patients and their relatives," *International Journal of Dermatology*, 35, 18–21 (1996).

9. Cucchi, M.L., Frattini, P., Santagostino, G., Orecchia, G., "Higher plasma catecholamine and metabolite levels in the early phase of nonsegmental vitiligo," *Pigment Cell Research,* 13(1), 28–32 (February 2000).

10. Schallreuter, K.U., Zachiesche, M., Moore, J., Panske, A., Hibberts, N.A., Herrmann, F.H., Metelmann, H.R., Sawatzki, J., "In vivo evidence for compromised phenylalanine metabolism in vitiligo," *Biochemical and Biophysical Research Communications,* 13, 243(2), 395–399 (February 1998).

11. Camacho, F., Mazuecos, J., "Treatment of vitiligo with oral and topical phenylalanine: 6 years of experience," *Archives of Dermatology,* 135, 216–217 (1999).

12. Juhlin, L., Olsson, M.J., "Improvement of vitiligo after oral treatment with vitamin B_{12} and folic acid and the importance of sun exposure," *Acta Dermatological et Venereologica (Stockholm),* 77, 460–462 (1997).

13. Hofer, A., Kerl, H., Wolf, P., "Long-term results in the treatment of vitiligo with oral khellin plus UVA," *European Journal of Dermatology,* 11(3), 225–229 (May–June 2001).

WASTING

1. Morley, J.E., Kraenzle,D., "Causes of weight loss in a community nursing home," *Journal of the American Geriatric Society,* 42, 583–585 (1994).

2. Pinchcofsky-Devin, G.D., Kaminski, M.V., Jr., "Correlation of pressure sores and nutritional status," *Journal of the American Geriatric Society,* 34, 435–440 (1986).

3. Morley, J.E., Silver, A.J., "Anorexia in the elderly," *Neurobiology of Aging,* 9, 9–16 (1988).

4. Harris,T., Cook, E.F., Garrison, R., Higgins, M., Kannel, W., Goldman, L., "Body mass index and mortality among nonsmoking older persons. The framingham heart study," *Journal of the American Medical Association,* 259, 1520–1524 (1988).

5. Roubenoff, R., Roubenoff, R.A., Selhub, J., Nadeau, M.R., Cannon, J.G., Freeman, L.M., Dinarello, C.A., Rosenberg, I.H., "Rheumatoid cachexia: cytokine-driven hypermetabolism accompanying reduced body cell mass in chronic inflammation," *Journal of Clinical Investigation,* 93, 2379–2386 (1994).

6. Groundwater, P., Beck, S.A., Barton, C., Tisdale, M.J., "Alternation of serum and urinary lipolytic activity with weight loss in cachetic cancer patients," *British Journal of Cancer,* 62, 816–821 (1990).

7. Todorov, P.T., McDevitt, T.M., Cariuk, P., Deacon, M., Tisdale, M.J., "Induction of muscle protein degradation and weight loss by a tumor product," *Cancer Research,* 56, 1256–1261 (1996).

8. Roubenoff, R., Roubenoff, R.A., Selhub, J., Nadeau, M.R., Cannon, J.G., Freeman, L.M., Dinarello, C.A., Rosenberg, I.H., ibid.

9. Moldawer, L.L., Rogy, M.A., Lowry, S.F., "The role of cytokines in cancer cachexia," *Journal of Parenteral and Enteral Nutrition,* 16 (Suppl), 43S–49S (1992).

10. Kinoshita, N., Suzuki, E., Yagi, G., Kato, R., Asai, M., "Il-1ß augments release of norepinephrine, dopamine, and serotonin in the rat anterior hypothalamus, "*Journal of Neuroscience,* 13, 3574–3581 (1993).

11. Wilder, R.L., "Interleukin-6 in autoimmune and inflammatory diseases." In Papanicolaou, D.A., moderator, "The pathophysiological roles of interleukin-6 in human disease," *Annals of Internal Medicine,* 128, 130–132 (1998).

12. Strassmann, G., Fong, M., Kenny, J.S., Jacob, C.O., "Evidence for the involvement of interleukin-6 in experimental cancer cachexia," *Journal of Clinical Investigation,* 89, 1681–1684 (1992).

13. Lemaire, I., Assinewe, V., Cano, P., Awang, D.V., Arnason, J.T., "Stimulation of interleukin-1 and -6 production in alveolar macrophages by the neotropical liana, *Uncaria tomentosa* (uña de gato)," *Journal of Ethnopharmacology,* 64(2), 109–115 (February 1999).

14. Kilter, D.B., Tierney, A.A., Culpepper-Morgan, J.A., Pierson, R.N., "Effect of home total parental nutrition on body composition in patients with acquired immunodeficiency syndrome," *Journal of Parenteral and Enteral Nutrition,* 14, 454–458 (1990).

15. Garter, R., Seefried, M., Vorlberding, P., "Dronabinol effects on weight in patients with HIV infections," *AIDS,* 6, 127 (1992).

16. Kaiser, F.E., Silver, A.J., Morley, J.E., "The effect of recombinant growth human growth hormone on malnourished older individuals," *Journal of the American Geriatric Society,* 39, 235–240 (1991).

17. Barber, M.D., "Cancer cachexia and its treatment with fish-oil-enriched nutritional supplementation," *Nutrition,* 17(9), 751–755 (September 2001).

18. Weglicki, W.B., Phillips, T.M., Mak, I.T., et al., "Cytokines, neuropeptides, and reperfusion injury during magnesium deficiency," *Annals of the New York Academy of Sciences,* 723, 246–257 (1994).

19. Rose, D., Oliveira, V., "Nutrient intakes of individuals from food-insufficient household in the United States," *American Journal of Public Health,* 87, 1956–1961 (1997).

20. Lissoni, P., Paolorossi, F., Tancini, G., Barni, S., Ardizzoia, A., Brivio, F., Zubelewicz, B., Chatikhine, V., "Is there a role for melatonin in the treatment of neoplastic cachexia?" *European Journal of Cancer,* 32A(8), 1340–1343 (July 1996).

21. Lissoni, P., Rovelli, F., Malugani, F., Bucovec, R., Conti, A., Maestroni, G.J., "Anti-angiogenic activity of melatonin in advanced cancer patients," *Neuroendocrinology Letters,* 22(1), 45–47 (2001).

22. Lissoni, P., "Is there a role for melatonin in supportive care?" *Supportive Care of Cancer,* 10(2), 110–116 (March 2002).

23. Sandoval, M., Charbonnet, R.M., Okuhama, N.N., Roberts, J., Krenova, Z., Trentacosti, A.M., Miller, M.J., "Cat's claw inhibits TNFalpha production and scavenges free radicals: role in cytoprotection," *Free Radicals in Biology and Medicine,* 29(1), 71–78 (1 July 2000).

24. Austgen, T.R., Chen, M.K., Dudrick, P.S., Dudrick, P.S., Copeland, E.M., Souba, W.W., "Cytokine regulation of intestinal glutamine utilization," *American Journal of Surgery,* 163, 174–179 (1992).

25. Brocker, P., Vellas, B., Albarede, J., Poynard, T. "A two centre, randomized, double-blind trial of ornithine oxoglutarate in 194 elderly, ambulatory, convalescent subjects," *Age and Aging,* 23, 303–306 (1994).

26. Pi-Sunyer, F.X., "Overnutrition and undernutrition as modifiers of metabolic processes in disease states," *American Journal of Clinical Nutrition,* 72(2), 533S-537S (August 2000).

WEIGHT CONTROL

1. Harper, M.E., Dent, R., Monemdjou, S., Bezaire, V., Van Wyck, L., Wells, G., Kavaslar, G.N., Gauthier, A., Tesson, F., McPherson, R., "Decreased mitochondrial proton leak and reduced expression of uncoupling protein 3 in skeletal muscle of obese diet-resistant women," *Diabetes,* 51(8), 2459–2466 (August 2002).

2. Willett, W.C., "Dietary fat plays a major role in obesity: no," *Obesity Review,* 3(2), 59–68 (May 2002).

3. Jequier, E., "Pathways to Obesity," *International Journal of Obesity and Related Metabolic Disorders,* 26 Suppl 2, 21–27 (September 2002).

4. Dulloo, A.G., Jacquet, J., Montani, J.P., "Pathways from weight fluctuations to metabolic diseases: focus on maladaptive thermogenesis during catch-up fat," *International Journal of Obesity and Related Metabolic Disorders,* 26 Suppl 2, 46–57 (September 2002).

5. Greenwood, M.R., Clearly, M.P., Green, R., et al., "Effect of (–) hydroxycitrate on development of obesity in the Zucker obese rat," *American Journal of Physiology,* 240, E72–E78 (1981).

6. Heymsfield, S.B., Allison, D.B., Vasseli, J.R., et al., "*Garcinia cambogia* (hydroxycitirc aicd) as a potential antiobesity agent: a randomized controlled trial," *Journal of the American Medical Association,* 280, 1596–1600 (1998).

7. Buck, S.H., Burks, T.F., "The neuropharmacology of capsaicin: review of some recent observations," *Pharmacology Review,* 38, 179–226 (1986).

WEST SYNDROME

1. Toribe, Y., "High-dose vitamin B(6) treatment in West syndrome," *Brain Development,* 23(7), 654–657 (November 2001).

WILSON'S DISEASE

1. Brewer, J.G., Yuzbasiyan-Gurkan, V., Lee, D-Y., Appelman, H., "Treatment of Wilson's disease with zinc. VI. Initial treatment studies," *Journal of Laboratory and Clinical Medicine,* 114, 633–638 (1989).

WRINKLES

1. Cross. E., van der Vliet, A., Louie, S., Thiele, J.J., Halliwell, B., "Oxidative stress and antioxidants at biosurfaces: plants, skin and respiratory tract surfaces," *Environmental Health Perspectives,* 106, 1241–1251 (1998).

2. Yin, L., Morita, A., Tsuji, T., "Alterations of extracellular matrix induced by tobacco smoke extract," *Archives of Dermatological Research,* 292(4), 188–194 (April 2000).

3. Clausen, W.W., "Carotinemia and resistance to infection," *Transactions of the American Pediatric Society,* 43, 27–30 (1931).

4. Carughim, A., Hooper, P.G., "Plasma carotenoid concentrations before and after supplementation with a carotenoid mixture," *American Journal of Clinical Nutrition,* 59, 896–899 (1994).

5. Ben-Amotz, A., Mokadya, S., Edelstein S, Avron, M., "Bioavailability of a natural isomer mixture as compared with synthetic all-trans-beta-carotene in rats and chicks," *Journal of Nutrition,* 119(7), 1013–1019 (July 1989).

6. Stampfer, M.J., Willett, W., Hennekens, C.H., "Carotene, carrots, and neutropenia," *Lancet,* II, 615 (1982).

7. Kemmann, E., Pasquale, S.A., Skaf, R., "Amenorrhea associated with carotenemia," *Journal of the American Medical Association,* 249, 926–929 (1983).

8. Lowe, N.J., DeQuoy, P.R., "Linoleic acid effects on epidermal DNA synthesis and cutaneous prostaglandin levels in essential fatty acids deficiency," *Journal of Investigational Dermatology,* 70, 200–203 (1978).

9. Prottey, C., "Investigation of functions of essential fatty acids in the skin," *British Journal of Dermatology,* 9, 29–38 (1977).

10. Ziboh, V.A., "Biochemical abnormalities in essential fatty acid deficiency," *Models in Dermatology,* 3, 106–111 (1987).

11. Haak, E., Usadel, K.H., Kusterer, K., Amini, P., Frommeyer, R., Tritschler, H.J., Haak, T., "Effect of alpha-lipoic acid on microcirculation in patients with peripheral diabetic neuropathy," *Experimental and Clinical Endocrinology and Diabetes,* 108(3), 168–174 (2000).

12. Bratman, S., "Vitamin C for Nicer Skin," TNP.com (06 April 2001).

13. Funasaka, Y., Sato, H., Usuki, A., Ohashi, A., Kotoya, H., Miyamoto, K., Hillebrand, G.G., Ichihashi, M., "The efficacy of glycolic acid for treating wrinkles: analysis using newly developed facial imaging systems equipped with fluorescent illumination," *Journal of Dermatological Science,* Suppl 1, S53–59 (August 2001).

14. Rosenblat, G., Perelman, N., Katzier, E., Gal-Or, S., Jonas, A., Nimni, M.E., Sorgente, N., Neeman, I., "Acylated ascorbate stimulates collagen synthesis in cultured human foreskin fibroblasts at lower doses than does ascorbic acid," *Connective Tissue Research,* 37(3–4), 303–311 (1998).

YELLOW NAIL SYNDROME

1. Williams, H.C., Buffham, R., du Vivier, A., "Successful use of topical vitamin E solution in the treatment of nail changes in yellow nail syndrome," *Archive of Dermatology,* 127, 1023–1028 (1991).

ZINC DEFICIENCY

1. Kury, S., Dreno, B., Bezieau, S., Giraudet, S., Kharfi, M., Kamoun, R., Moisan, J.P., "Identification of SLC39A4, a gene involved in acrodermatitis enteropathica," *Nature Genetics,* 31(3), 239–240 (July 2002).

2. Smith, K.J., Skelton, H., "Histopathologic features seen in Gianotti-Crosti syndrome secondary to Epstein-Barr virus," *Journal of the American Academy of Dermatology,* 43(6), 1076–1079 (December 2000).

3. Lebech, A.M., "Polymerase chain reaction in diagnosis of *Borrelia burgdorferi* infections and studies on taxonomic classification," *APMIS Supplement,* 105, 1–40 (2002).

4. Andiran, N., Senturk, G.B., Bukulmez, G., "Combined vaccination by measles and hepatitis B vaccines: a new cause of Gianotti-Crosti syndrome," *Dermatology,* 204(1), 75–76 (2002).

INDEX